Calculations for determining the amount of local anesthetic and/or vasoconstrictor in dental cartridges

Typical local anesthetic concentrations

Strength		*mg/ml Equivalent*
0.5%	=	5 mg/ml
1.5%	=	15 mg/ml
2.0%	=	20 mg/ml
3.0%	=	30 mg/ml
4.0%	=	40 mg/ml

Typical vasoconstrictor concentrations

Strength		*mg/ml (or µg/ml) Equivalent*
1:20,000	=	0.05 mg/ml (50 µg/ml)
1:50,000	=	0.02 mg/ml (20 µg/ml)
1:100,000	=	0.01 mg/ml (10 µg/ml)
1:200,000	=	0.005 mg/ml (5 µg/ml)

General calculation guidelines:

1) Convert % solution to mg/ml (or µg/ml) as shown above.
2) Multiply mg/ml (or µg/ml) × cartridge volume × number of cartridges = quantity of drug. *Note:* Cartridge volumes may vary between products.

Example: Two cartridges of a 2% lidocaine HCl and 1:100,000 epinephrine HCl solution were administered. The cartridge volume was 1.8 ml for each. What quantity of each drug was given?

Answer:

for lidocaine HCl: 20 mg × 1.8 ml × 2 cartridges = 72 mg

for epinephrine HCl: 0.01 mg/ml × 1.8 ml × 2 cartridges = 0.036 mg or 10 µg/ml × 1.8 ml × 2 cartridges = 36 µg

Mosby's
Dental Drug Reference

Mosby's Dental Drug Reference

Fifth Edition

Tommy W. Gage, RPh, DDS, PhD
Professor and Vice Chairman
Department of Oral and Maxillofacial
Surgery and Pharmacology
Baylor College of Dentistry
The Texas A&M University System Health Science Center
Dallas, Texas

Frieda Atherton Pickett, RDH, MS
Formerly, Associate Professor
Caruth School of Dental Hygiene
Baylor College of Dentistry
The Texas A&M University System Health Science Center
Dallas, Texas
Adjunct Associate Professor
Department of Dental Hygiene
East Tennessee State University
Johnson City, Tennessee

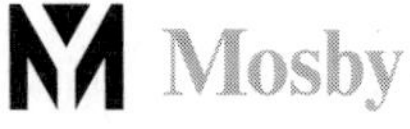

A Harcourt Health Sciences Company

St. Louis London Philadelphia Sydney Toronto

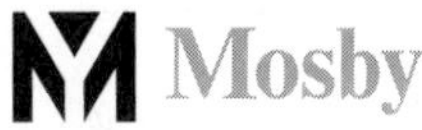

A Harcourt Health Sciences Company

Editor-in-Chief: John Schrefer
Editor: Penny Rudolph
Developmental Editor: Kimberly Frare
Project Manager: Linda McKinley
Production Editor: René Saller
Cover Design: Elizabeth Rohne Rudder

FIFTH EDITION

A NOTE TO THE READER

The authors and publisher have made every attempt to check dosages and dental content for accuracy. Because the science of pharmacology is continually advancing, our knowledge base continues to expand. Therefore we recommend that the reader always check product information for changes in dosage or administration before administering any medication. This is particularly important with new or rarely used drugs.

Mosby, Inc.
A Harcourt Health Sciences Company
11830 Westline Industrial Drive
St. Louis, Missouri 63146

Printed in the United States of America

International Standard Book Number 0-323-01196-9

00 01 02 03 04 GW/RDC 9 8 7 6 5 4 3 2 1

Editorial Review Board

Authors' Comments

Our goal of creating a quick and concise drug reference resource remains steadfast. We trust this revision will continue to provide essential information for assistance in patient evaluation, which involves many individual decisions customized to meet each patient's needs. Your acceptance of this drug information resource has been extremely gratifying and supports our vision of the need for such a volume. Because the book is revised every 2 years, new drug information is posted as periodic updates on Mosby's web site at http://www.mosby.com/dental. You are encouraged to access this web site for updated drug information and for information about new drugs approved after the publication date for this volume.

The pharmacologic and therapeutic index in the front section of this volume has been well accepted in assisting both users and patients in the identification of drugs. In addition to updating each monograph, a new section containing information about a limited number of herbal and nonherbal remedies was developed. We are working to keep the book as small as possible for convenience in handling, but the number of new drugs and drug products approved for marketing each year presents a considerable challenge. Our focus is on the most frequently prescribed medications and new products. Because of these reasons, not every drug that is available is listed in this edition. However, it does include the majority of new drugs marketed through December 1999.

This book is only as good as it enables the practitioner to quickly locate drug facts. The overwhelming acceptance of prior volumes and constructive feedback from the book's users are greatly appreciated. The authors are hopeful that this edition will be equally acceptable and useful. Your comments for improvements are solicited.

The authors wish to express their sincere gratitude for the contributions made by the members of the Editorial Review Board, who have been selected on the basis of their extensive experience and knowledge. A special word of appreciation goes to Mrs. Brigitte Wallaert Sims for her assistance in data entry, in the laborious task of printing the completed manuscript, and in putting up with our demands.

Preface

Mosby's Dental Drug Reference is designed to be used chairside in the dental office and by the student or resident as a quick, concise drug reference resource. Its purpose is to assist in the rapid identification of drugs patients may be taking as they present for dental care. The easy-to-use design provides rapid access to essential drug information to facilitate completion of the medical history review and patient evaluation.

This book is not intended to be a comprehensive drug compendium nor to make specific recommendations about selecting and prescribing dental drugs. It contains concise and easy-to-read "micro" drug monographs with basic information about each drug.

Selected herbal and nonherbal remedies have been placed in a special section to aid the dental practitioner in identifying dental implications of these products. Drugs are presented alphabetically by generic name in a succinctly ordered and standardized format with pertinent drug information for the dentist, dental hygienist, or dental assistant. A user-friendly cross index is the key to using the book for both brand and generic name identification. A second index based on a therapeutic and pharmacologic classification can also be used to identify the location of drug monographs, but in addition, will aid in identifying drugs when the patient cannot recall the name or spelling of a drug being taken. This index also groups drugs by classes or use so the reader can easily identify other drugs within a given class or application. Information is provided on more than 1600 drug products, including the most recently approved drugs and new drug products through 1999. Special features of this book are an emphasis on drug interactions of dental interest and the highlighting of oral side effects. The dental considerations section includes information that will be useful in developing patient management strategies. Useful fact tables are located on the inside covers and in the appendixes, with information about dose calculations. This volume also contains the 1997 ADA drug and dose recommendations for antibiotic prophylaxis for patients at risk for bacterial endocarditis and for those patients with prosthetic joints. We have also revised the tables listing drugs that can alter salivary flow and affect taste in some manner.

Each drug monograph is designed to include the following information:

GENERIC NAME of the drug
PRONUNCIATION of the generic name
COMMON BRAND NAMES for the generic drug as sold in the United States and Canada (drugs available in Canada only are designated by a maple leaf)
DRUG CLASS to facilitate drug identification
CONTROLLED SUBSTANCES schedule as appropriate for the United States and Canada
ACTION, with a brief description of the mechanism of action of the drug
USES or indications for the drug, including those approved by the FDA (unapproved uses are identified as appropriate for selected drugs)
DOSES AND ROUTES OF ADMINISTRATION to assist the dental professional in assessing the dose in relationship to the seriousness of the patient's disease and predicting potential side effects and drug interactions
SIDE EFFECTS/ADVERSE REACTIONS grouped according to body systems; common side effects listed in italics, and life-threatening reactions listed in boldface type; information regarding oral manifestations of side effects listed separately
CONTRAINDICATIONS identified for instances in which the medication should absolutely not be given or when risk-benefit criteria must be established
PRECAUTIONS to be considered when prescribing and using the drug and identification of pregnancy categories
PHARMACOKINETICS, with brief descriptions for each drug
DRUG INTERACTIONS OF CONCERN TO DENTISTRY listed for use in determining whether a given interaction is beneficial or harmful (clinical judgment must always be applied for each interaction listed)
DENTAL CONSIDERATIONS, including general information related to dental concerns in treating a patient taking a given drug, suggestions for medical consultations, and recommendations for the patient/family in preventing dental complications or disease

Appendixes following the drug monograph section include the following:

APPENDIX A Selected abbreviations

APPENDIX B	Drugs that cause dry mouth
APPENDIX C	Controlled substances chart
APPENDIX D	FDA pregnancy categories
APPENDIX E	Drugs that affect taste
APPENDIX F	Selected drug combination products
APPENDIX G	Dose calculations by weight
APPENDIX H	Herbal and nonherbal remedies
APPENDIX I	Selected references

Located on the inside cover pages are useful tables and drugs and doses for antibiotic prophylaxis.

Tommy W. Gage
Frieda Atherton Pickett

Contents

Therapeutic/Pharmacologic Index, *1*

Individual Drugs, *17*

Appendixes, *723*

A. Abbreviations, *725*
B. Drugs that cause dry mouth, *730*
C. Controlled substances chart, *734*
D. FDA pregnancy categories, *735*
E. Drugs that affect taste, *736*
F. Combination products, *739*
G. Dose calculations by weight, *751*
H. Herbal and nonherbal remedies, *752*
I. Selected references, *767*

Generic and Trade Name Index, *769*

Therapeutic/Pharmacologic Index

Drugs Classified by Usual Therapeutic/Pharmacologic Category

This section of the book features drugs classified by primary therapeutic or pharmacologic group, or both. Thus you can locate drugs by knowing their primary therapeutic use or general pharmacologic class. This arrangement makes it easy to find the matching drug monograph by using the generic name. The individual drug monographs are arranged by generic name in alphabetical order and can simply be found in the appropriate alphabet section. Colored tabs on the side of the book mark the alphabetical sections. An originator or common brand name is also listed for convenience and may help with identification. This arrangement allows the book user to see other drugs in the same classification that are included in this volume.

For example, take the case of a patient using a drug for depression and having difficulty recalling the drug name. Find the *Antidepressants* section. All of the antidepressants listed in this volume can be seen and may help the patient remember the exact drug currently used. Or if you want to know which drugs are calcium channel antagonists, go to the *Antihypertensives* section and find the subtopic of calcium channel antagonists. The calcium channel antagonists included in this volume are listed. As you identify the drug, use the generic name to quickly tab to the appropriate alphabet section.

ADRENERGIC AGONISTS

ephedrine
epinephrine (Adrenalin)
isoproterenol (Isuprel)

ALZHEIMER'S

donepezil (Aricept)
tacrine (Cognex)

AMINOGLYCOSIDES (TOPICALS)

gentamycin ophth. (Garamycin)
neomycin (Myciguent)
polymyxin B ophth. (Aerosporin)
tobramycin ophth. (Tobrex)

AMYOTROPHIC LATERAL SCLEROSIS

riluzole (Rilutek)

ANALGESICS (NONOPIOID)

acetaminophen
aspirin
salsalate (Anaflex)

ANALGESICS (NSAIDS)

(see nonsteroidal antiinflammatory drugs)

ANALGESICS (OPIOIDS)

codeine
fentanyl transdermal (Duragesic)
hydromorphone (Dilaudid)
meperidine (Demerol)
methadone (Dolophine)
morphine (MS Contin)
oxycodone (Roxicodone)
pentazocine (Talwin Nx)
propoxyphene hydrochloride (Darvon)
propoxyphene napsylate (Darvon-N)
tramadol (Ultram)

ANESTHETICS (LOCAL)

bupivacaine (Marcaine)
etidocaine (Duranest)
lidocaine (Xylocaine)
mepivacaine (Carbocaine)
prilocaine (Citanest)

ANESTHETICS (TOPICAL)

benzocaine (Hurricaine)
dyclonine HCl (Dyclone)
lidocaine (Xylocaine)
lidocaine transoral (DentiPatch)
tetracaine (Pontocaine)

ANESTHETICS (GENERAL)

midazolam (Versed)
propofol (Diprivan)

ANOREXIANTS

diethylpropion (Tenuate)
mazindol (Mazanor)
methamphetamine (Desoxyn)
phendimetrazine (Prelu-2)
phentermine (Ionamin)
sibutramine (Merida)

ANTACIDS

magaldrate (Riopan)

ANTAGONISTS

disulfiram (Antabuse)
flumazenil (Romazicon)
levomethadyl acetate (Orlaam)
nalmefene (Revex)
naloxone (Narcan)
naltrexone (ReVia)

ANTIANGINALS

Nitrates

isorbide dinitrate (Isordil)
isorbide mononitrate (ISMO)
nitroglycerin

Beta-adrenergic antagonists

atenolol (Tenormin)
metoprolol (Lopressor)

nadolol (Corgard)
propranolol (Inderal)

Calcium channel antagonists

amlodipine (Norvasc)
bepridil (Vascor)
diltiazem (Cardizem)
felodipine (Plendil)
nicardipine (Cardene)
nifedipine (Procardia)
verapamil (Calan)

ANTIANXIETY/SEDATIVE-HYPNOTICS

Barbiturates

pentobarbital (Nembutal)
phenobarbital (Luminal)
secobarbital (Seconal)

Benzodiazepines

alprazolam (Xanax)
chlordiazepoxide (Librium)
clorazepate dipotassium (Tranxene)
diazepam (Valium)
estazolam (ProSom)
flurazepam (Dalmane)
halazepam (Proxipam)
lorazepam (Ativan)
midazolam (Versed)
oxazepam (Serax)
quazepam (Doral)
temazepam (Restoril)
triazolam (Halcion)

Antihistamines

diphenhydramine (Benadryl)
hydroxyzine (Atarax, Vistaril)
promethazine (Phenergan)

Others

buspirone (BuSpar)
chloral hydrate (Aquachloral)
doxepin (Sinaquan)
meprobamate (Equanil, Miltown)
zaleplon (Sonata)
zolpidem (Ambien)

ANTIASTHMATICS

(see bronchodilators)

ANTICARIES

sodium fluoride

ANTICHOLELITHICS

chenodiol (Chenix)
ursodiol (Actigall)

ANTICHOLINERGICS

atropine (Sal-Tropine)
benztropine (Cogentin)
biperidin (Akineton)
clidinium (Quarzan)
dicyclomine (Bentyl)
ethopropazine (Parsidol)
glycopyrrolate (Robinul)
hyoscyamine (Levsin)
mepenzolate (Cantil)
methantheline (Banthine)
oxybutynin (Ditropan)
propantheline (Pro-Banthine)
scopolamine tolterodine (Detrol)

ANTICOAGULANTS

ardeparin (Normiflo)
dalteparin (Fragmin)
danaparoid (Orgaran)
enoxaparin (Lovenox)
heparin
warfarin (Coumadin)

ANTICONVULSANTS

acetazolamide (Diamox)
carbamazepine (Tegretol)
clonazepam (Klonopin)
diazepam (Valium)
divalproex (Depakote)
ethosuximide (Zarontin)
ethotoin (Peganone)
felbamate (Felbatol)
fosphenytoin (Cerebyx)
gabapentin (Neurontin)
lamotrigine (Lamictal)

levetiracetam (Keppra)
mephenytoin (Mesantoin)
mephobarbital (Mebaral)
methsuximide (Celontin)
phenobarbital (Luminal)
phensuximide (Milontin)
phenytoin (Dilantin)
primidone (Mysoline)
tiagabine (Gabitril)
topiramate (Topamax)
trimethadione (Tridione)
valproic acid (Depakene)

ANTIDEPRESSANTS

Atypical

bupropion (Wellbutrin)
nefazodone (Serzone)
trazodone (Desyrel)
venlafaxine (Effexor)

Monoamine oxidase inhibitors

isocarboxazid (Marplan)
phenelzine sulfate (Nardil)
tranylcypromine sulfate (Parnate)

Serotonin-specific reuptake inhibitors

citalopram (Celexa)
fluoxetine (Prozac)
fluvoxamine (Luvox)
paroxetine (Paxil)
sertraline (Zoloft)

Tetracyclics

maprotiline (Ludiomil)
mirtazapine (Remeron)

Tricyclics

amitriptyline (Elavil)
amoxapine (Asendin)
clomipramine (Anafranil)
desipramine (Norpramin)
doxepin (Sinequan)
imipramine (Tofranil)
nortriptyline (Pamelor)
protriptyline (Vivactil)
trimipramine (Surmontil)

ANTIDIABETICS

acarbose (Precose)
acetohexamide (Dymelor)
chlorpropamide (Diabinese)
glimepiride (Amaryl)
glipizide (Glucotrol)
glyburide (DiaBeta)
insulin
metformin (Glucophage)
miglitol (Glyset)
pioglitazone (Actos)
repaglinide (Prandin)
rosiglitazone (Avandia)
tolazamide (Tolinase)
tolbutamide (Orinase)
troglitazone (Rezulin)

ANTIDIARRHEALS

bismuth subsalicylate (Pepto-Bismol)
camphorated opium tincture (Paregoric)
difenoxin/atropine (Motofen)
diphenoxylate/atropine (Lomotil)
loperamide (Imodium-AD)

ANTIDYSRHYTHMICS (ANTIARRHYTHMICS)

amiodarone (Cordarone)
digitoxin (Crystodigin)
digoxin (Lanoxin)
disopyramide (Norpace)
flecainide acetate (Tambocor)
lidocaine (Xylocaine Cardiac)
mexiletine (Mexitil)
moricizine (Ethmozine)
procainamide (Pronestyl)
propafenone (Rythmol)
propranolol (Inderal)
quinidine (Quinaglute)
sotalol (Betapace)
tocainide (Tonocard)

ANTIEMETICS

chlorpromazine (Thorazine)
cyclizine (Merezine)
dimenhydrinate (Dramamine)
dolasetron (Anzemet)
meclizine (Bonine)
metoclopramide (Reglan)
odansetron (Zofran)
prochlorperazine (Compazine)
promethazine (Phenergan)
scopolamine (Transderm-Scop)
thiethylperazine (Torecan)
triflupromazine (Vesprin)
trimethobenzamide (Tigan)

ANTIFUNGALS (TOPICAL)

amphotericin B (Fungizone)
butenafine (Mentax)
butoconazole (Femstat)
ciclopirox (Loprox)
clotrimazole (Mycelex)
econazole (Spectazole)
itraconazole (Sporanox)
miconazole (Monistat, Micatin)
naftifine (Naftin)
nystatin (Mycostatin)
sulconazole (Exelderm)
terbinafine (Lamisil)
terconazole (Terazol)
tolnaftate (Tinactin)

ANTIFUNGALS (SYSTEMIC)

fluconazole (Diflucan)
flucytosine (Ancobon)
griseofulvin (Fulvicin)
itraconazole (Sporanox)
ketoconazole (Nizoral)
terbinafine (Lamisil)

ANTIGOUTS

allopurinol (Zyloprim)
colchicine

ANTIHISTAMINES (H_2) ANTAGONISTS

cimetidine (Tagamet)
famotidine (Pepcid)
nizatidine (Axid)
ranitidine (Zantac)

ANTIHISTAMINES (H_1) ANTAGONISTS

azatadine (Optimine)
azelastine (Astelin)
bropheniramine (Dimetane)
buclizine (Bucladin-S)
cetirizine (Zyrtec)
chlorpheniramine (Chlor-Trimeton)
clemastine fumarate (Tavist)
cyclizine (Marezine)
cyproheptadine (Periactin)
dexchlorpheniramine (Polaramine)
dimenhydrinate (Dramamine)
diphenhydramine (Benadryl)
emedastine (Emadine)
fexofenadine (Allegra)
hydroxyzine (Atarax, Vistaril)
ketotifen (Zaditor)
levocabastine (Livostin)
loratadine (Claritin)
meclizine (Bonine)
olopatadine (Patanol)
promethazine (Phenergan)
tripelennamine (PBZ)

ANTIHYPERCALCEMICS (OSTEOPOROSIS)

alendronate (Fosamax)
etidronate (Didronel)
calcitonin (Calcimar)
raloxifene (Evista)
risedronate (Actonel)
tilundronate (Skelid)

ANTIHYPERLIPIDEMICS

atorvastatin (Lipitor)
cerivastatin (Baycol)
cholestyramine (Questran)
clofibrate (Atromid-S)
colestipol (Colestid)
fenofibrate (Tricor)
fluvastatin (Lescol)
gemfibrozil (Lopid)
lovastatin (Mevacor)
niacin (Nia-Bid)
pravastatin (Pravachol)
simvastatin (Zocor)

ANTIHYPERTENSIVES

(also see diuretics)

Alpha-adrenergic antagonists

doxazosin (Cardura)
phenoxybenzamine (Dibenzyline)
phentolamine (Regitine)
prazosin (Minipress)
terazosin (Hytrin)

Alpha/beta-adrenergic antagonists

carvedilol (Coreg)
labetalol (Normodyne)

Angiotensin-converting enzyme inhibitors

benazepril (Lotensin)
captopril (Capoten)
enalapril (Vasotec)
fosinopril (Monopril)
lisinopril (Prinivil, Zestril)
moexipril (Univasc)
perindopril (Aceon)
quinapril (Accupril)
ramipril (Altace)
trandolopril (Mavik)

Angiotensin II receptor antagonists

candesartan (Atacand)
eprosartin (Teveten)
irbesartan (Avapro)
losartan (Cozaar)
telmisartan (Micardis)
valsartan (Diovan)

Beta-adrenergic antagonists

Selective

atenolol (Tenormin)
betaxolol (Kerlone)
bisoprolol (Zebeta)
carteolol (Cartrol)
metoprolol (Lopressor)
nadolol (Corgard)

Nonselective

penbutolol (Levatol)
pindolol (Visken)
propranolol (Inderal)
timolol (Blocadren)

Calcium channel antagonists

amlodipine (Norvasc)
bepridil (Vascor)
diltiazem (Cardizem)
felodipine (Plendil)
isradipine (DynaCirc)
mibefradil (Posicor)
nicardipine (Cardene)
nifedipine (Procardia XL)
nislodipine (Sular)
verapamil (Calan)

Centrally acting

clonidine (Catapres)
guanabenz (Wytensin)
guanfacine (Tenex)
methyldopa (Aldomet)

Other

quanadrel (Hylorel)
quanethidine (Ismelin)
hydralazine (Apresoline)
mecamylamine (Inversine)
minoxidil (Loniten)
reserpine (Serpasil)

ANTIINFECTIVES (TOPICAL)

chlorhexidine (Peridex, PerioGard)
erythromycin (Erytroderm)
mupirocin (Bactroban)
povidone-iodine (Betadine)

ANTIINFECTIVES (MISCELLANEOUS)

atovaquone (Mepron)
clofazimine (Lamprene)
dapsone metronidazole (Flagyl)
pentamidine (NebuPent)

ANTIINFECTIVES (SYSTEMIC)

(see specific class: penicillins, cephalosporins, etc.)

ANTIINFLAMMATORY ANTIARTHRITICS

allopurinol (Zyloprim)
aspirin
auranofin gold (Ridura)
aurothioglucose (Solganol)
celecoxib (Celebrex)
choline salicylate (Arthropan)
colchicine
diflunisal (Dolobid)
etanercept (Enbrel)
etodolac (Lodine)
fenoprofen (Nelfon)
gold sodium thiomalate (Myochrysine)
ibuprofen (Motrin)
indomethacin (Indocin)
ketoprofen (Orudus)
leflunomide (Arava)
methotrexate (Rheumatrex)
nabumetone (Relafen)
naproxen sodium (Anaprox)
naproxen (Naprosyn)
oxaprozin (Daypro)
piroxicam (Feldene)
probenecid (Benemid)
rofecoxib (Vioxx)
salsalate (Anaflex)
sulindac (Clinoril)
tolmetin (Tolectin)

ANTIMALARIALS

chloroquine (Aralen)
hydroxycloroquine (Plaquenil)
primaquine
quinine

ANTIPARKINSONIANS

amantadine (Symmetrel)
benztropine (Cogentin)
biperiden (Akineton)
bromocriptine (Parlodel)
diphenhydramine (Benadryl)
entacapone (Comtan)
ethopropazine (Parsidol)
levodopa (Larodopa)
levodopa/carbidopa (Sinemet)
pergolide (Permax)
pramipexole (Mirapex)
procyclidine (Kemadrin)
ropinirole (ReQuip)
selegiline (Eldepryl)
tolcapone (Tasmar)
trihexyphenidyl (Artane)

ANTIPSYCHOTICS

Phenothiazines

chlorpromazine (Thorazine)
fluphenazine (Prolixin)
mesoridazine (Serentil)
perphenazine (Trilafon)
prochlorperazine (Compazine)
promazine (Sparine)
thioridazine (Mellaril)
trifluoperazine (Stelazine)
triflupromazine (Vesprin)

Butyrophenone

haloperidol (Haldol)

Thioxanthene

thiothixene (Navane)

Others

clozapine (Clozaril)
loxapine (Loxitane)
molindone (Moban)
olanzapine (Zyprexa)
pimozide (Orap)
quetiapine (Seroquel)
risperidone (Risperdal)

Bipolar disease
lithium carbonate (Eskalith)
valproic acid (Depakene)

ANTITHYROIDS

methimazole (Tapazole)
propylthiouracil

ANTITUBERCULARS

cycloserine (Seromycin)
ethambutol (Myambutol)
ethionamide (Trecator)
isoniazid (Laniazid)
pyrazinamide
rifabutin (Mycobutin)
rifampin (Rifadin)
rifapentine (Priftin)

ANTITUSSIVES/ EXPECTORANTS

benzonatate (Tessalon)
codeine
dextromethorphan (Robitussin)
diphenhydramine (Benadryl)
guaifenesin (Humibid)
hydrocodone (Hycodan)

ANTIVIRALS (SYSTEMIC)

Herpes viruses
acyclovir (Zovirax)
famciclovir (Famvir)
foscarnet (Foscavir)
ganciclovir (Cytovene)
valacyclovir (Valtex)
Influenza viruses
amantadine (Symmetrel)
oseltamivir (Tamiflu)
rimantadine (Flumadine)
zanamivir (Relenza)
HIV—nonnucleoside analogs
delaviridine (Rescriptor)
efavirenz (Sustiva)
nevirapine (Viramune)
HIV—nucleoside analogs
abacavir (Ziagen)
didanosine (ddI) (Videx)
lamivudine (3TC) (Epivir)
stavudine (d4T) (Zerit)
zalcitabine (Hivid)
zidovudine (AZT) (Retrovir)
HIV—protease inhibitors
amprenavir (Agenerase)
indinavir (Crixivan)
nelfinavir (Viracept)
ritonavir (Norvir)
saquinavir (Invirase, Fortovase)

ANTIVIRALS (TOPICAL)

acyclovir (Zovirax)
idoxuridine (Herplex)
penciclovir (Denavir)
vidarabine (Vira-A)

APHTHOUS STOMATITIS

amlexanox (Aphthasol)
chlorhexidine (Peridex)

APPETITE SUPPRESSANTS

diethylpropion (Tenuate)
mazindol (Mazanor)
methamphetamine (Desoxyn)
orlistat (Xenical)
phendimetrazine (Prelu-2)
phentermine (Ionamin)
sibutramine (Merida)

ASTHMA TREATMENT

(see bronchodilators)

ASTHMA PREVENTION

montelukast (Singulair)
salmeterol (Serevent)
zafirlukast (Accolate)
zileuton (Zyflo)

BARBITURATES

pentobarbital (Nembutal)
phenobarbital (Luminal)
secobarbital (Seconal)

BRONCHODILATORS

albuterol (Proventil, Ventolin)
aminophylline (Somophyllin)
bitolterol (Tornalate)

dyphylline (Dilor)
ephedrine
epinephrine (Adrenalin)
epinephrine inhalation (Primatine)
ipratropium (Atrovent)
isoetharine (Bronkometer)
isoproterenol (Isuprel)
levalbuterol (Xopenex)
metaproterenol (Alupent)
oxitriphylline (Choledyl)
pirbuterol (Maxair)
terbutaline (Brethine)
theophylline (Theo-Dur)

CANCER CHEMOTHERAPY

aminogluthethimide (Cytadren)
bicalutamide (Casodex)
busulfan (Myleran)
chlorambucil (Leukeran)
cyclophosphamide (Cytoxan)
fluorouracil (Efudex)
flutamide (Eulexin)
hydroxyurea (Hydrea)
interferon alfa-2a (Roferon-A)
interferon alfa-2b (Intron-A)
leucovorin (Wellcovorin)
lomustine (CeeNu)
masoprocal (Actinex)
megestrol (Megace)
melphalan (Alkeran)
mercaptopurine (Purinethol)
methotrexate (Folex)
mitotane (Lysodren)
paclitaxel (Taxol)
procarbazine (Matulane)
tamoxifen (Novaldex)
tormifene (Fareston)

CARDIAC GLYCOSIDES

digoxin (Lanoxin)
digitoxin (Crystodigin)

CENTRAL NERVOUS SYSTEM STIMULANTS

dextroamphetamine (Dexedrine)
methylphenidate (Ritalin)
methamphetamine (Desoxyn)
modafinil (Provigil)
pimoline (Cylert)

CEPHALOSPORINS

cefaclor (Ceclor)
cefadroxil (Duricef)
cefazolin (Ancef)
cefdinir (Omnicef)
cefepime (Maxipime)
cefixime (Suprax)
cefpodoxime (Vantil)
cefprozil (Cefzil)
ceftibutin (Cedax)
cefuroxime (Ceftin)
cephalexin (Keflex)
cephadrine (Velosef)
loracarbef (Lorabid)

CHOLESTEROL LOWERING AGENTS

atorvastatin (Lipitor)
cerivastatin (Baycol)
fluvastatin (Lescol)
lovastatin (Mevacor)
pravastatin (Pravachol)

CHOLINERGIC AGONISTS

bethanechol (Urecholine)
pyridostigmine (Mestinon)

CHOLINESTRASE INHIBITORS

ambenonium (Mytelase)
neostigmine (Prostigmin)
pyridostigmine (Mestinon)

DECONGESTANTS

oxymetazoline (Afrin)
phenylephrine (Neo-Synephrine)
pseudoephedrine (Sudafed)

DEMENTIA/ALZHEIMER'S

donepezil (Aricept)
ergoloid mesylate (Hydergine)
tacrine (Cognex)

DERMATOLOGICS

acitretin (Soriatane)
alitretinoin (Panretin)
azelaic acid (Azelex)
capsaicin (Zostrix)
doxepin (Zonalon)
isotretinoin (Accutane)
methotrexate (Folex)
minoxidil (Rogaine)
tazarotene (Tazorac)
tretinoin (Retin-A)

DIURETICS

Loop diuretics
bumetanide (Bumex)
ethacrynate (Edecrin)
furosemide (Lasix)
torsemide (Demadex)

Potassium sparing
amiloride (Midamor)
spironolactone (Aldactone)
triamterene (Dyrenium)

Thiazides
chlorothiazide (Diuril)
hydrochlorothiazide (HydroDIURIL)
polythiazide (Renese)

Thiazide-like
chlorthalidone (Hygroton)
indapamide (Lozol)
metolazone (Zaroxolyn)

Others
acetazolamide (Diamox)
methazolamide (Neptazane)

ENDOCRINE

clomiphene (Clomid)
conjugated estrogens (Premarin)
conjugated estrogens, synthetic (Cenestin)
danizol (Danocrine)
desmopressin (DDAVP)
esterified estrogens (Estrab)
estradiol transdermal (Estraderm)
estradiol valerate (Estrace)
estripioate (Ogen)
estrogen substance conjugated (Premarin)
ethinyl estradiol (Estinyl)
finasteride (Proscar)
fluoxymesterone (Halotestin)
levonorgestrel (Norplant System)
levothyroxine (Synthroid)
liothyronine (Cytomel)
liotrix (Euthroid)
lypressin (Diapid)
medroxyprogesterone (Provera)
norethindrone (Aygestin)
norgestrel (Ovrette)
oral contraceptives (many brands)
oxandrolone (Oxandrin)
oxymetholone (Anadrol)
raloxifene (Evista)
stanozolol (Winstrol)
testosterone
thyroid

ERECTILE DYSFUNCTION

alprostadil (Caverject)
sildenafil (Viagra)

ERGOT ALKALOIDS

(see migraine)
ergotamine (Ergostat)

EXPECTORANT

guaifenesin (Humibid)

FLUOROQUINOLONES

alatrofloxacin (Trovan IV)
ciprofloxacin (Cipro)
enoxacin (Penetrex)
levofloxacin (Levaquin)
lomefloxacin (Maxaquin)
norfloxacin (Noroxin)
ofloxacin (Floxin)
sparfloxacin (Zagam)
trovafloxacin (Trovan)

FOLATE ANTAGONIST
trimetrexate (Neutrexin)

GASTROESOPHAGEAL REFLUX DISEASE
lansoprazole (Prevacid)
omeprazole (Prilosec)
rabeprazole (Aciphex)
ursodiol (Actigall)

GASTROINTESTINAL DRUGS
cisapride (Propulsid)
lansoprazole (Prevacid)
mesalamine (Asacol)
metoclopramide (Reglan)
misoprostol (Cytotec)
olsalazine (Dipentum)
pancrelipase (Cotazyme)
rabeprazole (Aciphex)
sucralfate (Carafate)
sulfasalazine (Azulfidine)

GLAUCOMA TREATMENT
acetazolamide (Diamox)
apraclonidine (Iopidine)
betaxolol (Betopic)
brimonidine (Alphagan)
brinzolamide (Azopt)
carteolol (Ocupress)
dipiverfrin (Propine C)
dorzolamide (Trusopt)
emedastine (Emadine)
latanoprost (Xalatan)
levobunolol (Betagan)
methazolamine (Neptazine)
pilocarpine (Isopto-Carpine)
timolol (Timoptic)

GLUCOCORTICOIDS
Inhalant sprays
beclomethasone (Vanceril Inh)
budesonide (Rhinocort Inh)
flunisolide (Aerobid Inh)
fluticasone (Flonase)
triamcinolone (Azmacort)

Systemic
betamethasone (Celestone)
cortisone (Cortone)
dexamethasone (Dexadron)
fludrocortisone (Florinef)
hydrocortisone (Cortef)
methylprednisolone (Medrol)
prednisolone (Delta-Cortef)
prednisone (Meticorten)
triamcinolone (Aristocort)

Topical
betamethasone (Diprolene)
clobetasol (Temovate)
clocortolone (Cloderm)
desonide (DesOwen)
desoximetasone (Topicort)
dexamethasone (Decaderm)
diflorasone (Florone)
fluocinonide (Lidex)
flurandrenolide (Cordran)
fluticasone (Cutivate)
halcinonide (Halog)
halobetasol (Ultravate)
hydrocortisone (Allercort)
hydrocortisone butaprate (Pandel)
loteprednol (Lotemax, Alrex)
prednicarbate (Dermatop)
rimexolone (Vexol)
triamcinolone topical (Kenalog)

HEMOSTATICS
absorbable gelatin sponge (Gelfoam)
aminocaproic acid (Amicar)
oxidized cellulose (Surgicel)
tranexamic acid (Cyklokapron)

IMMUNOMODULATORS
imiquimod (Aldara)
interferon alfa-2a (Roferon-A)
interferon alfa-2b (Intron-A)
interferon alfa-n_1 (Wellferon)
interferon alfa-n_3 (Alferon-N)
interferon beta-1a (Avonex)

interferon gamma-1b (Actimmune)
levamisole (Ergamisol)

IMMUNOSUPPRESSANTS
azathioprine (Imuran)
cyclosporine (Sandimmune)
daclizumab (Zenapax)
mycophenolate (CellCept)
prednisone (Meticorten)
tacrolimus (Prograf)

LEUKOTRIENE RECEPTOR ANTAGONIST
montelukast (Singulair)
zafirlukast (Accolate)

LEUKOTRIENE PATHWAY INHIBITOR
zileuton (Zyflo)

LINCOSAMIDES
clindamycin (Cleocin)
lincomycin (Lincocin)

MACROLIDES
azithromycin (Zithromax)
clarithromycin (Biaxin)
dirithromycin (DynaBac)
erythromycin (Erythrocin)

MALE PATTERN BALDNESS
finasteride (Propecia)
minoxidil (Rogaine)

MAST CELL STABILIZERS
cromolyn (Intal)
lodoxamide (Alomide)
nedocromil (Tilade)

MIGRAINE
(see ergot alkaloids)
divalproex (Depakote)
methysergide (Sansert)
naratriptan (Amerge)
propranolol (Inderal)
rizatriptan (Maxalt)
sumatriptan (Imitrex)
timolol (Blocadren)
zolmitripan (Zomig)

MINERALS
ferrous gluconate
ferrous sulfate (Feosol)
ferrous fumarate
potassium chloride (Micro-K)
sodium fluoride

MUCOLYTIC
dornase alpha (Pulmozyme)

MULTIPLE SCLEROSIS
tizanidine (Zanaflex)

MYASTHENIA GRAVIS
ambenonium (Mytelase)
neostigmine (Prostigmin)
pyridostigmine (Mestinon)

MYDRIATIC
atropine sulfate (optic) (Isopto Atropine)
homatropine hydrobromide (optic) (Isopto Homatropine)

NARCOTICS
(see analgesics [opioid])

NITROIMIDAZOLE
metronidazole (Flagyl)

NONSTEROIDAL ANTIINFLAMMATORY DRUGS
aspirin
celecoxib (Celebrex)
diclofenac (Voltaren)
diflunisal (Dolobid)
etodolac (Lodine)
fenoprofen (Nalfon)
flurbiprofen (Ansaid)
ibuprofen (Motrin)
indomethacin (Indocin)

ketoprofen (Orudis)
ketorolac (Toradol)
meclofenamate (Meclomen)
mefenamic acid (Ponstel)
nabumetone (Relafen)
naproxen (Naprosyn)
naproxen sodium (Anaprox)
oxaprozin (Daypro)
piroxicam (Feldene)
rofecoxib (Vioxx)
sulindac (Clinoril)
tolmetin (Tolectin)

OPHTHALMICS

atropine sulfate (optic) (Isopto Atropine)
betaxolol (Betoptic)
carteolol (Occupres)
dipivefrin (Propine)
erythromycin (Ilotycin)
flurbiprofen (Ocufen)
gentamicin (Garamycin)
homatropine hydrobromide (optic) (Isopto Homatropine)
idoxuridine (Herplex)
ketotifen (Zaditor)
levocabastine (Livostin)
loteprednol (lotemax, Alrex)
naphazoline (Naphcon)
ofloxacin (Ocuflox)
olopatadine (Patanol)
pilocarpine (Isopto Carpine)
polymyxin (Aerosporin)
sulfacetamide (Sulamyd)
timolol (Timoptic)
tobramycin (Tabrex)
trifluridine (Viroptic)
vidarabine (Vira-A)

PENICILLINS

amoxicillin (Amoxil)
amoxicillin/clavulanate (Augmentin)
ampicillin (Omnipen)
bacampicillin (Spectrobid)
cloxacillin (Tegopen)
dicloxacillin (Dynapen)
oxacillin (Prostaphlin)
penicillin G benzathine (Bi-cillin)
penicillin V potassium (V-Cillin K)

PEPTIDE ANTIINFECTIVE

vancomycin (Vancocin)

PERIODONTAL SPECIALTY PRODUCTS

chlorhexidine (PerioChip)
doxycycline (Atridox)
doxycycline (Periostat)

PERIPHERAL VASCULAR DISEASE

cilostazol (Pletal)
isoxsuprine (Vasodilan)
papaverine
pentoxifylline (Trental)

PLATELET AGGREGATION INHIBITORS

anagrelide (Agrylin)
aspirin clopidogrel (Plavix)
dipyradimole (Persantine)
ticlopidine (Ticlid)

PNEUMOCYSTIC PNEUMONITIS

atovaquone (Mepron)
pentamidine (Pentam 300)
sulfamethoxazole/trimethoprim (Bactrim)
trimetrexate (Neutrexin)

PROSTAGLANDIN

alprostadil (Caverject)
misoprostol (Cytotec)

PROSTATE HYPERPLASIA

finasteride (Proscar)
tamsulosin (Flomax)
terazosine (Hytrin)

SALIVARY STIMULANTS

cevimeline (Exovac)
pilocarpine (Salagen)

SKELETAL MUSCLE RELAXANTS

baclofen (Lioresal)
carisoprodol (Soma)
chlorphenesin (Maolate)
chlorzoxazone (Paraflex)
cyclobenzaprine (Flexeril)
dantrolene (Dantrium)
methocarbamol (Robaxin)
orphenadrine (Norflex)

SMOKING CESSATION

bupropion (Zyban)
nicotine polacrylex (Nicorette)
nicotine transdermal (Habitrol, ProStep)

SULFONAMIDES

sulfacetamide sodium (Sulamyd Sodium)
sulfamethizole (Thiosulfil Forte)
sulfamethoxazole/trimethoprim (Septra, Bactrim)
sulfamethoxazole (Gantanol)
sulfisoxazole (Gantrisin)

TETRACYCLINES

demeclocycline (Declomyin)
doxycycline (Atridox)
doxycycline (Periostat)
doxycycline (Vibramycin)
minocycline (Minocin)
tetracycline (Achromycin)
tetracycline fiber (Actisite)

URICOSURIC

aspirin probenecid (Benemid)
sulfinpyrazone (Anturane)

URINARY TRACT INFECTIONS

cinoxacin (Cinobac)
flavoxate (Uripas)
fosfomycin (Monurol)
methenamine (Hiprex)
nitrofurantoin (Furadantin)
phenazopyridine (Pyridium)
sulfamethizole (Thiosulfil Forte)
sulfamethoxazole (Gantanol)
sulfamethoxazole/trimethoprim (Bactrim, Septra)

VASOCONSTRICTOR

epinephrine (Adrenalin)
phenylephrine (Neo-Synephrine)

VITAMINS

ascorbic acid calcipotriene (Dovonex, D_3)
cyanocobalamin (Rubramin)
dihydrotachysterol (Hytakerol)
doxercalciferol (Hectorol)
folic acid (Folvite, B_9)
niacin (Nicolid)
phytonadione (Aqua MEPHYTON)
pyridoxine (B_6)
riboflavin (B_2)
thiamine (B_1)
vitamin A (Aquasol A)
vitamin D (Calciferol)
vitamin E (Aquasol E)

WOUND REPAIR

becaplermin (Regranex)

XANTHINES AND XANTHINE DERIVATIVES

aminophylline (Somophyllin)
dyphylline (Dilor)
oxitriphylline (Choledyl)
pentoxifylline (Trental)
theophylline (Theo-Dur)

Individual Drugs

abacavir sulfate

(a-bak'a-veer)

Ziagen

Drug class.: Antiviral, nucleoside analog

Action: Converted to active metabolite, carbovir, that inhibits reverse transcriptase enzymes in human immunodeficiency virus type 1 (HIV-1)

Uses: Used in combination with other antiviral drugs for treatment of HIV-1 infection

Dosage and routes:

• *Adult:* PO 300 mg bid in combination with other HIV-1 antiviral drugs

• *Child 3 mo-16 yr:* PO 8 mg/kg bid not to exceed adult dose; use with other antiviral drugs for HIV-1

Available forms include: Tabs 300 mg, oral sol 20 mg/ml in 240 ml vol

Side effects/adverse reactions:

▼*ORAL:* Mucous membrane lesions

CNS: Insomnia, fatigue, headache, asthenia, lethargy

CV: Edema

GI: Nausea, vomiting, diarrhea, anorexia, ***lactic acidosis***

RESP: Shortness of breath

INTEG: Rash, urticaria

META: Elevation of blood glucose, triglyceride elevation, alteration of liver enzymes

MS: Myalgia, arthralgia

MISC: ***Fatal hypersensitivity reactions****, fever*

Contraindications: Hypersensitivity

Precautions: Do not breast-feed, pregnancy category C, bone marrow depression, renal or hepatic impairment, use with other antivirals to avoid emergence of resistant viruses, avoid alcohol use

Pharmacokinetics:

PO: Bioavailability (83%), plasma protein binding (50%), hepatic metabolism (alcohol dehydrogenase), primarily renal excretion, fecal excretion (16%)

Drug interactions of concern to dentistry:

• None reported

DENTAL CONSIDERATIONS

General:

• Examine for oral manifestation of opportunistic infection.

• Patient on chronic drug therapy may rarely have symptoms of blood dyscrasias, which include infection, bleeding, and poor healing.

• Avoid dental light in patient's eyes; offer dark glasses for patient comfort.

• Place on frequent recall due to oral side effects.

• Consider semisupine chair position for patient comfort if GI side effects occur.

Consultations:

• In a patient with symptoms of blood dyscrasias, request a medical consult for blood studies and postpone treatment until normal values are reestablished.

• Medical consult may be required to assess disease control in the patient.

Teach patient/family:

• Importance of good oral hygiene to prevent soft tissue inflammation

• To prevent trauma when using oral hygiene aids

• To be alert for the possibility of secondary oral infection and the need to see dentist immediately if signs of infection occur

absorbable gelatin sponge

Gelfoam

Drug class.: Hemostatic, purified gelatin sponge

Action: Absorbs blood, provides area for clot formation

Uses: Hemostasis adjunct in dental surgery

Dosage and routes:

Dental use

• *Adult:* TOP can be applied dry or moistened with normal saline solution; blot on sterile gauze to remove excess solution, shape to fit with light finger compression; hold pressure on dry foam for 1-2 min

Available forms include: Dental packs, size 4 (2 × 2 cm)

Side effects/adverse reactions:

• *None reported*

Contraindications: Hypersensitivity, frank infection

Precautions: Avoid use in presence of infection, potential nidus of infection, do not resterilize product

Pharmacokinetics:

IMPLANT: Absorbed in 4-6 wk

DENTAL CONSIDERATIONS

Teach patient/family:

• To immediately report any sign of infection to the dentist

acarbose

(ay′car-bose)

Precose

♣ Prandase

Drug class.: Oral antidiabetic

Action: Inhibits α-glucosidase enzyme in the GI tract to delay the breakdown of carbohydrates to glucose, which results in lower postprandial plasma glucose levels

Uses: Use as single drug or in combination with insulin or other oral hypoglycemics in type 2 diabetes (NIDDM) when diet control is ineffective in controlling blood glucose levels

Dosage and routes:

• *Adult:* PO initial dose 25 mg tid at start of each meal; after testing may be increased to 50 mg tid at start of each meal; max dose >60 kg is 100 mg tid; max dose <60 kg is 50 mg bid

Caution: Doses must be individualized for each patient

Available forms include: Tabs 50, 100 mg

Side effects/adverse reactions:

GI: Bloating, flatulence, diarrhea, abdominal pain

META: Elevations of AST/ALT

Contraindications: Hypersensitivity, diabetic ketoacidosis, cirrhosis, inflammatory or obstructive GI disease

Precautions: Use glucose for hypoglycemia, monitor blood glucose levels, pregnancy category B, avoid use in lactation, children

Pharmacokinetics:

PO: Limited oral absorption, absorbed dose excreted in urine, metabolized in the GI tract and major portion of dose excreted in feces

Drug interactions of concern to dentistry:

• None reported; this is a new drug and information is lacking

DENTAL CONSIDERATIONS

General:

• Ensure that patient is following prescribed diet and takes medication regularly.

• Type 2 patients may also be using insulin. Should symptomatic hypoglycemia occur while taking this drug use dextrose rather than sucrose because of interference with sucrose metabolism.

- Place on frequent recall to evaluate healing response.
- Patients with diabetes may be more susceptible to infection and have delayed wound healing.
- Question the patient about self-monitoring the drug's antidiabetic effect.
- Consider semisupine chair position for patient comfort when GI side effects occur.

Consultations:

- Medical consult may be required to assess disease control and patient's ability to tolerate stress.

Teach patient/family:

- Importance of good oral hygiene to prevent soft tissue inflammation

---

acetaminophen

(a-seet-a-min′oh-fen)

Aspirin Free Anacin Maximum Strength, Aspirin Free Excedrin, Apacet, Dapa, Datril, Liquiprin, Panadol, Tempra, Tylenol, Tylenol Arthritis Extended Relief, Valadol, and many others

🍁 Abenol, Atasol, Robigesic, Rounax

Drug class.: Nonnarcotic analgesic

Action: Presumed to block the initiation of pain impulses by inhibition of prostaglandin synthesis; acts mainly in the CNS and to a lesser degree in peripheral nerves; antipyretic action results from inhibition of prostaglandin synthesis in the hypothalamic heat-regulating center

Uses: Mild-to-moderate pain, fever; also used in combination with other ingredients, including opioids

Dosage and routes:

- *Adult and child >12 yr:* PO 325-650 mg q4h prn or 1 g q6h, not to exceed 4 g/day; REC: 325-650 mg q4-6h prn, not to exceed 4 g/day
- *Adult:* PO for osteoarthritis, 1300 mg tid
- *Child 0-3 mo:* PO 40 mg/dose q4h
- *Child 4-12 mo:* PO 80 mg/dose q4h
- *Child 1-2 yr:* PO 120 mg/dose q4h
- *Child 2-4 yr:* PO/REC 160 mg/dose q4h
- *Child 4-6 yr:* PO/REC 240 mg/dose q4h
- *Child 6-9 yr:* PO/REC 320 mg/dose q4h
- *Child 9-11 yr:* PO/REC 320-400 mg/dose q4h
- *Child 11-12 yr:* PO/REC 320-480 mg/dose q4h

Available forms include: Rec supp 120, 125, 325, 650 mg; chew tab 80, 160 mg; tabs 325, 500, 650 mg; caps 500 mg; elix 120, 160, 325 mg/5 ml; liq 160 mg/5 ml, 500 mg/15 ml; sol (infant drops) 100 mg/1 ml, 120 mg/2.5 ml

Side effects/adverse reactions:

CNS: Stimulation, drowsiness

GI: ***Hepatotoxicity,*** nausea, vomiting, abdominal pain

HEMA: ***Leukopenia, neutropenia, hemolytic anemia*** (long-term use), ***thrombocytopenia, pancytopenia***

INTEG: ***Angioedema,*** rash, urticaria

TOXICITY: ***Cyanosis, anemia, neutropenia, jaundice, pancytopenia, CNS stimulation, delirium; then vascular collapse, convulsions, coma, death***

Contraindications: Hypersensitivity, chronic heavy alcohol use
Precautions: Anemia, hepatic disease, renal disease, chronic alcoholism, pregnancy category B
Pharmacokinetics:
PO: Onset 10-30 min, peak 0.5-2 hr, duration 4-6 hr, half-life 1-3 hr
REC: Slow, variable onset
For all routes, is metabolized in the liver, excreted by the kidneys, crosses the placenta, and found in breast milk
Drug interactions of concern to dentistry:
- Decreased effects: barbiturates
- Nephrotoxicity: NSAIDs, salicylates (chronic, high-dose concurrent use)
- Liver toxicity: chronic use of hydantoins, chronic alcohol use
- *Buffered acetaminophen:* Decreased absorption of tetracycline
- *When prescribed for dental pain:* Question patients about recent use of acetaminophen because acetaminophen has been shown to increase the INR to 4.0 or greater depending on the amount of acetaminophen taken. Obtain a new PT or INR value if surgical procedures are required.
- Data indicate that use of four regular strength acetaminophen tablets (325 mg) for 1 week can increase the risk of INR values greater than 6.0. If acetaminophen must be used for a long duration, it will be important to have INR values closely monitored. *JAMA* 279:657-662.

DENTAL CONSIDERATIONS
General:
- Avoid prolonged use with aspirin-containing products.
- Determine why the patient is taking the drug.
- Patients on chronic drug therapy may rarely have symptoms of blood dyscrasias, which can include infection, bleeding, and poor healing.

Consultations:
- In a patient with symptoms of blood dyscrasias, request a medical consult for blood studies, and postpone dental treatment until normal values are reestablished.

acetazolamide/ acetazolamide sodium

(a-set-a-zole'a-mide)
Ak-Zol, Dazamide, Diamox, Storzolamide
Acetazolam, Apo-Acetazolamide
Drug class.: Diuretic; carbonic anhydrase inhibitor

Action: Inhibits carbonic anhydrase activity in proximal renal tubular cells to decrease reabsorption of water, sodium, potassium, bicarbonate; decreases carbonic anhydrase in CNS, increasing seizure threshold; able to decrease aqueous humor in eye, which lowers intraocular pressure
Uses: Open-angle glaucoma, narrow-angle glaucoma (preoperatively, if surgery delayed), epilepsy (petit mal, grand mal, mixed), edema in CHF, drug-induced edema, acute altitude sickness
Dosage and routes:
Narrow-angle glaucoma
- *Adult:* PO/IM/IV 250 mg q4h, or 250 mg bid, to be used for short-term therapy; ext rel 500 mg bid

Open-angle glaucoma
- *Adult:* PO/IM/IV 250 mg to 1 g/day in divided doses for amounts over 250 mg

Available forms include: Tabs 125, 250 mg; sus rel caps 500 mg; inj IM/IV 500 mg

Side effects/adverse reactions:

▼ *ORAL:* Dry/burning mouth, tongue, lips; paresthesia; metallic taste; thirst

CNS: Drowsiness, paresthesia, anxiety, depression, headache, dizziness, confusion, stimulation, fatigue, seizures, sedation, nervousness

GI: Nausea, vomiting, anorexia, ***hepatic insufficiency,*** constipation, diarrhea, melena, weight loss

HEMA: ***Aplastic anemia, hemolytic anemia, leukopenia, agranulocytosis, thrombocytopenia, purpura, pancytopenia***

GU: Frequency, hypokalemia, ***uremia,*** polyuria, glucosuria, hematuria, dysuria

EENT: Myopia, tinnitus

INTEG: Rash, ***Stevens-Johnson syndrome,*** photosensitivity, pruritus, urticaria, fever

ENDO: Hyperglycemia

Contraindications: Hypersensitivity to sulfonamides, severe renal disease, severe hepatic disease, electrolyte imbalances (hyponatremia, hypokalemia), hyperchloremic acidosis, Addison's disease, long-term use in narrow-angle glaucoma, COPD

Precautions: Hypercalciuria, pregnancy category C; chronic use of oral sulfonylureas has been associated with increased risk of CV mortality; risk is controversial

Pharmacokinetics:

PO: Onset 1-1.5 hr, peak 1-3 hr, duration 6-12 hr

PO (SUS REL): Onset 2 hr, peak 8-12 hr, duration 18-24 hr

IV: Onset 2 min, peak 15 min, duration 4-5 hr

65% absorbed if fasting (oral), 75% absorbed if given with food; half-life 2.5-5.5 hr; excreted unchanged by kidneys (80% within 24 hr); crosses placenta

Drug interactions of concern to dentistry:

- Toxicity: salicylates (large doses)
- Hypokalemia: corticosteroids (systemic use)
- Crystalluria: ciprofloxacin

DENTAL CONSIDERATIONS:

General:

- Patients on chronic drug therapy may rarely have symptoms of blood dyscrasias, which can include infection, bleeding, and poor healing.
- Assess salivary flow as a factor in caries, periodontal disease, and candidiasis.
- Avoid drugs that may exacerbate glaucoma (e.g., anticholinergics).

Consultations:

- In a patient with symptoms of blood dyscrasias, request a medical consult for blood studies and postpone dental treatment until normal values are reestablished.
- Consult may be required to assess disease control in patient.

Teach patient/family:

- Importance of good oral hygiene to prevent soft tissue inflammation
- Caution to prevent injury when using oral hygiene aids

When chronic dry mouth occurs, advise patient:

- To avoid mouth rinses with high alcohol content due to drying effects
- To use daily home fluoride products for anticaries effect
- To use sugarless gum, frequent sips of water, or saliva substitutes

acetohexamide

(a-set-oh-hex'a-mide)
Dymelor
🍁 Dimelor

Drug class.: Sulfonylurea (first generation); antidiabetic

Action: Causes functioning beta cells in pancreas to release insulin, leading to drop in blood glucose levels; may improve binding between insulin and insulin receptors or increase number of insulin receptors; not effective if patient lacks functioning beta cells

Uses: Stable adult-onset diabetes mellitus (type 2)

Dosage and routes:

• *Adult:* PO 250 mg-1.5 g/day; usually given before breakfast, unless large dose is required, then dose is divided in two

Available forms include: Tabs 250, 500 mg scored

Side effects/adverse reactions:

CNS: Headache, weakness, tinnitus, fatigue, dizziness, vertigo

GI: ***Hepatotoxicity, jaundice,*** heartburn, nausea, vomiting, diarrhea

HEMA: ***Leukopenia, thrombocytopenia, agranulocytosis, aplastic anemia, hemolytic anemia,*** increased AST/ALT, alk phosphatase

INTEG: Rash, allergic reactions, pruritus, urticaria, eczema, photosensitivity, erythema

ENDO: ***Hypoglycemia***

Contraindications: Hypersensitivity to sulfonylureas, juvenile or brittle diabetes

Precautions: Pregnancy category C, elderly, cardiac disease, renal disease, hepatic disease, thyroid disease, severe hypoglycemic reactions

Pharmacokinetics:

PO: Onset 1 hr, peak 2-4 hr, duration 12-24 hr, half-life 6-8 hr; completely absorbed by GI route; metabolized in liver; excreted in urine (active metabolites, unchanged drug)

Drug interactions of concern to dentistry:

• Increased hypoglycemic effects: salicylates (large doses), NSAIDs, ketoconazole, miconazole
• Decreased action: corticosteroids
• Disulfiram-like reaction: alcohol

DENTAL CONSIDERATIONS

General:

• Monitor vital signs every appointment due to cardiovascular effects of diabetes.
• Patients on chronic drug therapy may rarely have symptoms of blood dyscrasias, which can include infection, bleeding, and poor healing.
• Place on frequent recall to evaluate healing response.
• Ensure that patient is following prescribed diet and takes medication regularly.
• Question patient about self-monitoring of drug's antidiabetic effect, including blood glucose values (SMBG) or finger-stick records.
• Avoid prescribing aspirin-containing products.
• Early morning appointments and a stress reduction protocol may be required for anxious patients.
• Patients with diabetes may be more susceptible to infection and have delayed wound healing.

Consultations:

• In a patient with symptoms of blood dyscrasias, request a medical

consult for blood studies and postpone dental treatment until normal values are reestablished.

• Medical consult may include data from patient's blood glucose monitoring, including glycosylated hemoglobin (GHb) or HbA_{1c} testing.

Teach patient/family:

• Importance of good oral hygiene to prevent soft tissue inflammation

• Caution to prevent injury when using oral hygiene aids

• To avoid mouth rinses with high alcohol content

---

acitretin

(a-si-tre'tin)

Soriatane

Drug class.: Systemic retinoid

Action: Unclear; may enhance the inflammatory response and accelerate reappearance of the stratum corneum

Uses: Severe psoriasis; unlabeled uses: nonpsoritic dermatoses, keratinization disorders

Dosage and routes:

• *Adult:* PO initial dose 25 mg to 50 mg qd taken with the main meal, adjust dose by patient response

Available forms include: Caps 10, 25 mg

Side effects/adverse reactions:

▼ *ORAL: Xerostomia (30%), ulcerative and nonulcerative stomatitis, taste perversion, cheilitis, gingival bleeding,* gingival hyperplasia

CNS: Fatigue, headache, dizziness, dysesthesia

CV: Flushing, ***pseudotumor cerebri***

GI: Abdominal pain, diarrhea, nausea, ***hepatitis, pancreatitis***

RESP: Sinusitis

HEMA: Thrombocytosis

EENT: Rhinitis, xerophthalmia, earache, tinnitus, dry eyes, dry nose, conjunctivitis, epistaxis, blurred vision, eye pain, photophobia

INTEG: Abnormal skin color, dry skin, alopecia, bulbous eruption, dermatitis, rash, purpura, skin fissures and ulcerations, photosensitivity

META: Elevation in serum transaminase, lipid disturbances, hyperglyceridemia

MS: Arthralgia, myalgia, spinal hyperostosis

MISC: Joint pains, asthenia, chills, diaphoresis

Contraindications: Hypersensitivity, hypersensitivity to etretinate, pregnancy, ethanol use, concurrent use with vitamin A, hepatic disease

Precautions: Women are advised to use effective contraception during use and for 2 years after use, renal impairment, lactation, pregnancy category X, hyperlipidemia, cardiovascular disease

Pharmacokinetics:

PO: Peak serum levels 2-5 hr; food enhances bioavailability, highly plasma protein bound (99.9%), hepatic metabolism, active metabolite; excreted in urine and bile

Drug interactions of concern to dentistry:

• Avoid vitamin preparations containing vitamin A

DENTAL CONSIDERATIONS

General:

• Determine why patient is taking the drug.

• Apply lubricant to dry lips for patient comfort before dental procedures.

• Assess salivary flow as factor in caries, periodontal disease, and candidiasis.
• Palliative medication may be required for management of oral side effects.
• Place on frequent recall due to oral side effects.
• Consider semisupine chair position for patient comfort if GI side effects occur.
• Avoid dental light in patient's eyes; offer dark glasses for patient comfort.

Consultations:
• Medical consult may be required to assess disease control in the patient.

Teach patient/family:
• Importance of good oral hygiene to prevent soft tissue inflammation
• Caution patient to prevent trauma when using oral hygiene aids
• To report oral lesions, soreness, or bleeding to dentist

When chronic dry mouth occurs, advise patient:
• To avoid mouth rinses with high alcohol content due to drying effects
• To use daily home fluoride products for anticaries effect
• To use sugarless gum, frequent sips of water, or saliva substitutes

---

acyclovir (topical)

(ay-sye'kloe-ver)
Zovirax

Drug class.: Antiviral

Action: Converted to acyclovir triphosphate by herpes simplex thymidine kinase thereby inhibiting viral DNA replication

Uses: Simple mucocutaneous herpes simplex, and in immunocompromised patients with initial herpes genitalis

Dosage and routes:
• *Adult and child:* TOP apply to all lesions q3h while awake, 6 × daily × 1 wk

Available forms include: TOP oint 5% (50 mg/g) in 3 g and 15 g tubes

Side effects/adverse reactions:
▼*ORAL:* Stinging sensation (lip application)
INTEG: Rash, urticaria, stinging, burning, pruritus, vulvitis

Contraindications: Hypersensitivity

Precautions: Pregnancy category C, lactation; cutaneous use only

DENTAL CONSIDERATIONS

General:
• Postpone dental treatment when oral herpetic lesions are present.

Teach patient/family:
• To dispose of toothbrush or other contaminated oral hygiene devices used during period of infection to prevent reinoculation of herpetic infection
• To apply with a finger cot or latex glove to prevent herpes infection on fingers
• To avoid mouth rinses with high alcohol content due to irritating effects

---

acyclovir sodium

(ay-sye'kloe-ver)
Zovirax
🍁 Avirax

Drug class.: Antiviral

Action: Converted to acyclovir triphosphate by herpes simplex thymidine kinase thereby inhibiting viral DNA replication

Uses: Mucocutaneous herpes simplex virus in immunocompromised patients, herpes genitalis (HSV-1, HSV-2), herpes zoster, varicella (chickenpox), herpes simplex encephalitis

Dosage and routes:

Herpes simplex (mucocutaneous)

• *Adult:* PO 200 mg to 400 mg 5 x daily for 10 days in immunocompromised patients

Genital herpes

• *Adult:* PO initial dose 200 mg q4h 5 × daily while awake for 10 days; recurrent 400 mg 2 × daily × 12 mo

Herpes zoster

• 800 mg q4h, 5 × daily for 7-10 days

Chickenpox

• *Child 2 yr age or older:* PO 20 mg/kg per dose (limit 800 mg), 4 × daily for 5 days; start at earliest sign of symptoms

• *Adults and children over 40 kg:* PO 800 mg 4 × daily × 5 days

Available forms include: Caps 200 mg; tabs 400 mg and 800 mg; powder for inj IV 500 mg and 1000 mg vials; susp 200 mg/5 ml

Side effects/adverse reactions:

▼ *ORAL:* Glossitis, medication taste

CNS: ***Convulsions,*** confusion, lethargy, hallucinations, dizziness, headache

GI: Nausea, vomiting, diarrhea, abdominal pain

HEMA: ***Thrombocytopenia, leukopenia***

GU: Elevated creatinine

INTEG: ***Erythema multiforme, toxic epidermal necrolysis,*** rash, urticaria, pruritus, phlebitis at IV site

META: Increased ALT/AST

Contraindications: Hypersensitivity

Precautions: Lactation, hepatic disease, renal disease, electrolyte imbalance, dehydration, pregnancy category B

Pharmacokinetics:

IV: Peak 1 hr, half-life 20 min to 3 hr (terminal); metabolized by liver; excreted by kidneys as unchanged drug (95%); crosses placenta

PO: Peak levels 1.5-2 hr, plasma half-life 2.5-3 hr; low protein binding

Drug interactions of concern to dentistry:

• None reported in otherwise uncompromised patients

DENTAL CONSIDERATIONS

General:

• Patients on chronic drug therapy may rarely have symptoms of blood dyscrasias, which can include infection, bleeding, and poor healing.

• Determine why the patient is taking the drug.

Consultations:

• In a patient with symptoms of blood dyscrasias, request a medical consult for blood studies and postpone dental treatment until normal values are reestablished.

• Medical consult may be required to assess disease control in the patient.

Teach patient/family:

• Importance of good oral hygiene to prevent soft tissue inflammation

• Caution to prevent injury when using oral hygiene aids

• To avoid mouth rinses with high alcohol content due to drying effects

• To dispose of toothbrush or other contaminated oral hygiene devices used during period of infection to prevent reinoculation of herpetic infection

albuterol

(al-byoo'ter-ole)

Airet, Gen-Salbutamol, Proventil, Proventil Repetabs, Proventil HFA, Ventodisk, Ventolin, Ventlin Nebules, Ventolin Rotacaps, Volmax

✤ Novo-Salmol

Drug class.: Adrenergic β_2-agonist

Action: Causes bronchodilation by action of β_2-receptors by increasing levels of cAMP, which relaxes smooth muscle with very little effect on heart rate

Uses: Prevention of exercise-induced asthma, bronchospasm with reversible obstructive airway disease, exercise-induced bronchospasm

Dosage and routes:

Asthma:

• *Adult:* INH 2 puffs 15 min before exercising; NEBULIZ/LPPB 5 mg tid-qid

Bronchospasm:

• *Adult:* INH 1-2 puffs q4-6h; PO 2-4 mg tid-qid, not to exceed 8 mg qid

• *Child ≥6 yr:* PO 2 mg tid or qid, max 24 hr dose 24 mg

Available forms include: Aerosol 90, 100 ✤ μ/actuation; tabs 2, 4 mg; ext rel tabs 4, 8 mg; syr 2 mg/5 ml; inhal sol 0.083%, 0.5%; cap inh 200 μ

Side effects/adverse reactions:

▼ *ORAL:* Taste changes, dry mouth, teeth discoloration

CNS: Tremors, anxiety, insomnia, headache, dizziness, stimulation, restlessness, hallucinations, flushing, irritability

CV: Palpitation, tachycardia, hypertension, angina, hypotension, dysrhythmias

GI: Heartburn, nausea, vomiting, diarrhea

*RESP: **Bronchospasm***

GU: Difficulty in urination

EENT: Dry nose, irritation of nose and throat

MS: Muscle cramps

Contraindications: Hypersensitivity to sympathomimetics, tachydysrhythmias, severe cardiac disease

Precautions: Lactation, pregnancy category C, cardiac disorders, hyperthyroidism, diabetes mellitus, hypertension, prostatic hypertrophy, narrow-angle glaucoma, seizures

Pharmacokinetics:

PO: Onset 0.5 hr, peak 2.5 hr, duration 4-6 hr, half-life 2.5 hr

INH: Onset 5-15 min, peak 0.5-2 hr, duration 3-6 hr, half-life 4 hr

Metabolized in the liver; excreted in urine; crosses placenta, breast milk, blood-brain barrier

Drug interactions of concern to dentistry:

• Increased dysrhythmias: halogenated hydrocarbon anesthetics

DENTAL CONSIDERATIONS

General:

• Monitor vital signs every appointment due to cardiovascular and respiratory side effects.

• Assess salivary flow as a factor in caries, periodontal disease, and candidiasis.

• Consider semisupine chair position for patients with respiratory disease.

• Midday appointments and a stress reduction protocol may be required for anxious patients.

• Be aware that aspirin or sulfite preservatives in vasoconstrictor-containing products can exacerbate asthma.

• Acute asthmatic episodes may be precipitated in the dental office. Sympathomimetic inhalants should be available for emergency use.

Consultations:

• Medical consult may be required to assess disease control in the patient.

• Medical consult may be required to assess patient's ability to tolerate stress.

Teach patient/family:

• For inhalation dosage forms, rinse mouth with water after each dose to prevent dryness

When chronic dry mouth occurs, advise patient:

• To avoid mouth rinses with high alcohol content due to drying effects

• To use daily home fluoride products for anticaries effect

• To use sugarless gum, frequent sips of water, or saliva substitutes

---

alendronate sodium

(a-len′droe-nate)

Fosamax

Drug class.: Amino biphosphonate

Action: Acts as a specific inhibitor of osteoclast-mediated bone resorption

Uses: Osteoporosis treatment and prevention in postmenopausal women, glucocorticoid-induced osteoporosis in men and women receiving glucocorticoids at daily dose of 7.5 mg prednisone, Paget's disease of bone

Dosage and routes:

Osteoporosis in postmenopause

• *Adult:* PO 10 mg/day; must be taken at least 30 min before first food, beverage, or other medication of the day; take with full glass of water and avoid lying down for 30 min after dose; supplemental calcium and vitamin D required for all patients if dietary intake is inadequate

Prevention in postmenopause

• *Adult:* PO 5 mg/day

Paget's disease

• *Adult:* PO 40 mg/day × 6 months; take as described above; supplemental calcium and vitamin D required for all patients if dietary intake is inadequate

Available forms include: Tabs 5, 10, 40 mg

Side effects/adverse reactions:

▼ *ORAL:* Taste alteration

CNS: Headache, nervousness

GI: Abdominal pain, nausea, constipation, diarrhea, acid regurgitation, gastritis, esophagitis

INTEG: Rash, erythema

MS: Pain, cramps

Contraindications: Hypersensitivity, hypocalcemia, esophageal abnormalities, inability to sit upright for 30 minutes

Precautions: Renal insufficiency, active upper GI disease, may see decrease in serum calcium/phosphate, pregnancy category C, lactation

Pharmacokinetics:

PO: Food, coffee, or juice reduces bioavailability; rapidly distributed to bone; not metabolized; almost complete urinary excretion

Drug interactions of concern to dentistry:

• Increased risk of GI side effects in doses >10 mg/day: Use NSAIDs, ASA with caution

• After administration, must wait at least 30 min before taking any other drug

DENTAL CONSIDERATIONS

General:

• Be aware of oral manifestations of Paget's disease (macrognathia, alveolar pain).

• Consider semisupine chair position for patient comfort due to pain experienced in osteoporosis and possible GI side effects of drug.

• Consider short appointments for patient comfort.

Consultations:

• Medical consult may be required to assess disease control and patient's ability to tolerate stress.

---

alitretinoin

(al-i-tra'ta-noyn)

Panretin

Drug class.: Topical retinoid

Action: Binds to all known intracellular retinoid receptor subtypes to function as a transcription factor in the regulation of gene expression that controls the process of cellular differentiation and proliferation in both normal and neoplastic cells

Uses: Topical treatment of cutaneous lesions in patients with AIDs-related Kaposi's sarcoma

Dosage and routes:

• *Adult:* TOP apply bid; can increase to tid or qid if application toxicity is not severe; apply enough gel to cover the lesion

Available forms include: Gel 0.1%, 60 g tube

Side effects/adverse reactions:

INTEG: Rash, pain, pruritus, erythema, edema, exfoliative dermatitis, vesiculation

Contraindications: Hypersensitivity, avoid application to mucous membranes and normal skin, hypersensitivity to retinoids

Precautions: Avoid pregnancy, pregnancy category D, discontinue breast feeding when used, safe use in children unknown, patients >65 years of age, occlusive dressings

Pharmacokinetics: No data

Drug interactions of concern to dentistry:

• Risk of photosensitivity reaction: tetracyclines, fluoroquinolones, other photosensitizing drugs

DENTAL CONSIDERATIONS

General:

• Patients will be taking antiviral drugs; note which drugs are being used, because some have potential for significant drug interactions.

• Take a complete medical history, including a current drug history with doses and duration of therapy.

---

allopurinol/allopurinol sodium

(al-oh-pure'i-nole)

Lopurin, Zyloprim

Alloprin, Apo-Allopurinol, Purinol

Drug class.: Antigout drug

Action: Inhibits the enzyme xanthine oxidase, reducing uric acid synthesis

Uses: Chronic gout, hyperuricemia associated with malignancies, recurrent calcium oxalate calculi, uric acid nephropathy

Dosage and routes:

Gout/hyperuricemia

• *Adult:* PO 100-600 mg qd depending on severity, not to exceed 800 mg/day

• *Child 6-10 yr:* 300 mg qd or 100 mg tid

• *Child <6 yr:* 50 mg tid

Available forms include: Tabs 100, 200 ✤, 300 mg

NOTE: Zyloprim for injection (allopurinol sodium) used only for patients with certain cancers for control of uric acid levels

Side effects/adverse reactions:

▼ *ORAL:* Metallic taste, stomatitis, lichenoid drug reaction, salivary gland swelling

CNS: Headache, drowsiness, neuritis, paresthesia

GI: Nausea, vomiting, anorexia, malaise, cramps, peptic ulcer, diarrhea

HEMA: ***Agranulocytosis, thrombocytopenia, aplastic anemia, pancytopenia, leukopenia, bone marrow depression, eosinophilia***

EENT: Retinopathy, cataracts, epistaxis

INTEG: Fever, chills, dermatitis, pruritus, purpura, erythema, ecchymosis, alopecia

MISC: Myopathy, arthralgia, hepatomegaly, ***cholestatic jaundice, renal failure***

Contraindications: Hypersensitivity

Precautions: Pregnancy category B, lactation, renal disease, hepatic disease, children

Pharmacokinetics:

PO: Peak 2-4 hr, half-life 1-2 hr; excreted in feces, urine

Drug interactions of concern to dentistry:

• Increased risk of rash: ampicillin, amoxicillin, bacampicillin, hetacillin

DENTAL CONSIDERATIONS

General:

• Patients on chronic drug therapy may rarely have symptoms of blood dyscrasias, which can include infection, bleeding, and poor healing.

Consultations:

• In a patient with symptoms of blood dyscrasias, request a medical consult for blood studies and postpone dental treatment until normal values are reestablished.

• Medical consult may be required to assess disease control in the patient.

Teach patient/family:

• Importance of good oral hygiene to prevent soft tissue inflammation

• To avoid mouth rinses with high alcohol content due to drying effects

---

alprazolam

(al-pray′zoe-lam)

Xanax

✤ Apo-Alpraz, Novo-Alprazol, Nu-Alpraz, Xanax TS

Drug class.: Benzodiazepine

Controlled Substance Schedule IV

Action: Produces CNS depression by interacting with benzodiazepine receptors to facilitate the action of the inhibitory neurotransmitter γ-aminobutyric acid (GABA)

Uses: Anxiety, panic disorders, anxiety with depressive symptoms

Dosage and routes:

• *Adult:* PO 0.25-0.5 mg tid, not to exceed 4 mg in divided doses/day

• *Geriatric:* PO 0.25 mg bid-tid

Available forms include: Tab 0.25, 0.5, 1, 2 mg

Side effects/adverse reactions:

▼ *ORAL:* Dry mouth

CNS: Dizziness, drowsiness, confu-

sion, headache, anxiety, tremors, stimulation, fatigue, depression, insomnia, hallucinations
CV: Orthostatic hypotension, ***ECG changes, tachycardia,*** hypotension
GI: Constipation, nausea, vomiting, anorexia, diarrhea
EENT: Blurred vision, tinnitus, mydriasis
INTEG: Rash, dermatitis, itching
Contraindications: Hypersensitivity to benzodiazepines, narrow-angle glaucoma, psychosis, pregnancy category D, child <18 yr, ketoconazole, itraconazole, ritonavir, indinavir
Precautions: Elderly, debilitated, hepatic disease, renal disease
Pharmacokinetics:
PO: Onset 30 min, peak 1-2 hr, duration 4-6 hr, half-life 12-15 hr; therapeutic response 2-3 days; metabolized by liver; excreted by kidneys; crosses placenta, breast milk
Drug interactions of concern to dentistry:
• Increased CNS depression: alcohol, other CNS depressants, clarithromycin, erythromycin, fluconazole, miconazole, fluoxetine, isoniazid
• Contraindicated with ketoconazole, itraconazole, ritonavir, indinavir

DENTAL CONSIDERATIONS
General:
• Monitor vital signs every appointment due to cardiovascular side effects.
• After supine positioning, have patient sit upright for at least 2 min to avoid orthostatic hypotension.
• Assess salivary flow as a factor in caries, periodontal disease, and candidiasis.
• Psychologic and physical dependence may occur with chronic administration.
Consultations:
• Medical consult may be required to assess disease control in the patient.
Teach patient/family:
When chronic dry mouth occurs, advise patient:
• To avoid mouth rinses with high alcohol content due to drying effects
• To use daily home fluoride products for anticaries effect
• To use sugarless gum, frequent sips of water, or saliva substitutes

alprostadil

(al-pros'ta-dil)
Caverject, Edex, Muse
Drug class.: Naturally occurring prostaglandin (E_1, PGE_1)

Action: Induces erection by relaxation of trabecular smooth muscle and by dilation of cavernosal arteries
Uses: Treatment of erectile dysfunction due to neurogenic, vasculogenic, psychogenic, or mixed etiology
(NOTE: Another alprostadil-containing product, Prostin VR Pediatric, is used to maintain ductus arteriosus patency in neonates until surgery can be performed.)
Dosage and routes:
Male gender
• *Adult:* Intracavernosal—initial dose must be in physician's office, individualized dose for each patient; initial doses range from 1.25 to 2.5 µg, titrate dose in increments of 5 to 10 µg erection for intercourse, doses over 60 µg are not

recommended; administer with supplied self-injection system by injecting into the corpora cavernosa; onset varies from 5-20 min; increase until suitable erection is achieved; using more than 3 times weekly is not recommended; alternate side and site of injection

• *Adult:* Intraurethral—follow dosing schedule because each patient must be individualized in the physician's office; no more than two doses in 24 hr

Available forms include: Vials 10 and 20 μg/ml as a powder with diluent and self-injection system; instructions for use and administration accompany package; pellets: 125, 250, 500, and 1000 μg

Side effects/adverse reactions:

CNS: Headache, dizziness

CV: Hypotension

RESP: Flulike syndrome, cough

GU: Penile pain, priapism, fibrosis, hematoma, rash or edema at site of injection, prostatic disorder, penile trauma

EENT: Nasal congestion, sinusitis

MS: Pain

Contraindications: Hypersensitivity, conditions predisposing to priapism (sickle cell anemia, sickle trait, multiple myeloma, or leukemia), penile deformation, penile implants, or Peyronie's disease

Precautions: Patients on anticoagulant therapy, use of sterile technique, care of syringe, physician instruction in use required, sexually transmitted disease

Pharmacokinetics: Rapidly metabolized and cleared from body by urinary excretion

Drug interactions of concern to dentistry:

• None reported

DENTAL CONSIDERATIONS

• None

amantadine HCl

(a-man'ta-deen)

Symadine, Symmetrel

Drug class.: Antiviral, antiparkinsonian agent

Action: Prevents uncoating of nucleic acid in viral cell, preventing penetration of virus to host; causes release of dopamine from neurons; may block reuptake of dopamine into presynaptic neurons

Uses: Prophylaxis or treatment of respiratory tract illness caused by influenza type A; extrapyramidal reactions; parkinsonism

Dosage and routes:

Influenza type A

• *Adult and child >12 yr:* PO 200 mg/day in single dose or divided bid

• *Adult >65 yr:* PO 200 mg daily

• *Child age 9-12 yr:* PO 100 mg q12h

• *Child 1-9 yr:* PO 2.2-4.4 mg/kg/day q12h, not to exceed 150 mg/day

Extrapyramidal reaction/parkinsonism

• *Adult:* PO 100 mg bid, up to 400 mg/day in EPS; give for 1 wk, then 100 mg as needed in parkinsonism

Available forms include: Caps 100 mg; syr 50 mg/5 ml

Side effects/adverse reactions:

▼ *ORAL: Dry mouth,* glossitis

CNS: ***Convulsions,*** headache, dizziness, drowsiness, fatigue, anxiety, psychosis, impaired concentration, insomnia, depression, hallucinations, tremors

CV: ***CHF,*** orthostatic hypotension

GI: Nausea, vomiting, constipation

HEMA: ***Leukopenia***
GU: Frequency, retention
EENT: Blurred vision
INTEG: Photosensitivity, dermatitis
Contraindications: Hypersensitivity, lactation, child <1 yr, pregnancy category C
Precautions: Epilepsy, CHF, orthostatic hypotension, psychiatric disorders, hepatic disease, renal disease (requires dose adjustment)
Pharmacokinetics:
PO: Onset 48 hr, half-life 24 hr; not metabolized; excreted in urine (90%) unchanged; crosses placenta; excreted in breast milk
Drug interactions of concern to dentistry:
• Increased anticholinergic response: anticholinergic drugs
• Increased CNS depression: alcohol, other CNS depressants

DENTAL CONSIDERATIONS
General:
• Monitor vital signs every appointment due to cardiovascular side effects.
• Assess salivary flow as a factor in caries, periodontal disease, and candidiasis.
• After supine positioning, have patient sit upright for at least 2 min to avoid orthostatic hypotension.
• Avoid dental light in patient's eyes; offer dark glasses for patient comfort.
• Short appointments and stress reduction protocol may be required for anxious patients.
• Consider semisupine chair position for patients with respiratory distress.
Teach patient/family:
• To avoid mouth rinses with high alcohol content due to drying effects
• To use electric toothbrush if patient has difficulty holding conventional devices

ambenonium chloride
(am-be-noe'nee-um)
Mytelase
Drug class.: Cholinesterase inhibitor

Action: An acetylcholinesterase inhibitor; inhibits destruction of acetylcholine, which increases concentration at sites in which acetylcholine is released; this facilitates transmission of impulses across the myoneural junction
Uses: Myasthenia gravis, when other drugs cannot be used
Dosage and routes:
• *Adult:* PO 5 mg tid or qid, then gradually increased q1-2d; 5 mg to 75 mg/dose is usually sufficient. Caution: doses more than 200 mg per day
Available forms include: Tabs 10 mg
Side effects/adverse reactions:
▼ *ORAL: Increased salivary secretions*
CNS: ***Paralysis, loss of consciousness, convulsions,*** drowsiness, dizziness, headache, weakness, incoordination
CV: ***Cardiac arrest,*** tachycardia, dysrhythmias, bradycardia, hypotension, AV block, ECG changes, syncope
GI: Nausea, diarrhea, vomiting, cramps, gastric secretions, dysphagia, increased peristalsis
RESP: ***Respiratory depression, bronchospasm, constriction, laryngospasm, respiratory arrest,*** increased secretions, dyspnea

GU: Frequency, incontinence, urgency
EENT: Miosis, blurred vision, lacrimation, visual changes
INTEG: Rashes, urticaria, sweating
Contraindications: Obstruction of intestine or renal system, hypersensitivity
Precautions: Seizure disorders, bronchial asthma, coronary occlusion, hyperthyroidism, dysrhythmias, peptic ulcer, megacolon, poor GI motility, pregnancy category C, bradycardia, hypotension, lactation, children
Pharmacokinetics:
PO: Onset 20-30 min, duration 3-8 hr
Drug interactions of concern to dentistry:
• Avoid drugs with anticholinergic activity and neuromuscular blocking agents
• Avoid systemic use of ester-type local anesthetics due to reduced plasma cholinesterase activity

DENTAL CONSIDERATIONS
General:
• Control excessive salivary flow with rubber dam and suction.
• Avoid drugs that reduce salivary flow, because they will antagonize this drug.
• Patient may be unable to keep mouth open for long periods due to disease; short appointments may be necessary.
• Monitor vital signs every appointment due to cardiovascular side effects. Evaluate respiration characteristics and rate.
• Consider semisupine chair position for patient comfort due to GI side effects of the drug.
• After supine positioning, have patient sit upright for at least 2 min to avoid orthostatic hypotension.

amiloride HCl
(a-mil'oh-ride)
Midamor
Drug class.: Potassium-sparing diuretic

Action: Acts primarily on distal tubule and secondarily by inhibiting reabsorption of sodium and increasing potassium retention
Uses: Edema in CHF in combination with other diuretics, for hypertension, adjunct with other diuretics to maintain potassium
Dosage and routes:
• *Adult:* PO 5 mg qd, may be increased to 10-20 mg qd if needed
Available forms include: Tab 5 mg
Side effects/adverse reactions:
▼ *ORAL:* Dry mouth, increased thirst
CNS: Headache, dizziness, fatigue, weakness, paresthesias, tremor, depression, anxiety
CV: Orthostatic hypotension
GI: Nausea, diarrhea, vomiting, anorexia, cramps, constipation, abdominal pain, jaundice, bleeding
*HEMA: **Agranulocytopenia, leukopenia, thrombocytopenia*** (rare)
GU: Polyuria, dysuria, frequency, impotence
EENT: Loss of hearing, tinnitus, blurred vision, nasal congestion, increased intraocular pressure
INTEG: Rash, pruritus, alopecia, urticaria
ELECT: Acidosis, hyponatremia, ***hyperkalemia,*** hypochloremia
MS: Cramps, joint pain

Contraindications: Anuria, hypersensitivity, hyperkalemia, impaired renal function

Precautions: Dehydration, pregnancy category B, diabetes, acidosis, lactation

Pharmacokinetics:

PO: Onset 2 hr, peak 6-10 hr, duration 24 hr, half-life 6-9 hr; excreted in urine, feces

Drug interactions of concern to dentistry:

- Decreased effects: corticosteroids, NSAIDs, indomethacin

DENTAL CONSIDERATIONS

General:

- Monitor vital signs every appointment due to cardiovascular side effects.
- Assess salivary flow as a factor in caries, periodontal disease, and candidiasis.
- After supine positioning, have patient sit upright for at least 2 min to avoid orthostatic hypotension.
- Patients on chronic drug therapy may rarely have symptoms of blood dyscrasias, which can include infection, bleeding, and poor healing.
- Limit use of sodium-containing products such as saline IV fluids for those patients with a dietary salt restriction.

Consultations:

- Medical consult may be required to assess patient's ability to tolerate stress.
- Medical consult may be required to assess disease control in the patient.
- In a patient with symptoms of blood dyscrasias, request a medical consult for blood studies and postpone dental treatment until normal values are reestablished.

Teach patient/family:

- Importance of good oral hygiene to prevent soft tissue inflammation
- Caution to prevent injury when using oral hygiene aids

When chronic dry mouth occurs, advise patient:

- To avoid mouth rinses with high alcohol content due to drying effects
- To use daily home fluoride products for anticaries effect
- To use sugarless gum, frequent sips of water, or saliva substitutes

---

aminocaproic acid

(a-mee-noe-ka-proe'ik)

Amicar

Drug class.: Hemostatic

Action: Inhibits fibrinolysis by inhibiting plasminogen activator substances

Uses: Hemorrhage from hyperfibrinolysis; adjunctive therapy in hemophilia; unapproved use for hemorrhages following dental surgery in hemophilia

Dosage and routes:

- *Adult:* PO/IV 5 g loading dose, then 1-1.25 g qh if needed, not to exceed 30 g/day

Available forms include: Inj IV 250 mg/ml; tab 500 mg; syr 250 mg/ml

Side effects/adverse reactions:

CNS: Headache, dizziness, ***convulsions,*** malaise, fatigue, hallucinations, delirium, psychosis, weakness

CV: ***Dysrhythmias,*** orthostatic hypotension, bradycardia

GI: Nausea, vomiting, abdominal cramps, diarrhea

HEMA: ***Thrombosis***

GU: ***Renal failure,*** dysuria, frequency, oliguria, ejaculatory failure, menstrual irregularities
EENT: Tinnitus, nasal congestion, conjunctival suffusion
INTEG: Rash
Contraindications: Hypersensitivity, abnormal bleeding, postpartum bleeding, DIC, upper urinary tract bleeding, new burns
Precautions: Neonates/infants, mild or moderate renal disease, hepatic disease, thrombosis, cardiac disease, pregnancy category C
Pharmacokinetics:
PO: Peak 2 hr, excreted by kidneys as unmetabolized drug, rapidly absorbed

DENTAL CONSIDERATIONS

General:
- Monitor vital signs every appointment due to cardiovascular side effects.
- After supine positioning, have patient sit upright for at least 2 min to avoid orthostatic hypotension.
- Consider additional local hemostasis measures to prevent excessive bleeding in patients with hemophilia.
- Determine why the patient is taking the drug.
- Avoid drugs such as aspirin; NSAIDs may have the potential to prolong bleeding.

Consultations:
- Medical consult may be required to assess disease control in the patient.
- Medical consult may be required to assess patient's ability to tolerate stress.

Teach patient/family:
- Importance of good oral hygiene to prevent soft tissue inflammation
- Caution to prevent injury when using oral hygiene aids

---

aminoglutethimide

(a-meen-noe-gloo-teth'i-mide)
Cytadren

Drug class.: Antineoplastic, adrenal steroid inhibitor

Action: Acts by inhibiting the enzymatic conversion of cholesterol to pregnenolone, thereby blocking synthesis of all adrenal steroids; also blocks conversion of androgens to estrogens in peripheral tissues
Uses: Suppression of adrenal function in Cushing's syndrome, metastatic breast cancer, adrenal cancer; unapproved use in prostate carcinoma
Dosage and routes:
- *Adult:* PO 250 mg bid or tid, may increase by 250 mg/day q1-2wk, not to exceed 2 g/day; monitor plasma cortisol

Available forms include: Tabs 250 mg
Side effects/adverse reactions:
CNS: Drowsiness, dizziness, headache, lethargy
CV: Hypotension, tachycardia, postural hypotension
GI: Nausea, vomiting, anorexia, ***hepatotoxicity***
HEMA: ***Neutropenia, leukopenia, pancytopenia, agranulocytosis*** (rare)
INTEG: Morbilliform skin rash, pruritus, hirsutism
Contraindications: Hypersensitivity, hypothyroidism, pregnancy category D, herpes infection
Precautions: Renal disease, hepatic disease, respiratory disease

Pharmacokinetics:
PO: Half-life 13 hr; metabolized in liver; excreted in urine; crosses placenta

Drug interactions of concern to dentistry:
• Accelerates metabolism of dexamethasone; if glucocorticoid replacement is needed, alternative steroid should be prescribed

DENTAL CONSIDERATIONS

General:
• Patients taking opioids for acute or chronic pain should be given alternative analgesics for dental pain.
• After supine positioning, have patient sit upright for at least 2 min to avoid orthostatic hypotension.
• Consider semisupine chair position for patient comfort if GI side effects occur.
• Patients on chronic drug therapy may rarely have symptoms of blood dyscrasias, which can include infection, bleeding, and poor healing.
• Monitor vital signs every appointment due to cardiovascular side effects.
• Drug may cause adrenocortical hypofunction, especially under conditions of stress, such as surgery, trauma, or acute illness. Patients should be carefully monitored and given hydrocortisone and mineralocorticoid supplements as needed.

Consultations:
• Medical consult may be required to assess disease control and patient's ability to tolerate stress.

Teach patient/family:
• Importance of good oral hygiene to prevent soft tissue inflammation
• That patient should use caution to prevent trauma when using oral hygiene aids
• That secondary oral infection may occur; need to see dentist immediately if infection occurs
• To report oral lesions, soreness, or bleeding to dentist
• Importance of updating health history/drug record if physician makes any changes in evaluations/drug regimens

---

aminophylline (theophylline ethylenediamine)

(am-in-off'i-lin)

Phyllocontin, Truphylline

♣ Phyllocontin-350

Drug class.: Xanthine

Action: Relaxes smooth muscle of respiratory system by blocking phosphodiesterase, which increases AMP

Uses: Bronchial asthma, bronchospasm, Cheyne-Stokes respirations

Dosage and routes:
• *Adult:* PO 6 mg/kg q6h, dose titrated to need in 3 or 4 doses/day; usually 300 mg/day (400-600 mg daily could be used if titrated and tolerated)
• *Child:* PO 7.5 mg/kg, then 3-6 mg/kg q6-8h; IV 7.5 mg/kg, then 3-6 mg/kg q6-8h injected over 5 min, do not exceed 25 mg/min, may give loading dose of 5.6 mg/kg over 1/2 hr; CONT IV 1 mg/kg/hr (maintenance)

Available forms include: Inj IV 250 mg/10 ml; IM/rectal supp 250, 500 mg; elix 250 mg/5 ml; oral liq 105 mg/5 ml; tabs 100, 200 mg; sus rel tabs 225 mg

Side effects/adverse reactions:

▼ *ORAL:* Bitter taste

CNS: Anxiety, restlessness, insomnia, dizziness, ***convulsions,*** headache, light-headedness, muscle twitching

CV: Palpitation, sinus tachycardia, hypotension, flushing, dysrhythmias

GI: Nausea, vomiting, anorexia, diarrhea, dyspepsia, anal irritation (suppositories), epigastric pain

RESP: Increased rate

GU: Urinary frequency

INTEG: Flushing, urticaria

Contraindications: Hypersensitivity to xanthines, tachydysrhythmias

Precautions: Elderly, CHF, cor pulmonale, hepatic disease, active peptic ulcer disease, diabetes mellitus, hyperthyroidism, hypertension, children, pregnancy category C, glaucoma, prostatic hypertrophy

Pharmacokinetics:

IV: Peak 30 min; 16 mg of anhydrous aminophylline provides a dose equivalent to 100 mg anhydrous theophylline

Drug interactions of concern to dentistry:

• Increased action: erythromycin (macrolides), ciprofloxacin

• Cardiac dysrhythmia: CNS stimulants, hydrocarbon inhalation aneshetics

• Decreased effects: barbiturates, carbamazepine

• Decreased effects of benzodiazepines

DENTAL CONSIDERATIONS

General:

• Monitor vital signs every appointment due to cardiovascular and respiratory side effects.

• Consider semisupine chair position for patient comfort due to respiratory disease and GI side effects of the drug.

• Midday appointments and a stress reduction protocol may be required for anxious patients.

• Be aware that aspirin or sulfite preservatives in vasoconstrictor-containing products can exacerbate asthma.

• Acute asthmatic episodes may be precipitated in the dental office. Sympathomimetic inhalants should be available for emergency use.

Consultations:

• Medical consult may be required to assess disease control in the patient.

---

amiodarone HCl

(a-mee'oh-da-rone)

Cordarone, Cordarone IV, Pacerone

Drug class.: Antidysrhythmic (Class III)

Action: Prolongs action potential duration and effective refractory period, noncompetitive α- and β-adrenergic receptor inhibition

Uses: Documented life-threatening ventricular tachycardia; unapproved: ventricular fibrillation not controlled by first-line agents

Dosage and routes:

• *Adult:* PO loading dose 800-1600 mg/day 1-3 wk, then 600-800 mg/day 1 mo; maintenance 200-600 mg/day

Available forms include: Tabs 200 mg; INJ 50 mg/ml

Side effects/adverse reactions:

▼ *ORAL:* Bitter taste sensation, dry mouth

CNS: Headache, dizziness, involuntary movement, tremors, peripheral neuropathy, malaise, fatigue, ataxia, paresthesias, insomnia

CV: Hypotension, bradycardia, ***si-***

nus arrest, CHF, dysrhythmias, SA node dysfunction

GI: ***Hepatotoxicity,*** nausea, vomiting, diarrhea, abdominal pain, anorexia, constipation

RESP: ***Pulmonary fibrosis,*** pulmonary inflammation

EENT: ***Corneal microdeposits,*** blurred vision, halos, photophobia, dry eyes

INTEG: Rash, photosensitivity, bluish-gray skin discoloration, rash, alopecia, spontaneous ecchymosis

ENDO: Hyperthyroidism or hypothyroidism

MS: Weakness, pain in extremities

MISC: Flushing, abnormal smell, edema, coagulation abnormalities

Precautions: Goiter, Hashimoto's thyroiditis, SN dysfunction, second- or third-degree AV block, electrolyte imbalances, pregnancy category C, bradycardia, lactation

Pharmacokinetics:

PO: Onset 1-3 wk, peak 3-7 hr, half-life 15-100 days; metabolized by liver; excreted by kidneys

Drug interactions of concern to dentistry:

- Bradycardia, hypotension: inhalation anesthetics, lidocaine, anticholinergics, vasoconstrictors
- Increased photosensitization: tetracyclines

DENTAL CONSIDERATIONS

General:

- Monitor vital signs every appointment due to cardiovascular and respiratory side effects.
- Assess salivary flow as a factor in caries, periodontal disease, and candidiasis.
- Avoid dental light in patient's eyes; offer dark glasses for patient comfort.
- After supine positioning, have patient sit upright for at least 2 min before standing to avoid orthostatic hypotension.
- Use vasoconstrictors with caution, in low doses, and with careful aspiration. Avoid gingival retraction cord with epinephrine.
- Stress from dental procedures may compromise cardiovascular function; determine patient risk.
- Delay or avoid dental treatment if patient shows signs of cardiac symptoms or respiratory distress.

Consultations:

- Medical consult may be required to assess patient's ability to tolerate stress.
- Medical consult may be required to assess disease control in the patient.

Teach patient/family:

When chronic dry mouth occurs, advise patient:

- To avoid mouth rinses with high alcohol content due to drying effects
- To use daily home fluoride products for anticaries effect
- To use sugarless gum, frequent sips of water, or saliva substitutes

---

amitriptyline HCl

(a-mee-trip'ti-leen)

Elavil, Endep

♣ Apo-Amitriptyline, Levate, Novotriptyn

Drug class.: Antidepressant—tricyclic

Action: Inhibits both norepinephrine and serotonin (5-HT) uptake in the brain, although the precise antidepressant mechanism remains unclear

Uses: Major depression; unapproved: enuresis and neurogenic pain

Dosage and routes:

• *Adult:* PO 75 mg/day in divided doses or 50-100 mg hs, may increase to 150 mg qd; IM 20-30 mg qid or 80-120 mg hs

• *Adolescent/geriatric:* PO 30 mg/day in divided doses, may be increased to 150 mg/day

Available forms include: Tabs 10, 25, 50, 75, 100, 150 mg; inj IM 10 mg/ml; syr 10 mg/5 ml ✱

Side effects/adverse reactions:

▼ *ORAL: Dry mouth, unpleasant taste,* stomatitis, salivary gland pain

CNS: Dizziness, drowsiness, confusion, headache, anxiety, tremors, stimulation, weakness, insomnia, nightmares, EPS (elderly), increased psychiatric symptoms, seizures, ataxia, paresthesias

CV: Orthostatic hypotension, ***ECG changes, tachycardia, hypertension,*** palpitation, syncope

GI: Diarrhea, ***paralytic ileus, hepatitis,*** increased appetite, cramps, epigastric distress, jaundice, nausea, vomiting

HEMA: ***Agranulocytosis, thrombocytopenia, eosinophilia, leukopenia***

GU: Retention

EENT: Blurred vision, tinnitus, mydriasis, ophthalmoplegia

INTEG: Rash, urticaria, sweating, pruritus, photosensitivity

Contraindications: Hypersensitivity to tricyclic antidepressants, recovery phase of MI

Precautions: Suicidal patients, convulsive disorders, prostatic hypertrophy, schizophrenia, psychotic disorders, severe depression, increased intraocular pressure, narrow-angle glaucoma, urinary retention, cardiac disease, hepatic disease, renal disease, hyperthyroidism, electroshock therapy, elective surgery, child <12 yr, pregnancy category C, elderly, MAO inhibitors

Pharmacokinetics:

PO/IM: Onset 45 min, peak 2-12 hr, therapeutic response 2-3 wk, half-life 10-50 hr; metabolized by liver; excreted in urine, feces, breast milk; crosses placenta

Drug interactions of concern to dentistry:

• Increased anticholinergic effects: muscarinic blockers, antihistamines, phenothiazines

• Increased effects of direct-acting sympathomimetics (epinephrine, levonordefrin)

• Possible risk of increased CNS depression: alcohol, barbiturates, benzodiazepines, CNS depressants

• Decreased antihypertensive effect: clonidine, guanadrel, guanethidine

DENTAL CONSIDERATIONS

General:

• Take vital signs every appointment due to cardiovascular side effects.

• Assess salivary flow as a factor in caries, periodontal disease, and candidiasis.

• Patients on chronic drug therapy may rarely have symptoms of blood dyscrasias, which can include infection, bleeding, and poor healing.

• After supine positioning, have patient sit upright for at least 2 min to avoid orthostatic hypotension.

• Use vasoconstrictors with caution, in low doses, and with careful aspiration. Avoid use of gingival retraction cord with epinephrine.

• Place on frequent recall due to oral side effects.

Consultations:

• In a patient with symptoms of blood dyscrasias, request a medical consult for blood studies and postpone dental treatment until normal values are reestablished.

• Medical consult may be required to assess disease control in the patient.

• Physician should be informed if significant xerostomic side effects occur (e.g., increased caries, sore tongue, problems eating or swallowing, difficulty wearing prosthesis) so a medication change can be considered.

Teach patient/family:

• Importance of good oral hygiene to prevent soft tissue inflammation

• Caution to prevent injury when using oral hygiene aids

When chronic dry mouth occurs, advise patient:

• To avoid mouth rinses with high alcohol content due to drying effects

• To use daily home fluoride products for anticaries effect

• To use sugarless gum, frequent sips of water, or saliva substitutes

---

amlexanox

(am-lex'an-ox)

Aphthasol

Drug class.: Topical antiinflammatory

Action: Mechanism of action is unknown; has antiinflammatory and antiallergic activities; accelerates the resolution of pain and healing of aphthous ulcers

Uses: Aphthous ulcers in patients with normal immune systems

Dosage and routes:

• *Adult:* TOP squeeze dab (0.5 cm) of paste onto fingertip and dab each ulcer qid, after oral hygiene, after each meal, and hs; use until ulcer heals

Available forms include: Oral paste 5%, 5 g tube

Side effects/adverse reactions:

▼ *ORAL:* Transient stinging and burning on application, contact mucositis

GI: Nausea, diarrhea

Contraindications: Hypersensitivity

Precautions: Wash hands immediately before and after each use; discontinue if mucositis appears, pregnancy category B, lactation, children

Pharmacokinetics:

TOP: Systemic absorption from GI tract if swallowed, drug and metabolites excreted in urine

Drug interactions of concern to dentistry:

• None reported

DENTAL CONSIDERATIONS

General:

• Recurrent aphthous ulcers may be associated with systemic conditions; evaluate as needed if healing has not occurred after 10 days.

Teach patient/family:

• To apply paste as directed and wash hands immediately before and after each use

• To report oral lesions or soreness to dentist

A

amlodipine besylate

(am-loe′di-peen)

Norvasc

Drug class.: Calcium channel blocker

Action: Inhibits calcium ion influx across cell membrane during cardiac depolarization; produces relaxation of coronary vascular smooth muscle; dilates coronary arteries; decreases SA/AV node conduction; dilates peripheral arteries

Uses: Hypertension as a single agent or in combination with other antihypertensives, chronic stable angina pectoris, vasospastic angina

Dosage and routes:

Hypertension

- *Adult:* PO 5 mg/day; max daily dose 10 mg
- *Geriatric or small, fragile adults:* PO 2.5 mg/day

Available forms include: Tabs 2.5, 5, 10 mg

Side effects/adverse reactions:

▼ *ORAL:* Dry mouth, altered taste; gingival overgrowth has been reported with other calcium channel blockers

CNS: Headache, fatigue, lethargy, somnolence, dizziness, light-headedness

CV: Peripheral edema, palpitation, syncope, CHF, tachycardia, chest pain

GI: Nausea, dyspepsia, discomfort, diarrhea, flatulence

RESP: Pulmonary edema

GU: Sexual difficulties

EENT: Diplopia, eye pain

INTEG: Petechiae, bruising, ecchymoses, purpura

MS: Muscle cramps, joint stiffness

Contraindications: Sick sinus syndrome, second- or third-degree heart block, hypotension less than 90 mm Hg systolic, cardiogenic shock, severe CHF

Precautions: Pregnancy category C, CHF, hypotension, hepatic injury, lactation, children, renal disease

Pharmacokinetics:

PO: Peak plasma levels 6-12 hr, half-life 30-50 hr; highly protein bound; metabolized in liver; excreted in urine

Drug interactions of concern to dentistry:

- Decreased effect: indomethacin, possibly other NSAIDs, phenobarbital
- Increased effect: parenteral and inhalational general anesthetics or other drugs with hypotensive actions

DENTAL CONSIDERATIONS

General:

- Monitor cardiac status; take vital signs at each appointment because of CV side effects. Consider a stress reduction protocol to prevent stress-induced angina during the dental appointment.
- After supine positioning, have patient sit upright for at least 2 min to avoid orthostatic hypotension.
- Limit use of sodium-containing products such as saline IV fluids for those patients with a dietary salt restriction.
- Assess salivary flow as a factor in caries, periodontal disease, and candidiasis.

Consultations:

- Medical consult may be required to assess disease control in the patient.

Teach patient/family:

• Need for frequent oral prophylaxis if gingival overgrowth should occur

When chronic dry mouth occurs, advise patient:

• To avoid mouth rinses with high alcohol content due to drying effects

• To use daily home fluoride products for anticaries effect

• To use sugarless gum, frequent sips of water, or artificial saliva

---

amoxapine

(a-mox'a-peen)

Asendin

Drug class.: Antidepressant—tricyclic

Action: Inhibits both norepinephrine and serotonin (5-HT) uptake in the brain, although the precise antidepressant mechanism remains unclear

Uses: Depression

Dosage and routes:

• *Adult:* PO 50 mg tid, may increase to 100 mg tid on third day of therapy, not to exceed 300 mg/day unless lower doses have been given for at least 2 wk; may be given daily dose hs, not to exceed 600 mg/day in hospitalized patients

Available forms include: Tabs 25, 50, 100, 150 mg

Side effects/adverse reactions:

▼ *ORAL: Dry mouth,* stomatitis

CNS: Dizziness, drowsiness, confusion, headache, anxiety, tremors, tardive dyskinesia, stimulation, weakness, insomnia, nightmares, EPS (elderly), increased psychiatric symptoms, paresthesia

CV: Orthostatic hypotension, ECG changes, tachycardia, ***hypertension,*** palpitation

GI: Diarrhea, constipation, ***paralytic ileus, hepatitis,*** nausea, vomiting, increased appetite, cramps, epigastric distress, jaundice

HEMA: ***Agranulocytosis, thrombocytopenia, eosinophilia, leukopenia***

GU: ***Acute renal failure,*** retention

EENT: Blurred vision, tinnitus, mydriasis, ophthalmoplegia

INTEG: Rash, urticaria, sweating, pruritus, photosensitivity

Contraindications: Hypersensitivity to tricyclic antidepressants, recovery phase of MI, convulsive disorders, prostatic hypertrophy

Precautions: Suicidal patients, severe depression, increased intraocular pressure, narrow-angle glaucoma, urinary retention, cardiac disease, hepatic disease, hyperthyroidism, electroshock therapy, elective surgery, elderly, pregnancy category C, MAO inhibitors

Pharmacokinetics:

PO: Peak blood levels 90 min, steady state 7 days, half-life 8 hr; metabolized by liver; excreted by kidneys; crosses placenta

Drug interactions of concern to dentistry:

• Increased anticholinergic effects: muscarinic blockers, antihistamines, phenothiazines

• Increased effects of direct-acting sympathomimetics (epinephrine, levonordefrin)

• Potential risk of increased CNS depression: alcohol, barbiturates, benzodiazepines, CNS depressants

• Decreased antihypertensive effect: clonidine, guanadrel, guanethidine

DENTAL CONSIDERATIONS

General:

• Take vital signs every appointment due to cardiovascular side effects.

• Assess salivary flow as a factor in caries, periodontal disease, and candidiasis.

• Patients on chronic drug therapy may rarely have symptoms of blood dyscrasias, which can include infection, bleeding, and poor healing.

• After supine positioning, have patient sit upright for at least 2 min to avoid orthostatic hypotension.

• Use vasoconstrictors with caution, in low doses, and with careful aspiration. Avoid use of gingival retraction cord with epinephrine.

• Place on frequent recall due to oral side effects.

Consultations:

• In a patient with symptoms of blood dyscrasias, request a medical consult for blood studies and postpone dental treatment until normal values are reestablished.

• Medical consult may be required to assess disease control in the patient.

• Physician should be informed if significant xerostomic side effects occur (e.g., increased caries, sore tongue, problems eating or swallowing, difficulty wearing prosthesis) so a medication change can be considered.

Teach patient/family:

• Importance of good oral hygiene to prevent soft tissue inflammation

• Caution to prevent injury when using oral hygiene aids

When chronic dry mouth occurs, advise patient:

• To avoid mouth rinses with high alcohol content due to drying effects

• To use daily home fluoride products for anticaries effect

• To use sugarless gum, frequent sips of water, or saliva substitutes

amoxicillin/clavulanate potassium

(a-mox-i-sil′in)/(klav′yoo-la-nate)

Augmentin

✤ Clavulin

Drug class.: Aminopenicillin with a β-lactamase inhibitor

Action: Interferes with cell-wall replication of susceptible organisms; the cell wall, rendered osmotically unstable, swells and bursts from osmotic pressure

Uses: Sinusitis, pneumonia, lower RTI, otitis media, skin and urinary tract infections caused by susceptible microorganisms that include β-lactamase–producing organisms

Dosage and routes:

• *Adult:* PO one 500 mg tab q12h or one 250 mg tab q8h depending on severity of infection

• *Child:* PO 20-40 mg/kg/day in divided doses q8h

*Do not use the 250/125 mg tab until child weighs at least 40 kg or more.

Severe and respiratory tract infections

• *Adult:* PO one 875 mg tab q12h or one 500 mg tab q8h

Available forms include: Amoxicillin/clavulate K amounts: Tabs 250/125, 500/125, 875/125 mg; chew tabs 125/31.25, 200/28.5, 250/62.5, 400/57 mg; powder for oral susp 125/31.25, 200/28.5, 250/62.5, 400/57 mg/5 ml when reconstituted; note that the single dose of clavulanate K should not exceed 125 mg. Augmentin 250 mg tab and Augmentin 250 mg chewable tab do not contain the same amount of clavulanic acid. They are not interchangeable.

Side effects/adverse reactions:
▼ *ORAL:* Discolored tongue, glossitis, increased thirst, candidiasis, stomatitis
CNS: Headache
GI: Nausea, diarrhea, vomiting, increased AST/ALT, abdominal pain, colitis, antibiotic-associated pseudomembraneous colitis
HEMA: ***Bone marrow depression, granulocytopenia, leukopenia, eosinophilia,*** thrombocytopenic purpura, anemia
GU: Vaginitis, moniliasis, ***glomerulonephritis,*** oliguria, proteinuria, hematuria
INTEG: Pemphigus-like reaction
META: Hyperkalemia, hypokalemia, alkalosis, hypernatremia
SYST: ***Anaphylaxis,*** pruritus, urticaria, angioedema, bronchospasm (allergy symptoms)

Contraindications: Hypersensitivity to penicillins; neonates, clavulanate K–associated cholestatic/hepatic dysfunction

Precautions: Pregnancy category B, hypersensitivity to cephalosporins, hepatic function impairment

Pharmacokinetics:
PO: Good oral absorption with or without food; peak 2 hr, duration 6-8 hr, half-life 1-1.33 hr; metabolized in liver; excreted in urine; crosses placenta; enters breast milk

Drug interactions of concern to dentistry:
• Decreased antimicrobial effectiveness: tetracyclines, erythromycins, lincomycins
• Increased amoxicillin concentrations: probenecid
• Increased risk of skin rashes: allopurinol
When used for dental infection:
• May reduce effectiveness of oral contraceptives

DENTAL CONSIDERATIONS

General:
• Take precautions regarding allergy to medication.
• Determine why the patient is taking the drug.

Consultations:
• Medical consult may be required to assess disease control in the patient.

Teach patient/family:
• Importance of good oral hygiene to prevent soft tissue inflammation
• Caution to prevent injury when using oral hygiene aids
When used for dental infection, advise patient:
• On birth control pill to use additional method of contraception for duration of cycle
• To report sore throat, oral burning sensation, fever, and fatigue, any of which could indicate superinfection
• To take at prescribed intervals and complete dosage regimen
• To immediately notify the dentist if signs or symptoms of infection increase

---

amoxicillin trihydrate

(a-mox-i-sil'in)
Amoxil, Polymox, Trimox, Wymox
🍁 Apo-Amoxi, Nova moxin, Nu-Amox

Drug class.: Aminopenicillin

Action: Interferes with cell wall replication of susceptible organisms; the cell wall, rendered osmotically unstable, swells and bursts from osmotic pressure

Uses: Sinus infections, pneumonia, otitis media, skin infections, urinary tract infections; effective for strains of *E. coli, P. mirabilis, H. influenzae, S. faecalis, S. pneumoniae;* unlabeled uses for chlamydia, *H. pylori*

Dosage and routes:

Systemic infections

• *Adult:* PO 250-500 mg q8h or q12h depending on severity of infection

• *Child:* PO 20-40 mg/kg/day in divided doses q8h; optional dose 200 mg q12h (in place of 125 mg q8h) or 400 mg q12h (in place of 250 mg q8h)

Bacterial endocarditis prophylaxis

• *Adult:* PO 2 g 1 hr before dental procedure

• *Children:* PO 50 mg/kg of body weight, not to exceed the adult dose, 1 hr before dental procedure

Prosthetic joint prophylaxis (when indicated)

• *Adult:* PO 2 g 1 hr before dental procedure

Available forms include: Caps 250, 500 mg; tabs 500, 875 mg; chew tabs 125, 250 mg; powder for oral susp 50 mg/ml and 125, 250 mg/5 ml

Side effects/adverse reactions:

▼ *ORAL:* Discolored tongue, glossitis, increased thirst, candidiasis, stomatitis

CNS: Headache

GI: Nausea, vomiting, diarrhea, increased AST/ALT, abdominal pain, colitis

HEMA: ***Bone marrow depression, granulocytopenia,*** anemia, increased bleeding time

INTEG: Pemphigus-like reaction

SYST: ***Anaphylaxis*** (allergy symptoms), pruritus, urticaria, angioedema, bronchospasm

Contraindications: Hypersensitivity to penicillins; neonates

Precautions: Pregnancy category B, hypersensitivity to cephalosporins

Pharmacokinetics:

PO: Peak 2 hr, duration 6-8 hr, half-life 1-1.33 hr; metabolized in liver; excreted in urine; crosses placenta; enters breast milk

Drug interactions of concern to dentistry:

• Decreased antimicrobial effectiveness: tetracyclines, erythromycins, lincomycins

• Increased amoxicillin concentrations: probenecid

• Suspected increase in methotrexate toxicity

When used for dental infection:

• May decrease effectiveness of oral contraceptives

DENTAL CONSIDERATIONS

General:

• Take precautions regarding allergy to medication.

• Determine why the patient is taking the drug.

Consultations:

• Medical consult may be required to assess disease control in the patient.

Teach patient/family:

• Importance of good oral hygiene to prevent soft tissue inflammation

• Caution to prevent injury when using oral hygiene aids

When used for dental infection, advise patient:

• On birth control pill to use additional method of contraception for duration of cycle

• To report sore throat, oral burning

sensation, fever, and fatigue, any of which could indicate superinfection
• To take at prescribed intervals and complete dosage regimen
• To immediately notify the dentist if signs or symptoms of infection increase

amphotericin B (topical)

(am-foe-ter′i-sin)
Fungizone Oral Suspension
Drug class.: Polyene antifungal

Action: Increases cell membrane permeability in susceptible organisms by binding to cell membrane sterols
Uses: Oral, mucocutaneous infections caused by *Candida*
Dosage and routes:
• *Adult and child:* SOL oral suspension rinse with 1 ml (100 mg) qid
Available forms include: Oral suspension 100 mg/ml in 24 ml dropper bottle
Side effects/adverse reactions:
GI: Nausea, vomiting, diarrhea
INTEG: Urticaria, angioedema (rare), ***Stevens-Johnson syndrome***
Contraindications: Hypersensitivity
Precautions: Pregnancy category C, lactation; not for systemic fungal infections
Pharmacokinetics: Topical rinse only, poorly absorbed if swallowed
Drug interactions of concern to dentistry:
• None reported
DENTAL CONSIDERATIONS
General:
• Determine why the patient is taking the drug.
• Broad-spectrum antibiotics may contribute to oral *Candida* infections.
Teach patient/family:
• That long-term therapy may be needed to clear infection; complete entire course of medication
• Not to use commercial mouthwashes for mouth infection unless prescribed by dentist
• That patient with removable dental appliance should soak appliance in antifungal agent overnight
• To prevent reinoculaton of *Canada* infection by disposing of toothbrush or other contaminated oral hygiene devices used during period of infection

ampicillin/ampicillin sodium/ampicillin trihydrate

(am-pi-sil′in)
Ampicillin sodium (parenteral): Omnipen-N, Polycillin-N, Totacillin-N; *ampicillin:* Marcillin, Omnipen, Polycillin, Principen, Totacillin
✦ *Ampicillin sodium (parenteral):* Ampicin, Penbri tin; ***ampicillin:*** Apo-Ampi, Novo-Ampicillin, Nu-Ampi
Drug class.: Aminopenicillin

Action: Interferes with cell wall replication of susceptible organisms; the cell wall, rendered osmotically unstable, swells and bursts from osmotic pressure
Uses: Sinus infections, pneumonia, otitis media, skin infections, UTIs; effective for strains of *E. coli, P. mirabilis, H. influenzae, S. faecalis, S. pneumoniae*

Dosage and routes:
Systemic infections
• *Adult:* PO 250-500 mg q6h depending on severity of infection; IV/IM 2-8 g qd in divided doses q4-6h
• *Child:* PO 50-100 mg/kg/day in divided doses q6h; IV/IM 100-200 mg/kg/day in divided doses q6h
Bacterial endocarditis prophylaxis
• *Adult:* IV or IM for patients unable to take oral medications and who are not allergic to penicillin 2 g within 30 min of dental procedure
• *Child:* IV or IM for patients unable to take oral medications and who are not allergic to penicillin 50 mg/kg of body weight not to exceed the adult dose
Prosthetic joint prophylaxis (when indicated)
• *Adult:* IV or IM for patients unable to take oral medications and who are not allergic to penicillin 2 g 1 hr before dental procedure
Available forms include: Powder for inj IV/IM 125, 250, 500 mg and 1, 2, 10 g; IV inf 500 mg and 1, 2 g; caps 250, 500 mg; powder for oral susp 100 mg/ml and 125, 250, 500 mg/5 ml
Side effects/adverse reactions:
▼ *ORAL:* Discolored tongue, glossitis, increased thirst, candidiasis, stomatitis
CNS: ***Coma, convulsions,*** lethargy, hallucinations, anxiety, depression, twitching
GI: Nausea, vomiting, diarrhea
HEMA: ***Bone marrow depression, granulocytopenia,*** anemia, increased bleeding time
GU: Vaginitis, moniliasis, ***glomerulonephritis,*** oliguria, proteinuria, hematuria
INTEG: Rash, urticaria
SYST: ***Anaphylaxis,*** pruritus, urticaria, angioedema, bronchospasm (allergy symptoms)
Contraindications: Hypersensitivity to penicillins
Precautions: Pregnancy category B; hypersensitivity to cephalosporins; neonates
Pharmacokinetics:
PO: Peak 2 hr
IV: Peak 5 min
IM: Peak 1 hr
Half-life 50-110 min; metabolized in liver; excreted in urine, bile, breast milk; crosses placenta
Drug interactions of concern to dentistry:
• Decreased antimicrobial effectiveness: tetracyclines, erythromycins, lincomycins
• Increased ampicillin concentrations: probenecid
When used for dental infection:
• May reduce effectiveness of oral contraceptives
DENTAL CONSIDERATIONS
General:
• Take precautions regarding allergy to medication.
• Determine why the patient is taking the drug.
Consultations:
• Medical consult may be required to assess disease control in the patient.
Teach patient/family:
• Importance of good oral hygiene to prevent soft tissue inflammation
• Caution to prevent injury when using oral hygiene aids
When used for dental infection, advise patient:
• On birth control pill to use additional method of contraception for duration of cycle
• To report sore throat, oral burning sensation, fever, and fatigue, any

of which could indicate superinfection
• To take at prescribed intervals and complete dosage regimen
• To immediately notify the dentist if signs or symptoms of infection increase

amprenavir

(am-pren'ah-veer)
Agenerase
Drug class.: Antiviral

Action: Inhibits human immunodeficiency virus (HIV) protease enzymes
Uses: HIV infection, in combination with other antiretroviral agents
Dosage and routes:
• *Adult:* PO 1200 mg bid in combination with other antiretroviral drugs
• *Child 13-16 yr:* PO 1200 mg bid in combination with other antiretroviral drugs
• *Child 4-12 yr or 13-16 yr weighing less than 50 kg:* PO 20 mg/kg bid or 15 mg/kg tid (max 2400 mg/day) in combination with other antiretroviral drugs
Oral solution
• *Child 4-12 yr or 13-16 yr weighing less than 50 kg:* PO 22.5 mg/kg (1.5 ml/kg) bid or 17 mg/kg (1.1 ml/kg) tid in combination with other antiretroviral drugs; max daily limit 2800 mg
Available forms include: Caps 50, 150 mg; oral sol 15 mg/ml in 240 ml
(NOTE: capsules and oral solution are not interchangeable on a mg per mg basis)
Side effects/adverse reactions:
▼ *ORAL: Perioral paresthesia, taste disorders*
CNS: Headache, peripheral paresthesia, depression
GI: Nausea, vomiting, diarrhea, abdominal pain
HEMA: ***Acute hemolytic anemia***
INTEG: Rash, ***Stevens-Johnson syndrome***
META: Hyperglycemia, hyperlipidemia, hypercholesterolemia
MISC: Fatigue
Contraindications: Concurrent use with midazolam, triazolam, bepridil, cisapride, and ergot-like drugs; hypersensitivity; serious reactions could occur with lidocaine (systemic) and tricyclic antidepressants; avoid use of drugs metabolized by CYP3A4 enzymes, lactation
Precautions: Exacerbation of diabetes, hyperglycemia, use of additional vitamin E, hemophilia, viral resistance, risk of cross allergy with sulfonamides, fat redistribution, pregnancy category C, children <4 yr, hepatic disease, patients on oral contraceptives, sildenafil
Pharmacokinetics:
PO: Rapid oral absorption (except with fatty meal), bioavailability of oral solutions is less than capsules, peak plasma concentration 1-2 hr, plasma protein binding 90%, hepatic metabolism (CYP450, CYP3A4), excreted in feces (75%) and urine
Drug interactions of concern to dentistry:
• Contraindicated with midazolam, triazolam, tricyclic antidepressants
• Increased plasma levels of erythromycin, clarithromycin, itraconazole, alprazolam, chlorazepate, diazepam, carbamazepine, loratadine, flurazepam, ketoconazole, lidocaine

DENTAL CONSIDERATIONS

General:

• Palliative medication may be required for management of oral side effects.

• Examine for oral manifestation of opportunistic infection.

• Patient on chronic drug therapy may rarely have symptoms of blood dyscrasias, which can include infection, bleeding, and poor healing.

• Consider semisupine chair position for patient comfort if GI side effects occur.

Consultations:

• In a patient with symptoms of blood dyscrasias, request a medical consult for blood studies and postpone treatment until normal values are reestablished.

• Medical consult may be required to assess disease control and patient's ability to tolerate stress.

Teach patient/family:

• Importance of good oral hygiene to prevent soft tissue inflammation

• To prevent trauma when using oral hygiene aids

• Importance of updating health and drug history if physician makes any changes in evaluation/drug regimens

• That secondary oral infection may occur; must see dentist immediately if infection occurs

---

anagrelide hydrochloride

(an-ag're-lide)

Agrylin

Drug class.: Platelet-reducing agent

Action: Unclear; may involve a reduction in megakaryocyte hypermaturation without affecting WBC count or coagulation, insignificant reduction in RBC count; platelet aggregation may be inhibited in larger doses

Uses: Treatment of essential thrombocythemia, polycythemia vera

Dosage and routes:

• *Adult:* PO (requires close medical supervision)—initial dose 0.5 mg qid or 1.0 mg bid; after 1 week adjust dose to maintain platelet count at 600,000/µl; limit dose increases to 0.5 mg/day; dose limit 10 mg/day and 2.5 mg per single dose

Available forms include: Tabs 0.5 mg and 1.0 mg

Side effects/adverse reactions:

▼ *ORAL:* Aphthous stomatitis

CNS: Headache, dizziness, paresthesia, seizures

CV: Palpitation, edema, tachycardia

GI: Diarrhea, abdominal pain, nausea, dyspepsia, flatulence, vomiting, anorexia, ***pancreatitis,*** ulceration

RESP: ***Pulmonary infiltrate, pulmonary hypertension***

EENT: Rash, urticaria

MS: Back pain

MISC: Asthenia, malaise

Precautions: Cardiac disease, renal impairment, hepatic impairment, monitor reduction in platelets, risk of thrombocytopenia especially while correct dose is being found, sudden discontinuance of use, pregnancy category C, lactation, children <16 yr

Pharmacokinetics:

PO: Extensive hepatic metabolism, urinary excretion, half-life 1.3 hr

Drug interactions of concern to dentistry:

• Possible risk of hemorrhage: NSAIDs, aspirin

DENTAL CONSIDERATIONS

General:

• Laboratory studies should include routine CBCs.

• Patients have risk of thrombohemorrhagic complications; prolonged bleeding time, anemia, or splenomegaly may occur in some patients with this disease. However, thrombosis may also occur in some patients.

• Mucosal bleeding can be a symptom of disease.

• Patients with severe symptoms may be taking chemotherapy.

• Monitor vital signs every appointment due to cardiovascular side effects.

• Consider semisupine chair position for patient comfort when GI side effects occur.

Consultations:

• Medical consult with hematologist or physician directing therapy is essential before dental treatment.

Teach patient/family:

• To inform dentist of unusual bleeding episodes following dental treatment

• Importance of updating health and drug history if physician makes any changes in evaluation/drug regimens

---

apraclonidine

(a-pra-kloe'ni-deen)

Iopidine

Drug class.: Selective α_2-adrenergic agonist

Action: Reduces elevated or normal intraocular pressure

Uses: Control or prevention of increases in intraocular pressure related to laser surgery of eye; short-term control of increased intraocular pressure as an adjunctive drug

Dosage and routes:

• *Adult:* TOP INSTILL 1 or 2 gtt (0.5% sol) tid; allow a 5 min interval between other required ophthalmic drops

• *Adult:* TOP prelaser surgery use 1 gtt (1% sol) 1 hr before surgery and 1 gtt when surgery is completed

Available forms include: Sterile ophthalmic sol 0.5% and 1.0%

Side effects/adverse reactions:

▼ *ORAL:* Dry mouth, taste alterations (both 1%)

CNS: Insomnia, paresthesia, headache, dizziness

CV: Bradycardia, vasovagal syncope, palpitation

GI: Abdominal pain, diarrhea, emesis, nausea

RESP: Dyspnea, asthma

EENT: Hyperemia, discomfort, edema, tearing, mydriasis, blurred vision

INTEG: Pruritus

MISC: Facial edema

Contraindications: Hypersensitivity to this drug or clonidine; concurrent use of monoamine oxidase inhibitors

Precautions: Tachyphylaxis, impaired renal or liver function, depression, pregnancy category A, lactation, children, cardiovascular disease

Pharmacokinetics:

TOP: Onset 1 hr, maximum effect 3-5 hr; some systemic absorption

Drug interactions of concern to dentistry:

• No drug interactions have been reported; this is a new drug and data are lacking

• Avoid using drugs that can exacerbate glaucoma: anticholinergic drugs

DENTAL CONSIDERATIONS

General:

• Protect patient's eyes from accidental spatter during dental treatment.

• Avoid dental light in patient's eyes; offer dark glasses for patient comfort.

• Determine why the patient is taking the drug.

• Assess salivary flow as a factor in caries, periodontal disease, and candidiasis.

Consultations:

• Medical consult may be required to assess disease control in the patient.

Teach patient/family:

When chronic dry mouth occurs, advise patient:

• To avoid mouth rinses with high alcohol content due to drying effects

• Need for daily home fluoride to prevent caries

• To use sugarless gum, frequent sips of water, or saliva substitutes

---

ardeparin sodium

(ar-dee-pa'rin)

Normiflo

Drug class.: Heparin-type anticoagulant

Action: A low-molecular-weight heparin that inhibits coagulation by binding to antithrombin III, thereby enhancing antithrombin III to inhibit serine proteases and factor X_a; also inhibits thrombin by binding to heparin cofactor II

Uses: Prevention of deep vein thrombosis following knee replacement surgery

Dosage and routes:

• *Adult:* SC 50 anti-X_a units/kg q12hr; start drug in evening or following morning after surgery and continue for 14 days or until patient is fully ambulatory, whichever is shorter

Available forms include: Tubex cartridge-needle units: 5000 anti-X_a units/0.5 ml and 10,000 anti-X_a units/0.5 ml

Side effects/adverse reactions:

GI: Nausea, constipation

HEMA: Hemorrhage, hematoma, ecchymosis, thrombocytopenia, anemia

EENT: Pruritus, rash

META: Alteration in triglyceride levels, elevation of AST and ALT

MISC: Fever

Contraindications: Hypersensitivity, thrombocytopenia (with positive in vitro test for antiplatelet antibodies), pork products hypersensitivity

Precautions: Product contains parabens and sulfites, thrombocytopenia, hemorrhagic stroke, cerebral aneurysm, bleeding disorders, severe liver disease, severe renal failure, pregnancy category C

Pharmacokinetics:

SC: Good absorption, bioavailability 90%; peak plasma levels 2-3 hr; activity declines to half after 6 hr; renal excretion, protein binding (70%-90%)

Drug interactions of concern to dentistry:

• Avoid concurrent use of aspirin, NSAIDs

DENTAL CONSIDERATIONS

General:

• Determine why patient is taking the drug.

• Consider local hemostasis measures to prevent excessive bleeding if dental procedures must be performed.

• Antibiotic prophylaxis before dental treatment may be required for joint prosthesis. See 1997 ADA guidelines.

• Avoid products that affect platelet function, such as aspirin and NSAIDs.

• Delay elective dental treatment until patient completes anticoagulant therapy.

Consultations:

• Medical consult should include routine blood counts, including platelet counts and bleeding time.

Teach patient/family:

• Importance of good oral hygiene to prevent soft tissue inflammation

• Caution patient to prevent trauma when using oral hygiene aids

• To report oral lesions, soreness, or bleeding to dentist

ascorbic acid (vitamin C)

(a-skor′bic)

Ascorbicap, Cebid, Cecon, Cemill, Cetane, Cevi-Bid, Vita-C, Dull-C, Flavorcee

♣ Apo-C

Drug class.: Vitamin C, water-soluble vitamin

Action: Needed for wound healing, collagen synthesis, antioxidant, carbohydrate metabolism

Uses: Vitamin C deficiency, scurvy, delayed wound and bone healing, chronic disease, urine acidification, before gastrectomy

Dosage and routes:

Scurvy

• *Adult:* PO/SC/IM/IV 100-500 mg qd, then 50 mg or more qd

• *Child:* PO/SC/IM/IV 100-300 mg qd, then 35 mg or more qd

Wound healing/chronic disease/fracture

• *Adult:* SC/IM/IV/PO 200-500 mg qd

• *Child:* SC/IM/IV/PO 100-200 mg added doses

Urine acidification

• *Adult:* SC/IM/IV/PO 4-12 g qd in divided doses

Available forms include: Tabs 50, 100, 250, 500, 1000, 1500 mg; effervescent tabs 1000 mg; chew tabs 100, 250, 500 mg; sus rel tabs 500, 750, 1000, 1500 mg; sus rel caps 500 mg; crys 4 g/tsp; powd 4 g/tsp; liq 35 mg/0.6 ml; sol 100 mg/ml; syr 20 mg/ml, 500 mg/5 ml; inj SC/IM/IV 100, 250, 500 mg/ml; loz 60 mg

Side effects/adverse reactions:

▼ *ORAL:* Enamel erosion, caries (chewable form, chronic use)

CNS: Headache, insomnia, dizziness, fatigue, flushing

GI: Nausea, vomiting, diarrhea, anorexia, heartburn, cramps

HEMA: ***Hemolytic anemia in patients with G6PD***

GU: Polyuria, urine acidification, oxalate or urate renal stones

Contraindications: None significant

Precautions: Gout, pregnancy category A

Pharmacokinetics:

PO/INJ: Metabolized in liver; unused amounts excreted in urine (unchanged) and metabolites; crosses placenta and excreted in breast milk

Drug interactions of concern to dentistry:

• Increased urinary excretion: salicylates, barbiturates

DENTAL CONSIDERATIONS

General:

- An increased incidence of caries and soft tissue injury has been reported with excessive use of chewable ascorbic acid tablets.

---

aspirin

(as'pir-in)

Arthritis Foundation Pain Reliever, ASA, Aspirin, Easprin, Ecotrin, Empirin, Genuine Bayer, Measurin

Combinations: Often combined with other analgesic drugs

🍁 Entrophen, Novasen, Sal-Adult, Sal-Infant, Supasa

Drug class.: Nonnarcotic analgesic salicylate

Action: Inhibits prostaglandin synthesis by interfering with cyclooxygenase needed for biosynthesis; possesses analgesic, antiinflammatory, antipyretic properties

Uses: Mild-to-moderate pain or fever, including arthritis, thromboembolic disorders, transient ischemic attacks in men, rheumatic fever, postmyocardial infarction

Dosage and routes:

Arthritis

- *Adult:* PO 2.6-5.2 g/day in divided doses q4-6h
- *Child:* PO 90-130 mg/kg/day in divided doses q4-6h

Pain/fever

- *Adult:* PO/REC 500 mg q3h, 325-650 mg q4h or 650-1000 mg q6h
- *Child 2-4 yr:* PO/REC 160 mg q4h
- *Child 4-6 yr:* PO/REC 240 mg q4h
- *Child 6-9 yr:* PO/REC 325 mg q4h
- *Child 9-11 yr:* PO/REC 320-400 mg q4h
- *Child 11-12 yr:* PO/REC 320-480 mg q4h

Thromboembolic disorders

- *Adult:* PO 325-650 mg/day or bid

Transient ischemic attacks in men

- *Adult:* PO 650 mg bid or 325 mg qid; lower daily doses of 160-325 mg have also been used

Available forms include: Tabs 65, 81, 325, 500, 650, 975 mg; chew tabs 81 mg; caps 325, 500 mg; con rel tabs 800 mg; time rel tabs 650 mg; supp 60, 120, 125, 130, 195, 200, 300, 325, 600, 650 mg, and 1.2 g; cream; gum 227.5 mg

Side effects/adverse reactions:

▼ *ORAL:* Increased bleeding (chronic, high doses)

CNS: ***Coma, convulsion,*** stimulation, drowsiness, dizziness, confusion, headache, flushing, hallucinations

CV: Rapid pulse, pulmonary edema

GI: Nausea, vomiting, ***GI bleeding, hepatitis,*** diarrhea, heartburn, anorexia

RESP: Wheezing, hyperpnea

HEMA: ***Thrombocytopenia, agranulocytosis, leukopenia, neutropenia, hemolytic anemia,*** increased pro-time, bleeding time

EENT: Tinnitus, hearing loss

INTEG: Rash, urticaria, bruising

ENDO: Hypoglycemia, hyponatremia, hypokalemia

Contraindications: Hypersensitivity to salicylates, GI bleeding, bleeding disorders, children <3 yr, children with flulike symptoms, pregnancy category C, lactation, vitamin K deficiency, peptic ulcer

Precautions: Anemia, hepatic disease, renal disease, Hodgkin's disease, preoperative, postoperative

Pharmacokinetics:
PO: Onset 15-30 min, peak 1-2 hr, duration 4-6 hr
REC: Onset slow, duration 4-6 hr, half-life 1-3.5 hr; metabolized by liver; excreted by kidneys; crosses placenta; excreted in breast milk

Drug interactions of concern to dentistry:
• Increased risk of GI complaints and occult blood loss: alcohol, NSAIDs, corticosteroids
Interactions when used as a dental drug:
• Increased risk of bleeding: oral anticoagulants, valproic acid, dipyridamole
• Increased risk of hypoglycemia: oral antidiabetics
• Increased risk of toxicity: methotrexate, lithium, zidovudine
• Decreased effects of probenecid, sulfinpyrazone
• Avoid prolonged or concurrent use with NSAIDs, corticosteroids, acetaminophen

DENTAL CONSIDERATIONS
General:
• Patients on chronic drug therapy may rarely have symptoms of blood dyscrasias, which can include infection, bleeding, and poor healing.
• Avoid prescribing buffered aspirin-containing products if patient is on a sodium-restricted diet.
• Chewable forms of aspirin should not be used for 7 days following oral surgery because of possible soft tissue injury.
• Evaluate allergic reactions: rash, urticaria; patients with allergy to salicylates may not be able to take NSAIDs; drug may need to be discontinued.
Consultations:
• In a patient with symptoms of blood dyscrasias, request a medical consult for blood studies and postpone dental treatment until normal values are reestablished.
• Take precautions if dental surgery is anticipated due to risk of increased bleeding; avoid prescribing aspirin before dental surgery.
• Tinnitus, ringing, roaring in ears after high-dose and long-term therapy requires referral for salicylism.
Teach patient/family:
• That aspirin or buffered aspirin tablets should not be placed directly on a tooth or mucosal surface due to the risk of chemical burn
• To read label on other OTC drugs; may contain aspirin
• To avoid alcohol ingestion; GI bleeding may occur

---

atenolol

(a-ten'oh-lole)
Tenormin
✦ Apo-Atenol, Novo-Atenolol
Drug class.: Antihypertensive, selective β_1-blocker

Action: This is a selective β_1-adrenergic antagonist. At higher doses selectivity may be lost with antagonism of β_2-receptors as well. The antihypertensive mechanism of action is unclear, but may include a reduction in cardiac output and inhibition of renin release by the renal juxtaglomerular apparatus. Peripheral resistance decreases with long-term use. The antianginal action (when indicated for this use) may be related to a decrease in myocardial oxygen demand and negative chronotropic and inotropic effects. The antiarrhythmic action (when indicated for this use) has been related to a reduction in spontaneous pacemaker firing and slowing of AV nodal conduction.

Uses: Mild-to-moderate hypertension, prophylaxis of angina pectoris

Dosage and routes:

• *Adult:* PO 50 mg qd, increasing q1-2wk to 100 mg qd; may increase to 200 mg qd for angina

Available forms include: Tabs 25, 50, 100 mg

Side effects/adverse reactions:

▼ *ORAL:* Dry mouth

CNS: Insomnia, fatigue, dizziness, mental changes, memory loss, hallucinations, depression, lethargy, drowsiness, strange dreams, catatonia

CV: ***Profound hypotension, bradycardia, CHF, cold extremities, postural hypotension, second- or third-degree heart block***

GI: Nausea, diarrhea, ***mesenteric arterial thrombosis, ischemic colitis,*** vomiting

RESP: ***Bronchospasm,*** dyspnea, wheezing

HEMA: ***Agranulocytosis, thrombocytopenia, purpura***

GU: Impotence

EENT: Sore throat, dry burning eyes

INTEG: Rash, fever, alopecia

ENDO: Hypoglycemia

Contraindications: Hypersensitivity to β-blockers, cardiogenic shock, second- or third-degree heart block, sinus bradycardia, CHF, cardiac failure

Precautions: Major surgery, pregnancy category C, lactation, diabetes mellitus, renal disease, thyroid disease, COPD, asthma, well-compensated heart failure

Pharmacokinetics:

PO: Peak 2-4 hr; half-life 6-7 hr; excreted unchanged in urine; protein binding 5%-15%; up to 50% excreted unchanged in feces as unabsorbed drug

Drug interactions of concern to dentistry:

• Decreased antihypertensive effects: NSAIDs, indomethacin

• May slow metabolism of lidocaine

• Decreased β-blocking effects (or decreased β-adrenergic effects) of epinephrine, levonordefrin, isoproterenol, and other sympathomimetics

DENTAL CONSIDERATIONS

General:

• Monitor vital signs every appointment due to cardiovascular and respiratory side effects.

• After supine positioning, have patient sit upright for at least 2 min before standing to avoid orthostatic hypotension.

• Patients on chronic drug therapy may rarely have symptoms of blood dyscrasias, which can include infection, bleeding, and poor healing.

• Assess salivary flow as a factor in caries, periodontal disease, and candidiasis.

• Stress from dental procedures may compromise cardiovascular function; determine patient risk.

• Short appointments and a stress reduction protocol may be required for anxious patients.

• Use vasoconstrictors with caution, in low doses, and with careful aspiration. Avoid use of gingival retraction cord with epinephrine.

Consultations:

• In a patient with symptoms of blood dyscrasias, request a medical

consult for blood studies and postpone dental treatment until normal values are reestablished.

• Medical consult may be required to assess disease control and stress tolerance of patient.

• Use precautions if general anesthesia is required for dental surgery.

Teach patient/family:

• Importance of good oral hygiene to prevent soft tissue inflammation

• Caution to prevent injury when using oral hygiene aids

When chronic dry mouth occurs, advise patient:

• To avoid mouth rinses with high alcohol content due to drying effects

• To use daily home fluoride products for anticaries effect

• To use sugarless gum, frequent sips of water, or saliva substitutes

---

atorvastatin calcium

(a-tore'va-sta-tin)

Lipitor

Drug class.: Cholesterol-lowering agent

Action: Inhibits HMG-CoA reductase enzyme, which reduces cholesterol synthesis

Uses: As an adjunct in primary hypercholesterolemia mixed hyperlipidemia (types IIa, IIIb); patient should first be placed on cholesterol-lowering diet; also approved to increase HDL cholesterol in patients with primary hypercholesterolemia and mixed dyslipidemia

Dosage and routes:

• *Adult:* PO initial 10 mg daily; dose can be modified according to lipid lab values at 2-4 wk; dose range 10-80 mg daily

Available forms include: Tabs 10, 20, 40 mg

Side effects/adverse reactions:

▼ *ORAL:* Angioneurotic edema, lichenoid reaction

CNS: Headache, insomnia

CV: Chest pain

GI: Flatulence, dyspepsia, abdominal pain, nausea

RESP: Bronchitis, rhinitis

EENT: Rash, pruritus

META: Elevated liver enzymes

MS: Myalgia, arthritis

MISC: Allergy, urinary tract infection, peripheral edema

Contraindications: Hypersensitivity, active liver disease, pregnancy, lactation

Precautions: Chronic alcohol liver disease, pregnancy X, monitor liver function and lipid levels

Pharmacokinetics:

PO: First-pass metabolism, half-life 14 hr, 98% protein bound

Drug interactions of concern to dentistry: Severe myopathy or rhabdomyolysis: erythromycin, niacin, itraconazole Increase in plasma levels: erythromycin, itraconazole

DENTAL CONSIDERATIONS

General:

• Consider semisupine chair position for patient comfort if GI side effects occur.

---

atovaquone

(a-toe'va-kwone)

Mepron

Drug class.: Antipneumocystic (antiprotozoal)

Action: Mechanism of action unknown; may inhibit synthesis of ATP and nucleic acids

Uses: Treatment and prevention of

P. carinii pneumonia in patients who are intolerant to trimethoprim-sulfamethoxazole

Dosage and routes:

• *Adults:* PO 750 mg bid × 21 days

Available forms include: Oral susp 750 mg/5 ml

Side effects/adverse reactions:

▼ *ORAL: Candidiasis,* taste alteration

CNS: Headache, insomnia, dizziness, anxiety

CV: Hypotension, hyponatremia

GI: Nausea, vomiting, abdominal pain, diarrhea, constipation

RESP: Cough

HEMA: ***Neutropenia,*** anemia

INTEG: Rash, sweating

MISC: Fever, hypoglycemia, asthenia

Contraindications: Hypersensitivity

Precautions: Pregnancy category C; lactation; children; elderly; GI diseases with malabsorption complications; must do CBC, ALT, and AST values; hepatic disease

Pharmacokinetics: Fatty meals enhance absorption; highly protein bound (99%); two peak plasma periods (first 1-8 hr, second 24-96 hr); metabolites excreted in urine

Drug interactions of concern to dentistry:

• Aspirin: There are no data on drug interactions related to specific dental medications; however, because of its high protein binding there is always a risk of diplacement when other highly protein bound drugs are administered

DENTAL CONSIDERATIONS

General:

• Examine patient for signs of oral manifestations of opportunistic infections.

• Place on frequent recall because of drug and disease oral side effects.

• Consider semisupine chair position due to GI side effects.

• Consider semisupine chair position for patients with respiratory disease.

• Patients on chronic drug therapy may rarely have symptoms of blood dyscrasias, which can include infection, bleeding, and poor healing.

Consultations:

• Medical consult may be required to assess disease control and stress tolerance in the patient.

• In a patient with symptoms of blood dyscrasias, request a medical consult for blood studies and postpone dental treatment until normal values are reestablished.

• Acute oral infection may require physican consult for coordination of antiinfective therapy.

Teach patient/family:

• Importance of good oral hygiene to prevent soft tissue inflammation

• Caution to prevent injury when using oral hygiene aids

• Importance of dietary suggestions to maintain oral and systemic health

• That secondary oral infections may occur; must see dentist immediately if infection occurs

atropine sulfate

(a'troe-peen)

Sal-Tropine

Drug class.: Anticholinergic

Action: Inhibits muscarinic actions of acetylcholine at postganglionic parasympathetic neuroeffector sites; dries secretions by antagonism of muscarinic cholinergic receptors

Uses: Reduction of salivary and bronchial secretions

Dosage and routes:

• *Adult:* PO 0.4 mg given 30-60 min before drying effect is required for dental procedure

• *Child:* PO >90 lb, 0.4 mg; 65-90 lb, 0.4 mg; 40-65 lb, 0.3 mg

Available forms include: Tabs 0.4 mg

Side effects/adverse reactions:

▼ *ORAL: Dry mouth,* burning sensation

CNS: Headache, dizziness, ***coma (toxic dose),*** involuntary movement, confusion, anxiety, flushing, drowsiness, insomnia

CV: Hypotension, paradoxic bradycardia, angina, PVCs, hypertension, tachycardia, ectopic ventricular beats

GI: Nausea, vomiting, abdominal pain, anorexia, constipation, ***paralytic ileus,*** abdominal distention

GU: Retention, hesitancy, impotence, dysuria

EENT: Blurred vision, photophobia, glaucoma, eye pain, pupil dilation, nasal congestion

INTEG: Rash, urticaria, contact dermatitis, dry skin, flushing

MISC: Suppression of lactation, decreased sweating

Contraindications: Hypersensitivity to belladonna alkaloids, angle-closure glaucoma, GI obstructions, myasthenia gravis, thyrotoxicosis, ulcerative colitis, prostatic hypertrophy, tachycardia/tachydysrhythmias, asthma

Precautions: Pregnancy category C, lactation, renal disease, CHF, hyperthyroidism, COPD, hepatic disease, child <6 yr, hypertension, geriatric

Pharmacokinetics:

PO: Onset 0.5-1 hr, moderate protein binding, duration of action 4-6 hr, renal excretion

Drug interactions of concern to dentistry:

• Increased anticholinergic effects: tricyclic antidepressants, antihistamines, opioid analgesics, antipsychotic medications, or other drugs with anticholinergic activity

• Decreased absorption of ketoconazole

DENTAL CONSIDERATIONS

General:

• Give PO dose 30-60 min before drying effects are required for dental procedures.

• Request that patient remove contact lenses before using due to possible drying effects in the eyes.

• Caution patients that they may feel a dry, burning sensation in the throat and experience blurred vision.

• This drug is intended for acute use, usually in single doses only; therefore chronic dry mouth should not be a concern.

• Avoid dental light in patient's eyes; offer dark glasses for patient comfort.

Consultations:

• Medical consult is advisable before using this drug in patients with a history of GI disease, cardiac disease, or glaucoma.

atropine sulfate (optic)

(a'troe-peen)

Atropair, Atropine Care, Atropine Sulfate S.O.P., Atropisol, Isopto Atropine, I-Tropine, Ocu-tropine

🍁 Mims Atropine

Drug class.: Mydriatic (anticholinergic)

Action: Blocks response of iris sphincter muscle and muscle of accommodation of ciliary body to cholinergic stimulation, resulting in dilation and paralysis of accommodation

Uses: Iritis, cycloplegic refraction

Dosage and routes:

• *Adult:* INSTILL SOL 1-2 gtt of a 1% sol qd-tid for iritis or 1 hr before refracting (cycloplegic refraction); INSTILL OINT bid-tid

• *Child:* INSTILL SOL 1-2 gtt of a 0.5% sol qd-tid for iritis or bid × 1-3 days before exam (cycloplegic refraction); INSTILL OINT qd-bid 2-3 days before exam

Available forms include: Oint 0.5%, 1%; sol 0.5%, 1%, 2%, 3%

Side effects/adverse reactions:

▼ *ORAL:* Dry mouth

SYST: Tachycardia, confusion, fever, flushing, dry skin, abdominal discomfort (infants: bladder distention, irregular pulse, respiratory depression)

Contraindications: Hypersensitivity, infants <3 mo, open- or narrow-angle glaucoma, conjunctivitis, Down syndrome

Pharmacokinetics:

INSTILL: Peak 30-40 min (mydriasis), 60-180 min (cycloplegia); duration of dilation up to 6-12 days

DENTAL CONSIDERATIONS

General:

• Avoid dental light in patient's eyes; offer dark glasses for patient comfort.

auranofin

(au-rane'oh-fin)

Ridaura

Drug class.: Gold salt

Action: Specific antiinflammatory action unknown; may decrease phagocytosis, lysosomal activity, concentration of rheumatoid factor or immunoglobulins

Uses: Rheumatoid arthritis, unapproved use for juvenile arthritis

Dosage and routes:

• *Adult:* PO 6 mg qd or 3 mg bid, may increase to 9 mg/day after 3 mo

Available forms include: Caps 3 mg

Side effects/adverse reactions:

▼ *ORAL: Stomatitis, lichenoid drug reaction,* metallic taste, glossitis, gingivitis

CNS: Dizziness, syncope

GI: Diarrhea, abdominal cramping, stomatitis, nausea, vomiting, enterocolitis, anorexia, flatulence, dyspepsia, jaundice, increased AST/ALT, melena, constipation

RESP: ***Interstitial pneumonitis, fibrosis,*** cough, dyspnea

HEMA: ***Thrombocytopenia, agranulocytosis, aplastic anemia, leukopenia, eosinophilia***

GU: Proteinuria, hematuria, increased BUN, creatinine, vaginitis

INTEG: Rash, pruritus, dermatitis, ***exfoliative dermatitis,*** urticaria, alopecia, photosensitivity

Contraindications: Hypersensi-

tivity to gold, necrotizing enterocolitis, bone marrow aplasia, child <6 yr, lactation, pulmonary fibrosis, exfoliative dermatitis, blood dyscrasias, recent radiation therapy

Precautions: Elderly, CHF, diabetes mellitus, allergic conditions, ulcerative colitis, renal disease, liver disease, pregnancy category C

Pharmacokinetics:

PO: Peak 2 hr; steady state 8-16 wk; 20%-25% absorbed by GI tract; excreted in urine and feces

DENTAL CONSIDERATIONS

General:

- Patients on chronic drug therapy may rarely have symptoms of blood dyscrasias, which can include infection, bleeding, and poor healing.
- Consider semisupine chair position for patients with arthritic disease.

Consultations:

- In a patient with symptoms of blood dyscrasias, request a medical consult for blood studies and postpone dental treatment until normal values are reestablished.

Teach patient/family:

- Importance of good oral hygiene to prevent soft tissue inflammation
- To avoid mouth rinses with high alcohol content due to drying and irritating effects

---

aurothioglucose/gold sodium thiomalate

(aur-oh-thye-oh-gloo'kose)

Solganal

Drug class.: Antiinflammatory gold compound

Action: Specific antiinflammatory action unknown; may decrease phagocytosis, lysosomal activity, prostaglandin synthesis

Uses: Rheumatoid arthritis; juvenile arthritis; unapproved: psoriatic arthritis, Felty's syndrome

Dosage and routes:

Aurothioglucose

- *Adult:* IM 10 mg, then 25 mg qwk × 2-3 wk, then 25-50 mg/wk until total of 800 mg to 1 g is administered, then 25-50 mg q3-4wk if there is improvement without toxicity; limit 50 mg/wk
- *Child 6-12 yr:* IM 2.5 mg × 1 wk, 6.25 mg qwk × 2-3 wk, then 12.5 mg/wk until total dose of 200-250 mg, then 6.25-12.5 mg q2-3wk

Gold sodium thiomalate

- *Adult:* IM 10 mg, then 25 mg after 1 wk, then 25-50 mg qwk for total of 1 g, then 25-50 mg q2wk × 20 wk, then 25-50 mg q3-4wk for maintenance
- *Child:* IM 10 mg × 1 wk, 1 mg/kg 2nd wk (limit 50 mg), then maintenance dose

Available forms include: IM inj 10, 25, 50 mg/ml

Side effects/adverse reactions:

▼ *ORAL:* Stomatitis, metallic taste

*CNS: Dizziness, **encephalitis,*** EEG abnormalities, confusion, hallucinations

CV: Bradycardia, rapid pulse

GI: ***Hepatitis,*** vomiting, nausea, jaundice, diarrhea, cramping, flatulence

RESP: ***Pulmonary fibrosis,*** interstitial pneumonitis, pharyngitis

HEMA: ***Thrombocytopenia, agranulocytosis, aplastic anemia, leukopenia, eosinophilia, neutropenia***

GU: Proteinuria, ***nephrosis, tubular necrosis,*** hematuria

EENT: Iritis, corneal ulcers

INTEG: Rash, pruritus, dermati-

*tis, **exfoliative dermatitis, angioedema,*** urticaria, alopecia, photosensitivity

MISC: ***Anaphylaxis***

Contraindications: Hypersensitivity to gold, SLE, uncontrolled diabetes mellitus, marked hypertension, recent radiation therapy, CHF, lactation, renal disease, liver disease

Precautions: Decreased tolerance in elderly, children, blood dyscrasias, pregnancy category C

Pharmacokinetics:

IM: Peak 4-6 hr; half-life 3-27 days; half-life increases up to 168 days with eleventh dose; excreted in urine and feces

Drug interactions of concern to dentistry:

- None reported

DENTAL CONSIDERATIONS

General:

- Patients on chronic drug therapy may rarely have symptoms of blood dyscrasias, which can include infection, bleeding, and poor healing.
- Palliative medication may be required for management of oral side effects.
- Consider semisupine chair position for patient comfort due to arthritic disease.

Consultations:

- Medical consult may be required to assess disease control and patient's ability to tolerate stress.
- In a patient with symptoms of blood dyscrasias, request a medical consult for blood studies and postpone dental treatment until normal values are reestablished.

Teach patient/family:

- Importance of good oral hygiene to prevent soft tissue inflammation
- Alert the patient to the possibility of secondary oral infection and the need to see dentist immediately if infection occurs
- To report oral lesions, soreness, or bleeding to dentist
- To avoid mouth rinses with high alcohol content due to drying effects

---

azatadine maleate

(a-za'ta-deen)

Optimine

Drug class.: Antihistamine, H_1-receptor antagonist

Action: Acts on blood vessels, GI system, and respiratory system by competing with histamine for H_1-receptor site; decreases allergic response by blocking histamine

Uses: Allergy symptoms, rhinitis, chronic urticaria, pruritus

Dosage and routes:

- *Adult:* PO 1-2 mg bid, not to exceed 4 mg/day

Available forms include: Tabs 1 mg

Side effects/adverse reactions:

▼ *ORAL:* Dry mouth

CNS: Dizziness, drowsiness, poor coordination, fatigue, anxiety, euphoria, confusion, paresthesia, neuritis, sweating, chills

CV: Hypotension, palpitation, tachycardia

GI: Constipation, nausea, vomiting, anorexia, diarrhea

RESP: Increased thick secretions, wheezing, chest tightness

HEMA: ***Thrombocytopenia, agranulocytosis, hemolytic anemia***

GU: Retention, dysuria, frequency, impotence

EENT: Blurred vision, dilated pupils, tinnitus, nasal stuffiness, dry nose/throat

INTEG: Rash, urticaria, photosensitivity

Contraindications: Hypersensitivity to H_1-receptor antagonist, acute asthma attack, lower respiratory tract disease, child <12 yr

Precautions: Increased intraocular pressure, renal disease, cardiac disease, bronchial asthma, seizure disorder, stenosed peptic ulcers, hyperthyroidism, prostatic hypertrophy, bladder neck obstruction, pregnancy category B, elderly, lactation

Pharmacokinetics:

PO: Peak 4 hr, half-life 9-12 hr; minimally bound to plasma proteins; metabolized in liver; excreted by kidneys; crosses placenta, blood-brain barrier

Drug interactions of concern to dentistry:

- Increased CNS depression: all CNS depressants, alcohol
- Increased anticholinergic effect: anticholinergics

DENTAL CONSIDERATIONS

General:

- Assess salivary flow as a factor in caries, periodontal disease, and candidiasis.
- Patients on chronic drug therapy may rarely have symptoms of blood dyscrasias, which can include infection, bleeding, and poor healing.
- Consider semisupine chair position for patient comfort due to respiratory disease.
- Monitor vital signs every appointment due to cardiovascular side effects.

Consultations:

- In a patient with symptoms of blood dyscrasia, request a medical consult for blood studies and postpone dental treatment until normal values are reestablished.

Teach patient/family:

- Importance of good oral hygiene to prevent soft tissue inflammation
- Caution to prevent injury when using oral hygiene aids

When chronic dry mouth occurs, advise patient:

- To avoid mouth rinses with high alcohol content due to drying effects
- To use daily home fluoride products for anticaries effect
- To use sugarless gum, frequent sips of water, or saliva substitutes

azathioprine

(ay-za-thye'oh-preen)

Imuran

Drug class.: Immunosuppressant

Action: Produces immunosuppression by inhibiting purine synthesis in cells, thereby preventing RNA and DNA synthesis

Uses: Renal transplants to prevent graft rejection, refractory rheumatoid arthritis, refractory ITP, glomerulonephritis, nephrotic syndrome, bone marrow transplant; unapproved: pemphigoid and pemphigus

Dosage and routes:

Prevention of rejection

- *Adult and child:* PO 3-5 mg/kg/day, then maintenance of at least 1-2 mg/kg/day

Refractory rheumatoid arthritis

- *Adult:* PO 1 mg/kg/day, may increase dose after 2 mo by 0.5 mg/kg/day, not to exceed 2.5 mg/kg/day

Unlabeled use in pemphigoid, pemphigus
• *Adult:* PO 1 mg/kg of body weight per day; can titrate dose after 6-8 weeks at 0.5 mg/kg of body weight per day. Maximum dose 2.5 mg/kg of body weight per day. Maintenance dose: determine the minimum effective dose by reducing dose at 0.5 mg/kg of body weight per day every 4-8 wk
Available forms include: Tabs 50 mg; inj IV 100 mg
Side effects/adverse reactions:
▼ *ORAL:* Stomatitis, oral ulceration
GI: ***Pancreatitis, hepatotoxicity, jaundice,*** nausea, vomiting, esophagitis
HEMA: ***Leukopenia, thrombocytopenia, anemia, pancytopenia***
INTEG: Rash
MS: Arthralgia, muscle wasting
Contraindications: Hypersensitivity, pregnancy category D
Precautions: Severe renal disease, severe hepatic disease
Pharmacokinetics: Metabolized in liver; excreted in urine (active metabolite); crosses placenta
Drug interactions of concern to dentistry:
• Increased blood dyscrasias: NSAIDs, especially phenylbutazone, dapsone, phenothiazines
• Increased immunosuppression, risk of infection: corticosteroids

DENTAL CONSIDERATIONS
General:
• Patients on chronic drug therapy may rarely have symptoms of blood dyscrasias, which can include infection, bleeding, and poor healing.
• To prevent infection if surgery or deep scaling is planned, prophylactic antibiotics may be indicated in patients who develop neutropenia.
• Determine why the patient is taking the drug.
• Alert the patient to the possibility of secondary oral infection; must see dentist immediately if infection occurs.
Consultations:
• In a patient with symptoms of blood dyscrasias, request a medical consult for blood studies and postpone dental treatment until normal values are reestablished.
• Medical consult may be required to assess disease control in the patient.
• Medical consult may be required to assess patient's ability to tolerate stress.
Teach patient/family:
• Importance of good oral hygiene to prevent soft tissue inflammation
• Caution to prevent injury when using oral hygiene aids
• To avoid mouth rinses with high alcohol content due to drying effects and irritation of mucous membranes

azelaic acid

(a-zel′ay-ik)
Azelex
Drug class.: A naturally occurring straight-chain dicarboxylic acid

Action: Exact mechanism unknown; has antimicrobial activity against *P. acnes* and *S. epidermidis*
Uses: Topical therapy of mild-to-moderate inflammatory acne vulgaris
Dosage and routes:
• *Adult and child <12 yr:* TOP wash skin and pat skin dry, apply thin film to affected area bid

Available forms include: Cream 20% in 30 g tube
Side effects/adverse reactions:
INTEG: Irritation, pruritus, burning, hypopigmentation
Contraindications: Hypersensitivity
Precautions: Prevent contact with eyes, pregnancy category B, child <12 yr, lactation
Pharmacokinetics:
TOP: Less than 4% systemic absorption
Drug interactions of concern to dentistry:
• None reported

DENTAL CONSIDERATIONS
General:
• Topical use rarely causes exacerbation of recurrent herpes labialis.
• Keep away from mouth and other mucous membranes; wash eyes if cream comes in contact; irritation can occur.

azelastine HCl

(a-zel'as-teen)
Astelin
Drug class.: H_1-receptor antogonist

Action: Acts by competitive antagonism of H_1-receptors to antagonize the wheal and flare responses and nasal hypersecretion; may also inhibit the release of other inflammatory mediators, including kinins and leukotrienes
Uses: Control of symptoms associated with seasonal allergic rhinitis or nonseasonal allergic rhinitis
Dosage and routes:
• *Adult and child >12 yr:* Nasal spray 2 sprays per nostril bid
Available forms include: Nasal spray unit, 137 μg per actuation
Side effects/adverse reactions:
▼ *ORAL: Bitter taste, dry mouth*
CNS: Somnolence, headache
GI: Nausea
RESP: Paroxysmal sneezing
EENT: Nasal burning
MISC: Fatigue
Contraindications: Hypersensitivity
Precautions: Child <12 yr, no data on pregnancy or lactation, renal impairment
Pharmacokinetics:
INH: Low absorption, metabolism to active metabolite, desmethylazelastine; excretion mostly in feces (75%), urine (25%)
Drug interactions of concern to dentistry:
• Increased risk of anticholinergic effects: anticholinergics
• Possible additive sedation: alcohol, anxiolytics, opioid analgesics

DENTAL CONSIDERATIONS
General:
• Assess salivary flow as factor in caries, periodontal disease, and candidiasis.
Teach patient/family:
When chronic dry mouth occurs, advise patient:
• To avoid mouth rinses with high alcohol content due to drying effects
• To use daily home fluoride products for anticaries effect
• To use sugarless gum, frequent sips of water, or saliva substitutes

azithromycin

(az-ith-roe-mye'sin)
Zithromax
Drug class.: Macrolide antibiotic

Action: Binds to 50S ribosomal subunits of susceptible bacteria and suppresses protein synthesis; similar spectrum of activity to erythromycin

Uses: Mild-to-moderate infections of the upper/lower respiratory tract; gonorrhea, chancroid, uncomplicated skin and skin structure infections caused by *M. catarrhalis, S. pneumoniae, S. pyogenes, S. aureus, S. agalactiae, H. influenzae, Clostridium, L. pneumophila;* nongonococcal urethritis; cervicitis due to *C. trachomatis;* otitis media due to *H. influenzae, S. pneumoniae, M. catarrhalis;* chlamydia; *M. avium* complex in HIV infection

Dosage and routes:

• *Adult:* PO 500 mg on day 1, then 250 mg qd on days 2-5 for a total dose of 1.5 g; do not take with meals; take 1 hr before or 2 hr after eating

Chlamydia/chancroid/urinary infections

• *Adult:* PO 1 g in a single dose

Gonorrhea

• *Adult:* PO 2 g in a single dose

Otitis media

• *Adult and child:* PO 10 mg/kg/day on day 1; then 5 mg/kg on days 2-5

Mycobacterium avium complex

• *Adult:* PO 1200 mg qwk

Bacterial endocarditis prophylaxis

• *Adult:* PO for patients allergic to amoxicillin, 500 mg 1 hr before dental procedure

• *Child:* PO for patients allergic to amoxicillin 15 mg/kg of body weight not to exceed the adult dose 1 hr before dental procedure

Available forms include: Tab 250 (Z-Pak 6 tabs), 600 mg; oral susp 100/5 ml (in 300 mg bottle), 200 mg/5 ml (in 600, 900, 1200 mg bottles)

Side effects/adverse reactions:

▼ *ORAL:* Stomatitis, candidiasis, angioedema (allergy)

CNS: Dizziness, headache, vertigo, somnolence, fatigue

CV: Palpitation, chest pain

GI: Nausea, vomiting, diarrhea, abdominal pain, ***hepatotoxicity,*** heartburn, dyspepsia, flatulence, melena

GU: Vaginitis, nephritis

INTEG: ***Cholestatic jaundice,*** rash, urticaria, pruritus (allergy), photosensitivity

Contraindications: Hypersensitivity to azithromycin or erythromycin

Precautions: Pregnancy category C; lactation; hepatic, renal, cardiac disease; elderly; child <16 yr

Pharmacokinetics:

PO: Peak 12 hr, duration 24 hr, half-life 11-57 hr; excreted in bile, feces, urine primarily as unchanged drug

Drug interactions of concern to dentistry:

• Increased serum levels: carbamazepine, cyclosporine

• Decreased action of clindamycin, penicillin, lincomycin, oral contraceptives

DENTAL CONSIDERATIONS

General:

• Alternative drug of choice for mild infection due to susceptible organisms in patients allergic to penicillin.

• Determine why the patient is taking the drug.

• Consider semisupine chair position for patient comfort if GI side effects occur.

Teach patient/family:

When used for dental infection, advise patient:

• Taking birth control pill to use

additional method of contraception for duration of cycle

• To report sore throat, oral burning sensation, fever, fatigue, any of which could indicate superinfection

• To take at prescribed intervals and complete dosage regimen

• To immediately notify the dentist if signs or symptoms of infection increase

bacampicillin HCl

(ba-kam-pi-sil′in)

Spectrobid

♣ Penglobe

Drug class.: Aminopenicillin

Action: Interferes with cell wall replication of susceptible organisms; the cell wall, rendered osmotically unstable, swells and bursts from osmotic pressure

Uses: Respiratory tract infections, skin infections, UTIs; effective for gram-positive cocci *(S. faecalis, S. pneumoniae),* gram-negative cocci *(N. gonorrhoeae),* gram-negative bacilli *(E. coli, H. influenzae, P. mirabilis)*

Dosage and routes:

• *Adult:* PO 400-800 mg q12h

• *Child:* PO 25-50 mg/kg/day in divided doses q12h

Available forms include: Tabs 400 mg; powder for oral susp 125 mg/ 5 ml

Side effects/adverse reactions:

▼ *ORAL:* Discolored tongue, glossitis, increased thirst, candidiasis, stomatitis

CNS: ***Coma, convulsions,*** lethargy, hallucinations, anxiety, depression, twitching

GI: Nausea, vomiting, diarrhea, increased AST/ALT, abdominal pain, colitis

HEMA: ***Bone marrow depression, granulocytopenia,*** anemia, increased bleeding time

GU: Vaginitis, moniliasis, ***glomerulonephritis,*** oliguria, proteinuria, hematuria

SYST: ***Anaphylaxis,*** pruritus, urticaria, angioedema, bronchospasm (allergy symptoms)

Contraindications: Hypersensitivity to penicillins; neonates

Precautions: Pregnancy category B, hypersensitivity to cephalosporins

Pharmacokinetics:

PO: Peak 30-60 min, duration 5-6 hr, half-life 0.5-1 hr; metabolized in liver; excreted in urine

Drug interactions of concern to dentistry:

• Decreased antimicrobial effectiveness: tetracyclines, erythromycins, lincomycins

• Increased bacampicillin concentrations: probenecid

When used for dental infection, advise patient:

• May reduce effectiveness of oral contraceptives

DENTAL CONSIDERATIONS:

General:

• Patients on chronic drug therapy may rarely have symptoms of blood dyscrasias, which can include infection, bleeding, and poor healing.

• Take precautions regarding allergy to medication.

• Determine why the patient is taking the drug.

Consultations:

• In a patient with symptoms of blood dyscrasias, request a medical

consult for blood studies and postpone dental treatment until normal values are reestablished.

• Medical consult may be required to assess disease control in the patient.

Teach patient/family:

• Importance of good oral hygiene to prevent soft tissue inflammation
• Caution to prevent injury when using oral hygiene aids

When used for dental infection, advise patient:

• Taking birth control pill to use additional method of contraception for duration of cycle
• To report sore throat, oral burning sensation, fever, fatigue, any of which could indicate superinfection
• To take at prescribed intervals and complete dosage regimen
• To immediately notify the dentist if signs or symptoms of infection increase

baclofen

(bak'loe-fen)

Lioresal

♣ Alpha-Baclofen, PMS-Baclofen

Drug class.: Skeletal muscle relaxant, central acting

Action: Precise mechanism of action is unknown; inhibits both monosynaptic and polysynaptic reflexes in the spinal cord and may act as an agonist for $GABA_B$ receptors; also causes some CNS depression

Uses: Skeletal muscle spasticity in multiple sclerosis, spinal cord injury; unapproved use in trigeminal neuralgia

Dosage and routes:

• *Adult:* PO 5 mg tid × 3 days, then 10 mg tid × 3 days, then 15 mg tid × 3 days, then 20 mg tid × 3 days, then titrated to response, not to exceed 80 mg/day

Available forms include: Tabs 10, 20 mg

Side effects/adverse reactions:

▼ *ORAL:* Dry mouth, taste alteration

CNS: Dizziness, weakness, fatigue, drowsiness, headache, disorientation, insomnia, paresthesias, tremors

CV: Hypotension, chest pain, palpitation, edema

GI: Nausea, constipation, vomiting, increased AST, alk phosphatase, abdominal pain, anorexia

GU: Urinary frequency

EENT: Nasal congestion, blurred vision, mydriasis, tinnitus

INTEG: Rash, pruritus

Contraindications: Hypersensitivity

Precautions: Peptic ulcer disease, renal disease, hepatic disease, stroke, seizure disorder, diabetes mellitus, pregnancy category C, elderly

Pharmacokinetics:

PO: Peak 2-3 hr, duration <8 hr, half-life 2.5-4 hr; partially metabolized in liver; excreted in urine (unchanged)

Drug interactions of concern to dentistry:

• Increased CNS depression: alcohol, all CNS depressants

When used in dentistry:

• Warn patient of sedative effects while taking medication

DENTAL CONSIDERATIONS:

General:

• Monitor vital signs every ap-

pointment due to cardiovascular side effects.

• Assess salivary flow as a factor in caries, periodontal disease, and candidiasis.

• After supine positioning, have patient sit upright for at least 2 min to avoid orthostatic hypotension.

Teach patient/family:

When chronic dry mouth occurs, advise patient:

• To avoid mouth rinses with high alcohol content due to drying effects

• To use daily home fluoride products for anticaries effect

• To use sugarless gum, frequent sips of water, or saliva substitutes

becaplermin

(bee-kap'ler-min)

Regranex Gel

Drug class.: Topical wound repair

Action: A recombinant human platelet-derived growth factor (rhPDGF-BB) that promotes chemotactic recruitment and proliferation of cells involved in wound repair and formation of granulation tissue

Uses: As an adjunct to good ulcer care practices in lower extremity diabetic, neuropathic ulcers that extend into subcutaneous tissues or beyond and have adequate blood supply

Dosage and routes:

• *Adult and child >16 yr:* TOP Calculate the amount of gel to apply by the area (L × W) of the ulcer according to maunfacturer's formula in gel package. Apply the gel once daily in a 1/16-inch-thick layer spread evenly on the ulcerated area. As the ulcer heals, the dose must be recalculated at weekly or biweekly intervals.

Available forms include: Gel 0.01% in 2, 7.5, and 15 g tubes

Side effects/adverse reactions:

INTEG: Erythematous rashes, pain, infection

Contraindications: Hypersensitivity, neoplasms at the site of application, ulcers due to vascular insufficiency

Precautions: Nonsterile, low-bioburden product that is not for use in ulcers that heal by primary intention, external use only, do not apply with fingers, pregnancy category C, lactation, children <16 yr

Drug interactions of concern to dentistry:

• Unknown

DENTAL CONSIDERATIONS:

General:

• Patients requiring use of this medication will probably be limited in activities or bedridden.

• Determine why patient is taking the drug.

• Question patient about self-monitoring of blood glucose values or finger-stick records.

• Diabetics may be more susceptible to infection and have delayed wound healing.

• Examine for oral manifestation of opportunistic infection.

• Patients with advanced diabetes should be questioned about any limitations in activities or stress tolerance. Some will also be receiving dialysis treatment if renal function is compromised. Dental treatment can usually be performed the day after dialysis.

Consultations:

• Medical consult may be required to assess disease control and patient's ability to tolerate stress.

• Medical consult may include data from patient's blood glucose monitoring, including glycosylated hemoglobin (GHb) or HbA_{1c} testing.
• Patients in dialysis may require antibiotic prophylaxis; determine need.

Teach patient/family:

• Importance of good oral hygiene to prevent soft tissue inflammation
• To prevent trauma when using oral hygiene aids
• Importance of updating health and drug history if physician makes any changes in evaluation/drug regimens

---

beclomethasone dipropionate

(be-kloe-meth'a-sone)

Oral inhalation: Beclovent, Vanceril, Vanceril 84 µg Double Strength

Nasal inhalation: Beconase AQ Nasal, Beconase Inhalation, Vancenase AQ, Vancenase AQ Forte, Vancenase Nasal, Vanceril DS

🍁 *Oral inhalation:* Beclodisk, Becloforte, Rota caps

Drug class.: Corticosteroid, synthetic

Action: Glucocorticoids have multiple actions that include antiinflammatory and immunosuppressant effects. They inhibit phospholipase A_2, interfering with or reducing the synthesis of prostaglandins and leukotrienes. They also bind to cytoplasmic glucocorticoid receptors (GRs) and enter the cell nucleus to bind with DNA. This results in the synthesis of various enzymes such as collagenase, elastase, and cytokines that play important roles in inflammation and immunosuppression. They also suppress the production of lymphocytes, monocytes, and eosinophils.

Uses: Chronic asthma, prevent recurrent nasal polyps, allergic and nonallergic rhinitis

Dosage and routes:

Oral inhalation:

• *Adult:* INH 2-4 puffs tid-qid, not to exceed 20 inhalations/day
• *Child 6-12 yr:* INH 1-2 puffs tid-qid, not to exceed 10 inhalations/day

Nasal inhalation:

• *Adult and child >6 yr:* INSTILL 1-2 sprays in each nostril bid-qid; 84 µg double strength is once-daily dosage

Available forms include: Aerosol 42, 84 µg/actuation in canisters containing 200 metered actuations

Side effects/adverse reactions:

▼ *ORAL:* Dry mouth, candidiasis (rare)

RESP: ***Bronchospasm***

EENT: Hoarseness, sore throat

Contraindications: Hypersensitivity; status asthmaticus (primary treatment); nonasthmatic bronchial disease; bacterial, fungal, or viral infections of mouth, throat, or lungs; child <3 yr

Precautions: Nasal disease/surgery, pregnancy category C

Pharmacokinetics:

INH: Onset 10 min, half-life 3-15 hr; crosses placenta; metabolized in lungs, liver, GI system; excreted in feces (metabolites)

DENTAL CONSIDERATIONS

General:

• Evaluate respiration characteristics and rate.
• Assess salivary flow as a factor in caries, periodontal disease, and candidiasis.

• Place on frequent recall due to oral side effects.

• Be aware that aspirin or sulfite preservatives in vasoconstrictor-containing products can exacerbate asthma.

• Acute asthmatic episodes may be precipitated in the dental office. Sympathomimetic inhalants should be available for emergency use.

• Midday appointments and a stress reduction protocol may be required for anxious patients.

Consultations:

• Medical consult may be required to assess patient's ability to tolerate stress.

Teach patient/family:

• That gargling and rinsing with water after each dose helps prevent candidiasis

When chronic dry mouth occurs, advise patient:

• To avoid mouth rinses with high alcohol content due to drying effects

• To use daily home fluoride products for anticaries effect

• To use sugarless gum, frequent sips of water, or saliva substitutes

---

benazepril

(ben-a'ze-pril)

Lotensin

Drug class.: Angiotensin-converting enzyme (ACE) inhibitor

Action: Selectively suppresses renin-angiotensin-aldosterone system; inhibits ACE; prevents conversion of angiotensin I to angiotensin II; results in dilation of arterial, venous vessels

Uses: Hypertension, alone or in combination with thiazide diuretics

Dosage and routes:

• *Adult:* PO 10 mg qd initially, then 20-40 mg/day divided bid or qd

Renal impairment: PO 5 mg qd with Ccr <30 ml/min/1.73 m^2, increase as needed to maximum of 40 mg/day

Available forms include: Tabs 5, 10, 20, 40 mg

Side effects/adverse reactions:

▼ *ORAL:* Angioedema, dry mouth (rare)

CNS: Anxiety, hypertonia, insomnia, paresthesia, headache, dizziness, fatigue

CV: Hypotension, postural hypotension, syncope, palpitation, angina

GI: Nausea, constipation, vomiting, gastritis, melena

RESP: Cough, asthma, bronchitis, dyspnea, sinusitis

HEMA: ***Neutropenia, agranulocytosis***

GU: Increased BUN, creatinine, decreased libido, impotence, UTI

INTEG: Rash, flushing, sweating

MS: Arthralgia, arthritis, myalgia

META: Hyperkalemia, hyponatremia

Contraindications: Hypersensitivity to ACE inhibitors, pregnancy category D, lactation, children

Precautions: Impaired renal or liver function, dialysis patients, hypovolemia, blood dyscrasias, CHF, COPD, asthma, elderly

Pharmacokinetics:

PO: Peak 0.5-1 hr, half-life 10-11 hr; serum protein binding 97%; metabolized by liver (metabolites); excreted in urine

Drug interactions of concern to dentistry:

• Increased hypotension: alcohol, phenothiazines

• Decreased hypotensive effects: indomethacin and possibly other NSAIDs, sympathomimetics

DENTAL CONSIDERATIONS:
General:

• Monitor vital signs every appointment due to cardiovascular and respiratory side effects.
• After supine positioning, have patient sit upright for at least 2 min to avoid orthostatic hypotension.
• Patients on chronic drug therapy may rarely have symptoms of blood dyscrasias, which can include infection, bleeding, and poor healing.
• Assess salivary flow as a factor in caries, periodontal disease, and candidiasis.
• Limit use of sodium-containing products such as saline IV fluids for those patients with a dietary salt restriction.
• Use vasoconstrictors with caution, in low doses, and with careful aspiration.
• Stress from dental procedures may compromise cardiovascular function; determine patient risk.
• Short appointments and a stress reduction protocol may be required for anxious patients.

Consultations:

• Medical consult may be required to assess disease control and patient's ability to tolerate stress.
• In a patient with symptoms of blood dyscrasias, request a medical consult for blood studies and postpone dental treatment until normal values are reestablished.
• Take precautions if dental surgery is anticipated and sedation or general anesthesia is required; there is risk of a hypotensive episode.

Teach patient/family:

• Importance of good oral hygiene to prevent soft tissue inflammation
• Caution to prevent injury when using oral hygiene aids

When chronic dry mouth occurs, advise patient:

• To avoid mouth rinses with high alcohol content due to drying effects
• To use daily home fluoride products for anticaries effect
• To use sugarless gum, frequent sips of water, or saliva substitutes

---

benzocaine (topical)

(ben'zoe-kane)

Benzocaine liquid 20%: Hurricaine, Maximum Strength Anbesol, Maximum Strength Orajel, Orajel Mouth Aid
Benzocaine gel 20%: Hurricaine, Maximum Strength Anbesol, Maximum Strength Orajel, Orajel Mouth-Aid
Benzocaine gel 15%: Orabase Gel
Benzocaine gel 10%: Baby Orajel Nighttime, Denture Orajel, Orajel
Benzocaine gel 7.5%: Baby Anbesol, Baby Orajel, Orabase Baby
Benzocaine gel 6%: ZilaDent
Benzocaine spray 20%: Hurricaine, Americaine
Benzocaine ointment/paste 20%: Benzodent, Orabase-B

Drug class.: Topical ester local anesthetic

Action: Inhibits conduction of nerve impulses from sensory nerves

Uses: Oral irritation, toothache, cold sore, canker sore, pain, teething pain, pain caused by dental prostheses or orthodontic appliances

Dosage and routes:
• *Adult and child >6 yr:* TOP apply to affected area according to manufacturer's labeled instructions
Available forms include: Liq 20%; gel 20%, 15%, 10%, 7.5%, 6%; spray 20%; oint 20%; paste 20%
Side effects/adverse reactions:
▼ *ORAL:* Numbness, tingling
EENT: Itching, irritation
INTEG: Rash, urticaria
Contraindications: Hypersensitivity
Precautions: Pregnancy category C
Pharmacokinetics:
TOP: Onset 1 min, duration 0.5-1 hr; esters metabolized by plasma esterases; excreted as urinary metabolites

DENTAL CONSIDERATIONS
General:
• Do not use for topical anesthesia if medical history reveals allergy to procaine, PABA, parabens, or other ester-type local anesthetics.
• Use smallest effective amount in infants and children.
• Avoid applying to large denuded areas of mucosa to prevent excessive systemic absorption and potential toxicity.

benzonatate

(ben-zoe′na-tate)
Tessalon
Drug class.: Antitussive, nonnarcotic

Action: Inhibits cough reflex by anesthetizing stretch receptors in respiratory system, lungs, and pleura
Uses: Nonproductive cough relief

Dosage and routes:
• *Adult and child:* PO 100 mg tid, not to exceed 600 mg/day
• *Child <10 yr:* PO 8 mg/kg in 3-6 divided doses
Available forms include: Perles 100 mg
Side effects/adverse reactions:
CNS: Dizziness, drowsiness, headache
CV: Increased BP, chest tightness, numbness
GI: Nausea, constipation, upset stomach
EENT: Nasal congestion, burning eyes
INTEG: Urticaria, rash, pruritus
Contraindications: Hypersensitivity
Precautions: Pregnancy category C, lactation
Pharmacokinetics:
PO: Onset 15-20 min, duration 3-8 hr; metabolized by liver; excreted in urine
Drug interactions of concern to dentistry:
• Increased CNS depression: slight risk of increased sedation with other CNS depressants

DENTAL CONSIDERATIONS
General:
• Elective dental treatment may not be possible with significant coughing episodes.

benztropine mesylate

(benz′troe-peen)
Cogentin
Apo-Benzotropine, PMS Benztropine
Drug class.: Anticholinergic, antidyskinetic

Action: Blockade of central acetylcholine receptors

Uses: Parkinson symptoms, extrapyramidal symptoms associated with neuroleptic drugs

Dosage and routes:

Drug-induced extrapyramidal symptoms

- *Adult:* IM/IV 1-2 ml 1-2 × daily; give PO dose as soon as possible; PO 1-4 mg qd-bid, increase by 0.5 mg q5-6d

Parkinson symptoms

- *Adult:* PO 0.5-1 mg qd, increased 0.5 mg q5-6d titrated to patient response

Available forms include: Tabs 0.5, 1, 2 mg; inj IM/IV 1 mg/ml

Side effects/adverse reactions:

▼ *ORAL: Dry mouth,* glossitis

CNS: Confusion, anxiety, restlessness, irritability, delusions, hallucinations, headache, sedation, depression, incoherence, dizziness, memory loss

CV: Palpitation, tachycardia, hypotension, bradycardia

GI: Constipation, ***paralytic ileus,*** nausea, vomiting, abdominal distress, epigastric distress

GU: Hesitancy, retention

EENT: Blurred vision, photophobia, dilated pupils, difficulty swallowing, dry eyes, mydriasis

INTEG: Rash, urticaria, dermatosis

MS: Muscular weakness, cramping

MISC: Increased temperature, flushing, decreased sweating, hyperthermia, heatstroke, numbness of fingers

Contraindications: Hypersensitivity, narrow-angle glaucoma, myasthenia gravis, GI/GU obstruction, child <3 yr, peptic ulcer, megacolon

Precautions: Pregnancy category C, elderly, lactation, tachycardia, prostatic hypertrophy, liver or kidney disease, drug abuse history, dysrhythmias, hypotension, hypertension, psychiatric patients

Pharmacokinetics:

IM/IV: Onset 15 min, duration 6-10 hr

PO: Onset 1 hr, duration 6-10 hr

Drug interactions of concern to dentistry:

- Increased anticholinergic effect: antihistamines, anticholinergics, and meperidine
- Decreased effects of phenothiazines

DENTAL CONSIDERATIONS

General:

- Monitor vital signs every appointment due to cardiovascular side effects.
- Assess salivary flow as a factor in caries, periodontal disease, and candidiasis.
- After supine positioning, have patient sit upright for at least 2 min to avoid orthostatic hypotension.
- Avoid dental light in patient's eyes; offer dark glasses for patient comfort.
- Do not use ingestible sodium bicarbonate products, such as the air polishing system (Prophy Jet), within 1 hr of taking benztropine.
- Place on frequent recall due to oral side effects.

Consultations:

- Medical consult may be required to assess disease control in the patient.
- Medical consult may be required to assess patient's ability to tolerate stress.

Teach patient/family:

- Importance of good oral hygiene to prevent soft tissue inflammation
- Use of electric toothbrush if patient has difficulty holding conventional devices

When chronic dry mouth occurs, advise patient:

- To avoid mouth rinses with high alcohol content due to drying effects
- To use daily home fluoride products for anticaries effect
- To use sugarless gum, frequent sips of water, or saliva substitutes

bepridil HCl

(be'pri-dil)

Bepadin, Vascor

Drug class.: Calcium channel blockers

Action: Inhibits calcium ion influx across cell membrane during cardiac depolarization; produces relaxation of coronary vascular smooth muscle; dilates coronary arteries; decreases SA/AV node conduction; dilates peripheral arteries

Uses: Stable angina, used alone or in combination with propranolol

Dosage and routes:

Angina

- *Adult:* PO 200 mg qd, can titrate to 300 mg or 400 mg qd; usual dose 200 mg/day

Available forms include: Film-coated tabs, PO 200, 300, 400 mg

Side effects/adverse reactions:

▼ *ORAL:* Dry mouth, taste changes (gingival overgrowth has been reported with other calcium channel blockers)

CNS: Headache, fatigue, drowsiness, dizziness, anxiety, depression, weakness, insomnia, confusion, light-headedness, nervousness

CV: Dysrhythmia, edema, CHF, bradycardia, hypotension, palpitation, AV block

GI: Nausea, vomiting, diarrhea, gastric upset, constipation, increased liver function studies

GU: Nocturia, polyuria

Contraindications: Sick sinus syndrome, second- or third-degree heart block, Wolff-Parkinson-White syndrome, hypotension less than 90 mm Hg (systolic), cardiogenic shock

Precautions: CHF, hypotension, hepatic injury, pregnancy category C, lactation, children, renal disease

Pharmacokinetics:

PO: Onset 60 min, peak 2-3 hr, half-life 42 hr; 99% plasma protein bound; completely metabolized in liver; excreted in urine and feces

Drug interactions of concern to dentistry:

- Decreased effect: indomethacin, possibly other NSAIDs, phenobarbital
- Increased effect: Parenteral and inhalational general anesthetics or other drugs with hypotensive actions
- Increased effects of carbamazepine

DENTAL CONSIDERATIONS

General:

- Monitor cardiac status; take vital signs at each appointment because of cardiovascular side effects. Consider a stress reduction protocol to prevent stress-induced angina during the dental appointment.
- After supine positioning, have patient sit upright for at least 2 min to avoid orthostatic hypotension.
- Limit use of sodium-containing products such as saline IV fluids for those patients with a dietary salt restriction.
- Assess salivary flow as a factor in caries, periodontal disease, and candidiasis.

Consultations:
• Medical consult may be required to assess disease control and stress tolerance of patient.

Teach patient/family:
• Need for frequent oral prophylaxis if gingival overgrowth occurs

When chronic dry mouth occurs, advise patient:
• To avoid mouth rinses with high alcohol content due to drying effects
• To use daily home fluoride products for anticaries effect
• To use sugarless gum, frequent sips of water, or saliva substitutes

betamethasone valerate/ betamethasone benzoate/ betamethasone dipropionate

(bay-ta-meth'a-sone)

Betamethasone dipropionate augmented cream 0.05%: Diprolene AF
Betamethasone dipropionate gel 0.05%: Diprolene
Betamethasone dipropionate oint 0.05%: Alphatrex, Diprolene, Diprosone, Maxivate
Betamethasone dipropionate lotion 0.05%: Alphatrex, Diprosone, Maxivate
Betamethasone valerate cream 0.1 or 0.01%: Betatrex, Beta-Val, Dermabet, Prevex B, Valisone, Valisone Reduced Strength, Valnac
🍁 *Betamethasone benzoate gel 0.025%:* Bepen
Betamethasone dipropionate augmented cream 0.05%: Diprolene
Betamethasone dipropionate oint 0.05%: Topilene, Topisone
Betamethasone dipropionate lotion 0.05%: Topisone
Betamethasone valerate cream 0.1 or 0.01%: Bentovate-1/2, Celestoderm-V/2, Ectosone Mild, Metaderm Mild, Metaderm Regular, NovoBetament
Drug class.: Topical corticosteroid

Action: Glucocorticoids have multiple actions that include antiinflammatory and immunosuppressant effects. They inhibit phospholipase A_2, interfering with or reducing the synthesis of prostaglandins and leukotrienes. They also bind to cytoplasmic glucocorticoid receptors (GRs) and enter the cell nucleus to bind with DNA. This results in the synthesis of various enzymes such as collagenase, elastase, betamethasone, and cytokines that play important roles in inflammation and immunosuppression. They also suppress the production of lymphocytes, monocytes, and eosinophils.

Uses: Psoriasis, eczema, contact dermatitis, pruritus, oral ulcerative inflammatory lesions

Dosage and routes:

• *Adult and child:* TOP apply to affected area qid

Available forms include: Oint 0.05%; cream 0.025% and 0.05%, lotion 0.1% and 0.01%, gel 0.05% (gel available in 15 and 45 g tubes)

Side effects/adverse reactions:

▼ *ORAL:* Thinning of mucosa, stinging sensation (oral application)

INTEG: Burning, dryness, itching, irritation, acne, folliculitis, hypertrichosis, perioral dermatitis, hypopigmentation, atrophy, striae, miliaria, allergic contact dermatitis, secondary infection

Contraindications: Hypersensitivity to corticosteroids, fungal infections

Precautions: Pregnancy category C, lactation, viral infections, bacterial infections

DENTAL CONSIDERATIONS

General:

• Place on frequent recall to evaluate healing response.

Teach patient/family:

• When used for oral lesions, advise patient to return for oral evaluation if response of oral tissues has not occurred in 7-14 days

• Importance of good oral hygiene to prevent soft tissue inflammation

• To apply at bedtime or after meals for maximum effect

• To apply with cotton-tipped applicator by pressing, not rubbing, paste on lesion

• That use on oral herpetic ulcerations is contraindicated

---

betamethasone/ betamethasone sodium phosphate/ betamethasone sodium phosphate and betamethasone acetate

(bay-ta-meth'a-sone)

Betamethasone oral: Celestone

Betamethasone sodium phosphate injection USP: Celestone Phosphate, Selestoject

Betamethasone sodium phosphate and betamethasone acetate USP: Celestone Soluspan

♣ *Betamethasone oral:* Betnelan, Betnesol, Celestone Extended Release

Drug class.: Glucocorticoid, long acting

Action: Glucocorticoids have multiple actions that include antiinflammatory and immunosuppressant effects. They inhibit phospholipase A_2, interfering with or reducing the synthesis of prostaglandins and leukotrienes. They also bind to cytoplasmic glucocorticoid receptors (GRs) and enter the cell nucleus to bind with DNA. This results in the synthesis of various enzymes such as collagenase, elastase, and cytokines that play important roles in inflammation and immunosuppression. They also suppress the production of lymphocytes, monocytes, and eosinophils.

Uses: Severe inflammation, shock, adrenal insufficiency, collagen disorders

Dosage and routes:

Betamethasone tablets or syrup

• *Adult:* PO 0.6 to 7.2 mg/day as a single dose or in divided doses; all doses must be individualized for the patient depending on the disease and patient response

• *Child:* 62.5 to 250 μg/kg of body weight in 3 or 4 divided doses daily for most indications; for adrenal cortical insufficiency: 17.5 μg/kg of body weight

Betamethasone sodium phosphate injection

• *Adult:* IM or IV up to 9 mg/day; intraarticular, intralesional, or soft tissue injection up to 9 mg as needed

Betamethasone sodium phosphate and betamethasone acetate suspension

• *Adult:* IM can be mixed with paraben-free 1% or 2% lidocaine for injection, 0.5-9 mg/day; intrabursal INJ 1.0 ml/0.6 mg; intraarticular INJ 0.5-2.0 mg (1.5-12 mg) depending on joint size; intradermal or intralesional INJ 1.2 mg/cm^2 of affected skin up to 6 mg at weekly intervals

Available forms include: Tabs 0.6 mg, effervescent tabs ♣ 0.5 mg; syrup 0.6 mg/5 ml; inj 4 mg betamethasone phosphate/ml in 5 ml vials; 3 mg betamethasone acetate with 3 mg betamethasone sodium phosphate in 5 ml vials

Side effects/adverse reactions:

▼ *ORAL:* Candidiasis, dry mouth

CNS: Depression, flushing, sweating, headache, mood changes

CV: Hypertension, ***circulatory collapse, thrombophlebitis, embolism,*** tachycardia, edema

GI: Diarrhea, nausea, abdominal distention, ***GI hemorrhage, pancreatitis,*** increased appetite

HEMA: ***Thrombocytopenia***

EENT: Fungal infections, increased intraocular pressure, blurred vision

INTEG: Acne, poor wound healing, ecchymosis, petechiae

MS: Fractures, osteoporosis, weakness

Contraindications: Psychosis, hypersensitivity, idiopathic thrombocytopenia, acute glomerulonephritis, amebiasis, fungal infections, nonasthmatic bronchial disease, child <2 yr, AIDS, TB

Precautions: Pregnancy category C, diabetes mellitus, glaucoma, osteoporosis, seizure disorders, ulcerative colitis, CHF, myasthenia gravis, renal disease, peptic ulcer, esophagitis

Pharmacokinetics:

PO: Peak 1-2 hr, duration 2.33 days

IM: Peak 8 hr, duration 6 days; half-life 3-4.5 hr

Drug interactions of concern to dentistry:

• Decreased action: barbiturates

• Increased GI side effects: alcohol, salicylates, and other NSAIDs

• Increased action: ketoconazole, macrolide antibiotics

DENTAL CONSIDERATIONS

General:

• Monitor vital signs every appointment due to cardiovascular side effects.

• Patients on chronic drug therapy

may rarely have symptoms of blood dyscrasias, which can include infection, bleeding, and poor healing.
• Symptoms of oral infections may be masked.
• Determine dose and duration of steroid therapy for each patient to assess risk for stress tolerance and immunosuppression.
• Avoid prescribing aspirin-containing products.
• Place on frequent recall to evaluate healing response.
• Prophylactic antibiotics may be indicated to prevent infection if surgery or deep scaling is planned.
• Patients who have been or are currently on chronic steroid therapy (>2 wk) may require supplemental steroids for dental treatment

Consultations:
• In a patient with symptoms of blood dyscrasias, request a medical consult for blood studies and postpone dental treatment until normal values are reestablished.
• Medical consult may be required to assess disease control in the patient.
• Consult may be required to confirm steroid dose and duration of use.

Teach patient/family:
• Importance of good oral hygiene to prevent soft tissue inflammation
• Caution to prevent injury when using oral hygiene aids

---

betaxolol HCl

(be-tax'oh-lol)
Kerlone

Drug class.: Antihypertensive, selective β_1-blocker

Action: This is a selective β_1-adrenergic antagonist. At higher doses selectivity may be lost with antagonism of β_2-receptors as well. The antihypertensive mechanism of action is unclear, but may include a reduction in cardiac output and inhibition of renin release by the renal juxtaglomerular apparatus. Peripheral resistance decreases with long-term use. The antianginal action (when indicated for this use) may be related to a decrease in myocardial oxygen demand and negative chronotropic and inotropic effects. The antiarrhythmic action (when indicated for this use) has been related to a reduction in spontaneous pacemaker firing and slowing of AV nodal conduction.

Uses: Hypertension

Dosage and routes:
• *Adult:* PO 10 mg qd, increasing to 20 mg qd if response is inadequate after 14 days

Available forms include: Tabs 10, 20 mg

Side effects/adverse reactions:
▼ *ORAL:* Dry mouth (less than 2%)
CNS: Dizziness, fatigue, lethargy, depression, headache
CV: Bradycardia, hypotension, dysrhythmias
GI: Nausea, dyspepsia, diarrhea
RESP: ***Bronchospasm,*** dyspnea, pharyngitis
GU: Impotence
EENT: Eye irritation, conjunctivitis, keratitis
INTEG: Rash, urticaria

Contraindications: Hypersensitivity to β-blockers, cardiogenic shock, second- or third-degree heart block, sinus bradycardia, CHF, cardiac failure

Precautions: Major surgery, pregnancy category C, lactation, diabetes mellitus, renal disease, thyroid disease, COPD, asthma, well-compensated heart failure, aortic or mitral valve disease

Pharmacokinetics:

PO: Peak 3-4 hr, half-life 14-22 hr; protein binding 50%; some hepatic metabolism; excreted in urine mostly unchanged

Drug interactions of concern to dentistry:

- Decreased antihypertensive effects: NSAIDs, indomethacin
- May slow metabolism of lidocaine
- Decreased β-blocking effects (or decreased β-adrenergic effects) of epinephrine, levonordefrin, isoproterenol, and other sympathomimetics

DENTAL CONSIDERATIONS

General:

- Monitor vital signs every appointment due to cardiovascular and respiratory side effects.
- After supine positioning, have patient sit upright for at least 2 min to avoid orthostatic hypotension.
- Assess salivary flow as a factor in caries, periodontal disease, and candidiasis.
- Stress from dental procedures may compromise cardiovascular function; determine patient risk.
- Short appointments and a stress reduction protocol may be required for anxious patients.
- Use vasoconstrictors with caution, in low doses, and with careful aspiration. Avoid use of gingival retraction cord with epinephrine.

Consultations:

- Medical consult may be required to assess disease control and stress tolerance of patient.
- Use precautions if general anesthesia is required for dental surgery.

Teach patient/family:

- Importance of good oral hygiene to prevent soft tissue inflammation
- Caution to prevent injury when using oral hygiene aids

When chronic dry mouth occurs, advise patient:

- To avoid mouth rinses with high alcohol content due to drying effects
- To use daily home fluoride products for anticaries effect
- To use sugarless gum, frequent sips of water, or saliva substitutes

betaxolol HCl (optic)

(be-tax'oh-lol)

Betoptic, Betoptic S

Drug class.: Selective β_1-blocker

Action: Reduces intraocular pressure by reducing production of aqueous humor

Uses: Chronic open-angle glaucoma, ocular hypertension

Dosage and routes:

- *Adult:* INSTILL 1-2 gtt bid

Available forms include: Susp 0.25%; sol 0.5%

Side effects/adverse reactions:

CNS: Insomnia, dizziness, headache, depression (all rarely occur)

CV: Bradycardia (rare)

RESP: ***Bronchospasm*** (rare)

EENT: Eye irritation, conjunctivitis, keratitis

Contraindications: Hypersensitivity, asthma, second- or third-degree heart block, right ventricular failure, congenital glaucoma (infants), COPD

Precautions: Pregnancy category C

Pharmacokinetics: Onset 30 min, maximum effect 2 hr, duration 12 hr

Drug interactions of concern to dentistry:

• Avoid use of anticholinergic drugs, atropine-like drugs, propantheline, and diazepam (benzodiazepines)

DENTAL CONSIDERATIONS

General:

• Monitor vital signs every appointment due to cardiovascular side effects.

• Check compliance of patient with prescribed drug regimen for glaucoma.

• Avoid dental light in patient's eyes; offer dark glasses for patient comfort.

Consultations:

• Consultation with physician may be needed if sedation or anesthesia is required.

bethanechol chloride

(be-than'e-kole)

Duvoid, Urabeth, Urecholine

Drug class.: Cholinergic stimulant

Action: Stimulates muscarinic ACh receptors directly; mimics effects of parasympathetic nervous system stimulation; stimulates gastric motility, stimulates ganglia

Uses: Urinary retention (postoperative, postpartum), neurogenic atony of bladder with retention; unapproved use: gastric atony

Dosage and routes:

• *Adult:* PO 10-50 mg bid-qid; SC 2.5-10 mg tid-qid prn

Available forms include: Tabs 5, 10, 25, 50 mg; inj SC 5 mg/ml

Side effects/adverse reactions:

ORAL: Increased salivation

CNS: ***Convulsions,*** dizziness, headache, confusion, weakness

CV: ***Cardiac arrest, circulatory collapse,*** hypotension, bradycardia, orthostatic hypotension, reflex tachycardia

GI: Nausea, bloody diarrhea, vomiting, cramps, fecal incontinence

RESP: ***Acute asthma, dyspnea***

GU: Frequency, incontinence

EENT: Miosis, lacrimation, blurred vision

INTEG: Rash, urticaria, flushing, increased sweating, hypothermia

Contraindications: Hypersensitivity, severe bradycardia, asthma, severe hypotension, hyperthyroidism, peptic ulcer, parkinsonism, seizure disorders, CAD, coronary occlusion, mechanical obstruction

Precautions: Hypertension, pregnancy category C, lactation, child <8 yr, urinary retention

Pharmacokinetics:

PO: Onset 30-90 min, duration 6 hr

SC: Onset 5-15 min, duration 2 hr; excreted by kidneys

Drug interactions of concern to dentistry:

• Decreased effects: anticholinergics

DENTAL CONSIDERATIONS

General:

• Monitor vital signs every appointment due to cardiovascular and respiratory side effects.

• After supine positioning, have patient sit upright for at least 2 min to avoid orthostatic hypotension.

Consultations:

• For excessive, troublesome salivation, reassure patient that treatment duration is usually limited to a few days; otherwise consult to lower bethanechol dose.

bicalutamide

(bye-ka-loo'ta-mide)

Casodex

Drug class.: Nonsteroidal antiandrogen, antineoplastic

Action: Competitively inhibits the action of androgens by binding to androgen receptors in target tissues

Uses: Combination therapy with a luteinizing hormone–releasing hormone (LHRH) analog for advanced prostate cancer

Dosage and routes:

- *Adult:* PO 50 mg daily with or without food

Available forms include: Tabs 50 mg

Side effects/adverse reactions:

▼ *ORAL:* Dry mouth (<5%)

CNS: Headache, dizziness, paresthesia, insomnia

CV: Hot flashes, hypertension, peripheral edema

GI: Diarrhea, abdominal pain, constipation, flatulence, vomiting

RESP: Dyspnea, cough

HEMA: Anemia

GU: Nocturia, hematuria, UTI, incontinence, inhibition of spermatogenesis

INTEG: Rash, sweating

ENDO: Gynecomastia, hyperglycemia

MS: Back pain, asthenia, bone pain

MISC: Breast pain, weight loss

Contraindications: Hypersensitivity, women who may become pregnant, pregnancy category X

Precautions: Hepatic impairment, lactation, children

Pharmacokinetics:

PO: Rapid absorption; 96% plasma protein binding; hepatic metabolism; excretion in feces and urine

Drug interactions of concern to dentistry:

- Avoid drugs that could exacerbate urinary retention, such as anticholinergics

DENTAL CONSIDERATIONS

General:

- Patients taking opioids for acute or chronic pain should be given alternative analgesics for dental pain.
- Palliative medication may be required for management of oral side effects.
- Assess salivary flow as a factor in caries, periodontal disease, and candidiasis.
- Monitor vital signs every appointment due to cardiovascular and respiratory side effects.
- Short appointments may be required for patient comfort.
- Consider semisupine chair position for patient comfort due to disease and drug side effects.

Consultations:

- Medical consult may be required to assess disease control and patient's ability to tolerate stress.

Teach patient/family:

- Place on frequent recall due to oral side effects
- Importance of updating medical/drug record if physician makes any changes in evaluations/drug regimens

When chronic dry mouth occurs, advise patient:

- To avoid mouth rinses with high alcohol content due to drying effects
- Of need for daily home fluoride to prevent caries
- To use sugarless gum, frequent sips of water, or saliva substitutes

biperiden HCl/ biperiden lactate

(bye-per'i-den)

Akineton

Drug class.: Anticholinergic

Action: Centrally acting competitive anticholinergic

Uses: Parkinson symptoms, extrapyramidal symptoms secondary to neuroleptic drug therapy

Dosage and routes:

Extrapyramidal symptoms

• *Adult:* PO 2-6 mg bid-tid; IM/IV 2 mg q30min, if needed, not to exceed 8 mg/24 hr

Parkinson symptoms

• *Adult:* PO 2 mg tid-qid

Available forms include: Tabs 2 mg; inj IM/IV 5 mg/ml (lactate)

Side effects/adverse reactions:

▼ *ORAL: Dry mouth,* glossitis

CNS: Confusion, anxiety, restlessness, irritability, delusions, hallucinations, headache, sedation, depression, incoherence, dizziness, euphoria, tremors, memory loss

CV: Palpitation, tachycardia, postural hypotension, bradycardia

GI: Constipation, ***paralytic ileus,*** nausea, vomiting, abdominal distress

GU: Hesitancy, retention

EENT: Blurred vision, photophobia, dilated pupils, difficulty swallowing, mydriasis

INTEG: Rash, urticaria, dermatosis

MS: Weakness, cramping

MISC: Increased temperature, flushing, decreased sweating, hyperthermia, heatstroke, numbness of fingers

Contraindications: Hypersensitivity, narrow-angle glaucoma, myasthenia gravis, GI/GU obstruction, megacolon, stenosing peptic ulcers

Precautions: Pregnancy category C, elderly, lactation, tachycardia, prostatic hypertrophy, dysrhythmias, liver or kidney disease, drug abuse, hypotension, hypertension, psychiatric patients, children

Pharmacokinetics:

IM/IV: Onset 15 min, duration 6-10 hr

PO: Onset 1 hr, duration 6-10 hr

Drug interactions of concern to dentistry:

• Increased anticholinergic effect: antihistamines, anticholinergic-acting drugs, meperidine

• Increased CNS depression: alcohol, CNS depressants

• Decreased effects of phenothiazines

DENTAL CONSIDERATIONS

General:

• Monitor vital signs every appointment due to cardiovascular side effects.

• After supine positioning, have patient sit upright at least 2 min to avoid orthostatic hypotension.

• Assess salivary flow as a factor in caries, periodontal disease, and candidiasis.

• Avoid dental light in patient's eyes; offer dark glasses for patient comfort.

Consultations:

• Medical consult may be required to assess disease control and patient's ability to tolerate stress.

Teach patient/family:

• To use electric toothbrush if patient has difficulty holding conventional devices

• Importance of good oral hygiene to prevent soft tissue inflammation

When chronic dry mouth occurs, advise patient:
• To avoid mouth rinses with high alcohol content due to drying effects
• To use daily home fluoride products for anticaries effect
• To use sugarless gum, frequent sips of water, or saliva substitutes

bismuth subsalicylate

(bis'meth)

Bismatrol, Bismatrol Extra Strength, Bismed, Helidac Chewable, Pepto-Bismol, Pepto-Bismol Maximum Strength

♣ PMS-bismuth subsalicylate

Drug class.: Antidiarrheal

Action: Mechanism of action is not known; may act through antisecretory, antimicrobial, or antiinflammatory effects

Uses: Diarrhea (cause undetermined), prevention of diarrhea when traveling; unapproved: gastritis, duodenal ulcer associated with *Helicobacter pylori*

Dosage and routes:
• *Adult:* PO 30 ml or 2 tabs q30-60 min, not to exceed 8 doses for >2 days
• *Child 10-14 yr:* PO 15 ml
• *Child 6-10 yr:* PO 10 ml
• *Child 3-6 yr:* PO 5 ml

Available forms include: Chew tabs 262 mg; susp 262 mg/15 ml

Side effects/adverse reactions:
▼ *ORAL:* Metallic taste, gray discoloration of tongue
CNS: Confusion, twitching
GI: Increased fecal impaction (high doses), dark stools
HEMA: Increased bleeding time
EENT: Hearing loss, tinnitus

Contraindications: Child <3 yr

Precautions: Anticoagulant therapy

Pharmacokinetics:
PO: Onset 1 hr, peak 2 hr, duration 4 hr

Drug interactions of concern to dentistry:
• Salicylate toxicity: other salicylates
• Decreased absorption of tetracyclines

DENTAL CONSIDERATIONS

General:
• Avoid prescribing aspirin-containing products for analgesia.

bisoprolol fumarate

(bis-oh'proe-lol)

Zebeta

Drug class.: Antihypertensive, selective β_1-blocker

Action: Produces fall in BP without reflex tachycardia or significant reduction in heart rate; acts to block β_1-adrenergic receptors; elevated plasma renins are reduced; blocks β_1-adrenergic receptors in bronchial and vascular smooth muscle only at high doses

Uses: Hypertension as a single agent or in combination with other antihypertensives; unapproved use for angina pectoris, PVCs, superventricular tachydysrhythmias

Dosage and routes:
• *Adult:* PO 5 mg/day, limit 20 mg/day
• *Geriatric:* PO 2.5 mg/day

Available forms include: Tabs 5, 10 mg

Side effects/adverse reactions:
▼ *ORAL:* Dry mouth
CNS: Insomnia, dizziness, ***depres-***

sion, mental changes, hallucinations, anxiety, headaches, nightmares, confusion, fatigue
CV: Bradycardia, palpitation, ***cardiac arrest, AV block,*** hypotension, dysrhythmias, CHF
GI: Hiccups, nausea, vomiting, colitis, cramps, diarrhea, constipation, flatulence
RESP: ***Bronchospasm,*** dyspnea, wheezing
HEMA: ***Agranulocytosis, eosinophilia, thrombocytopenic purpura***
GU: Impotence
EENT: Sore throat, dry burning eyes
INTEG: Rash, purpura, alopecia, dry skin, urticaria, pruritus
Contraindications: Hypersensitivity to β-blockers, cardiogenic shock, second- or third-degree heart block, sinus bradycardia, CHF, bronchial asthma
Precautions: Pregnancy category C, major surgery, lactation, diabetes mellitus, renal disease, thyroid disease, COPD, heart failure, CAD, nonallergic bronchospasm, hepatic disease
Pharmacokinetics:
PO: Half-life 9-12 hr; highly protein bound; 50% excreted unchanged in urine, rest as metabolites

Drug interactions of concern to dentistry:

- Decreased antihypertensive effects: NSAIDs, indomethacin, sympathomimetics
- May slow metabolism of lidocaine
- Decreased β-blocking effects (or decreased β-adrenergic effects) of epinephrine, levonordefrin, isoproterenol, and other sympathomimetics

DENTAL CONSIDERATIONS
General:

- Monitor vital signs every appointment due to cardiovascular side effects.
- After supine positioning, have patient sit upright for at least 2 min to avoid orthostatic hypotension.
- Patients on chronic drug therapy may rarely have symptoms of blood dyscrasias, which can include infection, bleeding, and poor healing.
- Assess salivary flow as a factor in caries, periodontal disease, and candidiasis.
- Stress from dental procedures may compromise cardiovascular function; determine patient risk.
- Short appointments and a stress reduction protocol may be required for anxious patients.
- Use vasoconstrictors with caution, in low doses, and with careful aspiration. Avoid use of gingival retraction cord with epinephrine.

Consultations:

- In a patient with symptoms of blood dyscrasias, request a medical consult for blood studies and postpone dental treatment until normal values are reestablished.
- Medical consult may be required to assess disease control and patient's ability to tolerate stress.
- Take precautions if general anesthesia is required for dental surgery.

Teach patient/family:
When chronic dry mouth occurs, advise patient:

- To avoid mouth rinses with high alcohol content due to drying effects
- To use daily home fluoride products for anticaries effect

• To use sugarless gum, frequent sips of water, or saliva substitutes

bitolterol mesylate

(bye-tole′ter-ole)
Tornalate
Drug class.: Adrenergic β_2-agonist

Action: Causes bronchodilation by action on β_2-receptors by increasing levels of cAMP, which relaxes smooth muscle with very little effect on heart rate
Uses: Treatment or prophylaxis of asthma, bronchitis, bronchospasm
Dosage and routes:
Treatment
• *Adult and child >12 yr:* INH 2 inhalations at intervals of 1-3 min, followed by third inhalation if needed; not to exceed 3 inh q6h or 2 inh q4h
Prophylaxis
• *Adult and child >12 yr:* INH 2 inhalations q8h
Available forms include: Aerosol 0.37 mg/actuation
Side effects/adverse reactions:
▼ *ORAL:* Taste change, dry mouth, discolored teeth
CNS: Tremors, anxiety, insomnia, *headache, dizziness,* stimulation, restlessness, flushing, irritability, hallucinations
CV: Palpitation, tachycardia, hypertension, angina, dysrhythmias, chest pain
GI: Heartburn, nausea, vomiting, diarrhea
RESP: ***Paradoxic bronchospasm***
GU: Difficult or painful urination
EENT: Dry nose, irritation of nose and throat
MS: Muscle cramps, twitching
Contraindications: Hypersensitivity to sympathomimetics, tachydysrhythmia, severe cardiac disease
Precautions: Lactation, pregnancy category C, cardiac disorders, hyperthyroidism, diabetes mellitus, hypertension, prostatic hypertrophy, narrow-angle glaucoma, pheochromocytoma, seizures
Pharmacokinetics:
INH: Onset 3-4 min, peak 0.5-1 hr, duration 5-8 hr
Drug interactions of concern to dentistry:
• Increased dysrhythmias: halogenated hydrocarbon anesthetics
• Increased CNS stimulation: cocaine and other CNS stimulants

DENTAL CONSIDERATIONS
General:
• Monitor vital signs every appointment due to cardiovascular and respiratory side effects.
• Assess salivary flow as a factor in caries, periodontal disease, and candidiasis.
• Consider semisupine chair position for patients with respiratory disease.
• Midday appointments and a stress reduction protocol may be required for anxious patients.
• Be aware that aspirin or sulfite preservatives in vasoconstrictor-containing products can exacerbate asthma.
• Acute asthmatic episodes may be precipitated in the dental office. Sympathomimetic inhalants should be available for emergency use.
Consultations:
• Medical consult may be required to assess disease control in the patient.
• Medical consult may be required to assess patient's ability to tolerate stress.

Teach patient/family:

• For inhalation dosage forms: rinse mouth with water after each dose to prevent dryness

When chronic dry mouth occurs, advise patient:

• To avoid mouth rinses with high alcohol content due to drying effects

• Of need for daily home fluoride to prevent caries

• To use sugarless gum, frequent sips of water, or saliva substitutes

brimonidine tartrate

(bri-moe'ni-deen)

Alphagan

Drug class.: α-adrenergic agonist

Action: Selective α_2-adrenergic agonist that reduces aqueous humor production and increases uveoscleral outflow

Uses: Lowering of intraocular pressure in open-angle glaucoma or ocular hypertension; prevention of postoperative intraocular pressure elevation after argon laser trabeculoplasty

Dosage and routes:

• *Adult:* OPTH 1 drop in affected eye(s) tid; at 8 hr intervals

Available forms include: Sol 0.2%; 5, 10 ml

Side effects/adverse reactions:

▼ *ORAL: Dry mouth,* abnormal taste

CNS: Headache, drowsiness, fatigue, insomnia, depression

CV: Hypertension, palpitation, syncope

EENT: Ocular hyperemia, burning, stinging, ocular allergy, blurring, foreign body reaction, photophobia

MS: Muscular pain

Contraindications: Hypersensitivity, MAO inhibitor

Precautions: Severe cardiovascular disease, hepatic or renal impairment, depression, cerebral or coronary insufficiency, Raynaud's phenomenon, orthostatic hypotension, thromboangiitis obliterans, pregnancy category B, lactation, children

Pharmacokinetics:

TOP: Peak plasma levels 1-4 hr; half-life 3 hr; hepatic metabolism, urinary excretion

Drug interactions of concern to dentistry:

Drug interactions have not been studied; however, the following possibilities exist:

• Increased CNS depression: opioids, sedatives, alcohol, and general anesthetics

• Possible risk of interference with lowering intraocular pressure: anticholinergic drugs or drugs with anticholinergic actions; tricyclic antidepressants

DENTAL CONSIDERATIONS

General:

• Assess salivary flow as factor in caries, periodontal disease, and candidiasis.

• Avoid dental light in patient's eyes; offer dark glasses for patient comfort.

• Question patient about compliance with prescribed drug regimen for glaucoma.

• Avoid drugs with anticholinergic activity, such as antihistamines, opioids, benzodiazepines, propantheline, atropine, and scopolamine.

• Monitor vital signs every appointment due to cardiovascular side effects.

Consultations:

• Consultation with physician may

be needed if sedation or general anesthesia is required.

Teach patient/family:

• Importance of updating health and drug history if physician makes any changes in evaluation/ drug regimens

When chronic dry mouth occurs, advise patient:

• To avoid mouth rinses with high alcohol content due to drying effects

• To use daily home fluoride products for anticaries effect

• To use sugarless gum, frequent sips of water, or saliva substitutes

brinzolamide (optic)

(brin-zoh'la-mide)

Azopt

Drug class.: Carbonic anhydrase inhibitor

Action: Reduces intraocular pressure through inhibition of carbonic anhydrase enzyme

Uses: Ocular hypertension, open-angle glaucoma

Dosage and routes:

• *Adult:* OPTH 1 gtt in affected eye tid

Available forms include: Ophthalmic suspension 1% in 2.5, 5, 10, 15 ml

Side effects/adverse reactions:

▼ *ORAL: Bitter taste,* dry mouth (>1%)

CNS: Headache, dizziness

GI: Diarrhea

EENT: Blurred vision, blepharides, dry eye, ocular pain, foreign body sensation

MISC: Allergy

Contraindications: Hypersensitivity

Precautions: Pregnancy category C, lactation, no pediatric data for use

Pharmacokinetics:

TOP: Some systemic absorption, active metabolite, plasma protein binding 60%, urinary excretion

Drug interactions of concern to dentistry:

• Avoid drugs that can exacerbate glaucoma (e.g., anticholinergics)

DENTAL CONSIDERATIONS

General:

• Avoid dental light in patient's eyes; offer dark glasses for patient comfort.

• Question patient about compliance with prescribed drug regimen for glaucoma.

Consultations:

• Medical consult may be required to assess disease control in the patient.

bromocriptine mesylate

(broe-moe-krip'teen)

Parlodel, Parlodel SnapTabs

♣ Alti-Bromocriptine, Apo-Bromocriptine

Drug class.: Dopamine receptor agonist; ovulation stimulant

Action: Inhibits prolactin release by activating postsynaptic dopamine receptors; activation of striatal dopamine receptors could be reason for improvement in Parkinson's disease

Uses: Female infertility, Parkinson's disease, prevention of postpartum lactation, amenorrhea caused by hyperprolactinemia, acromegaly

Dosage and routes:

Hyperprolactinemic indications

• *Adult:* PO 1.25-2.5 mg with

meals; may increase by 2.5 mg q3-7d; usual range 5-7.5 mg

Acromegaly

• *Adult:* PO 1.25-2.5 mg × 3 days hs, may increase by 1.25-2.5 mg q3-7d, usual range 20-30 mg/day

Postpartum lactation

• *Adult:* PO 2.5 mg qd-tid with meal × 14 or 21 days

Parkinson's disease

• *Adult:* PO 1.25 mg bid with meals, may increase q2-4wk by 2.5 mg/day, not to exceed 100 mg qd

Available forms include: Caps 5 mg; tabs 2.5 mg

Side effects/adverse reactions:

▼ *ORAL:* Dry mouth

CNS: Headache, ***convulsions,*** depression, restlessness, anxiety, nervousness, confusion, hallucinations, dizziness, fatigue, drowsiness, abnormal involuntary movements, psychosis

CV: ***Shock,*** orthostatic hypotension, decreased BP, palpitation, extra systole, dysrhythmias, bradycardia

GI: Nausea, vomiting, anorexia, cramps, constipation, diarrhea, hemorrhage

GU: Frequency, retention, incontinence, diuresis

EENT: Blurred vision, diplopia, burning eyes, nasal congestion

INTEG: Rash on face/arms, alopecia

Contraindications: Hypersensitivity to ergot, severe ischemic disease, pregnancy category D, severe peripheral vascular disease

Precautions: Lactation, hepatic disease, renal disease, children

Pharmacokinetics:

PO: Peak 1-3 hr, duration 4-8 hr, half-life 3 hr; 90%-96% protein bound; metabolized by liver (inactive metabolites); excreted in urine, feces

Drug interactions of concern to dentistry:

• Decreased action: phenothiazines, loxapine, haloperidol, droperidol, amitriptyline

DENTAL CONSIDERATIONS

General:

• Monitor vital signs every appointment due to cardiovascular side effects.

• After supine positioning, have patient sit upright for at least 2 min to avoid orthostatic hypotension.

• Assess salivary flow as a factor in caries, periodontal disease, and candidiasis.

• Short appointments may be required due to disease effects on musculature.

Consultations:

• Medical consult may be required to assess disease control in the patient.

Teach patient/family:

• To avoid mouth rinses with high alcohol content due to drying effects

---

brompheniramine maleate

(brome-fen-ir'a-meen)

Bromphen, Codimal-A, Conjec-B, Cophene-B, Dehist, Diamine TD, Dimetane, Dimetane Extentabs, Dimetapp Allergy, Histaject Modified, Oraminic II, Veltane

♣ Chlorphed, Nasahist-B, ND-Stat Revised

Drug class.: Antihistamine, H_1-receptor antagonist

Action: Acts on blood vessels, GI system, respiratory system by com-

peting with histamine for H_1-receptor sites; decreases allergic response by blocking histamine
Uses: Allergy symptoms, rhinitis
Dosage and routes:
• *Adult:* PO 4-8 mg tid-qid, not to exceed 36 mg/day; TIME REL 8-12 mg bid-tid, not to exceed 24 mg/day; IM/IV/SC 5-20 mg q6-12h, not to exceed 40 mg/day
• *Child >6 yr:* PO 2 mg tid-qid, not to exceed 12 mg/day; IM/IV/SC 0.5 mg/kg/day divided tid or qid
• *Child <6 yr:* Only as directed by physician
Available forms include: Tabs 4 mg; time rel tabs 8, 12 mg; elix 2 mg/5 ml; inj IM/SC/IV 10, 100 mg/ml
Side effects/adverse reactions:
▼ *ORAL:* Dry mouth
CNS: Dizziness, drowsiness, poor coordination, fatigue, anxiety, euphoria, confusion, paresthesia, neuritis
CV: Hypotension, palpitation, tachycardia
GI: Nausea, vomiting, anorexia, constipation, diarrhea
RESP: Increased thick secretions, wheezing, chest tightness
HEMA: ***Thrombocytopenia, agranulocytosis, hemolytic anemia***
GU: Retention, dysuria, frequency, impotence
EENT: Blurred vision, dilated pupils, tinnitus, nasal stuffiness, dry nose/throat
INTEG: Photosensitivity
Contraindications: Hypersensitivity to H_1-receptor antagonists, acute asthma attack, lower respiratory tract disease, child <6 yr
Precautions: Increased intraocular pressure, renal disease, cardiac disease, hypertension, bronchial asthma, seizure disorder, stenosed peptic ulcers, hyperthyroidism, prostatic hypertrophy, bladder neck obstruction, pregnancy category C
Pharmacokinetics:
PO: Peak 2-5 hr, duration to 48 hr, half-life 12-34 hr; metabolized in liver; excreted by kidneys
Drug interactions of concern to dentistry:
• Increased CNS depression: alcohol, all CNS depressants
• Additive photosensitization: tetracyclines
• Increased drying effect: anticholinergics
• Hypotension: general anesthetics
DENTAL CONSIDERATIONS
General:
• Assess salivary flow as a factor in caries, periodontal disease, and candidiasis.
• Consider semisupine chair position for patients with respiratory disease.
• Determine why the patient is taking the drug.
Teach patient/family:
• Importance of good oral hygiene to prevent soft tissue inflammation
• To avoid mouth rinses with high alcohol content due to drying effects

---

budesonide

(byoo-des'oh-nide)
Rhinocort Nasal Inhaler, Pulmacort Turbuhaler
Drug class.: Corticosteroid, synthetic

Action: Glucocorticoids have multiple actions that include antiinflammatory and immunosuppressant effects. They inhibit phospholipase A_2, interfering with or reducing the synthesis of prostaglandins and leukotrienes. They also bind to cytoplasmic glucocorticoid receptors (GRs) and enter the cell nucleus to bind with DNA. This results in the synthesis of various enzymes such as collagenase, elastase, and cytokines that play important roles in inflammation and immunosuppression. They also suppress the production of lymphocytes, monocytes, and eosinophils.

Uses: Management of symptoms of perennial allergic rhinitis in adults and children >6 years of age, perennial nonallergic rhinitis in adults

Dosage and routes:

For intranasal use only

• *Adult and child >6 yr:* INH 1 spray in each nostril AM and PM, up to 4 sprays in each nostril in AM, then reduce to smallest amount required for symptom control

Available forms include: Metered inhaler: 7 g canister (contains 200 doses); each actuation provides 32 µg

Side effects/adverse reactions:

▼ *ORAL: Dry mouth, alteration of taste*

CNS: Nervousness

GI: Nausea

RESP: Wheezing, dyspnea

EENT: Irritation of nasal membranes, sneezing, coughing, epistaxis, candidosis, altered smell, nasal septum injury

INTEG: Rash, pruritus, facial edema

MS: Myalgia, arthralgia

Contraindications: Hypersensitivity; bacterial, viral, or fungal infections of mouth, throat, or lungs

Precautions: Pregnancy category C, lactation, child age <6 yr with nonallergic rhinitis; larger doses may cause symptoms of hypercorticism and suppress HPA function

Pharmacokinetics: INH approximately 20% of inhaled dose is absorbed; highly protein bound; liver metabolism; urinary excretion

Drug interactions of concern to dentistry:

• None reported

DENTAL CONSIDERATIONS

General:

• Evaluate respiration characteristics and rate.

• Assess salivary flow as a factor in caries, periodontal disease, and candidiasis.

• Midday appointments suggested with stress reduction protocol for anxious patients.

• Place on frequent recall due to oral side effects.

• Acute asthmatic episodes may be precipitated in the dental office. Rapid-acting sympathomimetic inhalants should be available for emergency use. Budesonide is not a rapid-acting drug and is not intended for use in acute asthmatic attacks.

Consultations:

• Medical consult may be required to assess disease control in the patient.

Teach patient/family:

• Importance of good oral hygiene to prevent soft tissue inflammation

• That gargling and rinsing with water after each dose helps prevent fungal infection

When chronic dry mouth occurs, advise patient:

• To avoid mouth rinses with high alcohol content due to drying effects

• To use daily home fluoride products for anticaries effect

• To use sugarless gum, frequent sips of water, or artificial saliva substitutes

bumetanide

(byoo-met′a-nide)
Bumex

Drug class.: Loop diuretic

Action: Acts on loop of Henle to decrease the reabsorption of chloride and sodium with resultant diuresis

Uses: Edema in CHF, liver disease, renal disease (nephrotic syndrome), pulmonary edema, ascites (nephrotic syndrome), hypertension

Dosage and routes:

• *Adult:* PO 0.5-2.0 mg qd, may give second or third dose at 4-5 hr intervals, not to exceed 10 mg/day, may be given on alternate days or intermittently; IV/IM 0.5-1.0 mg/day, may give second or third dose at 2-3 hr intervals, not to exceed 10 mg/day

Available forms include: Tabs 0.5, 1, 2 mg; inj IV/IM 0.25 mg/ml

Side effects/adverse reactions:

▼ *ORAL:* Dry mouth, increased thirst

CNS: Headache, fatigue, weakness, vertigo

CV: ***Circulatory collapse,*** chest pain, hypotension, ECG changes

GI: Nausea, ***acute pancreatitis, jaundice,*** diarrhea, vomiting, anorexia, cramps, upset stomach, abdominal pain

HEMA: ***Thrombocytopenia, agranulocytosis, neutropenia***

GU: Polyuria, ***renal failure,*** glycosuria

EENT: Loss of hearing, ear pain, tinnitus, blurred vision

INTEG: Rash, pruritus, ***Stevens-Johnson syndrome,*** purpura, sweating, photosensitivity

ENDO: Hyperglycemia

ELECT: Hypokalemia, hypochloremic alkalosis, hypomagnesemia, hyperuricemia, hypocalcemia, hyponatremia

MS: Cramps, arthritis, stiffness

Contraindications: Hypersensitivity to sulfonamides, anuria, hepatic coma, hypovolemia, lactation, cisapride

Precautions: Dehydration, ascites, severe renal disease, pregnancy category C

Pharmacokinetics:

PO: Onset 0.5-1 hr, duration 4 hr
IM: Onset 40 min, duration 4 hr
IV: Onset 5 min, duration 2-3 hr; excreted by kidneys; crosses placenta; excreted by breast milk

Drug interactions of concern to dentistry:

• Decreased diuretic effect: NSAIDs, indomethacin

• Masked ototoxicity: phenothiazines

• Increased electrolyte imbalance: nondepolarizing skeletal muscle relaxants, corticosteroids

DENTAL CONSIDERATIONS

General:

• Monitor vital signs every appointment due to cardiovascular side effects.

• Patients on chronic drug therapy may rarely have symptoms of blood dyscrasias, which can include infection, bleeding, and poor healing.

• After supine positioning, have patient sit upright for at least 2 min to avoid orthostatic hypotension.

• Assess salivary flow as a factor in caries, periodontal disease, and candidiasis.

• Limit use of sodium-containing products such as saline IV fluids for patients with a dietary salt restriction.
• Patients on high-potency diuretics should be monitored for serum K^+ levels.

Consultations:
• In a patient with symptoms of blood dyscrasias, request a medical consult for blood studies and postpone dental treatment until normal values are reestablished.
• Medical consult may be required to assess disease control in the patient.

Teach patient/family:
• Importance of good oral hygiene to prevent soft tissue inflammation
• Caution to prevent injury when using oral hygiene aids

When chronic dry mouth occurs, advise patient:
• To avoid mouth rinses with high alcohol content due to drying effects
• To use daily home fluoride products for anticaries effect
• To use sugarless gum, frequent sips of water, or saliva substitutes

---

bupivacaine HCl (local)

(byoo-piv′a-kane)

Marcaine, Sensorcaine, Sensorcaine-MPF

With vasoconstrictor: Marcaine Hydrochloride with Epinephrine, Sensorcaine with Epinephrine, Sensorcaine-MPF with Epinephrine

Drug class.: Amide local anesthetic

Action: Inhibits ion fluxes across membranes, particularly sodium transport across cell membrane; decreases rise of depolarization phase of action potential; blocks nerve action potential

Uses: Local dental anesthesia, epidural anesthesia, peripheral nerve block, caudal anesthesia

Dosage and routes:

Dental injection: infiltration or conduction block
• *Bupivacaine 0.5% with epinephrine 1:200,000:* Max dose 1.3 mg/kg or 0.6 mg/lb; limit 90 mg* per dental appointment for healthy patients; doses must be adjusted downward for medically compromised, debilitated, or elderly and for each individual patient. **Always use the lowest effective dose, a slow injection rate, and careful aspiration technique.**

Example calculations illustrating amount of drug administered per dental cartridge

# of cartridges (1.8 ml)	mg of bupivacaine (0.5%)	mg(μ) of vasoconstrictor (1:200,000)
1	9	0.009 (9)
2	18	0.018 (18)
4	36	0.036 (36)
6	54	0.054 (54)
10	90	0.090 (90 g)

*Maximum dose is cited from the *USP-DI,* ed 16, 1996, US Pharmacopeial Convention, Inc. Doses may differ in other published reference resources.

• Package insert does not recommend bupivacaine for children <12 yr.

Available forms include: Inj 0.25%, 0.5%, 0.75%; inj with epinephrine 1:200,000 in 0.25%, 0.5%, 0.75%

Side effects/adverse reactions:
▼ *ORAL:* Numbness, tingling, trismus
CNS: ***Convulsions, loss of consciousness,*** drowsiness, disorientation, tremors, shivering, anxiety, restlessness
CV: ***Myocardial depression, cardiac arrest, dysrhythmias,*** bradycardia, hypotension, hypertension, fetal bradycardia
GI: Nausea, vomiting
RESP: ***Status asthmaticus, respiratory arrest, anaphylaxis***
EENT: Blurred vision, tinnitus, pupil constriction
INTEG: Rash, urticaria, allergic reactions, edema, burning, skin discoloration at injection site, tissue necrosis

Contraindications: Hypersensitivity, cross sensitivity between amides (rare), severe liver disease, 0.75% sol in dentistry

Precautions: Elderly, severe drug allergies, pregnancy category C, use in children (risk of local injury due to long duration of anesthesia)

Pharmacokinetics: INJ onset 4-17 min, duration 4-12 hr; excreted in urine (metabolites); metabolized by liver

Drug interactions of concern to dentistry:

- CNS depressants: may see increased risk of CNS depression with all CNS depressants, especially in children and when larger doses are used
- Avoid placing dental cartridges in disinfectant solutions with heavy metals or surface-active agents; may see release of metal ions into local anesthetic solutions, with tissue irritation following injection
- Avoid excessive exposure of dental cartridges to light or heat; it hastens deterioration of vasoconstrictor; color change in local anesthetic solution indicates breakdown of vasoconstrictor
- Risk of cardiovascular side effects: rapid intravascular administration of local anesthetic containing vasoconstrictor, either alone or in patients taking tricyclic antidepressants, MAO inhibitors, digitalis drugs, cocaine, phenothiazines, β-blockers and in the presence of halogenated hydrocarbon general anesthetics; always use the smallest effective vasoconstrictor dose and careful aspiration technique
- Avoid use of vasoconstrictors in patients with uncontrolled hyperthyroidism, diabetes, angina, or hypertension; refer these patients for medical treatment before elective dental procedures

DENTAL CONSIDERATIONS

General:

- Monitor vital signs every appointment due to cardiovascular and respiratory side effects.
- Lubricate dry lips before injection or dental treatment as required.

Teach patient/family:

- To use care to prevent injury while numbness exists; do not chew gum or eat following dental anesthesia
- That numbness with this drug is expected to last for a considerable period
- To report any signs of infection, muscle pain, or fever to dentist when oral sensations return

• To report any unusual soft tissue reactions

bupropion hydrochloride

(byoo-proe′pee-on)
Wellbutrin, Wellbutrin SR, Zyban
Drug class.: Antidepressant

Action: Weak uptake inhibitor of dopamine, serotonin, norepinephrine; antidepressant and smoking cessation mechanism unknown
Uses: Depression; smoking cessation treatment (Zyban)
Dosage and routes:
Depression
• *Adult:* PO 100 mg bid initially, then increase after third day to 100 mg tid if needed; may increase after 1 mo to 150 mg tid. Usual dose 300 mg/day in three equally divided doses; limit use of higher doses to 450 mg/day
Smoking cessation
• *Adult:* PO initial dose 150 mg/day × 3 days, can increase to 150 mg bid if required; max daily dose 300 mg; initiate dose while patient is still smoking to allow for steady-state blood levels; set stop smoking date within 2 wk of administration; continue doses for 7-12 wk; may be used in combination with nicotine transdermal system
Available forms include: Tabs 75, 100 mg; sus rel tabs 50, 100, 150 mg; Zyban sus rel tabs 100 and 150 mg
Side effects/adverse reactions:
▼ *ORAL: Dry mouth*
CNS: Headache, agitation, confusion, ***seizures,*** akathisia, delusions, insomnia, sedation, tremors
CV: Dysrhythmias, hypertension, palpitation, tachycardia, hypotension
GI: Nausea, vomiting, increased appetite, constipation
GU: Impotence, frequency, retention
EENT: Blurred vision, auditory disturbance
INTEG: Rash, pruritus, sweating
Contraindications: Hypersensitivity, seizure disorder, eating disorders (bulimia, anorexia), ritonavir, MAO inhibitors
Precautions: Renal and hepatic disease, recent MI, cranial trauma, pregnancy category B, lactation, children, low abuse potential
Pharmacokinetics:
PO: Onset 2-4 wk, half-life 12-14 hr, metabolized by liver
Drug interactions of concern to dentistry:
• Increased adverse reactions (seizures): tricyclic antidepressants, phenothiazines, benzodiazepines, alcohol, haloperidol, and trazodone

DENTAL CONSIDERATIONS
General:
• Assess salivary flow as a factor in caries, periodontal disease, and candidiasis.
• Short appointments and a stress reduction protocol may be required for anxious patients.
• See nicotine transdermal systems for additional smoking cessation considerations.
Consultations:
• Medical consult may be required to assess disease control and patient's ability to tolerate stress.
• Physician should be informed if significant xerostomic side effects occur (e.g., increased caries, sore tongue, problems eating or swal-

lowing, difficulty wearing prosthesis) so a medication change can be considered.

Teach patient/family:

When chronic dry mouth occurs, advise patient:

- To avoid mouth rinses with high alcohol content due to drying effects
- To use daily home fluoride products for anticaries effect
- To use sugarless gum, frequent sips of water, or saliva substitutes

buspirone HCl

(byoo-spye'rone)

BuSpar

Drug class.: Antianxiety agent

Action: Unknown; may act by inhibiting 5-HT receptors or dopamine receptors

Uses: Management and short-term relief of anxiety disorders

Dosage and routes:

- *Adult:* PO 5 mg tid, may increase by 5 mg/day q2-3d, not to exceed 60 mg/day

Available forms include: Tabs 5, 10 mg

Side effects/adverse reactions:

▼ *ORAL:* Dry mouth

CNS: Dizziness, headache, depression, stimulation, insomnia, nervousness, light-headedness, numbness, paresthesia, incoordination, tremors, excitement, involuntary movements, confusion, akathisia

CV: Tachycardia, palpitation, CVA, CHF, MI, hypotension, hypertension

GI: Nausea, diarrhea, constipation, flatulence, increased appetite, rectal bleeding

RESP: Hyperventilation, chest congestion, shortness of breath

GU: Frequency, hesitancy, menstrual irregularity, change in libido

EENT: Sore throat, tinnitus, blurred vision, nasal congestion, red/itching eyes, change in smell

INTEG: Rash, edema, pruritus, alopecia, dry skin

MS: Pain, weakness, muscle cramps, spasms

MISC: Sweating, fatigue, weight gain, fever

Contraindications: Hypersensitivity, child <18 yr

Precautions: Pregnancy category B, lactation, elderly, impaired hepatic/renal function

Pharmacokinetics:

PO: Peak plasma levels 30-60 min, highly protein bound; metabolized in liver; mainly renal excretion of metabolites, some fecal excretion; full antianxiety effects may not be seen until after 2 wk

Drug interactions of concern to dentistry:

- Increased sedation: alcohol, all CNS depressants

DENTAL CONSIDERATIONS

General:

- Monitor vital signs every appointment due to cardiovascular side effects.
- Assess salivary flow as a factor in caries, periodontal disease, and candidiasis.
- Short appointments and a stress reduction protocol may be required for anxious patients.
- Determine why the patient is taking the drug.

Consultations:

- Medical consult may be required to assess disease control in the patient.

Teach patient/family:

When chronic dry mouth occurs, advise patient:

- To avoid mouth rinses with high alcohol content due to drying effects
- To use daily home fluoride products for anticaries effect
- To use sugarless gum, frequent sips of water, or saliva substitutes

busulfan

(byoo-sul'fan)

Myleran

Drug class.: Antineoplastic

Action: Changes essential cellular ions to covalent bonding with resultant alkylation, which interferes with biologic function of DNA; activity is not phase specific; effect is due to myelosuppression

Uses: Chronic myelocytic leukemia, orphan drug in preparative therapy for malignancies treated with bone marrow transplant

Dosage and routes:

- *Adult:* PO 4-12 mg/day initially until WBC levels fall to 10,000/mm^3, then drug is stopped until WBC levels rise over 50,000/mm^3, then 1-3 mg/day
- *Child:* PO 0.06-0.12 mg/kg or 1.8-4.6 mg/m^2 day; dose is titrated to maintain WBC levels at 20,000/mm^3

Available forms include: Tabs 2 mg

Side effects/adverse reactions:

▼ *ORAL:* Dry mouth, cheilosis, stomatitis

CV: ***Endocardial fibrosis***

GI: Diarrhea, weight loss, nausea, vomiting, anorexia

RESP: ***Irreversible pulmonary fibrosis,*** pneumonitis

HEMA: ***Thrombocytopenia, leukopenia, pancytopenia, severe bone marrow depression,*** anemia

GU: ***Renal toxicity,*** impotence, sterility, amenorrhea, gynecomastia, hyperuremia, adrenal insufficiency–like syndrome

EENT: Cataracts

INTEG: Hyperpigmentation, dermatitis, alopecia

MISC: ***Chromosomal aberrations,*** weakness, fatigue

Contraindications: Radiation, chemotherapy, lactation, pregnancy category D, blastic phase of chronic myelocytic leukemia, hypersensitivity

Precautions: Childbearing-age men and women, leukopenia, thrombocytopenia, anemia, hepatotoxicity, renal toxicity

Pharmacokinetics:

PO: Well absorbed orally; hepatic metabolism, excreted in urine; crosses placenta; excreted in breast milk; long retention of metabolites in body

Drug interactions of concern to dentistry:

- May be an increased risk of bleeding with aspirin

DENTAL CONSIDERATIONS

General:

- Patients taking opioids for acute or chronic pain should be given alternative analgesics for dental pain.
- Consider semisupine chair position for patient comfort if GI side effects occur.
- Chlorhexidine mouth rinse before and during chemotherapy may reduce severity of mucositis.
- Patients on chronic drug therapy may rarely have symptoms of

blood dyscrasias, which can include infection, bleeding, and poor healing.

- Palliative medication may be required for management of oral side effects.
- Apply lubricant to dry lips for patient comfort before dental procedures.
- Assess salivary flow as factor in caries, periodontal disease, and candidiasis.
- Patients in active chemotherapy treatment should have adequate WBC count before completing dental procedures that may produce a wound. Consultation with the oncologist may be required to determine WBC values before treatment.

Consultations:

- Medical consult may be required to assess disease control and patient's ability to tolerate stress.
- In a patient with symptoms of blood dyscrasias, request a medical consult for blood studies and postpone dental treatment until normal values are reestablished.
- Consult oncologist; prophylactic antibiotics may be indicated to prevent infection if surgery or deep scaling is planned.

Teach patient/family:

- Importance of good oral hygiene to prevent soft tissue inflammation
- To prevent trauma when using oral hygiene aids
- To report oral lesions, soreness, or bleeding to dentist
- That secondary oral infection may occur; must see dentist immediately if infection occurs
- Importance of updating medical/drug record if physician makes any changes in evaluation or drug regimen

When chronic dry mouth occurs, advise patient:

- To avoid mouth rinses with high alcohol content due to drying effects
- To use daily home fluoride products for anticaries effect
- To use sugarless gum, frequent sips of water, or artificial saliva substitutes

butenafine

(byoo'ten-a-feen)

Mentax

Drug class.: Antifungal

Action: Inhibits epoxidation of squalene, thereby interfering with the synthesis of fungal cell membranes

Uses: Tinea pedis caused by *E. floccosum, T. mentagrophytes,* or *T. rubrum*

Dosage and routes:

- *Adult:* TOP apply to affected area and adjacent skin once daily for 4 weeks

Available forms include: Cream 1% in 2, 15, and 30 g sizes

Side effects/adverse reactions:

INTEG: Dermatitis, burning, stinging, erythema, itching

Contraindications: Hypersensitivity

Precautions: External use only, pregnancy category B, lactation, children <12 yr, not for oral use

Pharmacokinetics:

TOP: Some systemic absorption, hepatic metabolism

DENTAL CONSIDERATIONS

General:

- There are no dental drug interactions or relevant considerations to dentistry for this drug.

butoconazole nitrate

(byoo-toe-koe′na-zole)

Femstat, FemStat One, Femstat 3

Drug class.: Antifungal

Action: Binds sterols in fungal cell membrane, which increases permeability

Uses: Vulvovaginal infections caused by *Candida*

Dosage and routes:

• *Adult:* INTRA VAG 1 applicator × 6 days (second/third trimester pregnancy)

• *Three day treatment:* INTRAVAG insert 1 applicator for 3 days

Available forms include: Vaginal cream 2%

Side effects/adverse reactions:

GU: Rash, stinging, burning, vulvovaginal itching, soreness, swelling, discharge

Contraindications: Hypersensitivity

Precautions: Pregnancy category C, lactation

DENTAL CONSIDERATIONS

General:

• Examine oral mucous membranes for signs of yeast infection.

• Broad-spectrum antibiotics for dental infections may cause vaginal yeast infection.

calcipotriene

(kal-si-poe′try-een)

Dovonex

Drug class.: Vitamin D_3 derivative (synthetic)

Action: Regulation of skin cell production and development

Uses: Chronic, moderately severe scalp psoriasis

Dosage and routes:

• *Adult:* TOP: Apply small amount to skin bid, rub in gently

Available forms include: Ointment, cream 0.005%; 30, 60, 100 g

Side effects/adverse reactions:

INTEG: Local irritation, itching, burning, dry skin, dermatitis

Contraindications: Hypersensitivity

Precautions: Pregnancy category C, external use only, elderly >65 yr, lactation, children, hypercalcemia

Drug interactions of concern to dentistry:

• None reported

DENTAL CONSIDERATIONS

General:

• Be aware that psoriasis may have oral manifestations.

calcitonin (human)/ calcitonin (salmon)

(kal-si-toe′nin)

Calcitonin (human): Cibacalcin

Calcitonin (salmon): Calcimar, Miacalcin Nasal Spray

Drug class.: Synthetic polypeptide calcitonins

Action: Inhibits bone resorption; reduces osteoclast function; reduces serum calcium levels in hypercalcemia

Uses: Paget's disease, postmenopausal osteoporosis, hypercalcemia, unlabeled use in intractable bone pain

Dosage and routes:

Paget's disease

• *Adult:* SC/IM 50-100 IU (salmon) daily; monitor disease symptoms, serum alk phosphatase, and urinary hydroxyproline; maintenance dose of 50 IU qd-qod may be sufficient; or SC/IM 0.5 mg (human) daily, reducing to 0.5 mg 2-3× wk

Postmenopausal osteoporosis

• *Adult:* SC/IM 100 IU (salmon) daily with supplemental calcium and vitamin D; NASAL spray 200 IU daily

Hypercalcemia

• *Adult:* SC/IM 4 IU (salmon) q12h for 1-2 days, increasing if required to 8 IU (salmon) q12h; maximum dose 8 IU (salmon) q6-12h

Available forms include: Calcitonin (salmon) 100, 200 IU/ml; calcitonin (human) 0.5 mg/vial; nasal spray 2 ml

Side effects/adverse reactions:

▼ *ORAL:* Dry mouth, metallic taste (all infrequent)

CNS: Headache, dizziness, insomnia, anorexia, anxiety, depression

CV: Hypertension, angina pectoris, tachycardia, palpitation

GI: Nausea, vomiting, diarrhea, abdominal pain

RESP: URI, coughing, dyspnea, bronchospasm

HEMA: Lymphadenopathy, anemia

GU: Frequency of urination, cystitis, hematuria, renal calculus

EENT (NASAL SPRAY): Epistaxis, rhinitis, nasal irritation, dryness, sores, crusting, tinnitus

INTEG: Erythematous skin rashes, flushing face and hands, inflammation at injection site, pruritus

ENDO: Goiter, hyperthyroidism

MS: Myalgia, arthrosis

MISC: Fatigue, flulike symptoms, severe allergic reactions

Contraindications: Hypersensitivity (skin test before use)

Precautions: Allergy, hypocalcemic tetany, routine monitoring of urine sediment, osteogenic sarcoma in Paget's disease, pregnancy category C, lactation, children

Pharmacokinetics:

NASAL: Low bioavailability

IM/SC: Therapeutic response; see decrease in serum calcium in 2 hr, duration 6-8 hr; pain relief in bone may take 8-10 days; Paget's disease response may take several months; rapidly metabolized in kidney and other tissues; renal excretion

Drug interactions of concern to dentistry:

• Supplemental calcium and vitamin D may already be used; not to use additional amounts

DENTAL CONSIDERATIONS:

General:

• Consider semisupine chair position for patient comfort due to effects of disease.

• Consider semisupine chair position for patient comfort if GI side effects occur.

• Assess salivary flow as factor in caries, periodontal disease, and candidiasis.

Teach patient/family:

• Importance of good oral hygiene to prevent soft tissue inflammation

When chronic dry mouth occurs, advise patient:

• To avoid mouth rinses with high alcohol content due to drying effects

• To use daily home fluoride products for anticaries effect

• To use sugarless gum, frequent sips of water, or saliva substitutes

camphorated opium tincture

(oh'pee-um)

Paregoric

Drug class.: Antidiarrheal

Controlled Substance Schedule III, Canada N

Action: Antiperistaltic and analgesic with activity related to morphine content

Uses: Diarrhea

Dosage and routes:

• *Adult:* PO 5-10 ml qd-qid

• *Child:* PO 0.25-0.5 ml/kg qd-qid

Available forms include: Liq 2 mg morphine equivalent per 5 ml

Side effects/adverse reactions:

▼ *ORAL:* Dry mouth

CNS: ***CNS depression,*** dizziness, drowsiness, fainting, flushing, physical dependency

GI: Nausea, vomiting, constipation, abdominal pain

Contraindications: Hypersensitivity, severe ulcerative colitis, pseudomembranous colitis

Precautions: Liver disease, addiction-prone individuals, prostatic hypertrophy (severe), pregnancy category B

Pharmacokinetics:

PO: Duration 4 hr, half-life 2-3 hr; metabolized in liver; excreted in urine

Drug interactions of concern to dentistry:

• Increased action of both drugs: alcohol, all other CNS depressants

• Decreased peristalsis: anticholinergic drugs

DENTAL CONSIDERATIONS

General:

• Psychologic and physical dependence may occur with chronic administration.

• Determine why the patient is taking the drug.

Teach patient/family:

• To avoid mouth rinses with high alcohol content due to drying effects

candesartan cilexetil

(kan-de-sar'tan)

Atacand

Drug class.: Angiotensin II (AT_1) receptor antagonist

Action: Blocks the vasoconstrictor and aldosterone-releasing effects of angiotensin II

Uses: Hypertension, as a single drug or in combination with other antihypertensives

Dosage and routes:

• *Adult:* Usual starting dose 16 mg once a day when use as monotherapy if not volume depleted; can be given once or twice daily with total daily dose range 8-32 mg

Available forms include: Tabs 4, 8, 16, 32 mg

Side effects/adverse reactions:

CNS: Headache, dizziness, fatigue, anxiety

CV: Peripheral edema, chest pain, tachycardia, palpitation

GI: Dyspepsia

RESP: URI, bronchitis, cough

GU: Hematuria

EENT: Pharyngitis, rhinitis, sinusitis

INTEG: Rash, sweating

MS: Back pain, myalgia

Contraindications: Hypersensitivity

Precautions: Discontinue drug if pregnancy occurs, risk of fetal and neonatal injury, correct volume depletion if present, renal impairment, pregnancy category C (first trimester) and D (second and third trimesters), lactation

Pharmacokinetics:

PO: Pro-drug rapidly converted to candesartan on absorption, bioavailability 15%, peak serum levels 3-4 hr, highly plasma protein bound (99%), minor hepatic metabolism, 67% excreted in feces, 33% in urine

Drug interactions of concern to dentistry:

• Potential for increased hypotensive effects with other hypotensive and sedative drugs

DENTAL CONSIDERATIONS

General:

• Monitor vital signs at every appointment in patients with history of hypertension.

• Evaluate respiration characteristics and rate due to respiratory side effects.

• Consider semisupine chair position for patient comfort if GI side effects occur.

• Limit use of sodium-containing products such as saline IV fluids for those patients with a dietary salt restriction.

• Stress from dental procedures may compromise cardiovascular function; determine patient risk.

• Short appointments and a stress reduction protocol may be required for anxious patients.

• Use precaution if sedation or general anesthesia is required; risk of hypotensive episode.

Consultations:

• Medical consult may be required to assess disease control and patient's ability to tolerate stress.

Teach patient/family:

• Importance of updating health and drug history if physician makes any changes in evaluation/drug regimens

capsaicin

(kap'say-sin)

Capsin, Capzasin-P, No Pain-HP, Pain Doctor, Pain X, R-Gel, Zostrix, Zostrix-HP

Drug class.: Topical analgesic for selected pain syndromes

Action: Exact mechanism unknown; depletes and prevents reaccumulation of substance P in peripheral sensory neurons

Uses: Neuralgia associated with herpes zoster or diabetic neuropathy; pain of osteoarthritis and rheumatoid arthritis; unapproved use for postmastectomy pain, causalgia, and TMD pain

Dosage and routes:

• *Adult and child >2 yr:* TOP apply sparingly to affected area tid or qid; transient burning may occur

Available forms include: Cream 0.025% in 45, 90 g tubes; cream 0.075% in 30, 60 g tubes

Side effects/adverse reactions:

EENT: Coughing if inhaled

INTEG: Local burning sensation, stinging

Contraindications: Hypersensitivity, persons especially sensitive to hot peppers, children <2 yr

Precautions: Pregnancy category not reported, lactation, avoid use on broken skin

Drug interactions of concern to dentistry:

• None reported

DENTAL CONSIDERATIONS

General:

• Determine why the patient is taking the drug.

• Consider location of lesions and alter dental procedures accordingly.

Teach patient/family:

• To wash hands thoroughly after use and avoid contact with mouth or eyes

---

captopril

(kap'toe-pril)

Capoten

Drug class.: Angiotensin-converting enzyme (ACE) inhibitor

Action: Selectively suppresses renin-angiotensin-aldosterone system; inhibits ACE; prevents conversion of angiotensin I to angiotensin II; results in dilation of arterial, venous vessels

Uses: Hypertension, heart failure not responsive to conventional therapy; unapproved use: hypertension of scleroderma

Dosage and routes:

Hypertension

• *Initial dose:* 12.5 mg 2-3× daily; may increase to 50 mg bid-tid at 1-2 wk intervals; usual range 25-150 mg bid-tid; max 450 mg

CHF

• *Adult:* PO 12.5 mg 2-3× daily given with a diuretic, digitalis; may increase to 50 mg bid-tid, after 14 days; may increase to 150 mg tid if needed

Available forms include: Tabs 12.5, 25, 37.5, 50, 100 mg

Side effects/adverse reactions:

▼ *ORAL:* Dry mouth, glossitis, oral ulceration (Stevens-Johnson syndrome), angioedema, bleeding, lichenoid drug reaction

CNS: Fever, chills

CV: Hypotension

RESP: ***Bronchospasm,*** dyspnea, cough

HEMA: ***Neutropenia***

GU: ***Nephrotic syndrome, acute reversible renal failure,*** polyuria, oliguria, frequency, impotence, dysuria, nocturia, proteinuria

INTEG: Angioedema, rash, pemphigus-like reaction

META: Hyperkalemia

Contraindications: Hypersensitivity, pregnancy category D, lactation, heart block, children, K-sparing diuretics

Precautions: Dialysis patients, hypovolemia, leukemia, scleroderma, lupus erythematosus, blood dyscrasias, CHF, diabetes mellitus, renal disease, thyroid disease, COPD, asthma

Pharmacokinetics:

PO: Peak 1-1.5 hr, duration 2-6 hr, half-life 3 hr; metabolized by liver (metabolites); excreted in urine; crosses placenta; excreted in breast milk

Drug interactions of concern to dentistry:

• Increased hypotension: alcohol, phenothiazines

• Decreased hypotensive effects: indomethacin and possibly other NSAIDs, sympathomimetics

DENTAL CONSIDERATIONS

General:

• Monitor vital signs every appointment due to cardiovascular side effects.

• After supine positioning, have patient sit upright at least 2 min before standing to avoid orthostatic hypotension.

• Patients on chronic drug therapy may rarely have symptoms of

blood dyscrasias, which can include infection, bleeding, and poor healing.

• Assess salivary flow as a factor in caries, periodontal disease, and candidiasis.

• Limit use of sodium-containing products such as saline IV fluids for patients with a dietary salt restriction.

• Stress from dental procedures may compromise cardiovascular function; determine patient risk.

• Short appointments and a stress reduction protocol may be required for anxious patients.

Consultations:

• Medical consult may be required to assess patient's ability to tolerate stress.

• In a patient with symptoms of blood dyscrasias, request a medical consult for blood studies and postpone dental treatment until normal values are reestablished.

• Take precautions if dental surgery is anticipated and sedation or general anesthesia is required; there is risk of a hypotensive episode.

Teach patient/family:

• Importance of good oral hygiene to prevent soft tissue inflammation

• Caution to prevent injury when using oral hygiene aids

When chronic dry mouth occurs, advise patient:

• To avoid mouth rinses with high alcohol content due to drying effects

• To use daily home fluoride products for anticaries effect

• To use sugarless gum, frequent sips of water, or saliva substitutes

carbamazepine

(kar-ba-maz'e-peen)

Atretol, Epitol, Tegretol, Tegretol Chewtabs, Tegretol CR, Tegretol XR

♣ Apo-Carbamazepine, Novo-Carbamaz, Nu-Carbamazepine, PMS Carbamazepine

Drug class.: Anticonvulsant

Action: Inhibits nerve impulses by limiting influx of sodium ions across cell membrane in motor cortex

Uses: Tonic-clonic, complex-partial, mixed seizures; trigeminal neuralgia; unapproved use: neurogenic pain, some psychotic disorders

Dosage and routes:

Seizures

• *Adult and child >12 yr:* PO 200 mg bid, may be increased by 200 mg/day in divided doses q6-8h; adjustment is needed to minimum dose to control seizures; up to 1.6 g/day

• *Child <12 yr:* PO 10-20 mg/kg/day in 2-3 divided doses

Trigeminal neuralgia

• *Adult:* PO 100 mg bid, may increase 100 mg q12h until pain subsides, not to exceed 1.2 g/day; maintenance is 200-400 mg bid

Available forms include: Chew tabs 100 mg; tabs 200 mg; ext rel tabs 100, 200, 400 mg

Side effects/adverse reactions:

▼ *ORAL:* Dry mouth, oral ulceration, glossitis, lichenoid reaction

CNS: Drowsiness, ***paralysis,*** dizziness, confusion, fatigue, headache, hallucinations

CV: ***Hypertension, CHF,*** hypotension, aggravation of CAD

GI: Nausea, constipation, diarrhea, ***hepatitis,*** anorexia, vomiting, abdominal pain, increased liver enzymes

RESP: Pulmonary hypersensitivity (fever, dyspnea, pneumonitis)

HEMA: ***Thrombocytopenia, agranulocytosis, leukocytosis, neutropenia, aplastic anemia, eosinophilia,*** increased pro-time

GU: Frequency, retention, albuminuria, glycosuria, impotence

EENT: Tinnitus, blurred vision, diplopia, nystagmus, conjunctivitis

INTEG: Rash, ***Stevens-Johnson syndrome,*** urticaria

Contraindications: Hypersensitivity to carbamazepine or tricyclic antidepressants, bone marrow depression, concomitant use of MAO inhibitors

Precautions: Glaucoma, hepatic disease, renal disease, cardiac disease, psychosis, pregnancy category C, lactation, child <6 yr

Pharmacokinetics:

PO: Onset slow, peak 4-8 hr, half-life 14-16 hr; metabolized by liver; excreted in urine, feces; crosses placenta; excreted in breast milk; trigeminal neuralgia pain relief 8-72 hr

Drug interactions of concern to dentistry:

- Decreased metabolism, risk of toxicity: erythromycin, clarithromycin, propoxyphene, troleandomycin, metronidazole
- Increased serum levels: tricylic antidepressants, terfenadine, fluoxetine, fluvoxamine, nefazodone
- Increased CNS depression: haloperidol, phenothiazines
- Decreased half-life: doxycycline
- Decreased effects of phenobarbital, corticosteroids, benzodiazepines, doxycycline

DENTAL CONSIDERATIONS

General:

- Monitor vital signs every appointment due to cardiovascular side effects.
- Patients on chronic drug therapy may rarely have symptoms of blood dyscrasias, which can include infection, bleeding, and poor healing.
- Assess salivary flow as a factor in caries, periodontal disease, and candidiasis.
- Short appointments and a stress reduction protocol may be required for anxious patients.
- Talk with patient about type of epilepsy, seizure frequency, and quality of seizure control.

Consultations:

- In a patient with symptoms of blood dyscrasias, request a medical consult for blood studies and postpone dental treatment until normal values are reestablished.
- Medical consult may be required to assess disease control and patient's ability to tolerate stress.

Teach patient/family:

- Importance of good oral hygiene to prevent soft tissue inflammation
- Caution to prevent injury when using oral hygiene aids

When chronic dry mouth occurs, advise patient:

- To avoid mouth rinses with high alcohol content due to drying effects
- To use daily home fluoride products for anticaries effect
- To use sugarless gum, frequent sips of water, or saliva substitutes

carisoprodol

(kar-eye-soe-proe'dole)

Soma, Vanadom

Drug class.: Skeletal muscle relaxant, central acting

Action: May act by blocking interneuronal activity in spinal cord, produces nonspecific CNS sedation

Uses: Adjunct for relief of muscle spasm in musculoskeletal conditions

Dosage and routes:

• *Adult and child >12 yr:* PO 350 mg tid and hs

• *Child 5-12 yr:* PO 6.25 mg/kg qid

Available forms include: Tabs 350 mg

Side effects/adverse reactions:

▼ *ORAL:* Glossitis, swelling of lips

CNS: Dizziness, weakness, drowsiness, headache, tremor, depression, insomnia, ataxia, irritability

CV: Postural hypotension, tachycardia

GI: Nausea, vomiting, hiccups, epigastric discomfort

EENT: Diplopia, temporary loss of vision

INTEG: Rash, pruritus, fever, facial flushing

Contraindications: Hypersensitivity, intermittent porphyria

Precautions: Renal disease, hepatic disease, addictive personalities, pregnancy category C, elderly

Pharmacokinetics:

PO: Onset 0.5 hr, duration 4-6 hr, half-life 8 hr; metabolized by liver; excreted in urine; crosses placenta; excreted in breast milk (large amounts)

Drug interactions of concern to dentistry:

• Increased CNS depression: alcohol, all CNS depressants

DENTAL CONSIDERATIONS

General:

• When used in dentistry, may be more effective when used in combination with aspirin or NSAIDs.

Teach patient/family:

• To use electric toothbrush if patient has difficulty holding conventional devices

carteolol

carteolol

(kar-tee'oh-lole)

Cartrol

Drug class.: Nonselective β-adrenergic blocker

Action: This is a nonselective β_1- and β_2-adrenergic antagonist. The antihypertensive mechanism of action is unclear but may include a reduction in cardiac output and inhibition of renin release by the renal juxtaglomerular apparatus. Peripheral resistance decreases with long-term use. The antianginal action (when indicated for this use) may be related to a decrease in myocardial oxygen demand and negative chronotropic and inotropic effects. The antiarrhythmic action (when indicated for this use) has been related to a reduction in spontaneous pacemaker firing and slowing of AV nodal conduction.

Uses: Mild-to-moderate hypertension; unapproved for angina pectoris

Dosage and routes:

• *Adult:* PO 2.5 mg tid initially, may gradually increase to desired response up to 10 mg/day

Available forms include: Tabs 2.5, 5 mg

Side effects/adverse reactions:

▼ *ORAL:* Dry mouth

CNS: Dizziness, mental changes, drowsiness, fatigue, headache, catatonia, depression, anxiety, nightmares, paresthesia, lethargy, insomnia, decreased concentration

CV: ***Bradycardia, CHF, ventricular dysrhythmias, AV block, peripheral vascular insufficiency,*** palpitation, orthostatic hypotension

GI: Nausea, vomiting, diarrhea, flatulence, constipation, anorexia

RESP: ***Bronchospasm,*** dyspnea, wheezing, nasal stuffiness, pharyngitis

HEMA: ***Agranulocytosis, thrombocytopenic purpura*** (rare)

GU: Impotence, dysuria, ejaculatory failure, urinary retention

EENT: Tinnitus, visual changes, sore throat, double vision, dry/burning eyes

INTEG: Rash, alopecia, urticaria, pruritus, fever

MS: Joint pain, arthralgia, muscle cramps, pain

MISC: Facial swelling, decreased exercise tolerance, weight change, Raynaud's disease

Contraindications: Hypersensitivity to β-blockers, cardiogenic shock, second- or third-degree heart block, sinus bradycardia, CHF, bronchial asthma

Precautions: Major surgery, pregnancy category C, lactation, diabetes mellitus, renal disease, thyroid disease, COPD, well-compensated heart failure, CAD, nonallergic bronchospasm

Pharmacokinetics:

PO: Onset 1-2 hr, peak 2-4 hr, duration 8-12 hr, half-life 6-8 hr; metabolized by liver (metabolites inactive); crosses placenta; excreted in breast milk, urine, bile

Drug interactions of concern to dentistry:

• Hypertension, bradycardia: sympathomimetics (epinephrine, ephedrine)

• Slow metabolism of drug: lidocaine

• Increased hypotension, myocardial depression: fentanyl derivatives, hydrocarbon inhalation anesthetics

• Decreased hypotensive effect: indomethacin and other NSAIDs

DENTAL CONSIDERATIONS

General:

• Monitor vital signs every appointment due to cardiovascular side effects.

• Patients on chronic drug therapy may rarely have symptoms of blood dyscrasias, which can include infection, bleeding, and poor healing.

• After supine positioning, have patient sit upright for at least 2 min before standing to avoid orthostatic hypotension.

• Limit use of sodium-containing products such as saline IV fluids for patients with a dietary salt restriction.

• Assess salivary flow as a factor in caries, periodontal disease, and candidiasis.

• Stress from dental procedures may compromise cardiovascular function; determine patient risk.

• Short appointments and a stress reduction protocol may be required for anxious patients.

Consultations:

• In a patient with symptoms of blood dyscrasias, request a medical

consult for blood studies and postpone dental treatment until normal values are reestablished.

• Take precautions if dental surgery is anticipated and anesthesia is required.

• Medical consult may be required to assess disease control and patient's ability to tolerate stress.

Teach patient/family:

• Importance of good oral hygiene to prevent soft tissue inflammation

• Caution to prevent injury when using oral hygiene aids

When chronic dry mouth occurs, advise patient:

• To avoid mouth rinses with high alcohol content due to drying effects

• To use daily home fluoride products for anticaries effect

• To use sugarless gum, frequent sips of water, or saliva substitutes

carteolol HCl

(kar-tee'oe-lole)

Ocupress

Drug class.: β-adrenergic blocker

Action: Nonselective β-adrenergic blocking agent, reduces production of aqueous humor by unknown mechanisms

Uses: Chronic open-angle glaucoma, ocular hypertension

Dosage and routes:

• *Adult:* INSTILL 1 gtt in affected eye bid

Available forms include: Sol 1%

Side effects/adverse reactions:

CNS: Ataxia, dizziness, lethargy

CV: Bradycardia, hypotension, dysrhythmias

GI: Nausea

RESP: ***Bronchospasm***

EENT: Eye irritation, conjunctivitis

Contraindications: Hypersensitivity, asthma, second- and third-degree heart block, right ventricular failure, congenital glaucoma (infants), COPD

Precautions: Pregnancy category C, lactation, elderly, children

Pharmacokinetics: INSTILL: Onset 1 hr, peak effects 2 hr, duration of action 6-8 hr

Drug interactions of concern to dentistry:

• Avoid use of anticholinergic drugs, including atropine-like drugs, propantheline, and diazepam (benzodiazepine)

DENTAL CONSIDERATIONS

General:

• Check compliance of patient with prescribed drug regimen for glaucoma.

• Avoid dental light in patient's eyes; offer dark glasses for comfort.

Consultations:

• Consultation with physician may be needed if sedation or anesthesia is required.

carvedilol

(kar've-di-lole)

Coreg

Drug class.: Nonselective β-adrenergic blocking agent with α_1-blocking activity

Action: Produces fall in BP without reflex tachycardia or significant reduction in heart rate through mixture of α-blocking, β-blocking effects; elevated plasma renin reduced

Uses: Essential hypertension, alone or with other antihypertensives, CHF; unlabeled use in angina

Dosage and routes:

Essential hypertension

• *Adult:* PO initially 6.25 mg bid for 7-14 days, then 12.5 mg bid if required for 7-14 days, then 25 mg bid; take with food to minimize risk of orthostatic hypotension

CHF

• *Adult:* PO 3.125 mg bid for 2 wk, patients must be closely monitored by physician

Available forms include: Tabs 3.125, 6.25, 12.5, 25 mg

Side effects/adverse reactions:

▼ *ORAL:* Dry mouth (<1%)

CNS: Dizziness, insomnia, somnolence

CV: ***Heart block,*** *orthostatic hypotension, syncope, bradycardia,* peripheral edema, fatigue

GI: Diarrhea, hepatocellular injury, abdominal pain

RESP: ***Status asthmaticus,*** *rhinitis,* pharyngitis, dyspnea

HEMA: ***Thrombocytopenia***

GU: UTI, impotence

INTEG: Pruritus, rash

MS: Back pain

MISC: Hypertriglyceridemia

Contraindications: Class IV heart failure, bronchial asthma, bronchospastic diseases, second- or third-degree AV block, cardiogenic shock or severe bradycardia, hypersensitivity

Precautions: Elderly, hepatic impairment, renal impairment, pregnancy category C, lactation, child <18 yr

Pharmacokinetics:

PO: Rapid oral absorption, hepatic metabolism, metabolites excreted in feces, 98% plasma protein binding

Drug interactions of concern to dentistry:

• Decreased hypotensive effect: indomethacin, NSAIDs

• Increased hypotension, myocardial depression: hydrocarbon inhalation anesthetics

• Hypertension, bradycardia: sympathomimetics (epinephrine, ephedrine)

DENTAL CONSIDERATIONS

General:

• Monitor vital signs every appointment due to cardiovascular side effects.

• After supine positioning, have patient sit upright for at least 2 min before standing to avoid orthostatic hypotension.

• Assess salivary flow as a factor in caries, periodontal disease, and candidiasis.

• Patients on chronic drug therapy may rarely have symptoms of blood dyscrasias, which can include infection, bleeding, and poor healing.

• Limit use of sodium-containing products, such as saline IV fluids, for those patients with a dietary salt restriction.

• Stress from dental procedures may compromise cardiovascular function; determine patient risk.

• Short appointments and a stress reduction protocol may be required for anxious patients.

Consultations:

• In a patient with symptoms of blood dyscrasias, request a medical consult for blood studies and postpone dental treatment until normal values are reestablished.

• Medical consult may be required to assess disease control and patient's ability to tolerate stress.

Teach patient/family:

• To report oral lesions, soreness, or bleeding to dentist

When chronic dry mouth occurs, advise patient:

• To avoid mouth rinses with high alcohol content due to drying effects

• Of need for daily home fluoride to prevent caries

• To use sugarless gum, frequent sips of water, or saliva substitutes

cefaclor

(sef'a-klor)

Ceclor, Ceclor CD

✱ Apo-Cefaclor

Drug class.: Antibiotic, cephalosporin (second generation)

Action: Inhibits bacterial cell wall synthesis, which renders cell wall osmotically unstable

Uses: Gram-negative bacilli: *H. influenzae, E. coli, P. mirabilis, Klebsiella;* gram-positive organisms: *S. pneumoniae, S. pyogenes, S. aureus;* upper/lower respiratory tract, urinary tract, skin infections; otitis media; *Bacteroides* species and in vitro activity against *Peptococcus* and *Peptostreptococcus*

Dosage and routes:

• *Adult:* PO 250-500 mg q8h, not to exceed 4 g/day

• *Child >1 mo:* PO 20-40 mg/kg/qd in divided doses q8h, not to exceed 1 g/day

Available forms include: Caps 250, 500 mg; powder for oral susp 125, 187, 250, 375 mg/5 ml; ext rel tabs 375, 500 mg

Side effects/adverse reactions:

▼ *ORAL:* Candidiasis, glossitis

CNS: Headache, dizziness, weakness, paresthesia, fever, chills

GI: *Diarrhea, anorexia,* nausea, vomiting, pain, bleeding, increased AST/ALT, bilirubin, LDH, alk phosphatase, abdominal pain

RESP: Dyspnea

HEMA: ***Leukopenia, thrombocytopenia, agranulocytosis, neutropenia, lymphocytosis, eosinophilia, pancytopenia, hemolytic anemia,*** anemia

GU: ***Nephrotoxicity, renal failure,*** proteinuria, vaginitis, pruritus, candidiasis, increased BUN

INTEG: ***Anaphylaxis,*** rash, urticaria, dermatitis

Contraindications: Hypersensitivity to cephalosporins, infants <1 mo

Precautions: Hypersensitivity to penicillins, pregnancy category B, lactation, renal disease

Pharmacokinetics:

PO: Peak 0.5-1 hr, half-life 36-54 min; 25% bound by plasma proteins; 60%-85% eliminated unchanged in urine in 8 hr; crosses placenta; excreted in breast milk

Drug interactions of concern to dentistry:

• Decreased bactericidal effects: tetracyclines, erythromycins

• Increased and prolonged serum levels: probenecid

• May reduce effectiveness of oral contraceptives

DENTAL CONSIDERATIONS

General:

• Take precautions regarding allergy to medication.

• Determine why the patient is taking the drug.

Consultations:

• Medical consult may be required

to assess disease control in the patient.

Teach patient/family:

• Importance of good oral hygiene to prevent soft tissue inflammation

• To avoid mouth rinses with high alcohol content due to drying effects and possible drug-drug reaction

When used for dental infection, advise patient:

• Taking birth control pill to use additional method of contraception for duration of cycle

• To report sore throat, oral burning sensation, fever, fatigue, any of which could indicate superinfection

• To take at prescribed intervals and complete dosage regimen

• To immediately notify the dentist if signs or symptoms of infection increase

---

cefadroxil

(sef-a-drox'il)

Duricef

Drug class.: Cephalosporin (first generation)

Action: Inhibits bacterial cell wall synthesis, rendering cell wall osmotically unstable

Uses: Gram-negative bacilli: *E. coli, P. mirabilis, Klebsiella* (UTI only); gram-positive organisms: *S. pneumoniae, S. pyogenes, S. aureus;* upper/lower respiratory tract, urinary tract, skin infections; otitis media; tonsillitis; particularly for UTI

Dosage and routes:

• *Adult:* PO 500 mg-1 g q12h; dosage reduction indicated in renal impairment (CrCl <50 ml/min); limit 4 g/day

• *Child:* PO 30 mg/kg/day or 15 mg/kg q12h

Bacterial endocarditis prophylaxis

• *Adult:* PO 2 g 1 hr before dental procedure

• *Child:* PO 50 mg/kg of body weight not to exceed the adult dose 1 hr before dental procedure

Available forms include: Caps 500 mg; tabs 1 g; oral susp 125, 250, 500 mg/5 ml

Side effects/adverse reactions:

▼ *ORAL:* Candidiasis, glossitis

CNS: Headache, dizziness, weakness, paresthesia, fever, chills

GI: Diarrhea, anorexia, ***pseudomembranous colitis,*** nausea, vomiting, pain, bleeding, increased AST/ALT, bilirubin, LDH, alk phosphatase, abdominal pain

RESP: Dyspnea

HEMA: ***Leukopenia, thrombocytopenia, agranulocytosis, neutropenia, lymphocytosis, eosinophilia, pancytopenia, hemolytic anemia***

GU: ***Nephrotoxicity, renal failure,*** proteinuria, vaginitis, pruritus, candidiasis, increased BUN

INTEG: ***Anaphylaxis,*** rash, urticaria, dermatitis

Contraindications: Hypersensitivity to cephalosporins, infants <1 mo

Precautions: Hypersensitivity to penicillins, pregnancy category B, lactation, renal disease

Pharmacokinetics: PO: Peak 1-1.5 hr, half-life 1-2 hr; 20% bound by plasma proteins; crosses placenta; excreted in breast milk

Drug interactions of concern to dentistry:

• Decreased bactericidal effects: tetracyclines, erythromycins

• Increased and prolonged serum levels: probenecid

• May reduce effectiveness of oral contraceptives

DENTAL CONSIDERATIONS

General:

• Take precautions regarding allergy to medication.

• Determine why the patient is taking the drug.

Consultations:

• Medical consult may be required to assess disease control in the patient.

Teach patient/family:

• Importance of good oral hygiene to prevent soft tissue inflammation

• To avoid mouth rinses with high alcohol content due to drying effects and possible drug-drug reaction

When used for dental infection, advise patient:

• Taking birth control pill to use additional method of contraception for duration of cycle

• To report sore throat, oral burning sensation, fever, fatigue, any of which could indicate superinfection

• To take at prescribed intervals and complete dosage regimen

• To immediately notify the dentist if signs or symptoms of infection increase

---

cefazolin sodium

(sef-a'zoe-lin)

Ancef, Kefzol, Zolicef

♣ Gen-Cefazolin

Drug class.: Cephalosporin (first generation)

Action: Inhibits bacterial cell wall synthesis, rendering cell wall osmotically unstable

Uses: Gram-negative bacilli: *H. influenzae, E. coli, P. mirabilis, Klebsiella;* gram-positive organisms: *S. pneumoniae, S. pyogenes, S. aureus;* upper/lower respiratory tract, urinary tract, skin infections; bone, joint, biliary, genital infections; endocarditis; surgical prophylaxis; septicemia

Dosage and routes:

Life-threatening infections

• *Adult:* IM/IV 1-1.5 g q6h

• *Child >1 mo:* IM/IV 100 mg/kg in 3-4 equal doses

Mild-to-moderate infections

• *Adult:* IM/IV 250-500 mg q8h

• *Child >1 mo:* IM/IV 25-50 mg/kg in 3-4 equal doses

Dosage reduction indicated in renal impairment (CrCl < 54 ml/min)

Bacterial endocarditis prophylaxis

• *Adult:* IM or IV patients unable to take oral medications (caution allergy to amoxicillin) 1 g 30 min before dental procedure

• *Child:* IM or IV 25 mg/kg of body weight not to exceed the adult dose 30 min before dental procedure

Prosthetic joint prophylaxis (when indicated)

• *Adult:* IM or IV 1 g 1 hr before dental procedure

Available forms include: Inj IM/IV 250, 500 mg; 1, 5, 10 g

Side effects/adverse reactions:

▼ *ORAL:* Candidiasis

CNS: Headache, dizziness, weakness, paresthesia, fever, chills

GI: Diarrhea, anorexia, nausea, vomiting, pain, glossitis, bleeding, increased AST/ALT, bilirubin, LDH, alk phosphatase, abdominal pain

HEMA: ***Leukopenia, thrombocytopenia, agranulocytosis, anemia, neutropenia, lymphocytosis, eosinophilia, pancytopenia, hemolytic anemia***

GU: ***Nephrotoxicity, renal failure,*** proteinuria, vaginitis, pruritus, increased BUN
INTEG: ***Anaphylaxis,*** rash, urticaria, dermatitis
Contraindications: Hypersensitivity to cephalosporins, infants <1 mo
Precautions: Hypersensitivity to penicillins, pregnancy category B, lactation, renal disease
Pharmacokinetics:
IM: Peak 0.5-2 hr, half-life 1.5-2.25 hr
IV: Peak 10 min, eliminated unchanged in urine 70%-86% protein bound
Drug interactions of concern to dentistry:
• Decreased bactericidal effects: tetracyclines, erythromycins
• Increased and prolonged serum levels: probenecid
• May reduce effectiveness of oral contraceptives
DENTAL CONSIDERATIONS
General:
• Take precautions regarding allergy to medication.
• Determine why the patient is taking the drug.
Consultations:
• Medical consult may be required to assess disease control in the patient.
Teach patient/family:
• Importance of good oral hygiene to prevent soft tissue inflammation
• To avoid mouth rinses with high alcohol content due to drying effects and possible drug-drug reaction
When used for dental infection, advise patient:
• Taking birth control pill to use additional method of contraception for duration of cycle
• To report sore throat, oral burning sensation, fever, fatigue, any of which could indicate superinfection
• To take at prescribed intervals and complete dosage regimen
• To immediately notify the dentist if signs or symptoms of infection increase

---

cefdinir
(sef′di-ner)
Omnicef
Drug class.: Cephalosporin (third generation)

Action: Inhibits bacterial cell wall synthesis, rendering cell wall osmotically unstable
Uses: Infections caused by susceptible strains of organisms that cause community-acquired pneumonia, acute exacerbation of chronic bronchitis, pharyngitis, tonsillitis, uncomplicated skin and skin structure infections, acute maxillary sinusitis, and acute bacterial otitis media
Dosage and routes:
• *Adult and child <13 yr:* PO dose depends on type of infection and patient; range is from 300 mg every 12 hr to 600 mg every 24 hr for 5-10 days taken with or without food
• *Child <6 mo to 12 yr:* PO dose depends on type of infection and patient: range is from 7 mg/kg of body weight every 12 hr to 14 mg/kg of body weight every 24 hr for 5-10 days with or without food
Available forms include: Caps 300 mg; powder for oral suspension 125 mg/5 ml
Side effects/adverse reactions:
▼ *ORAL:* None reported, but most

antiinfectives carry a risk of opportunistic candidiasis
CNS: Dizziness, insomnia, somnolence
GI: Diarrhea, nausea, abdominal pain, ***antibiotic-associated pseudomembranous colitis***
RESP: Dyspnea
HEMA: Eosinophilia
GU: Vaginal candidiasis
INTEG: Rash, cutaneous candidiasis
META: Abnormal liver function tests, elevated AST/ALT, bilirubin, potassium, and urinary pH
MS: Asthenia, ***anaphylaxis***
Contraindications: Hypersensitivity
Precautions: Hypersensitivity to other cephalosporins, penicillins, or penicillamine; renal impairment (need dose reduction); ulcerative colitis, pseudomembranous colitis, bleeding disorders, renal impairment, hemodialysis, β-lactamase–resistant organisms, pregnancy category B, not detected in breast milk, child <6 mo
Pharmacokinetics:
PO: Slow absorption, peak serum levels 2-4 hr, bioavailability ranges from 16%-25%, depending on dose amd dose form, plasma protein binding 60%-70%, little to no metabolism, renal excretion
Drug interactions of concern to dentistry:
• Absorption retarded by iron salts, magnesium, or aluminum antacids: take antiinfective dose at least 2 hr before antacids or iron preparations
• Increased plasma levels: probenecid

DENTAL CONSIDERATIONS
General:
• Use precaution regarding allergy to medication.
• Determine why patient is taking the drug.
• Examine for oral manifestation of opportunistic infection.
Consultations:
• Medical consult may be required to assess disease control in the patient.
Teach patient/family:
• Importance of good oral hygiene to prevent soft tissue inflammation

---

cefepime

(sef′e-pim)
Maxipime
Drug class.: Cephalosporin (fourth generation)

Action: Inhibits bacterial cell wall synthesis
Uses: Urinary tract infections (uncomplicated and complicated), skin and soft tissue infections, complicated intraabdominal infections (in combination with metronidazole) and pneumonia caused by susceptible strains of microorganisms including *E. coli, K. pneumonia, P. mirabilis, S. aureus* (methicillin susceptible), *S. pneumoniae* and *S. pyogenes;* febrile neutropenia
Dosage and routes:
Mild to moderate infections
• *Adult:* IV/IM 0.5-1.0 g q12h depending on severity of the infection for 7-10 days; IM doses for mild infections only
Moderate to severe infections
• *Adult:* IV 1.0-2.0 g q12h for 10 days depending on severity of the infection; adjust all doses in patients with renal impairment
Available forms include: Powder for injection vials 500 mg, 1, 2 g

Side effects/adverse reactions:
▼ *ORAL:* Candidiasis
CNS: Headache, light-headedness
CV: ***Phlebitis***
GI: Diarrhea, pseudomembraneous colitis, vomiting, dyspepsia
GU: Vaginitis
EENT: Blurred vision
INTEG: Urticaria, pruritus, rash
META: Elevation of liver function tests
MISC: Local reactions, fever

Contraindications: Hypersensitivity to cephalosporins or penicillins

Precautions: Renal impairment, overgrowth of resistant organisms, colitis, monitor prothrombin, pregnancy category B, lactation, child <12 yr

Pharmacokinetics:
IV: Peak levels vary with dose and occur within 0.5-1 hr, protein binding 20%, urinary excretion (85% of dose), therapeutic serum levels up to 8 hr
IM: Peak levels 0.5-1.5 hr

Drug interactions of concern to dentistry:
- Increased risk of nephrotoxicity, ototoxicity: aminoglycosides in high doses, furosemide

DENTAL CONSIDERATIONS
General:
- Precaution regarding allergy to medication.
- Determine why patient is taking the drug.

Consultation: Medical consult may be required to assess disease control in the patient.

Teach patient/family:
- Importance of good oral hygiene to prevent soft tissue inflammation
- To report sore throat, oral burning sensation, fever, fatigue, any of which could indicate presence of a superinfection

cefixime
(sef-ix'eem)
Suprax
Drug class.: Cephalosporin (third generation)

Action: Inhibits bacterial cell wall synthesis, rendering cell wall osmotically unstable

Uses: Uncomplicated UTI *(E. coli, P. mirabilis),* pharyngitis and tonsillitis *(S. pyogenes),* otitis media *(H. influenzae, M. catarrhalis),* acute bronchitis, and acute exacerbations of chronic bronchitis *(S. pneumoniae, H. influenzae)*

Dosage and routes:
- *Adult:* PO 400 mg qd as a single dose or 200 mg q12h
- *Child >50 kg or >12 yr:* PO use adult dosage
- *Child <50 kg or <12 yr:* PO 8 mg/kg/day as a single dose or 4 mg/kg q12h

Available forms include: Tabs 200, 400 g; powder for oral susp 100 mg/5 ml

Side effects/adverse reactions:
▼ *ORAL:* Candidiasis, glossitis
CNS: Headache, dizziness, paresthesia, fever, chills, lethargy, fatigue, confusion
GI: Nausea, vomiting, diarrhea, anorexia, pain, bleeding, increased AST/ALT, bilirubin, LDH, alk phosphatase, heartburn, dysgeusia, flatulence
RESP: ***Bronchospasm,*** dyspnea, tight chest
HEMA: ***Leukopenia, thrombocytopenia, agranulocytosis, neutropenia, lymphocytosis, eosinophilia,***

pancytopenia, hemolytic anemia
GU: ***Proteinuria, nephrotoxicity, renal failure,*** pyuria, dysuria, vaginitis, pruritus, increased BUN
INTEG: ***Exfoliative dermatitis, anaphylaxis,*** rash, urticaria
Contraindications: Hypersensitivity to cephalosporins, infants <6 mo
Precautions: Hypersensitivity to penicillins, pregnancy category B, lactation, renal disease
Pharmacokinetics:
PO: Peak 1 hr, half-life 3-4 hr; 65% bound by plasma proteins, 50% eliminated unchanged in urine; crosses placenta; excreted in breast milk
Drug interactions of concern to dentistry:
• Decreased bactericidal effects: tetracyclines, erythromycins
• Increased and prolonged serum levels: probenecid
• May reduce effectiveness of oral contraceptives

DENTAL CONSIDERATIONS
General:
• Take precautions regarding allergy to medication.
• Determine why the patient is taking the drug.
Consultations:
• Medical consult may be required to assess disease control in the patient.
Teach patient/family:
• Importance of good oral hygiene to prevent soft tissue inflammation
• To avoid mouth rinses with high alcohol content due to drying effects and possible drug-drug reaction
When used for dental infection, advise patient:
• Taking birth control pill to use additional method of contraception for duration of cycle
• To report sore throat, oral burning sensation, fever, fatigue, any of which could indicate superinfection
• To take at prescribed intervals and complete dosage regimen
• To immediately notify the dentist if signs or symptoms of infection increase

cefpodoxime proxetil
(cef-pode-ox′eem)
Vantin
Drug class.: Cephalosporin (third generation)

Action: Inhibits bacterial cell wall synthesis, rendering cell wall osmotically unstable
Uses: Upper/lower respiratory tract infections, pharyngitis (tonsillitis), gonorrhea, UTI, uncomplicated skin and skin structure infections caused by susceptible organisms, otitis media
Dosage and routes:
• *Adult:* PO 100-200 mg q12h for 5 days; more severe infections 400 mg q12h
Otitis media
• *Child 2 mo to 12 yr:* PO 10 mg/kg/day in one dose (max daily dose 400 mg) or 5 mg/kg (max 200 mg/dose) bid for 5 days
Available forms include: Tabs 100, 200 mg; oral susp 50, 100 mg/5 ml
Side effects/adverse reactions:
▼ *ORAL:* Candidiasis, glossitis
CNS: Headache, dizziness, weakness, paresthesia, fever, chills
GI: Diarrhea, anorexia, nausea, vomiting, abdominal pain, bleed-

ing, increased AST/ALT, bilirubin, LDH, alk phosphatase

RESP: Dyspnea

HEMA: ***Leukopenia, thrombocytopenia, agranulocytosis, neutropenia, lymphocytosis, eosinophilia, pancytopenia, hemolytic anemia***

GU: ***Nephrotoxicity, renal failure,*** proteinuria, vaginitis, pruritus, candidiasis, increased BUN

INTEG: ***Anaphylaxis,*** rash, urticaria, dermatitis

Contraindications: Hypersensitivity to cephalosporins, infants <1 mo

Precautions: Hypersensitivity to penicillins, lactation, renal disease, pregnancy category not listed

Pharmacokinetics:

PO: Half-life 2-3 hr; excreted unchanged in urine; alter dose with renal impairment

Drug interactions of concern to dentistry:

- Decreased bactericidal effects: tetracyclines, erythromycins
- Increased and prolonged serum levels: probenecid
- May reduce effectiveness of oral contraceptives

DENTAL CONSIDERATIONS

General:

- Take precautions regarding allergy to medication.
- Determine why the patient is taking the drug.

Consultations:

- Medical consult may be required to assess disease control in the patient.

Teach patient/family:

- Importance of good oral hygiene to prevent soft tissue inflammation
- To avoid mouth rinses with high alcohol content due to drying effects and possible drug-drug reaction

When used for dental infection, advise patient:

- Taking birth control pill to use additional method of contraception for duration of cycle
- To report sore throat, oral burning sensation, fever, fatigue, any of which could indicate superinfection
- To take at prescribed intervals and complete dosage regimen
- To immediately notify the dentist if signs or symptoms of infection increase

---

cefprozil monohydrate

(sef-pro'zil)

Cefzil

Drug class.: Cephalosporin (second generation)

Action: Inhibits bacterial cell wall synthesis, which renders cell wall osmotically unstable

Uses: Pharyngitis/tonsillitis, otitis media, secondary bacterial infection of acute bronchitis, sinusitis; acute bacterial sinusitis; acute bacterial exacerbation of chronic bronchitis and uncomplicated skin and skin structure infections

Dosage and routes:

Upper respiratory infections

- *Adult:* PO 500 mg qd × 10 days

Otitis media

- *Child 6 mo to 12 yr:* PO 15 mg/kg q12h × 10 days

Lower respiratory infections

- *Adult:* PO 500 mg bid × 10 days

Skin/skin structure infections

- *Adult:* PO 250-500 mg q12h × 10 days

Available forms include: Tabs 250, 500 mg; susp 125, 250 mg/5ml

Side effects/adverse reactions:
▼ *ORAL:* Candidiasis, glossitis
CNS: Dizziness, headache, weakness, paresthesia, fever, chills
GI: ***Pseudomembranous colitis,*** diarrhea, nausea, vomiting, pain, anorexia, bleeding, increased AST/ALT, bilirubin, LDH, alk phosphatase, abdominal pain, flatulence
RESP: ***Anaphylaxis,*** dyspnea
HEMA: ***Leukopenia, thrombocytopenia, agranulocytosis, anemia, neutropenia, lymphocytosis, eosinophilia, pancytopenia, hemolytic anemia***
GU: ***Nephrotoxicity, proteinuria, increased BUN, renal failure, hematuria,*** vaginitis, genitoanal pruritus, candidiasis
INTEG: Rash, urticaria, dermatitis
Contraindications: Hypersensitivity to cephalosporins
Precautions: Pregnancy category B, lactation, elderly, hypersensitivity to penicillins, renal disease
Pharmacokinetics:
PO: Peak 6-10 hr, elimination half-life 25 hr; plasma protein binding 99%; extensively metabolized to an active metabolite
Drug interactions of concern to dentistry:
- Decreased bactericidal effects: tetracyclines, erythromycins
- Increased and prolonged serum levels: probenecid
- May reduce effectiveness of oral contraceptives

DENTAL CONSIDERATIONS
General:
- Take precautions regarding allergy to medication.
- Determine why the patient is taking the drug.
- Examine for evidence of oral manifestations of blood dyscrasia (infection, bleeding, poor healing) and superinfection.

Consultations:
- Medical consult may be required to assess disease control in the patient.

Teach patient/family:
- Importance of good oral hygiene to prevent soft tissue inflammation
- To avoid mouth rinses with high alcohol content due to drying effects and possible drug-drug reaction

When used for dental infection, advise patient:
- Taking birth control pill to use additional method of contraception for duration of cycle
- To report sore throat, oral burning sensation, fever, fatigue, any of which could indicate superinfection
- To take at prescribed intervals and complete dosage regimen
- To immediately notify the dentist if signs or symptoms of infection increase

---

ceftibuten
(sef-tye'byoo-ten)
Cedax
Drug class.: Cephalosporin (third generation)

Action: Inhibits bacterial cell wall synthesis, which renders cell wall osmotically unstable
Uses: Acute exacerbations of chronic bronchitis due to susceptible strains of *H. influenzae, M. catarrhalis, S. pneumoniae;* acute otitis media due to susceptible strains of *H. influenzae, M. catarrhalis, S. pyogenes;* pharyngitis and tonsillitis due to *S. pyogenes*

Dosage and routes:
- *Adult and child >12 yr:* PO 400 mg qd × 10 days
- *Child:* SUSP 9 mg/kg qd × 10 days, susp administered 2 hr before or 1 hr after a meal

Available forms include: Caps 400 mg; susp 90, 180 mg/5ml in 30, 60, 120 ml volumes

Side effects/adverse reactions:
▼ *ORAL:* Candidiasis, dry mouth (<1%)
CNS: Headache, dizziness, weakness, paresthesia, fever, chills
GI: Diarrhea, dyspepsia, nausea, vomiting, abdominal pain, bleeding, anorexia, increased AST/ALT, bilirubin, LDH, alk phosphatase, antibiotic-associated pseudomembraneous colitis
RESP: Dyspnea
HEMA: ***Leukopenia, thrombocytopenia, agranulocytosis, neutropenia, lymphocytosis, eosinophilia, pancytopenia, hemolytic anemia***
GU: ***Nephrotoxicity, renal failure,*** proteinuria, vaginitis, pruritus, candidiasis, increased BUN
INTEG: Rash, pruritus, ***anaphylaxis,*** urticaria, dermatitis

Contraindications: Hypersensitivity to cephalosporins

Precautions: Hypersensitivity to penicillins, lactation, renal impairment, pregnancy category B, lactation, infants <6 mo, pseudomembraneous colitis, oral suspension contains 1 g sucrose/5 ml

Pharmacokinetics:
PO: Half-life 2-3 hr; protein binding 6%, excreted mostly unchanged in urine; alter dose with renal impairment

Drug interactions of concern to dentistry:
- Decreased bactericidal effects: tetracyclines, erythromycins
- Increased and prolonged serum levels: probenecid
- May reduce effectiveness of oral contraceptives
- Aminoglycosides increase nephrotoxic potential

DENTAL CONSIDERATIONS

General:
- Take precautions regarding allergy to medication.
- Assess salivary flow as factor in caries, periodontal disease, and candidiasis.
- Oral suspension contains sucrose; patient should rinse mouth after use.
- Determine why the patient is taking the drug.

Consultations:
- Medical consult may be required to assess disease control in the patient.

Teach patient/family:
- Importance of good oral hygiene to prevent soft tissue inflammation

When used for dental infection, advise patient:
- Taking birth control pill to use additional method of contraception for duration of cycle
- To report sore throat, oral burning sensation, fever, fatigue, any of which could indicate superinfection
- To take at prescribed intervals and complete dosage regimen
- To immediately notify the dentist if signs or symptoms of infection increase

cefuroxime axetil

(sef-fyoor-ox'eem)
Ceftin

Drug class.: Cephalosporin (second generation)

Action: Inhibits bacterial cell wall synthesis, rendering cell wall osmotically unstable

Uses: Gram-negative bacilli *(H. influenzae, E. coli, Neisseria, P. mirabilis, Klebsiella);* gram-positive organisms *(S. pneumoniae, S. pyogenes, S. aureus);* serious lower respiratory tract, urinary tract, skin, gonococcal infections; septicemia; meningitis; early Lyme disease; acute bronchitis, acute bacterial maxillary sinusitis

Dosage and routes:

• *Adult and child:* PO 250 mg q12h, may increase to 500 mg q12h in serious infections

Urinary tract infections

• *Adult:* PO 125 mg q12h, may increase to 250 q12h if needed

Otitis media

• *Child <2 yr:* PO 125 mg bid
• *Child >2 yr:* PO 250 mg bid

Available forms include: Tabs 125, 250, 500 mg

Side effects/adverse reactions:

▼ *ORAL:* Candidiasis, glossitis

CNS: Headache, dizziness, weakness, paresthesia, fever, chills

GI: Nausea, vomiting, diarrhea, anorexia, **pseudomembranous colitis,** bleeding, increased AST/ALT, bilirubin, LDH, alk phosphatase, abdominal pain

RESP: ***Anaphylaxis***

HEMA: ***Leukopenia, thrombocytopenia, agranulocytosis, neutropenia, lymphocytosis, eosinophilia, pancytopenia, hemolytic anemia***

GU: ***Nephrotoxicity, renal failure,*** proteinuria, vaginitis, pruritus, candidiasis, increased BUN

INTEG: Rash, urticaria, dermatitis

Contraindications: Hypersensitivity to cephalosporins, infants <1 mo

Precautions: Hypersensitivity to penicillins, pregnancy category B, lactation, renal disease

Pharmacokinetics:

PO: Half-life 1-2 hr in normal renal function, 65% excreted unchanged in urine

Drug interactions of concern to dentistry:

• Decreased bactericidal effects: tetracyclines, erythromycins
• Increased and prolonged serum levels: probenecid
• May reduce effectiveness of oral contraceptives

DENTAL CONSIDERATIONS

General:

• Take precautions regarding allergy to medication.
• Determine why the patient is taking the drug.

Consultations:

• Medical consult may be required to assess disease control in the patient.

Teach patient/family:

• Importance of good oral hygiene to prevent soft tissue inflammation
• To avoid mouth rinses with high alcohol content due to drying effects and possible drug-drug reaction

When used for dental infection, advise patient:

• Taking birth control pill to use additional method of contraception for duration of cycle
• To report sore throat, oral burning

sensation, fever, fatigue, any of which could indicate superinfection
• To take at prescribed intervals and complete dosage regimen
• To immediately notify the dentist if signs or symptoms of infection increase

celecoxib

sel-e-cox'ib
Celebrex

Drug class.: Nonsteroidal antiinflammatory

Action: A selective inhibitor of cyclooxygenase 2 (COX 2) enzymes preventing the synthesis of prostaglandins

Uses: Relief of signs and symptoms of osteoarthritis and relief of signs and symptoms of rheumatoid arthritis in adults; also approved for reducing the number of intestinal polyps in patients with familial adenomatous polyposis

Dosage and routes:

Osteoarthritis
• *Adult:* PO 200 mg/day as a single dose or 100 mg bid

Rheumatoid arthritis
• *Adult:* PO 100 mg to 200 mg bid

Available forms include: Caps 100, 200 mg

Side effects/adverse reactions:

▼ *ORAL:* Dry mouth, stomatitis, taste alteration

CNS: Headache, dizziness, insomnia, anxiety

CV: May aggravate hypertension, palpitation, syncope, ***CHF***

GI: Abdominal pain, diarrhea, dyspepsia, flatulence, nausea, ***severe GI bleeding***

RESP: Pharyngitis, URI, aggravates bronchospasm

HEMA: Anemia, ecchymosis, ***thrombocytopenia***

GU: UTI, ***acute renal failure***

EENT: Rhinitis, sinusitis, tinnitus, deafness, blurred vision

INTEG: Skin rash, pruritus, urticaria

META: Hyperchloremia, hypophosphatemia, elevated BUN, elevated liver enzymes (SGOT, SGPT)

MS: Myalgia, arthralgia

MISC: Back pain

Contraindications: Hypersensitivity, allergy to sulfonamides, patients who have experienced asthma, urticaria, or allergic-type reactions to ASA or NSAIDs

Precautions: Geriatrics weighing <50 kg use lowest dose, children <18 yr, severe hepatic or renal impairment, upper active GI disease, GI bleeding, avoid in late pregnancy (category D after 34 wk), pregnancy category C, lactation, dehydrated patients, heart failure, hypertension, asthma

Pharmacokinetics:

PO: Fatty meal delays absorption, peak plasma levels 3 hr, half-life 11 hr, metabolism (CYP450 2C9), metabolites excreted in feces (57%) and urine (27%)

Drug interactions of concern to dentistry:
• Increased plasma levels: fluconazole
• Increased risk of GI bleeding: long-duration NSAIDs, aspirin (except low doses), oral glucocorticoids, alcoholism, smoking, older age, and generally poor health

DENTAL CONSIDERATIONS

General:
• Patients on chronic drug therapy may rarely have symptoms of

blood dyscrasias, which can include infection, bleeding, and poor healing.

- Assess salivary flow as a factor in caries, periodontal disease, and candidiasis.
- Consider semisupine chair position for patient comfort due to disease and GI side effects of drug.

Teach patient/family:

- Importance of good oral hygiene to prevent soft tissue inflammation
- Importance of updating health and drug history if physician makes any changes in evaluation/drug regimens
- Use of electric toothbrush if patient has difficulty holding conventional devices

When chronic dry mouth occurs, advise patient:

- To avoid mouth rinses with high alcohol content due to drying effects
- To use daily home fluoride products for anticaries effect
- To use sugarless gum, frequent sips of water, or saliva substitutes

cephalexin

(sef-a-lex'in)

Biocef, C-Lexin, Cefanex, Keflex, Keftab

✦ Apo-Cephalex, Novo-Lexin, Nu-Cephalex, PMS-Cephalexin

Drug class.: Cephalosporin (first generation)

Action: Inhibits bacterial cell wall synthesis, rendering cell wall osmotically unstable

Uses: Gram-negative bacilli: *H. influenzae, E. coli, P. mirabilis, Klebsiella;* gram-positive organisms: *S. pneumoniae, S. pyogenes, S. aureus;* upper/lower respiratory tract, urinary tract, skin, bone infections; otitis media

Dosage and routes:

- *Adult:* PO 250-500 mg q6h, up to 4 g/day
- *Child:* PO 6.25-50 mg/kg/day in 4 equal doses

Moderate skin infections

- 500 mg q12h

Severe infections

- *Adult:* PO 500 mg-1 g q6h
- *Child:* PO 50-100 mg/kg/day in 4 equal doses

Dosage reduction indicated in renal impairment (CrCl <50 ml/min)

Bacterial endocarditis prophylaxis:

- *Adult:* PO 2 g 1 hr before dental procedure for those patients unable to take amoxicillin
- *Child:* PO 50 mg/kg of body weight 1 hr before dental procedure, not to exceed the adult dose for those patients unable to take amoxicillin

Available forms include: Caps 250, 500 mg; tabs 250, 500; oral susp 125, 250 mg/5 ml; pediatric susp 100 mg/ml

Side effects/adverse reactions:

▼ *ORAL:* Candidiasis, glossitis

CNS: Headache, dizziness, weakness, paresthesia, fever, chills

GI: Nausea, vomiting, diarrhea, anorexia, ***pseudomembranous colitis,*** bleeding, increased AST/ALT, bilirubin, LDH, alk phosphatase, abdominal pain

RESP: ***Anaphylaxis,*** dyspnea

HEMA: ***Leukopenia, thrombocytopenia, agranulocytosis, neutropenia, lymphocytosis, eosinophilia, pancytopenia, hemolytic anemia***

GU: ***Nephrotoxicity, renal failure,*** proteinuria, vaginitis, pruritus, candidiasis, increased BUN

INTEG: Rash, urticaria, dermatitis
Contraindications: Hypersensitivity to cephalosporins, infants <1 mo
Precautions: Hypersensitivity to penicillins, pregnancy category B, lactation, renal disease
Pharmacokinetics:
PO: Peak 1 hr, duration 6-8 hr, half-life 30-72 min; 5%-15% bound by plasma proteins, 90%-100% eliminated unchanged in urine; crosses placenta; excreted in breast milk
Drug interactions of concern to dentistry:
• Decreased bactericidal effects: tetracyclines, erythromycins
• Increased and prolonged serum levels: probenecid
• May reduce effectiveness of oral contraceptives

DENTAL CONSIDERATIONS
General:
• Take precautions regarding allergy to medication.
• Determine why the patient is taking the drug.
Consultations:
• Medical consult may be required to assess disease control in the patient.
Teach patient/family:
• Importance of good oral hygiene to prevent soft tissue inflammation
• To avoid mouth rinses with high alcohol content due to drying effects and possible drug-drug reaction
When used for dental infection, advise patient:
• Taking birth control pill to use additional method of contraception for duration of cycle
• To report sore throat, oral burning sensation, fever, fatigue, any of which could indicate superinfection
• To take at prescribed intervals and complete dosage regimen
• To immediately notify the dentist if signs or symptoms of infection increase

cephradine
(sef'ra-deen)
Velosef
Drug class.: Cephalosporin (first generation)

Action: Inhibits bacterial cell wall synthesis, rendering cell wall osmotically unstable
Uses: Gram-negative bacilli: *H. influenzae, E. coli, P. mirabilis, Klebsiella;* gram-positive organisms: *S. pneumoniae, S. pyogenes, S. aureus;* serious respiratory tract, urinary tract, skin infections; otitis media
Dosage and routes:
• *Adult:* IM/IV 500 mg-1 g q4-6h, not to exceed 8 g/day; PO 250 mg-1 g q6-12h; limit PO dose to 4 g/day
• *Child >1 yr:* IM/IV 12-25 mg/kg q6h; PO 6-25 mg/kg q6h
Available forms include: Powder for inj IM/IV 250, 500 mg and 1, 2 g; caps 250, 500 mg; oral susp 125, 250 mg/5 ml
Side effects/adverse reactions:
▼ *ORAL:* Candidiasis, glossitis
CNS: Headache, dizziness, weakness, paresthesia, fever, chills
GI: Nausea, vomiting, diarrhea, anorexia, ***pseudomembranous colitis,*** bleeding, increased AST/ALT, bilirubin, LDH, alk phosphatase, abdominal pain
RESP: ***Anaphylaxis,*** dyspnea

HEMA: ***Leukopenia, thrombocytopenia, agranulocytosis, neutropenia, lymphocytosis, eosinophilia, pancytopenia, hemolytic anemia***
GU: ***Nephrotoxicity, renal failure,*** proteinuria, vaginitis, pruritus, candidiasis, increased BUN
INTEG: Rash, urticaria, dermatitis
Contraindications: Hypersensitivity to cephalosporins, infants <1 mo
Precautions: Hypersensitivity to penicillins, pregnancy category B, lactation, renal disease
Pharmacokinetics:
PO: Peak 1 hr
IV: Peak 5 min
IM: Peak 1 hr
Half-life 0.75-1.5 hr; 20% bound by plasma proteins, 80%-90% eliminated unchanged in urine; crosses placenta; excreted in breast milk

Drug interactions of concern to dentistry:
• Decreased bactericidal effects: tetracyclines, erythromycins
• Increased and prolonged serum levels: probenecid
• May reduce effectiveness of oral contraceptives

DENTAL CONSIDERATIONS
General:
• Take precautions regarding allergy to medication.
• Determine why the patient is taking the drug.
Consultations:
• Medical consult may be required to assess disease control in the patient.
Teach patient/family:
• Importance of good oral hygiene to prevent soft tissue inflammation
• To avoid mouth rinses with high alcohol content due to drying effects and possible drug-drug reaction
When used for dental infection, advise patient:
• Taking birth control pill to use additional method of contraception for duration of cycle
• To report sore throat, oral burning sensation, fever, fatigue, any of which could indicate superinfection
• To take at prescribed intervals and complete dosage regimen
• To immediately notify the dentist if signs or symptoms of infection increase

---

cerivastatin sodium

(se-riv′a-stat-in)
Baycol
Drug class.: Cholesterol-lowering agent

Action: Inhibits HMG-CoA reductase enzyme, which reduces cholesterol synthesis
Uses: Adjunct in primary hypercholesterolemia and mixed dyslipidemia (types IIa and IIb) when dietary restrictions or other pharmacologic measures also are inadequate, reduction of triglycerides and apolipoprotein B
Dosage and routes:
• *Adult:* PO 0.3 mg qd (renal impairment start dose at 0.2 mg); maximum daily dose 0.4 mg
Triglyceride reduction
• *Adult:* PO 0.4 mg qd
Available forms include: Tabs 0.2, 0.3, 0.4 mg
Side effects/adverse reactions:
▼ *ORAL:* Alteration of taste
CNS: Headache, dizziness, insomnia, tremors, peripheral nerve palsy, facial paresis
CV: Peripheral edema

GI: Abdominal pain, dyspepsia, diarrhea, flatulence, constipation
RESP: Pharyngitis, sinusitis, cough
GU: Myoglobinuria, UTI
EENT: Rhinitis
INTEG: Rash, skin discoloration; angioedema, ***anaphylaxis,*** Stevens-Johnson syndrome, lupus-like reaction (rare)
META: Elevation of serum transaminase (ALT, AST), creatine kinase
MS: Back pain, asthenia, leg pain, chest pain, arthralgia, ***rhabdomyolysis with acute renal failure,*** myopathy, myalgia
MISC: Flulike syndrome

Contraindications: Hypersensitivity, acute liver disease, or unexplained elevations of serum transaminases; pregnancy and lactation

Precautions: Use pretreatment liver function tests, liver disease, heavy alcohol use, pregnancy category X, children, renal insufficiency, liver disease

Pharmacokinetics:
PO: Bioavailability 60%, peak plasma levels 2.5 hr, highly plasma protein bound 99%, active metabolites, excretion in feces (70%) and urine (24%)

Drug interactions of concern to dentistry:
• Increased risk of myopathy: erythromycin, cyclosporine, niacin, azole antifungals (ketoconazole, itraconazole)

DENTAL CONSIDERATIONS
General:
• Consider semisupine chair position for patient comfort when respiratory or GI side effects occur.
• Evaluate respiration characteristics and rate.

cetirizine hydrochloride

(se-ti′ra-zeen)
Zyrtec
Reactine
Drug class.: Antihistamine

Action: Competitive antagonist for peripheral H_1-receptors

Uses: Treatment of symptoms of seasonal allergic rhinitis, perennial allergic rhinitis, chronic urticaria

Dosage and routes:
• Adult and child >6 yr: PO 5-10 mg bid, limit 20 mg/day
Available forms include: Tabs 5, 10 mg; syrup 5 mg/5 ml

Side effects/adverse reactions:
ORAL: Dry mouth (5%), taste alteration, tongue edema, orofacial dyskinesia (all rare)
CNS: Sedation, drowsiness, dizziness, headache, somnolence, depression
CV: Palpitation, tachycardia, hypertension, cardiac failure
GI: Constipation, diarrhea
HEMA: ***Hemolytic anemia, thrombocytopenia***
GU: Difficult urination, urinary retention, dysmenorrhea
EENT: Pharyngitis, dry nose or throat, tinnitus, earache
INTEG: Pruritus, rash, dry skin
MS: Myalgia, arthralgia
MISC: Photosensitivity

Contraindications: Hypersensitivity

Precautions: Renal impairment (requires dose reduction), elderly, glaucoma, urinary obstruction, pregnancy category not listed, lactation

Pharmacokinetics:
PO: Peak plasma levels 1 hr, duration up to 24 hr, half-life 8-11 hr;

highly protein bound; rapid oral absorption, minimal metabolism; excreted mostly unchanged in urine

Drug interactions of concern to dentistry:

• No drug interactions reported, but should be similar to other antihistamines; anticipate increased sedation with other CNS depressants and increased anticholinergic effects with anticholinergic drugs

DENTAL CONSIDERATIONS

General:

• Assess salivary flow as factor in caries, periodontal disease, and candidiasis.

Teach patient/family:

When chronic dry mouth occurs, advise patient:

• To avoid mouth rinses with high alcohol content due to drying effects

• To use daily home fluoride products for anticaries effect

• To use sugarless gum, frequent sips of water, or saliva substitutes

---

cevimeline

(ce-vi-me'leen)

Evoxac

Drug class.: Cholinergic (muscarinic) agonist

Action: Acts directly on cholinergic (muscarinic) receptor sites in the CNS and in exocrine glands (i.e., salivary glands); also binds to cholinergic receptors in the GI and GU tracts; derivative of acetylcholine; peripheral effects may resemble pilocarpine

Uses: Treatment of symptoms of dry mouth associated with Sjögren's syndrome

Dosage and routes:

• *Adult:* PO 30 mg tid (higher doses have not been demonstrated to provide greater effects)

Available forms include: Cap 30 mg

Side effects/adverse reactions:

▼ *ORAL: Salivation*

CNS: Confusion, headache, dizziness, fatigue, insomnia

CV: Palpitation, chest pain

GI: Diarrhea, nausea, abdominal pain, vomiting

GU: Urinary frequency, sinusitis, UTI, polyuria

RESP: Rhinitis, URI, *coughing*

EENT: Pharyngitis, conjunctivitis, bronchitis, abnormal vision, eye pain, ear pain, visual blurring, lacrimation

INTEG: Diaphoresis, rash, allergy

MS: Back pain, arthralgia

MISC: Asthenia, pain, skeletal pain

Contraindications: Hypersensitivity, uncontrolled asthma, acute iritis, narrow-angle glaucoma

Precautions: Has the potential to alter heart rate or cardiac conduction; use with care in cardiovascular disease, asthma, bronchitis, COPD, seizure disorders, Parkinson's disease, urinary tract/bladder obstruction, cholecystitis, cholangitis, biliary obstruction, GI ulcers, pregnancy category C, lactation, children (no data), history of adverse effects to other cholinergic agonists

Pharmacokinetics:

PO: Good oral absorption, peak concentration in 1.5-2 hr, <20% bound to plasma proteins, half-life 4-6 hr, hepatic metabolism by cytochrome P-450 (CYP2D6 and CYP3A/4), renal excretion (97%)

Drug interactions of concern to dentistry:

• Use with caution in patients taking β-adrenergic blockers: possible conduction disturbances.

• There are no specific data on dental drug interactions; however, use caution with other cholinergic agonist.

• There is always the possibility that a cholinergic antagonist could interfere with this drug's action.

• Although there are no supporting data, use with caution in patients taking drugs that inhibit cytochrome P-450 (CYP3A/4 and CYP2D6).

DENTAL CONSIDERATIONS

General:

• Assess salivary flow as a factor in caries, periodontal disease, and candidiasis.

• Monitor vital signs every appointment due to possible cardiovascular side effects.

• Place on frequent recall to assess effectiveness.

Consultations:

• Medical consult may be required to assess disease control in the patient.

• Medical consult may be necessary before prescribing for those patients with cardiovascular or respiratory disease.

Teach patient/family:

• That this drug may cause visual disturbances, especially with night driving, which may impair driving safety

• That the patient should drink extra fluids (water) to compensate for excessive sweating

When chronic dry mouth occurs, advise patient:

• To avoid mouth rinses with high alcohol content due to drying effects

• Of need for daily home fluoride to prevent caries

• To use sugarless gum, frequent sips of water, or saliva substitutes

---

chenodiol

(kee-noe-dye'ole)

Chenix

Drug class.: Antilithic

Action: Mechanism unclear; increases amount of bile acids in relation to cholesterol; may permit gradual solubilization of cholesterol from gallstones

Uses: Dissolving gallstones instead of surgery

Dosage and routes:

• *Adult:* PO 13-16 mg/kg bid; start with 250 mg bid × 2 wk, then increase by 250 mg/day qwk until max tolerated dose is attained; discontinue if no response in 18 mo

Available forms include: Tabs 250 mg

Side effects/adverse reactions:

GI: Diarrhea, ***hepatotoxicity,*** fecal urgency, heartburn, nausea, cramps, increased ALT/AST, LDH, vomiting, dysphagia, flatulence, dyspepsia

HEMA: ***Leukopenia***

Contraindications: Hypersensitivity, hepatic disease, bile duct obstruction, biliary GI fistula, pregnancy category X, radiopaque stones, gallbladder complications

Precautions: Lactation, children, atherosclerosis, elderly, requires periodic liver function tests

Pharmacokinetics:

PO: Metabolized by liver; excreted

in feces (metabolite/unchanged drug); crosses placenta

Drug interactions of concern to dentistry:

• None reported

DENTAL CONSIDERATIONS

General:

• Consider semisupine chair position for patient comfort if GI side effects occur.

• Determine why the patient is taking the drug.

• Patients on chronic drug therapy may rarely have symptoms of blood dyscrasias, which can include infection, bleeding, and poor healing.

Consultations:

• Medical consult may be required to assess disease control in the patient.

• In a patient with symptoms of blood dyscrasias, request a medical consult for blood studies and postpone dental treatment until normal values are reestablished.

Teach patient/family:

• To report any unusual or GI side effects following oral use of prescribed dental drugs

chloral hydrate

(klor-al hye′drate)

Aquachloral Supprettes

♣ Novo-Chlorhydrate, PMS-Chloral Hydrate

Drug class.: Sedative-hypnotic, chloral derivative

Controlled Substance Schedule IV, Schedule F

Action: Active metabolite, trichloroethanol, produces mild CNS depression

Uses: Sedation, insomnia

Dosage and routes:

Sedation

• *Adult:* PO/REC 250 mg tid pc; preoperative 500 mg-1 g 30 min before surgery

• *Child:* PO 25-50 mg/kg of body weight/day not to exceed 1 g/dose

Insomnia-hypnotic dose

• *Adult:* PO/REC 500 mg-1g 0.5 hr hs

Available forms include: Caps 250, 500 mg; syr 250, 500 mg/5 ml; supp 325, 500, 650 mg

Side effects/adverse reactions:

▼ *ORAL:* Unpleasant taste, mucosal irritation

CNS: Drowsiness, dizziness, stimulation, nightmares, ataxia, hangover (rare), light-headedness, headache, paranoia

CV: Hypotension, dysrhythmias

GI: Nausea, vomiting, flatulence, diarrhea, ***gastric necrosis***

RESP: ***Depression***

HEMA: ***Eosinophilia, leukopenia***

INTEG: Rash, urticaria, angioedema, fever, purpura, eczema

Contraindications: Hypersensitivity to this drug or triclofos, severe renal disease, severe hepatic disease, GI disorders (oral forms), gastritis

Precautions: Severe cardiac disease, depression, suicidal individuals, asthma, intermittent porphyria, pregnancy category C, lactation, elderly; no specific reversal agent available, use extreme caution in dose calculation when used in pediatric patients for sedation

Pharmacokinetics:

PO: Onset 0.5-1 hr, duration 4-8 hr

REC: Onset slow, duration 4-6 hr; metabolized by liver; excreted by kidneys (inactive metabolite) and in feces; crosses placenta; excreted in breast milk; metabolite is highly protein bound

Drug interactions of concern to dentistry:

• Increased action of both drugs: alcohol, all CNS depressants, including nitrous oxide

DENTAL CONSIDERATIONS

General:

• Consider semisupine chair position for patient comfort due to GI effects of drug.

• Administer syrup in juice or beverage to mask taste and reduce GI upset.

• Contraindicated for use in patients with GI ulcerative disease.

• Have someone drive patient to and from dental office when used for conscious sedation.

• Geriatric patients are more susceptible to drug effects; use lower dose.

• Psychologic and physical dependence may occur with chronic administration.

chlorambucil

(klor-am'byoo-sil)

Leukeran

Drug class.: Antineoplastic alkylating agent

Action: Alkylates DNA, RNA; inhibits enzymes that allow synthesis of amino acids in proteins

Uses: Chronic lymphocytic leukemia, Hodgkin's disease, other lymphomas, macroglobulinemia, nephrotic syndrome, breast carcinoma, choreocarcinoma, ovarian carcinoma

Dosage and routes:

• *Adult:* PO 0.1-0.2 mg/kg/day for 3-6 wk initially, then 2-6 mg/day; maintenance 0.2 mg/kg for 2-4 wk; course may be repeated at 2-4 wk intervals

• *Child:* PO 0.1-0.2 mg/kg/day in divided doses or 4.5 mg/m^2/day as 1 dose or in divided doses

Available forms include: Tabs 2 mg

Side effects/adverse reactions:

ORAL: Stomatitis, sore mouth, lips

CNS: ***Convulsions in children***

GI: Nausea, vomiting, diarrhea, weight loss

RESP: ***Fibrosis, pneumonitis***

HEMA: ***Thrombocytopenia, leukopenia, pancytopenia*** (prolonged use), ***permanent bone marrow depression***

GU: Hyperuremia

INTEG: Alopecia (rare), dermatitis, rash

Contraindications: Radiation therapy within 1 mo, chemotherapy within 1 mo, thrombocytopenia, smallpox vaccination, pregnancy category D (first trimester)

Precautions: *Pneumococcus* vaccination

Pharmacokinetics:

PO: Half-life 2 hr; well absorbed orally; metabolized in liver; excreted in urine

Drug interactions of concern to dentistry:

• Increased seizures: haloperidol, loxapine, phenothiazines, thioxanthenes

• Increased blood dyscrasia: NSAIDs, dapsone, phenothiazines

• Increased infection: corticosteroids

DENTAL CONSIDERATIONS

General:

• Patients on chronic drug therapy may rarely have symptoms of

blood dyscrasias, which can include infection, bleeding, and poor healing.

• Prophylactic antibiotics may be indicated to prevent infection if surgery or deep scaling is planned.

• Avoid prescribing NSAIDs or aspirin-containing products due to risk of GI bleeding.

• Determine why the patient is taking the drug.

• Patients receiving chemotherapy may require palliative treatment for stomatitis.

Consultations:

• In a patient with symptoms of blood dyscrasias, request a medical consult for blood studies and postpone dental treatment until normal values are reestablished.

• Medical consult may be required to assess disease control in the patient.

Teach patient/family:

• Importance of good oral hygiene to prevent soft tissue inflammation

• Caution to prevent injury when using oral hygiene aids

• To avoid mouth rinses with high alcohol content due to drying effects

---

chlordiazepoxide HCl

(klor-dye-az-e-pox′ide)

Libritabs, Librium

🍁 Apo-Chlordiazepoxide, Novo-Poxide

Drug class.: Benzodiazepine antianxiety

Controlled Substance Schedule IV

Action: Produces CNS depression by interacting with a benzodiazepine receptor to facilitate the action of the inhibitory neurotransmitter γ-aminobutyric acid (GABA)

Uses: Short-term management of anxiety, acute alcohol withdrawal, preoperatively for relaxation

Dosage and routes:

Mild anxiety

• *Adult:* PO 5-10 mg tid-qid

• *Child >6 yr:* PO 5 mg bid-qid, not to exceed 10 mg bid-tid

Severe anxiety

• *Adult:* PO 20-25 mg tid-qid

Preoperatively

• *Adult:* PO 5-10 mg tid-qid on day before surgery; IM 50-100 mg 1 hr before surgery

Alcohol withdrawal

• *Adult:* PO/IM/IV 50-100 mg, not to exceed 300 mg/day

Available forms include: Caps 5, 10, 25 mg; tabs 10, 25 mg; powder for IM inj 100 mg

Side effects/adverse reactions:

▼ *ORAL:* Dry mouth

CNS: Dizziness, drowsiness, confusion, headache, anxiety, tremors, stimulation, fatigue, depression, insomnia, hallucinations

CV: Orthostatic hypotension, ***ECG changes, tachycardia,*** hypotension

GI: Constipation, nausea, vomiting, anorexia, diarrhea

EENT: Blurred vision, tinnitus, mydriasis

INTEG: Rash, dermatitis, itching

Contraindications: Hypersensitivity to benzodiazepines, narrow-angle glaucoma, psychosis, pregnancy category D, child <18 yr; ritonavir, indinavir

Precautions: Elderly, debilitated, hepatic disease, renal disease

Pharmacokinetics:

PO: Onset 30 min, peak 30 min, duration 4-6 hr, half-life 5-30 hr;

metabolized by liver; excreted by kidneys; crosses placenta, breast milk

Drug interactions of concern to dentistry:

• Delayed elimination: erythromycin

• Increased CNS depression: CNS depressants, alcohol

• Increased serum levels and prolonged effects of benzodiazepines: ketoconazole, itraconazole, fluconazole, miconazole (systemic)

• Contraindicated with ritonavir, indinavir

DENTAL CONSIDERATIONS

General:

• After supine positioning, have patient sit upright for at least 2 min to avoid orthostatic hypotension.

• Assess salivary flow as a factor in caries, periodontal disease, and candidiasis.

• Psychologic and physical dependence may occur with chronic administration.

• Geriatric patients are more susceptible to drug effects; use lower dose.

• Have someone drive patient to and from dental office if used for conscious sedation.

Consultations:

• Medical consult may be required to assess disease control in the patient.

Teach patient/family:

• Importance of good oral hygiene to prevent soft tissue inflammation

• To avoid mouth rinses with high alcohol content due to drying effects

chlorhexidine gluconate

(klor-hex'i-deen)

Peridex, PerioGard

Drug class.: Antiinfective—oral rinse

Action: Adsorbed on tooth surfaces, dental plaque, and oral mucosa; a sustained reduction of plaque organisms occurs

Uses: Treatment of gingivitis; unlabeled use: acute aphthous ulcers and denture stomatitis

Dosage and routes:

Gingivitis

• *Adult:* Rinse 15 ml for 30 sec bid after brushing and flossing teeth; expectorate after rinsing

Denture stomatitis

• Soak dentures for 1-2 min bid, with patient following oral rinse instructions

Available forms include: Oral rinse, 0.12% in 16 oz bottles

Side effects/adverse reactions:

ORAL: Staining of teeth, tongue, and restorations; increased calculus formation; taste alteration; mucosal desquamation and irritation; transient parotitis

Contraindications: Hypersensitivity

Precautions: Pregnancy category B, lactation, efficacy not established for children <18 yr, not intended for periodontitis

Pharmacokinetics: Approximately 30% of chlorhexidine is retained in the oral cavity and slowly released; poorly absorbed orally

Drug interactions of concern to dentistry:

• Disulfiram-like effects due to alcohol content: Antabuse, metronidazole

DENTAL CONSIDERATIONS

General:

• Perform dental examination and prophylaxis/scaling/root planing before starting rinse.

• Place on frequent recall due to oral side effects.

• Use discretion when prescribing to patients with anterior facial restorations with rough surfaces or margins.

Teach patient/family:

• Instruct patient to eat, brush, and floss before using rinse

• Do not rinse with water after using chlorhexidine

• Inform patient of oral side effects

chlorhexidine gluconate chip

(klor-hex'i-deen)

PerioChip

Drug class.: Antiinfective

Action: Interferes with the integrity of the bacterial cell membrane, causing leakage of the intracellular components; penetrates into the cell, precipitates the cytoplasm, and the cell dies; effective against numerous supragingival and subgingival bacteria

Uses: Adjunct to scaling and root planing for reduction of the subgingival bacterial flora

Dosage and routes:

• *Adult:* Insert chip into a periodontal pocket with probing depth ≥5 mm. Up to eight chips may be inserted per single visit. Treatment recommended once every 3 mo in pockets ≥5 mm in depth. If chip dislodges within 48 hr of placement, replace with new chip. Do not replace chips lost after 48 hr, but reevaluate in 3 mo. If chip is dislodged 7 days or more after placement, consider this a full course of treatment.

Available forms include: CHIP 2.5 mg

Side effects/adverse reactions:

▼ *ORAL: Localized pain, tenderness, aching, throbbing, toothache*

NOTE: All other side effects reported did not differ from placebo chip

Contraindications: Hypersensitivity

Precautions: Not recommended for acutely abscessed periodontal pocket, pregnancy category C, use in children not established

Pharmacokinetics:

TOP: 40% of chlorhexidine released in first 24 hr, remainder released over 7-10 days; no detectable plasma levels

Drug interactions of concern to dentistry:

• None reported

DENTAL CONSIDERATIONS

General:

• Avoid brushing or use of dental floss at site of chip placement.

Teach patient/family:

• Notify dentist immediately if chip is dislodged or if pain, swelling, or other symptoms occur

chloroquine HCl/ chloroquine phosphate

(klor'oh-kwin)

Aralen HCl, Aralen Phosphate

Drug class.: Antimalarial

Action: Inhibits parasite replications, transcription of DNA to RNA by forming complexes with DNA of parasite; unapproved uses:

juvenile arthritis, rheumatoid arthritis, discoid or systemic lupus erythematosus, solar urticaria

Uses: Malaria caused by *P. vivax, P. malariae, P. ovale, P. falciparum* (some strains); rheumatoid arthritis; amebiasis

Dosage and routes:

Malaria suppression

• *Adult:* 500 mg on exactly the same day each week (500 mg phosphate = 300 mg base)

• *Child:* 5 mg/kg, calculated as base, on same day each week; not to exceed adult dose

Acute attack: PO initial 1 phosphate form, followed by 500 mg after 6-8 hr, then 500 mg/day on each of 2 following days

Rheumatoid arthritis

• *Adult:* PO up to 4 mg/kg/day

Available forms include: Tabs 250, 500 mg; inj IM 50 mg/ml

Side effects/adverse reactions:

▼ *ORAL:* Stomatitis, discolored mucosa, lichenoid drug reaction

CNS: ***Convulsion,*** headache, stimulation, fatigue, irritability, bad dreams, dizziness, confusion, psychosis, decreased reflexes

CV: Hypotension, heart block, asystole with syncope, ECG changes

GI: Nausea, vomiting, anorexia, diarrhea, cramps, weight loss

HEMA: ***Thrombocytopenia, agranulocytosis, hemolytic anemia, leukopenia***

EENT: Blurred vision, corneal changes, retinal changes, difficulty focusing, tinnitus, vertigo, deafness, photophobia, corneal edema

INTEG: ***Exfoliative dermatitis,*** alopecia, pruritus, pigmentary changes, skin eruptions, lichenoid eruptions, eczema

Contraindications: Hypersensitivity, retinal field changes, porphyria, children (long-term use)

Precautions: Pregnancy category C, children, blood dyscrasias, severe GI disease, neurologic disease, alcoholism, hepatic disease, G6PD deficiency, psoriasis, eczema

Pharmacokinetics:

PO: Peak 1-2 hr, half-life 3-5 days; metabolized in the liver; excreted in urine, feces, breast milk; crosses placenta

Drug interactions of concern to dentistry:

• Hepatotoxicity: alcohol, hepatotoxic drugs

DENTAL CONSIDERATIONS

General:

• Patients on chronic drug therapy may rarely have symptoms of blood dyscrasias, which can include infection, bleeding, and poor healing.

• Avoid dental light in patient's eyes; offer dark glasses for patient comfort.

• Determine why the patient is taking the drug.

Consultations:

• In a patient with symptoms of blood dyscrasias, request a medical consult for blood studies and postpone dental treatment until normal values are reestablished.

Teach patient/family:

• Importance of good oral hygiene to prevent soft tissue inflammation

• To avoid mouth rinses with high alcohol content due to drying effects

chlorothiazide

(klor-oh-thye′a-zide)
Diuril
Drug class.: Thiazide diuretic

Action: Acts on distal tubule by increasing excretion of water, sodium, chloride, potassium
Uses: Edema, hypertension, diuresis
Dosage and routes:
Edema, hypertension
• *Adult:* PO/IV 500 mg-2 g qd in 2 divided doses
Diuresis
• *Child >6 mo:* PO 20 mg/kg/day in divided doses
• *Child <6 mo:* PO up to 30 mg/kg/day in 2 divided doses
Available forms include: Tabs 250, 500 mg; oral susp 250 mg/5 ml; inj 500 mg
Side effects/adverse reactions:
▼ *ORAL: Dry mouth, increased thirst,* lichenoid drug reaction
CNS: Dizziness, fatigue, weakness, drowsiness, paresthesia, anxiety, depression, headache
CV: Irregular pulse, orthostatic hypotension, palpitation, volume depletion
GI: Nausea, vomiting, anorexia, ***hepatitis,*** constipation, diarrhea, cramps, pancreatitis, GI irritation
HEMA: ***Aplastic anemia, hemolytic anemia, leukopenia, agranulocytosis, thrombocytopenia, neutropenia***
GU: Frequency, ***uremia,*** polyuria, glucosuria
EENT: Blurred vision
INTEG: Rash, urticaria, purpura, photosensitivity, fever
META: Hyperglycemia, hyperuricemia, hypomagnesemia, increased creatinine, BUN
ELECT: Hypokalemia, hypercalcemia, hyponatremia, hypochloremia
Contraindications: Hypersensitivity to thiazides or sulfonamides, anuria, renal decompensation, pregnancy category D
Precautions: Hypokalemia, renal disease, hepatic disease, gout, COPD, lupus erythematosus, diabetes mellitus, elderly
Pharmacokinetics:
PO: Onset 2 hr, peak 4 hr, duration 6-12 hr; crosses placenta; excreted in breast milk
Drug interactions of concern to dentistry:
• Increased photosensitization: tetracyclines
• Decreased hypotensive response, nephrotoxicity: indomethacin and other NSAIDs

DENTAL CONSIDERATIONS
General:
• Monitor vital signs every appointment due to cardiovascular side effects.
• After supine positioning, have patient sit upright for at least 2 min before standing to avoid orthostatic hypotension.
• Patients on chronic drug therapy may rarely have symptoms of blood dyscrasias, which can include infection, bleeding, and poor healing.
• Assess salivary flow as a factor in caries, periodontal disease, and candidiasis.
• Limit use of sodium-containing products such as saline IV fluids for patients with a dietary salt restriction.
• Stress from dental procedures may compromise cardiovascular function; determine patient risk.

• Short appointments and a stress reduction protocol may be required for anxious patients.
• Patients taking diuretics should be monitored for serum K^+ levels.

Consultations:
• In a patient with symptoms of blood dyscrasias, request a medical consult for blood studies and postpone dental treatment until normal values are reestablished.
• Medical consult may be required to assess disease control and patient's ability to tolerate stress.
• Physician should be informed if significant xerostomic side effects occur (increased caries, sore tongue, problems eating or swallowing, difficulty wearing prosthesis) so a medication change can be considered.

Teach patient/family:
• Importance of good oral hygiene to prevent soft tissue inflammation
• Caution to prevent injury when using oral hygiene aids

When chronic dry mouth occurs, advise patient:
• To avoid mouth rinses with high alcohol content due to drying effects
• To use daily home fluoride products for anticaries effect
• To use sugarless gum, frequent sips of water, or saliva substitutes

---

chlorphenesin carbamate

(klor-fen′e-sin)

Maolate

Drug class.: Skeletal muscle relaxant, central acting

Action: Unknown; may be related to sedative properties; does not directly relax muscle or depress nerve conduction

Uses: Adjunct for relieving pain in acute, painful musculoskeletal conditions

Dosage and routes:
• *Adult:* PO 800 mg tid, maintenance 400 mg qid, not to exceed 8 wk

Available forms include: Tabs 400 mg

Side effects/adverse reactions:
CNS: Dizziness, weakness, drowsiness, headache, tremor, depression, insomnia, confusion
CV: Postural hypotension, tachycardia
GI: Nausea, vomiting, hiccups
HEMA: ***Blood dyscrasias, leukopenia, thrombocytopenia, agranulocytosis***
EENT: Diplopia, temporary loss of vision
INTEG: Rash, pruritus, fever, facial flushing
SYST: ***Anaphylaxis,*** drug fever

Contraindications: Hypersensitivity, child <12 yr, intermittent porphyria, carbamate derivatives

Precautions: Renal disease, hepatic disease, addictive personality, pregnancy category unknown, elderly, lactation, using for >8 wk, impairment of mental alertness

Pharmacokinetics:
PO: Onset 0.5 hr, peak 1-2 hr, duration 4-6 hr, half-life 4 hr; metabolized by liver; excreted in urine; crosses placenta; excreted in breast milk (large amounts)

Drug interactions of concern to dentistry:
• Increased CNS depression: alcohol, tricyclic antidepressants, narcotics, barbiturates, sedatives, hypnotics

DENTAL CONSIDERATIONS
General:
• Patients on chronic drug therapy may rarely have symptoms of blood dyscrasias, which can include infection, bleeding, and poor healing.
• After supine positioning, have patient sit upright for at least 2 min to avoid orthostatic hypotension.
• Consider semisupine chair position for patient comfort if GI side effects occur.
Consultations:
• In a patient with symptoms of blood dyscrasias, request a medical consult for blood studies and postpone dental treatment until normal values are reestablished.
Teach patient/family:
• Importance of good oral hygiene to prevent soft tissue inflammation
• Caution to prevent trauma when using oral hygiene aids
• To report oral lesions, soreness, or bleeding to dentist

chlorpheniramine maleate

(klor-fen-eer'a-meen)

Aller-Chlor, Chlo-Amine, Chlorate, Chlor-Trimeton, Gen-Allerate, Pedia Care Allergy Formula, Phenetron, Telachlor, Teldrin

♣ Chlor-Tripolon, Novo-Pheniram

Drug class.: Antihistamine, H_1-receptor antagonist

Action: Acts on blood vessels, GI system, respiratory system by competing with histamine for H_1-receptor site; decreases allergic response by blocking histamine
Uses: Allergy symptoms, rhinitis
Dosage and routes:
• *Adult:* PO 2-4 mg tid-qid, not to exceed 36 mg/day; time rel 8-12 mg bid-tid, not to exceed 36 mg/day; IM/IV/SC 5-40 mg/day
• *Child 6-12 yr:* PO 2 mg q4-6h, not to exceed 12 mg/day; sus rel 8 mg hs or qd, sus rel not recommended for child <6 yr
• *Child 2-5 yr:* PO 1 mg q4-6h, not to exceed 4 mg/day
Available forms include: Chew tabs 2 mg; tabs 4 mg; time rel tabs 8, 12 mg; time rel caps 8, 12 mg; syr 2 mg/5 ml; inj IM/SC/IV 10, 100 mg/ml
Side effects/adverse reactions:
▼ *ORAL:* Dry mouth
CNS: Dizziness, drowsiness, poor coordination, fatigue, anxiety, euphoria, confusion, paresthesia, neuritis
GI: Nausea, anorexia, diarrhea
RESP: Increased thick secretions, wheezing, chest tightness
HEMA: ***Thrombocytopenia, agranulocytosis, hemolytic anemia***
GU: Retention, dysuria, frequency
EENT: Blurred vision, dilated pupils, tinnitus, nasal stuffiness, dry nose, throat
INTEG: Photosensitivity
Contraindications: Hypersensitivity to H_1-receptor antagonists, acute asthma attack, lower respiratory tract disease
Precautions: Increased intraocular pressure, renal disease, cardiac disease, hypertension, bronchial asthma, seizure disorder, stenosed peptic ulcers, hyperthyroidism, prostatic hypertrophy, bladder neck obstruction, pregnancy category B, elderly
Pharmacokinetics:
PO: Onset 20-60 min, duration

8-12 hr, half-life 20-24 hr; detoxified in liver; excreted by kidneys (metabolites/free drug)

Drug interactions of concern to dentistry:

• Increased CNS depression: alcohol, all CNS depressants

• Increased anticholinergic effect: other anticholinergics, phenothiazines, tricyclic antidepressants

DENTAL CONSIDERATIONS

General:

• Assess salivary flow as a factor in caries, periodontal disease, and candidiasis.

• Consider semisupine chair position for patients with respiratory disease.

• Determine why the patient is taking the drug.

Teach patient/family:

• Importance of good oral hygiene to prevent soft tissue inflammation

• Caution to prevent injury when using oral hygiene aids

When chronic dry mouth occurs, advise patient:

• To avoid mouth rinses with high alcohol content due to drying effects

• To use daily home fluoride products for anticaries effect

• To use sugarless gum, frequent sips of water, or saliva substitutes

chlorpromazine HCl

(klor-proe'ma-zeen)

Largactil, Ormazine, Thorazine, Thor-Prom

Chlorpromanyl, Novo-Chlorpromazine

Drug class.: Phenothiazine antipsychotic

Action: Blocks neurotransmission at dopaminergic synapses in the cerebral cortex, hypothalamus, and limbic system; exhibits strong peripheral α-adrenergic, anticholinergic blocking action; mechanism for antipsychotic effects is unclear

Uses: Psychotic disorders, mania, schizophrenia, anxiety, intractable hiccups, nausea, vomiting, preoperatively for relaxation, acute intermittent porphyria, behavioral problems in children

Dosage and routes:

Psychiatry

• *Adult:* PO 10-50 mg q1-4h initially, then increase up to 2000 mg/day if necessary; IM 10-50 mg q1-4h

• *Child:* PO 0.25 mg/lb q4-6h or 0.5 mg/kg; IM 0.25 mg/lb q6-8h or 0.5 mg/kg; REC 0.5 mg/lb q6-8h or 1 mg/kg

Nausea and vomiting

• *Adult:* PO 10-25 mg q4-6h prn; IM 25-50 mg q3h prn; REC 50-100 mg q6-8h prn, not to exceed 400 mg/day; IV 25-50 mg qd-qid

• *Child:* PO 0.25 mg/lb q4-6h prn; IM 0.25 mg/lb q6-8h prn not to exceed 40 mg/day (<5 yr) or 75 mg/day (5-12 yr); REC 0.5 mg/lb q6-8h prn; IV 0.55 mg/kg q6-8h

Intractable hiccups

• *Adult:* PO 25-50 mg tid-qid; IM 25-50 mg (used only if PO dose does not work); IV 25-50 mg in 500-1000 ml saline (only for severe hiccups)

Available forms include: Tabs 10, 25, 50, 100, 200 mg; time rel caps 30, 75, 150, 200, 300 mg; syr 10 mg/5 ml; conc 30, 100 mg/ml; supp 25, 100 mg; inj IM/IV 25 mg/ml

Side effects/adverse reactions:

▼ *ORAL: Dry mouth,* lichenoid reaction

CNS: Extrapyramidal symptoms:

pseudoparkinsonism, akathisia, dystonia, tardive dyskinesia, seizures, headache
CV: Orthostatic hypotension, ***cardiac arrest, tachycardia,*** hypertension, ECG changes
GI: Nausea, vomiting, anorexia, constipation, diarrhea, jaundice, weight gain
RESP: ***Laryngospasm, respiratory depression,*** dyspnea
HEMA: ***Leukopenia, leukocytosis, agranulocytosis,*** anemia
GU: Urinary retention, urinary frequency, enuresis, impotence, amenorrhea, gynecomastia, breast engorgement
EENT: Blurred vision, glaucoma, dry eyes
INTEG: Rash, photosensitivity, dermatitis

Contraindications: Hypersensitivity, circulatory collapse, liver damage, cerebral arteriosclerosis, coronary disease, severe hypertension/hypotension, blood dyscrasias, coma, child <2 yr, brain damage, bone marrow depression, alcohol and barbiturate withdrawal states

Precautions: Pregnancy category C, lactation, seizure disorders, hypertension, hepatic disease, cardiac disease, elderly

Pharmacokinetics:
PO: Onset erratic, peak 2-4 hr, duration may be detected for up to 6 mo after last dose
IM: Onset 15-30 min, peak 15-20 min, duration may be detected for up to 6 mo after last dose
IV: Onset 5 min, peak 10 min, duration may be detected for up to 6 mo after last dose
REC: Onset erratic, peak 3 hr, elimination half-life 10-30 hr; 95% bound to plasma proteins; metabolized by liver; excreted in urine (metabolites); crosses placenta; enters breast milk

Drug interactions of concern to dentistry:
- Increased sedation: other CNS depressants, alcohol, barbiturate anesthetics, opioid analgesics
- Hypotension, tachycardia: epinephrine (systemic)
- Increased extrapyramidal effects: related drugs such as haloperidol, droperidol, and metoclopramide
- Additive photosensitization: tetracyclines
- Increased anticholinergic effects: anticholinergics

DENTAL CONSIDERATIONS

General:
- Monitor vital signs every appointment due to cardiovascular side effects.
- Patients on chronic drug therapy may rarely have symptoms of blood dyscrasias, which can include infection, bleeding, and poor healing.
- After supine positioning, have patient sit upright for at least 2 min before standing to avoid orthostatic hypotension.
- Assess salivary flow as a factor in caries, periodontal disease, and candidiasis.
- Avoid dental light in patient's eyes; offer dark glasses for patient comfort.
- Assess for presence of extrapyramidal motor symptoms, such as tardive dyskinesia and akathisia. Extrapyramidal motor activity may complicate dental treatment.
- Geriatric patients are more susceptible to drug effects; use a lower dose.

Consultations:
- In a patient with symptoms of

blood dyscrasias, request a medical consult for blood studies and postpone dental treatment until normal values are reestablished.

• Take precautions if dental surgery is anticipated, anesthesia required.

• If signs of tardive dyskinesia or akathisia are present, refer to physician.

• Physician should be informed if significant xerostomic side effects occur (increased caries, sore tongue, problems eating or swallowing, difficulty wearing prosthesis) so a medication change can be considered.

Teach patient/family:

• Importance of good oral hygiene to prevent soft tissue inflammation

• Caution to prevent injury when using oral hygiene aids

• To use electric toothbrush if patient has difficulty holding conventional devices

When chronic dry mouth occurs, advise patient:

• To avoid mouth rinses with high alcohol content due to drying effects

• To use daily home fluoride products for anticaries effect

• To use sugarless gum, frequent sips of water, or saliva substitutes

---

chlorpropamide

(klor-proe′pa-mide)

Diabinese

✤ Apo-Chlorpromaide, Novopropamide

Drug class.: Antidiabetic, sulfonylurea (first generation)

Action: Causes functioning β-cells in pancreas to release insulin, leading to drop in blood glucose levels; may improve insulin binding to insulin receptors or increase the number of insulin receptors; not effective if patient lacks functioning β-cells

Uses: Stable adult-onset diabetes mellitus (type 2)

Dosage and routes:

• *Adult:* PO 100-250 mg qd, initially, then 100-500 mg maintenance according to response; not to exceed 750 mg/day

Available forms include: Tabs 100, 250 mg

Side effects/adverse reactions:

▼ *ORAL:* Lichenoid drug reaction

CNS: Headache, weakness, dizziness, drowsiness, tinnitus, fatigue, vertigo

GI: ***Hepatotoxicity, cholestatic jaundice,*** nausea, vomiting, diarrhea, heartburn

HEMA: ***Leukopenia, thrombocytopenia, agranulocytosis, aplastic anemia, pancytopenia, hemolytic anemia***

INTEG: Rash, allergic reactions, pruritus, urticaria, eczema, photosensitivity, erythema

ENDO: ***Hypoglycemia***

Contraindications: Hypersensitivity to sulfonylureas, juvenile or brittle diabetes, pregnancy category D

Precautions: Elderly, cardiac disease, thyroid disease, renal disease, hepatic disease, severe hypoglycemic reactions

Pharmacokinetics:

PO: Completely absorbed by GI route, onset 1 hr, peak 3-6 hr, duration 60 hr, half-life 36 hr; 90%-95% is plasma protein bound; metabolized in liver; excreted in urine (metabolites and unchanged drug), breast milk

Drug interactions of concern to dentistry:
- Increased hypoglycemic effects: salicylates, NSAIDs, ketoconazole, miconazole
- Decreased action: corticosteroids, sympathomimetics

DENTAL CONSIDERATIONS

General:
- Patients on chronic drug therapy may rarely have symptoms of blood dyscrasias, which can include infection, bleeding, and poor healing.
- Short appointments and a stress reduction protocol may be required for anxious patients.
- Question patient about self-monitoring of drug's antidiabetic effect, including blood glucose values or finger-stick records.
- Ensure that patient is following prescribed diet and regularly takes medication.
- Determine if medication controls disease. Patients with diabetes may be more susceptible to infection and have delayed wound healing.
- Question patient about self-monitoring of drug's antidiabetic effect.
- Avoid prescribing aspirin-containing products.

Consultations:
- In a patient with symptoms of blood dyscrasias, request a medical consult for blood studies and postpone dental treatment until normal values are reestablished.
- Medical consult may be required to assess disease control in the patient.
- Medical consult may include data from patient's blood glucose monitoring, including glycosylated hemoglobin or HbA_{1c} testing.

Teach patient/family:
- Importance of good oral hygiene to prevent soft tissue inflammation
- Caution to prevent injury when using oral hygiene aids
- To avoid mouth rinses with high alcohol content due to drying effects

C

---

chlorthalidone

(klor-thal′i-done)

Hygroton, Thalitone

🍁 Apo-Chlorthalidone, Novo-Thalidone, Uridon

Drug class.: Diuretic with thiazide-like effects

Action: Acts on distal tubule by increasing excretion of water, sodium, chloride, potassium

Uses: Edema, hypertension, diuresis, CHF

Dosage and routes:
- *Adult:* PO 25-100 mg/day or 100 mg qod
- *Child:* PO 2 mg/kg 3 × weekly

Available forms include: Tabs 25, 50, 100 mg

Side effects/adverse reactions:

▼ *ORAL: Dry mouth, increased thirst*

CNS: Dizziness, fatigue, weakness, drowsiness, paresthesia, anxiety, depression, headache

CV: Irregular pulse, orthostatic hypotension, palpitation, volume depletion

GI: Nausea, vomiting, anorexia, ***hepatitis,*** constipation, diarrhea, cramps, pancreatitis, GI irritation

HEMA: ***Aplastic anemia, hemolytic anemia, leukopenia, agranulocytosis, thrombocytopenia, neutropenia***

GU: Frequency, ***uremia,*** glucosuria, polyuria

EENT: Blurred vision
INTEG: Rash, urticaria, purpura, photosensitivity, fever
META: Hyperglycemia, hyperuremia, increased creatinine, BUN
ELECT: Hypokalemia, hypomagnesemia, hypercalcemia, hyponatremia, hypochloremia
Contraindications: Hypersensitivity to thiazides or sulfonamides, anuria, renal decompensation
Precautions: Hypokalemia, renal disease, pregnancy category C, hepatic disease, gout, diabetes mellitus, elderly
Pharmacokinetics:
PO: Onset 2 hr, peak 6 hr, duration 24-72 hr, half-life 40 hr; excreted unchanged by kidneys; crosses placenta; enters breast milk
Drug interactions of concern to dentistry:
• Increased photosensitization: tetracyclines
• Decreased hypotensive response, nephrotoxicity: NSAIDs, indomethacin

DENTAL CONSIDERATIONS
General:
• Monitor vital signs every appointment due to cardiovascular side effects.
• After supine positioning, have patient sit upright for at least 2 min before standing to avoid orthostatic hypotension.
• Patients on chronic drug therapy may rarely have symptoms of blood dyscrasias, which can include infection, bleeding, and poor healing.
• Assess salivary flow as a factor in caries, periodontal disease, and candidiasis.
• Limit use of sodium-containing products such as saline IV fluids for those patients with a dietary salt restriction.
• Short appointments and a stress reduction protocol may be required for anxious patients.
• Stress from dental procedures may compromise cardiovascular function; determine patient risk.
Consultations:
• In a patient with symptoms of blood dyscrasias, request a medical consult for blood studies and postpone dental treatment until normal values are reestablished.
• Medical consult may be required to assess disease control and patient's ability to tolerate stress.
Teach patient/family:
• Importance of good oral hygiene to prevent soft tissue inflammation
• Caution to prevent injury when using oral hygiene aids
When chronic dry mouth occurs, advise patient:
To avoid mouth rinses with high alcohol content due to drying effects
To use daily home fluoride products for anticaries effect
To use sugarless gum, frequent sips of water, or saliva substitutes

chlorzoxazone

(klor-zox'a-zone)
EZE-DS, Paraflex, Parafon Forte DSC, Relaxazone, Remular, Remular-S, Strifton Forte DSC
Drug class.: Skeletal muscle relaxant, centrally acting

Action: Depresses multisynaptic pathways in the spinal cord

Uses: Adjunct for relief of muscle spasm in musculoskeletal conditions

Dosage and routes:

• *Adult:* PO 250-750 mg tid-qid

• *Child:* PO 20 mg/kg/day in divided doses tid-qid

Available forms include: Tabs 250, 500 mg (DSC)

Side effects/adverse reactions:

CNS: Dizziness, drowsiness, headache, insomnia, stimulation, malaise

GI: Nausea, ***hepatotoxicity, jaundice,*** vomiting, anorexia, diarrhea, constipation

HEMA: ***Granulocytopenia, anemia***

GU: Urine discoloration

INTEG: ***Angioedema,*** rash, pruritus, petechiae, ecchymoses

SYST: ***Anaphylaxis***

Contraindications: Hypersensitivity, impaired hepatic function

Precautions: Pregnancy category C, lactation, hepatic disease, elderly

Pharmacokinetics:

PO: Onset 1 hr, peak 3-4 hr, duration 6 hr, half-life 1 hr; metabolized in liver; excreted in urine (metabolites)

Drug interactions of concern to dentistry:

• Increased CNS depression: alcohol, narcotics, barbiturates, sedatives, hypnotics

DENTAL CONSIDERATIONS

General:

• Determine why the patient is taking the drug.

• Consider semisupine chair position if back is involved.

• When used for dental-related problems, consider aspirin or NSAIDs to improve response.

cholestyramine

(koe-less-teer'a-meen)

Questran, Questran Lite, Prevalite

Drug class.: Antihyperlipidemic

Action: Absorbs, combines with bile acids to form insoluble complex that is excreted through feces; loss of bile acids lowers cholesterol levels

Uses: Primary hypercholesterolemia, pruritus associated with biliary obstruction, diarrhea caused by excess bile acid, digitalis toxicity, xanthomas

Dosage and routes:

• *Adult:* PO 4 g once or twice daily ac; maintenance dose 8-24 g in 2-6 divided doses

• *Child:* PO 4 g/day in 2 divided doses; administer with food or drink

Available forms include: Powder 5 g, 5.5 g, and 9 g

Side effects/adverse reactions:

CNS: Headache, dizziness, drowsiness, vertigo, tinnitus

GI: Constipation, abdominal pain, nausea, fecal impaction, hemorrhoids, flatulence, vomiting, steatorrhea, peptic ulcer

HEMA: ***Hyperchloremic acidosis; bleeding;*** decreased pro-time, decreased vitamin A, D, K; red cell folate content

INTEG: Rash; irritation of perianal area, tongue, skin

MS: Muscle, joint pain

Contraindications: Hypersensitivity, biliary obstruction

Precautions: Pregnancy category C, lactation, children

Pharmacokinetics:
PO: Excreted in feces, max effect in 2 wk

Drug interactions of concern to dentistry:
• Decreased absorption of tetracyclines, cephalexin, phenobarbital, corticosteroids, clindamycin, penicillins; administer doses several hours apart

DENTAL CONSIDERATIONS
General:
• Consider semisupine chair position for patient comfort due to GI effects of disease.

---

choline salicylate

(koe'leen)
Arthropan
Drug class.: Salicylate analgesic

Action: Inhibits prostaglandin synthesis by interfering with cyclooxygenase need for biosynthesis; possesses analgesic, antipyretic, and antiinflammatory properties

Uses: Mild-to-moderate pain or fever, arthritis, juvenile rheumatoid arthritis

Dosage and routes:
Arthritis
• *Adult:* PO 870-1740 mg qid

Pain/fever
• *Adult and child >12 yr:* PO 870 mg q3-4h prn; maximum 6 doses/day
• *Child 3-6 yr:* PO 107-133 mg, kg of body weight in divided doses

Available forms include: Liq 870 mg/5 ml (salicylate equivalent to 650 mg aspirin)

Side effects/adverse reactions:
CNS: ***Coma, convulsions,*** stimulation, drowsiness, dizziness, confusion, headache, flushing, hallucinations
CV: Rapid pulse, pulmonary edema
GI: Nausea, vomiting, GI bleeding, diarrhea, heartburn, **hepatitis,** anorexia
RESP: Wheezing, hyperpnea
HEMA: ***Thrombocytopenia, agranulocytosis, leukopenia, neutropenia, hemolytic anemia,*** increased pro-time
EENT: Tinnitus, hearing loss
INTEG: Rash, urticaria, bruising
ENDO: Hypoglycemia, hyponatremia, hypokalemia

Contraindications: Hypersensitivity to salicylates, GI bleeding, bleeding disorders, child <3 yr, vitamin K deficiency, child with flulike symptoms

Precautions: Anemia, hepatic disease, renal disease, Hodgkin's disease, pregnancy category C, lactation, geriatric patients

Pharmacokinetics:
PO: Onset 15-30 min; metabolized by liver; excreted by kidneys; crosses placenta; excreted in breast milk

Drug interactions of concern to dentistry:
• Increased risk of hypoglycemia: oral hypoglycemics
• Increased risk of GI complaints: alcohol, NSAIDs, steroids
• Avoid prolonged or concurrent use with ASA, NSAIDs, corticosteroids, acetaminophen
• Increased effects of anticoagulants, valproic acid, methotrexate, dipyridamole
• Decreased effects of probenecid, sulfinpyrazone

DENTAL CONSIDERATIONS
General:
• Patients on chronic drug therapy may rarely have symptoms of

blood dyscrasias, which can include infection, bleeding, and poor healing.
• Consider semisupine chair position for patient comfort if GI side effects occur.
• Determine why the patient is taking the drug.
• Evaluate allergic reactions: rash, urticaria; patients with allergy to salicylates may not be able to take NSAIDs. Drug may need to be discontinued.
• Consider semisupine chair position for patient comfort due to arthritic disease.

Consultations:
• In a patient with symptoms of blood dyscrasias, request a medical consult for blood studies and postpone dental treatment until normal values are reestablished.
• Medical consult may be required to assess disease control and patient's ability to tolerate stress.
• Tinnitus, ringing, roaring in ears after high dose and long-term therapy requires referral for evaluation for salicylism.

Teach patient/family:
• Importance of good oral hygiene to prevent soft tissue inflammation
• Caution to prevent trauma when using oral hygiene aids
• To read label on other OTC drugs; many contain aspirin
• To report oral lesions, soreness, or bleeding to dentist
• To avoid alcohol ingestion; GI bleeding may occur

ciclopirox olamine (topical)

(sye-kloe-peer′ox)
Loprox

Drug class.: Topical antifungal

Action: Interferes with fungal cell membrane, which increases permeability, leaking of cell nutrients
Uses: Tinea cruris, tinea corporis, tinea pedis, tinea versicolor, cutaneous candidiasis
Dosage and routes:
• *Adult and child >10 yr:* TOP rub into affected area bid
Available forms include: Cream 1%, lotion 1%
Side effects/adverse reactions:
INTEG: Rash, urticaria, stinging, burning, pruritus, pain
Contraindications: Hypersensitivity
Precautions: Pregnancy category B, lactation, child <10 yr

DENTAL CONSIDERATIONS
General:
• There are neither dental drug interactions nor relevant considerations to dentistry for this drug.

cilostazol

(sil′os-tah-zol)
Pletal

Drug class.: Phosphodiesterase inhibitor

Action: Inhibits phosphodiesterase III enzymes, decreasing cAMP degradation to increase cAMP in platelets and blood vessels; inhibits platelet aggregation and causes vasodilation in vascular beds
Uses: Reduction of symptoms of

intermittent claudication (leg pain on walking)

Dosage and routes:

• *Adult:* PO 100 mg bid at least 30 min before or 2 hr after breakfast and dinner

NOTE: With inhibitors of CYP3A4, give 50 mg bid

Available forms include: Tabs 50, 100 mg

Side effects/adverse reactions:

▼ *ORAL:* Glossitis, gingival bleeding

CNS: Headache, palpitation, dizziness, vertigo, tachycardia

CV: Peripheral edema

GI: Diarrhea, abdominal pain, dyspepsia, nausea, flatulence, vomiting

RESP: Bronchitis

HEMA: Anemia, purpura, ecchymosis

GU: UTI

EENT: Pharyngitis, rhinitis

INTEG: Dry skin, urticaria

META: Increased creatinine, hyperlipidemia, hyperuricemia

MS: Arthralgia, leg cramps

MISC: Infection, malaise, asthenia

Contraindications: Hypersensitivity, CHF

Precautions: Pregnancy category C, lactation, children

Pharmacokinetics:

PO: High-fat meal enhances absorption; metabolized by cytochrome P-450 enzymes (3A4); active metabolites, peak plasma levels 2-3 hr; highly protein bound (95%-98%)

Drug interactions of concern to dentistry:

• Risk of interaction with other platelet aggregation inhibitors possible, not established

• Risk of drug interaction with cytochrome P-450 3A4 inhibitors: erythromycin, ketoconazole, itraconazole, diltiazem, grapefruit juice

DENTAL CONSIDERATIONS

General:

• Determine why patient is taking the drug.

• Avoid products that affect platelet function, such as aspirin and NSAIDs.

Consultations:

• Consultation with physician may be needed if excessive bleeding occurs during dental treatment

• Consult should include data on bleeding time.

Teach patient/family:

• Importance of updating health and drug history if physician makes any changes in evaluation/drug regimens

• To inform dentist of unusual bleeding episodes following dental treatment

• To prevent trauma when using oral hygiene aids

• Importance of good oral hygiene to prevent soft tissue inflammation

cimetidine

(sye-met'i-deen)

Nu-Cimet, Peptol, Tagamet, Tagamet HB (OTC), Tagamet HB 200 (OTC)

🍁 Apo-Cimetidine, Gen-Cimetidine, Novo-Cimetidine, PMS-Cimetidine

Drug class.: H_2 histamine receptor antagonist

Action: Inhibits histamine at H_2-receptor site in parietal cells, which inhibits gastric acid secretion

Uses: Short-term treatment of duodenal and gastric ulcers and maintenance

Dosage and routes:

• *Adult and child >16 yr:* PO 300 mg qid with meals, hs × 8 wk or 400 mg bid, 800 mg hs; after 8 wk give hs dose only; IV bol 300 mg/20 ml 0.9% NaCl over 1-2 min q6h; IV inf 300 mg/50 ml D_5W over 15-20 min; IM 300 mg q6h, not to exceed 2400 mg

OTC dose: PO 200 mg qd-bid

Prophylaxis of duodenal ulcer

• *Adult and child >16 yr:* 400 mg hs

Available forms include: Tabs (100, 200 mg OTC) 300, 400, 800 mg; liq 300 mg/5 ml; inj IV 300 mg/2 ml, 300 mg/50 ml 0.9% NaCl; susp 200 mg

Side effects/adverse reactions:

▼ *ORAL:* Lichenoid reaction

CNS: Confusion, headache, ***convulsions,*** depression, dizziness, anxiety, weakness, psychosis, tremors

CV: Bradycardia, tachycardia

GI: Diarrhea, ***paralytic ileus, jaundice,*** abdominal cramps

HEMA: ***Agranulocytosis, thrombocytopenia, neutropenia, aplastic anemia,*** increase in pro-time

GU: Gynecomastia, galactorrhea, impotence, increase in BUN, creatinine

INTEG: ***Exfoliative dermatitis,*** urticaria, rash, alopecia, sweating, flushing

Contraindications: Hypersensitivity

Precautions: Pregnancy category B, lactation, child <16 yr, organic brain syndrome, hepatic disease, renal disease

Pharmacokinetics:

PO: Peak 1-1.5 hr, half-life 1.5 hr; metabolized by liver; excreted in urine (unchanged); crosses placenta; enters breast milk

Drug interactions of concern to dentistry:

• GI ulceration, bleeding: aspirin, NSAIDs

• Decreased absorption: sodium bicarbonate

• Decreased absorption of fluconazole, ketoconazole, tetracycline (take doses 2 hr apart)

• Increased blood levels of metronidazole, alcohol, lidocaine, narcotic analgesics

DENTAL CONSIDERATIONS

General:

• Monitor vital signs every appointment due to cardiovascular side effects.

• Consider semisupine chair position for patient comfort due to GI effects of disease.

• Avoid prescribing aspirin or NSAID-containing products in patients with active upper GI disease; there is a risk of irritation and ulceration.

• Sodium bicarbonate products can be used 1 hr before or 1 hr after cimetidine dose.

Teach patient/family:

• Importance of good oral hygiene to prevent soft tissue inflammation

• Caution to prevent injury when using oral hygiene aids

---

cinoxacin

(sin-ox'a-sin)

Cinobac

Drug class.: Urinary tract antibacterial

Action: Interferes with DNA replication

Uses: UTIs caused by *E. coli, Klebsiella, Enterobacter, P. mirabilis, P. vulgaris, P. morganii, Serratia, Citrobacter*

Dosage and routes:

• *Adult and child >12 yr:* PO 1 g/day in 2-4 divided doses × 1-2 wk

Available forms include: Caps 250, 500 mg

Side effects/adverse reactions:

CNS: Dizziness, headache, agitation, insomnia, confusion

GI: Nausea, vomiting, anorexia, abdominal cramps, diarrhea

EENT: Sensitivity to light, visual disturbances, blurred vision, tinnitus

INTEG: Pruritus, rash, urticaria, photosensitivity, edema

Contraindications: Hypersensitivity to this drug, anuria, CNS damage

Precautions: Renal disease, hepatic disease, pregnancy category C, lactation

Pharmacokinetics:

PO: Duration 6-8 hr, half-life 1.5 hr; excreted in urine (unchanged/inactive metabolites)

DENTAL CONSIDERATIONS

General:

• Be aware that the patient has a UTI.

Consultations:

• May need to consult with physician when it is necessary to prescribe antiinfectives for a dental infection.

---

ciprofloxacin

(sip-roe-flox'a-sin)

Cipro, Cipro IV

Drug class.: Fluoroquinolone antiinfective

Action: A broad-spectrum bactericidal agent that inhibits the enzyme DNA gyrase needed for bacterial DNA replication

Uses: Adult UTIs (including complicated) caused by *E. coli, E. cloacae, P. mirabilis, K. pneumoniae, C. freundi, S. epidermidis,* and others; lower respiratory tract infections caused by *H. parainfluenzae, H. influenzae, K. pneumoniae, E. coli, E. cloacae;* chronic bacterial prostatitis; skin and skin structure infections, bone/joint infections caused by *E. cloacae, S. marcescens, P. aeruginosa,* infectious diarrhea, typhoid fever, STDs, and acute uncomplicated cystitis in females

Dosage and routes:

Uncomplicated UTIs

• *Adult:* PO 250 mg q12h; IV 200 mg q12h for 7-14 days; 3-day regimen: PO 100 mg bid q3d

Complicated/severe UTIs/nosocomial pneumonia

• *Adult:* PO 500 mg q12h for 7-14 days; IV 400 mg q12h

Lower respiratory tract infections (mild to moderate)

• *Adult:* PO 500 mg q12h, IV 400 mg q12h

Bone and joint infections

• *Adult:* PO 500-750 mg q12h for 4-6 wk

Available forms include: Tabs 100, 250, 500, 750 mg; IV 200 mg/100 ml D_5W, 400 mg/200 ml D_5W; 200, 400 mg vial

Side effects/adverse reactions:

▼ *ORAL:* Candidiasis, unpleasant taste

CNS: Headache, dizziness, fatigue, insomnia, depression, restlessness, tremors, confusion, hallucinations

GI: Nausea, vomiting, diarrhea, abdominal pain, constipation, increased ALT/AST, flatulence, insomnia, heartburn, dysphagia, pseudomembranous colitis

INTEG: Rash, pruritus, urticaria, photosensitivity, flushing, fever, chills
GU: Vaginitis
EENT: Blurred vision, diplopia, tinnitus, phototoxicity
MS: Tendinitis, tendon rupture, arthralgia
META: Elevation of liver enzymes ALT, AST
MISC: ***Anaphylaxis***
Contraindications: Hypersensitivity to quinolines
Precautions: Pregnancy category C, lactation, children, renal disease, tendon ruptures of shoulder, hand, and Achilles tendons, epilepsy, severe cerebral arteriosclerosis
Pharmacokinetics:
PO: Peak 1 hr, half-life 3-4 hr; steady state 2 days; excreted in urine as active drug, metabolites
Drug interactions of concern to dentistry:
• Decreased absorption: divalent, trivalent antacids, iron and zinc salts
• Increased serum levels: probenecid, warfarin (monitor)
• Serious adverse effects with theophylline

DENTAL CONSIDERATIONS
General:
• Determine why the patient is taking the drug.
• Avoid dental light in patient's eyes; offer dark glasses for patient comfort.
• Minimize exposure to sunlight and wear sunscreen if sun exposure is planned.
• Ruptures of the shoulder, hand, and Achilles tendon that required surgical repair or resulted in prolonged disability have been reported with this drug.
Consultations:
• Consult with patient's physician if an acute dental infection occurs and another antiinfective is required.
Teach patient/family:
• To discontinue treatment and inform dentist immediately if patient experiences pain or inflammation of a tendon, and to rest and refrain from exercise

---

citalopram hydrobromide

(ce'tal-o-pram)
Celexa
Drug class.: Antidepressant

Action: Selectively inhibits the reuptake of serotonin
Uses: Major depression
Dosage and routes:
• *Adult:* PO initial 20 mg once daily; can increase dose in 20 mg increments at intervals of at least 1 wk; doses above 40 mg once daily generally not recommended
Elderly or hepatic impairment
• *Elderly:* PO 20 mg qd/daily limit
Available forms include: Tabs 20, 40 mg; oral sol 10 mg/5 ml
Side effects/adverse reactions:
▼ *ORAL: Dry mouth,* unspecified dysphagia, teeth grinding, gingivitis
CNS: Dizziness, insomnia, somnolence, agitation, fatigue, anxiety, decreased libido
CV: Tachycardia, postural hypotension, hypotension
GI: Nausea, vomiting, dyspepsia, abdominal pain
RESP: URI, cough
HEMA: Purpura, anemia

GU: Ejaculation disorder, impotence
EENT: Rhinitis, sinusitis
INTEG: Rash, pruritus
MS: Asthenia, tremor, arthralgia, myalgia
MISC: Sweating, fever, alcohol intolerance

Contraindications: Hypersensitivity, concurrent use of MAO inhibitor

Precautions: Activation of mania, hypomania, seizure disorders, hepatic impairment, pregnancy category C, lactation, safe use in children unknown, reduce doses in elderly

Pharmacokinetics:
PO: Peak blood levels approximately 4 hr, bioavailability 80%, hepatic metabolism, three active metabolites, enterohepatic circulation, fecal and renal excretion

Drug interactions of concern to dentistry:
• Possibly increased CNS depression: all CNS depressants, alcohol
• Decrease in plasma levels: carbamazepine
• Increase in plasma levels: macrolide antibiotics, ketoconazole, itraconazole, omeprazole

DENTAL CONSIDERATIONS
General:
• Evaluate for TMJ therapy if bruxism causes symptoms of pain.
• Assess salivary flow as a factor in caries, periodontal disease, and candidiasis.
• Monitor vital signs every appointment due to cardiovascular and respiratory side effects.
• After supine positioning, have patient sit upright for 2 min or more to avoid orthostatic hypotension.
• Consider semisupine chair position for patient comfort due to GI side effects of drug.
• Short appointments and a stress reduction protocol may be required for anxious patients.

Consultations:
• Medical consult may be required to assess disease control and patient's ability to tolerate stress.
• Physician should be informed if significant xerostomic side effects occur (e.g., increased caries, sore tongue, problems eating or swallowing, difficulty wearing prosthesis) so a medication change can be considered.

Teach patient/family:
• Importance of good oral hygiene to prevent soft tissue inflammation
• Use of electric toothbrush if patient has difficulty holding conventional devices

When chronic dry mouth occurs, advise patient:
• To avoid mouth rinses with high alcohol content due to drying effects
• To use daily home fluoride products for anticaries effect
• To use sugarless gum, frequent sips of water, or saliva substitutes

clarithromycin

(kla-rith'roe-mye-sin)
Biaxin

Drug class.: Macrolide antibiotic

Action: Binds to 50S ribosomal subunits of susceptible bacteria and suppresses protein synthesis

Uses: Mild-to-moderate infections of the upper/lower respiratory tract; uncomplicated skin and skin structure infections caused by *S. pneumoniae, M. pneumoniae, C.*

diphtheriae, B. pertussis, L. monocytogenes, H. influenzae, S. pyogenes, S. aureus; otitis media; maxillary sinusitis; middle ear infection; disseminated MAC (mycobacterium avium complex); unlabeled use with omeprazole or ranitidine for *H. pylori* duodenal ulcer

Dosage and routes:

• *Adult:* PO 250-500 mg bid for 7-14 days

Bacterial endocarditis prophylaxis

• *Adult:* PO for patients allergic to amoxicillin, 500 mg 1 hr before dental procedure

• *Child:* PO for patients allergic to amoxicillin, 15 mg/kg of body weight not to exceed the adult dose 1 hr before dental procedure

Eradicating H. pylori (double therapy)

• *Adult:* PO (days 1-14) 500 mg clarithromycin tid plus omeprazole 20 mg bid every morning; days 15-28 omeprazole 20 mg every morning

Eradicating H. pylori (triple therapy)

• *Adult:* PO 500 mg clarithromycin plus 30 mg lansoprazole plus 1 g amoxicillin q12h for 14 days

Available forms include: Tabs 250, 500 mg; susp 125 mg/5 ml and 250 mg/ml in 50, 100 ml

Side effects/adverse reactions:

▼ *ORAL: Abnormal taste,* candidiasis, stomatitis

GI: Nausea, abdominal pain, diarrhea, ***hepatotoxicity,*** heartburn, anorexia, vomiting

GU: Vaginitis, moniliasis

INTEG: Rash, urticaria, pruritus

MISC: Headache

Contraindications: Hypersensitivity, cisapride, indinavir

Precautions: Pregnancy category C, lactation, hepatic and renal disease

Pharmacokinetics:

PO: Peak 2 hr, duration 12 hr, half-life 4-6 hr; metabolized by the liver; excreted in bile, feces

Drug interactions of concern to dentistry:

• Decreased effect: anticholinergic drugs

• Increased effects of cyclosporine, warfarin

• Decreased action of clindamycin, penicillins, lincomycin, oral contraceptives, rifabutin, rifampin, zidovudine

• Increased serum levels of carbamazepine, theophylline, digoxin

• Contraindicated with indinavir, cisapride

DENTAL CONSIDERATIONS

General:

• Determine why the patient is taking the drug.

• May prove to be an alternative drug of choice for mild infections due to a susceptible organism in patients who are allergic to penicillin.

Teach patient/family:

• Importance of good oral hygiene to prevent soft tissue inflammation

When used for dental infection, advise patient:

• Taking birth control pill to use additional method of contraception for duration of cycle

• To report sore throat, oral burning sensation, fever, fatigue, any of which could indicate superinfection

• To take at prescribed intervals and complete dosage regimen

• To immediately notify the dentist if signs or symptoms of infection increase

clemastine fumarate

(klem'as-teen)

Antihist-1, Tavist-1

♣ Tavist

Drug class.: Antihistamine, H_1-receptor antagonist

Action: Acts on blood vessels, GI, respiratory system by competing with histamine for H_1-receptor site; decreases allergic response by blocking histamine

Uses: Allergy symptoms, rhinitis, angioedema, urticaria, common cold

Dosage and routes:

• *Adult and child >12 yr:* PO 1.34-2.68 mg bid-tid, not to exceed 8.04 mg/day

Available forms include: Tabs 1.34, 2.68 mg; syr 0.67 mg/5 ml

Side effects/adverse reactions:

▼ *ORAL:* Dry mouth

CNS: Dizziness, drowsiness, poor coordination, fatigue, anxiety, euphoria, confusion, paresthesia, neuritis

CV: Hypotension, palpitation, tachycardia

GI: Constipation, nausea, vomiting, anorexia, diarrhea

RESP: Increased thick secretions, wheezing, chest tightness

HEMA: ***Thrombocytopenia, agranlocytosis, hemolytic anemia***

GU: Retention, dysuria, frequency

EENT: Blurred vision, dilated pupils, tinnitus, nasal stuffiness, dry nose/throat

INTEG: Rash, urticaria, photosensitivity

Contraindications: Hypersensitivity to H_1-receptor antagonists, acute asthma attack, lower respiratory tract disease

Precautions: Increased intraocular pressure, renal disease, cardiac disease, hypertension, bronchial asthma, seizure disorder, stenosed peptic ulcers, hyperthyroidism, prostatic hypertrophy, bladder neck obstruction, pregnancy category B, elderly

Pharmacokinetics:

PO: Peak 5-7 hr, duration 10-12 hr or more; metabolized in liver; excreted by kidneys

Drug interactions of concern to dentistry:

• Increased CNS depression: all CNS depressants, alcohol

• Increased anticholinergic effect of anticholinergics, phenothiazines, tricyclic antidepressants

DENTAL CONSIDERATIONS

General:

• Assess salivary flow as a factor in caries, periodontal disease, and candidiasis.

• Determine why the patient is taking the drug.

Teach patient/family:

• Importance of good oral hygiene to prevent soft tissue inflammation

• Caution to prevent injury when using oral hygiene aids

When chronic dry mouth occurs, advise patient:

• To avoid mouth rinses with high alcohol content due to drying effects

• To use daily home fluoride products for anticaries effect

• To use sugarless gum, frequent sips of water, or saliva substitutes

clidinium bromide

(kli-di'nee-um)

Quarzan

Drug class.: GI anticholinergic

Action: Inhibits muscarinic actions

of acetylcholine at postganglionic parasympathetic neuroeffector sites

Uses: Treatment of peptic ulcer disease in combination with other drugs

Dosage and routes:

• *Adult:* PO 2.5-5 mg tid-qid ac, hs
• *Elderly:* PO 2.5 mg tid ac

Available forms include: Caps 2.5, 5 mg

Side effects/adverse reactions:

▼ *ORAL: Dry mouth,* taste alteration

CNS: Confusion, stimulation in elderly, headache, insomnia, dizziness, drowsiness, anxiety, weakness, hallucinations

CV: Palpitation, tachycardia

GI: Constipation, ***paralytic ileus,*** heartburn, nausea, vomiting, dysphagia

GU: Hesitancy, retention, impotence

EENT: Blurred vision, photophobia, mydriasis, cycloplegia, increased ocular tension

INTEG: Urticaria, rash, pruritus, anhidrosis, fever, allergic reactions

Contraindications: Hypersensitivity to anticholinergics, narrow-angle glaucoma, GI obstruction, myasthenia gravis, paralytic ileus, GI atony, toxic megacolon

Precautions: Hyperthyroidism, coronary artery disease, dysrhythmias, CHF, ulcerative colitis, hypertension, hiatal hernia, hepatic disease, renal disease, pregnancy category C, urinary retention, prostatic hypertrophy, elderly

Pharmacokinetics:

PO: Onset 1 hr, duration 3 hr; excreted in urine

Drug interactions of concern to dentistry:

• Increased anticholinergic effect: atropine, scopolamine, tricyclic antidepressants, antihistamines, opioid analgesics, and other drugs with anticholinergic actions
• Decreased effects of: ketoconazole

DENTAL CONSIDERATIONS

General:

• Assess salivary flow as a factor in caries, periodontal disease, and candidiasis.
• Avoid dental light in patient's eyes; offer dark glasses for patient comfort.

Consultations:

• Physician should be informed if significant xerostomic side effects occur (increased caries, sore tongue, problems eating or swallowing, difficulty wearing prosthesis) so a medication change can be considered.

Teach patient/family:

• Importance of good oral hygiene to prevent soft tissue inflammation

When chronic dry mouth occurs, advise patient:

• To avoid mouth rinses with high alcohol content due to drying effects
• Of need for daily home fluoride to prevent caries
• To use sugarless gum, frequent sips of water, or saliva substitutes

---

clindamycin HCl/ clindamycin palmitate HCl/clindamycin phosphate

(klin-da-mye'sin)

Cleocin, Cleocin Pediatric

♣ Dalacin C Flavored Granules

Drug class.: Lincomycin derivative antiinfective

Action: Binds to 50S subunit of

bacterial ribosomes, suppresses protein synthesis

Uses: Infections caused by staphylococci, streptococci, pneumococci, *Rickettsia, Fusobacterium, Actinomyces, Peptococcus, Clostridium, Bacteroides, Peptostreptococcus*

Dosage and routes:

• *Adults:* PO 150-450 mg q6h; IM/IV 300 mg q6-12h, not to exceed 4800 mg/day

• *Child >1 mo:* PO 8-25 mg/kg/day in divided doses q6-8h; IM/IV 15-40 mg/kg/day in divided doses q6-8h 3-4 equal doses

PID

• *Adult:* IV 600 mg qid plus gentamicin

Bacterial endocarditis prophylaxis

• *Adult:* PO in patients allergic to amoxicillin, 600 mg 1 hr before dental procedure; IV for patients unable to take oral medications, 600 mg 1 hr before dental procedure

• *Child:* PO in patients allergic to amoxicillin, 20 mg/kg of body weight, not to exceed the adult dose, 1 hr before dental procedure; IV for patients unable to take oral medications, 20 mg/kg of body weight, not to exceed the adult dose, 1 hr before dental procedure

Prosthetic joint prophylaxis (when indicated)

• *Adult:* PO 600 mg 1 hr before dental procedure; IV for patients unable to take oral medications, 600 mg 1 hr before dental procedure

Available forms include: Inj 300 mg/ml, 2, 4, 6 ml; caps 75, 150, 300 mg; oral sol 75 mg/ml

Side effects/adverse reactions:

▼ *ORAL:* Candidiasis

GI: Nausea, vomiting, abdominal pain, diarrhea, ***pseudomembranous colitis,*** anorexia, weight loss

HEMA: ***Leukopenia, eosinophilia, agranulocytosis, thrombocytopenia***

GU: Vaginitis, increased AST/ALT, bilirubin, alk phosphatase, jaundice, urinary frequency

EENT: Rash, urticaria, pruritus, erythema, pain, abscess at injection site

Contraindications: Hypersensitivity to this drug or lincomycin, ulcerative colitis/enteritis, infants <1 mo

Precautions: Renal disease, liver disease, GI disease, elderly, pregnancy category B, lactation, tartrazine sensitivity

Pharmacokinetics:

PO: Peak 45 min, duration 6 hr

IM: Peak 3 hr, duration 8-12 hr, half-life 2.5 hr; metabolized in liver; excreted in urine, bile, feces as active/inactive metabolites; crosses placenta; excreted in breast milk

Drug interactions of concern to dentistry:

• Decreased action: erythromycin

• Increased effects of nondepolarizing muscle relaxants, hydrocarbon inhalation anesthetics

• Avoid antiperistaltic drugs if diarrhea occurs

DENTAL CONSIDERATIONS

General:

• Determine why the patient is taking the drug.

Consultations:

• Medical consult may be required to assess disease control in the patient.

Teach patient/family:

• Importance of good oral hygiene to prevent soft tissue inflammation

• Caution to prevent injury when using oral hygiene aids

When used for dental infection, advise patient:

• Taking birth control pill to use additional method of contraception for duration of cycle

• To report sore throat, oral burning sensation, fever, fatigue, any of which could indicate superinfection

• To take at prescribed intervals and complete dosage regimen

• To immediately notify the dentist if signs or symptoms of infection increase

clobetasol propionate

(klo-bay'ta-sol)

Dermovate, Temovate, Temovate Emollient Cream, Temovate Gel

Drug class.: Topical corticosteroid, group I potency

Action: Glucocorticoids have multiple actions that include antiinflammatory and immunosuppressant effects. They inhibit phospholipase A_2, interfering with or reducing the synthesis of prostaglandins and leukotrienes. They also bind to cytoplasmic glucocorticoid receptors (GRs) and enter the cell nucleus to bind with DNA. This results in the synthesis of various enzymes such as collagenase, elastase, and cytokines that play important roles in inflammation and immunosuppression. They also suppress the production of lymphocytes, monocytes, and eosinophils.

Uses: Psoriasis, eczema, contact dermatitis, pruritus, symptomatic relief of ulcerative inflammatory lesions; usually reserved for severe dermatoses that have not responded to less potent formulations

Dosage and routes:

• *Adult and child:* TOP apply to affected area bid

Available forms include: Oint 0.05%; cream 0.05% in 15, 30, 45 g; gel 0.05% in 15, 30, 60 g

Side effects/adverse reactions:

INTEG: Burning, dryness, itching, irritation, acne, folliculitis, hypertrichosis, perioral dermatitis, hypopigmentation, atrophy, striae, miliaria, allergic contact dermatitis, secondary infection

Contraindications: Hypersensitivity to corticosteroids, fungal infections, viral infections

Precautions: Pregnancy category C, lactation, bacterial infections

DENTAL CONSIDERATIONS

General:

• Place on frequent recall to evaluate healing response.

• Topical adrenocorticosteroids are not indicated for treating plaque-related gingivitis, which should be treated by removal of local irritants and improved oral hygiene.

Teach patient/family:

• Importance of good oral hygiene to prevent soft tissue inflammation

• That use on oral herpetic ulcerations is contraindicated

• To apply at bedtime or after meals for maximum effect

• To apply with cotton-tipped applicator by pressing, not rubbing, paste on lesion

• When used for oral lesions, advise patient to return for oral evaluation if response of oral tissues has not occurred in 7-14 days

clocortolone pivalate

(klo-kort′o-lone)

Cloderm

Drug class.: Topical corticosteroid, group III medium potency

Action: Glucocorticoids have multiple actions that include antiinflammatory and immunosuppressant effects. They inhibit phospholipase A_2, interfering with or reducing the synthesis of prostaglandins and leukotrienes. They also bind to cytoplasmic glucocorticoid receptors (GRs) and enter the cell nucleus to bind with DNA. This results in the synthesis of various enzymes such as collagenase, elastase, and cytokines that play important roles in inflammation and immunosuppression. They also suppress the production of lymphocytes, monocytes, and eosinophils.

Uses: Psoriasis, eczema, contact dermatitis, pruritus

Dosage and routes:

• *Adult and child:* Apply to affected area tid or qid

Available forms include: Cream 0.1%

Side effects/adverse reactions:

▼ *ORAL:* Perioral dermatitis

INTEG: Burning, dryness, itching, irritation, acne, folliculitis, hypertrichosis, hypopigmentation, atrophy, striae, miliaria, allergic contact dermatitis, secondary infection

Contraindications: Hypersensitivity to corticosteroids, fungal infections

Precautions: Pregnancy category C, lactation, viral infections, bacterial infections

DENTAL CONSIDERATIONS

General:

• Determine why the patient is taking the drug.

• Place on frequent recall to evaluate healing response if used on a chronic basis.

• Apply lubricant to dry lips for patient comfort before dental procedures.

clofazimine

(kloe-fa′zi-meen)

Lamprene

Drug class.: Leprostatic

Action: Inhibits mycobacterial growth, binds to mycobacterial DNA

Uses: Lepromatous leprosy, dapsone-resistant leprosy, lepromatous leprosy complicated by erythema nodosum leprosum

Dosage and routes:

Erythema nodosum leprosum

• *Adult:* PO 100-200 mg qd × 3 mo, then taper dosage to 100 mg when disease is controlled, do not exceed 300 mg/day

Dapsone-related leprosy

• *Adult:* PO 100 mg/day in combination with at least one other antileprosy drug × 3 yr, then 100 mg qd clofazimine (only)

Available forms include: Caps 50, 100 mg

Side effects/adverse reactions:

▼ *ORAL:* Stomatitis (rarely)

CNS: Dizziness, headache, fatigue, drowsiness

GI: Diarrhea, nausea, vomiting, abdominal pain, intolerance, ***GI bleeding, obstruction, hepatitis,*** anorexia, constipation, jaundice

EENT: Pigmentation of cornea, conjunctiva, drying, burning, itching, irritation
INTEG: Pink or brown discoloration, dryness, pruritus, rash, photosensitivity, acne, monilial cheilosis
MISC: Discolored urine, feces, sputum, sweat
Precautions: Pregnancy category C, lactation, children, abdominal pain, diarrhea, depression
Pharmacokinetics:
PO: Half-life 70 days; deposited in fatty tissue, reticuloendothelial system; small amount excreted in feces, sputum, sweat
Drug interactions of concern to dentistry:
• None reported
DENTAL CONSIDERATIONS
General:
• Develop awareness of the patient's disease.
Teach patient/family:
• Importance of good oral hygiene to prevent soft tissue inflammation
• To avoid mouth rinses with high alcohol content due to drying effects

clofibrate

(kloe-fye'brate)
Abitrate, Atromid-S
✱ Claripex, Novofibrate
Drug class.: Antihyperlipidemic

Action: Inhibits biosynthesis of VLDL and LDL, which are responsible for triglyceride development; mobilizes triglycerides from tissue; increases excretion of neutral sterols
Uses: Hyperlipidemia (types III, IV, V)
Dosage and routes:
• *Adult:* PO 1.5-2 g/day in 2-4 divided doses
Available forms include: Caps 500 mg, 1 g
Side effects/adverse reactions:
▼ *ORAL:* Stomatitis
CNS: Fatigue, weakness, drowsiness, dizziness
CV: ***Pulmonary emboli,*** angina, dysrhythmias, thrombophlebitis
GI: Nausea, vomiting, dyspepsia, increased liver enzymes, flatulence
HEMA: ***Leukopenia, eosinophilia,*** anemia, bleeding
GU: ***Hematuria,*** decreased libido, impotence, dysuria, proteinuria, oliguria
INTEG: Rash, urticaria, pruritus, dry hair and skin, alopecia
MS: Myalgias, arthralgias
MISC: Polyphagia, weight gain
Contraindications: Severe hepatic disease, severe renal disease, primary biliary cirrhosis, pregnancy, lactation, children
Precautions: Peptic ulcer, pregnancy category C
Pharmacokinetics:
PO: Peak 2-6 hr, half-life 6-25 hr; plasma protein binding >90%; metabolized in liver; excreted in urine
DENTAL CONSIDERATIONS
General:
• Consider semisupine chair position for patient comfort if GI side effects occur.
• Patients on chronic drug therapy may rarely have symptoms of blood dyscrasias, which can include infection, bleeding, and poor healing.
• No dental drug interactions have been reported.
Consultations:
• In a patient with symptoms of blood dyscrasias, request a medical

consult for blood studies and postpone treatment until normal values are reestablished.

Teach patient/family:

• Importance of good oral hygiene to prevent soft tissue inflammation

clomiphene citrate

(kloe'mi-feen)

Clomid, Milophene, Serophene

Drug class.: Nonsteroidal ovulatory stimulant

Action: Binds to estrogen receptors, resulting in increase of LH and FSH release from the pituitary, which increases maturation of ovarian follicle, ovulation, and development of corpus luteum

Uses: Female infertility

Dosage and routes:

• *Initial adult:* PO 50 mg qd × 5 days; may be repeated until conception occurs or 3-4 cycles of therapy have been completed

• *Second trial adult:* PO 100 mg/day × 5 days, can repeat third time

Available forms include: Tabs 50 mg

Side effects/adverse reactions:

CNS: Headache, depression, restlessness, anxiety, nervousness, fatigue, insomnia, dizziness, flushing

CV: Vasomotor flushing, phlebitis, deep vein thrombosis

GI: Nausea, vomiting, constipation, abdominal pain, bloating

GU: Polyuria, frequency, birth defects, spontaneous abortions, multiple ovulation, breast pain, oliguria, abnormal uterine bleeding

EENT: Blurred vision, diplopia, photophobia

INTEG: Rash, dermatitis, urticaria, alopecia

Contraindications: Hypersensitivity, pregnancy category X, hepatic disease, undiagnosed vaginal bleeding

Precautions: Hypertension, depression, convulsions, diabetes mellitus

Pharmacokinetics:

PO: Metabolized in liver, excreted in feces

DENTAL CONSIDERATIONS

General:

• Consider semisupine chair position for patient comfort due to GI effects of drug.

• Avoid dental light in patient's eyes; offer dark glasses for patient comfort.

• Be aware that patient may be in early stage of pregnancy.

clomipramine

(kloe-mi'pra-meen)

Anafranil

Drug class.: Tricyclic antidepressant

Action: Inhibits both norepinephrine and serotinin (5-HT) uptake in the brain, although the precise antidepressant mechanism remains unclear

Uses: Obsessive-compulsive disorder; unapproved use: depression, panic disorder, narcolepsy, and neurogenic pain

Dosage and routes:

Obsessive-compulsive disorder

• *Adult:* PO 25 mg hs; increase gradually over 4 wk to a dose of 75-300 mg/day in divided doses

• *Child 10-18 yr:* PO 50 mg/day gradually increased; not to exceed 200 mg/day

Depression

• *Adult:* PO 50-150 mg/day in a single or divided dose

Anxiety/agoraphobia
• *Adult:* PO 25-75 mg/day
Available forms include: Caps 25, 50, 75 mg; tabs 10, 25, 50 mg
Side effects/adverse reactions:
▼ *ORAL: Dry mouth, unpleasant taste,* bleeding
CNS: Dizziness, tremors, mania, ***seizures,*** aggressiveness
CV: ***Cardiac arrest,*** hypotension, tachycardia
GI: Constipation
HEMA: ***Agranulocytosis, neutropenia, pancytopenia***
GU: Delayed ejaculation, anorgasmy, retention
INTEG: Diaphoresis
ENDO: Galactorrhea, hyperprolactinemia
META: Hyponatremia
Contraindications: Pregnancy category C, hypersensitivity
Precautions: Seizures, suicidal patients, elderly, MAO inhibitors
Pharmacokinetics:
PO: Half-life: 21 hr parent compound, 36 hr metabolite; extensively bound to tissue and plasma proteins; demethylated in liver (active metabolites); excreted in urine (metabolites)
Drug interactions of concern to dentistry:
• Increased anticholinergic effects: muscarinic blockers, antihistamines, phenothiazines
• Increased effects of direct-acting sympathomimetics (epinephrine, levonordefrin)
• Potential risk of CNS depression: alcohol, barbiturates, benzodiazepines, and other CNS depressants
• Decreased antihypertensive effects: clonidine, guanadrel, guanethidine

DENTAL CONSIDERATIONS
General:
• Take vital signs every appointment due to cardiovascular side effects.
• Assess salivary flow as a factor in caries, periodontal disease, and candidiasis.
• Patients on chronic drug therapy may rarely have symptoms of blood dyscrasias, which can include infection, bleeding, and poor healing.
• After supine positioning, have patient sit upright for at least 2 min before standing to avoid orthostatic hypotension.
• Use vasoconstrictor with caution, in low doses, and with careful aspiration. Avoid use of gingival retraction cord with epinephrine.
• Place on frequent recall due to oral side effects.
• A stress reduction protocol may be required.
Consultations:
• In a patient with symptoms of blood dyscrasias, request a medical consult for blood studies and postpone dental treatment until normal values are reestablished.
• Physician should be informed if significant xerostomic side effects occur (increased caries, sore tongue, problems eating or swallowing, difficulty wearing prosthesis) so a medication change can be considered.
• Medical consult may be required to assess disease control in the patient.
Teach patient/family:
• Importance of good oral hygiene to prevent soft tissue inflammation
• Caution to prevent injury when using oral hygiene aids

When chronic dry mouth occurs, advise patient:
- To avoid mouth rinses with high alcohol content due to drying effects
- To use daily home fluoride products for anticaries effect
- To use sugarless gum, frequent sips of water, or saliva substitutes

clonazepam

(kloe-na'zi-pam)
Klonopin, Syn-Clonazepam
♣ Apo-Clonazepam, Alti-Clonazepam, Clonapam, Gen-Clonazepam, PMS-Clonazepam, Rivotril

Drug class.: Anticonvulsant, benzodiazepine derivative

Controlled Substance Schedule IV

Action: Inhibits spike and wave formation in absence seizures (petit mal); decreases amplitude, frequency, duration, spread of discharge in minor motor seizures; acts on benzodiazepine receptors in the CNS

Uses: Absence, atypical absence, akinetic, myoclonic seizures; panic disorder

Dosage and routes:

Seizures
- *Adult:* PO not to exceed 1.5 mg/day in 3 divided doses; may be increased 0.5-1 mg q3d until desired response; not to exceed 20 mg/day
- *Child <10 yr or 30 kg:* PO 0.01-0.03 mg/kg/day in divided doses q8h, not to exceed 0.05 mg/kg/day; may be increased 0.25-0.5 mg q3d until desired response, not to exceed 0.1-0.2 mg/kg/day

Panic disorder
- *Adult:* PO 1-2 mg/day to a maximum of 4 mg

Available forms include: Tabs 0.125, 0.25, 0.5, 1, 2 mg

Side effects/adverse reactions:

▼ *ORAL:* Dry mouth or increased salivation, bleeding

CNS: Drowsiness, dizziness, confusion, behavioral changes, tremors, insomnia, headache, suicidal tendencies, slurred speech

CV: Palpitation, bradycardia

GI: Nausea, constipation, polyphagia, anorexia, xerostomia, diarrhea, gastritis

RESP: ***Respiratory depression,*** dyspnea, congestion

HEMA: ***Thrombocytopenia, leukocytosis, eosinophilia***

GU: Dysuria, enuresis, nocturia, retention

EENT: Nystagmus, diplopia, abnormal eye movements

INTEG: Rash, alopecia, hirsutism

Contraindications: Hypersensitivity to benzodiazepines, acute narrow-angle glaucoma, ritonavir

Precautions: Open-angle glaucoma, chronic respiratory disease, pregnancy category C, renal, hepatic disease, elderly

Pharmacokinetics:

PO: Peak 1-2 hr, half-life 18-50 hr; metabolized by liver; excreted in urine

Drug interactions of concern to dentistry:
- Increased sedation: alcohol, all CNS depressants, indinavir

DENTAL CONSIDERATIONS

General:
- Patients on chronic drug therapy may rarely have symptoms of blood dyscrasias, which can include infection, bleeding, and poor healing.

• Assess salivary flow as a factor in caries, periodontal disease, and candidiasis.
• Psychologic and physical dependence may occur with chronic administration.
• Geriatric patients are more susceptible to drug effects; use lower dose.
• Ask about type of epilepsy, seizure frequency, and quality of seizure control.

Consultations:
• Medical consult may be required to assess disease control in the patient.
• In a patient with symptoms of blood dyscrasias, request a medical consult for blood studies and postpone dental treatment until normal values are reestablished.

Teach patient/family:
• Importance of good oral hygiene to prevent soft tissue inflammation
• Caution to prevent injury when using oral hygiene aids

When chronic dry mouth occurs, advise patient:
• To avoid mouth rinses with high alcohol content due to drying effects
• To use daily home fluoride products for anticaries effect
• To use sugarless gum, frequent sips of water, or saliva substitutes

clonidine HCl/clonidine transdermal

(kloe'ni-deen)

Catapres, Catapres-TTS
♣ Dixarit

Drug class.: Antihypertensive, central α-adrenergic agonist

Action: Inhibits sympathetic vasomotor center in CNS, which reduces impulses in sympathetic nervous system; decreases blood pressure, pulse rate, and cardiac output

Uses: Hypertension; unapproved uses: opioid abstinence syndrome, nicotine withdrawal, vascular headache

Dosage and routes:

Hypertension
• *Adult:* PO/TRANS 0.1 mg bid, then increase by 0.1 mg/day or 0.2 mg/day until desired response; range 0.2-0.8 mg/day in divided doses

Available forms include: Tabs 0.1, 0.2, 0.3 mg; transderm sys 2.5, 5, 7.5 mg delivering 0.1, 0.2, 0.3 mg/24 hr, respectively

Side effects/adverse reactions:
▼ *ORAL:* Dry mouth, taste changes, salivary pain or swelling
CNS: Drowsiness, sedation, headache, fatigue, nightmares, insomnia, mental changes, anxiety, depression, hallucinations, delirium
CV: Orthostatic hypotension, palpitation, ***CHF,*** ECG abnormalities
GI: Nausea, vomiting, malaise, constipation
GU: Impotence, nocturia, dysuria, gynecomastia
EENT: Parotid pain
INTEG: Rash, alopecia, facial pallor, pruritus, hives, edema, burning papules, excoriation (transdermal patches)
ENDO: Hyperglycemia
MS: Muscle/joint pain, leg cramps

Contraindications: Hypersensitivity

Precautions: MI (recent), diabetes mellitus, chronic renal failure, Raynaud's disease, thyroid disease, depression, COPD, child <12 yr (patches), asthma, pregnancy category C, lactation, elderly

Pharmacokinetics:
PO: Peak 3-5 hr, half-life 12-16 hr; metabolized by liver (metabolites); excreted in urine (unchanged, inactive metabolites), feces; crosses blood-brain barrier; excreted in breast milk

Drug interactions of concern to dentistry:

- Increased CNS depression: alcohol, all CNS depressants
- Decreased hypotensive effects: NSAIDs, especially indomethacin, sympathomimetics, tricyclic antidepressants

DENTAL CONSIDERATIONS

General:

- Monitor vital signs every appointment due to cardiovascular side effects.
- After supine positioning, have patient sit upright for at least 2 min before standing to avoid orthostatic hypotension.
- Limit use of sodium-containing products such as saline IV fluids for patients with a dietary salt restriction.
- Assess salivary flow as a factor in caries, periodontal disease, and candidiasis.
- Stress from dental procedures may compromise cardiovascular function; determine patient risk.
- Short appointments and a stress reduction protocol may be required for anxious patients.
- Consider drug in diagnosis of taste alterations.

Consultations:

- Medical consult may be required to assess disease control in the patient.

Teach patient/family:

When chronic dry mouth occurs, advise patient:

- To avoid mouth rinses with high alcohol content due to drying effects
- To use daily home fluoride products for anticaries effect
- To use sugarless gum, frequent sips of water, or saliva substitutes

---

clopidogrel bisulfate

(kloe-pid-o′grel)

Plavix

Drug class.: Platelet aggregation inhibitor

Action: Irreversibly inhibits adenosine diphosphate–induced platelet aggregation

Uses: Adjunctive treatment in MI, ischemic stroke, and peripheral vascular disease in patients with atherosclerosis

Dosage and routes:

- *Adult:* PO 75 mg qd with or without food

Available forms include: Tabs 75 mg

Side effects/adverse reactions:

GI: Diarrhea, abdominal pain, nausea, gastritis with bleeding, dyspepsia

RESP: RTI, bronchitis, coughing

EENT: Epistaxis, rhinitis

HEMA: Bleeding, neutropenia (rare)

INTEG: Rash, urticaria, purpura, pruritus

META: Liver function abnormalities, hepatotoxicity, hyperchlosterolemia

MS: Arthralgia, back pain

Contraindications: Hypersensitivity, active bleeding, bleeding disorders, anticoagulants, antiplatelet agents

Precautions: Hepatic impairment, renal impairment, hypertension,

history of bleeding disorders, major surgery, pregnancy category B
Pharmacokinetics:
PO: Well absorbed, peak levels <1 hr, hepatic metabolism, active metabolite, plasma protein binding 94%-98%, excreted in both urine and feces, maximal effect on bleeding time 5-7 days
Drug interactions of concern to dentistry:
• Avoid prescribing aspirin; caution in use with NSAIDs
DENTAL CONSIDERATIONS
General:
• Effects on platelet aggregation return to normal in 5 to 7 days.
• Patient on chronic drug therapy may rarely have symptoms of blood dyscrasias, which can include infection, bleeding, and poor healing.
• Consider local hemostasis measures to prevent excessive bleeding.
Consultations:
• Medical consult may be required to assess disease control and patient's ability to tolerate stress.
• Consult should include data on bleeding time.
• In a patient with symptoms of blood dyscrasias, request a medical consult for blood studies and postpone treatment until normal values are reestablished.
Teach patient/family:
• Importance of updating health and drug history if physician makes any changes in evaluation/drug regimens
• Caution to prevent trauma when using oral hygiene aids
• To report any unusual or prolonged bleeding episodes after dental treatment

clorazepate dipotassium

(klor-az'e-pate)
Gen-Xene, Traxene T-Tab, Tranxene-SD
♣ Apo-Chlorazepate, Novo-Clopate, Tranxene
Drug class.: Benzodiazepine

Controlled Substance Schedule IV
Action: Produces CNS depression by interaction with a benzodiazepine receptor to facilitate the action of the inhibitory neurotransmitter γ-aminobutyric acid (GABA)
Uses: Anxiety, acute alcohol withdrawal
Dosage and routes:
Anxiety
• *Adult:* PO 15-60 mg/day
Alcohol withdrawal
• *Adult:* PO 30 mg, then 30-60 mg in divided doses; day 2, 45-90 mg in divided doses; day 3, 22.5-45 mg in divided doses; day 4, 15-30 mg in divided doses; then reduce daily dose to 7.5-15 mg
Available forms include: Caps 3.75, 7.5, 15 mg; tabs 3.75, 7.5, 15 mg, single-dose tab 11.25, 22.5 mg
Side effects/adverse reactions:
▼ *ORAL:* Dry mouth
CNS: Dizziness, drowsiness, confusion, headache, anxiety, tremors, stimulation, fatigue, depression, insomnia, hallucinations
CV: Orthostatic hypotension, ***ECG changes, tachycardia,*** hypotension
GI: Constipation, nausea, vomiting, anorexia, diarrhea
EENT: Blurred vision, tinnitus, mydriasis
INTEG: Rash, dermatitis, itching
Contraindications: Hypersensi-

tivity to benzodiazepines, narrow-angle glaucoma, psychosis, pregnancy category D, child <18 yr; ritonavir

Precautions: Elderly, debilitated, hepatic disease, renal disease

Pharmacokinetics:

PO: Onset 15 min, peak 1-2 hr, duration 4-6 hr, half-life 30-100 hr; metabolized by liver; excreted by kidneys; crosses placenta, excreted in breast milk

Drug interactions of concern to dentistry:

• Increased effects: CNS depressants, alcohol, opioid analgesics, general anesthetics, indinavir

• Increased serum levels and prolonged effect of benzodiazepines: fluconazole, ketoconazole, itraconazole, miconazole (systemic)

DENTAL CONSIDERATIONS

General:

• Monitor vital signs every appointment due to cardiovascular side effects.

• Assess salivary flow as a factor in caries, periodontal disease, and candidiasis.

• After supine positioning, have patient sit upright for at least 2 min to avoid orthostatic hypotension.

• Psychologic and physical dependence may occur with chronic administration.

• Geriatric patients are more susceptible to drug effects; use a lower dose.

Consultations:

• Medical consult may be required to assess disease control in the patient.

Teach patient/family:

When chronic dry mouth occurs, advise patient:

• To avoid mouth rinses with high alcohol content due to drying effects

• To use daily home fluoride products for anticaries effect

• To use sugarless gum, frequent sips of water, or saliva substitutes

---

clotrimazole

(kloe-trim'a-zole)

Canesten Combi-Pak, Clotriaderm, FemCare, Femizole, Gyne-Lotrimin, Gyne-Lotrimin Combination Pack, Gyne-Lotrimin 3, Lotrimin, Mycelex-G, Mycelex Lozenges, Mycelex Twin Pack, Mycelex-7

✤ Canesten, Myclo-Gyne

Drug class.: Imidazole antifungal

Action: Interferes with fungal DNA replication; binds sterols in fungal cell membrane, which increases permeability, leaking of cell nutrients; fungicidal

Uses: Tinea pedis; tinea cruris; tinea corporis; tinea versicolor; *C. albicans* infection of the vagina, vulva, throat, mouth

Dosage and routes:

• *Adult and child:* TOP rub into affected area bid × 1-8 wk; TROCHE dissolve in mouth 5× daily × 2 wk; INTRA VAG 1 applicator/1 tab × 1-2 wk hs; ORAL TROCHE 10 mg 5× daily × 14 days; 3-DAY REGIMEN insert tab qd × 3 days, apply cream externally prn

Available forms include: Cream, sol, lotion 1%; vag tabs 100, 500 mg; vag cream 1%; troches 10 mg

Side effects/adverse reactions:

INTEG: Rash, urticaria, stinging, burning, peeling, blistering

MISC: Abdominal cramps, bloating, urinary frequency, dyspareunia

Contraindications: Hypersensitivity

Precautions: Pregnancy category B, lactation

Drug interactions of concern to dentistry:

• None reported

DENTAL CONSIDERATIONS

General:

• Determine why the patient is taking the drug.

• Examine oral mucous membranes for signs of fungal infection.

Teach patient/family:

• If used for oral infection: to soak full or partial dentures in an antifungal solution overnight until lesions are absent; prolonged infections may require fabrication of new prosthesis

• To dispose of toothbrush used during oral infection after oral lesions are absent to prevent reinoculation

• That long-term therapy may be needed to clear infection; to complete entire course of medication

cloxacillin sodium

(klox-a-sil′in)

Cloxapen, Tegopen

Apo Cloxi, Novo-Cloxin, Nu-Cloxi, Orbenin

Drug class.: Penicillinase-resistant penicillin

Action: Interferes with cell wall replication of susceptible organisms; the cell wall, rendered osmotically unstable, swells and bursts from osmotic pressure

Uses: Effective for gram-positive cocci *(S. aureus, S. pyogenes, E. pyogenes, S. pneumoniae),* when penicillinase-producing organisms are confirmed pathogens

Dosage and routes:

• *Adult:* PO 1-4 g/day in divided doses q6h

• *Child <40 kg:* PO 50-100 mg/kg in divided doses q6h

Available forms include: Caps 250, 500 mg; powder for oral susp 250 mg/5 ml; inj 250, 500 mg and 1, 2, 4, 10 g

Side effects/adverse reactions:

ORAL: Discolored tongue, candidiasis, glossitis

CNS: ***Coma, convulsions,*** lethargy, hallucinations, anxiety, depression, twitching

GI: Nausea, vomiting, diarrhea, increased AST/ALT, abdominal pain, colitis

HEMA: ***Bone marrow depression, granulocytopenia,*** anemia, increased bleeding time

GU: Vaginitis, moniliasis, ***glomerulonephritis,*** oliguria, proteinuria, hematuria

META: Pruritus, urticaria, angioedema, bronchospasm, anaphylaxis (allergy symptoms)

Contraindications: Hypersensitivity to penicillins; neonates

Precautions: Pregnancy category B, hypersensitivity to cephalosporins

Pharmacokinetics:

PO: Peak 1 hr, duration 6 hr, half-life 0.5-1 hr; metabolized in liver; excreted in urine, bile, breast milk; crosses placenta

Drug interactions of concern to dentistry:

• Decreased antimicrobial effectiveness: tetracyclines, erythromycins

• Increased cloxacillin concentrations: probenecid

When used for dental infections:

• Decreased effectiveness of oral contraceptives

DENTAL CONSIDERATIONS

General:

• Use precautions regarding allergy to medication.

• Determine why the patient is taking the drug.

Consultations:

• Medical consult may be required to assess disease control in the patient.

Teach patient/family:

• Importance of good oral hygiene to prevent soft tissue inflammation

• Caution to prevent injury when using oral hygiene aids

When used for dental infection, advise patient:

• Taking birth control pill to use additional method of contraception for duration of cycle

• To report sore throat, oral burning sensation, fever, fatigue, any of which could indicate superinfection

• To take at prescribed intervals and complete dosage regimen

• To immediately notify the dentist if signs or symptoms of infection increase

---

clozapine

(klo'za-pin)

Clozaril, Leponex

Drug class.: Antipsychotic, atypical

Action: Interferes with binding of dopamine at D_1 and D_2 receptors with lack of extrapyramidal symptoms; also acts as an adrenergic, cholinergic, histaminergic, and serotonergic antagonist

Uses: Management of psychotic symptoms in schizophrenic patients for whom other antipsychotics have failed

Dosage and routes:

• *Adult:* PO 25 mg qd or bid, may increase by 25-50 mg/day; normal range 300-450 mg/day after 2 wk; do not increase dose more than 2 × weekly; do not exceed 900 mg/day; use lowest dose to control symptoms

Available forms include: Tabs 25, 100 mg

Side effects/adverse reactions:

▼ *ORAL: Dry mouth, increased salivation,* glossitis

CNS: Sedation, dizziness, headache, tremors, sleep problems, akinesia, fever, ***seizures,*** sweating, akathisia, confusion, fatigue, insomnia, depression, slurred speech, anxiety

CV: Tachycardia, hypotension, hypertension, chest pain, ECG changes

GI: Constipation, nausea, abdominal discomfort, vomiting, diarrhea, anorexia

RESP: Dyspnea, nasal congestion, throat discomfort

HEMA: ***Leukopenia, neutropenia, agranulocytosis, eosinophilia***

GU: Urinary abnormalities, incontinence, ejaculation dysfunction, frequency, urgency, retention

MS: Weakness; pain in back, neck, legs; spasm

Contraindications: Hypersensitivity, myeloproliferative disorders, severe granulocytopenia, CNS depression, coma, narrow-angle glaucoma

Precautions: Pregnancy category B; lactation; children <16 yr; hepatic, renal, cardiac disease; seizures; prostatic enlargement; elderly

Pharmacokinetics:

PO: Steady state 2.5 hr, half-life 8-12 hr; 95% protein bound; completely metabolized by the liver; excreted in urine and feces (metabolites)

Drug interactions of concern to dentistry:

• Increased anticholinergic effects: anticholinergics

• Increased CNS depression: alcohol, all CNS depressant drugs

• Increased serum concentration, leukocytosis: erythromycin base

DENTAL CONSIDERATIONS

General:

• Monitor vital signs every appointment due to cardiovascular and respiratory side effects.

• Patients on chronic drug therapy may rarely have symptoms of blood dyscrasias, which can include infection, bleeding, and poor healing.

• After supine positioning, have patient sit upright for at least 2 min before standing to avoid orthostatic hypotension.

• Assess salivary flow as a factor in caries, periodontal disease, and candidiasis.

• Determine why the patient is taking the drug.

• Place on frequent recall due to oral side effects.

Consultations:

• In a patient with symptoms of blood dyscrasias, request a medical consult for blood studies and postpone dental treatment until normal values are reestablished.

• Medical consult may be required to assess disease control and stress tolerance of patient.

• Physician should be informed if significant xerostomic side effects occur (increased caries, sore tongue, problems eating or swallowing, difficulty wearing prosthesis) so a medication change can be considered.

Teach patient/family:

• Importance of good oral hygiene to prevent soft tissue inflammation

• Caution to prevent injury when using oral hygiene aids

• To use electric toothbrush if patient has difficulty holding conventional devices

When chronic dry mouth occurs, advise patient:

• To avoid mouth rinses with high alcohol content due to drying effects

• To use daily home fluoride products for anticaries effect

• To use sugarless gum, frequent sips of water, or saliva substitutes

---

codeine sulfate/ codeine phosphate

(koe'deen)

generic codeine

Drug class.: Narcotic analgesic

Controlled Substance Schedule II, Canada N

Action: Depresses pain impulse transmission in CNS by interacting with opioid receptors

Uses: Mild-to-moderate pain, nonproductive cough

Dosage and routes:

Pain

• *Adult:* PO 15-60 mg q4h prn; IM/SC 15-60 mg q4h prn

• *Child:* PO 3 mg/kg/day in divided doses q4h prn

Cough

• *Adult:* PO 10-20 mg q4-6h, not to exceed 120 mg/day

• *Child:* PO 1-1.5 mg/kg/day in 4 divided doses, not to exceed 60 mg/day

Available forms include: Inj IM/SC 15, 30, 60 mg/ml; tabs 15, 30, 60 mg

Side effects/adverse reactions:

▼ *ORAL:* Dry mouth, lichenoid reaction

CNS: Drowsiness, sedation, dizziness, agitation, dependency, lethargy, restlessness

CV: Bradycardia, palpitation, orthostatic hypotension, tachycardia

GI: Nausea, vomiting, anorexia, constipation

RESP: ***Respiratory depression, respiratory paralysis***

GU: Urinary retention

INTEG: Flushing, rash, urticaria

Contraindications: Hypersensitivity to opiates, respiratory depression, increased intracranial pressure, seizure disorders, severe respiratory disorders

Precautions: Elderly, cardiac dysrhythmias, pregnancy category C

Pharmacokinetics:

PO: Onset 15-30 min, peak 1-2 hr, duration 4-6 hr, half-life 2.5-4 hr; metabolized by liver; excreted by kidneys; crosses placenta; excreted in breast milk

Drug interactions of concern to dentistry:

• Increased sedation with other CNS depressants and alcohol

• Increased effects of anticholinergics

DENTAL CONSIDERATIONS

General:

• Monitor vital signs every appointment due to cardiovascular and respiratory side effects.

• After supine positioning, have patient sit upright for at least 2 min to avoid orthostatic hypotension.

• Assess salivary flow as a factor in caries, periodontal disease, and candidiasis.

• Psychologic and physical dependence may occur with chronic administration.

Teach patient/family:

When chronic dry mouth occurs, advise patient:

• To avoid mouth rinses with high alcohol content due to drying effects

• To use daily home fluoride products for anticaries effect

• To use sugarless gum, frequent sips of water, or saliva substitutes

colchicine

(kol'chi-seen)

generic colchicine

Drug class.: Antigout agent

Action: Inhibits deposition of ureate crystals in soft tissues; mechanism unclear

Uses: Gout, gouty arthritis (prevention, treatment), to arrest progression of neurologic disability in multiple sclerosis

Dosage and routes:

Prevention

• *Adult:* PO 0.5-1.8 mg qd depending on severity; IV 0.5-1 mg 1-2 × daily

Treatment

• *Adult:* PO 0.5-1.2 mg, then 0.5-1.2 mg q1h until pain decreases or side effects occur; IV 2 mg, 0.5 mg q6h, not to exceed 4 mg/24 hr

Available forms include: Tabs 0.5, 0.6 mg; inj IV 1 mg/2 ml

Side effects/adverse reactions:

▼ *ORAL:* Metallic taste, lichenoid reaction

GI: Nausea, vomiting, anorexia, malaise, cramps, peptic ulcer, diarrhea

HEMA: ***Agranulocytosis, thrombo-***

cytopenia, aplastic anemia, pancytopenia
GU: Hematuria, oliguria, renal damage
INTEG: Chills, dermatitis, pruritus, purpura, erythema
MISC: Myopathy, alopecia, reversible azoospermia, peripheral neuritis
Contraindications: Hypersensitivity; serious GI, renal, hepatic, cardiac disorders; blood dyscrasias
Precautions: Severe renal disease, blood dyscrasias, pregnancy category C, hepatic disease, elderly, lactation, children
Pharmacokinetics:
PO: Peak 0.5-2 hr, half-life 20 min; deacetylates in liver; excreted in feces (metabolites/active drug)
Drug interactions of concern to dentistry:
• Increased risk of GI side effects: NSAIDs, aspirin

DENTAL CONSIDERATIONS
General:
• Consider drug in diagnosis of taste alteration.
• Patients on chronic drug therapy may rarely have symptoms of blood dyscrasias, which can include infection, bleeding, and poor healing.
• Avoid prescribing aspirin-containing products.
Consultations:
• Medical consult may be required to assess disease control in the patient.
• In a patient with symptoms of blood dyscrasias, request a medical consult for blood studies and postpone dental treatment until normal values are reestablished.
Teach patient/family:
• Importance of good oral hygiene to prevent soft tissue inflammation
• Caution to prevent injury when using oral hygiene aids
• To avoid mouth rinses with high alcohol content due to drying effects

C

colestipol HCl
(koe-les'ti-pole)
Colestid
Drug class.: Antihyperlipidemic

Action: Absorbs, combines with bile acids to form insoluble complex that is excreted through feces; loss of bile acids lowers cholesterol levels
Uses: Primary hypercholesterolemia, xanthomas, digitalis toxicity, pruritus due to biliary obstruction, diarrhea due to bile acids
Dosage and routes:
• *Adult:* PO 5-30 g/day in 2-4 divided doses
Available forms include: Tabs 1 g, granules for oral suspension 5 g/ 7.5 g powder
Side effects/adverse reactions:
ORAL: Glossitis
GI: Constipation, abdominal pain, nausea, fecal impaction, hemorrhoids, flatulence, vomiting, steatorrhea, peptic ulcer
HEMA: Decreased vitamins A, D, K red folate content; ***hyperchloremic acidosis;*** bleeding; decreased protime
INTEG: Rash, irritation of perianal area, skin
Contraindications: Hypersensitivity, biliary obstruction
Precautions: Pregnancy category B, lactation, children, bleeding disorders
Pharmacokinetics:
PO: Excreted in feces

Drug interactions of concern to dentistry:

- Decreased absorption of tetracyclines, cephalexin, phenobarbital, corticosteroids, clindamycin, penicillins; administer doses several hours apart

DENTAL CONSIDERATIONS

General:

- Consider semisupine chair position for patient comfort due to GI effects of disease.

cortisone acetate

(kor'ti-sone)

Cortone

Drug class.: Glucocorticoid, short-acting

Action: Glucocorticoids have multiple actions that include antiinflammatory and immunosuppressant effects. They inhibit phospholipase A_2, interfering with or reducing the synthesis of prostaglandins and leukotrienes. They also bind to cytoplasmic glucocorticoid receptors (GRs) and enter the cell nucleus to bind with DNA. This results in the synthesis of various enzymes such as collagenase, elastase, and cytokines that play important roles in inflammation and immunosuppression. They also suppress the production of lymphocytes, monocytes, and eosinophils.

Uses: Inflammation, severe allergy, adrenal insufficiency, collagen disorders, respiratory, dermatologic disorders

Dosage and routes:

- *Adult:* PO 25-300 mg qd or q2d, titrated to patient response

Available forms include: Tabs 5, 10, 25 mg

Side effects/adverse reactions:

▼ *ORAL:* Dry mouth, poor wound healing, petechiae, candidiasis

CNS: Depression, flushing, sweating, headache, mood changes

CV: Hypertension, ***circulatory collapse, thrombophlebitis, embolism, necrotizing angiitis, CHF,*** tachycardia, edema

GI: Diarrhea, nausea, abdominal distention, ***GI hemorrhage, pancreatitis,*** increased appetite

HEMA: ***Thrombocytopenia***

EENT: Fungal infections, increased intraocular pressure, blurred vision

INTEG: Acne, poor wound healing, ecchymosis, bruising, petechiae

MS: Fractures, osteoporosis, weakness

Contraindications: Psychosis, hypersensitivity, idiopathic thrombocytopenia, acute glomerulonephritis, amebiasis, fungal infections, nonasthmatic bronchial disease, child <2 yr, AIDS, TB

Precautions: Pregnancy category C, diabetes mellitus, glaucoma, osteoporosis, seizure disorders, ulcerative colitis, CHF, myasthenia gravis, renal disease, esophagitis, peptic ulcer, rifampin

Pharmacokinetics:

PO: Peak 2 hr, duration 1.5 days

IM: Peak 20-48 hr, duration 1.5 days

Drug interactions of concern to dentistry:

- Decreased action: barbiturates, rifabutin, rifampin
- Increased GI side effects: alcohol, salicylates, NSAIDs
- Increased action: ketoconazole, macrolide antibiotics
- Hepatotoxicity: acetaminophen (chronic, high doses)

DENTAL CONSIDERATIONS

General:

• Monitor vital signs every appointment due to cardiovascular side effects.
• Patients on chronic drug therapy may rarely have symptoms of blood dyscrasias, which can include infection, bleeding, and poor healing.
• Assess salivary flow as a factor in caries, periodontal disease, and candidiasis.
• Avoid prescribing aspirin-containing products.
• Symptoms of oral infections may be masked.
• Place on frequent recall to evaluate healing response.
• Prophylactic antibiotics may be indicated to prevent infection if surgery or deep scaling is planned.
• Determine dose and duration of steroid therapy for each patient to assess risk for stress tolerance and immunosuppression.
• Patients who have been or are currently on chronic steroid therapy (>2 wk) may require supplemental steroids for dental treatment.
• Determine why the patient is taking the drug.

Consultations:

• In a patient with symptoms of blood dyscrasias, request a medical consult for blood studies and postpone dental treatment until normal values are reestablished.
• Medical consult may be required to assess disease control and stress tolerance of patient.
• Consult may be required to confirm steroid dose and duration of use.

Teach patient/family:

• Importance of good oral hygiene to prevent soft tissue inflammation
• Caution to prevent injury when using oral hygiene aids

When chronic dry mouth occurs, advise patient:

• To avoid mouth rinses with high alcohol content due to drying effects
• To use daily home fluoride products for anticaries effect
• To use sugarless gum, frequent sips of water, or saliva substitutes

---

cromolyn sodium (disodium cromoglycate)

(kroe′moe-lin)

Gastrocrom, Intal, Nasalcrom

✤ Novo-Cromolyn, PMS-Sodium Chromglycate, Rynacrom

Drug class.: Antiasthmatic, mast cell stabilizer

Action: Stabilizes the membrane of the sensitized mast cell, preventing release of chemical mediators after an antigen-IgE interaction

Uses: Allergic rhinitis, severe perennial bronchial asthma, exercise-induced bronchospasm (prevention), prevention of acute bronchospasm induced by environmental pollutants, mastocytosis

Dosage and routes:

Allergic rhinitis

• *Adult and child >6 yr:* NASAL SOL 1 spray in each nostril tid-qid, not to exceed 6 doses/day

Bronchospasm

• *Adult and child >5 yr:* INH 20 mg <1 hr before exercise

Bronchial asthma

• *Adult and child >5 yr:* INH 20 mg qid; NEBULIZ 20 mg qid by nebulization

Mastocytosis

• *Adult:* PO 200 mg qid 30 min ac and hs

• *Child 2-12 yr:* PO 100 mg qid 30 min ac and hs

• *Child <2 yr:* PO 20 mg/kg of body weight per day in 4 divided doses

Available forms include: Sol 40 mg/ml; caps for inh 20 mg/2 ml; neb sol 20 mg; aerosol 800 μ/actuation; oral conc 5 ml/100 mg

Side effects/adverse reactions:

▼ *ORAL:* Dry, burning mouth, bitter taste (aerosol)

GI: Nausea, vomiting, anorexia

GU: Frequency, dysuria

INTEG: Rash, urticaria, angioedema

MS: Joint pain/swelling

Contraindications: Hypersensitivity to this drug or lactose, status asthmaticus

Precautions: Pregnancy category B, lactation, renal disease, hepatic disease, child <5 yr

Pharmacokinetics:

INH: Peak 15 min, duration 4-6 hr, half-life 80 min; excreted unchanged in feces

DENTAL CONSIDERATIONS

General:

• Assess salivary flow as a factor in caries, periodontal disease, and candidiasis.

• Consider semisupine chair position for patients with respiratory disease.

• A stress reduction protocol may be required.

• Midday appointments and a stress reduction protocol may be required for anxious patients.

• Be aware that aspirin or sulfite preservatives in vasoconstrictor-containing products can exacerbate asthma.

Consultations:

• Consider drug in diagnosis of taste alteration and burning mouth syndrome.

• Medical consult may be required to assess disease control and stress tolerance of patient.

Teach patient/family:

• For inhalation dosage forms, rinse mouth with water after each dose to prevent dryness

When chronic dry mouth occurs, advise patient:

• To avoid mouth rinses with high alcohol content due to drying effects

• To use daily home fluoride products for anticaries effect

• To use sugarless gum, frequent sips of water, or saliva substitutes

---

cyanocobalamin (vitamin B_{12})/ hydroxocobalamin (vitamin $B_{12}a$)

(sye-an-oh-koe-bal'a-min)

Cobex, Crystamine, Crysti-12, Cyanoject, Cyomin, Neuroforte-R, Primabalt, Rubesol, Rubramin PC, Shovite, Vibal, Vibedoz, and Vitabee

🍁 Anacobin, Bedoz

Drug class.: Vitamin B_{12}, water-soluble vitamin

Action: Needed for adequate nerve functioning, protein and carbohydrate metabolism, normal growth, RBC development, cell reproduction

Uses: Vitamin B_{12} deficiency, pernicious anemia, vitamin B_{12} malabsorption syndrome, Schilling test, increased requirements with pregnancy thyrotoxicosis, hemolytic anemia, hemorrhage, renal and hepatic disease

Dosage and routes:

• *Adult:* PO 25 µg qd × 5-10 days, maintenance 100-200 mg IM qmo; IM/SC 30-100 µg qd × 5-10 days, maintenance 100-200 µg IM qmo

• *Child:* PO 1 µg qd × 5-10 days, maintenance 60 µg IM qmo or more; IM/SC 1-30 µg qd × 5-10 days, maintenance 60 µg IM qmo or more

Pernicious anemia/malabsorption syndrome

• *Adult:* IM 100-1000 µg qd × 2 wk, then 100-1000 µg IM qmo

• *Child:* IM 100-500 µg over 2 wk or more given in 100-500 µg doses, then 60 µg IM/SC qmo

Schilling test

• *Adult and child:* IM 1000 µg in one dose

Available forms include: Tabs 25, 50, 100, 250, 500, 1000 µg; inj IM 100, 120, 1000 µg/ml

Side effects/adverse reactions:

CNS: Flushing, optic nerve atrophy

CV: ***CHF, pulmonary edema,*** peripheral vascular thrombosis

GI: Diarrhea

INTEG: Itching, rash, pain at site

META: Hypokalemia

Contraindications: Hypersensitivity, optic nerve atrophy

Precautions: Pregnancy category A, lactation, children

Pharmacokinetics:

PO: Stored in liver, kidneys, stomach; 50%-90% excreted in urine; crosses placenta, excreted in breast milk

Drug interactions of concern to dentistry:

• Increased absorption: prednisone

DENTAL CONSIDERATIONS

General:

• Deficiency in B_{12} and other B-complex vitamins may cause oral symptomatology.

---

cyclizine HCl/cyclizine lactate

(sye'kli-zeen)

Marezine

Drug class.: Antiemetic, antihistaminic, anticholinergic

Action: May act centrally by blocking chemoreceptor trigger zone, which in turn acts on vomiting center; also antagonizes histamine peripherally

Uses: Motion sickness, prevention of postoperative vomiting

Dosage and routes:

Vomiting

• *Adult:* IM 50 mg 0.5 hr before termination of surgery, then q4-6h prn (lactate)

• *Child:* IM 3 mg/kg divided in 3 equal doses (lactate)

Motion sickness

• *Adult:* PO 50 mg, then q4-6h prn, not to exceed 200 mg/day (HCl)

• *Child:* PO 25 mg q4-6h prn

Available forms include: Tabs 50 mg; inj 50 mg/ml

Side effects/adverse reactions:

▼ *ORAL:* Dry mouth

CNS: Drowsiness, dizziness, convulsions in children, vertigo, fatigue, restlessness, headache, insomnia, hallucinations (auditory/visual)

GI: Nausea, anorexia
EENT: Blurred vision, tinnitus
Contraindications: Hypersensitivity to cyclizines, shock
Precautions: Children, narrow-angle glaucoma, urinary retention, lactation, prostatic hypertrophy, elderly, pregnancy category B, lactation
Pharmacokinetics:
PO: Duration 4-6 hr, other pharmacokinetics not known
Drug interactions of concern to dentistry:
• Increased CNS depression: alcohol, all CNS depressants
• May increase effect of anticholinergic drugs
DENTAL CONSIDERATIONS
General:
• Monitor vital signs every appointment due to cardiovascular side effects.
• Assess salivary flow as a factor in caries, periodontal disease, and candidiasis.
Teach patient/family:
When chronic dry mouth occurs, advise patient:
• To avoid mouth rinses with high alcohol content due to drying effects
• To use daily home fluoride products for anticaries effect
• To use sugarless gum, frequent sips of water, or saliva substitutes

---

cyclobenzaprine HCl
(sye-kloe-ben′za-preen)
Cycoflex, Flexeril
Drug class.: Skeletal muscle relaxant, centrally acting tricyclic

Action: Unknown; may be related to antidepressant effects, has actions similar to those of tricyclic antidepressants
Uses: Adjunct for relief of muscle spasm and pain in musculoskeletal conditions
Dosage and routes:
• *Adult:* PO 10 mg tid × 1 wk, not to exceed 60 mg/day × 3 wk
Side effects/adverse reactions:
▼ *ORAL:* Dry mouth, unpleasant taste
CNS: Dizziness, weakness, drowsiness, headache, tremor, depression, insomnia, confusion, paresthesia
CV: Postural hypotension, tachycardia, dysrhythmias
GI: Nausea, vomiting, hiccups
GU: Urinary retention, frequency, change in libido
EENT: Diplopia, temporary loss of vision
INTEG: Rash, pruritus, fever, facial flushing, sweating
Contraindications: Acute recovery phase of MI, dysrhythmias, heart block, CHF, hypersensitivity, child <12 yr, intermittent porphyria, thyroid disease
Precautions: Renal disease, hepatic disease, addictive personalities, pregnancy category B, elderly
Pharmacokinetics:
PO: Onset 1 hr, peak 3-8 hr, duration 12-24 hr, half-life 1-3 days; metabolized by liver; excreted in urine; crosses placenta; excreted in breast milk
Drug interactions of concern to dentistry:
• Increased CNS depression: alcohol, narcotics, barbiturates, sedatives, hypnotics
• Increased effects of anticholinergic drugs

• Increased effects of direct-acting sympathomimetics (epinephrine, levonordefrin)

DENTAL CONSIDERATIONS

General:

• Monitor vital signs every appointment due to cardiovascular side effects.

• Assess salivary flow as a factor in caries, periodontal disease, and candidiasis.

• After supine positioning, have patient sit upright for at least 2 min to avoid orthostatic hypotension.

• Use vasoconstrictors with caution, in low doses, and with careful aspiration. Avoid use of gingival retraction cord with epinephrine.

• Place on frequent recall due to oral side effects.

• Consider drug in diagnosis of taste alterations.

Consultations:

• Medical consult may be required to assess disease control in the patient.

Teach patient/family:

When chronic dry mouth occurs, advise patient:

• To avoid mouth rinses with high alcohol content due to drying effects

• To use daily home fluoride products for anticaries effect

• To use sugarless gum, frequent sips of water, or saliva substitutes

---

cyclophosphamide

(sye-kloe-foss'fa-mide)

Cytoxan, Neosar

♣ Procytox

Drug class.: Antineoplastic alkylating agent

Action: Alkylates DNA, RNA; inhibits enzymes that allow synthesis of amino acids in proteins; is also responsible for cross-linking DNA strands

Uses: Hodgkin's disease; lymphomas; leukemia; cancer of female reproductive tract, lung, prostate; multiple myeloma; neuroblastoma, retinoblastoma; Ewing's sarcoma

Dosage and routes:

• *Adult:* PO initially 1-5 mg/kg over 2-5 days, maintenance 1-5 mg/kg; IV initially 40-50 mg/kg in divided doses over 2-5 days, maintenance 10-15 mg/kg q7-10d or 3-5 mg/kg q3d

• *Child:* PO/IV 2-8 mg/kg or 60-250 mg/m^2 in divided doses for at least 6 days; maintenance 10-15 mg/kg q7-10d or 30 mg/kg q3-4wk; dose should be reduced by half when bone marrow depression occurs

Available forms include: Powder for inj IV 100, 200, 500 mg and 1, 2 g; tabs 25, 50 mg

Side effects/adverse reactions:

▼ *ORAL:* Stomatitis, swelling of lips, tongue

CNS: Headache, dizziness

CV: ***Cardiotoxicity*** (high doses)

GI: *Nausea, vomiting, diarrhea, weight loss,* **hepatotoxicity,** colitis

RESP: ***Fibrosis***

HEMA: ***Thrombocytopenia, leukopenia, pancytopenia, myelosuppression***

GU: ***Hemorrhagic cystitis, hematuria, neoplasms,*** amenorrhea, azoospermia, impotence, sterility, ovarian fibrosis

INTEG: *Alopecia,* dermatitis

ENDO: Syndrome of inappropriate antidiuretic hormone (SIADH)

Contraindications: Lactation, pregnancy category D

Precautions: Radiation therapy

Pharmacokinetics:
PO: Half-life 4-6.5 hr; 50% bound to plasma proteins; metabolized by liver; excreted in urine

Drug interactions of concern to dentistry:

- Increased blood dyscrasia: NSAIDs, dapsone, phenothiazines, corticosteroids
- Increased metabolism: phenobarbital

DENTAL CONSIDERATIONS

General:

- Monitor vital signs every appointment due to cardiovascular and respiratory side effects.
- Patients on chronic drug therapy may rarely have symptoms of blood dyscrasias, which can include infection, bleeding, and poor healing.
- Avoid prescribing aspirin-containing products.
- Prophylactic antibiotics may be indicated to prevent infection if surgery or deep scaling is planned due to leukopenic drug side effects.
- Patients receiving chemotherapy may require palliative treatment for stomatitis.

Consultations:

- In a patient with symptoms of blood dyscrasias, request a medical consult for blood studies and postpone dental treatment until normal values are reestablished.
- Take precautions if dental surgery is anticipated and anesthesia is required.

Teach patient/family:

- Importance of good oral hygiene to prevent soft tissue inflammation
- Caution to prevent injury when using oral hygiene aids

cycloserine

(sye-kloe-ser'een)
Seromycin Pulvules
Drug class.: Antitubercular

Action: Inhibits cell wall synthesis, analog of D-alanine
Uses: Pulmonary TB, extrapulmonary as adjunctive
Dosage and routes:

- *Adult:* PO 250 mg q12h × 14 days, then 250 mg q8h × 2 wk if there are no signs of toxicity, then 250 mg q6h if there are no signs of toxicity, not to exceed 1 g/day
- *Child:* PO 10-20 mg/kg/day (max 0.75-1 g) individual doses

Available forms include: Caps 250 mg
Side effects/adverse reactions:
CNS: ***Convulsions,*** headache, anxiety, drowsiness, tremors, lethargy, depression, confusion, psychosis, aggression
CV: ***CHF***
HEMA: ***Megaloblastic anemia,*** vitamin B_{12} deficiency, folic acid deficiency, leukocytosis
INTEG: Dermatitis, photosensitivity
Contraindications: Hypersensitivity, seizure disorders, renal disease, alcoholism (chronic), depression, severe anxiety, lactation, anemia
Precautions: Pregnancy category C, children
Pharmacokinetics:
PO: Peak 3-8 hr; excreted unchanged in urine; crosses placenta; excreted in breast milk

Drug interactions of concern to dentistry:

- Seizures: alcohol
- Drowsiness is a common side

effect; although no drug interactions with sedatives are reported, increased drowsiness might be possible

DENTAL CONSIDERATIONS
General:
• Patients on chronic drug therapy may rarely have symptoms of blood dyscrasias, which can include infection, bleeding, and poor healing.
• Examine for evidence of oral signs of disease.
• Determine why the patient is taking the drug (for preventive or therapeutic therapy).
Consultation:
• Medical consult may be required to assess patient's ability to tolerate stress.
• In a patient with symptoms of blood dyscrasias, request a medical consult for blood studies and postpone dental treatment until normal values are reestablished.
Determine that noninfectious status exists by ensuring that:
• Anti-TB drugs have been taken more than 3 wk
• Culture confirms antibiotic susceptibility to TB microorganism
• Patient has had three consecutive negative sputum smears
• Patient is not in the coughing stage
Teach patient/family:
• To avoid mouth rinses with high alcohol content
• Caution to prevent injury when using oral hygiene aids
• Importance of good oral hygiene to prevent soft tissue inflammation
• Importance of taking medication for full length of prescribed therapy to ensure effectiveness of treatment and prevent the emergence of resistant forms of microbe

C

cyclosporine
(sye'kloe-spor-een)
Neoral, Sandimmune, Sandimmune SGC, SangCya
Drug class.: Immunosuppressant

Action: Produces immunosuppression by inhibiting lymphocytes (T)
Uses: To prevent rejection of tissues/organ transplants; severe recalcitrant psoriasis; rheumatoid arthritis
Dosage and routes:
• *Adult and child:* PO 15 mg/kg several hours before surgery, daily for 2 wk, reduce dosage by 2.5 mg/kg/wk to 5-10 mg/kg/day; IV 5-6 mg/kg several hours before surgery, daily, switch to PO form as soon as possible
Available forms include: Oral sol 100 mg/ml; inj IV 50 mg/ml
Side effects/adverse reactions:
▼ *ORAL: Candidiasis, gingival overgrowth*
CNS: Tremors, headache
CV: Hypertension
GI: ***Hepatotoxicity,*** nausea, vomiting, diarrhea, pancreatitis
GU: ***Albuminuria, hematuria, proteinuria, renal failure***
INTEG: Hirsutism, rash, acne
Contraindications: Hypersensitivity
Precautions: Severe renal disease, severe hepatic disease, pregnancy category C
Pharmacokinetics:
PO: Peak 4 hr, half-life (biphasic) 1.2 hr, 25 hr; highly protein bound;

metabolized in liver; crosses placenta; excreted in feces, breast milk

Drug interactions of concern to dentistry:

• Hepatotoxicity/nephrotoxicity: erythromycin, miconazole, ketoconazole, NSAIDs

• Decreased action: barbiturates

• Increased infection and immunosuppression: corticosteroids

• A single case reported elevated cyclosporine levels: ketoconazole

DENTAL CONSIDERATIONS

General:

• Monitor vital signs every appointment due to cardiovascular side effects.

• Patients on chronic drug therapy may rarely have symptoms of blood dyscrasias, which can include infection, bleeding, and poor healing.

• Place on frequent recall to evaluate gingival condition and healing response.

• Monitor time since organ/tissue transplant.

Consultations:

• Antibiotic prophylaxis is usually recommended in patients with organ transplants and immunosuppression.

• In a patient with symptoms of blood dyscrasias, request a medical consult for blood studies and postpone dental treatment until normal values are reestablished.

• Request baseline blood pressure in renal transplant patients for patient evaluation before dental treatment.

Teach patient/family:

• Importance of good oral hygiene to prevent soft tissue inflammation

• Caution to prevent injury when using oral hygiene aids

cyproheptadine HCl

(si-proe-hep′ta-deen)

Periactin

PMS-Cyproheptadine

Drug class.: Antihistamine, H_1-receptor antagonist

Action: Acts on blood vessels, GI, respiratory system by competing with histamine for H_1 receptor site; decreases allergic response by blocking histamine

Uses: Allergy symptoms, rhinitis, pruritus, cold urticaria

Dosage and routes:

• *Adult:* PO 4 mg tid-qid, not to exceed 0.5 mg/kg/day

• *Child 7-14 yr:* PO 4 mg bid-tid, not to exceed 16 mg/day

• *Child 2-6 yr:* PO 2 mg bid-tid, not to exceed 12 mg/day

Available forms include: Tabs 4 mg; syr 2 mg/5 ml

Side effects/adverse reactions:

ORAL: Dry mouth

CNS: Dizziness, drowsiness, poor coordination, fatigue, anxiety, euphoria, confusion, paresthesia, neuritis

CV: Hypotension, palpitation, tachycardia

GI: Constipation, nausea, vomiting, anorexia, diarrhea, weight gain

RESP: Increased thick secretions, wheezing, chest tightness

GU: Retention, dysuria, frequency, increased appetite

EENT: Blurred vision, dilated pupils, tinnitus, nasal stuffiness, dry nose/throat

INTEG: Rash, urticaria, photosensitivity

Contraindications: Hypersensitivity to H_1-receptor antagonist, acute asthma attack, lower respiratory tract disease

Precautions: Increased intraocular pressure, renal disease, cardiac disease, hypertension, bronchial asthma, seizure disorder, stenosed peptic ulcers, hyperthyroidism, prostatic hypertrophy, bladder neck obstruction, pregnancy category B, elderly

Pharmacokinetics:

PO: Duration 4-6 hr; metabolized in liver; excreted by kidneys; excreted in breast milk

Drug interactions of concern to dentistry:

• Increased CNS depression: alcohol, CNS depressants

• Increased effect of anticholinergic drugs

DENTAL CONSIDERATIONS

General:

• Assess salivary flow as a factor in caries, periodontal disease, and candidiasis.

• Determine why the patient is taking the drug.

Teach patient/family:

When chronic dry mouth occurs, advise patient:

• To avoid mouth rinses with high alcohol content due to drying effects

• To use daily home fluoride products for anticaries effect

• To use sugarless gum, frequent sips of water, or saliva substitutes

daclizumab

(da-klik′si-mab)

Zenapax

Drug class.: Immunosuppresive monoclonal antibody

Action: Saturates the Tac subunit of interleukin-2 (IL-2) receptor for approximately 120 days after transplant

Uses: Prophylaxis of acute organ rejection in patients with renal transplants; use in combination with cyclosporine and glucocorticoids

Dosage and routes:

• *Adult:* IV infusion; 1 mg/kg of body weight as an initial dose no more than 24 hours before transplant surgery and an additional 4 doses given at intervals of 14 days

Available forms include: Vials 25 mg/5 ml

Side effects/adverse effects:

CNS: Tremor, headache, dizziness, insomnia

CV: Peripheral edema, aggravated hypertension

GI: Diarrhea, vomiting, constipation, abdominal pain

RESP: Cough, dyspnea, pulmonary edema

HEMA: Bleeding, lymphocele

GU: Oliguria, dysuria, urinary tract bleeding

EENT: Blurred vision

INTEG: Impaired wound healing, acne, pruritus, rash

MS: Myalgia, back pain

MISC: Fever, pain, fatigue

Contraindications: Hypersensitivity

Precautions: Risk of lymphoproliferative disease and opportunistic infections, anaphylaxis risk unknown, long-term effects unknown, pregnancy category C, lactation, children, geriatric patients

Pharmacokinetics:

IV: Required serum levels for Tac saturation 5-10 μg/ml, terminal elimination half-life 20 days with a range of 11-38 days, renal clearance

Drug interactions of concern to dentistry:
- None reported

DENTAL CONSIDERATIONS:
General:
- This is a hospital-type drug, but because some dosing is continued, patients may appear in the dental office while receiving this drug.
- Transplant patients may also be taking cyclosporine and glucorticoids; review each transplant patient's medications.
- Short appointments and a stress reduction protocol may be required for anxious patients.

Consultations:
- Antibiotic prophylaxis is usually recommended in patients with organ transplants and immunosuppression.
- Medical consult may be required to assess disease control and patient's ability to tolerate stress.

Teach patient/family:
- Importance of good oral hygiene to prevent soft tissue inflammation
- To prevent trauma when using oral hygiene aids
- Importance of updating health and drug history if physician makes any changes in evaluation/drug regimens

dalteparin sodium

(dal-te′pa-rin)

Fragmin

Drug class.: Heparin-type anticoagulant

Action: Low-molecular-weight heparin having antithrombotic actions with higher anti-Factor X_a activity compared with anti-Factor II_a

Uses: Prevention of deep vein thrombosis following abdominal surgery, treatment of life-threatening conditions such as unstable angina, non–Q-wave MI; prevention of ischemia complications due to blood clot formation in patients on aspirin therapy; in combination with warfarin in deep vein thrombosis with or without pulmonary embolism

Dosage and routes:
- *Adult:* SC 2500 IU each day starting 1-2 hr before surgery and repeated once daily for 5-10 days postoperatively

Available forms include: Prefilled syringes: 16 mg/0.2 ml and 32 mg/0.2 ml

Side effects/adverse reactions:

HEMA: *Bleeding after surgery, thrombocytopenia*

INTEG: Skin necrosis

MISC: Local pain, irritation, ***anaphylaxis*** (rare)

Contraindications: Hypersensitivity, active major bleeding, thrombocytopenia, IM administration

Precautions: Hemorrhage, cannot be used interchangeably with other forms of heparin, pregnancy category B, lactation, children, requires monitoring, GI bleeding

Pharmacokinetics:

SC INJ ONLY: Good absorption, peak levels of anti-Factor X_a activity 4 hr, renal excretion

Drug interactions of concern to dentistry: Avoid concurrent use of aspirin, NSAIDS, dipyridamole, and sulfinpyrazone

DENTAL CONSIDERATIONS:
General:
- Product may be used in outpatient therapy. Delay elective dental treatment until patient completes anticoagulant therapy.

• Determine why patient is taking the drug.
• Consider local hemostasis measures to prevent excessive bleeding.
• Avoid prescribing aspirin-containing products.

Consultations:
• Medical consult should include routine blood counts, including platelet counts and bleeding time.

Teach patient/family:
• Importance of good oral hygiene to prevent soft tissue inflammation
• To prevent trauma when using oral hygiene aids
• To report oral lesions, soreness, or bleeding to dentist

---

danaparoid

(da-nap′a-roid)

Orgaran

Drug class.: Heparin-type anticoagulant

Action: Low-molecular-weight heparin having antithrombotic actions with higher anti-Factor X_a activity compared with anti-Factor II_a

Uses: Prevention of deep vein thrombosis following hip or knee replacement surgery; unapproved use in thromboembolism, hemodialysis, and cardiovascular surgery

Dosage and routes:
• *Adult:* SC 750 anti-Factor X_a units bid; 1-4 hr preoperatively and not sooner than 2 hr after surgery; may be used for 7-12 days

Available forms include: Inj 750 anti-Factor X_a U/0.6 ml, amps and prefilled syringes

Side effects/adverse reactions:
CNS: Insomnia, headache, dizziness
CV: Peripheral edema
GI: Nausea, vomiting, constipation
HEMA: Bleeding after surgery, anemia
GU: UTI, urinary retention
INTEG: Rash, pruritus
MS: Asthenia
MISC: Fever, injection site pain, joint disorder

Contraindications: Hypersensitivity, severe bleeding disorders, type II thrombocytopenia, IM administration

Precautions: Cannot interchange with heparin, hemorrhage, thrombocytopenia, renal or hepatic impairment, pregnancy category B, lactation, children, antidotes not available, GI bleeding

Pharmacokinetics:
SC INJ ONLY: Bioavailability 100%, maximum activity 2-5 hr; renal excretion; half-life based on plasma anti-X_a activity is 18-28 hr

Drug interactions of concern to dentistry:
• Avoid concurrent use of platelet aggregation antagonist such as aspirin, NSAIDs, dipyridamole

DENTAL CONSIDERATIONS

General:
• Determine why patient is taking the drug.
• Consider local hemostasis measures to prevent excessive bleeding if dental treatment must be performed.
• Antibiotic prophylaxis before dental treatment may be required for joint prosthesis. See 1997 ADA guidelines.
• Delay elective dental treatment until patient completes danaparoid therapy.

Consultations:
• Medical consult should include routine blood counts, including platelet counts and bleeding time.

D

Teach patient/family:

• Importance of good oral hygiene to prevent soft tissue inflammation

• Caution to prevent trauma when using oral hygiene aids

• To report oral lesions, soreness, or bleeding to dentist

danazol

(da'na-zole)

Danocrine

🍁 Cyclomen

Drug class.: Androgen, α-ethinyl testosterone derivative

Action: Decreases FSH and LH output, which are controlled by pituitary; this leads to amenorrhea/anovulation

Uses: Endometriosis, prevention of hereditary angioedema, fibrocystic breast disease

Dosage and routes:

Endometriosis

• *Adult:* PO initial dose 800 mg bid, then decreased to 200-400 mg bid × 3-9 mo

Fibrocystic breast disease

• *Adult:* PO 100-400 mg qd in 2 divided doses × 2-6 mo

Hereditary angioedema

• *Adult:* PO 200 mg bid-tid until desired response, then decrease dose to 100 mg at 1-3 mo intervals

Available forms include: Caps 50, 100, 200 mg

Side effects/adverse reactions:

▼ *ORAL:* Gingival bleeding (rare), stomatitis, Stevens-Johnson syndrome (rare)

CNS: Dizziness, headache, fatigue, tremors, paresthesia, flushing, sweating, anxiety, lability, insomnia

CV: Increased BP

GI: Cholestatic jaundice, nausea, vomiting, constipation, weight gain

GU: Hematuria, amenorrhea, atrophic vaginitis, decreased libido, decreased breast size, clitoral hypertrophy, testicular atrophy

EENT: Carpal tunnel syndrome, conjunctional edema, nasal congestion

INTEG: Rash, acneiform lesions, oily hair/skin, flushing, sweating, acne vulgaris, alopecia, hirsutism

ENDO: Abnormal GTT

MS: Cramps, spasms

Contraindications: Severe renal disease, severe cardiac disease, severe hepatic disease, hypersensitivity, genital bleeding (abnormal)

Precautions: Migraine headaches, seizure disorders, pregnancy category X

Pharmacokinetics: Limited data available; oral absorption variable; metabolized in the liver

Drug interactions of concern to dentistry:

• Increased serum concentration of carbamazepine; consider avoiding use of concurrent administration

DENTAL CONSIDERATIONS

General:

• Patients on chronic drug therapy may rarely have symptoms of blood dyscrasias, which can include infection, bleeding, and poor healing.

Consultations:

• In a patient with symptoms of blood dyscrasias, request a medical consult for blood studies and postpone dental treatment until normal values are reestablished.

Teach patient/family:

• Importance of good oral hygiene to prevent soft tissue inflammation

• To avoid mouth rinses with high alcohol content due to drying and irritating effects

dantrolene sodium

(dan'troe-leen)

Dantrium, Dantrium Intravenous

Drug class.: Skeletal muscle relaxant, direct acting

Action: Interferes with intracellular release of the calcium necessary to initiate contraction

Uses: Spasticity in multiple sclerosis, stroke, spinal cord injury, cerebral palsy, malignant hyperthermia

Dosage and routes:

Spasticity

• *Adult:* PO 25 mg/day; may increase by 25-100 mg bid-qid, not to exceed 400 mg/day × 1 wk

• *Child:* PO 1 mg/kg/day given in divided doses bid-tid; may increase gradually, not to exceed 100 mg qid

Malignant hyperthermia

• *Adult and child:* IV 1 mg/kg, may repeat to total dose of 10 mg/kg; PO 4-8 mg/kg/day in 4 divided doses × 3 days to prevent further hyperthermia

Available forms include: Caps 25, 50, 100 mg; powder for inj IV 20 mg/vial

Side effects/adverse reactions:

▼ *ORAL:* Alteration of taste

CNS: Dizziness, weakness, fatigue, drowsiness, headache, disorientation, insomnia, paresthesia, tremors

CV: Hypotension, chest pain, palpitation

GI: Nausea, constipation, vomiting, increased AST, alk phosphatase, abdominal pain, anorexia, hepatitis

HEMA: ***Eosinophilia***

GU: Urinary frequency, nocturia, impotence, crystalluria

EENT: Nasal congestion, blurred vision, mydriasis

INTEG: Rash, pruritus, photosensitivity

Contraindications: Hypersensitivity, compromised pulmonary function, active hepatic disease, impaired myocardial function

Precautions: Peptic ulcer disease, renal disease, hepatic disease, stroke, seizure disorder, diabetes mellitus, pregnancy category C, elderly

Pharmacokinetics:

PO: Peak 5 hr, half-life 8 hr; highly protein bound; metabolized in liver; excreted in urine (metabolites)

Drug interactions of concern to dentistry:

• Increased CNS depression: alcohol, other CNS depressants

DENTAL CONSIDERATIONS

General:

• Monitor vital signs every appointment due to cardiovascular and respiratory side effects.

• Patients on chronic drug therapy may rarely have symptoms of blood dyscrasias, which can include infection, bleeding, and poor healing.

• Requires proficiency in IV administration technique when used for emergency treatment of malignant hyperthermia.

Consultations:

• In a patient with symptoms of blood dyscrasias, request a medical consult for blood studies and postpone dental treatment until normal values are reestablished.

Teach patient/family:
• Importance of good oral hygiene to prevent soft tissue inflammation
• To avoid mouth rinses with high alcohol content due to drying effects

dapsone (DDS)

(dap′sone)

♣ Avlosulfon

Drug class.: Leprostatic, antibacterial

Action: Bactericidal and bacteriostatic against *M. leprae;* may also be immunosuppressant

Uses: Leprosy (Hansen's disease); dermatitis herpetiformis; unapproved for cicatricial pemphigoid, LE, pemphigoid, malaria, *P. carinii*

Dosage and routes:

Leprosy
• *Adult:* PO 50-100 mg qd with rifampin 600 mg qd × 6 mo

Dermatitis herptiformis
• *Adult:* PO initial dose 50 mg d; can increase by 50 mg every 1-2 wk until remission; dose limit 500 mg/day; gradually reduce dose to lowest effective maintenance dose

Available forms include: Tabs 25, 100 mg

Side effects/adverse reactions:
▼ *ORAL:* Oral ulceration (erythema multiforme), lichenoid drug reaction
CNS: ***Convulsions,*** peripheral neuropathy, headache, anxiety, drowsiness, tremors, lethargy, depression, confusion, psychosis, aggression
GI: Nausea, vomiting, abdominal pain, anorexia
HEMA: ***Megaloblastic anemia***
GU: Proteinuria, nephrotic syndrome, renal papillary necrosis
EENT: Blurred vision, optic neuritis, photophobia
INTEG: ***Exfoliative dermatitis,*** photosensitivity

Contraindications: Hypersensitivity to sulfones, severe anemia

Precautions: Renal disease, hepatic disease, G6PD deficiency, pregnancy category C, lactation

Pharmacokinetics:
PO: Half-life 10-50 hr; rapid complete absorption; highly bound to plasma protein; metabolized in liver; excreted in urine

DENTAL CONSIDERATIONS

General:
• Patients on chronic drug therapy may rarely have symptoms of blood dyscrasias, which can include infection, bleeding, and poor healing.
• Avoid dental light in patient's eyes; offer dark glasses for patient comfort.

Consultations:
• In a patient with symptoms of blood dyscrasias, request a medical consult for blood studies and postpone dental treatment until normal values are reestablished.

Teach patient/family:
• Importance of good oral hygiene to prevent soft tissue inflammation
• Caution to prevent injury when using oral hygiene aids

delavirdine mesylate

(de-la-vir′deen)

Rescriptor

Drug class.: Antiviral, nonnucleoside

Action: Inhibits HIV-I reverse transcriptase enzymes; inhibits both DNA- and RNA-directed polymerase activity

Uses: HIV infection in combination with zidovudine or didanosine or both

Dosage and routes:

• *Adult:* PO 400 mg tid; may be given with or without food

Available forms include: Tabs 100, 200 mg

Side effects/adverse reactions:

▼ *ORAL:* Dry mouth (<2%), stomatitis, mouth ulcers, taste perversion

CNS: Headache, fatigue, agitation, confusion

CV: Bradycardia, palpitation, orthostatic hypotension, syncope

GI: Nausea, vomiting, abdominal pain, dyspepsia, diarrhea

RESP: Cough, congestion

HEMA: Neutropenia, leukopenia, thrombocytopenia, anemia, granulocytopenia

GU: Proteinuria

EENT: Dry eyes, conjunctivitis, diplopia

INTEG: Skin rash, pruritus

META: Altered liver function tests, elevated serum creatinine, alcohol intolerance

MS: Myalgia, cramps

Contraindications: Hypersensitivity, cisipride

Precautions: Modify dose in liver disease; children <16 yr, pregnancy category C, lactation

Pharmacokinetics:

PO: Peak plasma levels 1.0 hr, highly protein bound (99%), hepatic metabolism, excreted in both urine and feces, plasma half-life 2-11 hr

Drug interactions of concern to dentistry:

• Reduced absorption: antacids, cimetidine

• Increased plasma levels of alprazolam, triazolam, clarithromycin, midazolam

• Avoid coadministration with carbamazepine, phenobarbital, cisapride, ketoconazole

DENTAL CONSIDERATIONS

General:

• Examine for oral manifestation of opportunistic infection.

• Patient on chronic drug therapy may rarely have symptoms of blood dyscrasias, which can include infection, bleeding, and poor healing.

• Assess salivary flow as factor in caries, periodontal disease, and candidiasis.

• After supine positioning, have patient sit upright for at least 2 min before standing to avoid orthostatic hypotension.

• Do not use ingestible sodium bicarbonate products, such as the air polishing system (ProphyJet), within 2 hr of drug use.

Consultations:

• In a patient with symptoms of blood dyscrasias, request a medical consult for blood studies and postpone treatment until normal values are reestablished.

• Medical consult may be required to assess disease control and patient's ability to tolerate stress.

Teach patient/family:

• Importance of good oral hygiene to prevent soft tissue inflammation

• Caution to prevent trauma when using oral hygiene aids

• That secondary oral infection may occur; must see dentist immediately if infection occurs

When chronic dry mouth occurs advise patient:

• To avoid mouth rinses with high

alcohol content due to drying effects

• To use daily home fluoride products for anticaries effect

• To use sugarless gum, frequent sips of water, or saliva substitutes

demeclocycline HCl

(dem-e-kloe-sye'kleen)

Declomycin

Drug class.: Tetracycline

Action: Inhibits protein synthesis and phosphorylation in microorganisms by binding to 30S ribosomal subunits, reversibly binding to 50S ribosomal subunits; bacteriostatic

Uses: Uncommon gram-positive/gram-negative bacteria, protozoa, *Rickettsia, Mycoplasma*

Dosage and routes:

• *Adult:* PO 150 mg q6h or 300 mg q12h

• *Child >8 yr:* PO 6-12 mg/kg/day in divided doses q6-12h

Gonorrhea

• *Adult:* PO 600 mg, then 300 mg q12h × 4 days, total 3 g

Syndrome of inappropriate antidiuretic hormone

• *Adult:* PO 600-1200 mg/day in divided doses

Available forms include: Tabs 150, 300 mg; caps 150 mg

Side effects/adverse reactions:

▼ *ORAL:* Candidiasis, tooth discoloration, increased thirst, discolored tongue, lichenoid reaction

CNS: Fever, headache, paresthesia

CV: Pericarditis

GI: Nausea, vomiting, diarrhea, ***hepatotoxicity, pseudomembranous colitis,*** anorexia, enterocolitis, flatulence, abdominal cramps, epigastric burning

HEMA: ***Eosinophilia, neutropenia, thrombocytopenia, leukocytosis, hemolytic anemia***

GU: Increased BUN, ***renal failure, nephrotoxicity***, polyuria, polydipsia

EENT: Dysphagia, abdominal pain

INTEG: Rash, urticaria, photosensitivity, increased pigmentation, ***exfoliative dermatitis,*** pruritus, angioedema

Contraindications: Hypersensitivity to tetracyclines, children <8 yr, pregnancy category D

Precautions: Renal disease, hepatic disease, lactation, nephrogenic diabetes insipidus

Pharmacokinetics:

PO: Peak 3-6 hr, duration 48-72 hr, half-life 10-17 hr; 36%-91% bound to serum protein; crosses placenta; excreted in urine, breast milk

Drug interactions of concern to dentistry:

• Decreased effect of penicillins, cephalosporins, oral contraceptives

• When used for dental infections: decreased effects of oral contraceptives

DENTAL CONSIDERATIONS

General:

• Examine oral cavity for side effects if on long-term drug therapy.

• Determine why the patient is taking the drug.

• Do not prescribe during pregnancy or before age 8 yr due to tooth discoloration.

• Absorption is reduced by dairy products, metals, and antacids.

Consultations:

• Medical consult may be required to assess disease control in the patient.

Teach patient/family:

• Importance of good oral hygiene to prevent soft tissue inflammation

• Caution to prevent injury when using oral hygiene aids

When used for dental infection, advise patient:

• Taking birth control pill to use additional method of contraception for duration of cycle

• To report sore throat, oral burning sensation, fever, fatigue, any of which could indicate superinfection

• To take at prescribed intervals and complete dosage regimen

• To immediately notify the dentist if signs or symptoms of infection increase

desipramine HCl

(des-ip′ra-meen)

Norpramin, Pertofrane

Drug class.: Antidepressant, tricyclic

Action: Inhibits both norepinephrine and serotonin (5-HT) uptake in the brain, although the precise antidepressant mechanism remains unclear

Uses: Depression; unapproved use: neurogenic pain

Dosage and routes:

• *Adult:* PO 75-150 mg/day in divided doses, may increase to 300 mg/day or may give daily dose hs

• *Adolescent/geriatric:* PO 25-50 mg/day, may increase to 100 mg/day

Available forms include: Tabs 10, 25, 50, 75, 100, 150 mg; caps 25, 50 mg

Side effects/adverse reactions:

▼ *ORAL: Dry mouth, unpleasant taste,* bleeding, stomatitis

CNS: Dizziness, drowsiness, confusion, headache, anxiety, tremors, stimulation, weakness, insomnia, nightmares, EPS (elderly), increased psychiatric symptoms, paresthesia

CV: Orthostatic hypotension, ECG changes, tachycardia, ***hypertension,*** palpitation

GI: Diarrhea, ***paralytic ileus, hepatitis,*** increased appetite, cramps, epigastric distress, jaundice, nausea, vomiting

HEMA: ***Agranulocytosis, thrombocytopenia, eosinophilia, leukopenia***

GU: Retention, ***acute renal failure***

EENT: Blurred vision, tinnitus, mydriasis, ophthalmoplegia

INTEG: Rash, urticaria, sweating, pruritus, photosensitivity

Contraindications: Hypersensitivity to tricyclic antidepressants, recovery phase of MI, narrow-angle glaucoma, convulsive disorders, prostatic hypertrophy, child <12 yr

Precautions: Suicidal patients, severe depression, increased intraocular pressure, narrow-angle glaucoma, elderly, pregnancy category C, MAO inhibitors

Pharmacokinetics:

PO: Steady state 2-11 days, half-life 14-62 hr; metabolized by liver; excreted by kidneys; crosses placenta

Drug interactions of concern to dentistry:

• Increased anticholinergic effects: muscarinic blockers, antihistamines, phenothiazines

• Increased effects of direct-acting sympathomimetics: epinephrine, levonordefrin

• Potential risk for increased CNS depression: alcohol, barbiturates, benzodiazepines, and other CNS depressants

• Decreased antihypertensive effects: clonidine, guanadrel, guanethidine
• At higher tricyclic doses, serum levels of fluconazole and ketoconazole may be elevated

DENTAL CONSIDERATIONS
General:
• Take vital signs every appointment due to cardiovascular side effects.
• Assess salivary flow as a factor in caries, periodontal disease, and candidiasis.
• Patients on chronic drug therapy may rarely have symptoms of blood dyscrasias, which can include infection, bleeding, and poor healing.
• After supine positioning, have patient sit upright for at least 2 min to avoid orthostatic hypotension.
• Use vasoconstrictors with caution, in low doses, and with careful aspiration. Avoid use of gingival retraction cord with epinephrine.
• Place on frequent recall due to oral side effects.

Consultations:
• In a patient with symptoms of blood dyscrasias, request a medical consult for blood studies and postpone dental treatment until normal values are reestablished.
• Medical consult may be required to assess disease control in the patient.
• Physician should be informed if significant xerostomic side effects occur (increased caries, sore tongue, problems eating or swallowing, difficulty wearing prosthesis) so a medication change can be considered.

Teach patient/family:
• Importance of good oral hygiene to prevent soft tissue inflammation
• Caution to prevent injury when using oral hygiene aids

When chronic dry mouth occurs, advise patient:
• To avoid mouth rinses with high alcohol content due to drying effects
• To use daily home fluoride products for anticaries effect
• To use sugarless gum, frequent sips of water, or saliva substitutes

---

desmopressin acetate

(des-moe-press'in)
DDAVP, DDAVP Nasal Spray, Stimate, Stimate Nasal Spray
♣ DDAVP Rhinal Tube, DDAVP Rhinyl Nasal Solution, DDAVP Spray, Octosim

Drug class.: Synthetic antidiuretic hormone (a synthetic analog of vasopressin)

Action: Promotes reabsorption of water by action on renal tubular epithelium; also causes an increase in Factor VIII levels

Uses: Primary nocturnal enuresis, hemophilia A with Factor VIII levels >5%, von Willebrand's disease, neurogenic diabetes insipidus, renal concentration capacity

Dosage and routes:
Diabetes insipidus
• *Adult:* INTRANASAL 0.1-0.4 ml qd in divided doses; IV/SC 0.5-1 ml qd in divided doses
• *Adult:* PO initial dose 0.05 mg bid, increase to 0.1-1.2 mg in divided doses as required
• *Child 3 mo-12 yr:* INTRANASAL 0.05-0.3 ml qd in divided doses

Hemophilia/von Willebrand's disease
• *Adult and child:* IV 0.3 μg/kg in

NaCl over 15-30 min; may repeat if needed

Available forms include: Nasal sol 1.5 mg/ml; nasal spray pump 0.1 mg/ml; intranasal test 0.1 mg/ml; inj IV/SC 4, 15 μg/ml; tab 0.1 and 0.2 mg

Side effects/adverse reactions:

CNS: Headache, drowsiness, lethargy, flushing

CV: Increased BP

GI: Nausea, *mild abdominal cramps,* heartburn

GU: Vulval pain

EENT: Nasal irritation, congestion, rhinitis

Contraindications: Hypersensitivity, nephrogenic diabetes insipidus

Precautions: Pregnancy category B, CAD, lactation, hypertension

Pharmacokinetics:

NASAL: Onset 1 hr, peak 1-2 hr, duration 8-20 hr, half-life 8 min, 76 min (terminal)

Drug interactions of concern to dentistry:

• Decreased antidiuretic effects: demeclocycline

• Increased antidiuretic effects: carbamazepine

DENTAL CONSIDERATIONS

General:

• Monitor vital signs every appointment due to cardiovascular side effects.

• Avoid prescribing aspirin-containing products if treatment is for bleeding disorder.

• Consider local hemostasis measures to prevent excessive bleeding.

• Determine why the patient is taking the drug.

• Consider semisupine chair position for patient comfort due to GI effects of disease.

Consultations:

• Medical consult may be required to assess disease control in the patient; definite consult in patients with chronic bleeding disorders.

• Medical consult should include partial prothrombin or prothrombin times.

Teach patient/family:

• To advise dentist if excessive bleeding occurs or continues after dental treatment

desonide

(dess'oh-nide)

DesOwen, Tridesilon

Drug class.: Topical corticosteroid, group IV low potency

Action: Glucocorticoids have multiple actions that include antiinflammatory and immunosuppressant effects. They inhibit phospholipase A_2, interfering with or reducing the synthesis of prostaglandins and leukotrienes. They also bind to cytoplasmic glucocorticoid receptors (GRs) and enter the cell nucleus to bind with DNA. This results in the synthesis of various enzymes such as collagenase, elastase, and cytokines that play important roles in inflammation and immunosuppression. They also suppress the production of lymphocytes, monocytes, and eosinophils.

Uses: Psoriasis, eczema, contact dermatitis, pruritus

Dosage and routes:

• *Adult and child:* TOP apply to affected area bid-tid

Available forms include: Cream 0.05%; oint 0.05%; lotion 0.05%

Side effects/adverse reactions:

ORAL: Perioral dermatitis

INTEG: Burning, dryness, itching, irritation, acne, folliculitis, hypertrichosis, hypopigmentation, atrophy, striae, miliaria, allergic contact dermatitis, secondary infection

Contraindications: Hypersensitivity to corticosteroids, fungal infections

Precautions: Pregnancy category C, lactation, viral infections, bacterial infections

DENTAL CONSIDERATIONS

General:

• Determine why the patient is taking the drug.

• Place on frequent recall to evaluate healing response if used on chronic basis.

• Apply lubricant to dry lips for patient comfort before dental procedures.

---

desoximetasone

(des-ox-i-met'a-sone)

Topicort, Topicort LP

✤ Topicort Mild

Drug class.: Topical corticosteroid, group II potency (0.25%), group III potency (0.05%)

Action: Glucocorticoids have multiple actions that include antiinflammatory and immunosuppressant effects. They inhibit phospholipase A_2, interfering with or reducing the synthesis of prostaglandins and leukotrienes. They also bind to cytoplasmic glucocorticoid receptors (GRs) and enter the cell nucleus to bind with DNA. This results in the synthesis of various enzymes such as collagenase, elastase, and cytokines that play important roles in inflammation and immunosuppression. They also suppress the production of lymphocytes, monocytes, and eosinophils.

Uses: Psoriasis, eczema, contact dermatitis, pruritus

Dosage and routes:

• *Adult and child:* TOP apply to affected area bid-tid

Available forms include: Cream 0.05% (LP), 0.25%; oint 0.25%; gel 0.05% in 15 and 60 g tubes

Side effects/adverse reactions:

▼ *ORAL:* Thinning of mucosa, stinging sensation (oral application)

INTEG: Burning, dryness, itching, irritation, acne, folliculitis, hypertrichosis, perioral dermatitis, hypopigmentation, atrophy, striae, miliaria, allergic contact dermatitis, secondary infection

Contraindications: Hypersensitivity to corticosteroids, fungal infections

Precautions: Pregnancy category C, lactation, viral infections, bacterial infections

DENTAL CONSIDERATIONS

General:

• Gel formulations are used in the treatment of oral lichen planus lesions when the diagnosis has been confirmed by immunofluorescent biopsy testing.

• Place on frequent recall to evaluate healing response.

Teach patient/family:

• When used for oral lesions, to return for oral evaluation if response of oral tissues has not occurred in 7-14 days

• Importance of good oral hygiene to prevent soft tissue inflammation

• That use on oral herpetic ulcerations is contraindicated

• To apply at bedtime or after meals for maximum effect
• To apply with cotton-tipped applicator, dabbing gently, not rubbing medication on lesion

dexamethasone/ dexamethasone sodium phosphate

(dex-a-meth'a-sone)

Aeroseb-Dex, Decaderm, Decadron Phosphate, Decaspray

Drug class.: Synthetic topical corticosteroid

Action: Glucocorticoids have multiple actions that include antiinflammatory and immunosuppressant effects. They inhibit phospholipase A_2, interfering with or reducing the synthesis of prostaglandins and leukotrienes. They also bind to cytoplasmic glucocorticoid receptors (GRs) and enter the cell nucleus to bind with DNA. This results in the synthesis of various enzymes such as collagenase, elastase, and cytokines that play important roles in inflammation and immunosuppression. They also suppress the production of lymphocytes, monocytes, and eoinophils.

Uses: Corticosteroid-responsive dermatoses, oral ulcerative inflammatory lesions

Dosage and routes:

• *Adult and child:* TOP apply to affected area bid-qid

Available forms include: Gel 0.1%; aerosol 0.01%, 0.04%; cream 0.1%

Side effects/adverse reactions:

▼ *ORAL:* Thinning of mucosa, stinging sensation (oral application)

INTEG: Burning, dryness, itching, irritation, acne, folliculitis, hypertrichosis, perioral dermatitis, hypopigmentation, atrophy, striae, miliaria, allergic contact dermatitis, secondary infection

Contraindications: Hypersensitivity to corticosteroids, fungal infections, viral infections

Precautions: Pregnancy category C, lactation, viral infections, bacterial infections

DENTAL CONSIDERATIONS

General:

• Place on frequent recall to evaluate healing response.

Teach patient/family:

• When used for oral lesions, to return for oral evaluation if response of oral tissues has not occurred in 7-14 days
• Importance of good oral hygiene to prevent soft tissue inflammation
• To apply approximately 0.25 inch; measure and apply with cotton-tipped applicator by gently dabbing, not rubbing, medication on lesion
• To apply at bedtime or after meals for maximum effect
• That use on oral herpetic ulcerations is contraindicated

dexamethasone/ dexamethasone acetate/ dexamethasone sodium phosphate

(dex-a-meth'a-sone)

Dexamethasone oral tab: Decadron, Decadron DosePak, Dexaone, Hexadrol, Hexadrol Therapeutic Pack

🍁 Deronil, Dexasone, Oradexan

Dexamethasone elixir: Decadron, Hexadrol, Mymethasone

Dexamethasone acetate (long-lasting injection NOT FOR IV USE): Dalalaone DP, Dalalone LA, Decadron LA, Decaject-LA, Dexacen LA-8, Dexasone-LA, Dexone LA, Solurex-LA

Dexamethasone sodium phosphate (inj): AK-Dex, Dalaone, Decadrol, Decadron Phosphate, Decaject, Dexacen-4, Dexone, Hexadrol Phosphate, Solurex

Drug class.: Glucocorticoid, long acting

Action: Decreases inflammation by suppression of macrophage and leukocyte migration; reduces capillary permeability and inhibits lysosomal enzymes and phagocytosis; may have some effects on mediators of inflammation

Uses: Inflammation, allergies, neoplasms, cerebral edema, shock, collagen disorders

Dosage and routes:

Inflammation

• *Adult:* PO 0.25-4 mg bid-qid; IM 4-16 mg q1-3wk (acetate)

Shock

• *Adult:* IV 1-6 mg/kg or 40 mg q2-6h (phosphate)

Cerebral edema

• *Adult:* IV 10 mg, then 4-6 mg q6h × 2-4 days, then taper over 1 wk

• *Child:* PO 0.2 mg/kg/day in divided doses

Available forms include: Tabs 0.25, 0.5, 0.75, 1, 1.5, 2, 4, 6 mg; inj IM acetate 8, 16 mg/ml; inj IV phosphate 4, 10, 20, 24 mg/ml; elix 0.5 mg/5 ml; oral sol 0.5 mg/5 ml, 0.5 mg/1 ml

Side effects/adverse reactions:

▼ *ORAL: Candidiasis,* dry mouth

CNS: Depression, flushing, sweating, headache, mood changes

CV: Hypertension, ***circulatory collapse, thrombophlebitis, embolism,*** tachycardia, edema

GI: Diarrhea, nausea, abdominal distention, ***GI hemorrhage, pancreatitis,*** increased appetite

HEMA: ***Thrombocytopenia***

EENT: Fungal infections, increased intraocular pressure, blurred vision

INTEG: Acne, poor wound healing, ecchymosis, petechiae

MS: Fractures, osteoporosis, weakness

Contraindications: Psychosis, hypersensitivity, idiopathic thrombocytopenia, acute glomerulonephritis, amebiasis, fungal infections, nonasthmatic bronchial disease, child <2 yr, AIDS, TB

Precautions: Pregnancy category C, diabetes mellitus, glaucoma, osteoporosis, seizure disorders, ulcerative colitis, CHF, myasthenia gravis, renal disease, peptic ulcer, esophagitis

Pharmacokinetics:

PO: Peak 1-2 hr, duration 2.33 days

IM: Peak 8 hr, duration 6 days

Half-life 3-4.5 hr

Drug interactions of concern to dentistry:

• Decreased action: barbiturates

• Increased side effects: alcohol, salicylates, and other NSAIDs
• Increased action: ketoconazole, macrolide antibiotics

DENTAL CONSIDERATIONS
General:
• Monitor vital signs every appointment due to cardiovascular side effects.
• Patients on chronic drug therapy may rarely have symptoms of blood dyscrasias, which can include infection, bleeding, and poor healing.
• Symptoms of oral infections may be masked.
• Patients who have been or are currently on chronic steroid therapy (>2 wk) may require supplemental steroids for dental treatment.
• Avoid prescribing aspirin-containing products.
• Place on frequent recall to evaluate healing response.
• Prophylactic antibiotics may be indicated to prevent infection if surgery or deep scaling is planned.
Consultations:
• In a patient with symptoms of blood dyscrasias, request a medical consult for blood studies and postpone dental treatment until normal values are reestablished.
• Medical consult may be required to assess disease control in the patient.
• Consult may be required to confirm steroid dose and duration of use.
Teach patient/family:
• Importance of good oral hygiene to prevent soft tissue inflammation
• Caution to prevent injury when using oral hygiene aids
• To avoid mouth rinses with high alcohol content due to drug interaction

dexchlorpheniramine maleate

(dex-klor-fen-eer′a-meen)
Dexchlor, Polaramine, Polaramine Repetabs
Drug class.: Antihistamine

Action: Acts on blood vessels, GI system, respiratory system by competing with histamine for H_1-receptor site; decreases allergic response by blocking histamine
Uses: Allergy symptoms, rhinitis, pruritus, contact dermatitis
Dosage and routes:
• *Adult:* PO 1-2 mg tid-qid; repeat action 4-6 mg tid
• *Child 6-11 yr:* PO 1 mg q4-6h; time rel 4 mg hs
• *Child 2-5 yr:* PO 0.5 mg q4-6h; do not use repeat-action form
Available forms include: Tabs 2 mg; repeat-action tab 4, 6 mg; syr 2 mg/5 ml
Side effects/adverse reactions:
▼ *ORAL:* Dry mouth
CNS: Dizziness, drowsiness, poor coordination, fatigue, anxiety, euphoria, confusion, paresthesia, neuritis
CV: Hypotension, palpitations, tachycardia
GI: Constipation, nausea, vomiting, anorexia, diarrhea
RESP: Increased thick secretions, wheezing, chest tightness
GU: Retention, dysuria, frequency
EENT: Blurred vision, dilated pupils, tinnitus, nasal stuffiness, dry nose/throat
INTEG: Rash, urticaria, photosensitivity
Contraindications: Hypersensitivity to H_1-receptor antagonist;

D

acute asthma attack, lower respiratory tract disease

Precautions: Increased intraocular pressure, renal disease, cardiac disease, hypertension, bronchial asthma, seizure disorder, stenosed peptic ulcers, hyperthyroidism, prostatic hypertrophy, bladder neck obstruction, pregnancy category B, elderly

Pharmacokinetics:

PO (EXCEPT EXTENDED-ACTION DOSE FORMS): Onset 15 min, peak 3 hr, duration 3-6 hr; metabolized in liver; excreted by kidneys (inactive metabolites); excreted in breast milk (small amounts)

Drug interactions of concern to dentistry:

- Increased CNS depression: barbiturates, narcotics, hypnotics, tricyclic antidepressants, alcohol
- Increased anticholinergic effect: anticholinergic drugs

DENTAL CONSIDERATIONS

General:

- Assess salivary flow as a factor in caries, periodontal disease, and candidiasis.
- Consider semisupine chair position for patient comfort due to respiratory effects of disease.

Teach patient/family:

When chronic dry mouth occurs, advise patient:

- To avoid mouth rinses with high alcohol content due to drying effects
- To use sugarless gum, frequent sips of water, or saliva substitutes
- To use daily home fluoride products for anticaries effect

dextroamphetamine sulfate

(dex-troe-am-fet'a-meen)

Dexedrine, Dexedrine Spansules, DextroStat

Drug class.: Amphetamine

Controlled Substance Schedule II, Canada G

Action: Increases release of norepinephrine, dopamine in cerebral cortex to reticular activating system

Uses: Narcolepsy, attention deficit disorder with hyperactivity

Dosage and routes:

Narcolepsy

- *Adult:* PO 5-60 mg qd in divided doses
- *Child >12 yr:* PO 10 mg qd, increasing by 10 mg/day at weekly intervals, limit usually 40 mg/day
- *Child 6-12 yr:* PO 5 mg qd increasing by 5 mg/wk

Attention deficit disorder

- *Child >6 yr:* PO 5 mg qd-bid increasing by 5 mg/day at weekly intervals
- *Child 3-6 yr:* PO 2.5 mg qd increasing by 2.5 mg/day at weekly intervals

Available forms include: Tabs 5, 10 mg; sus rel caps 5, 10, 15 mg

Side effects/adverse reactions:

▼ *ORAL:* Dry mouth, metallic taste

CNS: Hyperactivity, insomnia, restlessness, talkativeness, dizziness, headache, chills, stimulation, dysphoria, irritability, aggressiveness, tremor

CV: Palpitation, tachycardia, hypertension, decrease in heart rate, dysrhythmias

GI: Anorexia, diarrhea, constipation, weight loss
GU: Impotence, change in libido
INTEG: Urticaria
Contraindications: Hypersensitivity to sympathomimetic amines, hyperthyroidism, hypertension, glaucoma hypertrophy, severe arteriosclerosis, drug abuse, cardiovascular disease, anxiety, MAO inhibitors or within 14 days of MAO inhibitor use
Precautions: Gilles de la Tourette's syndrome, pregnancy category C, lactation, child <3 yr
Pharmacokinetics:
PO: Onset 30 min, peak 1-3 hr, duration 4-20 hr, half-life 10-30 hr; metabolized by liver; urine excretion pH dependent; crosses placenta, excreted in breast milk
Drug interactions of concern to dentistry:
• Increased risk of serious side effects: meperidine, propoxyphene, tricyclic antidepressants

DENTAL CONSIDERATIONS
General:
• Monitor vital signs every appointment due to cardiovascular side effects.
• Assess salivary flow as a factor in caries, periodontal disease, and candidiasis.
• Psychologic and physical dependence may occur with chronic administration.
Consultations:
• Medical consult may be required to assess disease control in the patient.
Teach patient/family:
When chronic dry mouth occurs, advise patient:
• To avoid mouth rinses with high alcohol content due to drying effects
• To use daily home fluoride products for anticaries effect
• To use sugarless gum, frequent sips of water, or saliva substitutes

dextromethorphan hydrobromide
(dex-troe-meth-or′fan)
Benylin Adult, Benylin Pediatric, Drixoral Cough, Mediquell, Pertussin CS and ES, Robitussin Pediatric, and many other brands
♣ DM Syrup, Robidex, Sedatuss
Drug class.: Antitussive, nonnarcotic

Action: Depresses cough center in medulla
Uses: Nonproductive cough
Dosage and routes:
• *Adult:* PO 10-20 mg q4h or 30 mg q6-8h, not to exceed 120 mg/day; con rel liq 60 mg bid, not to exceed 120 mg/day
• *Child 6-12 yr:* PO 5-10 mg q4h; con rel liq 30 mg bid, not to exceed 60 mg/day
• *Child 2-6 yr:* PO 2.5-5 mg q4h or 7.5 mg q6-8h, not to exceed 30 mg/day
Available forms include: Loz 5 mg; sol 5, 7.5, 10, 15 mg/5 ml
Side effects/adverse reactions:
CNS: Dizziness
GI: Nausea
Contraindications: Hypersensitivity, asthma/emphysema, productive cough, MAO inhibitor
Precautions: Nausea, vomiting, increased temperature, persistent headache, pregnancy category C

Pharmacokinetics:
PO: Onset 15-30 min, duration 3-6 hr

DENTAL CONSIDERATIONS
General:
• Consider semisupine chair position for patients with respiratory disease.

---

diazepam

(dye-az′e-pam)
Diastat, Diazemuls, Diazepam Intensol, Diazc, Valium
♣ Apo-Diazepam, Novo-Dipam, PMS Diazepam, Vivol
Drug class.: Benzodiazepine, anxiolytic

Controlled Substance Schedule IV

Action: Produces CNS depression by interacting with a benzodiazepine receptor to facilitate the action of the inhibitory neurotransmitter γ-aminobutyric acid (GABA)

Uses: Anxiety, acute alcohol withdrawal, adjunct in seizure disorders, skeletal muscle spasm; unapproved use: conscious sedation

Dosage and routes:

Anxiety/convulsive disorders/sedation
• *Adult:* PO 2-10 mg tid-qid; ext rel 15-30 mg qd
• *Child >6 mo:* PO 1-2.5 mg tid-qid

Tetanic muscle spasms
• *Child >5 yr:* IM/IV 5-10 mg q3-4h prn
• *Infant >30 days:* IM/IV 1-2 mg q3-4h prn

Status epilepticus
• *Adult:* IV BOLUS 5-20 mg, 2 mg/min; may repeat q5-10 min, not to exceed 60 mg; may repeat in 30 min if seizures reappear
• *Child:* IV BOLUS 0.1-0.3 mg/kg (1 mg/min over 3 min); may repeat q15min × 2 doses

Available forms include: Tabs 2, 5, 10 mg; ext rel caps 15 mg; IM/IV inj 5 mg/ml; oral sol 5 mg/ml

Side effects/adverse reactions:
▼ *ORAL:* Dry mouth, ulcerations
CNS: Dizziness, drowsiness, confusion, headache, anxiety, tremors, stimulation, fatigue, depression, insomnia, hallucinations
CV: Orthostatic hypotension, ***ECG changes, tachycardia,*** hypotension
GI: Constipation, nausea, vomiting, anorexia, diarrhea
EENT: Blurred vision, tinnitus, mydriasis
INTEG: Rash, dermatitis, itching

Contraindications: Hypersensitivity to benzodiazepines, narrow-angle glaucoma, psychosis, pregnancy category D, child <18 yr, ritonavir, indinavir

Precautions: Elderly, debilitated, hepatic disease, renal disease

Pharmacokinetics:
PO: Onset 30 min, duration 2-3 hr
IM: Onset 15-30 min, duration 1-1.5 hr
IV: Onset 1-5 min, duration 15 min, half-life 20-50 hr; metabolized by liver; excreted by kidneys; crosses placenta, excreted in breast milk; more effective by mouth

Drug interactions of concern to dentistry:
• Increased effects of diazepam: alcohol, all CNS depressants
• Increased serum levels and prolonged effect of benzodiazepines: erythromycin, clarithromycin, ketoconazole, itraconazole, fluconazole, miconazole (systemic)

DENTAL CONSIDERATIONS
General:
• Assess salivary flow as a factor in

caries, periodontal disease, and candidiasis.
• After supine positioning, have patient sit upright for at least 2 min before standing to avoid orthostatic hypotension.
• Psychologic and physical dependence may occur with chronic administration.
• Geriatric patients are more susceptible to drug effects; use lower dose.
• Have someone drive patient to and from dental appointment when used for conscious sedation.
• Provide assistance when escorting patient to and from dental chair when dizziness occurs.
• Avoid the use of this drug in a patient with a history of drug abuse or alcoholism.

Teach patient/family:
• Importance of good oral hygiene to prevent soft tissue inflammation

When chronic dry mouth occurs, advise patient:
• To avoid mouth rinses with high alcohol content due to drying effects
• To use daily home fluoride products for anticaries effect
• To use sugarless gum, frequent sips of water, or saliva substitutes

diclofenac

(dye-kloe'fen-ak)

Diclofenac potassium: Cataflam

♣ Difenac, Voltaren Rapide

Diclofenac sodium delayed release: Voltaren, Voltarin XR

Diclofenac sodium: Novo-Difenac

♣ Apo-Diclo, Nu-Diclo, Voltaren Suppositories

Diclofenac extended release: Voltarten SR

♣ Novo-Difenac SR

Drug class.: Nonsteroidal antiinflammatory

Action: Inhibits prostaglandin synthesis by interfering with cyclooxygenase needed for biosynthesis; possesses analgesic, antiinflammatory, antipyretic properties

Uses: Acute, chronic rheumatoid arthritis, osteoarthritis, ankylosing spondylitis

Dosage and routes:

Osteoarthritis (immediate or delayed release tablets)
• *Adult:* PO 100-150 mg/day in divided doses; chronic therapy 100 mg/day

Rheumatoid arthritis (immediate or delayed release tablets)
• *Adult:* PO 150-200 mg/day in divided doses; chronic therapy 100 mg/day

Ankylosing spondylitis (delayed release tablets)
• *Adult:* PO 100-125 mg/day; give 25 mg qid and 25 mg hs if needed

Analgesia and dysmenorrhea (immediate release tablets)
• *Adult:* PO 50 mg tid or 100 mg first dose followed by 50 mg with a daily first day limit of 200 mg; do not exceed 150 mg/day thereafter

Available forms include: Enteric-coated tabs 25, 50, 75 mg; ext rel tabs 100 mg

Side effects/adverse reactions:

▼ *ORAL:* Dry mouth, stomatitis, bitter taste, lichenoid reaction

CNS: Dizziness, drowsiness, fatigue, tremors, confusion, insomnia, anxiety, depression, nervousness, paresthesia, muscle weakness

CV: ***CHF, dysrhythmias,*** tachycardia, peripheral edema, palpitation, hypotension, hypertension, fluid retention

GI: ***Jaundice, cholestatic hepatitis*** constipation, flatulence, cramps, peptic ulcer, GI bleeding, nausea, anorexia, vomiting, diarrhea

RESP: ***Bronchospasm, laryngeal edema,*** rhinitis, shortness of breath, dyspnea, hemoptysis, pharyngitis

HEMA: ***Blood dyscrasias,*** epistaxis, bruising

GU: ***Nephrotoxicity: dysuria, hematuria, oliguria, azotemia, cystitis, UTI***

EENT: Tinnitus, hearing loss, blurred vision

INTEG: Purpura, rash, pruritus, sweating, erythema, petechiae, photosensitivity, alopecia

Contraindications: Hypersensitivity to aspirin, iodides, other nonsteroidal antiinflammatory agents, asthma

Precautions: Pregnancy category B (first, second trimester), lactation, children, bleeding disorders, GI disorders, cardiac disorders, hypersensitivity to other antiinflammatory agents

Pharmacokinetics:

PO: Peak 2-3 hr, elimination half-life 1-2 hr; 90% bound to plasma proteins; metabolized in liver to metabolite; excreted in urine

Drug interactions of concern to dentistry:

• GI ulceration, bleeding: aspirin, alcohol, corticosteroids

• Nephrotoxicity: acetaminophen (prolonged use)

• Possible risk of decreased renal function: cyclosporine

When prescribed for dental pain:

• Risk of increased effects: oral anticoagulants, oral antidiabetics, lithium, methotrexate

• Decreased antihypertensive effects of diuretics, β-adrenergic blockers, and ACE inhibitors

DENTAL CONSIDERATIONS

General:

• Patients on chronic drug therapy may rarely have symptoms of blood dyscrasias, which can include infection, bleeding, and poor healing.

• Assess salivary flow as a factor in caries, periodontal disease, and candidiasis.

• Avoid prescribing for dental use in last trimester of pregnancy.

• Avoid prescribing aspirin-containing products.

• Consider semisupine chair position for patients with rheumatic disease.

Consultations:

• In a patient with symptoms of blood dyscrasias, request a medical consult for blood studies and postpone dental treatment until normal values are reestablished.

• Medical consult may be required to assess disease control in the patient.

Teach patient/family:

• Importance of good oral hygiene to prevent soft tissue inflammation

• Caution to prevent injury when using oral hygiene aids

When chronic dry mouth occurs, advise patient:

• To avoid mouth rinses with high alcohol content due to drying effects

• To use daily home fluoride products for anticaries effect

• To use sugarless gum, frequent sips of water, or saliva substitutes

dicloxacillin sodium

(dye-klox-a-sil'in)

Dycill, Dynapen, Pathocil

Drug class.: Penicillinase-resistant penicillin

Action: Interferes with cell wall replication of susceptible organisms; the cell wall, rendered osmotically unstable, swells and bursts from osmotic pressure

Uses: Infections caused by penicillinase-producing *Staphylococcus*

Dosage and routes:

• *Adult:* PO 500 mg-1 g q4-6h

• *Child: PO 12.5-25 mg/kg in divided doses q6h (up to 40 kg)*

Available forms include: Caps 125, 250, 500 mg; powder for oral susp 250 mg/5 ml

Side effects/adverse reactions:

▼ *ORAL: Candidiasis* (superinfection)

CNS: ***Coma, convulsions,*** lethargy, hallucinations, anxiety, depression, twitching

GI: Nausea, vomiting, diarrhea, increased AST/ALT, abdominal pain, colitis

HEMA: ***Bone marrow depression, granulocytopenia,*** anemia, increased bleeding time

GU: ***Oliguria, proteinuria, hematuria, vaginitis, moniliasis, glomerulonephritis***

Contraindications: Hypersensitivity to penicillins; neonates

Precautions: Hypersensitivity to cephalosporins, pregnancy category B

Pharmacokinetics:

PO: Peak 1 hr, duration 4-6 hr; metabolized in liver; excreted in urine, bile, breast milk; crosses placenta

Drug interactions of concern to dentistry:

• Decreased antimicrobial effectiveness: tetracyclines, erythromycins

When prescribed for dental infection:

• Decreased effect of oral contraceptives

• Increased dicloxacillin concentration: probenecid

DENTAL CONSIDERATIONS

General:

• Take precautions regarding allergy to medication.

• Determine why the patient is taking the drug.

Consultations:

• Concern for drug of choice if dental infection is also present.

Teach patient/family:

• Importance of good oral hygiene to prevent soft tissue inflammation

• Caution to prevent trauma when using oral hygiene aids

When used for dental infection, advise patient:

• Taking birth control pill to use additional method of contraception for duration of cycle

• To report sore throat, oral burning sensation, fever, fatigue, any of which could indicate superinfection

• To take at prescribed intervals and complete dosage regimen
• To immediately notify the dentist if signs or symptoms of infection increase

dicyclomine HCl

(dye-sye'kloe-meen)
Antispas, Bentyl
♣ A-Spas, Bentylol, Formulex, Spasmoban
Drug class.: GI anticholinergic

Action: Inhibits muscarinic actions of acetylcholine at postganglionic parasympathetic neuroeffector sites
Uses: Treatment of peptic ulcer disease in combination with other drugs; infant colic
Dosage and routes:
• *Adult:* PO 10-20 mg tid-qid; IM 20 mg q4-6h
• *Child >6 yr:* PO 10 mg tid-qid
Available forms include: Caps 10, 20 mg; tabs 20 mg; syr 10 mg/5 ml; inj IM 10 mg/ml
Side effects/adverse reactions:
▼ *ORAL: Dry mouth*
CNS: Confusion, stimulation in elderly, ***seizures, coma*** (child <3 mo), headache, insomnia, dizziness, drowsiness, anxiety, weakness, hallucination
CV: Palpitation, tachycardia
GI: Constipation, ***paralytic ileus,*** heartburn, nausea, vomiting, dysphagia
GU: Hesitancy, retention, impotence
EENT: Blurred vision, photophobia, mydriasis, cycloplegia, increased ocular tension
SYST: Urticaria, rash, pruritus, anhidrosis, fever, allergic reactions
Contraindications: Hypersensitivity to anticholinergics, narrow-angle glaucoma, GI obstruction, myasthenia gravis, paralytic ileus, GI atony, toxic megacolon
Precautions: Hyperthyroidism, CAD, dysrhythmias, CHF, ulcerative colitis, hypertension, hiatal hernia, hepatic disease, renal disease, pregnancy category B, urinary retention, prostatic hypertrophy
Pharmacokinetics:
PO: Onset 1-2 hr, duration 3-4 hr; metabolized by liver; excreted in urine
Drug interactions of concern to dentistry:
• Increased anticholinergic effect: atropine, scopolamine, other anticholinergics and meperidine
• Decreased effect of ketoconazole

DENTAL CONSIDERATIONS

General:
• Assess salivary flow as a factor in caries, periodontal disease, and candidiasis.
• Avoid dental light in patient's eyes; offer dark glasses for patient comfort.
Consultation:
• Physician should be informed if significant xerostomic side effects occur (increased caries, sore tongue, problems eating or swallowing, difficulty wearing prosthesis) so a medication change can be considered.
Teach patient/family:
• Importance of good oral hygiene to prevent soft tissue inflammation
When chronic dry mouth occurs, advise patient:
• To avoid mouth rinses with high alcohol content due to drying effects
• To use daily home fluoride products for anticaries effect

• To use sugarless gum, frequent sips of water, or saliva substitutes

didanosine

(dye-dan'o-seen)

Videx (also called ddI, dideoxyinosine)

Drug class.: Synthetic antiviral, nucleoside analog

Action: Converted by cellular enzymes to active form, which acts as an antimetabolite to inhibit HIV reverse transcriptase and viral replication

Uses: Advanced HIV infections in adults and children who have been unable to use zidovudine or who have not responded to treatment

Dosage and routes:

• *Adult:* PO >75 kg: 300 mg bid tabs or 375 mg bid buffered powder; tabs must be chewed or crushed in water; 50-74 kg: 200 mg bid tabs or 250 mg bid buffered powder; 35-49 kg: 125 mg bid tabs or 167 mg bid buffered powder; or 400 mg once daily

• *Child:* PO 1.1-1.4 m^2, 100 mg bid tabs or 125 mg bid pedi powder; 0.8-1.0 m^2, 75 mg bid tabs or 94 mg bid pedi powder; 0.5-0.7 m^2, 50 mg bid tabs or 62 mg bid pedi powder; <0.4 m^2, 25 mg bid tabs or 31 mg bid pedi powder

Available forms include: Tabs, buffered, chewable/dispersible 25, 50, 100, 150, 200 mg; powder for oral sol, buffered 100, 167, 250, 375 mg; powder for oral sol, pedi 2, 4 g

Side effects/adverse reactions:

▼ *ORAL:* Stomatitis, dry mouth, taste perversion, candidiasis

CNS: ***Peripheral neuropathy, seizures, CNS depression,*** confusion, anxiety, hypertonia, abnormal thinking, asthenia, insomnia, pain, dizziness, chills, fever, headache

CV: Hypertension, vasodilation, dysrhythmia, syncope, CHF, palpitation

GI: ***Pancreatitis,*** diarrhea, nausea, vomiting, abdominal pain, constipation, dyspepsia, liver abnormalities, flatulence, melena, increased ALT/AST, alk phosphatase, amylase

RESP: Cough, pneumonia, dyspnea, asthma, epistaxis, hypoventilation, sinusitis

HEMA: ***Leukopenia, granulocytopenia, thrombocytopenia, anemia***

GU: Increased bilirubin, uric acid

EENT: Ear pain, otitis, photophobia, visual impairment

INTEG: Rash, pruritus, alopecia, ecchymosis, hemorrhage, petechiae, sweating

MS: Myalgia, arthritis, myopathy, muscular atrophy

Contraindications: Hypersensitivity

Precautions: Renal disease, hepatic disease, pregnancy category B, lactation, children, sodium-restricted diets; pancreatitis (in combination with stavudine)

Pharmacokinetics:

PO: Elimination half-life 1.62 hr; extensive metabolism is thought to occur; administration within 5 min of food decreases absorption

Drug interactions of concern to dentistry:

• Decreased absorption: ketoconazole, dapsone, itraconazole, tetracyclines, fluoroquinolone antibiotics

• Increased risk of pancreatitis: metronidazole, sulfonamides, sulindac, tetracyclines

• Increased risk of peripheral neuropathy: metronidazole, nitrous oxide

DENTAL CONSIDERATIONS
General:

• Monitor vital signs every appointment due to cardiovascular side effects.

• Avoid dental light in patient's eyes; offer dark glasses for patient comfort.

• Patients on chronic drug therapy may rarely have symptoms of blood dyscrasias, which can include infection, bleeding, and poor healing.

Consultations:

• Medical consult may be required to assess patient's ability to tolerate stress.

• In a patient with symptoms of blood dyscrasias, request a medical consult for blood studies and postpone dental treatment until normal values are reestablished.

Teach patient/family:

• Importance of good oral hygiene to prevent soft tissue inflammation

• Caution to prevent injury when using oral hygiene aids

When chronic dry mouth occurs, advise patient:

• To avoid mouth rinses with high alcohol content due to drying effects

• To use daily home fluoride products for anticaries effect

• To use sugarless gum, frequent sips of water, or saliva substitutes

diethylpropion HCl

(dye-eth-il-proe'pee-on)

Tenuate Dospan, Tenuate, Ten-Tab, Tepanil

Drug class.: Anorexiant, amphetamine-like

Controlled Substance Schedule IV

Action: Stimulates satiety center by acting on adrenergic pathways

Uses: Exogenous obesity

Dosage and routes:

• *Adult:* PO 25 mg/1 hr ac; con rel 75 mg qd midmorning

Available forms include: Tabs 25 mg; susp rel tabs 75 mg

Side effects/adverse reactions:

▼ *ORAL:* Dry mouth, unpleasant taste

CNS: Hyperactivity, restlessness, anxiety, insomnia, dizziness, dysphonia, depression, tremors, headache, blurred vision, incoordination, fatigue, malaise, euphoria, depression, tremor, confusion

CV: Palpitation, tachycardia, hypertension, dysrhythmias, pulmonary hypertension, ECG changes

GI: Nausea, vomiting, anorexia, diarrhea, constipation

HEMA: ***Bone marrow depression,*** leukopenia, agranulocytosis

GU: Impotence, change in libido, menstrual irregularities, dysuria, polyuria

INTEG: Urticaria

Contraindications: Hypersensitivity, hyperthyroidism, hypertension, glaucoma, angina pectoris, drug abuse, cardiovascular disease, children <12 yr, severe arteriosclerosis, agitated states

Precautions: Convulsive disorders, pregnancy category B, lactation

Pharmacokinetics:

PO: Duration 4 hr

CON REL: Duration 10-14 hr, half-life 1-3.5 hr; metabolized by liver; excreted by kidneys; crosses placenta, excreted in breast milk

Drug interactions of concern to dentistry:

• Dysrhythmia: hydrocarbon inhalation anesthetics

• Decreased effects: barbiturates, tricyclic antidepressants, phenothiazines

DENTAL CONSIDERATIONS

General:

• Monitor vital signs every appointment due to cardiovascular and respiratory side effects.

• Examine for evidence of oral manifestations of blood dyscrasias (infection, bleeding, poor healing).

• Assess salivary flow as a factor in caries, periodontal disease, and candidiasis.

• Psychologic and physical dependence may occur with chronic administration.

• Consider semisupine chair position for patient comfort due to GI effects of disease.

Consultations:

• Medical consult for blood studies (CBC); leukopenic or thrombocytopenic side effects may result in infection, delayed healing, and excessive bleeding. Postpone dental treatment until normal values are maintained.

Teach patient/family:

• Importance of good oral hygiene to prevent soft tissue inflammation

• Caution in use of oral hygiene aids to prevent injury

When chronic dry mouth occurs, advise patient:

• To avoid mouth rinses with high alcohol content due to drying effects

• To use daily home fluoride products for anticaries effect

• To use sugarless gum, frequent sips of water, or saliva substitutes

difenoxin HCl with atropine sulfate

(dye-fen-ox'in)

Motofen

Drug class.: Antidiarrheal

Controlled Substance Schedule IV

Action: Inhibits gastric motility by acting on mucosal receptors responsible for peristalsis

Uses: Acute nonspecific and acute exacerbations of chronic functional diarrhea

Dosage and routes:

• *Adult:* PO 2 mg, then 1 mg after each loose stool; or 1 mg q3-4h as needed, not to exceed 8 mg/24 hr

Available forms include: Tab 1 mg difenoxin HCl with 0.025 mg atropine sulfate

Side effects/adverse reactions:

▼ *ORAL: Dry mouth*

CNS: Dizziness, drowsiness, headache, fatigue, nervousness, insomnia, confusion

GI: Nausea, vomiting, epigastric distress, constipation

EENT: Burning eyes, blurred vision

Contraindications: Hypersensitivity, pseudomembranous enterocolitis, jaundice, glaucoma, child <2 yr, severe electrolyte imbalances, diarrhea associated with organisms that penetrate intestinal mucosa, MAO inhibitor

Precautions: Hepatic disease, renal disease, ulcerative colitis, pregnancy category C, lactation, severe liver disease

Pharmacokinetics:

PO: Peak 40-60 min, duration 3-4 hr, terminal half-life 12-14 hr; metabolized in liver to inactive metabolite; excreted in urine, feces

Drug interactions of concern to dentistry:

• Increased effects of alcohol: all CNS depressants, opioid analgesics, and anticholinergics

DENTAL CONSIDERATIONS

General:

• This drug product is normally used only for a few doses for acute problems; however, some patients may have to take it for longer time periods as dictated by a contributing disease.

• Assess salivary flow as a factor in caries, periodontal disease, and candidiasis.

Teach patient/family:

When chronic dry mouth occurs, advise patient:

• To avoid mouth rinses with high alcohol content due to drying effects

• To use daily home fluoride products for anticaries effect

• To use sugarless gum, frequent sips of water, or saliva substitutes

diflorasone diacetate

(die-floor'a-sone)

Florone, Florone E, Maxiflor, Psorcon

Drug class.: Topical corticosteroid, group II high potency

Action: Glucocorticoids have multiple actions that include antiinflammatory and immunosuppressant effects. They inhibit phospholipase A_2, interfering with or reducing the synthesis of prostaglandins and leukotrienes. They also bind to cytoplasmic glucocorticoid receptors (GRs) and enter the cell nucleus to bind with DNA. This results in the synthesis of various enzymes such as collagenase, elastase, and cytokines that play important roles in inflammation and immunosuppression. They also suppress the production of lymphocytes, monocytes, and eosinophils.

Uses: Psoriasis, eczema, contact dermatitis, pruritus

Dosage and routes:

• *Adult and child:* Apply to affected area qd-tid

Available forms include: Cream 0.05%; oint 0.05%

Side effects/adverse reactions:

▼ *ORAL:* Perioral dermatitis (not intraoral)

INTEG: Burning, dryness, itching, irritation, acne, folliculitis, hypertrichosis, hypopigmentation, atrophy, striae, miliaria, allergic contact dermatitis, secondary infection

Contraindications: Hypersensitivity to corticosteroids, fungal infections

Precautions: Pregnancy category C, lactation, viral infections, bacterial infections

DENTAL CONSIDERATIONS

General:

• Determine why the patient is taking the drug.

• Apply lubricant to dry lips for patient comfort before dental procedures.

• Place on frequent recall to evaluate healing response if used on chronic basis.

diflunisal

(dye-floo'ni-sal)

Dolobid

♣ Apo-Diflunisal, Novo-Diflunisal

Drug class.: Salicylate derivative, nonsteroidal antiinflammatory

Action: Inhibits prostaglandin synthesis by interfering with cyclooxygenase needed for biosynthesis; possesses analgesic, antiinflammatory, antipyretic properties

Uses: Mild-to-moderate pain, symptoms of rheumatoid arthritis and osteoarthritis

Dosage and routes:

Pain/fever

• *Adult:* PO loading dose 1 g, then 500-1000 mg/day in 2 divided doses q12h, not to exceed 1500 mg/day

Available forms include: Tabs 250, 500 mg

Side effects/adverse reactions:

▼ *ORAL:* Dry mouth, lichenoid reaction

CNS: ***Convulsions,*** stimulation, drowsiness, dizziness, confusion, headache, flushing, hallucinations, coma

CV: ***Pulmonary edema,*** rapid pulse

GI: Nausea, vomiting, GI bleeding, diarrhea, heartburn, ***hepatitis,*** anorexia

RESP: Wheezing, hyperpnea

HEMA: ***Thrombocytopenia, agranulocytosis, leukopenia, neutropenia, hemolytic anemia,*** increased pro-time

EENT: Blurred vision, decreased acuity, corneal deposits

INTEG: Rash, urticaria, bruising

ENDO: Hypoglycemia, hyponatremia, hypokalemia

Contraindications: Hypersensitivity to salicylates, GI bleeding, bleeding disorders, children <3 yr, vitamin K deficiency

Precautions: Anemia, hepatic disease, renal disease, Hodgkin's disease, pregnancy category C, lactation

Pharmacokinetics:

PO: Onset 15-30 min, peak 2-3 hr, half-life up to 6 hr; 99% protein bound; metabolized by liver; excreted by kidneys; crosses placenta; excreted in breast milk

Drug interactions of concern to dentistry:

• Increased risk of GI ulceration and bleeding: aspirin, steroids, alcohol, indomethacin, and other NSAIDs

• Hepatotoxicity, nephrotoxicity: acetaminophen (prolonged use)

DENTAL CONSIDERATIONS

General:

• Patients on chronic drug therapy may rarely have symptoms of blood dyscrasias, which can include infection, bleeding, and poor healing.

• Assess salivary flow as a factor in caries, periodontal disease, and candidiasis.

• Avoid prescribing for dental use in first and last trimester of pregnancy.

Consultations:

• Medical consult may be required to assess disease control in the patient.

• In a patient with symptoms of blood dyscrasias, request a medical consult for blood studies and postpone dental treatment until normal values are reestablished.

Teach patient/family:

• Importance of good oral hygiene to prevent soft tissue inflammation

• Caution to prevent injury when using oral hygiene aids

When chronic dry mouth occurs, advise patient:

• To avoid mouth rinses with high alcohol content due to drying effects

• To use daily home fluoride products for anticaries effect

• To use sugarless gum, frequent sips of water, or saliva substitutes

---

digitoxin

(di-ji-tox′in)

Crystodigin

♣ Digitaline

Drug class.: Cardiac glycoside

Action: Acts by inhibiting the sodium-potassium ATPase, which makes more calcium available for contractile proteins, resulting in increased cardiac contractility and cardiac output

Uses: CHF, atrial fibrillation, paroxysmal atrial flutter, atrial tachycardia, rapid digitalization in these disorders

Dosage and routes:

• *Adult:* PO rapid digitalization 0.6 mg initially, then 0.4 mg after 4-6 hr, and 0.2 mg after another 4 hr period, then maintenance dose; slow digitalization 0.2 mg bid × 4 days, followed by maintenance dose

Maintenance dose: PO 0.05 to 0.3 mg qd

Available forms include: Tabs 0.05, 0.1 mg

Side effects/adverse reactions:

▼ *ORAL:* Sensitive gag reflex

CNS: Headache, drowsiness, apathy, confusion, disorientation, fatigue, depression, hallucinations

CV: ***Dysrhythmias, hypotension,*** bradycardia, AV block

GI: Nausea, vomiting, anorexia, abdominal pain, diarrhea

EENT: Blurred vision, yellowish-green halos, photophobia, diplopia

MS: Muscular weakness

Contraindications: Hypersensitivity to digitalis, ventricular fibrillation, ventricular tachycardia, carotoid sinus syndrome, second- or third-degree heart block

Precautions: Hepatic disease, acute MI, AV block, hypokalemia, hypomagnesemia, sinus node disease, lactation, severe respiratory disease, hypothyroidism, elderly, pregnancy category C

Pharmacokinetics:

PO: Onset 0.5-2 hr, peak 4-12 hr, duration 2-3 wk, half-life 4-20 days; metabolized in liver; excreted in urine

Drug interactions of concern to dentistry:

• Hypokalemia: corticosteroids

• Increased blood levels: erythromycin

• Cardiac dysrhythmias: adrenergic agonists, succinylcholine

DENTAL CONSIDERATIONS

General:

• Monitor vital signs every appointment due to cardiovascular side effects.

• After supine positioning, have patient sit upright for at least 2 min to avoid orthostatic hypotension.

• Avoid dental light in patient's eyes; offer dark glasses for patient comfort.

• An increased gag reflex may make dental procedures, such as obtaining radiographs or impressions, difficult.

• Use vasoconstrictors with caution, in low doses, and with careful aspiration. Exercise caution when using dental retraction cord with epinephrine.

Consultations:

• Stress from dental procedures may compromise cardiovascular function; determine patient risk.

• Medical consult may be required to assess disease control and stress tolerance of patient.

---

digoxin

(di-jox′in)

Lanoxicaps, Lanoxin

♣ Novo-digoxin

Drug class.: Cardiac glycoside

Action: Acts by inhibiting the sodium-potassium ATPase, which makes more calcium available for contractile proteins, resulting in increased cardiac contractility and cardiac output

Uses: CHF, atrial fibrillation, atrial flutter, paroxysmal atrial tachycardia, rapid digitalization in these disorders

Dosage and routes:

• *Adult:* IV 0.5 mg given over >5 min, then PO 0.125-0.5 mg qd in divided doses q4-6h as needed

• *Elderly:* PO 0.125 qd maintenance

• *Child >2 yr:* PO 0.02-0.04 mg/kg divided q8h over 24 hr; maintenance 0.006-0.012 mg/kg qd in divided doses q12h; IV loading dose 0.015-0.035 mg/kg over >5 min

• *Child 1 mo-2 yr:* IV 0.03-0.05 mg/kg in divided doses over >5 min q4-8h; change to PO as soon as possible; PO 0.035-0.060 mg/kg divided in 3 doses over 24 hr; maintenance 0.01-0.02 mg/kg in divided doses q12h

• *Neonates:* IV loading dose 0.02-0.03 mg/kg over >5 min in divided doses q4-8h; change to PO as soon as possible; PO loading dose 0.035 mg/kg divided q8h over 24 hr; maintenance 0.01 mg/kg in divided doses q12h

• *Premature infants:* IV 0.015-0.025 mg/kg divided in 3 doses over 24 hr, given over >5 min; maintenance 0.003-0.009 mg/kg in divided doses q12h

Available forms include: Caps 0.05, 0.1, 0.2 mg; elix 0.05 mg/ml; tabs 0.125, 0.25, 0.50 mg; inj 0.1, 0.25 mg/ml

Side effects/adverse reactions:

▼ *ORAL:* Sensitive gag reflex

CNS: Headache, drowsiness, apathy, confusion, disorientation, fatigue, depression, hallucinations

CV: ***Dysrhythmias, hypotension,*** bradycardia, ***AV block***

GI: Nausea, vomiting, anorexia, abdominal pain, diarrhea

EENT: Blurred vision, yellowish-green halos, photophobia, diplopia

MS: Muscular weakness

Contraindications: Hypersensitivity to digitalis, ventricular fibrillation, ventricular tachycardia, carotid sinus syndrome, second- or third-degree heart block

Precautions: Renal disease, acute MI, AV block, severe respiratory disease, hypothyroidism, elderly, pregnancy category C, sinus nodal disease, lactation, hypokalemia

Pharmacokinetics:

IV: Onset 5-30 min, peak 1-5 hr, duration variable, half-life 1.5 days; excreted in urine

Drug interactions of concern to dentistry:
- Hypokalemia: corticosteroids
- Increased digoxin blood levels: erythromycin, clarithromycin, tetracyclines
- Cardiac dysrhythmias: adrenergic agonists, succinylcholine

DENTAL CONSIDERATIONS

General:
- Monitor vital signs every appointment due to cardiovascular side effects.
- After supine positioning, have patient sit upright for at least 2 min to avoid orthostatic hypotension.
- Avoid dental light in patient's eyes; offer dark glasses for patient comfort.
- An increased gag reflex may make dental procedures such as taking radiographs or impressions difficult.
- Use vasoconstrictors with caution, in low doses, and with careful aspiration. Avoid use of gingival retraction cord with epinephrine.

Consultations:
- Stress from dental procedures may compromise cardiovascular function; determine patient risk.
- Medical consult may be required to assess disease control and stress tolerance of patient.

---

dihydrotachysterol (DHT)

(dye-hye-droe-tak-iss'ter-ole)

DHT Intensol, DHT Oral Solution, Hytakerol

Drug class.: Vitamin D analog

Action: Increases intestinal absorption of calcium for bones, increases renal tubular absorption of phosphate

Uses: Nutritional supplement, rickets, hypoparathyroidism, pseudohypoparathyroidism, familial hypophosphatemia, postoperative tetany

Dosage and routes:

Hypophosphatemia
- *Adult and child:* PO 0.5-2 mg qd; maintenance 0.2-1.5 mg qd

Hypoparathyroidism/pseudohypoparathyroidism
- *Adult:* PO 0.8-2.4 mg qd × 1 wk; maintenance 0.2-1 mg qd regulated by serum Ca levels
- *Child:* PO 1-5 mg qd × 1 wk; maintenance 0.2-1 mg qd regulated by serum Ca levels

Available forms include: Tabs 0.125, 0.2, 0.4 mg; caps 0.125 mg; oral sol 0.2, 0.25 mg/ml

Side effects/adverse reactions:

▼ *ORAL:* Dry mouth, metallic taste

CNS: Drowsiness, headache, vertigo, fever, lethargy

GI: Nausea, diarrhea, vomiting, jaundice, anorexia, constipation, cramps

GU: ***Polyuria, hematuria,*** hypercalciuria, hyperphosphatemia

EENT: Tinnitus

MS: Myalgia, arthralgia, decreased bone development

Contraindications: Hypersensitivity, renal disease, hyperphosphatemia, hypercalcemia

Precautions: Pregnancy category C, renal calculi, lactation, cardiovascular disease

Pharmacokinetics:

PO: Onset 2 wk; metabolized by liver; excreted in feces (active/inactive)

Drug interactions of concern to dentistry:
- Decreased effect of dihydro-

tachysterol: prolonged use of corticosteroids, barbiturates

DENTAL CONSIDERATIONS

General:

• Consider semisupine chair position for patient comfort due to GI effects of drug.

• Assess salivary flow as a factor in caries, periodontal disease, and candidiasis.

Teach patient/family:

When chronic dry mouth occurs, advise patient:

• To avoid mouth rinses with high alcohol content due to drying effects

• Of need for daily home fluoride to prevent caries

• To use sugarless gum, frequent sips of water, or saliva substitutes

---

diltiazem HCl

(dil-tye'a-zem)

Cardizem, Cardizem CD, Cardizem SR, Cartia XT, Dilacor XR, Tiazac, Tiamate

♣ Apo-Diltaz, Novo-Diltiazem, Nu-Dilitaz, Syn-Diltiazem

Drug class.: Calcium channel blocker

Action: Inhibits calcium ion influx across cell membrane during cardiac depolarization; produces relaxation of coronary vascular smooth muscle; dilates coronary arteries; slows SA/AV node conduction; dilates peripheral arteries

Uses: Chronic stable angina pectoris, vasospastic angina, coronary artery spasm, hypertension, supraventricular tachydysrhythmias

Dosage and routes:

• *Adult:* PO 30 mg qid, increasing dose gradually to 180-360 mg/day in divided doses or 60-120 mg bid; may increase to 240-360 mg/day

• *Adult:* PO sus rel in hypertension 180-240 mg once daily; angina initial dose 120 mg, range may vary from 180-480 mg/day

Available forms include: Tabs 30, 60, 90, 120 mg; sus rel 60, 90, 120, 180, 240, 300 mg; inj 5 mg/ml in 5 ml, 10 ml vials

Side effects/adverse reactions:

▼ *ORAL:* Dry mouth, gingival overgrowth, altered taste, ulcers

CNS: Headache, fatigue, drowsiness, dizziness, depression, weakness, insomnia, tremor, paresthesia

CV: Dysrhythmia, edema, ***CHF,*** bradycardia, hypotension, palpitation, heart block, peripheral edema, angina

GI: Nausea, vomiting, diarrhea, gastric upset, constipation, increased liver function studies

GU: ***Acute renal failure,*** nocturia, polyuria

INTEG: Rash, pruritus, flushing, photosensitivity

Contraindications: Sick sinus syndrome, second- or third-degree heart block, hypotension <90 mm Hg systolic, acute MI, pulmonary congestion

Precautions: CHF, hypotension, hepatic injury, pregnancy category C, lactation, children, renal disease

Pharmacokinetics:

PO: Onset 30-60 min, peak 2-3 hr (immediate rel), 6-11 hr (sus rel), half-life 3.5-9 hr; metabolized by liver; excreted in urine (96% as metabolites)

Drug interactions of concern to dentistry:

• Decreased effect: indomethacin, possibly other NSAIDs, phenobarbital

• Increased effect: parenteral and

inhalational general anesthetics or other drugs with hypotensive actions
• Increased effects of carbamazepine, midazolam, triazolam

DENTAL CONSIDERATIONS

General:
• Monitor cardiac status; take vital signs at each appointment because of CV side effects. Consider a stress reduction protocol to prevent stress-induced angina during the dental appointment.
• After supine positioning, have patient sit upright for at least 2 min to avoid orthostatic hypotension.
• Place on frequent recall to monitor gingival condition.
• Limit use of sodium-containing products such as saline IV fluids for patients with a dietary salt restriction.
• Assess salivary flow as a factor in caries, periodontal disease, and candidiasis.
• Consider drug in diagnosis of taste alterations.

Consultations:
• Medical consult may be required to assess disease control in the patient.

Teach patient/family:
• Importance of good oral hygiene to prevent soft tissue inflammation and to minimize gingival overgrowth
• Need for frequent oral prophylaxis if gingival overgrowth occurs

When chronic dry mouth occurs, advise patient:
• To avoid mouth rinses with high alcohol content due to drying effects
• To use daily home fluoride products for anticaries effect
• To use sugarless gum, frequent sips of water, or saliva substitutes

dimenhydrinate

(dye-men-hye'dri-nate)

Calm-X, Dinate, Dramanate, Dramamine, Hydrate, PMS-Dimenhydrinate, Traveltabs, Triptone Caplets, Vertab

♣ Apo-Dimenhydrinate, Gravol, Gravol L/A, Novo-Dimenate

Drug class.: H_1-receptor antagonist

Action: Acts on blood vessels, GI system, respiratory system by competing with histamine for H_1-receptor site; decreases allergic response by blocking histamine

Uses: Motion sickness, nausea, vomiting

Dosage and routes:
• *Adult:* PO 50-100 mg q4h; REC 100 mg qd or bid; IM/IV 50 mg as needed
• *Child:* IM/PO 5 mg/kg divided in 4 equal doses

Available forms include: Tabs 50 mg; inj 500 mg/ml; liq 12.5/4 ml; supp 50, 100 mg

Side effects/adverse reactions:

▼ *ORAL: Dry mouth*

CNS: Drowsiness, ***convulsions*** (young children), restlessness, headache, dizziness, insomnia, confusion, nervousness, tingling, vertigo, hallucinations

CV: Hypertension, hypotension, palpitation

GI: Nausea, anorexia, diarrhea, vomiting, constipation

EENT: Blurred vision, diplopia, nasal congestion, photosensitivity

SYST: Rash, urticaria, fever, chills, flushing

Contraindications: Hypersensitivity to narcotics, shock

Precautions: Children, cardiac

dysrhythmias, elderly, asthma, pregnancy category B, prostatic hypertrophy, bladder neck obstruction, narrow-angle glaucoma, stenosing peptic ulcer, pyloroduodenal obstruction

Pharmacokinetics:

IM/PO: Duration 4-6 hr

Drug interactions of concern to dentistry:

- Increased photosensitization: tetracycline
- Increased effects of alcohol, other CNS depressants, anticholinergics

DENTAL CONSIDERATIONS

General:

- Assess salivary flow as a factor in caries, periodontal disease, and candidiasis.

Teach patient/family:

When chronic dry mouth occurs, advise patient:

- To avoid mouth rinses with high alcohol content due to drying effects
- To use daily home fluoride products for anticaries effect
- To use sugarless gum, frequent sips of water, or saliva substitutes

---

diphenhydramine HCl

(dye-fen-hye′dra-meen)

AllerMax, AllerMed, Banophen, Benadryl, Benylin Cough, Bydramine, Compoz, Diphen, Diphenhist, Genahist, Hydramine, Hydril, Nervine SleepAid, Nytol Quickcaps, Phendry, Siladryl, Sleep-Eze-D, Sominex Formula, Tusstat, Uni-Bent Unisom, and others

♣ Allerdryl

Drug class.: Antihistamine, H_1-receptor antagonist

Action: Acts on blood vessels, GI system, respiratory system by competing with histamine for H_1-receptor site; decreases allergic response by blocking histamine

Uses: Allergy symptoms, rhinitis, motion sickness, antiparkinsonism, nighttime sedation, infant colic, nonproductive cough; unlabeled use for dental local anesthesia

Dosage and routes:

- *Adult:* PO 25-50 mg q4-6h, not to exceed 400 mg/day; IM/IV 10-50 mg, not to exceed 400 mg/day
- *Child >12 kg:* PO/IM/IV 5 mg/kg/day in 4 divided doses, not to exceed 300 mg/day
- *Local anesthetic (unapproved use):* INTRAORAL INJ use *only* the 10 mg/ml solution and never more than 1.5 ml per injection per patient; risk of tissue irritation if more is used; must use sterile technique at all times; no data to support combined use with vasoconstrictor

Available forms include: Caps 25, 50 mg; tabs 50 mg; elix 12.5 mg/5 ml; syr 12.5 mg/5 ml; inj IM/IV 10, 50 mg/ml

Side effects/adverse reactions:

▼ *ORAL:* Dry mouth

CNS: Dizziness, drowsiness, poor coordination, fatigue, anxiety, euphoria, confusion, paresthesia, neuritis

GI: Nausea, anorexia, diarrhea

RESP: Increased thick secretions, wheezing, chest tightness

HEMA: ***Thrombocytopenia, agranulocytosis, hemolytic anemia***

GU: Retention, dysuria, frequency

EENT: Blurred vision, dilated pupils, tinnitus, nasal stuffiness, dry nose/throat

INTEG: Photosensitivity

Contraindications: Hypersensi-

tivity to H_1-receptor antagonist, acute asthma attack, lower respiratory tract disease

Precautions: Increased intraocular pressure, renal disease, cardiac disease, hypertension, bronchial asthma, seizure disorder, stenosed peptic ulcers, hyperthyroidism, prostatic hypertrophy, bladder neck obstruction, pregnancy category C

Pharmacokinetics:

PO: Peak 1-3 hr, duration 4-7 hr

IM: Onset 0.5 hr, peak 1-4 hr, duration 4-7 hr

IV: Onset immediate, duration 4-7 hr, half-life 2-7 hr

Metabolized in liver; excreted by kidneys; crosses placenta; excreted in breast milk

Drug interactions of concern to dentistry:

- Increased CNS depression: all CNS depressants, alcohol
- Increased anticholinergic effect: anticholinergics

DENTAL CONSIDERATIONS

General:

- Patients on chronic drug therapy may rarely have symptoms of blood dyscrasias, which can include infection, bleeding, and poor healing.
- Assess salivary flow as a factor in caries, periodontal disease, and candidiasis.
- Consider semisupine chair position for patients with respiratory disease.

Consultations:

- In a patient with symptoms of blood dyscrasias, request a medical consult for blood studies and postpone dental treatment until normal values are reestablished.

Teach patient/family:

- Importance of good oral hygiene to prevent soft tissue inflammation
- Caution to prevent injury when using oral hygiene aids

When chronic dry mouth occurs, advise patient:

- To avoid mouth rinses with high alcohol content due to drying effects
- To use daily home fluoride products for anticaries effect
- To use sugarless gum, frequent sips of water, or saliva substitutes

diphenoxylate HCl with atropine sulfate

(dye-fen-ox'i-late)

Lofene, Logen, Lomocort, Lomotil, Lonox, Vi-Atrol

Drug class.: Antidiarrheal (opioid with atropine)

Controlled Substance Schedule V

Action: Inhibits gastric motility by acting on mucosal receptors responsible for peristalsis

Uses: Simple diarrhea

Dosage and routes:

- *Adult:* PO 2.5-5 mg qid, titrated to patient response
- *Child 2-12 yr:* PO 0.3-0.4 mg/kg/day in divided doses

Available forms include: Tabs 2.5 mg

Side effects/adverse reactions:

▼ *ORAL:* Dry mouth

CNS: Drowsiness, headache, sedation, depression, weakness, lethargy, flushing, hyperthermia

CV: Tachycardia

GI: Nausea, vomiting, ***paralytic ileus, toxic megacolon,*** abdominal pain, colitis

GU: Urinary retention
EENT: Blurred vision, nystagmus, mydriasis
SYST: ***Angioneurotic edema,*** rash, urticaria, pruritus
Contraindications: Hypersensitivity, severe liver disease, pseudomembranous enterocolitis, glaucoma, child <2 yr, electrolyte imbalances
Precautions: Hepatic disease, renal disease, ulcerative colitis, pregnancy category C, lactation, elderly
Pharmacokinetics:
PO: Onset 45-60 min, peak 2 hr, duration 3-4 hr, half-life 2.5 hr, terminal half-life 12-14 hr; metabolized in liver to active form; excreted in urine, feces, breast milk
Drug interactions of concern to dentistry:
• Contraindication: MAO inhibitors
• Increased effects of alcohol, all CNS depressants, opioid analgesics, anticholinergics

DENTAL CONSIDERATIONS
General:
• Assess salivary flow as a factor in caries, periodontal disease, and candidiasis.
• Psychologic and physical dependence may occur with chronic administration.
• Consider semisupine chair position for patient comfort due to GI effects of disease.
• This drug product is normally used only for a few doses for acute problems; however, some patients may have to take it for longer time periods as dictated by a contributing disease.
Teach patient/family:
• To avoid mouth rinses with high alcohol content due to drying effects

---

dipivefrin HCl
(dye-pi′ve-frin)
AKPro, DPE, Propine C Cap B.I.D., Ophtho-Dipivefrin
Drug class.: Adrenergic agonist

Action: Converted to epinephrine, which decreases aqueous production and increases outflow
Uses: Open-angle glaucoma
Dosage and routes:
• *Adult:* Instill 1 gtt q12h
Available forms include: Sol 0.1%
Side effects/adverse reactions:
CV: Hypertension, tachycardia, dysrhythmias
EENT: Burning, stinging, mydriasis, photophobia
Contraindications: Hypersensitivity, narrow-angle glaucoma
Precautions: Pregnancy category B, lactation, children, aphakia
Pharmacokinetics:
INSTILL: Onset 30 min, peak 1 hr, duration 12 hr
Drug interactions of concern to dentistry:
• Avoid use of anticholinergics such as atropine, scopolamine, and propantheline; use benzodiazepines with caution

DENTAL CONSIDERATIONS
General:
• Avoid dental light in patient's eyes; offer dark glasses for patient comfort.

dipyridamole

(dye-peer-id'a-mole)

Dipridacot, Persantine

♣ Apo-Dipyridamole, Novodipiradol

Drug class.: Platelet aggregation inhibitor

Action: Specific action unclear; inhibits ability of platelets to aggregate, possibly through effects on adenosine, cAMP, or thromboxane A_2

Uses: Prevention of transient ischemic attack (TIA), inhibition of platelet aggregation to prevent MI, thromboembolism, with warfarin in prosthetic heart valves, prevention of coronary bypass graft occlusion with aspirin

Dosage and routes:

TIA

• *Adult:* PO 75-100 mg qid, 1 hr ac, not to exceed 400 mg qd

Inhibition of platelet aggregation

• *Adult:* PO 50-75 mg qid in combination with aspirin *or* Coumadin, but not both

Available forms include: Tabs 25, 50, 75 mg

Side effects/adverse reactions:

▼ *ORAL:* Gingival bleeding

CNS: Headache, dizziness, weakness, fainting, syncope

CV: Postural hypotension

GI: Nausea, vomiting, anorexia, diarrhea

INTEG: Rash, flushing

Contraindications: Hypersensitivity, hypotension

Precautions: Pregnancy category B, children <12 yr

Pharmacokinetics:

PO: Peak 2-2.5 hr, duration 6 hr; therapeutic response may take several months; metabolized in liver; excreted in bile; undergoes enterohepatic recirculation

Drug interactions of concern to dentistry:

• Additive antiplatelet effects: aspirin and other NSAIDs

DENTAL CONSIDERATIONS

General:

• Monitor vital signs every appointment due to cardiovascular side effects.

• After supine positioning, have patient sit upright for at least 2 min to avoid orthostatic hypotension.

• Avoid prescribing aspirin-containing products.

• Evaluate for clotting ability during gingival instrumentation, because inhibition of platelet aggregation may occur.

• Consider local hemostatic measures to prevent excessive bleeding during instrumentation.

Consultations:

• Medical consult should include partial prothrombin or prothrombin times.

• Medical consult may be required to assess disease control in the patient.

Teach patient/family:

• Importance of good oral hygiene to prevent gingival inflammation

dirithromycin

(dye-rith'roe-mye-sin)

Dynabac

Drug class.: Macrolide antibiotic

Action: Active product (erythromycylamine) binds to 50S ribosomal subunits of susceptible bacteria to inhibit bacterial growth

Uses: Treatment of acute and secondary bacterial infection of acute bronchitis, community-acquired pneumonia, streptococcal pharyngitis, and uncomplicated skin and skin structure infections

Dosage and routes:

• *Adult and child >12 yr:* PO 500 mg/day for 7-14 days; give with food or within 1 hr of eating; do not crush or chew tablets

Available forms include: Tabs 250 mg

Side effects/adverse reactions:

▼ *ORAL:* Dry mouth, taste alteration, mouth ulcers (all <1%); although not documented, it is reasonable to assume opportunistic oral candidiasis

CNS: Headache, somnolence, dizziness, insomnia

GI: Diarrhea, abdominal pain, nausea, dyspepsia, pseudomembranous colitis

RESP: Dyspnea, cough

GU: Vaginal candidiasis

INTEG: Rash, pruritus, urticaria

MS: Asthenia

Contraindications: Hypersensitivity to macrolide antibiotics

Precautions: Not for *H. influenzae* or *S. pyogenes* infections, pregnancy category C, lactation, child <12 yr

Pharmacokinetics:

PO: Half-life 30-44 hr; after absorption, parent drug is converted to erythromycylamine; plasma protein binding low (15%-30%); excreted in bile

Drug interactions of concern to dentistry:

• Potential for dysrhythmias with terfenadine, astemizole is unknown; avoid combinations until more data are available

• Other drug interactions: data are limited; antacids and histamine H_2 antagonists tend to enhance absorption; refer to erythromycin for potential interacting drugs

DENTAL CONSIDERATIONS

General:

• Do not use in patients at risk for bacteremias due to inadequate serum levels.

• Potential value in dental infections is unknown.

• Determine why the patient is taking the drug.

• Examine for oral manifestations of opportunistic infections.

Consultations:

• Medical consult may be required to assess disease control in the patient.

Teach patient/family:

• Alert the patient to the possibility of secondary oral infection and the need to see dentist immediately if infection occurs

disopyramide/ disopyramide phosphate

(dye-soe-peer'a-mide)

Norpace, Norpace CR

✤ Rythmodan, Rythmodan-LA

Drug class.: Antidysrhythmic (Class IA)

Action: Prolongs action potential duration and effective refractory period; reduces disparity in refractoriness between normal and infarcted myocardium

Uses: PVCs, ventricular tachycardia, atrial flutter, fibrillation

Dosage and routes:

• *Adult:* PO 100-200 mg q6h, in renal dysfunction 100 mg q6h; sus rel caps 200 mg q12h

• *Child 12-18 yr:* PO 6-15 mg/kg/day, in divided doses q6h

• *Child 4-12 yr:* PO 10-15 mg/kg/day, in divided doses q6h
• *Child 1-4 yr:* PO 10-20 mg/kg/day, in divided doses q6h
• *Child <1 yr:* PO 10-30 mg/kg/day, in divided doses q6h

Available forms include: Caps 100, 150 mg (as phosphate); sus rel caps 100, 150 mg

Side effects/adverse reactions:

▼ *ORAL: Dry mouth*

CNS: Headache, dizziness, psychosis, fatigue, depression, paresthesia, anxiety, insomnia

CV: Hypotension, bradycardia, ***CHF, cardiac arrest,*** angina, PVCs, tachycardia, increase in QRS and QT segments, edema, weight gain, AV block, syncope, chest pain

GI: Constipation, nausea, anorexia, flatulence, diarrhea, vomiting

HEMA: ***Thrombocytopenia, agranulocytosis,*** anemia (rare), decreased hemoglobin, hematocrit

GU: Retention, hesitancy, impotence, urinary frequency, urgency

EENT: Blurred vision, dry nose/throat/eyes, narrow-angle glaucoma

INTEG: Rash, pruritus, urticaria

MS: Weakness, pain in extremities

META: Hypoglycemia

Contraindications: Hypersensitivity, second- or third-degree heart block, cardiogenic shock, CHF (uncompensated), sick sinus syndrome, QT prolongation

Precautions: Pregnancy category C, lactation, diabetes mellitus, renal disease, children, hepatic disease, myasthenia gravis, narrow-angle glaucoma, cardiomyopathy, conduction abnormalities

Pharmacokinetics:

PO: Peak 30 min-3 hr, duration 6-12 hr, half-life 4-10 hr; metabolized in liver; excreted in feces, urine, breast milk; crosses placenta

Drug interactions of concern to dentistry:

• Increased effects: erythromycin
• Increased side effects: anticholinergics, alcohol
• Decreased effects: barbiturates, corticosteroids

DENTAL CONSIDERATIONS

General:

• Monitor vital signs every appointment due to cardiovascular side effects.
• After supine positioning, have patient sit upright for at least 2 min before standing to avoid orthostatic hypotension.
• Patients on chronic drug therapy may rarely have symptoms of blood dyscrasias, which can include infection, bleeding, and poor healing.
• Assess salivary flow as a factor in caries, periodontal disease, and candidiasis.

Consultations:

• In a patient with symptoms of blood dyscrasias, request a medical consult for blood studies and postpone dental treatment until normal values are reestablished.
• Medical consult may be required to assess disease control and patient's ability to tolerate stress.

Teach patient/family:

• Importance of good oral hygiene to prevent soft tissue inflammation

When chronic dry mouth occurs, advise patient:

• To avoid mouth rinses with high alcohol content due to drying effects
• To use daily home fluoride products for anticaries effect
• To use sugarless gum, frequent sips of water, or saliva substitutes

disulfiram

(dye-sul'fi-ram)

Antabuse

Drug class.: Aldehyde dehydrogenase inhibitor

Action: Blocks oxidation of alcohol at acetaldehyde stage; accumulation of acetaldehyde produces the disulfiram-alcohol reaction

Uses: Chronic alcoholism (as adjunct)

Dosage and routes:

• *Adult:* PO 250-500 mg qd × 1-2 wk, then 125-500 mg qd

Available forms include: Tabs 250, 500 mg

Side effects/adverse reactions:

▼ *ORAL:* Metallic taste

CNS: Headache, drowsiness, restlessness, dizziness

CV: ***Dysrhythmias,*** tachycardia, chest pain, hypotension

GI: ***Hepatotoxicity,*** nausea, vomiting

RESP: ***Respiratory depression,*** hyperventilation, dyspnea

INTEG: Rash, dermatitis, urticaria

Disulfiram-alcohol reaction: Flushing, throbbing, headache, respiratory difficulty, nausea, vomiting, sweating, thirst, chest pain, palpitation, dyspnea, hyperventilation, tachycardia, confusion, CV collapse, MI, CHF, convulsions, death

Contraindications: Hypersensitivity, alcohol intoxication, psychoses, CV disease, pregnancy category not listed

Precautions: Hypothyroidism, hepatic disease, diabetes mellitus, seizure disorders, nephritis, cerebral damage

Pharmacokinetics:

PO: Onset 1-2 hr; oxidized by liver; excreted unchanged in feces; can affect alcohol metabolism for 1-2 wk after last dose

Drug interactions of concern to dentistry:

• Increased CNS depression: long-acting benzodiazepines

• Increased disulfiram reaction: alcohol

• Risk of psychosis: metronidazole (do not use), tricyclic antidepressants

DENTAL CONSIDERATIONS

General:

• Be aware of the needs of patients who are in recovery from substance abuse.

• Avoid other drugs that are also addicting, including opioids and benzodiazepines.

Consultations:

• Medical consult may be required to assess disease control in the patient.

Teach patient/family:

• To avoid mouth rinses with high alcohol content due to drying effects and drug-drug interaction

dolasetron mesylate

(dol-a'se-tron)

Anzemet

Drug class.: Antinauseant and antiemetic

Action: Acts as an antagonist for serotonin ($5HT_3$) receptors in the CNS; may also reduce afferent stimulus from GI tract

Uses: Control of nausea and vomiting associated with cancer chemotherapy and prevention of postoperative nausea and vomiting

Dosage and routes:
Cancer chemotherapy
• *Adult:* PO 100 mg given within 1 hr of chemotherapy
• *Child 2-16 yr:* PO 1.8 mg/kg given within 1 hr of chemotherapy not to exceed 100 mg
Parenteral chemotherapy
• *Adult:* IV 1.8 mg/kg as a single dose about 30 min before chemotherapy, alternatively for most patients, a fixed dose of 100 mg can be given over 30 seconds
• *Child 2-16 yr:* IV 1.8 mg/kg as a single dose approximately 30 min before chemotherapy up to a maximum of 100 mg
Prevention of postoperative nausea and vomiting
• *Adult:* IV 12.5 mg as a single dose 15 min before the end of anesthesia or as soon as nausea and vomiting are evident
• *Child 2-16 yr:* IV 0.35 mg/kg with a maximum dose of 12.5 mg (single dose) approximately 15 min before cessation of anesthesia or as soon as nausea and vomiting are present
Available forms include: Tabs 50, 100 mg; inj 12.5 mg/0.625 ml, 100 mg/5ml
Side effects/adverse reactions:
▼ *ORAL: Taste alteration*
CNS: Headache, fatigue, sedation, dizziness, light-headedness, nervousness, paresthesia
CV: Bradycardia, tachycardia, alteration of ECG, orthostatic hypotension, hypertension
GI: Increased appetite, nausea, constipation, diarrhea, dyspepsia, flatulence
EENT: Blurred vision
INTEG: Pruritus
META: Elevation of aminotransferases
MISC: Fever, chills
Contraindications: Hypersensitivity
Precautions: Previous hypersensitivity to other 5-HT_3 antagonists, cardiovascular disease, seizure disorders, ECG changes, hypokalemia, hypomagnesemia, diuretics, antiarrhythmics, pregnancy category B, lactation
Pharmacokinetics:
IV: Metabolized to active metabolite, peak plasma concentrations 1 hr, urinary excretion mostly, some fecal excretion
PO: Well absorbed, rapidly metabolized to active metabolite
Drug interactions of concern to dentistry:
• Does not influence anesthesia recovery time

DENTAL CONSIDERATIONS
General:
• Monitor patients in recovery to avoid untoward events.
• Patients taking opioids for acute or chronic pain should be given alternative analgesics for dental pain.
• Chlorhexidine mouth rinse before and during chemotherapy may reduce severity of mucositis.
• Palliative medication may be required for management of oral side effects.
Teach patient/family:
• To be aware of oral side effects
• To report excessive nausea and vomiting to dentist for patients recovering from anesthesia after dental treatment

donepezil HCl

(doe-nep'e-zeel)

Aricept

Drug class.: Cholinesterase inhibitor

Action: A centrally acting reversible inhibitor of choline esterase enzyme

Uses: Mild to moderate dementia associated with Alzheimer's disease

Dosage and routes:

• *Adult:* PO initial 5 mg/day; can increase to 10 mg/day after 4-6 wk evaluation at 5 mg dose; take dose in evening just before retiring

Available forms include: Tabs 5, 10 mg

Side effects/adverse reactions:

▼ *ORAL:* Toothache (1%), dry mouth, bad taste, gingivitis, tongue edema, coated tongue

CNS: Insomnia, anorexia, headache, dizziness, depression, abnormal dreams

CV: Syncope, hot flashes, hypotension, hypertension

GI: Nausea, diarrhea, vomiting, anorexia

RESP: Dyspnea

HEMA: Thrombocytopenia, ecchymosis, anemia

GU: Frequency of urination

EENT: Sore throat, dry eyes, blurred vision, earache, tinnitus

INTEG: Pruritus, urticaria

META: Weight decrease, dehydration

MS: Muscle cramps, arthritis

MISC: Fatigue, generalized pain

Contraindications: Hypersensitivity

Precautions: Bradycardia, sick sinus syndrome, GI ulcer disease, bladder obstruction, seizures, asthma, obstructive pulmonary disease, pregnancy category C, lactation, children, hepatic impairment

Pharmacokinetics:

PO: Bioavailability 100%, peak plasma levels 3-4 hr, 96% bound to plasma proteins, hepatic metabolism, active metabolites, urinary excretion

Drug interactions of concern to dentistry:

• Enhanced succinylcholine muscle relaxation during anesthesia

• Risk of GI side effects: NSAIDs

• Action may be inhibited by anticholinergic drugs or enhanced by cholinergic agonists

• Ketoconazole may inhibit metabolism of donepezil

DENTAL CONSIDERATIONS

General:

• Determine why patient is taking the drug.

• Monitor vital signs every appointment due to cardiovascular side effects.

• After supine positioning, have patient sit upright for at least 2 min before standing to avoid orthostatic hypotension.

• Use precaution if sedation or general anesthesia is required.

• Patient on chronic drug therapy may rarely have symptoms of blood dyscrasias, which can include infection, bleeding, and poor healing.

• Drug is used early in the disease; ensure patient or caregiver understands informed consent.

• Place on frequent recall because early attention to dental health is important for Alzheimer's patients.

• Assess salivary flow as factor in caries, periodontal disease, and candidiasis.

D

• Consider semisupine chair position for patient comfort if GI side effects occur.
• Consultation with physician may be needed if sedation or general anesthesia is required.

Consultations:
• Medical consult may be required to assess disease control and patient's ability to tolerate stress.
• In a patient with symptoms of blood dyscrasias, request a medical consult for blood studies and postpone treatment until normal values are reestablished.

Teach patient/family:
• Importance of good oral hygiene to prevent soft tissue inflammation
• To prevent trauma when using oral hygiene aids
• Use of electric toothbrush if patient has difficulty holding conventional devices

When chronic dry mouth occurs, advise patient:
• To avoid mouth rinses with high alcohol content due to drying effects
• To use daily home fluoride products for anticaries effect
• To use sugarless gum, frequent sips of water, or saliva substitutes

dornase alfa

(dor'nase)
Pulmozyme

Drug class.: Recombinant human deoxyribonuclease (DNase)

Action: Reduces sputum viscosity by hydrolyzing extracellular DNA in sputum

Uses: Cystic fibrosis; reduces incidence of pulmonary infections; improves pulmonary function

Dosage and routes:
• *Adult and child >5 yr:* INH inhale 2.5 mg once daily with recommended nebulizer

Available forms include: INH 1.0 mg/ml in 2.5 ml ampules

Side effects/adverse reactions:
CV: Chest pain, ***cardiac failure***
GI: Intestinal obstruction, abdominal pain
RESP: Apnea, bronchitis, dyspnea, coughing
EENT: Pharyngitis, laryngitis, conjunctivitis, voice alteration, sinusitis
INTEG: Rash, urticaria
MISC: Flulike symptoms, malaise, weight loss

Contraindications: Hypersensitivity, allergy to Chinese Hamster Ovary cell products

Precautions: Pregnancy category B, lactation, child <5 yr

Pharmacokinetics:
INH: Peak sputum levels 15 min

Drug interactions of concern to dentistry:
• None documented

DENTAL CONSIDERATIONS

General:
• Consider semisupine chair position for patients with respiratory disease.
• Monitor vital signs every appointment due to respiratory and cardiovascular side effects.
• A stress reduction protocol may be required.

Consultations:
• A medical consult may be required to assess disease control in the patient.

Teach patient/family:
• Importance of good oral hygiene to prevent soft tissue inflammation

dorzolamide HCl

(dor-zole'a-mide)
Trusopt

Drug class.: Carbonic anhydrase inhibitor

Action: Reduces intraocular pressure through inhibition of carbonic anhydrase enzyme

Uses: Ocular hypertension, open-angle glaucoma

Dosage and routes:

• *Adult:* Instill 1 gtt in affected eye(s) tid; if other ophthalmic drug products are also used, give the drugs at least 10 min apart

Available forms include: Sol 2% in 5, 10 ml

Side effects/adverse reactions:

▼ *ORAL: Bitter taste*

CNS: Headache

GI: Nausea

EENT: Ocular burning, stinging, conjunctivitis, lid reactions, keratitis, blurred vision, photophobia

INTEG: Skin rashes

Contraindications: Hypersensitivity

Precautions: Allergy to sulfonamides, renal or hepatic impairment, pregnancy category C, lactation, children, oral carbonic anhydrase inhibitors, contact lenses

Pharmacokinetics: Systemically absorbed from the eye

Drug interactions of concern to dentistry:

• Avoid drugs that may exacerbate glaucoma (anticholinergic drugs)

• High-dose salicylates to avoid systemic toxicity

DENTAL CONSIDERATIONS

General:

• Avoid dental light in patient's eyes; offer dark glasses for patient comfort.

• Protect patient's eyes from accidental spatter during dental treatment.

• Check compliance of patient with prescribed drug regimen for glaucoma.

Consultations:

• Medical consult may be required to assess disease control in the patient.

D

doxazosin mesylate

(dox-ay'zoe-sin)
Cardura

Drug class.: Peripheral α-adrenergic blocker

Action: Peripheral blood vessels dilated; peripheral resistance lowered; reduction in blood pressure results from α-adrenergic receptors being blocked

Uses: Hypertension, unlabeled use in benign prostatic hypertrophy

Dosage and routes:

• *Adult:* PO 1 mg qd, increasing up to 16 mg qd if required; usual range 4-16 mg/day

Available forms include: Tabs 1, 2, 4, 8 mg

Side effects/adverse reactions:

▼ *ORAL:* Dry mouth

CNS: Dizziness, headache, weakness, fatigue, asthenia, drowsiness, anxiety, depression, vertigo

CV: Palpitation, orthostatic hypotension, tachycardia, edema, dysrhythmias, chest pain

GI: Nausea, vomiting, diarrhea, constipation, abdominal pain

GU: Incontinence, polyuria

EENT: Epistaxis, tinnitus, red sclera, pharyngitis, rhinitis

INTEG: Lichen planus

Contraindications: Hypersensitivity to quinazolines

Precautions: Pregnancy category B, children, lactation, hepatic disease

Pharmacokinetics:

PO: Onset 2 hr, peak 2-6 hr, duration 24 hr, half-life 22 hr; extensively protein bound (98%); metabolized in liver; excreted via bile, feces (<63%) and in urine (9%)

Drug interactions of concern to dentistry:

- Increased hypotensive effects: all CNS depressants
- Reduced effects with indomethacin, NSAIDs, sympathomimetics

DENTAL CONSIDERATIONS

General:

- Monitor vital signs every appointment due to cardiovascular side effects.
- After supine positioning, have patient sit upright for at least 2 min before standing to avoid orthostatic hypotension.
- Assess salivary flow as a factor in caries, periodontal disease, and candidiasis.

Consultations:

- Medical consult may be required to assess disease control and patient's ability to tolerate stress.

Teach patient/family:

When chronic dry mouth occurs, advise patient:

- To avoid mouth rinses with high alcohol content due to drying effects
- To use daily home fluoride products for anticaries effect
- To use sugarless gum, frequent sips of water, or saliva substitutes

doxepin HCl (topical)

(dox'e-pin)

Zonalon

Drug class.: Topical antipruritic (tricyclic antidepressant)

Action: Antipruritic mechanism unknown; has antihistaminic activity; also produces drowsiness

Uses: Pruritus associated with eczema, atopic dermatitis, lichen simplex chronicus

Dosage and routes:

- *Adult:* TOP apply to affected area qid with intervals of 3-4 days between applications for up to 8 days

Available forms include: Cream 5% in 30 g tube

Side effects/adverse reactions:

▼ *ORAL: Dry mouth, taste alteration, dry lips*

CNS: Drowsiness, headache, fatigue, dizziness, anxiety

INTEG: Burning, stinging, dryness of skin, edema, paresthesia

MISC: Fever

Contraindications: Hypersensitivity, untreated glaucoma, tendency for urinary retention

Precautions: Pregnancy category B, lactation, children, for external use only, caution in driving car, current use with alcohol or MAO inhibitor

Pharmacokinetics:

TOP: Variable absorption, half-life 28-52 hr; hepatic metabolism; widely distributed; renal excretion

Drug interactions of concern to dentistry:

- Potential for interactions depends on how much drug is absorbed and duration of use (>8 days)
- Increased anticholinergic effects:

anticholinergics, antihistamines, phenothiazines, other tricyclic antidepressants
• Potential risk for increased CNS depression: all CNS depressants
• Increased effects of direct-acting sympathomimetics: epinephrine, levonordefrin

DENTAL CONSIDERATIONS
General:
• Doxepin may be absorbed and produce typical systemic side effects of tricyclic drugs.
• Monitor vital signs every appointment due to cardiovascular side effects.
• Use vasoconstrictors with caution, in low doses, and with careful aspiration.
• Place on frequent recall due to oral side effects.
• Apply lubricant to dry lips for patient comfort before dental procedures.
• Assess salivary flow as a factor in caries, periodontal disease, and candidiasis.

Consultations:
• Medical consult may be required to assess disease control in the patient.

Teach patient/family:
• To avoid mouth rinses with high alcohol content due to interaction with alcohol (see precautions) and drying effects

When chronic dry mouth occurs, advise patient:
• Of need for daily home fluoride for anticaries effect
• To use sugarless gum, frequent sips of water, or saliva substitutes

doxepin HCl

(dox′e-pin)
Sinequan
🍁 Novo-Doxepin, Triadapin

Drug class.: Antidepressant, tricyclic

Action: Inhibits both norepinephrine and serotonin (5-HT) reuptake in synapses in the brain, but the precise antidepressant mechanism remains unclear

Uses: Major depression, anxiety; unapproved use: panic disorders

Dosage and routes:
• *Adult:* PO 50-75 mg/day in divided doses; may increase to 150 mg/day or may give daily dose hs; severe depression up to 300 mg

Available forms include: Caps 10, 25, 50, 75, 100, 150 mg; oral conc 10 mg/ml

Side effects/adverse reactions:
▼ *ORAL: Dry mouth, unpleasant taste,* bleeding, stomatitis, lichenoid reaction

CNS: Dizziness, drowsiness, confusion, headache, anxiety, tremors, stimulation, weakness, insomnia, nightmares, EPS (elderly), increased psychiatric symptoms, paresthesia

CV: Orthostatic hypotension, ECG changes, tachycardia, ***hypertension,*** palpitation

GI: Diarrhea, ***paralytic ileus, hepatitis,*** increased appetite, cramps, epigastric distress, jaundice, nausea, vomiting

HEMA: ***Agranulocytosis, thrombocytopenia, eosinophilia, leukopenia***

GU: Retention, ***acute renal failure***

EENT: Blurred vision, tinnitus, mydriasis, ophthalmoplegia
INTEG: Rash, urticaria, sweating, pruritus, photosensitivity
Contraindications: Hypersensitivity to tricyclic antidepressants, urinary retention, narrow-angle glaucoma, prostatic hypertrophy
Precautions: Suicidal patients, elderly, pregnancy category C, MAO inhibitors
Pharmacokinetics:
PO: Steady state 2-8 days, half-life 8-24 hr; metabolized by liver; excreted by kidneys; crosses placenta; excreted in breast milk
Drug interactions of concern to dentistry:
• Increased anticholinergic effects: anticholinergic blockers, antihistamines, phenothiazines
• Increased effects of direct-acting sympathomimetics (epinephrine, levonordefrin)
• Potential risk of increased CNS depression: alcohol, barbiturates, benzodiazepines, and other CNS depressants
• Decreased antihypertensive effects: clonidine, guanadrel, guanethidine

DENTAL CONSIDERATIONS
General:
• Take vital signs every appointment due to cardiovascular side effects.
• Assess salivary flow as a factor in caries, periodontal disease, and candidiasis.
• Patients on chronic drug therapy may rarely have symptoms of blood dyscrasias, which can include infection, bleeding, and poor healing.
• After supine positioning, have patient sit upright for at least 2 min before standing to avoid orthostatic hypotension.
• Use vasoconstrictors with caution, in low doses, and with careful aspiration. Avoid use of gingival retraction cord with epinephrine.
• Place on frequent recall due to oral side effects.
Consultations:
• In a patient with symptoms of blood dyscrasias, request a medical consult for blood studies and postpone dental treatment until normal values are reestablished.
• Medical consult may be required to assess disease control in the patient.
• Physician should be informed if significant xerostomic side effects occur (increased caries, sore tongue, problems eating or swallowing, difficulty wearing prosthesis) so a medication change can be considered.
Teach patient/family:
• Importance of good oral hygiene to prevent soft tissue inflammation
When chronic dry mouth occurs, advise patient:
• To avoid mouth rinses with high alcohol content due to drying effects
• To use daily home fluoride products for anticaries effect
• To use sugarless gum, frequent sips of water, or saliva substitutes

doxycycline hyclate (dental—systemic)

(dox-i-sye'kleen)
Periostat
Drug class.: Tetracycline derivative for nonantibacterial use

Action: Reduces elevated collagenase activity in gingival crevicular fluid of patients with adult periodontitis; no antibacterial effect reported at this dose

Uses: Adjunct to scaling and root planing to promote attachment level gain and reduce pocket depth in adult periodontitis

Dosage and routes:

• *Adult:* PO 20 mg bid as an adjunct to scaling and root planing; may be administered for up to 9 mo; exceeding the recommended dosage may increase risk of side effects, including the development of resistant organisms

Available forms include: Caps 20 mg

Side effects/adverse reactions:

NOTE: In a clinical study of 428 patients there was little to no difference in the incidence of side effects reported between this drug and a placebo. See doxycycline hyclate monograph for typical side effects associated with oral administration. Whether these side effects would occur at doses used in this product is unknown.

Contraindications: Hypersensitivity to tetracyclines

Precautions: Not to be used for antimicrobial effect in periodontitis, in children <8 yr, pregnant and nursing mothers, predisposition to oral or vaginal candidiasis, pregnancy category D

Pharmacokinetics: No data available

Drug interactions of concern to dentistry:

• No data reported for this dose form; see doxycycline hyclate monograph for drug interactions reported with tetracyclines

DENTAL CONSIDERATIONS

General:

• Examine for oral manifestation of opportunistic infection

• Should be administered at least 1 hr before morning or evening meals

Teach patient/family:

• To avoid using ingestible sodium bicarbonate products, such as the air polishing system (ProphyJet), within 2 hr of drug use

---

doxycycline hyclate/ doxycycline calcium

(dox-i-sye'kleen)

Doxycycline calcium: Vibramycin

Doxycycline hyclate: BioTab, Doryx, Doxy-Caps, Doxycin, Dynacin, Monodox, Novodoxylin, Vibramycin, Vibra-Tabs

🍁 Apo-Doxy

Drug class.: Tetracycline, broad-spectrum antiinfective

Action: Inhibits protein synthesis and phosphorylation in microorganisms by binding to 30S ribosomal subunits, reversibly binding to 50S ribosomal subunits; bacteriostatic

Uses: Syphilis, *C. trachomatis,* gonorrhea, lymphogranuloma venereum, uncommon gram-negative/positive organisms, necrotizing ulcerative gingivostomatitis

Dosage and routes:

• *Adult:* PO 100 mg q12h on day 1, then 100 mg/day; IV 200 mg in 1-2 inf on day 1, then 100-200 mg/day

• *Child >8 yr:* PO/IV 4.4 mg/kg/day in divided doses q12h on day 1, then 2.2-4.4 mg/kg/day

Gonorrhea (uncomplicated)

• *Adult:* PO 200 mg, then 100 mg hs and 100 mg bid × 3 days or 300 mg, then 300 mg in 1 hr

• *Disseminated:* 100 mg PO bid × at least 7 days

Chlamydia trachomatis

• *Adult:* PO 100 mg bid × 7 days

Syphilis

• *Adult:* PO 300 mg/day in divided doses × 10 days

Available forms include: Tabs 50, 100 mg; caps 50, 100 mg; syr 50 mg/ml; powder for inj IV 100, 200 mg; powder for oral susp 25 mg/5 ml

Side effects/adverse reactions:

▼ *ORAL:* Candidiasis, tooth discoloration, tongue discoloration, dry mouth

CNS: Fever

CV: Pericarditis

GI: Nausea, abdominal pain, vomiting, diarrhea, ***hepatotoxicity,*** anorexia, enterocolitis, flatulence, abdominal cramps, gastric burning, pancreatitis

HEMA: ***Depression of plasma prothrombin activity, eosinophilia, neutropenia, thrombocytopenia, hemolytic anemia***

EENT: Dysphagia

INTEG: Rash, urticaria, photosensitivity, increased pigmentation, ***exfoliative dermatitis, angioedema,*** pruritus

Contraindications: Hypersensitivity to tetracyclines, children <8 yr, pregnancy category D

Precautions: Hepatic disease, lactation

Pharmacokinetics:

PO: Peak 1.5-4 hr, half-life 15-22 hr; 25%-93% protein bound; excreted in bile

Drug interactions of concern to dentistry:

• Decreased absorption: $NaHCO_3$, other antacids

• Increased rate of metabolism: barbiturates, carbamazepine, hydantoins

• Decreased effect of penicillins, cephalosporins

• May increase the effectiveness of anticoagulants

When used in dental infections:

• May reduce the effectiveness of birth control pills

DENTAL CONSIDERATIONS

General:

• Determine why the patient is taking tetracycline.

• Broad-spectrum antibiotics may promote oral or vaginal *Candida* infection.

Consultations:

• Medical consult may be required to assess disease control in the patient.

Teach patient/family:

• Can take with milk, food; take with a full glass of water

• To take tetracycline doses 1 hr before or 2 hr after air polishing device (ProphyJet), if used

When used for dental infection, advise patient:

• Taking birth control pill to use additional method of contraception for duration of cycle

• To report sore throat, oral burning sensation, fever, fatigue, any of which could indicate superinfection

• To take at prescribed intervals and complete dosage regimen

• To immediately notify the dentist if signs or symptoms of infection increase

doxycycline hyclate gel

(dox-i-sye'kleen)
Atridox

Drug class.: Tetracycline antiinfective

Action: Inhibits bacterial protein synthesis due to disruption of transfer RNA and messenger RNA
Uses: For adjunctive treatment of chronic adult periodontitis to increase clinical attachment, reduce probing depth, and reduce bleeding on probing
Dosage and routes:
• *Adult:* TOP mix contents of syringes according to detailed instructions, completing 100 cycles; attach blunt cannula to syringe A and fill the pocket; after it becomes firm, the mixture may be packed further into the pocket with a dental instrument
Available forms include: Syringe 50 mg and delivery system syringe (450 mg), blunt cannula; refrigerate
Side effects/adverse reactions:
▼ *ORAL: Gingival discomfort, pain, loss of attachment, toothache, periodontal abscess, exudate, infection, drainage, swelling, thermal tooth sensitivity, extreme mobility, localized allergic reaction*
CNS: Headache
CV: High blood pressure
GI: Diarrhea
GU: PMS
EENT: Skin infection, photosensitivity
MS: Muscle aches, backache
MISC: Common cold
Contraindications: Hypersensitivity
Precautions: Pregnancy category D, children (tooth staining), lactation, photosensitivity, predisposition to candidiasis
Pharmacokinetics: Gingival crevicular fluid levels peak 2 hr, sustained levels up to 18 hr and decline over 7 days; low serum levels not exceeding 0.1 g/ml
Drug interactions of concern to dentistry:
• None specifically identified for this product; unknown whether typical tetracycline interactions occur
DENTAL CONSIDERATIONS
General:
• Advise patient if dental drugs prescribed have a potential for photosensitivity.
• Examine for oral manifestation of opportunistic infection.
• Use additional method of contraception for duration of cycle if taking birth control pills
Teach patient/family:
• To be alert to the possibility of secondary oral infection and the need to see dentist immediately if signs of infection occur
• Caution against oral hygiene procedures in treated areas of mouth for 7 days to avoid dislodging product

dronabinol

(droe-nab'i-nol)
Marinol

Drug class.: Antiemetic; appetite stimulant

Controlled Substance Schedule III, Canada N
Action: Orally active cannabinoid (delta-9-tetrahydrocannabinol) with varying effects in the CNS; exact mechanism unknown, may

be due to inhibition of vomiting control mechanism in medulla oblongata

Uses: Control nausea, vomiting in selected patients receiving emetogenic cancer chemotherapy; stimulate appetite in AIDS-associated anorexia

Dosage and routes:

Chemotherapy prophylaxis for emesis

• *Adult:* PO 5 mg/m^2 1-3 hr before chemotherapy, then q2-4h for total of 6 doses per day; dose may be increased by 2.5 mg/m^2 if response is not adequate; do not exceed 15 mg/m^2 per dose

Appetite stimulant

• *Adult:* PO initially 2.5 mg bid, before lunch and supper, or 2.5 mg single dose in PM or hs; max dose 20 mg/day; 5 mg doses may be given if tolerated

Available forms include: Gelcaps 2.5, 5, 10 mg

Side effects/adverse reactions:

▼ *ORAL:* Dry mouth

CNS: Dizziness, drowsiness, poor concentration, ataxia, confusion, paranoid reactions, unsteadiness, restlessness, sleep disturbances, psychotomimetic effects

CV: Palpitation, tachycardia, flushing, orthostatic hypotension

GI: Nausea, vomiting, abdominal pain, diarrhea

EENT: Blurred vision, changes in vision

MS: Asthenia, myalgia

MISC: Abstinence syndrome (hot flashes, sweating, rhinorrhea, loose stools, hiccups, anorexia)

Contraindications: Hypersensitivity: marijuana, sesame oil

Precautions: Pregnancy category C, lactation, children, elderly; cardiac disorders, drug abuse, alcoholism, hypertension, manic or depressive state, schizophrenia

Pharmacokinetics:

PO: 90%-95% absorbed after single dose, only 10%-20% reaches systemic circulation due to first-pass hepatic metabolism and high lipid solubility; protein binding (97%); half-life alpha 4 hr; effects 4-24 hr; fecal elimination

Drug interactions of concern to dentistry:

• Increased CNS depression: alcohol, CNS depressants

• Additive hypertension, tachycardia, possible cardiotoxicity: amphetamines, other sympathomimetics

• Additive tachycardia, drowsiness: atropine, scopolamine, antihistamines, anticholinergic drugs

DENTAL CONSIDERATIONS

General:

• Monitor vital signs every appointment due to cardiovascular side effects.

• After supine positioning, have patient sit upright for at least 2 min to avoid orthostatic hypotension.

• Patients taking opioids for acute or chronic pain should be given alternative analgesics for dental pain.

• Assess salivary flow as a factor in caries, periodontal disease, and candidiasis.

• Consider semisupine chair position for patient comfort if GI side effects occur.

Teach patient/family:

When chronic dry mouth occurs, advise patient:

• To avoid mouth rinses with high alcohol content due to drying effects

• To use daily home fluoride products for anticaries effect
• To use sugarless gum, frequent sips of water, or saliva substitutes

dyclonine hydrochloride

(dye'kloe-neen)
Dyclone

Drug class.: Topically acting local anesthetic (ketone)

Action: Inhibits nerve impulses from sensory nerves, which produces local anesthesia; nerve impulses are blocked as a result of decreased nerve membrane permeability to sodium influx

Uses: Topical anesthesia of mucous membranes of mouth, pharynx, larynx, trachea, esophagus, and urethra before a variety of procedures; 0.5% solution may be used to block the gag reflex to relieve the pain of oral ulcers or stomatitis secondary to antineoplastic chemotherapy or radiation

Dosage and routes:
• *Adult:* TOP individualized dose depending on disease or patient need; use lowest effective dose; max recommended dose is 30 ml of a 1% solution (300 mg); usual dosage range is 4-20 ml; reduced dosage is recommended for elderly and pediatric patients

Available forms include: Topical solution 0.5%, 1.0% in 30 ml bottles

(NOTE: Astra no longer makes this product.)

Side effects/adverse reactions:
INTEG: Allergic reactions (urticaria, edema, contact dermatitis)
MISC: ***Anaphylaxis***

More severe systemic reactions can be observed if excessive absorption leads to toxic doses

Contraindications: Hypersensitivity

Precautions: Do not inject or apply to nasal or conjunctival mucous membranes, pregnancy category C, lactation, children <12 yr

Pharmacokinetics:
TOP: Rapid onset and relatively short duration of action

DENTAL CONSIDERATIONS
General:
• Low incidence of side effects following topical application.
• Expectorate excess solution when used topically.
• Limit area of application, especially in inflamed or denuded areas.
• Dry mucous membranes in area of application before applying solution.
• Symptoms of systemic toxicity include nervousness, nausea, excitement followed by drowsiness, convulsions, and cardiac and respiratory depression.
• Symptoms may vary because they depend on the amount of drug actually absorbed.

Teach patient/family
• To prevent injury while numbness is present
• To avoid chewing gum or eating after dental treatment

dyphylline

(dye'fi-lin)
Dilor, Dilor-400, Lufyllin, Lufyllin-400

Drug class.: Xanthine derivative

Action: Relaxes smooth muscle of respiratory system by blocking phosphodiesterase, which increases intracellular AMP

Uses: Bronchial asthma, bronchospasm in chronic bronchitis, COPD, emphysema

Dosage and routes:

- *Adult:* PO 200-800 mg q6h; IM 250-500 mg q6h injected slowly
- *Child >6 yr:* PO 4-7 mg/kg/day in 4 divided doses

Available forms include: Tabs 200, 400 mg; elix 100, 160 mg/15 ml; inj IM 250 mg/ml

Side effects/adverse reactions:

▼ *ORAL:* Bitter taste

CNS: Anxiety, restlessness, insomnia, dizziness, ***convulsions,*** headache, light-headedness, muscle twitching

CV: Palpitation, sinus tachycardia, hypotension, flushing, dysrhythmias

GI: Nausea, vomiting, anorexia, dyspepsia, epigastric pain

RESP: Tachypnea

INTEG: Flushing, urticaria

MISC: ***Albuminuria,*** fever, dehydration, hyperglycemia

Contraindications: Hypersensitivity to xanthines, tachydysrhythmias

Precautions: Elderly, CHF, cor pulmonale, hepatic disease, active peptic ulcer disease, diabetes mellitus, hyperthyroidism, hypertension, children, renal disease, pregnancy category C, glaucoma

Pharmacokinetics:

PO: Peak 1 hr, half-life 2 hr; excreted in urine unchanged

Drug interactions of concern to dentistry:

- Increased action: erythromycin, ciprofloxacin
- Increased risk of cardiac dysrhythmia: halothane-inhalation anesthesia, CNS stimulants
- Decreased effect: barbiturates, carbamazepine, ketoconazole
- May decrease sedative effects of benzodiazepines

DENTAL CONSIDERATIONS

General:

- Monitor vital signs every appointment due to cardiovascular and respiratory side effects.
- Consider semisupine chair position for patients with respiratory disease.

econazole nitrate (topical)

(e-kone'a-zole)

Ecostatin, Spectazole

Drug class.: Local antifungal

Action: Interferes with fungal cell membrane, which increases permeability, leaking of cell nutrients

Uses: Tinea pedis, tinea cruris, tinea corporis, tinea versicolor, cutaneous candidiasis

Dosage and routes:

- *Adult and child:* TOP apply to affected area bid-qid depending on condition

Available forms include: Cream 1%

Side effects/adverse reactions:

INTEG: Rash, urticaria, stinging, burning, pruritus

Contraindications: Hypersensitivity

Precautions: Pregnancy category C, lactation

DENTAL CONSIDERATIONS

- None

efavirenz

(ef-a-vir'enz)

Sustiva

Drug class.: Antiviral (nonnucleoside)

Action: Acts as a reverse transcriptase inhibitor in HIV-1

Uses: For use in HIV-1 infection only in combination with another antiviral agent for HIV-1 infection that the patient has not previously taken

Dosage and routes:

• *Adult:* PO 600 mg qd in combination with a protease inhibitor or nucleoside reverse transcriptase inhibitor or both; avoid high-fat meals with dosing

• *Child 3 yr or older weighing 10-40 kg:*

PO:

Weight (kg)	Dose (daily)
10-<15	200 mg
15-<20	250 mg
20-<25	300 mg
25-<32.5	350 mg
32.5-<40	400 mg

Available forms include: Caps 50, 100, 200 mg

Side effects/adverse reactions:

▼ *ORAL:* Dry mouth, altered taste

CNS: Dizziness, somnolence, insomnia, abnormal dreams, confusion, abnormal thinking, impaired concentration, amnesia, agitation, depersonalization, hallucinations, euphoria

CV: Flushing, palpitation, tachycardia, thrombophlebitis

GI: Nausea, vomiting, diarrhea

RESP: Cough, asthma

EENT: Tinnitus, blurred vision

INTEG: Rash, eczema, urticaria

META: Elevation of AST and ALT enzymes

MS: Arthralgia, myalgia

MISC: Fever, fatigue, alcohol intolerance

Contraindications: Hypersensitivity: concurrent use with astemizole, cisapride, midazolam triazolam, or ergot derivatives

Precautions: Must not be used as a single agent for HIV, avoid pregnancy with use, pregnancy category C, lactation, mental illness, substance abuse, caution with alcohol or psychotropic drugs, driving or other hazardous tasks, monitor cholesterol, hepatic impairment

Pharmacokinetics:

PO: Peak plasma levels 5 hr, avoid high-fat meals, hepatic metabolism by cytochrome P-450 enzymes, excreted in both urine and feces; high plasma protein binding (99%)

Drug interactions of concern to dentistry:

• Contraindicated drugs: astemizole, midazolam, triazolam

• Decreased plasma levels of clarithromycin

• Potential for increased levels with ketoconazole, itraconazole (no studies)

• Increased risk of CNS side effects with CNS depressants

DENTAL CONSIDERATIONS

General:

• Examine for oral manifestation of opportunistic infection.

• Monitor vital signs every appointment due to cardiovascular and respiratory side effects

• Consider semisupine chair position for patient comfort due to GI side effects of drug

• Assess salivary flow as a factor in caries, periodontal disease, and candidiasis

• Short appointments and a stress reduction protocol may be required for anxious patients

Consultations:

• Medical consult may be required to assess disease control in the patient

Teach patient/family:
• To prevent trauma when using oral hygiene aids
• Importance of good oral hygiene to prevent soft tissue inflammation
• To be alert for the possibility of secondary oral infection and to see dentist immediately if signs of infection occur
When chronic dry mouth occurs, advise patient:
• To avoid mouth rinses with high alcohol content due to drying effects
• To use daily home fluoride products for anticaries effect
• To use sugarless gum, frequent sips of water, or saliva substitutes

emedastine difumarate (optic)

(em-e-das'teen)
Emadine

Drug class.: Ophthalmic antihistamine

Action: Selective H_1-antagonist
Uses: Temporary relief of signs and symptoms of allergic conjunctivitis
Dosage and routes:
• *Adult:* Ophth 1 gtt in affected eye up to 4 times daily
Available forms include: Ophth sol 0.05% in 5 ml
Side effects/adverse reactions:
▼ *ORAL:* Bad taste
CNS: Headache, abnormal dreams
EENT: Blurred vision, burning, stinging, corneal staining, dry eyes, rhinitis, sinusitis, tearing
INTEG: Dermatitis, pruritus
MS: Asthenia
Contraindications: Hypersensitivity
Precautions: Avoid wearing contact lens if eye is red, wait at least 10 min after application to insert contact lens, pregnancy category B, lactation, no data for use in children <3yr
Pharmacokinetics:
TOP: Systemic absorption below level for assay; any absorbed drug is metabolized and excreted in urine
Drug interactions of concern to dentistry:
• None reported
DENTAL CONSIDERATIONS
General:
• Protect patient's eyes from accidental spatter during dental treatment.

enalapril maleate

(e-nal'a-pril)
Vasotec, Vasotec IV

Drug class.: Angiotensin-converting enzyme (ACE) inhibitor

Action: Selectively suppresses renin-angiotensin-aldosterone system; inhibits ACE; prevents conversion of angiotensin I to angiotensin II, leading to dilation of arterial and venous vessels
Uses: Hypertension, heart failure adjunct
Dosage and routes:
• *Adult:* PO 5 mg/day; may increase or decrease to desired response range 10-40 mg/day; lower initial dose with a diuretic
Hypertension
• *Adult:* IV 1.25 mg q6h over 5 min
Patients on diuretics
• *Adult:* IV 0.625 over 5 min; may give additional doses of 1.25 mg q6h

Renal impairment

• *Adult:* 1.25 mg q6h with CrCl <3 mg/dl or 0.625 mg if CrCl >3 mg/dl

Available forms include: Tabs 2.5, 5, 10, 20 mg; inj 1.25 mg/ml

Side effects/adverse reactions:

▼ *ORAL:* Loss of taste, oral ulceration (Stevens-Johnson syndrome, rare), dry mouth, angioedema (lips, tongue, mucous membranes), lichenoid drug reaction

CNS: Insomnia, dizziness, paresthesia, headache, fatigue, anxiety

CV: Hypotension, chest pain, tachycardia, dysrhythmias

GI: Nausea, vomiting, colitis, cramps, diarrhea, constipation, pancreatitis, flatulence

RESP: Dyspnea, cough, rales, angioedema

HEMA: ***Agranulocytosis, neutropenia***

GU: ***Proteinuria, renal failure,*** increased frequency of polyurea or oliguria

INTEG: Rash, purpura, alopecia

META: Hyperkalemia

Contraindications: Pregnancy category D; can cause serious reactions in second and third trimester; lactation

Precautions: Renal disease, hyperkalemia

Pharmacokinetics:

PO: Peak 1 hr, half-life 11 hr; metabolized by liver to active metabolite; excreted in urine

IV: Onset 5-15 min, peak up to 4 hr

Drug interactions of concern to dentistry:

• Increased hypotension: alcohol, phenothiazines

• Decreased hypotensive effects: indomethacin and possibly other NSAIDs, sympathomimetics

DENTAL CONSIDERATIONS

General:

• Monitor vital signs every appointment due to cardiovascular side effects.

• After supine positioning, have patient sit upright for at least 2 min before standing to avoid orthostatic hypotension.

• Patients on chronic drug therapy may rarely have symptoms of blood dyscrasias, which can include infection, bleeding, and poor healing.

• Assess salivary flow as a factor in caries, periodontal disease, and candidiasis.

• Limit use of sodium-containing products such as saline IV fluids for those patients with a dietary salt restriction.

• Use vasoconstrictors with caution, in low doses, and with careful aspiration.

• Stress from dental procedures may compromise cardiovascular function; determine patient risk.

• Short appointments and a stress reduction protocol may be required for anxious patients.

Consultations:

• Medical consult may be required to assess patient's ability to tolerate stress.

• In a patient with symptoms of blood dyscrasias, request a medical consult for blood studies and postpone dental treatment until normal values are reestablished.

• Take precautions if dental surgery is anticipated and sedation or general anesthesia is required; risk of hypotensive episode.

Teach patient/family:

• Importance of good oral hygiene to prevent soft tissue inflammation

When chronic dry mouth occurs, advise patient:
• To avoid mouth rinses with high alcohol content due to drying effects
• To use daily home fluoride products for anticaries effect
• To use sugarless gum, frequent sips of water, or saliva substitutes

---

enoxacin

(en-ox'a-sin)
Penetrex

Drug class.: Fluoroquinolone anti-infective

Action: A broad-spectrum bactericidal agent that inhibits the enzyme DNA gyrase needed for the replication of bacterial DNA

Uses: Uncomplicated urethral or cervical gonorrhea, uncomplicated and complicated UTIs

Dosage and routes:

Gonorrhea
• *Adult:* PO 400 mg as a single dose

Uncomplicated UTI
• *Adult:* PO 200 mg bid × 7 days

Complicated UTI
• *Adult:* PO 400 mg bid × 14 days

Available forms include: Tabs 200, 400 mg

Side effects/adverse reactions:

▼ *ORAL:* Candidiasis, dry mouth, unusual taste

CNS: Dizziness, headache, fatigue, somnolence, depression, insomnia

GI: Diarrhea, *nausea, vomiting,* anorexia, flatulence, heartburn, increased AST/ALT, ***pseudomembraneous colitis***

EENT: Visual disturbances, phototoxicity

INTEG: Rash

MS: Tendinitis

Contraindications: Hypersensitivity to quinolones

Precautions: Pregnancy category C, lactation, children, elderly, renal disease, seizure disorders

Pharmacokinetics:

PO: Peak 1-3 hr, steady state 2 days, half-life 3-6 hr; excreted in urine as unchanged drug, metabolites

Drug interactions of concern to dentistry:
• Decreased absorption of enoxacin: sodium bicarbonate
• Increased action of caffeine, cyclosporine

DENTAL CONSIDERATIONS

General:
• Due to drug interaction, do not use ingestible sodium bicarbonate products, such as the air polishing system (Prophy Jet), unless 2 hr have passed since enoxacin was taken.
• Assess salivary flow as a factor in caries, periodontal disease, and candidiasis.
• Use caution in prescribing caffeine-containing analgesics.
• Avoid dental light in patient's eyes; offer dark glasses for patient comfort.
• Determine why the patient is taking the drug.

Consultations:
• Consult with patient's physician if an acute dental infection occurs and another antiinfective is required.

Teach patient/family:
• Importance of good oral hygiene to prevent gingival inflammation
• To discontinue treatment and inform dentist immediately if patient experiences pain or inflammation of a tendon, and to rest and refrain from exercise

When chronic dry mouth occurs, advise patient:

- To avoid mouth rinses with high alcohol content due to drying effects
- To use daily home fluoride products for anticaries effect
- To use sugarless gum, frequent sips of water, or artificial saliva substitutes

enoxaparin sodium

(ee-nox-a-pa'rin)

Lovenox

Drug class.: Heparin-type anticoagulant

Action: Low-molecular-weight heparin having antithrombotic actions with higher anti-Factor X_a activity compared with anti-Factor II_a

Uses: Prevention and treatment of deep vein thrombosis following hip or knee replacement surgery; also used in abdominal and gynecologic surgery; (with aspirin) prevention of ischemic complications of unstable angina and non–Q-wave MI; in combination with warfarin for deep vein thrombosis with or without pulmonary embolism

Dosage and routes:

- *Adult:* SC 30 mg bid with first dose given 12-24 hr after surgery; or SC 40 mg qd with first dose given 2 hr before surgery

Available forms include: Prefilled syringes 30 mg/0.3ml, 40 mg/0.4 ml

Side effects/adverse reactions:

CNS: Confusion

GI: Nausea

HEMA: Bleeding after surgery, ***thromocytopenia,*** hemorrhage, anemia

INTEG: Edema, hematoma, erythema

MISC: Local pain, irritation, fever

Contraindications: Hypersensitivity, active major bleeding, thrombocytopenia, IM administration

Precautions: Hemorrhage, thrombocytopenia, renal impairment, elderly, pregnancy category B, lactation, children, requires monitoring, GI bleeding

Pharmacokinetics:

SC INJ ONLY: Maximum anti-Factor X_a and antithrombin effect 3-5 hr, activity lasts up to 12 hr; renal excretion

Drug interactions of concern to dentistry:

- Avoid concurrent use of aspirin, NSAIDs, dipyridamole, sulfinpyrazone

DENTAL CONSIDERATIONS

General:

- Determine why patient is taking the drug.
- Product may be used in outpatient therapy. Delay elective dental treatment until patient completes enoxaparin therapy.
- Consider local hemostasis measures to prevent excessive bleeding if dental treatment must be performed.
- Avoid products that affect platelet function, such as aspirin and NSAIDs.
- Antibiotic prophylaxis before dental treatment may be required for joint prosthesis. See 1997 ADA guidelines.

Consultations:

- Medical consult should include routine blood counts, including platelet counts and bleeding time.

Teach patient/family:

- Importance of good oral hygiene to prevent soft tissue inflammation

• Caution to prevent trauma when using oral hygiene aids
• To report oral lesions, soreness, or bleeding to dentist

entacapone

(en-tak'a-pone)
Comtan
Drug class.: Antiparkinsonian

Action: Inhibits catechol-O-methyltransferase (COMT), decreases peripheral conversion of levodopa to 3-O-methyldopa
Uses: Adjunct to levodopa/carbidopa in the treatment of Parkinson's disease, not used alone
Dosage and routes:
• *Adult:* PO 200 mg with each levodopa/carbidopa dose not to exceed 8 times daily; adjust dose down as symptoms improve
Available forms include: Tabs 200 mg
Side effects/adverse reactions:
▼ *ORAL:* Taste alteration, dry mouth (1%)
CNS: Dyskinesia, hyperkinesia, psychiatric reactions, hallucinations, aggravation of Parkinson's symptoms, hypokinesia, dizziness, anxiety
CV: Orthostatic hypotension, syncope
GI: Nausea, diarrhea, abdominal pain
RESP: Dyspnea
HEMA: Purpura
GU: Discolored urine (brown-orange)
INTEG: Sweating
META: May decrease serum iron levels
MS: ***Rhabdomyolysis,*** back pain, fatigue
Contraindications: Hypersensitivity, nonselective MAO inhibitors
Precautions: Enhanced orthostatic hypotension with levodopa/carbidopa, hepatic impairment, caution in driving, pregnancy category C, lactation, children
Pharmacokinetics:
PO: Rapid absorption, bioavailability 35%, highly plasma protein bound (98%), hepatic metabolism, metabolites excreted mostly (90%) in feces
Drug interactions of concern to dentistry:
• Increased heart rate, arrhythmias, hypertension: with epinephrine, norepinephrine, levonordefrin, or other sympathomimetics metabolized by COMT

DENTAL CONSIDERATIONS

General:
• Monitor vital signs every appointment due to cardiovascular side effects.
• Short appointments and a stress reduction protocol may be required for anxious patients.
• Consider semisupine chair position for patient comfort if GI side effects occur.
• Use vasoconstrictor with caution, in low doses and with careful aspiration. Avoid using gingival retraction cord containing epinephrine.
• Assess for presence of extrapyramidal motor symptoms, such as tardive dyskinesia and akathisia. Extrapyramidal motor activity may complicate dental treatment.
• After supine positioning, have patient sit upright for at least 2 min to avoid orthostatic hypotension.
• Assess salivary flow as a factor in caries, periodontal disease, and candidiasis.

Consultations:
• Medical consult may be required to assess disease control and patient's ability to tolerate stress.
Teach patient/family:
• Use of electric toothbrush if patient has difficulty holding conventional devices
• Importance of updating health and drug history if physician makes any changes in evaluation/ drug regimens
When chronic dry mouth occurs, advise patient:
To avoid mouth rinses with high alcohol content due to drying effects
To use daily home fluoride products for anticaries effect
To use sugarless gum, frequent sips of water, or saliva substitutes

---

ephedrine sulfate
(e-fed'rin)
generic
Drug class.: Adrenergic, mixed direct and indirect effects

Action: Causes increased contractility and heart rate by acting on β-receptors in the heart; also acts on α-receptors, causing vasoconstriction in blood vessels
Uses: Shock, increased perfusion, hypotension, bronchodilation
Dosage and routes:
• *Adult:* IM/SC 25-50 mg, not to exceed 150 mg/24 hr; IV 10-25 mg, not to exceed 150 mg/24 hr
• *Child:* SC/IV 3 mg/kg/day in divided doses q4-6h
Bronchodilation
• *Adult:* PO 12.5-50 mg bid-qid, not to exceed 400 mg/day
• *Child:* PO 2-3 mg/kg/day in 4-6 divided doses
Available forms include: Inj IM/ SC/IV 25, 50 mg/ml; caps 25, 50 mg; syr 11, 20 mg/5 ml
Side effects/adverse reactions:
▼ *ORAL:* Dry mouth
CNS: Tremors, anxiety, ***convulsions, CNS depression,*** insomnia, headache, dizziness, confusion, hallucinations
CV: ***Dysrhythmias,*** palpitation, tachycardia, hypertension, chest pain
GI: Anorexia, nausea, vomiting
GU: Dysuria, urinary retention
Contraindications: Hypersensitivity to sympathomimetics, narrow-angle glaucoma
Precautions: Pregnancy category C, cardiac disorders, hyperthyroidism, diabetes mellitus, prostatic hypertrophy
Pharmacokinetics:
PO: Onset 15-60 min, duration 2-4 hr
IV: Onset 5 min, duration 2 hr
Metabolized in liver; excreted in urine (unchanged); crosses blood-brain barrier, placenta, excreted in breast milk
Drug interactions of concern to dentistry:
• Decreased pressor effect: haloperidol, phenothiazines, thioxanthenes
• Dysrhythmia: halogenated general anesthetics
DENTAL CONSIDERATIONS
General:
• Monitor vital signs every appointment due to cardiovascular side effects.
• Assess salivary flow as a factor in caries, periodontal disease, and candidiasis.
• Consider semisupine chair position for patients with respiratory disease.

• Consider short appointments and a stress reduction protocol for anxious patients.

Consultations:

• Medical consult may be required to assess disease control and patient's tolerance for stress.

Teach patient/family:

When chronic dry mouth occurs, advise patient:

• To avoid mouth rinses with high alcohol content due to drying effects

• To use daily home fluoride products for anticaries effect

• To use sugarless gum, frequent sips of water, or saliva substitutes

---

epinephrine/ epinephrine bitartrate/ epinephrine HCl

(ep-i-nef'rin)

Epinephrine HCl inj: Adrenalin Chloride, EpiPen Jr., EpiPen Auto-Injector, Sus-Phrine Suspension

Epinephrine HCl inh: Adrenalin, Bronkaid Mist, Primatine Mist

♣ Bronkaid Mistometer

Epinephrine bitartrate inh: AsthmaHaler, Bronitin Mist, Medihalder-Epi, Primatene Mist Suspension

Racemic epinephrine: Asthma Nefrin, Dey-Dos Racepinephrine, Vaponefrin

Epinephrine HCl ophthalmic: Epiferin, Glaucon

Epinephrine borate ophthalmic: Epinal, Eppy/N

Drug class.: Adrenergic agonist, catecholamine

Action: β_1- and β_2-agonist, causing increased levels of cAMP and producing bronchodilation and cardiac stimulation; large doses cause vasoconstriction; small doses can cause vasodilation via β_2-vascular receptors

Uses: Acute asthmatic attacks, hemostasis, bronchospasm, anaphylaxis, allergic reactions, cardiac arrest, vasopressor

Dosage and routes:

• *Adult:* IM/SC 0.1-0.5 ml of 1:1000 sol, may repeat q10-15min; IV 0.1-0.25 ml of 1:1000 sol

• *Child:* SC 0.01 ml of 1:1000/kg, may repeat q20min to q4h; INH 0.005 ml/kg of 1:200 solution, may repeat q8-12h

Asthma

• *Adult and child:* INH 1-2 puffs of 1:100 or 2.25% racemic q15min

Hemostasis

• *Adult:* TOP 1:50,000-1:1000 applied as needed to stop bleeding

Cardiac arrest

• *Adult:* IC/IV endotracheal 0.1-1 mg, repeat q5min prn

• *Child:* IC/IV endotracheal 5-10 μg q5min, may use 0.1 μg/kg/min IV inf after initial dose

Available forms include: Aerosol 0.16, 0.2, 0.25 mg/spray; inj IM/IV/SC 1:1000 (1 mg/ml), 1:200 (5 mg/ml), 0.01 mg/ml (1:100,000), 0.1 mg/ml (1:10,000), 0.5 mg/ml (1:2,000); sol for nebuliz 1:100, 1.25% 2.25% (base)

Side effects/adverse reactions:

CNS: Tremors, anxiety, ***cerebral hemorrhage,*** insomnia, headache, dizziness, confusion, hallucinations

CV: ***Dysrhythmias,*** palpitations, tachycardia, hypertension, increased T wave

GI: Anorexia, nausea, vomiting

RESP: Dyspnea

GU: Urinary retention

Contraindications: Hypersensitivity to sympathomimetics, narrow-angle glaucoma

Precautions: Pregnancy category C, cardiac disorders, hyperthyroidism, diabetes mellitus, prostatic hypertrophy

Pharmacokinetics:

SC: Onset 3-5 min, duration 20 min

PO/INH: Onset 1 min

Drug interactions of concern to dentistry:

• Hypotension, tachycardia: haloperidol, loxapine, phenothiazines, thioxanthenes

• Ventricular dysrhythmia: hydrocarbon-inhalation anesthetics, CNS stimulants, tricyclic antidepressants

• With larger doses of epinephrine risk of hypertension followed by bradycardia with β-adrenergic antagonists

DENTAL CONSIDERATIONS

General:

• Monitor vital signs every appointment due to cardiovascular side effects.

• Assess salivary flow as a factor in caries, periodontal disease, and candidiasis.

• Consider semisupine chair position for patients with respiratory disease.

• Acute asthmatic episodes may be precipitated in the dental office. Sympathomimetic inhalants should be available for emergency use; a stress reduction protocol may be required.

---

eprosartan

(ep-roe-sar′tan)

Teveten

Drug class.: Antihypertensive, angiotensin II receptor (AT_1) antagonist

---

Note: Although approved in 1997, its marketing was delayed until 1999

Action: A selective antagonist for angiotensin II receptor sites (AT_1); antagonizes the vasoconstrictor and aldosterone secreting effects of angiotensin

Uses: Hypertension as a single drug or in combination with other antihypertensive drugs; may also be used in congestive heart failure or chronic renal failure

Dosage and route:

• *Adult:* PO 600-800 mg qd has been reported

Available forms include: Unknown

Side effects/adverse reactions: Information was not available. However, side effects reported with other angiotensin receptor antagonists have included taste alterations, insomnia, dizziness, a low incidence of palpitation, peripheral edema, hypotension, cough, and urinary frequency. The relationship of these side effects to this drug is unknown.

Contraindications: Hypersensitivity

Precautions: This group of drugs has a general warning about their use during the second and third trimesters of pregnancy

Pharmacokinetics: Not metabolized by cytochrome P-450 isoenzyme system

Drug interactions of concern to dentistry: Unknown, but ketoconazole may inhibit the metabolism of other similar drugs

DENTAL CONSIDERATIONS:

General:

• Monitor vital signs every appointment due to cardiovascular side effects.

• Stress from dental procedures may compromise cardiovascular function; determine patient risk.
• Limit use of sodium-containing products such as saline IV fluids for those patients with a dietary salt restriction.
• Short appointments and a stress reduction protocol may be required for anxious patients.
• Use precaution if sedation or general anesthesia is required; risk of hypotensive episode.

Consultations:
• Medical consult may be required to assess disease control and patient's ability to tolerate stress.

Teach patient/family:
• Importance of updating health and drug history if physician makes any changes in evaluation/drug regimens

ergoloid mesylate

(er'goe-loid mess'i-late)

Gerimal, Hydergine, Hydergine LC

Drug class.: Ergot alkaloids

Action: May increase cerebral metabolism and blood flow

Uses: Senile dementia, Alzheimer's dementia, multiinfarct dementia, primary progressive dementia

Dosage and routes:
• *Adult:* PO/SL 1 mg tid; may increase to 4.5-12 mg/day

Available forms include: Tabs SL 0.5, 1 mg; tabs 0.5, 1 mg; caps 1 mg; liq 1 mg/ml

Side effects/adverse reactions:
▼ *ORAL:* Sublingual irritation (SL tablet)
CNS: Dizziness, syncope, headache, anorexia
CV: Bradycardia, orthostatic hypotension
GI: Nausea, vomiting
EENT: Blurred vision, nasal stuffiness
INTEG: Skin rash, flushing

Contraindications: Hypersensitivity to ergot preparations; psychosis

Precautions: Acute intermittent porphyria, pregnancy category C

Pharmacokinetics:
PO: Peak 1 hr, half-life 3.5 hr; metabolized in liver; excreted as metabolites in feces; crosses blood-brain barrier

DENTAL CONSIDERATIONS

General:
• Monitor vital signs every appointment due to cardiovascular side effects.
• After supine positioning, have patient sit upright for at least 2 min before standing to avoid orthostatic hypotension.
• Consider semisupine chair position for patient comfort due to GI effects of drug.

Teach patient/family:
• Use of electric toothbrush if patient is unable to carry out oral hygiene procedures

ergotamine tartrate

(er-got'a-meen)

Ergomar, Ergostat, Medihaler-Ergotamine
♣ Gynergen

Drug class.: α-adrenergic blocker

Action: By a direct action, constricts vascular smooth muscle in peripheral and cranial blood vessels; relaxes uterine muscle

Uses: Vascular headache (migraine or histamine), cluster headache
Dosage and routes:
• *Adult:* 2 mg, then 1-2 mg qh or q0.5h for SL, not to exceed 6 mg/day or 10 mg/wk; inh 1 puff, may repeat in 5 min, not to exceed 6 per 24 hr
Available forms include: SL tabs 2 mg; tabs 1 mg; oral inh 360 μg/dose
Side effects/adverse reactions:
CNS: Numbness in fingers/toes, headache, weakness, visual changes
CV: Transient tachycardia, chest pain, bradycardia, edema, claudication, increase or decrease in BP
GI: Nausea, vomiting
MS: Muscle pain
Contraindications: Hypersensitivity to ergot preparations, occlusion (peripheral, vascular), CAD, hepatic disease, renal disease, peptic ulcer, hypertension, pregnancy category X
Precautions: Lactation, children, anemia
Pharmacokinetics:
PO: Peak 30 min-3 hr; metabolized in liver; excreted as metabolites in feces; crosses blood-brain barrier; excreted in breast milk
Drug interactions of concern to dentistry:
• Increased vasoconstriction: vasoconstrictor in local anesthetics
• Suspected increased risk of ergotism: erythromycin, clarithromycin, troleandomycin
• Use anticholinergic with caution in the elderly
DENTAL CONSIDERATIONS
General:
• Monitor vital signs every appointment due to cardiovascular side effects.
Teach patient/family:
• Use of electric toothbrush if patient has difficulty holding conventional devices

erythromycin (ophthalmic)

(er-ith-roe-mye'sin)
Ilotycin Ophthalmic
Drug class.: Antiinfective

Action: Inhibits bacterial protein synthesis
Uses: Infection of external eye, prophylaxis of neonatal conjunctivitis and ophthalmia neonatorium
Dosage and routes:
• *Adult and child:* Oint apply qd-qid as needed
Ophthalmia neonatorum
• *Neonates:* Apply oint to conjunctival sacs immediately after delivery
Available forms include: Oint 0.5%
Side effects/adverse reactions:
EENT: Poor corneal wound healing, temporary visual haze, irritation, overgrowth of nonsusceptible organisms, irritation
Contraindications: Hypersensitivity
Precautions: Antibiotic hypersensitivity, pregnancy category B, lactation
DENTAL CONSIDERATIONS
General:
• Avoid dental light in patient's eyes; offer dark glasses for patient comfort.
• Protect patient's eyes from accidental spatter during dental treatment.

erythromycin (topical)

(er-ith-roe-mye'sin)

Akne-mycin, A/T/S, Benzamycin, Del-Mycin, Erycette, Erygel, Erymax, Ery-sol, Erythra-Derm, Romyin, Staticin, Theramycin-Z, T-Stat

Drug class.: Macrolide antibacterial (topical)

Action: Interferes with bacterial protein synthesis to inhibit bacterial growth

Uses: Acne vulgaris

Dosage and routes:

• *Adult and child >12 yr:* Top apply to affected area bid

Available forms include: Top sol 1.5%, 2%; oint 2%; gel 2%; benzoyl peroxide in gel 30 mg/g

Side effects/adverse reactions:

INTEG: Rash, urticaria, stinging, burning, pruritus, dry/scaly/oily skin

EENT: Eye irritation, tenderness

Contraindications: Hypersensitivity

Precautions: Pregnancy category C, lactation

DENTAL CONSIDERATIONS

• None indicated

erythromycin base/ erythromycin estolate/ erythromycin ethylsuccinate/ erythromycin gluceptate/ erythromycin lactobionate/ erythromycin stearate

(er-ith-roe-mye'sin)

Erythromycin base: E-Base, E-Mycin, Eryc, Ery-Tab, Erythromycin Filmtabs, Ilotycin, PCE Dispertab

♣ Apo-Erythro, Apo-Erythro-EC, Erybid, Erythromid, Novo-Rythro EnCap

♣ *Erythromycin estolate:* Novo-Erythro

Erythromycin stearate: Erythrocin Stearate, Erythrocot, My-E, Wintrocin

♣ Apo-Erythro-S

Erythromycin ethylsuccinate: EES 400, EES 200, EES Granules, EryPed, Erythro

♣ Apo-Erythro-ES, Novo-Rythro

Erythromycin lactobionate inj: Erythrocin

Erythromycin glucepate inj: Ilotycin

Drug class.: Macrolide antibiotic

Action: Binds to 50S ribosomal subunits of susceptible bacteria and suppresses protein synthesis

Uses: Infections caused by *N. gonorrhoeae;* mild-to-moderate respiratory tract, skin, soft tissue infections caused by *S. pneumoniae, M. pneumoniae, C. diphtheriae, B. pertussis, L. monocytogenes, S. pyogenes;* syphilis; legionnaire's disease; *C. trachomatis; H. influenzae;* endocarditis prophylaxis

Dosage and routes:
Soft tissue infections
• *Adult:* PO 250-500 mg q6h (base, estolate, stearate); PO 400-800 mg q6h (ethylsuccinate); IV inf 15-20 mg/kg/day (lactobionate)
• *Child:* PO 30-50 mg/kg/day in divided doses q6h (salts); IV 15-20 mg/kg/day in divided doses q4-6h (lactobionate)

Available forms include: Base: enteric-coated tabs 250, 333, 500 mg; film-coated tabs 250, 500 mg; estolate: tabs 250, 500 mg; caps 250 mg; susp 125, 250 mg/5 ml; stearate: film-coated tabs 250, 500 mg; ethylsuccinate: chew tabs 200 mg; 100 mg/2.5 ml, 200, 400 mg/5 ml; susp 200, 400 mg powder for susp 100 mg/2.5 ml; 200 and 400 mg/5 ml powder for inj; 500 mg and 1 g (lactobionate)

Side effects/adverse reactions:
▼ *ORAL:* Candidiasis, lichenoid reaction
GI: Nausea, vomiting, diarrhea, ***hepatotoxicity,*** abdominal pain, heartburn, anorexia, pruritus ani, pseudomembranous colitis
GU: Vaginitis, moniliasis
EENT: Hearing loss, tinnitus
INTEG: Rash, urticaria, pruritus, thrombophlebitis (IV site), hypersensitivity

Contraindications: Hypersensitivity, erythromycin estolate in preexisting hepatic disease, cisipride, sparfloxacin, pimozide

Precautions: Pregnancy category B, hepatic disease, lactation

Pharmacokinetics:
PO: Peak 4 hr, duration 6 hr, half-life 1-3 hr; metabolized in liver; excreted in bile, feces

Drug interactions of concern to dentistry:
• Increased duration of alfentanil, cyclosporine
• Increased serum levels: indinavir, digoxin
• Decreased action of clindamycin, penicillins, lincomycin, oral contraceptives
• Increased serum levels of alfentanil, carbamazepine, theophylline (and other methylxanthines) and felodipine (possibly with other calcium blockers in the dihydropyridine class), ergotamine, oral anticoagulants
• Risk of rhabdomyolysis: HMG-CoA reductase inhibitors
• Contraindicated with cisapride
• May increase the effects of certain benzodiazepines: alprazolam, diazepam, midazolam, and triazolam

DENTAL CONSIDERATIONS

General:
• Alternate drug of choice for mild infection due to a susceptible organism in patients who are allergic to penicillin.
• Determine why the patient is taking the drug.
• Estolate salt form not indicated for adults due to risk of cholestatic jaundice.

Teach patient/family:
• To take oral drug with full glass of water; take with food if GI symptoms occur (estolate, ethylsuccinate, and coated tabs only)

When used for dental infection, advise patient:
• Taking birth control pill to use additional method of contraception for duration of cycle
• To report sore throat, oral burning

sensation, fever, fatigue, any of which could indicate superinfection
• To take at prescribed intervals and complete dosage regimen
• To immediately notify the dentist if signs or symptoms of infection increase

estazolam

(es-ta'zoe-lam)

ProSom

Drug class.: Benzodiazepine, sedative-hypnotic

Controlled Substance Schedule IV (US)

Action: Produces CNS depression by interacting with a benzodiazepine receptor to facilitate the action of the inhibitory neurotransmitter γ-aminobutyric acid (GABA)

Uses: Insomnia

Dosage and routes:
• *Adult:* PO 1-2 mg hs

Available forms include: Tabs 1, 2 mg

Side effects/adverse reactions:

ORAL: Dry mouth, taste alteration, oral ulceration

CNS: Lethargy, drowsiness, daytime sedation, dizziness, confusion, light-headedness, headache, anxiety, irritability, weakness, tremors, depression, lack of coordination

CV: Chest pain, pulse changes, palpitation, tachycardia

GI: Nausea, vomiting, diarrhea, heartburn, abdominal pain, constipation, anorexia

HEMA: ***Leukopenia, granulocytopenia*** (rare)

INTEG: Dermatitis, allergy, sweating, flushing, pruritus

MISC: Joint pain, congestion

Contraindications: Hypersensitivity to benzodiazepines, pregnancy category X, sleep apnea, ritonavir

Precautions: Hepatic disease, renal disease, suicidal individuals, drug abuse, elderly, psychosis, child <18 yr, lactation, depression, pulmonary insufficiency, narrow-angle glaucoma

Pharmacokinetics:

PO: Onset 15-45 min, peak 1.5-2 hr, duration 7-8 hr; metabolized by liver; excreted by kidneys (inactive/active metabolites); crosses placenta; excreted in breast milk

Drug interactions of concern to dentistry:
• Increased CNS depression: alcohol, all CNS depressants
• Increased serum levels and prolonged effect of benzodiazepines: ketoconazole, itraconazole, fluconazole, and miconazole (systemic), indinavir

DENTAL CONSIDERATIONS

General:
• Psychologic and physical dependence may occur with chronic administration.
• Geriatric patients are more susceptible to drug effects; use lower dose.
• Avoid the use of this drug in a patient with a history of drug abuse or alcoholism.

Teach patient/family:
• To avoid mouth rinses with high alcohol content due to drying effects

esterified estrogens

Estratab, Menest

♣ Neo-Estrone

Drug class.: Synthetic estrogen

Action: Required for the development, maintenance, and adequate function of the female reproductive system by increasing synthesis of DNA, RNA, and selected proteins; decreases the release of gonadotropin-releasing hormone; inhibits ovulation and helps maintain bone structure

Uses: Menopause, breast cancer, prostatic cancer, hypogonadism, ovariectomy, primary ovarian failure, osteoporosis prevention

Dosage and routes:

Menopause

• *Adult:* PO 0.30-3.75 mg qd 3 wk on, 1 wk off

Hypogonadism/ovariectomy/ovarian failure

• *Adult:* PO 2.5 mg qd-tid 3 wk on, 1 wk off

Prostatic cancer

• *Adult:* PO 1.25-2.50 mg tid

Breast cancer

• *Adult:* PO 10 mg tid × 3 mo or longer

Available forms include: Tabs 0.3, 0.625, 1.25, 2.5 mg

Side effects/adverse reactions:

▼ *ORAL:* Exacerbates gingivitis, bleeding

CNS: Dizziness, headache, migraines, depression

CV: ***Thromboembolism, stroke, pulmonary embolism, MI,*** hypertension, thrombophlebitis, edema

GI: Nausea, **cholestatic jaundice,** vomiting, diarrhea, anorexia, pancreatitis, cramps, constipation, increased appetite, increased weight

GU: Gynecomastia, testicular atrophy, impotence, amenorrhea, cervical erosion, breakthrough bleeding, dysmenorrhea, vaginal candidiasis, breast changes

EENT: Contact lens intolerance, increased myopia, astigmatism

INTEG: Rash, urticaria, acne, hirsutism, alopecia, oily skin, seborrhea, purpura, melasma

META: Folic acid deficiency, hypercalcemia, hyperglycemia

Contraindications: Breast cancer, thromboembolic disorders, reproductive cancer, vaginal bleeding (abnormal, undiagnosed), pregnancy category X

Precautions: Hypertension, asthma, blood dyscrasias, gallbladder disease, CHF, diabetes mellitus, bone disease, depression, migraine headache, convulsive disorders, hepatic disease, renal disease, family history of cancer of breast or reproductive tract

Pharmacokinetics:

PO: Degraded in liver, excreted in urine, crosses placenta, excreted in breast milk

Drug interactions of concern to dentistry:

• Increased action of corticosteroids

DENTAL CONSIDERATIONS

General:

• Place on frequent recall to evaluate gingival condition.

• Monitor vital signs every appointment due to cardiovascular side effects.

Teach patient/family:

• Importance of good oral hygiene to prevent gingival inflammation

estradiol/estradiol cypionate/estradiol valerate

(es-tra-dye'ole)

Depo-Estradiol, Depogen, Dura Estrin, E-Cypronate, Estrace, Estragyn LA, Estro-Cyp, Estrofem, Gynogen, Valergen

🍁 Dioval, Estroject-LA/Delestrogen, Femogex

Drug class.: Estrogen

Action: Required for the development, maintenance, and adequate function of the female reproductive system by increasing synthesis of DNA, RNA, and selected proteins; decreases the release of gonadotropin-releasing hormone; inhibits ovulation and helps maintain bone structure

Uses: Menopause, breast cancer, prostatic cancer, atrophic vaginitis, kraurosis vulvae, hypogonadism, ovariectomy, primary ovarian failure, prevention of osteoporosis and menopause-related vasomotor symptoms

Dosage and routes:

Menopause/hypogonadism/ovariectomy/ovarian failure

• *Adult:* PO 1-2 mg qd 3 wk on, 1 wk off or 5 days on, 2 days off; IM 0.2-1 mg qwk

Prostatic cancer

• *Adult:* IM 30 mg q1-2wk (valerate); PO 1-2 mg tid (oral estradiol)

Breast cancer

• *Adult:* PO 10 mg tid × 3 mo or longer

Atropic vaginitis

• *Adult:* Vag cream 2-4 g qd × 1-2 wk, then 1 g 1-3× weekly

Kraurosis valvae

• *Adult:* IM 1-1.5 mg 1-2× weekly

Available forms include: Estradiol—tabs 1, 2 mg; top 0.025, 0.05, 0.1 mg; cypionate—inj IM 1, 5 mg/ml; valerate—inj IM 10, 20, 40 mg/ml

Side effects/adverse reactions:

▼ *ORAL:* Exacerbates gingivitis, bleeding

CNS: Dizziness, headache, migraines, depression

CV: ***Thromboembolism, stroke, pulmonary embolism, MI,*** hypertension, thrombophlebitis, edema

GI: Nausea, ***cholestatic jaundice,*** vomiting, diarrhea, anorexia, pancreatitis, cramps, constipation, increased appetite, increased weight

GU: Gynecomastia, testicular atrophy, impotence, amenorrhea, cervical erosion, breakthrough bleeding, dysmenorrhea, vaginal candidiasis, breast changes

EENT: Contact lens intolerance, increased myopia, astigmatism

INTEG: Rash, urticaria, acne, hirsutism, alopecia, oily skin, seborrhea, purpura, melasma

META: Folic acid deficiency, hypercalcemia, hyperglycemia

Contraindications: Breast cancer, thromboembolic disorders, reproductive cancer, vaginal bleeding (abnormal, undiagnosed), pregnancy category X

Precautions: Hypertension, asthma, blood dyscrasias, gallbladder disease, CHF, diabetes mellitus, bone disease, depression, migraine headache, convulsive disorders, hepatic disease, renal disease, family history of cancer of breast or reproductive tract

Pharmacokinetics:

PO: Well absorbed; moderate-to-high protein binding; hepatic metabolism with primary renal excretion

Drug interactions of concern to dentistry:

- Increased action of corticosteroids

DENTAL CONSIDERATIONS

General:

- Place on frequent recall to evaluate gingival condition.
- Monitor vital signs due to cardiovascular side effects.

Teach patient/family:

- Importance of good oral hygiene to prevent gingival inflammation

---

estradiol transdermal system

(es-tra-dye'ole)

Alora, Climara, Esclim, Estraderm, FemPatch, Vivelle-Dot

Vivelle

Drug class.: Estrogen

Action: Required for the development, maintenance, and adequate function of the female reproductive system by increasing synthesis of DNA, RNA, and selected proteins; decreases the release of gonadotropin-releasing hormone; inhibits ovulation and helps maintain bone structure

Uses: Menopause, breast cancer, prostatic cancer, abnormal uterine bleeding, hypogonadism, ovariectomy, primary ovarian failure, osteoporosis

Dosage and routes:

Menopause

- *Adult:* 0.05 mg twice weekly; apply patch to skin

Postmenopausal bone loss

- *Adult:* 0.05 mg daily (one patch weekly)

Available forms include: Transdermal system patches with release rates of 0.025, 0.0375, 0.05, 0.075, 0.1 mg/24 hr

Side effects/adverse reactions:

ORAL: Exacerbates gingivitis, bleeding

CNS: Dizziness, headache, migraines, depression

CV: ***Thromboembolism, stroke, pulmonary embolism, MI,*** hypertension, thrombophlebitis, edema

GI: Nausea, ***cholestatic jaundice,*** vomiting, diarrhea, anorexia, pancreatitis, cramps, constipation, increased appetite, increased weight

GU: Gynecomastia, testicular atrophy, impotence, amenorrhea, cervical erosion, breakthrough bleeding, dysmenorrhea, vaginal candidiasis, breast changes

EENT: Contact lens intolerance, increased myopia, astigmatism

INTEG: Rash, urticaria, acne, hirsutism, alopecia, oily skin, seborrhea, purpura, melasma

META: Folic acid deficiency, hypercalcemia, hyperglycemia

Contraindications: Breast cancer, thromboembolic disorders, reproductive cancer, genital bleeding (abnormal, undiagnosed), pregnancy category X

Precautions: Hypertension, asthma, blood dyscrasias, gallbladder disease, CHF, diabetes mellitus, bone disease, depression, migraine headache, convulsive disorders, hepatic disease, renal disease, family history of cancer of the breast or reproductive tract

Pharmacokinetics:

TOP: Absorbed through the skin at a release rate of 0.05 or 1.0 mg/24 hr; hepatic metabolism and renal excretion; serum levels in 4 hr

Drug interactions of concern to dentistry:

- Increased action of corticosteroids

DENTAL CONSIDERATIONS

General:

- Place on frequent recall to evaluate gingival condition.
- Monitor vital signs due to cardiovascular side effects.

Teach patient/family:

- Importance of good oral hygiene to prevent gingival inflammation

estrogenic substances, conjugated

Premarin

✤ CES, Congest, Conjugated Estrogen CDS

Drug class.: Estrogen

Action: Required for the development, maintenance, and adequate function of the female reproductive system by increasing synthesis of DNA, RNA, and selected proteins; decreases the release of gonadotropin-releasing hormone; inhibits ovulation and helps maintain bone structure

Uses: Menopause, breast cancer, prostatic cancer, abnormal uterine bleeding, hypogonadism, ovariectomy, primary ovarian failure, osteoporosis

Dosage and routes:

Menopause

- *Adult:* PO 0.3-1.25 mg qd 3 wk on, 1 wk off

Prostatic cancer

- *Adult:* PO 1.25-2.5 mg tid

Breast cancer

- *Adult:* PO 10 mg tid × 3 mo or longer

Abnormal uterine bleeding

- *Adult:* IV/IM 25 mg, repeat in 6-12 hr

Ovariectomy/primary ovarian failure/osteoporosis

- *Adult:* PO 1.25 mg qd 3 wk on, 1 wk off

Hypogonadism

- *Adult:* PO 2.5 mg bid-tid × 20 days/mo

Available forms include: Tabs 0.3, 0.625, 0.9, 1.25, 2.5 mg

Side effects/adverse reactions:

▼ *ORAL:* Exacerbates gingivitis, bleeding

CNS: Dizziness, headache, migraine, depression

CV: ***Thromboembolism, stroke, pulmonary embolism, MI,*** hypertension, thrombophlebitis, edema

GI: Nausea, ***cholestatic jaundice,*** vomiting, diarrhea, anorexia, pancreatitis, cramps, constipation, increased appetite, increased weight

GU: Gynecomastia, testicular atrophy, impotence, amenorrhea, cervical erosion, breakthrough bleeding, dysmenorrhea, vaginal candidiasis, breast changes

EENT: Contact lens intolerance, increased myopia, astigmatism

INTEG: Rash, urticaria, acne, hirsutism, alopecia, oily skin, seborrhea, purpura, melasma

META: Folic acid deficiency, hypercalcemia, hyperglycemia

Contraindications: Breast cancer, thromboembolic disorders, reproductive cancer, vaginal bleeding (abnormal, undiagnosed), pregnancy category X, lactation

Precautions: Hypertension, asthma, blood dyscrasias, gallbladder disease, CHF, diabetes mellitus, bone disease, depression, migraine headache, convulsive disorders, hepatic disease, renal disease, fam-

ily history of cancer of breast or reproductive tract
Pharmacokinetics:
PO: Well absorbed; moderate-to-high protein binding; hepatic metabolism with primary renal excretion
Drug interactions of concern to dentistry:
• Increased action of corticosteroids
DENTAL CONSIDERATIONS
General:
• Place on frequent recall to evaluate gingival condition.
• Monitor vital signs due to cardiovascular side effects.
Teach patient/family:
• Importance of good oral hygiene to prevent gingival inflammation

estrogens A, conjugated synthetic

(es'troe-jenz)

Cenestin

Drug class.: Estrogens (nine synthetic estrogens expressed as alphabetical A for this combination)

Action: Reacts with estrogenic receptors; responsible for development and maintenance of female reproductive system and secondary sex characteristics, acts to reduce elevated levels of LH and FSH in postmenopausal women
Uses: Control of vasomotor symptoms, such as hot flashes and sweating in menopausal women
Dosage and routes:
• *Adult:* PO initial dose 0.625 mg; doses can be titrated to 1.25 mg; reassess use q3-6mo; discontinue as soon as possible
Available forms include: Tabs 0.625, 0.9 mg
Side effects/adverse reactions:
CNS: Headache
CV: Depression, insomnia, dizziness, nervousness, paresthesia
GI: Abdominal pain, flatulence, nausea, diarrhea
GU: Metrorrhagia, vagal bleeding changes
MS: Back pain, myalgia
MISC: Breast pain
Contraindications: Undiagnosed genital bleeding, breast cancer, estrogen-dependent neoplasm, active thrombophlebitis or thromboembolic disorders; pregnancy
Precautions: Endometrial cancer risk, venous thromboembolism, gallbladder disease, elevated BP, hyperlipoproteinemia, impaired liver function, lactation, pediatric patients, hypercalcemia
Pharmacokinetics:
PO: Well absorbed, maximum plasma levels in 4-16 hr; metabolized in liver, enterohepatic circulation
Drug interactions of concern to dentistry:
• None reported for dental drugs
DENTAL CONSIDERATIONS
General:
• Consider semisupine chair position for patient comfort if GI side effects occur.
Teach patient/family:
• Importance of good oral hygiene to prevent soft tissue inflammation

estropipate

(es'troe-pih-pate)

Ogen, Ortho-Est

Drug class.: Estrogen (piperazine estrone sulfate)

Action: Required for the development, maintenance, and adequate function of the female reproductive system by increasing synthesis of DNA, RNA, and selected proteins; decreases the release of gonadotropin-releasing hormone; inhibits ovulation and helps maintain bone structure

Uses: Vasomotor symptoms of menopause, atrophic vaginitis, primary female hypogonadism, primary ovarian failure, estrogen imbalance, advanced prostatic carcinoma, ovariectomy

Dosage and routes:

Menopause

• *Adult:* 0.625-5 mg daily

Hypogonadism

• *Adult:* 1.25-7.5 mg/day × 3 wk; rest 8-10 days

Available forms include: Tabs 0.625, 1.25, 2.5, 5 mg

Side effects/adverse reactions:

▼ *ORAL:* Exacerbates gingivitis, bleeding

CNS: Dizziness, headache, migraine, depression

CV: ***Thromboembolism, stroke, pulmonary embolism, MI,*** hypertension, thrombophlebitis, edema

GI: Nausea, ***cholestatic jaundice,*** vomiting, diarrhea, anorexia, pancreatitis, cramps, constipation, increased appetite, increased weight

GU: Gynecomastia, testicular atrophy, impotence, amenorrhea, cervical erosion, breakthrough bleeding, dysmenorrhea, vaginal candidiasis, breast changes

EENT: Contact lens intolerance, increased myopia, astigmatism

INTEG: Rash, urticaria, acne, hirsutism, alopecia, oily skin, seborrhea, purpura, melasma

META: Folic acid deficiency, hypercalcemia, hyperglycemia

Contraindications: Breast cancer, thromboembolic disorders, reproductive cancer, vaginal bleeding (abnormal, undiagnosed), pregnancy category X, lactation

Precautions: Hypertension, asthma, blood dyscrasias, gallbladder disease, CHF, diabetes mellitus, bone disease, depression, migraine headache, convulsive disorders, hepatic disease, renal disease, family history of cancer of breast or reproductive tract

Pharmacokinetics:

PO: Well absorbed; moderate-to-high protein binding; hepatic metabolism with primary renal excretion

Drug interactions of concern to dentistry:

• Increased action of corticosteroids

DENTAL CONSIDERATIONS

General:

• Place on frequent recall to evaluate gingival condition.

• Monitor vital signs due to cardiovascular side effects.

Teach patient/family:

• Importance of good oral hygiene to prevent gingival inflammation

---

etanercept

(e-tan′er-cept)

Enbrel

Drug class.: Antinflammatory and immunomodulator; biologic response modifier

Action: This drug consists of the extracellular ligand binding protein of tumor necrosis factor (TNF) receptor linked to the Fc portion of human IgG1 that specifically binds to TNF and blocks its interaction with cell surfaces.

Uses: Reduction in signs and symptoms of moderately to severely active rheumatoid arthritis in patients with an inadequate response to one or more disease-modifying antirheumatic drugs

Dosage and routes:

• *Adult:* SC 25 mg twice weekly; can be given with other drugs used in rheumatoid arthritis treatment

• *Child:* Limited use in children at doses of 0.4 mg/kg (limit 25 mg) 2 × weekly × 3 mo; no official dose listed

Available forms include: 25 mg single-use vial kit

Side effects/adverse reactions:

CNS: Headache, dizziness, asthenia

CV: ***MI, myocardial ischemia, cerebral ischemia*** (all rare but life-threatening reactions)

GI: Abdominal pain, vomiting in children

RESP: Sinusitis, URI, cough, pharyngitis, rhinitis

INTEG: Injection site reactions, rash

MISC: Infections, positive ANA readings, allergic reactions

Contraindications: Hypersensitivity, use of live vaccines

Precautions: Risk of new malignancies and infrequent severe cardiovascular events, discontinue if serious infection occurs, immunosuppression risk, pregnancy category B, lactation, viral infections, children <4 yr

Pharmacokinetics:

SC: Half-life 115 hr, maximum plasma levels 72 hr, no information on metabolism or excretion

Drug interactions of concern to dentistry:

• No studies have been conducted.

DENTAL CONSIDERATIONS

General:

• Monitor vital signs every appointment due to potential cardiovascular side effects

• Consider semisupine chair position for patient comfort due to GI side effects of drug

• If acute oral infection occurs, inform physician.

• Note elevated ANA levels if diagnosing Sjögren's syndrome.

Consultations:

• Consult if needed.

Teach patient/family:

• Importance of good oral hygiene to prevent soft tissue inflammation

• Use of electric toothbrush if patient has difficulty holding conventional devices

ethacrynate sodium/ ethacrynic acid

(eth-a-kri'nate)

Edecrin, Edecrin Sodium

Drug class.: Loop diuretic

Action: Acts on loop of Henle by increasing excretion of chloride, sodium

Uses: Pulmonary edema, edema in CHF, liver disease, nephrotic syndrome, ascites, hypertension

Dosage and routes:

• *Adult:* PO 50-200 mg/day; may give up to 200 mg bid

• *Child:* PO 25 mg, increased by 25 mg/day until desired effect occurs

Pulmonary edema

• *Adult:* IV 50 mg given over several minutes or 0.5-1.0 mg/kg

Available forms include: Tabs 25, 50 mg; powder for inj 50 mg

Side effects/adverse reactions:

▼ *ORAL:* Dry mouth, increased thirst

CNS: Headache, fatigue, weakness, vertigo

CV: ***Circulatory collapse,*** chest

pain, hypotension, ECG changes
GI: ***GI bleeding, severe diarrhea, acute pancreatitis,*** nausea, vomiting, anorexia, cramps, upset stomach, abdominal pain, jaundice
HEMA: ***Thrombocytopenia, agranulocytosis, leukopenia, neutropenia***
GU: Polyuria, renal failure, glycosuria
EENT: ***Loss of hearing,*** ear pain, tinnitus, blurred vision
INTEG: Rash, pruritus, ***Stevens-Johnson syndrome,*** sweating, purpura, photosensitivity
ENDO: Hyperglycemia
MS: Cramps, arthritis, stiffness
ELECT: Hypokalemia, hypochloremic alkalosis, hypomagnesemia, hyperuricemia, hypocalcemia, hyponatremia

Contraindications: Hypersensitivity to sulfonamides, anuria, hypovolemia, lactation, electrolyte depletion, infants; cisapride

Precautions: Dehydration, ascites, severe renal disease, pregnancy category D, hypoproteinemia

Pharmacokinetics:
PO: Onset 0.5 hr, peak 2 hr, duration 6-8 hr
IV: Onset 5 min, peak 15-30 min, duration 2 hr
Half-life 30-70 min, excreted by kidneys, crosses placenta

Drug interactions of concern to dentistry:
- Masked ototoxicity: phenothiazines
- Decreased antihypertensive effect: NSAIDs, especially indomethacin

DENTAL CONSIDERATIONS
General:
- Monitor vital signs every appointment due to cardiovascular side effects.
- Patients on chronic drug therapy may rarely have symptoms of blood dyscrasias, which can include infection, bleeding, and poor healing.
- Assess salivary flow as a factor in caries, periodontal disease, and candidiasis.
- After supine positioning, have patient sit upright for at least 2 min before standing to avoid orthostatic hypotension.
- Patients on high-potency diuretics should be monitored for serum K^+ levels.

Consultations:
- In a patient with symptoms of blood dyscrasias, request a medical consult for blood studies and postpone dental treatment until normal values are reestablished.
- Medical consult may be required to assess disease control in the patient.

Teach patient/family:
- Importance of good oral hygiene to prevent gingival inflammation

When chronic dry mouth occurs, advise patient:
- To avoid mouth rinses with high alcohol content due to drying effects
- To use daily home fluoride products for anticaries effect
- To use sugarless gum, frequent sips of water, or saliva substitutes

ethambutol HCl
(e-tham'byoo-tole)
Myambutol
Etibi
Drug class.: Antitubercular

Action: Inhibits RNA synthesis, decreases tubercle bacilli replication

Uses: Pulmonary TB, as an adjunct

Dosage and routes:

• *Adult and child >13 yr:* PO 15 mg/kg/day as a single dose

Re-treatment

• *Adult and child >13 yr:* PO 25 mg/kg/day as single dose × 2 mo with at least one other drug, then decrease to 15 mg/kg/day as single dose

Available forms include: Tabs 100, 400 mg

Side effects/adverse reactions:

▼ *ORAL:* Lichenoid reaction

CNS: Headache, confusion, fever, malaise, dizziness, disorientation, hallucinations, peripheral neuritis

GI: Abdominal distress, anorexia, nausea, vomiting

EENT: Blurred vision, optic neuritis, photophobia, decreased visual acuity

INTEG: Dermatitis, pruritus

META: Elevated uric acid, acute gout, liver function impairment

MISC: ***Thrombocytopenia,*** joint pain

Contraindications: Hypersensitivity, optic neuritis, child <13 yr

Precautions: Pregnancy category D, renal disease, diabetic retinopathy, cataracts, ocular defects, hepatic disorders, hematopoietic disorders

Pharmacokinetics:

PO: Peak 2-4 hr, half-life 3 hr; metabolized in liver; excreted in urine (unchanged drug/inactive metabolites); excreted unchanged in feces

DENTAL CONSIDERATIONS

General:

• Examine for evidence of oral signs of disease.

• Avoid dental light in patient's eyes; offer dark glasses for patient comfort.

• Determine why the patient is taking the drug.

Consultations:

• Medical consult is required to assess patient's current status; avoid elective dental procedures in active infections.

Determine that noninfectious status exists by ensuring the following:

• Anti-TB drugs have been taken for longer than 3 wk.

• Culture confirms antibiotic susceptibility to TB microorganisms.

• Patient has had 3 consecutive negative sputum smears.

• Patient is not in the coughing stage.

Teach patient/family:

• Importance of taking medication for full length of prescribed therapy to ensure effectiveness of treatment and to prevent the emergence of resistant forms of microbes

E

ethinyl estradiol

(eth'in-il ess-tra-dye'ole)

Estinyl

Drug class.: Nonsteroidal synthetic estrogen

Action: Needed for adequate functioning of female reproductive system; affects release of pituitary gonadotropins; inhibits ovulation; promotes adequate calcium use in bone structures

Uses: Menopause, prostatic cancer, breast cancer, hypogonadism, estrogen deficiency, postmenopausal osteoporosis; unapproved use: postcoital contraceptive

Dosage and routes:

Menopause

• *Adult:* PO 0.02-0.5 mg qd 3wk on, 1 wk off

Prostatic cancer
• *Adult:* PO 0.15-2 mg qd
Hypogonadism
• *Adult:* PO 0.05 mg qd-tid × 2 wk/mo, then 2 wk progesterone, then 3-6 mo cycles, then 2 mo off
Breast cancer
• *Adult:* PO 1 mg tid
Available forms include: Tabs 0.02, 0.05, 0.5 mg
Side effects/adverse reactions:
ORAL: Exacerbates gingivitis, bleeding
CNS: Dizziness, headache, migraine, depression
CV: ***Thromboembolism, stroke, pulmonary embolism, MI,*** hypertension, thrombophlebitis, edema
GI: Nausea, ***cholestatic jaundice,*** vomiting, diarrhea, anorexia, pancreatitis, cramps, constipation, increased appetite, increased weight
GU: Gynecomastia, testicular atrophy, impotence, amenorrhea, cervical erosion, breakthrough bleeding, dysmenorrhea, vaginal candidiasis, breast changes
EENT: Contact lens intolerance, increased myopia, astigmatism
INTEG: Rash, urticaria, acne, hirsutism, alopecia, oily skin, seborrhea, purpura, melasma
META: Folic acid deficiency, hypercalcemia, hyperglycemia
Contraindications: Breast cancer, thromboembolic disorders, reproductive cancer, vaginal bleeding (abnormal, undiagnosed), pregnancy category X
Precautions: Hypertension, asthma, blood dyscrasias, gallbladder disease, CHF, diabetes mellitus, bone disease, depression, migraine headache, convulsive disorders, hepatic disease, renal disease, family history of cancer of the breast or reproductive tract

Pharmacokinetics:
PO: Degraded in liver; excreted in urine; crosses placenta; excreted in breast milk
Drug interactions of concern to dentistry:
• Increased action of corticosteroids

DENTAL CONSIDERATIONS
General:
• Place on frequent recall to evaluate gingival condition.
• Monitor vital signs due to cardiovascular side effects.
Teach patient/family:
• Importance of good oral hygiene to prevent gingival inflammation

ethionamide

(e-thye-on-am′ide)
Trecator-SC
Drug class.: Antitubercular

Action: Bacteriostatic against *M. tuberculosis;* may inhibit protein synthesis
Uses: Pulmonary, extrapulmonary tuberculosis when other antitubercular drugs have failed
Dosage and routes:
• *Adult:* PO 500 mg-1 g qd in divided doses, with another antitubercular drug and pyridoxine
• *Child:* PO 15-20 mg/kg/day in 3-4 doses, not to exceed 1 g
Available forms include: Tabs 250 mg
Side effects/adverse reactions:
ORAL: Metallic taste, stomatitis, salivation
CNS: Anorexia, ***convulsions,*** headache, drowsiness, tremors, depression, psychosis, dizziness, peripheral neuritis
CV: Severe postural hypotension

GI: Anorexia, nausea, vomiting, diarrhea, hepatitis, jaundice, hypoglycemia
HEMA: ***Thrombocytopenia,*** purpura
EENT: Blurred vision, optic neuritis
INTEG: Dermatitis, alopecia, acne
MS: Asthenia
MISC: Gynecomastia, impotence, menorrhagia, difficulty managing diabetes mellitus, hypothyroidism

Contraindications: Hypersensitivity, severe hepatic disease

Precautions: Pregnancy category D, renal disease, diabetic retinopathy, cataracts, ocular defects, child <13 yr

Pharmacokinetics:
PO: Peak 3 hr, duration 9 hr, half-life 3 hr; metabolized in liver; excreted in urine (unchanged drug/inactive); crosses placenta

Drug interactions of concern to dentistry:
• None reported

DENTAL CONSIDERATIONS

General:
• Monitor vital signs every appointment due to cardiovascular side effects.
• After supine positioning, have patient sit upright for at least 2 min before standing to avoid orthostatic hypotension.
• Consider semisupine chair position for patient comfort due to GI effects of disease.
• Evaluate for clotting ability during gingival instrumentation.
• Examine for evidence of oral manifestations of blood dyscrasias (infection, bleeding, poor healing).
• Palliative treatment may be required for oral side effects.
• Examine for evidence of oral signs of disease.

Consultations:
• Medical consult for blood studies (CBC); leukopenic or thrombocytopenic side effects may result in infection, delayed healing, and excessive bleeding. Postpone elective dental treatment until normal values are maintained. Instruct patient to take with meals to decrease GI symptoms.
• Medical consult may be required to assess disease control in the patient and determine infectious nature of disease.

Teach patient/family:
• Importance of good oral hygiene to prevent soft tissue inflammation
• Caution in use of oral hygiene aids to prevent injury

ethopropazine
(eth-oh-pro′pa-zeen)

Parsidol
♣ Parsitan

Drug class.: Anticholinergic, antidyskinetic

Action: Blockade of central acetylcholine receptors

Uses: Parkinson symptoms, extrapyramidal drug reactions

Dosage and routes:
• *Adult:* PO initial 50 mg qd-bid, can increase to 100-400 mg with mild to moderate symptoms or up to 500-600 mg daily for severe symptoms

Available forms include: Tabs 10, 50 mg

Side effects/adverse reactions:
ORAL: Dry mouth, glossitis
CNS: Confusion, anxiety, restlessness, irritability, delusions, hallucinations, headache, sedation, depression, incoherence, dizziness, euphoria, tremors, memory loss

CV: Palpitation, tachycardia, postural hypotension, bradycardia
GI: Constipation, ***paralytic ileus,*** nausea, vomiting, abdominal distress
GU: Hesitancy, retention
EENT: Blurred vision, photophobia, dilated pupils, difficulty swallowing, mydriasis
INTEG: Rash, urticaria, dermatosis
MS: Weakness, cramping
MISC: Increased temperature, flushing, decreased sweating, hyperthermia, heatstroke, numbness of fingers

Contraindications: Hypersensitivity, angle-closure glaucoma, duodenal obstruction, prostatic hypertrophy, myasthenia gravis, and megacolon

Precautions: Pregnancy category C, lactation, pediatrics, elderly

Pharmacokinetics:
PO: Duration of action 4 hr

Drug interactions of concern to dentistry:

- May increase sedative effects: CNS depressants
- May increase anticholinergic responses: anticholinergics

DENTAL CONSIDERATIONS

General:

- Monitor vital signs every appointment due to cardiovascular side effects.
- After supine positioning, have patient sit upright at least 2 min before standing to avoid orthostatic hypotension.
- Assess salivary flow as a factor in caries, periodontal disease, and candidiasis.
- Avoid dental light in patient's eyes; offer dark glasses for patient comfort.

Consultations:

- Medical consult may be required to assess disease control and patient's ability to tolerate stress.

Teach patient/family:

- To use electric toothbrush if patient has difficulty holding conventional devices
- Importance of good oral hygiene to prevent soft tissue inflammation
- Caution about driving or performing other tasks requiring alertness

When chronic dry mouth occurs, advise patient:

- To avoid mouth rinses with high alcohol content due to drying effects
- To use daily home fluoride products for anticaries effect
- To use sugarless gum, frequent sips of water, or saliva substitutes

---

ethosuximide

(eth-oh-sux'i-mide)

Zarontin

Drug class.: Anticonvulsant

Action: Supresses spike and wave formation in absence seizures (petit mal); decreases amplitude, frequency, duration, spread of discharge in minor motor seizures

Uses: Absence seizures (petit mal); unapproved for use in complex partial seizures

Dosage and routes:

- *Adult and child >6 yr:* PO 250 mg bid initially; may increase by 250 mg q4-7d, not to exceed 1.5 g/day
- *Child 3-6 yr:* PO 250 mg/day or 125 mg bid; may increase by 250 mg q4-7d, not to exceed 1.5 g/day

Available forms include: Caps 250 mg; syr 250 mg/5 ml

Side effects/adverse reactions:
▼ *ORAL:* Gingival bleeding, ulcerations (Stevens-Johnson syndrome); swelling of tongue and gingival enlargement (rare)
CNS: Drowsiness, dizziness, fatigue, euphoria, lethargy, anxiety, aggressiveness, irritability, depression, insomnia, headache
GI: Nausea, vomiting, heartburn, anorexia, diarrhea, abdominal pain, cramps, constipation, hiccups, weight loss
HEMA: ***Agranulocytosis, aplastic anemia, thrombocytopenia, leukocytosis, eosinophilia, pancytopenia***
GU: ***Hematuria, renal damage,*** vaginal bleeding
EENT: Myopia
INTEG: ***Stevens-Johnson syndrome,*** urticaria, pruritic erythema, hirsutism
Contraindications: Hypersensitivity to succinimide derivatives, blood dyscrasias
Precautions: Lactation, pregnancy category not established, hepatic disease, renal disease
Pharmacokinetics:
PO: Peak 1-7 hr, steady state 4-7 days, half-life 24-60 hr; metabolized by liver; excreted in urine, bile, feces
Drug interactions of concern to dentistry:
• Enhanced CNS depression: CNS depressants, alcohol
• Decreased effects: phenothiazines, thioxanthenes, barbiturates

DENTAL CONSIDERATIONS
General:
• Patients on chronic drug therapy may rarely have symptoms of blood dyscrasias, which can include infection, bleeding, and poor healing.
• Talk with patient to ascertain seizure frequency and how well seizures are controlled. A stress reduction protocol may be required.
Consultations:
• In a patient with symptoms of blood dyscrasias, request a medical consult for blood studies and postpone dental treatment until normal values are reestablished.
• Medical consult may be required to assess disease control and patient's ability to tolerate stress.
Teach patient/family:
• Importance of good oral hygiene to prevent gingival inflammation
• To avoid mouth rinses with high alcohol content due to drying effects

---

ethotoin

(eth′oh-toyin)
Peganone
Drug class.: Hydantoin derivative anticonvulsant

Action: Inhibits spread of seizure activity in motor cortex
Uses: Generalized tonic-clonic or complex-partial seizures
Dosage and routes:
• *Adult:* PO 250 mg qid initially; may increase over several days to 3 g/day in divided doses
• *Child:* PO 250 mg bid; may increase to 250 mg qid, not to exceed 3 g/day
Available forms include: Tabs 250, 500 mg
Side effects/adverse reactions:
▼ *ORAL:* Gingival overgrowth (rare), gingival bleeding
CNS: Fatigue, insomnia, numbness, fever, headache, dizziness
CV: Chest pain
GI: Nausea, vomiting, diarrhea

HEMA: ***Agranulocytosis, thrombocytopenia, leukopenia, pancytopenia, megaloblastic anemia,*** lymphadenopathy
EENT: Nystagmus, diplopia
INTEG: Rash

Contraindications: Hypersensitivity to hydantoins, blood dyscrasias, hematologic disease, hepatic disease

Precautions: Pregnancy category C, lactation, geriatric patients

Pharmacokinetics:
PO: Half-life 3-9 hr, rapid oral absorption; metabolized by liver; excreted in urine

Drug interactions of concern to dentistry:
• Decreased effects: barbiturates, carbamazepine
• Increased effects: ketoconazole, fluconazole, metronidazole
• Hepatotoxicity: acetaminophen (chronic, high doses only)
• Decreased effects of corticosteroids, doxycycline

DENTAL CONSIDERATIONS

General:
• Patients on chronic drug therapy may rarely have symptoms of blood dyscrasias, which can include infection, bleeding, and poor healing.
• Place on frequent recall to evaluate gingival condition and self-care.
• Short appointments and a stress reduction protocol may be required for anxious patients.
• Determine type of epilepsy, seizure frequency, and quality of seizure control. A stress reduction protocol may be required.
• Consider semisupine chair position for patient comfort if GI side effects occur.

Consultations:
• In a patient with symptoms of blood dyscrasias, request a medical consult for blood studies and postpone dental treatment until normal values are reestablished.
• Medical consult may be required to assess disease control and patient's ability to tolerate stress.

Teach patient/family:
• Importance of good oral hygiene to prevent soft tissue inflammation and minimize gingival overgrowth
• Caution patient to prevent trauma when using oral hygiene aids

etidocaine HCl (local)

(et-ee'doe-kane)
Duranest, Duranest MPF
With vasoconstrictor: Duranest with Epinephrine, Duranest MPF
Drug class.: Amide, local anesthetic

Action: Inhibits ion fluxes across membranes, particularly sodium transport across cell membrane; decreases rise of depolarization phase of action potential; blocks nerve action potential

Uses: Local dental anesthetic, peripheral nerve block, caudal anesthetic, central neural block, vaginal block

Dosage and routes:
Dental injection: infiltration or conduction block
• *Etidocaine 1.5% with epinephrine 1:200,000:* Max dose limit recommended is 5.5 mg/kg, not to exceed 400 mg max dose for healthy patients; doses must be adjusted downward for medically compromised, debilitated, or elderly patients and for each individual patient. The package insert

indicates that 0.5 to 2.5 dental cartridges are usually adequate. **Always use the lowest effective dose, a slow injection technique, and a careful aspiration technique.**

Example calculations illustrating amount of drug administered per dental cartridge

# of cartridges (1.8 ml)	mg of etidocaine (1.5%)	mg (μg) of vasoconstrictor (1:200,000)
1	27 mg	0.009 mg (9 μg)
2	54 mg	0.018 mg (18 μg)
4	108 mg	0.036 mg (36 μg)
6	162 mg	0.054 mg (54 μg)

Maximum dose is cited from the *USP-DI,* ed 16, 1996, US Pharmacopeial Convention, Inc. Doses may differ in other published reference resources.

• Package insert does not list approved doses for pediatric patients

Available forms include: Inj 1%, 1.5%; inj with epinephrine 1:200,000 1%, 1.5%

Side effects/adverse reactions:

▼ *ORAL:* Numbness, tingling, trismus

CNS: ***Convulsions, loss of consciousness,*** drowsiness, disorientation, tremors, shivering, anxiety, restlessness

CV: ***Myocardial depression, cardiac arrest, dysrhythmias,*** bradycardia, hypotension, hypertension, fetal bradycardia

GI: Nausea, vomiting

RESP: ***Status asthmaticus, respiratory arrest, anaphylaxis***

EENT: Blurred vision, tinnitus, pupil constriction

INTEG: Rash, urticaria, allergic reactions, edema, burning, skin discoloration at injection site, tissue necrosis

Contraindications: Hypersensitivity, cross-sensitivity with other amides rare, child <12 yr, elderly, severe liver disease

Precautions: Elderly, severe drug allergies, pregnancy category B, children (risk of injury due to long duration)

Pharmacokinetics:

INJ: Onset 2-8 min, duration 1.5-9 hr; metabolized by liver; excreted in urine (metabolites)

Drug interactions of concern to dentistry:

• CNS depressants: may see increased risk of CNS depression with all CNS depressants, especially in children and when larger doses are used; avoid placing dental cartridges in disinfectant solutions with heavy metals or surface-active agents; after injection, may see release of metal ions into local anesthetic solutions with tissue irritation

• Avoid excessive exposure of dental cartridges to light or heat; hastens deterioration of vasoconstrictor; color change in local anesthetic solution indicates breakdown of vasoconstrictor

• Risk of cardiovascular side effects: rapid intravascular administration of local anesthetic containing vasoconstrictor, either alone or in patients taking tricyclic antidepressants, MAO inhibitors, digitalis drugs, cocaine, phenothiazines, β-blockers, and in the presence of halogenated-hydrocarbon general anesthetics; use small-

est effective vasoconstrictor dose and careful aspiration techniques
• Avoid use of vasoconstrictors in patients with uncontrolled hyperthyroidism, diabetes, angina, or hypertension; refer these patients for medical treatment before elective dental procedures

DENTAL CONSIDERATIONS
General:
• Monitor vital signs every appointment due to cardiovascular side effects.
• Lubricate dry lips before injection or dental treatment as required.

Teach patient/family:
• To use care to prevent injury while numbness exists by not chewing gum or eating after dental anesthesia
• That numbness with this drug is expected to last for a considerable period
• To report any signs of infection, muscle pain, or fever to dentist when feeling returns
• To report any unusual soft tissue reactions

etidronate disodium

(e-ti-droe'nate)
Didronel, Didronel IV

Drug class.: Antihypercalcemic

Action: Decreases bone resorption and new bone development (accretion)

Uses: Paget's disease, heterotopic ossification, hypercalcemia of malignancy

Dosage and routes:
Paget's disease
• *Adult:* PO 5-10 mg/kg/day 2 hr ac with water, not to exceed 20 mg/kg/day, max 6 mo

Heterotropic ossification
• *Adult:* PO 20 mg/kg qd × 2 wk, then 10 mg/kg/day for 10 wk, total 12 wk

Available forms include: Tabs 200, 400 mg; inj 50 mg/ml

Side effects/adverse reactions:
▼ *ORAL:* Altered taste (parenteral administration)
GI: Nausea, diarrhea
MS: Bone pain, hypocalcemia, decreased mineralization of nonaffected bones

Contraindications: Pathologic fractures, children, colitis, severe renal disease with creatinine >5 mg/dl, cardiac failure

Precautions: Pregnancy category C, renal disease, lactation, restricted vitamin D/calcium

Pharmacokinetics: Therapeutic response: 1-3 mo; not metabolized; excreted in urine, feces

DENTAL CONSIDERATIONS
General:
• Be aware of the oral manifestations of Paget's disease (macrognathia, alveolar pain).

Consultations:
• Medical consult may be required to assess disease control in the patient.

etodolac

(e-toe-doe'lack)
Lodine, Lodine XL

Drug class.: Nonsteroidal antiinflammatory

Action: Inhibits prostaglandin synthesis by interfering with cyclooxygenase needed for biosynthesis; possesses analgesic, antiinflammatory, antipyretic properties

Uses: Mild-to-moderate pain, osteoarthritis, rheumatoid arthritis

Dosage and routes:
Osteoarthritis
• *Adult:* PO 800-1200 mg/day in divided doses initially, then adjust dose to 600-1200 mg/day in divided doses; do not exceed 1200 mg/day; patients <60 kg, not to exceed 20 mg/kg; ext rel 400-1200 mg qd
Analgesia
• *Adult:* PO initial dose 400 mg, then 200-400 q6-8h prn for acute pain; do not exceed 1200 mg/day; patients <60 kg, not to exceed 20 mg/kg
Available forms include: Caps 200, 300, 400 mg; ext rel tabs 400, 500, 600 mg
Side effects/adverse reactions:
ORAL: Stomatitis, lichenoid reaction, dry mouth, bitter taste
CNS: Dizziness, headache, drowsiness, fatigue, tremors, confusion, insomnia, anxiety, depression, light-headedness, vertigo
CV: Tachycardia, peripheral edema, fluid retention, palpitation, dysrhythmias, CHF
GI: Nausea, anorexia, ***cholestatic hepatitis, GI bleeding,*** vomiting, diarrhea, jaundice, constipation, flatulence, cramps, peptic ulcer, dyspepsia
RESP: Bronchospasm
HEMA: ***Blood dyscrasias***
GU: ***Nephrotoxicity: dysuria, hematuria, oliguria, azotemia,*** cystitis, UTI
EENT: Tinnitus, hearing loss, blurred vision
INTEG: Erythema, urticaria, purpura, rash, pruritus, sweating, angioedema
Contraindications: Hypersensitivity; patients in whom aspirin, iodides, or other nonsteroidal antiinflammatories have produced asthma, rhinitis, urticaria, nasal polyps, angioedema, bronchospasm
Precautions: Pregnancy category C, lactation, children, bleeding disorders, GI disorders, cardiac disorders, elderly, renal, hepatic disorders
Pharmacokinetics:
PO: Onset 30 min, peak 1-2 hr, half-life 7 hr; serum protein binding >90%; metabolized by liver (metabolites excreted in urine)
Drug interactions of concern to dentistry:
• GI ulceration, bleeding: aspirin, alcohol, corticosteroids
• Decreased action: salicylates
• Nephrotoxicity: acetaminophen (prolonged use)
• Possible risk of decreased renal function: cyclosporine
When prescribed for dental pain:
• Risk of increased effects: oral anticoagulants, oral antidiabetics, lithium, methotrexate
• Decreased effects of diuretics

DENTAL CONSIDERATIONS
General:
• Patients on chronic drug therapy may rarely have symptoms of blood dyscrasias, which can include infection, bleeding, and poor healing.
• Assess salivary flow as a factor in caries, periodontal disease, and candidiasis.
• Avoid prescribing for dental use in last trimester of pregnancy.
• Avoid prescribing aspirin-containing products.
• Consider semisupine chair position for patients with arthritic disease.
Consultations:
• In a patient with symptoms of blood dyscrasias, request a medical

consult for blood studies and postpone dental treatment until normal values are reestablished.

• Medical consult may be required to assess disease control in the patient.

Teach patient/family:

• To avoid mouth rinses with high alcohol content due to drying effects

famciclovir

(fam-sye'kloe-veer)

Famvir

Drug class.: Antiviral

Action: Converted to active metabolite, penciclovir triphosphate, which inhibits DNA viral synthesis and replication

Uses: Acute herpes zoster (shingles) infection; recurrent genital herpes; recurrent herpes simplex virus infections in HIV-infected patients

Dosage and routes:

Shingles

• *Adult:* PO 500 mg tid × 7 days, start soon after symptoms appear; reduce doses in renal impairment

Recurrent genital herpes

• *Adult:* PO 125 mg bid/5 days; initiate therapy at first sign or symptom

Available forms include: Tabs 125, 250, 500 mg

Side effects/adverse reactions:

CNS: Headache, fatigue, dizziness, paresthesia

GI: Nausea, diarrhea, vomiting

EENT: Sinusitis, pharyngitis

INTEG: Pruritus

MS: Arthralgia, back pain

MISC: Fever

Contraindications: Hypersensitivity

Precautions: Pregnancy category B, children <18 yr, lactation, elderly, hepatic and renal function impairment

Pharmacokinetics:

PO: Peak plasma levels less than 1 hr; after PO absorption, converted to penciclovir; low plasma protein binding (20%-25%); renal excretion

Drug interactions of concern to dentistry:

• None reported in otherwise uncompromised patients

DENTAL CONSIDERATIONS

General:

• Determine why the patient is taking the drug.

• Consider semisupine chair position for patient comfort due to GI effects of drug.

• Awareness of general discomfort associated with shingles; acute symptoms may preclude patient's routine dental visit or mandate short appointments.

Consultations:

• Medical consult may be required to assess patient's ability to tolerate stress.

• Medical consult may be required to assess disease control in the patient.

famotidine

(fa-moe'te-deen)

Pepcid, Pepcid IV, Pepcid RPD

♣ Acid Control, Apo-Famotidine, Dysep HB, Gen-Famotidine, Nu-Famotidine, Ulcidine-HB

Over-the-counter agents: Pepcid AC Acid Controller, Mylanta-AR

Drug class.: H_2 histamine receptor antagonist

Action: Inhibits histamine at H_2-receptor site in parietal cells, which inhibits gastric acid secretion

Uses: Short-term treatment of active duodenal ulcer, maintenance therapy for duodenal ulcer, Zollinger-Ellison syndrome, multiple endocrine adenomas, gastric ulcers

Dosage and routes:

Duodenal ulcer

• *Adult:* PO 40 mg qd hs × 4-8 wk, then 20 mg qd hs if needed (maintenance); IV 20 mg q12h if unable to take PO

Hypersecretory conditions

• *Adult:* PO 20 mg q6h, may give 160 mg q6h if needed; IV 20 mg q12h if unable to take PO

Gastric distress (OTC):

• *Adult and child >12 yr:* PO prophylaxis 10 mg 15 min ac; treatment 10 mg once or twice daily (limit 20 mg/day)

Available forms include: Tabs 10 mg (OTC) and 20, 40 mg; powder for oral susp 40 mg/5 ml; oral disintegrating tab, inj IV 10 mg/ml; tabs chewable 10 mg

Side effects/adverse reactions:

▼ *ORAL: Dry mouth,* taste changes

CNS: Headache, dizziness, paresthesia, seizure, depression, anxiety, somnolence, insomnia, fever

GI: Constipation, nausea, vomiting, anorexia, cramps, abnormal liver enzymes

RESP: ***Bronchospasm***

HEMA: ***Thrombocytopenia***

EENT: Tinnitus, orbital edema

INTEG: Rash

MS: Myalgia, arthralgia

Contraindications: Hypersensitivity

Precautions: Pregnancy category B, lactation, children, severe renal disease, severe hepatic function, elderly

Pharmacokinetics:

PO: Peak 1-3 hr, half-life 2.5-3.5 hr; plasma protein binding 15%-20%; metabolized in liver (active metabolites); excreted by kidneys

Drug interactions of concern to dentistry:

• Decreased absorption of ketoconazole or itraconazole (take doses 2 hr apart)

DENTAL CONSIDERATIONS

General:

• Avoid prescribing aspirin-containing products in patients with active GI disease.

• Consider semisupine chair position for patient comfort due to GI effects of disease.

• Assess salivary flow as a factor in caries, periodontal disease, and candidiasis.

Teach patient/family:

• Importance of good oral hygiene to prevent gingival inflammation

When chronic dry mouth occurs, advise patient:

• To avoid mouth rinses with high alcohol content due to drying effects

• To use daily home fluoride products for anticaries effect

F

To use sugarless gum, frequent sips of water, or saliva substitutes

felbamate

(fel'ba-mate)

Felbatol

Drug class.: Anticonvulsant (carbamate derivative)

Action: Anticonvulsant action is unclear

Uses: Used alone or as adjunct therapy in partial seizures; also for partial seizures associated with Lennox-Gastaut syndrome in children

Dosage and routes:

• *Adult and child >14 yr:* PO (used alone) 1200 mg/day in 3 or 4 divided doses; increase dose by 600 mg increments q2wk; 3600 mg/day usual dose

• *Child 2-14 yr:* PO with Lennox-Gastaut syndrome (adjunctive) 15 mg/kg/day in 3-4 divided doses; reduce dose of other anticonvulsant drugs by 20%; increase dose by 15 mg/kg/day up to 45 mg/kg/day while further reducing the dose of other anticonvulsant drugs

Adjunctive therapy: PO reduce doses of other anticonvulsants by one third; then 1200 mg/day in 3 or 4 divided doses with 1200 mg increments to 3600 mg; doses of other anticonvulsants must be further reduced

Available forms include: Tabs 400, 600 mg; susp 600 mg/5 ml in 240, 960 ml sizes

Side effects/adverse reactions:

▼ *ORAL: Facial edema,* buccal mucous membrane swelling (rare), dry mouth

CNS: Insomnia, headache, somnolence, dizziness, ataxia, fatigue, anorexia, abnormal gait

CV: Palpitation, tachycardia

GI: Vomiting, diarrhea, nausea, constipation, dyspepsia

RESP: Dyspnea, upper respiratory infection, rhinitis

HEMA: ***Aplastic anemia,*** lymphadenopathy, leukopenia, thrombocytopenia, agranulocytosis, granulocytopenia

GU: UTI, incontinence (children)

EENT: Blurred vision

INTEG: Acne, rash, pruritus, photosensitivity reaction

MS: Tremor, abnormal gait

Contraindications: Hypersensitivity

Precautions: Pregnancy category C, lactation

Pharmacokinetics:

PO: Peak plasma levels 1-3 hr; 20%-25% protein bound; up to 40% excreted in urine unchanged

Drug interactions of concern to dentistry:

• Decreased effects of carbamazepine

DENTAL CONSIDERATIONS

General:

• Examine for evidence of oral manifestations of blood dyscrasia (infection, bleeding, poor healing).

• Short appointments and a stress reduction protocol may be required for anxious patients.

• Determine type of epilepsy, seizure frequency, and quality of seizure control. A stress reduction protocol may be required.

• Assess salivary flow as a factor in caries, periodontal disease, and candidiasis.

• Monitor vital signs every appointment due to cardiovascular side effects.

Consultations:
• Medical consult may be required to assess disease control in the patient.
• Medical consult may be required to assess patient's ability to tolerate stress.

Teach patient/family:
• Importance of good oral hygiene to prevent soft tissue inflammation
• Caution to prevent injury when using oral hygiene aids
• Use of electric toothbrush if patient has difficulty holding conventional devices

When chronic dry mouth occurs, advise patient:
• To avoid mouth rinses with high alcohol content due to drying effects
• To use daily home fluoride products for anticaries effect
• To use sugarless gum, frequent sips of water, or saliva substitutes

---

felodipine

(fel-loe'di-peen)
Plendil
✦ Renedil

Drug class.: Calcium channel blocker

Action: Inhibits calcium ion influx across cell membrane during cardiac depolarization; produces relaxation of coronary vascular smooth muscle, dilates coronary arteries, decreases SA/AV node conduction, dilates peripheral arteries

Uses: Essential hypertension, alone or with other antihypertensives, chronic angina pectoris

Dosage and routes:
• *Adult:* PO 5 mg qd initially, usual range 5-10 mg qd; do not exceed 20 mg qd; do not adjust dosage at intervals of <2 wk

Available forms include: Ext rel tabs 2.5, 5, 10 mg

Side effects/adverse reactions:
▼ *ORAL:* Gingival enlargement, dry mouth
CNS: Headache, fatigue, drowsiness, dizziness, anxiety, depression, nervousness, insomnia, lightheadedness, paresthesia, tinnitus, psychosis, somnolence
CV: ***MI, pulmonary edema,*** dysrhythmia, edema, CHF, hypotension, palpitation, tachycardia, syncope, AV block, angina
GI: Nausea, vomiting, diarrhea, gastric upset, constipation, increased liver function studies
HEMA: Anemia
GU: Nocturia, polyuria
INTEG: Rash, pruritus
MISC: Flushing, sexual difficulties, cough, nasal congestion, shortness of breath, wheezing, epistaxis, respiratory infection, chest pain

Contraindications: Hypersensitivity, sick sinus syndrome, second- or third-degree heart block

Precautions: CHF, hypotension <90 mm Hg systolic, hepatic injury, pregnancy category C, lactation, children, renal disease, elderly

Pharmacokinetics:
PO: Peak plasma levels 2.5-5 hr, elimination half-life 11-16 hr; highly protein bound; >99% metabolized in liver; 0.5% excreted unchanged in urine

Drug interactions of concern to dentistry:
• Decreased effect: indomethacin, possibly other NSAIDs, phenobarbital
• Increased effect: parenteral and

inhalational general anesthetics or other drugs with hypotensive actions
• Increased effects of nondepolarizing muscle relaxants
• Increased effects of carbamazepine
• Increased plasma levels of itraconazole

DENTAL CONSIDERATIONS

General:

• Monitor cardiac status; take vital signs at each appointment because of CV side effects. Consider a stress reduction protocol to prevent stress-induced angina during the dental appointment.
• After supine positioning, have patient sit upright for at least 2 min before standing to avoid orthostatic hypotension at dismissal.
• Place on frequent recall to monitor gingival condition.
• Limit use of sodium-containing products such as saline IV fluids for patients with a dietary salt restriction.
• Assess salivary flow as a factor in caries, periodontal disease, and candidiasis.
• Use vasoconstrictors with caution, in low doses, and with careful aspiration. Avoid use of gingival retraction cord with epinephrine.

Consultations:

• Medical consult may be required to assess disease control in the patient.

Teach patient/family:

• Importance of good oral hygiene to prevent gingival inflammation and minimize hyperplasia
• Need for frequent oral prophylaxis if hyperplasia occurs

When chronic dry mouth occurs, advise patient:

• To avoid mouth rinses with high alcohol content due to drying effects
• To use daily home fluoride products for anticaries effect
• To use sugarless gum, frequent sips of water, or saliva substitutes

---

fenofibrate (micronized)

(fen-o-fye'brate)

TriCor

Drug class.: Antihyperlipidemic

Action: Inhibits biosynthesis of triglyceride synthesis, reducing VLDL, and stimulates the catabolism of triglyceride-rich lipoprotein (ULDL); reduces serum uric acid levels

Uses: Hyperlipidemia, types IV and V, as an adjunct to diet therapy

Dosage and routes:

• *Adult:* PO initial dose 67 mg daily in conjunction with triglyceride-lowering diet; max dose 67 mg tid
• *Elderly:* Keep dose at 67 mg daily

Available forms include: Caps 67 mg

Side effects/adverse reactions:

CNS: Headache, dizziness, paresthesia, insomnia, increased appetite

CV: Arrhythmia

GI: Dyspepsia, flatulence, nausea, vomiting, abdominal pain, constipation, diarrhea, pancreatitis

RESP: Flulike syndrome, cough

HEMA: ***Thrombocytopenia, agranulocytosis*** (very rare)

GU: Decreased libido, polyuria, vaginitis

EENT: Rhinitis, sinusitis, earache, blurred vision, photosensitivity

INTEG: Pruritus, rash

MS: Asthenia, myositis, rhabdomyolysis (rare)
MISC: Fatigue, localized pain, hypersensitivity
Contraindications: Hypersensitivity, hepatic or severe renal dysfunction, primary biliary cirrhosis, preexisting gallbladder disease
Precautions: Monitor liver function; may lead to cholelithiasis; can be associated with myositis, myopathy, or rhabdomyolysis; pregnancy category C, avoid if lactating; safe use in children unknown; discontinue use if no response in 2 mo; increased anticoagulant effect with oral anticoagulants
Pharmacokinetics:
PO: Well absorbed, increased absorption with food, peak plasma levels 6-8 hr, highly plasma protein bound (99%), hepatic metabolism, active metabolite, excreted largely in urine (60%)
Drug interactions of concern to dentistry:
• No dental drug interactions reported
DENTAL CONSIDERATIONS
General:
• Monitor vital signs every appointment due to cardiovascular and respiratory side effects.
• Consider semisupine chair position for patient comfort due to GI side effects of drug.
• Patients on chronic drug therapy may rarely have symptoms of blood dyscrasias, which can include infection, bleeding, and poor healing.
• Avoid dental light in patient's eyes; offer dark glasses for patient comfort.
Consultations:
• In a patient with symptoms of blood dyscrasias, request a medical consult for blood studies and postpone treatment until normal values are reestablished.
Teach patient/family:
• Use of electric toothbrush if patient has difficulty holding conventional devices
• To prevent trauma when using oral hygiene aids

F

fenoprofen calcium

(fen-oh-proe'fen)
Nalfon, Nalfon 200
Drug class.: Nonsteroidal antiinflammatory, propionic acid derivative

Action: Inhibits prostaglandin synthesis by interfering with cyclooxygenase needed for biosynthesis; possesses analgesic, antiinflammatory, antipyretic properties
Uses: Mild-to-moderate pain, osteoarthritis, rheumatoid arthritis, acute gout, arthritis, ankylosing spondylitis, nonrheumatic inflammation, dysmenorrhea
Dosage and routes:
Pain (mild to moderate)
• *Adult:* PO 200 mg q4-6h as needed
Arthritis
• *Adult:* PO 300-600 mg qid, not to exceed 3.2 g/day
Available forms include: Caps 200, 300 mg; tabs 600 mg
Side effects/adverse reactions:
▼ *ORAL:* Dry mouth, bleeding, stomatitis, lichenoid reaction
CNS: Dizziness, headache, drowsiness, fatigue, tremors, confusion, insomnia, anxiety, depression
CV: Tachycardia, peripheral edema, palpitation, dysrhythmias
GI: ***Cholestatic hepatitis,*** nausea, anorexia, vomiting, diarrhea, jaun-

dice, constipation, flatulence, cramps, peptic ulcer

HEMA: ***Blood dyscrasias,*** increased bleeding time

GU: ***Nephrotoxicity: dysuria, hematuria, oliguria, azotemia***

EENT: Tinnitus, hearing loss, blurred vision

INTEG: Purpura, rash, pruritus, sweating

Contraindications: Hypersensitivity, asthma, severe renal disease, severe hepatic disease

Precautions: Pregnancy category not established (use not recommended); lactation, children, bleeding disorders, GI disorders, cardiac disorders, hypersensitivity to other antiinflammatory agents

Pharmacokinetics:

PO: Peak 2 hr, half-life 3-3.5 hr; 99% plasma protein binding; metabolized in liver; excreted in urine (metabolites), breast milk

Drug interactions of concern to dentistry:

• GI bleeding, ulceration: salicylates, alcohol, corticosteroids, other NSAIDs

• May decrease effects of fenoprofen: phenobarbital

• Nephrotoxicity: acetaminophen (prolonged use)

• Possible risk of decreased renal function: cyclosporine

DENTAL CONSIDERATIONS

General:

• Assess salivary flow as a factor in caries, periodontal disease, and candidiasis.

• Avoid prescribing for dental use in pregnancy.

• Possibility of cross-allergenicity when patient is allergic to aspirin.

Consultations:

• Medical consult may be required to assess disease control in the patient.

Teach patient/family:

• Importance of good oral hygiene to prevent gingival inflammation

• Caution to prevent injury when using oral hygiene aids

When chronic dry mouth occurs, advise patient:

• To avoid mouth rinses with high alcohol content due to drying effects

• To use daily home fluoride products for anticaries effect

• To use sugarless gum, frequent sips of water, or saliva substitutes

fentanyl transdermal system

(fen'ta-nil)

Duragesic 25, 50, 75, 100 Transdermal Patches

Oral transmucosal fentanyl citrate: Actiq (lozenges)

Drug class.: Narcotic analgesics

Controlled Substance Schedule II, Canada N

Action: Interacts with opioid receptors in the CNS to alter pain perception

Uses: Management of chronic pain when opioids are necessary; transmucosal form: only for management of breakthrough cancer pain in patients with malignancies who are using or tolerant to opioids

Dosage and routes:

Chronic pain

• *Adult only:* One patch every 72 hr; dose depends on need for pain control; titrate as required

Transmucosal form:

• *Adult only:* Dose must be titrated starting with lowest dose size

(must be kept secure from children)

Available forms include: Number on patch 25, 50, 75 and 100 refers to µg/hr/fentanyl-release rate; lozenges, transmucosal matrix attached to a radiopaque holder to be dissolved in mouth 200, 400, 600, 800, 1200, 1600 µg

Side effects/adverse reactions:

▼ *ORAL:* Dry mouth

CNS: Dizziness, delirium, euphoria

CV: ***Bradycardia, arrest,*** hypotension or hypertension

GI: Nausea, vomiting

RESP: ***Respiratory depression, arrest, laryngospasm***

EENT: Blurred vision, miosis

MS: Muscle rigidity

Contraindications: Hypersensitivity to opiates, myasthenia gravis

Precautions: Elderly, respiratory depression, increased intracranial pressure, seizure disorders, severe respiratory disorders, cardiac dysrhythmias, pregnancy category C

Pharmacokinetics:

TD: Dosage adjusted according to opioid tolerance if patient has been taking opioids (2.5 mg of transdermal fentanyl is equivalent to approximately 90 mg oral morphine in 24 hr); peak serum levels take up to 24 hr after applied; liver metabolism; renal excretion of metabolites

Drug interactions of concern to dentistry:

- Effects may be increased with other CNS depressants: alcohol, narcotics, sedative/hypnotics, skeletal muscle relaxants, chlorpromazine
- Additive hypotension: nitrous oxide, benzodiazepines, phenothiazines
- Increased anticholinergic effect: anticholinergics
- Contraindication: MAO inhibitors

DENTAL CONSIDERATIONS

General:

- Monitor vital signs every appointment due to cardiovascular and respiratory side effects.
- After supine positioning, have patient sit upright for at least 2 min before standing to avoid orthostatic hypotension.
- Assess salivary flow as a factor in caries, periodontal disease, and candidiasis.
- Psychologic and physical dependence may occur with chronic administration.
- Determine why the patient is taking the drug.
- Consider alternative drugs to opioids and NSAIDs for management of dental pain.

Consultations:

- Medical consult may be required to assess disease control in the patient.

Teach patient/family:

- Importance of good oral hygiene to prevent gingival inflammation
- To avoid mouth rinses with high alcohol content due to drying effects

F

ferrous fumarate/ ferrous gluconate/ ferrous sulfate

(fer'us fyoo'ma-rate; gloo'koe-nate)

Femiron, Feosol, Feostat, Fergon, Fero-Gradumet, Ferospace, Ferralet, Ferralyn, Fumasorb, Fumerin, Hemocyte, Ircon, Irospan, Mol-Iron, Neofer, Palmiron, Simiron, Fer-in-Sol, Slow-Fe

🍁 Fero-Grad, Fertinic, Nephro-Fer, Novoferrogluc, Novoferrosulfa, Novofumar, Palafer

Drug class.: Hematinic, iron preparation

Action: Replaces iron stores needed for red blood cell development, energy and O_2 transport, utilization

Uses: Iron deficiency anemia, prophylaxis for iron deficiency in pregnancy

Dosage and routes:

Fumarate

- *Adult:* PO 200 mg tid-qid
- *Child 2-12 yr:* PO 3 mg/kg/day (elemental iron) tid-qid
- *Child 6 mo-2 yr:* PO up to 6 mg/kg/day (elemental iron) tid-qid
- *Infants:* PO 10-25 mg/day (elemental iron) tid-qid

Gluconate

- *Adult:* PO 200-600 mg tid
- *Child 6-12 yr:* 300-900 mg qd
- *Child <6 yr:* 100-300 mg qd

Sulfate

- *Adult:* PO 0.750-1.5 g/day in divided doses tid
- *Child 6-12 yr:* 600 mg/day in divided doses

Pregnancy

- *Adult:* PO 300-600 mg/day in divided doses

Available forms include:

- *Fumarate:* Tabs 63, 195, 200, 324, 325 mg; chew tabs 100 mg; con rel tabs 300 mg; oral susp 100 mg/5 ml, 45 mg/0.6 ml
- *Gluconate:* Tabs 300, 320, 325 mg; caps 86, 325, 435 mg; film-coated tabs 300 mg; elix 300 mg/5 ml
- *Sulfate:* Tabs, 195, 300, 325 mg; enteric-coated tabs 325 mg; ext rel tabs, time rel caps, 525 mg

Side effects/adverse reactions:

▼ *ORAL:* Extrinsic stain on teeth (liquid form)

GI: Nausea, constipation, epigastric pain, black and red tarry stools, vomiting, diarrhea

Contraindications: Hypersensitivity, ulcerative colitis/regional enteritis, hemosiderosis/hemochromatosis, peptic ulcer disease, hemolytic anemia, cirrhosis

Precautions: Long-term anemia, pregnancy category A

Pharmacokinetics:

PO: Excreted in feces, urine, skin, breast milk; enters bloodstream; bound to transferrin; crosses placenta

Drug interactions of concern to dentistry:

- Decreased absorption of tetracycline, zinc, ciprofloxacin

DENTAL CONSIDERATIONS

Teach patient/family:

- If patient is using hydrogen peroxide as a dentifrice to remove extrinsic stain, caution against frequent use to avoid peroxide-related soft tissue injury

• That liquid iron preparation taken through straw followed by rinsing mouth can reduce staining

fexofenadine HCl

(fex-oh-fen'a-deen)
Allegra

Drug class.: Antihistamine, nonsedating

Action: Antagonist for histamine (H_1) receptors; active metabolite of terfenadine

Uses: Seasonal allergic rhinitis

Dosage and routes:

• *Adult and child >12 yr:* PO 60 mg bid

• *Adult >65 yr:* PO 60 mg qd

Available forms include: Caps 60 mg

Side effects/adverse reactions:

CNS: Drowsiness, headache

GI: Nausea, dyspepsia

GU: Dysmenorrhea

EENT: Throat irritation

MISC: Fatigue

Contraindications: Hypersensitivity; troglitazone

Precautions: Reduce dose in elderly, renally impaired, pregnancy category C, lactation, child <12 yr

Pharmacokinetics:

PO: Well absorbed, peak plasma levels 2.6 hr; excreted mainly in feces, only 5% of dose is metabolized, 60%-70% plasma protein bound

Drug interactions of concern to dentistry:

• Elevated plasma levels with erythromycin, ketoconazole

DENTAL CONSIDERATIONS
General:

• Consider semisupine chair position for patient comfort due to GI effects of drug.

finasteride

(fi-nas'teer-ide)
Proscar
Propecia (hair growth product)

Drug class.: Synthetic steroid

Action: Competitive inhibitor of type II 5-α-reductase, an enzyme that converts testosterone to 5-α-dihydrotestosterone; this enzyme is found in the liver, skin, and scalp

Uses:

Proscar: Symptomatic benign prostatic hyperplasia, reduce risk for acute urinary retention and surgery

Propecia: Treatment of male pattern baldness in men ages 18-41

Dosage and routes:

Prostatic hypertrophy

• *Adult:* PO 5 mg day up to 6 mo or longer

Male pattern baldness

• *Adult:* PO 1 mg daily; several months of therapy may be required

Available forms include: Tabs 1 and 5 mg

Side effects/adverse reactions:

GU: Impotence, decreased libido, decreased ejaculate volume

INTEG: Skin rash

MISC: Gynecomastia, allergic reactions

Contraindications: Hypersensitivity, pregnancy, lactation, children, prostate cancer, obstructive urinary disease

Precautions: Pregnancy category X, lactation, lower PSA levels do not suggest absence of prostate cancer; women should avoid drug/semen contact

Pharmacokinetics:
PO: Peak levels 1-2 hr, half-life 6 hr; highly protein bound; liver metabolism; metabolites excreted in feces, urine

Drug interactions of concern to dentistry:
• Opioids and anticholinergic drugs may enhance urinary retention; use alternative analgesics (NSAIDs)

DENTAL CONSIDERATIONS
Consultations:
• Determine why patient is taking the drug; for prostatic hyperplasia or male pattern baldness.
• Medical consult may be required to assess disease control in the patient.

flavoxate HCl

(fla-vox′ate)
Urispas

Drug class.: Antispasmatic

Action: Relaxes smooth muscles in urinary tract
Uses: Relief of nocturia, incontinence, suprapubic pain, dysuria, frequency associated with urologic conditions (symptomatic only)
Dosage and routes:
• *Adult and child >12 yr:* PO 100-200 mg tid-qid
Available forms include: Tabs 100, 200 mg
Side effects/adverse reactions:
▼ *ORAL: Dry mouth*
CNS: Anxiety, restlessness, dizziness, **convulsions,** headache, drowsiness, confusion, decreased concentration
CV: Palpitation, sinus tachycardia, hypotension
GI: Nausea, vomiting, anorexia, abdominal pain, constipation
HEMA: ***Leukopenia, eosinophilia***
GU: Dysuria
EENT: Blurred vision, increased intraocular tension, dry throat
INTEG: Urticaria, dermatitis
Contraindications: Hypersensitivity, GI obstruction, GI hemorrhage, GU obstruction
Precautions: Pregnancy category B, lactation, suspected glaucoma, children <12 yr
Pharmacokinetics: Excreted in urine

Drug interactions of concern to dentistry:
• Increased anticholinergic effect: anticholinergic drugs

DENTAL CONSIDERATIONS
General:
• Assess salivary flow as a factor in caries, periodontal disease, and candidiasis.
Teach patient/family:
• Importance of good oral hygiene to prevent gingival inflammation
• To avoid mouth rinses with high alcohol content due to drying effects

flecainide acetate

(fle-kay′nide)
Tambocor

Drug class.: Antidysrhythmic (Class IC)

Action: Decreases conduction in all parts of the heart, with greatest effect on His-Purkinje system, which stabilizes cardiac membrane
Uses: Life-threatening ventricular dysrhythmias, sustained supraventricular tachycardia
Dosage and routes:
• *Adult:* PO 100 mg q12h, may increase q4d by 50 mg q12h to

desired response, not to exceed 400 mg/day

Available forms include: Tabs 50, 100, 150 mg

Side effects/adverse reactions:

▼ *ORAL:* Changes in taste, dry mouth

CNS: Headache, dizziness, involuntary movement, confusion, psychosis, restlessness, irritability, paresthesia, ataxia, flushing, somnolence, depression, anxiety, malaise

CV: Hypotension, bradycardia, ***heart block, cardiovascular collapse, cardiac arrest,*** dysrhythmias, CHF, fatal ventricular tachycardia, angina, PVC

GI: Nausea, vomiting, anorexia, constipation, abdominal pain, flatulence

RESP: ***Respiratory depression,*** dyspnea

HEMA: ***Leukopenia, thrombocytopenia***

GU: Impotence, decreased libido, polyuria, urinary retention

EENT: Blurred vision, hearing loss, tinnitus

INTEG: Rash, urticaria, edema, swelling

Contraindications: Hypersensitivity, severe heart block, cardiogenic shock, nonsustained ventricular dysrhythmias, frequent PVCs, non–life-threatening dysrhythmias

Precautions: Pregnancy category C, lactation, children, renal disease, liver disease, CHF, respiratory depression, myasthenia gravis

Pharmacokinetics:

PO: Peak 3 hr, half-life 12-27 hr; metabolized by liver; excreted unchanged by kidneys (10%); excreted in breast milk

Drug interactions of concern to dentistry:

• No specific interactions are reported with dental drugs; however, any drug that could affect the cardiac action of flecainide (other local anesthetics, vasoconstrictors, and anticholinergics) should be used in the least effective dose.

DENTAL CONSIDERATIONS

General:

• Monitor vital signs every appointment due to cardiovascular and respiratory side effects.

• Assess salivary flow as a factor in caries, periodontal disease, and candidiasis.

• Stress from dental procedures may compromise cardiovascular function; determine patient risk.

• Use vasoconstrictors with caution, in low doses, and with careful aspiration. Avoid use of gingival retraction cord with epinephrine.

Consultations:

• Medical consult may be required to assess disease control and patient's ability to tolerate stress.

Teach patient/family:

• Importance of good oral hygiene to prevent gingival inflammation

• To avoid mouth rinses with high alcohol content due to drying effects

---

fluconazole

(floo-koe′na-zole)

Diflucan

Drug class.: Antifungal

Action: Inhibits ergosterol biosynthesis, causes direct damage to membrane phospholipids

Uses: Oropharyngeal candidiasis,

chronic mucocutaneous candidiasis, urinary candidiasis, cryptococcal meningitis

Dosage and routes:

Oropharyngeal candidiasis

• *Adult:* PO 200 mg first day, then 100 mg daily

Serious fungal infections

• *Adult:* IV 400 mg initially, then 200 mg/day; adjust dose downward for renal impairment

• *Adult:* PO 400 mg daily; or 400 mg first day, then 200 mg daily × 4 wk

Vaginal candidiasis

• *Adult:* PO 150 mg as a single dose

Available forms include: Tabs 50, 100, 150, 200 mg; IV inj 200, 400 mg

Side effects/adverse reactions:

GI: Nausea, vomiting, diarrhea, cramping, flatus, increased AST/ALT

INTEG: Skin rash, exfoliative skin disorders (Stevens-Johnson syndrome, rare)

META: Rare abnormal liver function

Contraindications: Hypersensitivity, cisapride

Precautions: Renal disease, pregnancy category C

Pharmacokinetics:

PO/IV: Bioavailability more than 90%, peak plasma levels 1-2 hr, with loading doses see quicker steady-state levels, low plasma protein binding (12%), minimal metabolism, 80% excreted unchanged in urine

Drug interactions of concern to dentistry:

• Use with caution in patients taking astemizole or terfenadine; risk of dysrhythmias is unknown

• Increased plasma levels of oral hypoglycemics: theophylline, cyclosporine

• Inhibits metabolism of certain benzodiazepines: alprazolam, chlordiazepoxide, clonazepam, clorazepate, diazepam, estazolam, flurazepam, halazepam, midazolam, triazolam, quazepam, zolpidem

• May inhibit metabolism of warfarin

• Contraindicated with cisapride

DENTAL CONSIDERATIONS

General:

• Culture may be required to confirm fungal organism.

Teach patient/family:

• That long-term therapy may be needed to clear infection

• To prevent reinoculation of *Candida* infection, dispose of toothbrush or other contaminated oral hygiene devices used during period of infection

---

flucytosine

(floo-sye'toe-seen)

Ancobon

♣ Ancotil

Drug class.: Antifungal

Action: Converted to fluorouracil after entering fungi, which inhibits DNA and RNA synthesis

Uses: *Candida* infections (septicemia, endocarditis, pulmonary and urinary tract infections), *Cryptococcus* (meningitis, pulmonary and urinary tract infections)

Dosage and routes:

• *Adult and child >50 kg:* PO 50-150 mg/kg/day q6h

Available forms include: Caps 250, 500 mg

Side effects/adverse reactions:
▼ *ORAL:* Bleeding (if bone marrow depression occurs), stomatitis
CNS: Headache, confusion, dizziness, sedation
GI: Nausea, vomiting, anorexia, ***bowel perforation*** (rare), diarrhea, cramps, enterocolitis, increased AST/ALT, alk phosphatase
RESP: ***Respiratory arrest,*** chest pain, dyspnea
HEMA: ***Thrombocytopenia, agranulocytosis, anemia, leukopenia, pancytopenia***
GU: Increased BUN, creatinine
INTEG: Rash, photosensitivity, urticaria
Contraindications: Hypersensitivity
Precautions: Renal disease, bone marrow depression, blood dyscrasias, radiation/chemotherapy, pregnancy category C
Pharmacokinetics:
PO: Peak 2.5-6 hr, half-life 3-6 hr; excreted in urine (unchanged); well distributed to CSF, aqueous humor, joints
Drug interactions of concern to dentistry:
• None

DENTAL CONSIDERATIONS
General:
• Patients on chronic drug therapy may rarely have symptoms of blood dyscrasias, which can include infection, bleeding, and poor healing.
• Examine for evidence of oral *Candida* infection.
Consultations:
• Medical consult may be required to assess disease control in the patient.
• In a patient with symptoms of blood dyscrasias, request a medical consult for blood studies and postpone dental treatment until normal values are reestablished.
Teach patient/family:
• Importance of good oral hygiene to prevent gingival inflammation

fludrocortisone acetate
(floo-droe-kor′ti-sone)
Florinef Acetate
Drug class.: Glucocorticoid and mineralocorticoid

Action: Glucocorticoids have multiple actions that include antiinflammatory and immunosuppressant effects. They inhibit phospholipase A_2, interfering with or reducing the synthesis of prostaglandins and leukotrienes. They also bind to cytoplasmic glucocorticoid receptors (GRs) and enter the cell nucleus to bind with DNA. This results in the synthesis of various enzymes such as collagenase, elastase, and cytokines that play important roles in inflammation and immunosuppression. They also suppress the production of lymphocytes, monocytes, and eosinophils.
Uses: Adrenal insufficiency, salt-losing adrenogenital syndrome
Dosage and routes:
• *Adult:* PO 0.1-0.2 mg
• *Pediatric:* PO 0.05-0.10 mg/day
Available forms include: Tabs 0.1 mg
Side effects/adverse reactions:
CNS: Flushing, sweating, headache
CV: Hypertension, ***circulatory collapse, thrombophlebitis, embolism,*** tachycardia, edema, enlargement of heart
MS: Fractures, osteoporosis, weakness

Contraindications: Hypersensitivity, acute glomerulonephritis, amebiasis

Precautions: Pregnancy category C, osteoporosis, CHF

Pharmacokinetics:

PO: Half-life 3.5 hr, duration 1-2 days; highly protein bound; metabolized by liver; excreted in urine

Drug interactions of concern to dentistry:

- Decreased action: barbiturates
- Increased side effects: sodium-containing food or sodium-containing polishing devices
- Decreased effects of salicylates

DENTAL CONSIDERATIONS

General:

- Patients with Addison's disease are more susceptible to stress and may require supplemental systemic glucocorticoids before dental treatment.
- Patients who have been or are currently on chronic steroid therapy (>2 wk) may require supplemental steroids for dental treatment.
- Evaluate vital signs at each appointment due to nature of disease.
- Short appointments and a stress reduction protocol may be required for anxious patients.
- Patients with Addison's disease must be evaluated closely for presence of oral infection.
- Do not use ingestible sodium bicarbonate products, such as the air polishing system (Prophy Jet), or IV saline fluids for patients on a salt-restriction regimen.
- Place on frequent recall to evaluate healing response.
- Use precautions if dental surgery is anticipated and conscious sedation or general anesthesia is required.
- Monitor patient for any signs of inadequate management of disease such as potassium depletion, muscle weakness, paresthesia, fatigue, nausea, depression, polyuria, and edema.

Consultations:

- Medical consult is required to assess disease control and stress tolerance of the patient.
- Consult may be required to confirm steroid dose and duration of use.

Teach patient/family:

- That identification as a steroid user should be carried
- To report to the dental office any signs that might indicate an oral infection

---

flumazenil

(floo-may'ze-nil)

Anexate, Romazicon

Drug class.: Benzodiazepine receptor antagonist

Action: Antagonizes the actions of benzodiazepines on the CNS; competitively inhibits the activity at the benzodiazepine recognition site on the GABA/benzodiazepine receptor complex

Uses: Reversal of the sedative effects of benzodiazepines

Dosage and routes:

Reversal of conscious sedation or in general anesthesia

- *Adult:* IV 0.2 mg (2 ml) given over 15-30 sec; wait 45-60 sec for desired response, then give 0.2 mg (2 ml) if consciousness does not occur; may be repeated at 60 sec intervals as needed, up to 4 additional times (max total dose 1 mg); dose is to be individualized

Management of suspected benzodiazepine overdose

• *Adult:* IV 0.2 mg (2 ml) given over 15-30 sec; wait 45-60 sec for desired response, then give 0.2 mg (2 ml) over 30 sec if consciousness does not occur; further doses of 0.5 mg (5 ml) can be given over 30 sec at intervals of 1 min up to cumulative dose of 3 mg in 1 hr

Available forms include: Inj 0.1 mg/ml

Side effects/adverse reactions:

CNS: ***Convulsions,*** dizziness, agitation, emotional lability, confusion, somnolence

CV: Hypertension, palpitation, cutaneous vasodilation, dysrhythmias, bradycardia, tachycardia, chest pain

GI: Nausea, vomiting, hiccups

EENT: Abnormal vision, blurred vision, tinnitus

SYST: Headache, injection site pain, increased sweating, fatigue, rigors

Contraindications: Hypersensitivity to this drug or benzodiazepines, serious cyclic antidepressant overdose, patients given benzodiazepine for control of life-threatening condition

Precautions: Pregnancy category C, lactation, children, elderly, renal disease, seizure disorders, head injury, labor and delivery, hepatic disease, hypoventilation, panic disorder, drug and alcohol dependency, ambulatory patients

Pharmacokinetics:

IV: Terminal half-life 41-79 min; metabolized in liver

Drug interactions of concern to dentistry:

• May not be effective: mixed drug overdosage

DENTAL CONSIDERATIONS

General:

• Monitor vital signs every appointment due to cardiovascular side effects.

• Monitor for resedation; duration of antagonism is short compared with benzodiazepines.

Teach patient/family:

• To be alert for possible resedation when discharged from office

F

flunisolide

(floo-niss'oh-lide)

Oral inh aerosol: Aerobid, Aerobid-M

✤ Bronalide

Nasal inh sol: Nasalide

✤ Rhinalar

Drug class.: Synthetic glucocorticoid

Action: Glucocorticoids have multiple actions that include antiinflammatory and immunosuppressant effects. They inhibit phospholipase A_2, interfering with or reducing the synthesis of prostaglandins and leukotrienes. They also bind to cytoplasmic glucocorticoid receptors (GRs) and enter the cell nucleus to bind with DNA. This results in the synthesis of various enzymes such as collagenase, elastase, and cytokines that play important roles in inflammation and immunosuppression. They also suppress the production of lymphocytes, monocytes, and eosinophils.

Uses: Rhinitis (seasonal or perennial)

Dosage and routes:

• *Adult:* Instill 2 sprays in each nostril bid, then increase to tid if needed; not to exceed 8 sprays in each nostril per day

• *Child 6-14 yr:* Instill 1 spray in each nostril tid or 2 sprays bid; not to exceed 4 sprays in each nostril per day

Available forms include: Aerosol 25 μg/spray

Side effects/adverse reactions:

▼ *ORAL:* Dry mouth, candidiasis, loss of taste sensation

CNS: Headache, dizziness

EENT: Nasal irritation, dryness, rebound congestion, epistaxis, sneezing

INTEG: Urticaria

SYST: ***CHF, convulsions,*** increased sodium, hypertension

Contraindications: Hypersensitivity, child <12 yr, fungal, bacterial infection of nose

Precautions: Lactation, pregnancy category C

Pharmacokinetics:

AERO: Effective response time 1-4 wk; metabolized in liver; excreted in urine and feces

DENTAL CONSIDERATIONS

General:

• Examine oral cavity for evidence of drug side effects.

• Assess salivary flow as a factor in caries, periodontal disease, and candidiasis.

• Evaluate respiration characteristics and rate.

• Consider semisupine chair position for patients with respiratory disease.

• Determine dose and duration of steroid therapy for each patient to assess risk for stress tolerance and immunosuppression.

• Acute asthmatic episodes may be precipitated in the dental office. Sympathomimetic inhalants should be available for emergency use. A stress reduction protocol may be required.

• Consider the drug in the diagnosis of taste alterations.

Consultations:

• Medical consult may be required to assess disease control in the patient.

Teach patient/family:

• Importance of good oral hygiene to prevent soft tissue inflammation

• Caution to prevent injury when using oral hygiene aids

• Importance of gargling, rinsing mouth with water, and expectorating after each aerosol dose

When chronic dry mouth occurs, advise patient:

• To use daily home fluoride products for anticaries effect

• To avoid mouth rinses with high alcohol content due to drying effects

• To use sugarless gum, frequent sips of water, or saliva substitutes

---

fluocinonide

(floo-oh-sin'oh-nide)

Cream: Fluonex, Lidex, Lidex-E, Fluocin, Licon

♣ Lidemol, Lyderm

Ointment: Lidex

Solution: Lidex

Gel: Lidex

♣ Topsyn

Drug class.: Topical corticosteroid, synthetic fluorinated agent, group II potency

Action: Glucocorticoids have multiple actions that include antiinflammatory and immunosuppressant effects. They inhibit phospholipase A_2, interfering with or

reducing the synthesis of prostaglandins and leukotrienes. They also bind to cytoplasmic glucocorticoid receptors (GRs) and enter the cell nucleus to bind with DNA. This results in the synthesis of various enzymes such as collagenase, elastase, and cytokines that play important roles in inflammation and immunosuppression. They also suppress the production of lymphocytes, monocytes, and eosinophils.
Uses: Psoriasis, eczema, contact dermatitis, pruritus, oral lichen planus lesions
Dosage and routes:
• *Adult and child:* Apply to affected area tid-qid
Available forms include: Oint 0.5%; cream 0.05%; sol 0.05%; gel 0.05% in 15, 30, 60, and 120 g tubes
Side effects/adverse reactions:
▼ *ORAL:* Thinning of mucosa, stinging sensation (oral application)
INTEG: Burning, dryness, itching, irritation, acne, folliculitis, hypertrichosis, perioral dermatitis, hypopigmentation, atrophy, striae, miliaria, allergic contact dermatitis, secondary infection
Contraindications: Hypersensitivity to corticosteroids, fungal infections
Precautions: Pregnancy category C, lactation, viral infections, bacterial infections
DENTAL CONSIDERATIONS
General:
• Place on frequent recall to evaluate healing response.
Teach patient/family:
• When used for oral lesions, to return for oral evaluation if response of oral tissues has not occurred in 7-14 days
• That use on oral herpetic ulcerations is contraindicated
• Importance of good oral hygiene to prevent soft tissue inflammation
• To apply at bedtime or after meals for maximum effect
• To apply with cotton-tipped applicator by pressing, not rubbing, paste on lesion

F

fluorouracil (topical)

(flure-oh-yoor'a-sil)
Efudex, Fluoroplex, 5-FU
Drug class.: Topical antineoplastic

Action: Inhibits synthesis of DNA and RNA in susceptible cells
Uses: Keratosis (multiple/actinic), basal cell carcinoma
Dosage and routes:
• *Adult and child:* TOP apply to affected area bid
Available forms include: Sol 1%, 2%, 5%; cream 1%, 5%
Side effects/adverse reactions:
▼ *ORAL:* Stomatitis, medicinal taste, lichenoid reaction
CNS: Insomnia, irritability
EENT: Lacrimation, soreness
*INTEG: **Pain, burning, pruritus,*** contact dermatitis, scaling, swelling, soreness, hyperpigmentation
Contraindications: Hypersensitivity, pregnancy
Precautions: Pregnancy category X, occlusive dressings, lactation, children, excessive exposure to sunlight
Pharmacokinetics:
TOP: No significant absorption, onset 2-3 days; treatment may last

up to 12 wk; healing may be delayed for 1-2 mo

Drug interactions of concern to dentistry:

• None reported, but limit drugs that may also produce photosensitivity reaction

DENTAL CONSIDERATIONS

General:

• Be aware of patient's disease and avoid treated areas to prevent further irritation.

---

fluoxetine

(floo-ox′e-teen)

Prozac

Drug class.: Antidepressant

Action: Inhibits CNS neuron uptake of serotonin, but not norepinephrine

Uses: Major depressive disorder, bulimia, obsessive-compulsive disorder, premenstrual tension, geriatric depression in patients >65 yr

Dosage and routes:

Depression

• *Adult:* PO 20 mg qd in AM; after several weeks if no clinical improvement is noted, dose may be increased to 20 mg bid, not to exceed 80 mg/day

Obsessive-compulsive disorder

• *Adult:* PO initial 20 mg qd in AM; if no improvement after several weeks dose may be increased to 20 mg bid, not to exceed 80 mg/day

Bulimia

• *Adult:* PO 60 mg qd in AM; can start with lower dose and gradually increase to 60 mg/day

Available forms include: Capsules 10, 20 mg, tabs 10, 20 mg

Side effects/adverse reactions:

ORAL: Dry mouth, taste changes

CNS: Headache, nervousness, insomnia, drowsiness, anxiety, tremor, dizziness, fatigue, sedation, poor concentration, abnormal dreams, agitation, convulsions, apathy, euphoria, hallucinations, delusions, psychosis

CV: Hot flashes, palpitation, ***MI,*** angina pectoris, hemorrhage, tachycardia, first-degree AV block, bradycardia, thrombophlebitis

GI: Nausea, diarrhea, anorexia, dyspepsia, constipation, cramps, vomiting, flatulence, decreased appetite

RESP: Infection, pharyngitis, nasal congestion, sinus headache, sinusitus, cough, dyspnea, bronchitis, asthma, hyperventilation, pneumonia

GU: Dysmenorrhea, decreased libido, abnormal ejaculation, urinary frequency, UTI, amenorrhea, cystitis, impotence

EENT: Visual changes, ear/eye pain, photophobia, tinnitus

INTEG: Sweating, rash, pruritus, acne, alopecia, urticaria

MS: Pain, arthritis, twitching

SYST: Asthenia, viral infection, fever, allergy, chills

Contraindications: Hypersensitivity, MAO inhibitors

Precautions: Pregnancy category B, lactation, children, elderly

Pharmacokinetics:

PO: Peak 6-8 hr, half-life 2-7 days; metabolized in liver; excreted in urine

Drug interactions of concern to dentistry:

• Increased CNS depression: alcohol, all CNS depressants

• Increased side effects: highly protein-bound drugs (aspirin)

• Increased half-life of diazepam

DENTAL CONSIDERATIONS

General:

• Monitor vital signs every appointment due to cardiovascular side effects.

• Assess salivary flow as a factor in caries, periodontal disease, and candidiasis.

Consultations:

• Medical consult may be required to assess disease control and patient's ability to tolerate stress.

• Physician should be informed if significant xerostomic side effects occur (increased caries, sore tongue, problems eating or swallowing, difficulty wearing prosthesis) so a medication change can be considered.

Teach patient/family:

• To use electric toothbrush if patient has difficulty holding conventional devices

When chronic dry mouth occurs, advise patient:

• To avoid mouth rinses with high alcohol content due to drying effects

• To use daily home fluoride products for anticaries effect

• To use sugarless gum, frequent sips of water, or saliva substitutes

---

fluoxymesterone

(floo-ox-i-mes′te-rone)

Android-F, Halotestin

Drug class.: Androgenic anabolic steroid

Controlled Substance Schedule III

Action: Increases weight by building body tissue; increases potassium, phosphorus, chloride, nitrogen levels; increases bone development

Uses: Impotence from testicular deficiency, hypogonadism, breast engorgement, palliative treatment of female breast cancer

Dosage and routes:

Hypogonadism/impotence

• *Adult:* PO 2-20 mg qd

Breast engorgement

• *Adult:* PO 2.5 mg qd, then 5-10 mg qd × 5 days

Breast cancer

• *Adult:* PO 10-40 mg qd in divided doses until therapeutic effect occurs; dosage should then be reduced

Available forms include: Tabs 2, 5, 10 mg

Side effects/adverse reactions:

▼ *ORAL:* Reddish spots on mucosa (high dose)

CNS: Dizziness, headache, fatigue, tremors, paresthesia, flushing, sweating, anxiety, lability, insomnia

CV: Increased BP

GI: ***Cholestatic jaundice,*** nausea, vomiting, constipation, weight gain

GU: ***Hematuria,*** amenorrhea, vaginitis, decreased libido, decreased breast size, clitoral hypertrophy, testicular atrophy

EENT: Carpal tunnel syndrome, conjunctional edema, nasal congestion

INTEG: Rash, acneiform lesions, oily hair/skin, flushing, sweating, acne vulgaris, alopecia, hirsutism

ENDO: Abnormal GTT

MS: Cramps, spasms

Contraindications: Severe renal disease, severe cardiac disease, severe hepatic disease, hypersensitivity, pregnancy category X, lactation, genital bleeding (abnormal)

Precautions: Diabetes mellitus, CV disease, MI

Pharmacokinetics:
PO: Metabolized in liver; excreted in urine; crosses placenta; excreted in breast milk

Drug interactions of concern to dentistry:
• Edema: corticosteroids

DENTAL CONSIDERATIONS

General:
• Monitor vital signs every appointment due to cardiovascular side effects.
• Patients receiving chemotherapy may require palliative treatment for stomatitis.

Teach patient/family:
• Importance of good oral hygiene to prevent soft tissue inflammation
• Caution the patient in use of dental hygiene aids to prevent trauma

fluphenazine decanoate/ fluphenazine enanthate/ fluphenazine HCl

(floo-fen'a-zeen)

Permitil, Permitil Concentrate HCl, Prolixin Concentrate, Prolixin Decanoate, Prolixin Enanthate

Apo-Fluphenazine, Modecate, Modecate concentrate, Moditen Enanthate, Moditen HCl

Drug class.: Phenothiazine antipsychotic

Action: Blocks neurotransmission at dopaminergic synapses in the cerebral cortex, hypothalamus, and limbic system; exhibits strong peripheral α-adrenergic, anticholinergic blocking action; mechanism for antipsychotic effects is unclear

Uses: Psychotic disorders, schizophrenia; unapproved use: adjunct to tricyclic antidepressants in neurogenic pain

Dosage and routes:

Enanthate, decanoate
• *Adult and child >12 yr:* SC 12.5-25 mg q1-3wk

HCl
• *Adult:* PO 2.5-10 mg in divided doses q6-8h, not to exceed 20 mg qd; IM initially 1.25 mg, then 2.5-10 mg in divided doses q6-8h

Available forms include: HCl—tabs 1, 2.5, 5, 10 mg; elix 2.5 mg/5 ml; conc 5 mg/ml; inj IM 2.5 mg/ml; enanthate, decanoate—inj SC/IM 25 mg/ml

Side effects/adverse reactions:

▼ *ORAL: Dry mouth,* lichenoid reaction

CNS: Extrapyramidal symptoms: pseudoparkinsonism, akathisia, dystonia, tardive dyskinesia, drowsiness, headache, ***neuroleptic malignant syndrome,*** seizures

CV: Orthostatic hypotension, ***cardiac arrest, tachycardia,*** hypertension, ECG changes

GI: ***Paralytic ileus, hepatitis,*** nausea, vomiting, anorexia, constipation, diarrhea, jaundice, weight gain

RESP: ***Respiratory depression,*** laryngospasm, dyspnea

HEMA: ***Leukopenia, leukocytosis, agranulocytosis,*** anemia

GU: Urinary retention, urinary frequency, enuresis, impotence, amenorrhea, gynecomastia

EENT: Blurred vision, glaucoma, dry eyes

INTEG: Rash, photosensitivity, dermatitis

Contraindications: Hypersensitivity, circulatory collapse, liver damage, cerebral arteriosclerosis, coronary disease, severe hypertension/hypotension, blood dyscrasias, coma, child <12 yr, brain damage, bone marrow depression, alcohol and barbiturate withdrawal states

Precautions: Pregnancy category not established, lactation, seizure disorders, hypertension, hepatic disease, cardiac disease

Pharmacokinetics:

PO/IM: HCl—onset 1 hr, peak 2-4 hr, duration 6-8 hr

SC: Enanthate—onset 1-2 days, peak 2-3 days, duration 1-3 wk, half-life 3.5-4 days; decanoate—onset 1-3 days, peak 1-2 days, duration >4 wk, half-life (single dose) 6.8-9.6 days, (multiple dose) 14.3 days; metabolized by liver; excreted in urine (metabolites); crosses placenta; excreted in breast milk

Drug interactions of concern to dentistry:

- Increased sedation: other CNS depressants, alcohol, barbiturate anesthetics, opioid analgesics
- Hypotension, tachycardia: epinephrine
- Increased extrapyramidal effects: phenothiazines and related drugs (haloperidol, droperidol), metoclopramide
- Additive photosensitization: tetracyclines
- Increased anticholinergic effects: anticholinergics

DENTAL CONSIDERATIONS

General:

- Monitor vital signs every appointment due to cardiovascular side effects.
- Patients on chronic drug therapy may rarely have symptoms of blood dyscrasias, which can include infection, bleeding, and poor healing.
- After supine positioning, have patient sit upright for at least 2 min before standing to avoid orthostatic hypotension.
- Assess salivary flow as a factor in caries, periodontal disease, and candidiasis.
- Avoid dental light in patient's eyes; offer dark glasses for patient comfort.
- Assess for presence of extrapyramidal motor symptoms, such as tardive dyskinesia and akathisia. Extrapyramidal motor activity may complicate dental treatment.
- Geriatric patients are more susceptible to drug effects; use a lower dose.
- Use vasoconstrictors with caution, in low doses, and with careful aspiration.

Consultations:

- In a patient with symptoms of blood dyscrasias, request a medical consult for blood studies and postpone dental treatment until normal values are reestablished.
- Take precautions if dental surgery is anticipated and anesthesia is required.
- If signs of tardive dyskinesia or akathisia are present, refer to physician.
- Physician should be informed if significant xerostomic side effects occur (increased caries, sore tongue, problems eating or swallowing, difficulty wearing prosthesis) so a medication change can be considered.

Teach patient/family:

- Importance of good oral hygiene to prevent soft tissue inflammation

• Caution to prevent injury when using oral hygiene aids
• To use electric toothbrush if patient has difficulty holding conventional devices

When chronic dry mouth occurs, advise patient:

• To avoid mouth rinses with high alcohol content due to drying effects
• To use daily home fluoride products for anticaries effect
• To use sugarless gum, frequent sips of water, or saliva substitutes

flurandrenolide

(flure-an-dren'oh-lide)
Cordran, Cordran SP
♣ Drenison, Dreison-1/4

Drug class.: Topical corticosteroid, group III medium potency

Action: Glucocorticoids have multiple actions that include antiinflammatory and immunosuppressant effects. They inhibit phospholipase A_2, interfering with or reducing the synthesis of prostaglandins and leukotrienes. They also bind to cytoplasmic glucocorticoid receptors (GRs) and enter the cell nucleus to bind with DNA. This results in the synthesis of various enzymes such as collagenase, elastase, and cytokines that play important roles in inflammation and immunosuppression. They also suppress the production of lymphocytes, monocytes, and eosinophils.

Uses: Corticosteroid-responsive dermatoses, pruritus

Dosage and routes:

• *Adult and child:* TOP apply to affected area tid-qid; apply tape q12-24h

Available forms include: Oint 0.025%, 0.05%; cream 0.025%, 0.05%; lotion 0.05%; tape 4 μg/cm^2

Side effects/adverse reactions:

▼ *ORAL:* Perioral dermatitis

INTEG: Burning, dryness, itching, irritation, acne, folliculitis, hypertrichosis, hypopigmentation, atrophy, striae, miliaria, allergic contact dermatitis, secondary infection

Contraindications: Hypersensitivity to corticosteroids, fungal infections, viral infections

Precautions: Pregnancy category C, lactation, viral infections, bacterial infections

DENTAL CONSIDERATIONS

General:

• Determine why the patient is taking the drug.
• Apply lubricant to dry lips for patient comfort before dental procedures.
• Place on frequent recall to evaluate healing response when used on chronic basis.

flurazepam HCl

(flur-az'e-pam)
Dalmane
♣ Apo-Flurazepam, Novoflupam, Somnol

Drug class.: Benzodiazepine, sedative-hypnotic

Controlled Substance Schedule IV

Action: Produces CNS depression by interacting with a benzodiazepine receptor to facilitate the action of the inhibitory neurotransmitter γ-aminobutyric acid (GABA)

Uses: Insomnia

Dosage and routes:
• *Adult:* PO 15-30 mg hs, may repeat dose once if needed
• *Geriatric:* PO 15 mg hs, may increase if needed
Available forms include: Caps 15, 30 mg
Side effects/adverse reactions:
▼ *ORAL:* Dry mouth (infrequent)
CNS: Lethargy, drowsiness, daytime sedation, dizziness, confusion, light-headedness, headache, anxiety, irritability
CV: Chest pain, pulse changes
GI: Nausea, vomiting, diarrhea, heartburn, abdominal pain, constipation
HEMA: ***Leukopenia, granulocytopenia*** (rare)
Contraindications: Hypersensitivity to benzodiazepines, pregnancy category X, lactation, intermittent porphyria, uncontrolled pain, ritonavir
Precautions: Anemia, hepatic disease, renal disease, suicidal individuals, drug abuse, elderly, psychosis, child <15 yr
Pharmacokinetics:
PO: Onset 15-45 min, duration 7-8 hr, half-life 47-100 hr, additional 100 hr for active metabolites; metabolized by liver; excreted by kidneys (inactive/active metabolites); crosses placenta; excreted in breast milk
Drug interactions of concern to dentistry:
• Increased sedation: alcohol, CNS depressants
• Increased serum levels and prolonged effect of benzodiazepines: ketoconazole, itraconazole, fluconazole, and miconazole (systemic), indinavir

DENTAL CONSIDERATIONS
General:
• Assess salivary flow as a factor in caries, periodontal disease, and candidiasis.
• Psychologic and physical dependence may occur with chronic administration.
• Geriatric patients are more susceptible to drug effects; use lower dose.
Consultations:
• Medical consult may be required to assess disease control in the patient.
Teach patient/family:
• To avoid mouth rinses with high alcohol content due to drying effects

F

---

flurbiprofen
(flure-bi'proe-fen)
Ansaid
✤ Apo-Flurbiprofen, Froben, Froben SR, Nu-Flurbiprofen, Novo-Flurbiprofen
Drug class.: Nonsteroidal antiinflammatory

Action: Inhibits prostaglandin synthesis by interfering with cyclooxygenase needed for biosynthesis; possesses analgesic, antiinflammatory, antipyretic properties
Uses: Acute, long-term treatment of rheumatoid arthritis, osteoarthritis; unapproved use: mild-to-moderate pain
Dosage and routes:
• *Adult:* PO 200-300 mg daily in divided doses bid, tid, or qid
Available forms include: Tabs 50, 100 mg
Side effects/adverse reactions:
▼ *ORAL:* Dry mouth, stomatitis, lichenoid reaction

CNS: Dizziness, drowsiness, fatigue, tremors, confusion, anxiety, myalgia, insomnia, depression, convulsions, malaise, nervousness, paresthesias

CV: Tachycardia, peripheral edema, palpitation, chest pain

GI: ***Jaundice, cholestatic hepatitis,*** nausea, anorexia, vomiting, diarrhea, constipation, flatulence, cramps, peptic ulcer, dyspepsia, indigestion

RESP: ***Bronchospasm,*** dyspnea, hemoptysis, rhinitis, shortness of breath

HEMA: ***Blood dyscrasias, bone marrow depression***

GU: ***Nephrotoxicity: dysuria, hematuria, oliguria, azotemia, cystitis, UTI, nocturia, renal insufficiency***

EENT: Tinnitus, hearing loss, blurred vision

INTEG: Purpura, rash, pruritus, erythema, urticaria, petechiae, ecchymosis, photosensitivity, exfoliative dermatitis, alopecia, eczema

Contraindications: Hypersensitivity, hypersensitivity to other antiinflammatory agents

Precautions: Pregnancy category B, first or second trimester, lactation, children, bleeding disorders, GI disorders, cardiac disorders, severe renal disease, severe hepatic disease

Pharmacokinetics:

PO: Peak 1.5 hr, half-life 6 hr; metabolized in liver; excreted in urine (metabolites), breast milk

Drug interactions of concern to dentistry:

- GI ulceration, bleeding: aspirin, alcohol, corticosteroids
- Decreased action: salicylates
- Nephrotoxicity: acetaminophen (prolonged use)

When prescribed for dental pain:

- Risk of increased effects: oral anticoagulants, oral antidiabetics, lithium, methotrexate
- Decreased effects of diuretics

DENTAL CONSIDERATIONS

General:

- Patients on chronic drug therapy may rarely have symptoms of blood dyscrasias, which can include infection, bleeding, and poor healing.
- Assess salivary flow as a factor in caries, periodontal disease, and candidiasis.
- Avoid prescribing for dental use in last trimester of pregnancy.
- Avoid prescribing aspirin-containing products.
- Consider semisupine chair position for patients with arthritic disease.

Consultations:

- Medical consult may be required to assess disease control in the patient.
- In a patient with symptoms of blood dyscrasias, request a medical consult for blood studies and postpone dental treatment until normal values are reestablished.

Teach patient/family:

- Importance of good oral hygiene to prevent soft tissue inflammation
- Caution to prevent injury when using oral hygiene aids

When chronic dry mouth occurs, advise patient:

- To avoid mouth rinses with high alcohol content due to drying effects
- To use daily home fluoride products for anticaries effect
- To use sugarless gum, frequent sips of water, or saliva substitutes

flurbiprofen sodium

(flure-bi′proe-fen)
Ocufen

Drug class.: Nonsteroidal antiinflammatory ophthalmic

Action: Inhibits enzyme system necessary for biosynthesis of prostaglandins; inhibits miosis
Uses: Inhibition of intraoperative miosis, corneal edema
Dosage and routes:
• *Adult:* 1 gtt q0.5h 2 hr before surgery (4 gtt total)
Available forms include: Sol 0.03%
Side effects/adverse reactions:
EENT: Burning, stinging in the eye, eye irritation/bleeding/redness
Contraindications: Hypersensitivity, epithelial herpes simplex keratitis
Precautions: Pregnancy category C, lactation, child, aspirin or nonsteroidal antiinflammatory drug hypersensitivity, allergy, bleeding disorder
DENTAL CONSIDERATIONS
General:
• Avoid dental light in patient's eyes; offer dark glasses for patient comfort.

flutamide

(floo′ta-mide)
Eulexin
✤ Euflex

Drug class.: Antineoplastic

Action: Interferes with testosterone at the cellular level; inhibits androgen uptake by inhibiting nuclear binding or by interfering with androgen in target tissues
Uses: Metastatic prostatic carcinoma, stage D2; early-stage prostate cancer, stages B2 and C, in combination with LHRH agonistic analogs (leuprolide) and radiation
Dosage and routes:
• *Adult:* PO 250 mg q8h, for a daily dose of 750 mg
Available forms include: Cap 125 mg
Side effects/adverse reactions:
CNS: Hot flashes, drowsiness, confusion, depression, anxiety
GI: Diarrhea, nausea, vomiting, ***hepatitis,*** increased liver function studies, anorexia
GU: Decreased libido, impotence, gynecomastia
INTEG: Irritation at site, rash, photosensitivity
MISC: Edema, hematopoietic symptoms, neuromuscular and pulmonary symptoms, hypertension
Contraindications: Hypersensitivity, severe hepatic impairment, pregnancy category D
Precautions: Liver toxicity, monitoring requirements for hepatic injury, women
Pharmacokinetics: Rapidly and completely absorbed, half-life 6 hr, geriatric half-life 8 hr; 94% bound to plasma proteins; excreted in urine and feces as metabolites
DENTAL CONSIDERATIONS
General:
• Talk with patient about any pain medication being taken.
• Avoid drugs (anticholinergics) that could exacerbate urinary retention (if present).

fluticasone propionate

(floo-tik'a-sone)
Cutivate (topical), Flonase (nasal spray), Flovent (inhaler)
Drug class.: Synthetic corticosteroid, medium potency

Action: Glucocorticoids have multiple actions that include antiinflammatory and immunosuppressant effects. They inhibit phospholipase A_2, interfering with or reducing the synthesis of prostaglandins and leukotrienes. They also bind to cytoplasmic glucocorticoid receptors (GRs) and enter the cell nucleus to bind with DNA. This results in the synthesis of various enzymes such as collagenase, elastase, and cytokines that play important roles in inflammation and immunosuppression. They also suppress the production of lymphocytes, monocytes, and eosinophils.
Uses: Topical for inflammation of corticosteroid-responsive skin disorders, eczema; spray for seasonal and perennial allergic rhinitis; inhaler for asthma
Dosage and routes:
• *Adult:* TOP apply to affected areas bid, 0.05% cream once daily dosing; instill nasal spray, 2 sprays in each nostril once daily; initial dose can also be given in 2 equal doses bid; reduce to 1 spray for maintenance; inh 1 puff bid
• *Child >12 yr:* Instill nasal spray, 1 spray in each nostril
Available forms include: Oint 0.005%; cream 0.05%; nasal spray 50 μg per actuation; inhaler 44, 110, 220 μg per puff
Side effects/adverse reactions:
INTEG: Burning, dryness, itching, irritation, acne, folliculitis, hypertrichosis, perioral dermatitis, hypopigmentation, atrophy, striae, miliaria, allergic contact dermatitis, secondary infections
Contraindications: Hypersensitivity, viral and fungal infections
Precautions: Pregnancy category C, lactation, bacterial infections; avoid spray in child <12 yr
DENTAL CONSIDERATIONS
General:
• Examine oral cavity for evidence of opportunistic candidiasis in patients using the spray.
• Allergic rhinitis may be a factor in mouth breathing and drying of oral tissues.
Teach patient/family:
• That use of topical preparations on herpetic ulcerations is contraindicated
• Importance of gargling, rinsing mouth with water, and expectorating after each aerosol use

fluvastatin sodium

(floo'va-sta-tin)
Lescol
Drug class.: Cholesterol-lowering agent, antihyperlipidemic

Action: Inhibits HMG-CoA reductase enzyme, which reduces cholesterol synthesis
Uses: As an adjunct in primary hypercholesterolemia (types IIa and IIb); slow progression of coronary atherosclerosis
Dosage and routes:
• *Adult:* PO 20 mg hs; dosage range 20-80 mg/day; new approved dosing 40 mg bid

Available forms include: Caps 20, 40 mg
Side effects/adverse reactions:
▼ *ORAL:* Taste alteration (rare)
CNS: Fatigue, headache, dizziness, insomnia
GI: Nausea, diarrhea, dyspepsia, abdominal pain, constipation, flatulence, elevated transaminase levels
RESP: Upper respiratory infection, bronchitis, coughing
GU: Decreased libido
EENT: Rhinitis, sinusitis, pharyngitis
INTEG: Rash, pruritus
MS: Muscle pain, back pain, arthropathy, ***rhabdomyolysis,*** myopathy
MISC: Photosensitivity, ***anaphylaxis***
Contraindications: Hypersensitivity, active liver disease, pregnancy, lactation, child <18 yr
Precautions: Pregnancy category X; liver dysfunction; alcoholism; severe acute infection; metabolic, endocrine, or electrolyte disorders; uncontrolled seizures; alterations in liver function tests may be observed with use
Pharmacokinetics:
PO: Good absorption; first-pass metabolism; highly protein bound, hepatic metabolism; excreted in feces
Drug interactions of concern to dentistry:
• No specific interactions reported but (as with other drugs in this class) should not be used with erythromycin, itraconazole, or cyclosporine
DENTAL CONSIDERATIONS
General:
• Consider semisupine chair position for patient comfort due to GI, musculoskeletal, and respiratory side effects.

fluvoxamine maleate

(floo-vox′a-meen)
✤ Luvox
Drug class.: Selective serotonin reuptake inhibitor, antidepressant

Action: Selectively inhibits the reuptake of serotonin in CNS neurons
Uses: Obsessive-compulsive disorder and panic disorder
Dosage and routes:
• *Adult:* PO initial dose 50 mg hs, increase by 50 mg increments slowly q4-7d as required in 2 divided doses; limit 300 mg/day
Available forms include: Tabs 25, 50, 100 mg
Side effects/adverse reactions:
▼ *ORAL: Dry mouth,* dysphagia, increased salivation (rare)
CNS: Somnolence, asthenia, nervousness, dizziness, headache, agitation, anxiety, suicidal ideation, anorexia
CV: Postural hypotension, palpitation, hypertension, syncope, tachycardia
GI: Nausea, dyspepsia, diarrhea
GU: Sexual dysfunction
RESP: Dyspnea
MS: Dystonic symptoms
Contraindications: Hypersensitivity, MAO inhibitors, terfenadine, astemizole, alcohol
Precautions: Pregnancy category C, lactation, renal and hepatic impairment, epilepsy
Pharmacokinetics:
PO: Rapid absorption, peak plasma levels 5 hr; plasma protein binding

77%; hepatic metabolism; urinary excretion

Drug interactions of concern to dentistry:

• Increased plasma levels of tricyclic antidepressants, carbamazepine, benzodiazepines, terfenadine, astemizole; reduce doses of alprazolam, diazepam, midazolam, and triazolam by one half

DENTAL CONSIDERATIONS

General:

• After supine positioning, have patient sit upright for at least 2 min to avoid orthostatic hypotension.

• Assess salivary flow as a factor in caries, periodontal disease, and candidiasis.

• Consider semisupine chair position for patient comfort due to GI effects of drug.

Consultations:

• Medical consult may be required to assess patient's ability to tolerate stress.

• Physician should be informed if significant xerostomic side effects occur (increased caries, sore tongue, problems eating or swallowing, difficulty wearing prosthesis) so a medication change can be considered.

Teach patient/family:

When chronic dry mouth occurs, advise patient:

• To avoid mouth rinses with high alcohol content due to drying effects

• To use daily home fluoride products for anticaries effect

• To use sugarless gum, frequent sips of water, or saliva substitutes

folic acid (vitamin B_9)

(foe'lic)

Folvite

Apo-Folic, Novo-Folacid

Drug class.: Water-soluble B vitamin

Action: Needed for erythropoiesis; increases RBC, WBC, and platelet formation in megaloblastic anemias

Uses: Megaloblastic or macrocytic anemia caused by folic acid deficiency; liver disease; alcoholism; hemolysis; intestinal obstruction; pregnancy

Dosage and routes:

Chemical supplement

• *Adult:* PO/IM/SC 0.1 mg qd

• *Child:* PO 0.05 mg qd

Megaloblastic/macrocytic anemia

• *Adult and child >4 yr:* PO/SC/IM 1 mg qd × 4-5 days

• *Child <4 yr:* PO/SC/IM 0.3 mg or less qd

• *Pregnancy/lactation:* PO/SC/IM 0.8 mg qd

Prevention of megaloblastic/macrocytic anemia

• *Pregnancy:* PO/SC/IM 1 mg qd

Available forms include: Tabs 0.1, 0.4, 0.8, 1 mg; inj SC/IM 5, 10 mg/ml

Side effects/adverse reactions:

RESP: ***Bronchospasm*** (rare allergic reaction)

Contraindications: Hypersensitivity, anemias other than megaloblastic/macrocytic anemia, vitamin B_{12} deficiency anemia

Precautions: Pregnancy category A

Pharmacokinetics:

PO: Peak 0.5-1 hr; bound to plasma proteins; excreted in breast milk;

methylated in liver; excreted in urine (small amounts)

Drug interactions of concern to dentistry:

• Increased metabolism of phenobarbital

DENTAL CONSIDERATIONS

General:

• Deficiency in folic acid; glossitis may be a symptom of folic acid deficiency.

foscarnet sodium/ phosphonoformic acid

(foss-car′net)

Foscavir

Drug class.: Antiviral

Action: Antiviral activity is produced by selective inhibition at the pyrophosphate binding site of viral DNA polymerase, preventing replication of herpes simplex virus (HSV)

Uses: Treatment of cytomegalovirus (CMV) retinitis in AIDS; unapproved use: life-threatening CMV disease, acyclovir-resistant herpes simplex I mucocutaneous diseases and acyclovir-resistant HSV in immunocompromised patients

Dosage and routes:

• *Adult:* IV inf 60 mg/kg given over at least 1 hr q8h × 2-3 wk initially, then 90-120 mg/kg/day over 2 hr

HSV

• *Adult:* IV inf 40 mg/kg bid × 3 wk

Available forms include: Inj 24 mg/ml in 250, 500 ml bottles

Side effects/adverse reactions:

▼ *ORAL:* Glossitis, stomatitis, facial edema, dry mouth, ulcerative stomatitis, taste perversion

CNS: ***Seizures, coma, paralysis, tetany,*** fever, dizziness, headache, fatigue, neuropathy, tremor, ataxia, dementia, stupor, EEG abnormalities, vertigo, abnormal gait, hypertonia, extrapyramidal disorders, hemiparesis, hyperreflexia paraplegia, hyporeflexia, neuralgia, neuritis, cerebral edema, paresthesia, depression, confusion, anxiety, insomnia, somnolence, amnesia, hallucinations, agitation

CV: ***Cardiac arrest,*** hypertension, palpitations, ECG abnormalities, first-degree AV block, nonspecific ST-T segment changes, hypotension, cerebrovascular disorder, cardiomyopathy, bradycardia, dysrhythmias

GI: ***Pseudomembranous colitis, paralytic ileus, esophageal ulceration, hepatitis,*** nausea, vomiting, anorexia, abdominal pain, constipation, dysphagia, rectal hemorrhage, melena, flatulence, pancreatitis, enteritis, enterocolitis, proctitis, increased amylases, gastroenteritis, duodenal ulcer, abnormal A-G ratio, increased AST/ALT, cholecystitis, dyspepsia, tenesmus, hepatosplenomegaly, jaundice

RESP: ***Pulmonary infiltration, pneumothorax, hemoptysis, bronchospasm, respiratory depression, pleural effusion, pulmonary hemorrhage,*** rhinitis, coughing, dyspnea, pneumonia, sinusitis, pharyngitis, bronchitis, stridor

HEMA: ***Granulocytopenia, leukopenia, thrombocytopenia, thrombosis, pulmonary embolism, coagulation disorders, decreased prothrombin, hypochromic anemia, pancytopenia, hemolysis, leukocytosis,*** lymphadenopathy, epistaxis, lymphopenia, anemia, platelet abnormalities

GU: ***Acute renal failure, glomeru-***

lonephritis, toxic nephropathy, nephrosis, renal tubular disorders, pyelonephritis, uremia, hematuria, albuminuria, dysuria, polyuria, decreased CCr, increased serum creatinine

EENT: Visual field defects, vocal cord paralysis, speech disorders, eye pain, conjunctivitis, tinnitus, otitis

INTEG: Rash, sweating, pruritus, skin ulceration, seborrhea, skin discoloration, alopecia, acne, dermatitis, pain/inflammation at injection site, facial edema, dry skin, urticaria

MS: Arthralgia, myalgia

SYST: ***Sepsis, death, ascites,*** hypokalemia, hypocalcemia, hypomagnesemia, increased alk phosphatase, LDH, BUN, acidosis, hypophosphatemia, hyperphosphatemia, dehydration, glycosuria, increased creatine phosphokinase, hypervolemia, infection, hyponatremia, hypochloremia, hypercalcemia

Contraindications: Hypersensitivity

Precautions: Pregnancy category C, lactation, children, elderly, renal disease, seizure disorders, electrolyte/mineral imbalances, severe anemia

Pharmacokinetics:

IV: Half-life 2-8 hr in normal renal function; 14%-17% plasma protein bound

Drug interactions of concern to dentistry:

- No specific interactions, but nephrotoxic drugs (acyclovir) should be avoided

DENTAL CONSIDERATIONS

General:

- Examine for oral manifestations of opportunistic infections.
- Examine for evidence of oral manifestations of blood dyscrasias (infection, bleeding, poor healing).
- Consider local hemostasis measures to prevent excessive bleeding.
- Assess salivary flow as a factor in caries, periodontal disease, and candidiasis.
- Monitor vital signs every appointment due to cardiovascular and respiratory side effects.
- Place on frequent recall to evaluate healing response.

Consultations:

- Medical consult for blood studies (CBC); leukopenic or thrombocytopenic side effects may result in infection, delayed healing, and excessive bleeding. Postpone elective dental treatment until normal values are maintained.
- Medical consult may be required to assess disease control in the patient.

Teach patient/family:

- Caution in use of oral hygiene aids to prevent injury
- That secondary oral infection may occur; must see dentist immediately if infection occurs
- Importance of good oral hygiene to prevent soft tissue inflammation
- Use of electric toothbrush if patient has difficulty holding conventional devices due to extrapyramidal side effects

When chronic dry mouth occurs, advise patient:

- To avoid mouth rinses with high alcohol content due to drying effects
- To use daily home fluoride products for anticaries effect
- To use sugarless gum, frequent sips of water, or saliva substitutes

fosfomycin tromethamine

(fos-foe-mye'sin)
Monurol

Drug class.: Antiinfective (phosphonic acid derivative)

Action: Broad-spectrum and bactericidal against a wide range of gram-positive aerobic microorganisms associated with GU infections; inactivates the enzyme diphosphate acetylglucosamine to interfere with cell wall synthesis
Uses: Uncomplicated UTIs in women due to susceptible strains of *E. coli* and *Enterococcus faecalis*
Dosage and routes:
• *Women >18 yr:* PO one sachet with or without food; mix contents of one sachet with water to take
Available forms include: Sachet 3 g
Side effects/adverse reactions:
▼ *ORAL:* Dry mouth (<1%)
CNS: Headache, dizziness, migraine, somnolence
GI: Diarrhea, nausea, dyspepsia
RESP: Asthma (rare)
HEMA: ***Angioedema (rare), aplastic anemia***
GU: Vaginitis
EENT: Rhinitis, pharyngitis
INTEG: Rash
ENDO: Menstrual disorder
MS: Asthenia, myalgia
MISC: Fever
Contraindications: Hypersensitivity
Precautions: Renal impairment, one dose per single episode of cystitis, pregnancy category B, lactation, children <12 yr
Pharmacokinetics:
PO: Peak plasma levels >2 hr; not plasma protein bound; widely distributed to GU tissues; excreted unchanged in urine and feces
Drug interactions of concern to dentistry:
• Lowered serum concentrations: metoclopramide
DENTAL CONSIDERATIONS
General:
• Determine why patient is taking the drug.
• Consider semisupine chair position for patient comfort if GI side effects occur.
Teach patient/family:
When chronic dry mouth occurs, advise patient:
• To avoid mouth rinses with high alcohol content due to drying effects
• To use daily home fluoride products for anticaries effect
• To use sugarless gum, frequent sips of water, or saliva substitutes

fosinopril

(foe-sin'oh-pril)
Monopril

Drug class.: Angiotension-converting enzyme (ACE) inhibitor

Action: Selectively suppresses renin-angiotensin-aldosterone system; inhibits ACE; prevents conversion of angiotensin I to angiotensin II; results in dilation of arterial, venous vessels
Uses: Hypertension, alone or in combination with thiazide diuretics
Dosage and routes:
• *Adult:* PO 10 mg qd initially, then 20-40 mg/day divided bid or qd
Available forms include: Tabs 10, 20 mg

Side effects/adverse reactions:
▼ *ORAL:* Taste disturbances, angioedema (lips, tongue), dry mouth
CNS: Insomnia, paresthesia, headache, dizziness, fatigue, memory disturbance, tremor, mood change
CV: Hypotension, chest pain, palpitation, angina, orthostatic hypotension
GI: Nausea, constipation, vomiting, diarrhea
RESP: ***Bronchospasm,*** cough, sinusitis, dyspnea
HEMA: ***Eosinophilia, leukopenia, neutropenia,*** decreased Hct/Hgb
GU: ***Proteinuria,*** increased BUN/creatinine, decreased libido
INTEG: ***Angioedema,*** rash, flushing, sweating, photosensitivity, pruritus
MS: Arthralgia, myalgia
META: Hyperkalemia

Contraindications: Hypersensitivity to ACE inhibitors, pregnancy category D, lactation, children

Precautions: Impaired liver function, hypovolemia, blood dyscrasias, CHF, COPD, asthma, elderly

Pharmacokinetics:
PO: Onset 1 hr, peak 3 hr, half-life 12 hr; serum protein binding 97%; metabolized by liver (metabolites excreted in urine, feces)

Drug interactions of concern to dentistry:
- Increased hypotension: alcohol, phenothiazines
- Decreased hypotensive effects: indomethacin and possibly other NSAIDs, sympathomimetics

DENTAL CONSIDERATIONS

General:
- Monitor vital signs every appointment due to cardiovascular and respiratory side effects.
- After supine positioning, have patient sit upright for at least 2 min before standing to avoid orthostatic hypotension.
- Patients on chronic drug therapy may rarely have symptoms of blood dyscrasias, which can include infection, bleeding, and poor healing.
- Assess salivary flow as a factor in caries, periodontal disease, and candidiasis.
- Limit use of sodium-containing products such as saline IV fluids for patients with a dietary salt restriction.
- Stress from dental procedures may compromise cardiovascular function; determine patient risk.
- Short appointments and a stress reduction protocol may be required for anxious patients.

Consultations:
- Medical consult may be required to assess disease control and patient's ability to tolerate stress.
- In a patient with symptoms of blood dyscrasias, request a medical consult for blood studies and postpone dental treatment until normal values are reestablished.
- Take precautions if dental surgery is anticipated and sedation or general anesthesia is required (risk of hypotensive episode).

Teach patient/family:
- Importance of good oral hygiene to prevent soft tissue inflammation
- Caution to prevent injury when using oral hygiene aids

When chronic dry mouth occurs, advise patient:
- To avoid mouth rinses with high alcohol content due to drying effects
- To use daily home fluoride products for anticaries effect

• To use sugarless gum, frequent sips of water, or saliva substitutes

fosphenytoin sodium

(fos'fen-i-toyn)
Cerebyx

Drug class.: Hydantoin-anticonvulsant

Action: Prodrug converted to phenytoin after injection; phenytoin inhibits spread of seizure activity in motor cortex

Uses: Control of generalized convulsive status epilepticus; prevention and treatment of seizures during neurosurgery; short-term substitute for oral phenytoin

Dosage and routes:

• *Adult:* IV loading dose, 15-20 mg phenytoin sodium equivalents (PE/kg) at 100-150 mg PE/min; effect is not immediate, may require use of IV benzodiazepine

• *Adult:* IV maintenance dose, IM 4-6 mg/PE/kg per day

Substitution for oral phenytoin

• *Adult:* IV, IM at the same total daily dose for phenytoin

Available forms include: Inj 10 ml (750 mg of fosphenytoin sodium equivalent to 500 mg phenytoin); 2 ml (150 mg of fosphenytoin equivalent to 100 mg of phenytoin)

Side effects/adverse reactions:

▼ *ORAL:* Dry mouth, taste perversion, gingival overgrowth

CNS: Nystagmus, dizziness, paresthesia, headache, somnolence, ataxia, tremor, extrapyramidal syndrome

CV: Hypotension, bradycardia, vasodilation, tachycardia

GI: Nausea, vomiting, constipation

HEMA: ***Thrombocytopenia, anemia, leukopenia,*** petechia

EENT: Tinnitus, diplopia

INTEG: Pruritus, rash

MS: Asthenia, back pain

META: Hypokalemia

Contraindications: Hypersensitivity to hydantoin drugs; sinus bradycardia, S-A block, second- and third-degree AV block; Adams-Stokes syndrome, abrupt discontinuation

Precautions: IV—do not exceed injection rate of 150 mg PE/min, risk of seizures with abrupt withdrawal; hypotension, severe myocardial insufficiency, phosphate restriction; thyroid, renal, or hepatic disease; elderly, pregnancy category D, lactation, pediatric use

Pharmacokinetics:

IV: Highly protein bound (95%-99%); converted to phenytoin; metabolized in liver; renal excretion

IM: Completely bioavailable, peak levels 30 min

Drug interactions of concern to dentistry:

• Increased phenytoin levels: benzodiazepines (chlordiazepoxide, diazepam), halothane, salicylates

• Increased CNS depression: benzodiazepines, H_1-blocker antihistamines, opiate agonists

• Decreased phenytoin levels: carbamazepine

• Decreased effectiveness of corticosteroids

DENTAL CONSIDERATIONS

General:

• This drug is intended for short-term use in an emergency department or hospital setting. Patient will probably return to oral phenytoin or other anticonvulsant after hospital care.

• Use precaution if sedation or general anesthesia is required; risk of hypotensive episode.

Consultations:

• Determine type of epilepsy, seizure frequency, and quality of seizure control. A stress reduction protocol may be required.

• Medical consult may be required to assess disease control and patient's ability to tolerate stress.

Teach patient/family:

• Importance of updating health and drug history if physician makes any changes in evaluation/drug regimens

---

furosemide

(fur-oh'se-mide)

Furoside, Lasix, Lasix Special, Myrosemide

✤ Apo-Furosemide, Novosemide, Uritol

Drug class.: Loop diuretic

Action: Acts on loop of Henle to decrease the reabsorption of chloride and sodium with resultant diuresis

Uses: Pulmonary edema, edema in CHF, liver disease, nephrotic syndrome, ascites, hypertension

Dosage and routes:

• *Adult:* PO 20-80 mg/day in AM, may give another dose in 6 hr, up to 600 mg/day; IM/IV 20-40 mg, increased by 20 mg q2h until desired response

• *Child:* PO/IM/IV 2 mg/kg, may increase by 1-2 mg/kg q6-8h up to 6 mg/kg

Pulmonary edema

• *Adult:* IV 40 mg given over several minutes, repeated in 1 hr; increase to 80 mg if needed

Available forms include: Tabs 20, 40, 80 mg; oral sol 10 mg/ml; inj IM/IV 10 mg/ml

Side effects/adverse reactions:

▼ *ORAL:* Dry mouth, increased thirst, lichenoid drug reaction

CNS: Headache, fatigue, weakness, vertigo, paresthesia

CV: ***Circulatory collapse,*** orthostatic hypotension, chest pain, ECG changes

GI: Nausea, diarrhea, vomiting, anorexia, cramps, gastric irritations, pancreatitis

HEMA: ***Thrombocytopenia, agranulocytosis, leukopenia, neutropenia, anemia***

GU: Polyuria, ***renal failure,*** glycosuria

EENT: Loss of hearing, ear pain, tinnitus, blurred vision

INTEG: Rash, pruritus, ***Stevens-Johnson syndrome,*** purpura, sweating, photosensitivity, urticaria

ENDO: Hyperglycemia

MS: Cramps, arthritis, stiffness

ELECT: Hypokalemia, hypochloremic alkalosis, hypomagnesemia, hyperuricemia, hypocalcemia, hyponatremia

Contraindications: Hypersensitivity to sulfonamides, anuria, hypovolemia, infants, lactation, electrolyte depletion; cisapride

Precautions: Diabetes mellitus, dehydration, ascites, severe renal disease, pregnancy category C

Pharmacokinetics:

PO: Onset 1 hr, peak 1-2 hr, duration 6-8 hr

IV: Onset 5 min, peak 0.5 hr, duration 2 hr

Excreted in urine, feces, breast milk; crosses placenta

Drug interactions of concern to dentistry:

• Increased electrolyte imbalance: corticosteroids

• Masked ototoxicity: phenothiazines
• Decreased antihypertensive effect: NSAIDs, especially indomethacin

DENTAL CONSIDERATIONS

General:

• Monitor vital signs every appointment due to cardiovascular side effects.
• Patients on chronic drug therapy may rarely have symptoms of blood dyscrasias, which can include infection, bleeding, and poor healing.
• Assess salivary flow as a factor in caries, periodontal disease, and candidiasis.
• After supine positioning, have patient sit upright for at least 2 min before standing to avoid orthostatic hypotension.
• Patients on high-potency diuretics should be monitored for serum K^+ levels.

Consultations:

• In a patient with symptoms of blood dyscrasias, request a medical consult for blood studies and postpone dental treatment until normal values are reestablished.
• Medical consult may be required to assess disease control in the patient.

Teach patient/family:

• Importance of good oral hygiene to prevent soft tissue inflammation
• Caution to prevent injury when using oral hygiene aids

When chronic dry mouth occurs, advise patient:

• To use daily home fluoride products for anticaries effect
• To avoid mouth rinses with high alcohol content due to drying effects
• To use sugarless gum, frequent sips of water, or saliva substitutes

gabapentin

(ga'ba-pen-tin)
Neurontin

Drug class.: Anticonvulsant

Action: Anticonvulsant action is unclear

Uses: Adjunctive therapy in adults with partial seizures; unlabeled use: neuropathic pain

Dosage and routes:

• *Adult and child >12 yr:* PO titration to 900-1800 mg/day in 3 equal doses; start 300 mg on day 1, 300 mg bid on day 2, 300 mg tid on day 3, can be increased to 1800 mg/day with titration of doses; doses up to 3600 mg/day have been used

Available forms include: Caps 100, 300, 400 mg

Side effects/adverse reactions:

▼ *ORAL:* Dry mouth, glossitis, gingivitis, stomatitis (infrequent)
CNS: Somnolence, dizziness, ataxia, fatigue, nystagmus
CV: Hypertension, palpitation, tachycardia
GI: Dyspepsia, constipation
RESP: Pharyngitis, coughing
HEMA: Leukopenia, purpura
GU: Impotence
EENT: Rhinitis, blurred vision
INTEG: Pruritus
MS: Myalgia
MISC: Edema

Contraindications: Hypersensitivity

Precautions: Pregnancy category C, lactation, renal function impairment, children <12 yr, elderly

Pharmacokinetics: Bioavailability decreases as dose increases; low protein binding 3%; renal excretion primary

Drug interactions of concern to dentistry:

• None reported at this time, but, because CNS side effects are common, the use of anxiolytic sedative drugs may potentially increase the CNS side effects.

DENTAL CONSIDERATIONS

General:

• Early-morning appointments and a stress reduction protocol may be required for anxious patients.

• Place on frequent recall due to oral side effects.

• Monitor vital signs every appointment due to cardiovascular side effects.

• Assess salivary flow as a factor in caries, periodontal disease, and candidiasis.

• Determine type of epilepsy and quality of seizure control.

Consultations:

• Medical consult may be required to assess disease control in the patient.

• Medical consult may be required to assess patient's ability to tolerate stress.

Teach patient/family:

• Importance of good oral hygiene to prevent soft tissue inflammation

• Caution in use of oral hygiene aids to prevent injury

When chronic dry mouth occurs, advise patient:

• To avoid mouth rinses with high alcohol content due to drying effects

• To use daily home fluoride products for anticaries effect

• To use sugarless gum, frequent sips of water, or saliva substitutes

---

ganciclovir

(gan-sye'kloe-veer)

Cytovene, Cytovene IV, DHPG, Vitrasert implant

Drug class.: Antiviral, nucleoside analog

Action: Inhibits replication of most herpes viruses in vitro; phosphorylated by CMV protein kinase to triphosphate forms; inhibits viral DNA polymerase and is incorporated into viral DNA, resulting in termination of elongation of viral DNA

Uses: Prevention and treatment of CMV retinitis in patients with AIDS or organ transplants; unapproved use: life-threatening CMV disease and CMV polyradiculopathy in patients with AIDS

Dosage and routes:

Induction treatment

• *Adult:* IV 5 mg/kg given over 1 hr, q12h × 2-3 wk

Maintenance treatment

• *Adult:* IV inf 5 mg/kg given over 1 hr, qd × 7 days/wk; or 6 mg/kg qd × 5 days/wk; dosage must be reduced in renal impairment

• *Adult:* PO 1000 mg tid with food or 500 mg q3h (for 6 doses) during waking hours and with food

Available forms include: Caps 250 mg; vials 500 mg; intraocular implant

Side effects/adverse reactions:

CNS: Fever, ***coma,*** chills, confusion, abnormal thoughts, dizziness, bizarre dreams, headache, psychosis, tremors, somnolence, paresthesia

CV: Dysrhythmia, hypertension/hypotension

GI: Abnormal LFTs, ***hemorrhage,*** nausea, vomiting, anorexia, diarrhea, abdominal pain
RESP: Dyspnea
HEMA: ***Granulocytopenia, thrombocytopenia, irreversible neutropenia, anemia, eosinophilia***
GU: ***Hematuria,*** increased creatinine/BUN
EENT: Retinal detachment in CMV retinitis
INTEG: Rash, alopecia, pruritus, urticaria, pain at site, phlebitis
Contraindications: Hypersensitivity to acyclovir or ganciclovir
Precautions: Preexisting cytopenias, renal function impairment, pregnancy category C, lactation, children <6 mo, elderly, platelet count <25,000/mm^3
Pharmacokinetics:
PO/IV: Half-life 3-4.5 hr; excreted by the kidneys (unchanged drug); crosses blood-brain barrier
Drug interactions of concern to dentistry:
• Increased risk of blood dyscrasias: dapsone, carbamazepine, phenothiazines
• Increased risk of seizures: imipenem/cilastatin (Primaxin)
• Low platelet counts may prevent the use of aspirin, NSAIDs

DENTAL CONSIDERATIONS
General:
• Examine for oral manifestations of opportunistic infection.
• Examine for evidence of oral manifestations of blood dyscrasias (infection, bleeding, poor healing).
• Place on frequent recall to evaluate healing response.
• Consider local hemostasis measures to prevent excessive bleeding.
• Monitor vital signs every appointment due to cardiovascular and respiratory side effects.
Consultations:
• Medical consult for blood studies (CBC); leukopenic or thrombocytopenic side effects may result in infection, delayed healing, and excessive bleeding. Postpone elective dental treatment until normal values are maintained.
• Medical consult may be required to assess disease control in the patient.
Teach patient/family:
• Caution in use of oral hygiene aids to prevent injury
• That secondary oral infection may occur; must see dentist immediately if infection occurs
• Importance of good oral hygiene to prevent soft tissue inflammation

gemfibrozil

(jem-fi'broe-zil)
Lopid, Nu-Gemfibrozil
🍁 Apo-Gemfibrozil, Gen-Fibro, Novo-Gemfibrozil
Drug class.: Antihyperlipidemic

Action: Reduces plasma triglyceride and very-low-density lipoprotein (VLDL) levels, possibly through inhibition of peripheral lypolysis and decreased hepatic extraction of free fatty acids; HDL levels increase
Uses: Type IIb, IV, V hyperlipidemia
Dosage and routes:
• *Adult:* PO 1200 mg in divided doses bid 30 min before meals
Available forms include: Tabs 600 mg, caps 300 mg

Side effects/adverse reactions:
CNS: Dizziness, blurred vision
GI: Nausea, vomiting, dyspepsia, diarrhea, abdominal pain
HEMA: ***Leukopenia, anemia, eosinophilia***
INTEG: Rash, urticaria, pruritus
Contraindications: Severe hepatic disease, preexisting gallbladder disease, severe renal disease, primary biliary cirrhosis, hypersensitivity
Precautions: Monitor hematologic and hepatic function, pregnancy category B, lactation
Pharmacokinetics:
PO: Peak 1-2 hr, half-life 1.5 hr; plasma protein binding >90%; excreted in urine; metabolized in liver
DENTAL CONSIDERATIONS
General:
• Patients on chronic drug therapy may rarely have symptoms of blood dyscrasias, which can include infection, bleeding, and poor healing.
Consultations:
• In a patient with symptoms of blood dyscrasias, request a medical consult for blood studies and postpone dental treatment until normal values are reestablished.

---

gentamicin sulfate (ophthalmic)

(jen-ta-mye'sin)
Garamycin Ophthalmic, Genoptic, Genoptic SOP, Gentacidin, Gentak
Drug class.: Aminoglycoside anti-infective ophthalmic

Action: Inhibits bacterial protein synthesis
Uses: Infection of external eye
Dosage and routes:
• *Adult and child:* Instill 1 gtt q4h; top apply oint to conjunctival sac bid (can use 1 gtt qh for severe infections)
Available forms include: Oint, sol 3%
Side effects/adverse reactions:
EENT: Poor corneal wound healing, temporary visual haze, overgrowth of nonsusceptible organisms
Contraindications: Hypersensitivity
Precautions: Antibiotic hypersensitivity, pregnancy category C
DENTAL CONSIDERATIONS
General:
• Avoid dental light in patient's eyes; offer dark glasses for patient comfort.
• Protect patient's eyes from accidental spatter during dental treatment.

---

glimepiride

(glye'me-pye-ride)
Amaryl
Drug class.: Oral antidiabetic (second generation)

Action: Causes functioning β-cells in pancreas to release insulin, leading to drop in blood glucose levels; may also play a role in increased sensitivity of peripheral tissues to insulin
Uses: Stable adult-onset diabetes mellitus (type II); may also be used with insulin or metformin where diet and exercise are not effective in controlling hyperglycemia
Dosage and routes:
• *Adult:* PO usual initial dose 1-2 mg once daily with breakfast or first meal of the day; maintenance

dose range 1-4 mg daily; max daily dose 8 mg; adjust dose increments at no more than 2 mg every 1-2 wk

Insulin supplementation

• *Adult:* PO 8 mg daily with first main meal; start low-dose insulin and adjust dose according to patient response

Available forms include: Tabs 1, 2, 4 mg

Side effects/adverse reactions:

CNS: Dizziness, headache

GI: Nausea, abdominal pain, cholestatic jaundice, vomiting, diarrhea

HEMA: ***Leukopenia, agranulocytosis, thrombocytopenia, hemolytic anemia, pancytopenia***

EENT: Blurred vision, changes in accommodation

INTEG: Pruritus, erythema, urticaria, rash, photosensitivity

META: Hyponatremia, hypoglycemia

MISC: Asthenia

Contraindications: Hypersensitivity, diabetic ketoacidosis

Precautions: Malnourished; adrenal, pituitary, or hepatic insufficiency; hypoglycemia recognition in elderly or in those taking β-blockers; increased risk of cardiovascular mortality has been reported in patients using oral hypoglycemics; alcohol use; pregnancy category C, lactation; children

Pharmacokinetics:

PO: Good oral absorption, peak plasma levels 2-3 hr; plasma protein binding 99.5%; extensive hepatic metabolism; excreted in urine (60%) and feces (40%)

Drug interactions of concern to dentistry:

• Risk of potentiation of hypoglycemic effects: NSAIDs, salicylates, sulfonamides, β-adrenergic blockers

DENTAL CONSIDERATIONS

General:

• Short appointments and a stress reduction protocol may be required for anxious patients.

• Question patient about self-monitoring of drug's antidiabetic effect, including blood glucose values or finger-stick records.

• Ensure that patient is following prescribed diet and regularly takes medication.

• Patients on chronic drug therapy may rarely have symptoms of blood dyscrasias, which can include infection, bleeding, and poor healing.

• Diabetics may be more susceptible to infection and have delayed wound healing.

• Place on frequent recall to evaluate healing response.

• Advise patient if dental drugs prescribed have a potential for photosensitivity.

Consultations:

• Medical consult may be required to assess disease control in the patient.

• In a patient with symptoms of blood dyscrasias, request a medical consult for blood studies and postpone treatment until normal values are reestablished.

• Medical consult may include data from patient's blood glucose monitoring, including glycosylated hemoglobin or HbA_{1c} testing.

Teach patient/family:

• Importance of good oral hygiene to prevent soft tissue inflammation

• Caution to prevent trauma when using oral hygiene aids

• Importance of updating health

and drug history if physician makes any changes in evaluation/ drug regimens

glipizide

(glip'i-zide)

Glucotrol, Glucotrol XL

Drug class.: Oral antidiabetic (second generation)

Action: Causes functioning β-cells in pancreas to release insulin, leading to drop in blood glucose levels; may improve insulin binding to insulin receptors or increase the number of insulin receptors; not effective if patient lacks functioning β-cells

Uses: Stable adult-onset diabetes mellitus (type II)

Dosage and routes:

• *Adult:* PO 5 mg initially, then increased to desired response; max 15 mg once-a-day dose, 40 mg/day in divided doses

• *Elderly:* PO 2.5 mg initially, then increased to desired response; max 40 mg/day in divided doses or 15 mg once-a-day dose

Available forms include: Tabs 5, 10 mg; ext rel 5, 10 mg

Side effects/adverse reactions:

CNS: Headache, weakness, dizziness, drowsiness, tinnitus, fatigue, vertigo

GI: ***Hepatotoxicity, cholestatic jaundice,*** nausea, vomiting, diarrhea, heartburn

HEMA: ***Leukopenia, thrombocytopenia, agranulocytosis, aplastic anemia, pancytopenia, hemolytic anemia,*** increased AST/ALT, alk phosphatase

INTEG: Rash, allergic reactions, pruritus, urticaria, eczema, photosensitivity, erythema

ENDO: ***Hypoglycemia***

Contraindications: Hypersensitivity to sulfonylureas, juvenile or brittle diabetes

Precautions: Pregnancy category C, elderly, cardiac disease, severe renal disease, severe hepatic disease, thyroid disease

Pharmacokinetics:

PO: Completely absorbed by GI route, onset 1-1.5 hr, duration 10-24 hr, half-life 2-4 hr; 90%-95% is plasma protein bound; metabolized in liver; excreted in urine

Drug interactions of concern to dentistry:

• Increased hypoglycemic effects: salicylates, ketoconazole

• Decreased action of glipizide: corticosteroids

• Disulfiram-like reaction: alcohol

DENTAL CONSIDERATIONS

General:

• Monitor vital signs every appointment due to cardiovascular side effects.

• Patients on chronic drug therapy may rarely have symptoms of blood dyscrasias, which can include infection, bleeding, and poor healing.

• Short appointments and a stress reduction protocol may be required for anxious patients.

• Place on frequent recall to evaluate healing response.

• Diabetics may be more susceptible to infection and have delayed wound healing.

• Question patient about self-monitoring of drug's antidiabetic effect, including blood glucose values or finger-stick records.

• Ensure that patient is following prescribed diet and regularly takes medication.
• Avoid prescribing aspirin-containing products.

Consultations:

• In a patient with symptoms of blood dyscrasias, request a medical consult for blood studies and postpone dental treatment until normal values are reestablished.
• Medical consult may be required to assess disease control in the patient.
• Medical consult may include data from patient's blood glucose monitoring, including glycosylated hemoglobin or HbA_{1c} testing.

Teach patient/family:

• Importance of good oral hygiene to prevent soft tissue inflammation
• Caution to prevent injury when using oral hygiene aids
• To avoid mouth rinses with high alcohol content due to drying effects

---

glyburide

(glye'byoor-ide)

DiaBeta, Glynase PresTab, Micronase

🍁 Albert Glyburide, Apo-Glyburide, Euglucon, Gen-Glybe, Novo-Glyburide, Nu-Glyburide

Drug class.: Oral antidiabetic (second generation)

Action: Causes functioning β-cells in pancreas to release insulin, leading to drop in blood glucose levels; may improve insulin binding to insulin receptors and increase number of insulin receptors; not effective if patient lacks functioning β-cells

Uses: Stable adult-onset diabetes mellitus (type II)

Dosage and routes:

• *Adult:* PO 2.5-5 mg initially, then increased to desired response; limit 20 mg/day
• *Elderly:* PO 1.25 mg initially, then increased to desired response; max 20 mg/day; maintenance 1.25-20 mg qd

Available forms include: Tabs 1.25, 1.5, 2.5, 3, 5, 6 mg

Side effects/adverse reactions:

CNS: Headache, weakness, paresthesia, tinnitus, fatigue, vertigo
GI: ***Hepatotoxicity, cholestatic jaundice,*** nausea, fullness, heartburn, vomiting, diarrhea
HEMA: ***Leukopenia, thrombocytopenia, agranulocytosis, aplastic anemia,*** increased AST/ALT, alk phosphatase
INTEG: Rash, allergic reactions, pruritus, urticaria, eczema, photosensitivity, erythema
ENDO: ***Hypoglycemia***
MS: Joint pains

Contraindications: Hypersensitivity to sulfonylureas, juvenile or brittle diabetes

Precautions: Pregnancy category B, elderly, cardiac disease, severe renal disease, severe hepatic disease, thyroid disease, severe hypoglycemia reactions

Pharmacokinetics:

PO: Completely absorbed by GI route, onset 2-4 hr, peak 2-8 hr, duration 24 hr, half-life 10 hr; 90%-95% is plasma protein bound; metabolized in liver; excreted in urine, feces (metabolites); crosses placenta

Drug interactions of concern to dentistry:

• Increased hypoglycemic effects:

NSAIDs, salicylates, ketoconazole
• Decreased action of glyburide: corticosteroids
• Disulfiram-like reaction: alcohol

DENTAL CONSIDERATIONS

General:

• Monitor vital signs every appointment due to cardiovascular side effects.
• Patients on chronic drug therapy may rarely have symptoms of blood dyscrasias, which can include infection, bleeding, and poor healing.
• Place on frequent recall to evaluate healing response.
• Ensure that patient is following prescribed diet and regularly takes medication.
• Short appointments and stress reduction protocol may be required for anxious patients.
• Patients with diabetes may be more susceptible to infection and have delayed wound healing.
• Question patient about self-monitoring of drug's antidiabetic effect, including blood glucose values or finger-stick records.
• Avoid prescribing aspirin-containing products.

Consultations:

• In a patient with symptoms of blood dyscrasias, request a medical consult for blood studies and postpone dental treatment until normal values are reestablished.
• Medical consult may be required to assess disease control in the patient.
• Medical consult may include data from patient's blood glucose monitoring, including glycosylated hemoglobin or HbA_{1c} testing.

Teach patient/family:

• Importance of good oral hygiene to prevent soft tissue inflammation
• Caution to prevent injury when using oral hygiene aids
• To avoid mouth rinses with high alcohol content due to drying effects

---

glycopyrrolate

(glye-koe-pye'roe-late)

Robinul, Robinul Forte

Drug class.: Anticholinergic

Action: Inhibits acetylcholine at receptor sites in autonomic nervous system, which controls secretions, free acids in stomach

Uses: Decreased secretions before surgery, reversal of neuromuscular blockade, peptic ulcer disease, irritable bowel syndrome

Dosage and routes:

Preoperatively

• *Adult:* IM 0.002 mg/lb 0.5-1 hr before surgery
• *Child 2-12 yr:* IM 0.002-0.004 mg/lb
• *Child <2 yr:* IM 0.004 mg/lb

Reversal of neuromuscular blockage

• *Adult:* IV 0.2 mg for each 1 mg of neostigmine or 5 mg IV of pyridostigmine simultaneously

GI disorders

• *Adult:* PO 1-2 mg bid-tid; IM/IV 0.1-0.2 mg tid-qid, titrated to patient response

Available forms include: Tabs 1, 2 mg; inj 0.2 mg/ml

Side effects/adverse reactions:

▼ *ORAL: Dry mouth*

CNS: Confusion, anxiety, restlessness, irritability, delusions, halluci-

nations, headache, sedation, depression, incoherence, dizziness, lethargy, flushing, weakness
CV: Palpitation, tachycardia, postural hypotension, paradoxic bradycardia
GI: Constipation, nausea, vomiting, abdominal distress, paralytic ileus
GU: Hesitancy, retention, impotence
EENT: Blurred vision, photophobia, dilated pupils, difficulty swallowing, increased intraocular pressure, mydriasis, cycloplegia
INTEG: Urticaria, allergic reactions
MISC: Suppression of lactation, nasal congestion, decreased sweating
Contraindications: Hypersensitivity, narrow-angle glaucoma, myasthenia gravis, GI/GU obstruction, child <3 yr, tachycardia, myocardial ischemia, hepatic disease, ulcerative colitis, toxic megacolon
Precautions: Pregnancy category C, elderly, lactation, prostatic hypertrophy, renal disease, CHF, pulmonary disease, hyperthyroidism
Pharmacokinetics:
PO: Peak 1 hr, duration 6 hr
IM: Peak 30-45 min, duration 7 hr
IV: Peak 10-15 min, duration 4 hr, excreted in urine, bile, feces (unchanged)

Drug interactions of concern to dentistry:

• Increased anticholinergic effect: antihistamines, phenothiazines, meperidine, haloperidol, scopolamine, atropine
• Do not mix with diazepam, pentobarbital, in syringe or solution
• Constipation, urinary retention: opioid analgesics
• Reduced absorption of ketoconazole

DENTAL CONSIDERATIONS
General:
• Avoid dental light in patient's eyes; offer dark glasses for patient comfort.
• Assess salivary flow as a factor in caries, periodontal disease, and candidiasis.
Consultation:
• Physician should be informed if significant xerostomic side effects occur (increased caries, sore tongue, problems eating or swallowing, difficulty wearing prosthesis) so a medication change can be considered.
Teach patient/family:
When chronic dry mouth occurs, advise patient:
• To avoid mouth rinses with high alcohol content due to drying effects
• To use daily home fluoride products for anticaries effect
• To use sugarless gum, frequent sips of water, or saliva substitutes

griseofulvin microsize/ griseofulvin ultramicrosize

(gri-see-oh-ful'vin)
Fulvicin U/F, Fulvicin P/G, Grifulvin V, Grisactin Ultra, Gris-PEG
♣ Grisovin-FP
Drug class.: Antifungal

Action: Arrests fungal cell division at metaphase; binds to human keratin, making it resistant to disease
Uses: Mycotic infections: tinea corporis, tinea pedis, tinea cruris, tinea barbae, tinea capitis, tinea

unguium if caused by *Epidermophyton, Microsporum, Trichophyton*
Dosage and routes:
• *Adult:* PO 250-500 mg qd in single or divided doses (microsize), 125-375 mg bid (ultramicrosize)
• *Child:* PO 10 mg/kg/day or 300 mg/m^2/day (microsize) or 5 mg/kg/day (ultramicrosize)
Available forms include: Microcaps 125, 250 mg; tabs 250, 500 mg; oral susp 125 mg/ml; ultratabs 125, 165, 250, 330 mg
Side effects/adverse reactions:
▼ *ORAL:* Dry mouth, candidiasis, furry tongue, lichenoid lesions, taste alteration
CNS: Headache, peripheral neuritis, paresthesia, confusion, dizziness, fatigue, insomnia, psychosis
GI: Nausea, vomiting, anorexia, diarrhea, cramps, flatulence
HEMA: ***Leukopenia, granulocytopenia, neutropenia, monocytosis***
GU: Proteinuria, cylindruria, precipitate porphyria
EENT: Blurred vision, transient hearing loss
INTEG: Rash, urticaria, photosensitivity, lichen planus, angioedema
Contraindications: Hypersensitivity, porphyria, hepatic disease, lupus erythematosus
Precautions: Penicillin sensitivity, pregnancy category C
Pharmacokinetics:
PO: Peak 4 hr, half-life 9-24 hr; metabolized in liver; excreted in urine (inactive metabolites), feces, perspiration
Drug interactions of concern to dentistry:
• Decreased absorption: barbiturates
• Additive photosensitization: tetracycline
• Potentiation of alcohol

DENTAL CONSIDERATIONS
General:
• Assess salivary flow as a factor in caries, periodontal disease, and candidiasis.
Teach patient/family:
When chronic dry mouth occurs, advise patient:
• To use daily home fluoride products for anticaries effect
• To avoid mouth rinses with high alcohol content due to drying effects
• To use sugarless gum, frequent sips of water, or saliva substitutes

guaifenesin

(gwye-fen'e-sin)
Anti-Tuss, Breonesin, Benylin-E, Genatuss, GG-Cen, GeeGee, Glycotuss, Glytuss, Guiatuss, Gylate, Fenesin, Humibid LA, Humibid Sprinkle, Hytuss, Hytuss 2X, Organidin NR, Robitussin
♣ Balminil, Resyl
Drug class.: Expectorant

Action: Acts as an expectorant by stimulating a mucosal reflex to increase the production of less viscous lung mucus
Uses: Dry, nonproductive cough
Dosage and routes:
• *Adult:* PO 200-400 mg q4-6h, not to exceed 1-2 g/day
• *Child 6-12 yr:* PO 100-200 mg q4h; max dose 1200 mg day
Available forms include: Tabs 100, 200 mg; caps 200 mg; syr 100 mg/5 ml; ext rel cap 300 mg
Side effects/adverse reactions:
CNS: Drowsiness
GI: Nausea, anorexia, vomiting
Contraindications: Hypersensitivity, persistent cough

Precautions: Pregnancy category C

DENTAL CONSIDERATIONS

General:

- Consider semisupine chair position for patients with respiratory disease.
- Elective dental treatment may be precluded by significant coughing episodes.

---

guanabenz acetate

(gwahn'a-benz)

Wytensin

Drug class.: Centrally acting antihypertensive

Action: Stimulates central α_2-adrenergic receptors, resulting in decreased sympathetic outflow from brain

Uses: Hypertension

Dosage and routes:

- *Adult:* PO 4 mg bid, increasing in increments of 4-8 mg/day q1-2wk, not to exceed 32 mg bid

Available forms include: Tabs 4, 8mg

Side effects/adverse reactions:

▼ *ORAL: Dry mouth*

CNS: Drowsiness, dizziness, sedation, headache, depression, weakness

CV: ***Severe rebound hypertension,*** chest pain, dysrhythmias, palpitation

GI: Nausea, diarrhea, constipation

GU: Impotence

EENT: Nasal congestion, blurred vision

Contraindications: Hypersensitivity to guanabenz

Precautions: Pregnancy category C, lactation, children <12 yr, severe coronary insufficiency, recent MI, cerebrovascular disease, severe hepatic or renal failure

Pharmacokinetics:

PO: Peak 2-4 hr, half-life 6 hr; excreted in urine

Drug interactions of concern to dentistry:

- Increased CNS depression: alcohol, all CNS depressants
- Decreased hypotensive effects: NSAIDs, especially indomethacin, sympathomimetics

DENTAL CONSIDERATIONS

General:

- Monitor vital signs every appointment due to cardiovascular side effects.
- Limit use of sodium-containing products such as saline IV fluids for patients with a dietary salt restriction.
- Assess salivary flow as a factor in caries, periodontal disease, and candidiasis.
- Stress from dental procedures may compromise cardiovascular function; determine patient risk.
- Short appointments and a stress reduction protocol may be required for anxious patients.

Consultations:

- Medical consult may be required to assess disease control and patient's ability to tolerate stress.

Teach patient/family:

When chronic dry mouth occurs, advise patient:

- To avoid mouth rinses with high alcohol content due to drying effects
- To use daily home fluoride products for anticaries effect
- To use sugarless gum, frequent sips of water, or saliva substitutes

guanadrel sulfate

(gwahn'a-drel)
Hylorel
Drug class.: Antihypertensive

Action: Inhibits sympathetic vasoconstriction by inhibiting release of norepinephrine; depletes norepinephrine stores in adrenergic nerve endings
Uses: Hypertension
Dosage and routes:
• *Adult:* PO 5 mg bid, adjusted to desired response, may need 20-75 mg/day in divided doses
Available forms include: Tabs 10, 25 mg
Side effects/adverse reactions:
▼ *ORAL:* Dry mouth
CNS: Drowsiness, fatigue, weakness, feeling of faintness, insomnia, dizziness, mental changes, memory loss, hallucinations, *depression,* anxiety, *confusion, paresthesias, headache*
CV: Orthostatic hypotension, bradycardia, ***CHF,*** palpitation, chest pain, tachycardia, dysrhythmias
GI: Nausea, cramps, diarrhea, constipation, anorexia, indigestion
RESP: ***Bronchospasm,*** dyspnea, cough, rales, shortness of breath
GU: Ejaculation failure, impotence, dysuria, nocturia, frequency
EENT: Nasal stuffiness, tinnitus, visual changes, sore throat, double vision, dry/burning eyes
INTEG: Rash, purpura, alopecia
MS: Leg cramps, aching, pain, inflammation
Contraindications: Hypersensitivity, pregnancy category B, pheochromocytoma, lactation, CHF, child <18 yr
Precautions: Elderly, bronchial asthma, peptic ulcer, electrolyte imbalances, vascular disease
Pharmacokinetics:
PO: Onset 0.5-2 hr, peak 1.5-2 hr, duration 4-14 hr, half-life 10-12 hr; excreted in urine (50% unchanged)
Drug interactions of concern to dentistry:
• Increased orthostatic hypotension: alcohol, opioid analgesics, barbiturates, phenothiazines, haloperidol
• Decreased hypotensive effect: ephedrine, sympathomimetics, NSAIDs, indomethacin, tricylic antidepressants

DENTAL CONSIDERATIONS

General:
• Monitor vital signs every appointment due to cardiovascular side effects.
• After supine positioning, have patient sit upright for at least 2 min before standing to avoid orthostatic hypotension.
• Limit use of sodium-containing products such as saline IV fluids for patients with a dietary salt restriction.
• Stress from dental procedures may compromise cardiovascular function; determine patient risk.
• Short appointments and a stress reduction protocol may be required for anxious patients.
• Assess salivary flow as a factor in caries, periodontal disease, and candidiasis.
Consultations:
• Medical consult may be required to assess disease control and patient's ability to tolerate stress.
Teach patient/family:
When chronic dry mouth occurs, advise patient:
• To avoid mouth rinses with high

alcohol content due to drying effects
• To use daily home fluoride products for anticaries effect
• To use sugarless gum, frequent sips of water, or saliva substitutes

guanethidine sulfate

(gwahn-eth'i-deen)
Ismelin
♣ Apo-Guanethidine
Drug class.: Antihypertensive

Action: Inhibits norepinephrine release, depleting norepinephrine stores in adrenergic nerve endings
Uses: Moderate-to-severe hypertension
Dosage and routes:
• *Adult:* PO 10 mg qd, increase by 10 mg qwk at monthly intervals; may require 25-50 mg qd
• *Adult (hospitalized):* 25-50 mg; may increase by 25-50 mg/day or qod
• *Child:* PO 200 μg/kg/day; increase q7-10d; not to exceed 3000 μg/kg/24 hr
Available forms include: Tabs 10, 25 mg
Side effects/adverse reactions:
▼ *ORAL:* Dry mouth, salivary gland pain or swelling
CNS: Depression
CV: Orthostatic hypotension, dizziness, weakness, lassitude, bradycardia, ***CHF,*** fatigue, angina, heart block, chest paresthesia
GI: Nausea, vomiting, *diarrhea,* constipation, weight gain, anorexia
RESP: Dyspnea
HEMA: ***Thrombocytopenia, leukopenia***
GU: Ejaculation failure, impotence, nocturia, edema, retention, increased BUN
EENT: Nasal congestion, ptosis, blurred vision
INTEG: Dermatitis, loss of scalp hair
Contraindications: Hypersensitivity, pheochromocytoma, recent MI, CHF, cardiac failure, sinus bradycardia
Precautions: Pregnancy category B, lactation, peptic ulcer, asthma
Pharmacokinetics:
PO: Therapeutic level 1-3 wk, half-life 5 days; metabolized by liver; excreted in urine (metabolites), breast milk
Drug interactions of concern to dentistry:
• Increased orthostatic hypotension: alcohol, opioid analgesics, barbiturates, phenothiazines, haloperidol
• Decreased hypotensive effect: ephedrine, NSAIDs, indomethacin, sympathomimetics, tricyclic antidepressants

DENTAL CONSIDERATIONS
General:
• Monitor vital signs every appointment due to cardiovascular and respiratory side effects.
• Patients on chronic drug therapy may rarely have symptoms of blood dyscrasias, which can include infection, bleeding, and poor healing.
• Assess salivary flow as a factor in caries, periodontal disease, and candidiasis.
• After supine positioning, have patient sit upright for at least 2 min before standing to avoid orthostatic hypotension.
• Limit use of sodium-containing products such as saline IV fluids for patients with a dietary salt restriction.
• Stress from dental procedures

may compromise cardiovascular function; determine patient risk.
• Short appointments and a stress reduction protocol may be required for anxious patients.
• Use vasoconstrictors with caution, in low doses, and with careful aspiration. Avoid using gingival retraction cord with epinephrine.
• Consider semisupine chair position for patients with respiratory distress.

Consultations:
• Medical consult may be required to assess disease control and patient's ability to tolerate stress.
• In a patient with symptoms of blood dyscrasias, request a medical consult for blood studies and postpone dental treatment until normal values are reestablished.

Teach patient/family:
• Importance of good oral hygiene to prevent soft tissue inflammation
• Caution to prevent injury when using oral hygiene aids

When chronic dry mouth occurs, advise patient:
• To avoid mouth rinses with high alcohol content due to drying effects
• To use daily home fluoride products for anticaries effect
• To use sugarless gum, frequent sips of water, or saliva substitutes

---

guanfacine HCl

(gwahn'fa-seen)
Tenex

Drug class.: Antihypertensive

Action: Stimulates central α-adrenergic receptors, resulting in decreased sympathetic outflow from brain

Uses: Hypertension in individuals using a thiazide diuretic; unapproved use: to suppress symptoms in heroin withdrawal

Dosage and routes:
• *Adult:* PO 1 mg/day hs, may increase dose in 2-3 wk to 2-3 mg/day

Available forms include: Tabs 1, 2, and 3 mg

Side effects/adverse reactions:
▼ *ORAL: Dry mouth,* taste changes
CNS: Somnolence, dizziness, headache, fatigue
CV: Bradycardia, chest pain
GI: Constipation, cramps, nausea, diarrhea
RESP: Dyspnea
GU: Impotence, urinary incontinence
EENT: Tinnitus, vision change, rhinitis
INTEG: Dermatitis, pruritus, purpura
MS: Leg cramps

Contraindications: Hypersensitivity

Precautions: Pregnancy category B, lactation, children <12 yr, severe coronary insufficiency, recent MI, renal or hepatic disease, CVA

Pharmacokinetics: Peak 1-4 hr, half-life 17 hr; 70% bound to plasma proteins; eliminated via kidney unchanged and as metabolites

Drug interactions of concern to dentistry:
• Increased CNS depression: alcohol, all CNS depressants
• Decreased hypotensive effects: NSAIDs, especially indomethacin, sympathomimetics

DENTAL CONSIDERATIONS

General:
• Monitor vital signs every ap-

pointment due to cardiovascular side effects.

• Limit use of sodium-containing products such as saline IV fluids for patients with a dietary salt restriction.

• Assess salivary flow as a factor in caries, periodontal disease, and candidiasis.

• Stress from dental procedures may compromise cardiovascular function; determine patient risk.

• Short appointments and a stress reduction protocol may be required for anxious patients.

Consultations:

• Medical consult may be required to assess disease control and patient's tolerance for stress.

Teach patient/family:

When chronic dry mouth occurs, advise patient:

• To avoid mouth rinses with high alcohol content due to drying effects

• To use daily home fluoride products for anticaries effect

• To use sugarless gum, frequent sips of water, or saliva substitutes

halazepam

(hal-az'e-pam)

Paxipam

Drug class.: Benzodiazepine

Controlled Substance Schedule IV

Action: Produces CNS depression by interacting with a benzodiazepine receptor to facilitate the action of the inhibitory neurotransmitter γ-aminobutyric acid (GABA)

Uses: Anxiety

Dosage and routes:

• *Adult:* PO 20-40 mg tid-qid

• *Geriatric:* PO 20 mg qd-bid

Available forms include: Tabs 20, 40 mg

Side effects/adverse reactions:

▼ *ORAL:* Dry mouth

CNS: Dizziness, drowsiness, confusion, headache, anxiety, tremors, stimulation, fatigue, depression, insomnia, hallucinations

CV: Orthostatic hypotension, ***ECG changes, tachycardia,*** hypotension

GI: Constipation, nausea, vomiting, anorexia, diarrhea

EENT: Blurred vision, tinnitus, mydriasis

INTEG: Rash, dermatitis, itching

Contraindications: Hypersensitivity to benzodiazepines, narrow-angle glaucoma, psychosis, pregnancy category D, child <18 yr; ritonavir

Precautions: Elderly, debilitated, hepatic disease, renal disease

Drug interactions of concern to dentistry:

• Increased effects of halazepam: alcohol, CNS depressants

• Increased serum levels and prolonged effect of benzodiazepines: ketoconazole, itraconazole, fluconazole, miconazole (systemic), indinavir

DENTAL CONSIDERATIONS

General:

• Assess salivary flow as a factor in caries, periodontal disease, and candidiasis.

• Monitor vital signs every appointment due to cardiovascular side effects.

• Psychologic and physical dependence may occur with chronic use.

• Geriatric patients are more susceptible to drug effects; use lower dose.

• After supine positioning, have patient slowly sit upright for at

H

least 2 min before standing to avoid orthostatic hypotension.

Teach patient/family:

When chronic dry mouth occurs, advise patient:

• To avoid mouth rinses with high alcohol content due to drying effects

• Of need for daily home fluoride to prevent caries

• To use sugarless gum, frequent sips of water, or saliva substitutes

halcinonide

(hal-sin'oh-nide)

Halog, Halog-E

Drug class.: Corticosteroid, synthetic topical

Action: Glucocorticoids have multiple actions that include antiinflammatory and immunosuppressant effects. They inhibit phospholipase A_2, interfering with or reducing the synthesis of prostaglandins and leukotrienes. They also bind to cytoplasmic glucocorticoid receptors (GRs) and enter the cell nucleus to bind with DNA. This results in the synthesis of various enzymes such as collagenase, elastase, and cytokines that play important roles in inflammation and immunosuppression. They also suppress the production of lymphocytes, monocytes, and eosinophils.

Uses: Inflammation of corticosteroid-responsive dermatoses

Dosage and routes:

• *Adult:* TOP apply to affected area bid-tid

Available forms include: Cream 0.025%, 0.1%; oint 0.1%; sol 0.1%

Side effects/adverse reactions:

▼ *ORAL:* Thinning of mucosa, stinging sensation (local application)

INTEG: Acne, atrophy, epidermal thinning, purpura, striae

Contraindications: Hypersensitivity, viral infections, fungal infections

Precautions: Pregnancy category C

DENTAL CONSIDERATIONS

General:

• Place on frequent recall to evaluate healing response when used on chronic basis.

Teach patient/family:

• Importance of good oral hygiene to prevent soft tissue inflammation

• When used for oral lesions, to return for oral evaluation if response of oral tissues has not occurred in 7-14 days

• To apply at bedtime or after meals for maximum effect

• To apply with cotton-tipped applicator by pressing, not rubbing, paste on lesion

• That use on oral herpetic ulcerations is contraindicated

halobetasol propionate

(hal-oh-bay'ta-sol)

Ultravate

Drug class.: Topical corticosteroid, group VI potency

Action: Glucocorticoids have multiple actions that include antiinflammatory and immunosuppressant effects. They inhibit phospholipase A_2, interfering with or reducing the synthesis of prostaglandins and leukotrienes. They also bind to cytoplasmic glucocorticoid receptors (GRs) and enter the cell nucleus to bind with DNA.

This results in the synthesis of various enzymes such as collagenase, elastase, and cytokines that play important roles in inflammation and immunosuppression. They also suppress the production of lymphocytes, monocytes, and eosinophils.

Uses: Psoriasis, eczema, contact dermatitis, pruritus

Dosage and routes:

• *Adult and child:* Apply to affected area tid-qid

Available forms include: Cream 0.05%; oint 0.005%

Side effects/adverse reactions:

INTEG: Burning, dryness, itching, irritation, acne, folliculitis, hypertrichosis, perioral dermatitis, hypopigmentation, atrophy, striae, miliaria, allergic contact dermatitis, secondary infection

Contraindications: Hypersensitivity to corticosteroids, fungal infections

Precautions: Pregnancy category C, lactation, viral infections, bacterial infections

DENTAL CONSIDERATIONS

Teach patient/family:

• That use on oral herpetic ulcerations is contraindicated

---

haloperidol/haloperidol decanoate

(ha-loe-per′i-dole)

Haldol, Haldol LA

♣ Apo-Haloperidol, Novoperidol, Peridol, PMS Haloperidol

Drug class.: Antipsychotic/butyrophenone

Action: Blocks neurotransmission at dopaminergic synapses in the cerebral cortex, hypothalamus, and limbic system; exhibits strong peripheral α-adrenergic and anticholinergic blocking action; mechanism for antipsychotic effects is unclear

Uses: Psychotic disorders, control of tics and vocal utterances in Tourette's syndrome, short-term treatment of hyperactive children showing excessive motor activity; unapproved use: autism and chemotherapy-induced nausea and vomiting

Dosage and routes:

Psychosis

• *Adult:* PO 0.5-5 mg bid or tid initially, depending on severity of condition, dose is increased to desired dose, max 100 mg/day; IM 2-5 mg q1-8h

• *Child 3-12 yr:* PO/IM 0.05-0.15 mg/kg/day

• *Decanoate:* Initial dose IM is 10-15× daily PO dose q4wk; do not administer IV; not to exceed 100 mg

Chronic schizophrenia

• *Adult:* IM 10-15× PO dose q4wk (decanoate)

• *Child 3-12 yr:* PO/IM 0.05-0.15 mg/kg/day

Tics/vocal utterances

• *Adult:* PO 0.5-5 mg bid or tid, increased until desired response occurs

• *Child 3-12 yr:* PO 0.05-0.075 mg/kg/day

Hyperactive children

• *Child 3-12 yr:* PO 0.05-0.075 mg/kg/day

Available forms include: Tabs 0.5, 1, 2, 5, 10, 20 mg; conc 2 mg/ml; inj IM 5 mg/ml

Side effects/adverse reactions:

▼ *ORAL: Dry mouth, tardive dyskinesia (tongue, lip movements),* sore throat, mouth

CNS: Extrapyramidal symptoms: pseudoparkinsonism, akathisia,

dystonia, tardive dyskinesia, drowsiness, headache, ***seizures, neuroleptic malignant syndrome,*** confusion
CV: Orthostatic hypotension, ***cardiac arrest, tachycardia,*** hypertension, ECG changes
GI: Nausea, vomiting, anorexia, constipation, ***ileus, hepatitis,*** diarrhea, jaundice, weight gain
RESP: ***Laryngospasm, respiratory depression,*** dyspnea
GU: Urinary retention, urinary frequency, enuresis, impotence, amenorrhea, gynecomastia
EENT: Blurred vision, glaucoma, dry eyes
INTEG: Rash, photosensitivity, dermatitis

Contraindications: Hypersensitivity, blood dyscrasias, coma, child <3 yr, brain damage, bone marrow depression, alcohol and barbiturate withdrawal states, Parkinson's disease, angina, epilepsy, urinary retention, narrow-angle glaucoma

Precautions: Pregnancy category C, lactation, seizure disorders, hypertension, hepatic disease, cardiac disease

Pharmacokinetics:
PO: Onset erratic, peak 2-6 hr, half-life 24 hr
IM: Onset 15-30 min, peak 15-20 min, half-life 21 hr
IM: Decanoate—peak 4-11 days, half-life 3 wk
Metabolized by liver; excreted in urine, bile; crosses placenta; excreted in breast milk

Drug interactions of concern to dentistry:
- Increased sedation: other CNS depressants, alcohol, barbiturate anesthetics, opioid analgesics
- Hypotension, tachycardia: epinephrine
- Increased extrapyramidal effects: phenothiazines and related drugs (haloperidol, droperidol), metoclopramide
- Additive photosensitization: tetracyclines
- Increased anticholinergic effects: anticholinergics

DENTAL CONSIDERATIONS

General:
- Monitor vital signs every appointment due to cardiovascular side effects.
- After supine positioning, have patient sit upright for at least 2 min before standing to avoid orthostatic hypotension.
- Assess salivary flow as a factor in caries, periodontal disease, and candidiasis.
- Avoid dental light in patient's eyes; offer dark glasses for patient comfort.
- Assess for presence of extrapyramidal motor symptoms, such as tardive dyskinesia and akathisia. Extrapyramidal motor activity may complicate dental treatment.
- Geriatric patients are more susceptible to drug effects; use lower dose.
- Use vasoconstrictors with caution, in low doses, and with careful aspiration. Avoid use of gingival retraction cord with epinephrine.

Consultations:
- Take precautions if dental surgery is anticipated and anesthesia is required.
- If signs of tardive dyskinesia or akathisia are present, refer to physician.
- Physician should be informed if significant xerostomic side effects occur (increased caries, sore

tongue, problems eating or swallowing, difficulty wearing prosthesis) so a medication change can be considered.

Teach patient/family:

• Importance of good oral hygiene to prevent soft tissue inflammation

• Caution to prevent injury when using oral hygiene aids

• To use electric toothbrush if patient has difficulty holding conventional devices

When chronic dry mouth occurs, advise patient:

• To avoid mouth rinses with high alcohol content due to drying effects

• To use daily home fluoride products for anticaries effect

• To use sugarless gum, frequent sips of water, or saliva substitutes

---

heparin/heparin calcium/heparin sodium

(hep′a-rin)

Heparin: Hep Lock, Hep-Lock U/P, generic

✤ *Heparin calcium:* Calciparine, Calcilean

Heparin sodium: Liquaemin Sodium, Liquamenin Sodium PF

✤ Heparin-Leo

Drug class.: Anticoagulant

Action: Acts in combination with antithrombin III (heparin cofactor) to inhibit thrombosis; inactivates Factor Xa and inhibits conversion of prothrombin to thrombin; affects both intrinsic and extrinsic clotting pathways

Uses: Anticoagulant in thrombosis, embolism (both prevention and treatment), coagulopathies, deep vein thrombosis, prevention of clotting when extracorporeal circulation is required (cardiac surgery), dialysis, maintenance of patency of indwelling IV lines

Dosage and routes: General doses listed, all doses must be individualized to patient and circumstance

• *Adult:* SC 10,000-20,000 U (USP) initially, then 8000-10,000 U q8h or 15,000 U q12h; IV 10,000 U initially, then 5000-10,000 U q4-6h; IV infusion 20,000-40,000 U in 1 L of normal saline over 24 hr

• *Child:* IV 50 U/kg initially, then 100 U/kg by IV drip q4h or 20,000 U/m^2 over 24 hr by continuous infusion

Available forms include: Amps 1000, 5000, 10,000 U/ml; vials 1000, 5000, 10,000, 20,000, 40,000 U/ml; unit dose 1000, 2500, 5000, 7500, 10,000, 20,000 U/dose; heparin lock flush 10, 100 U/ml; heparin calcium 5000 U/dose

Side effects/adverse reactions:

▼ *ORAL:* Bleeding, stomatitis

CNS: Fever, chills

GI: Diarrhea, ***hepatitis,*** nausea, vomiting, anorexia, abdominal cramps

GU: ***Hematuria***

HEMA: ***Hemorrhage, thrombocytopenia***

INTEG: Rash, hives, itching, allergies

Contraindications: Hypersensitivity, hemophilia, leukemia with bleeding, peptic ulcer disease, thrombocytopenic purpura, hepatic disease (severe), renal disease (severe), blood dyscrasias, pregnancy, severe hypertension, subacute bacterial endocarditis, acute nephritis

Precautions: Hematoma (IM); elderly; pregnancy category C; lactation; hyperkalemia; monitor APTT, PTT, WBC, ACT; endocarditis;

H

trauma; alcoholism; prolongs intrinsic clotting pathway approximately 4-6 hr after each dose

Pharmacokinetics:

IV: Peak 5 min, duration 2-6 hr

SC: Onset 20-60 min, duration 8-12 hr

Half-life 1.5 hr (variable depending on dose); 95% bound to plasma proteins; excreted in urine

Drug interactions of concern to dentistry:

- Increased risk of bleeding: salicylates, NSAIDs, parenteral penicillins, glucocorticoids, certain cephalosporins (cefamandole, cefoperazone, cefotetan)

DENTAL CONSIDERATIONS

General:

- Heparin is used only in hospitalized patients or during dialysis. A medical consult is necessary if oral and maxillofacial surgery or trauma treatment is required. May need to defer treatment.
- Avoid products that affect platelet function, such as aspirin and NSAIDs.
- Consider local hemostasis measures to prevent excessive bleeding.
- Take precautions if dental surgery or intubation for general anesthesia is anticipated.

Consultations:

- Medical consult may be required to assess disease control and patient's ability to tolerate stress.
- Medical consult should include ACT, partial prothrombin, and prothrombin times.

Teach patient/family:

- Caution to prevent trauma when using oral hygiene aids
- Importance of good oral hygiene to prevent soft tissue inflammation
- To report oral lesions, soreness, or bleeding

homatropine hydrobromide (optic)

(hoe-ma'troe-peen)

AK-Homatropine, Isopto Homatropine, L-Homatropine, Spectro-Homatropine

Minims Homatropine

Drug class.: Mydriatic (topical)

Action: Blocks response of iris sphincter muscle and muscle of accommodation of ciliary body to cholinergic stimulation, resulting in dilation and paralysis of accommodation

Uses: Cycloplegic refraction, uveitis, mydriatic lens opacities

Dosage and routes:

- *Adult and child:* Instill 1 gtt, repeat in 5-10 min for refraction or 1 gtt bid or tid for uveitis

Available forms include: Sol 2%, 5%

Side effects/adverse reactions:

CNS: Confusion, somnolence, flushing, fever

CV: Tachycardia

EENT: Blurred vision, photophobia, increased intraocular pressure, irritation, edema

Contraindications: Hypersensitivity, children <6 yr, narrow-angle glaucoma, increased intraocular pressure, infants

Precautions: Children, elderly, hypertension, hyperthyroidism, diabetes, pregnancy category C

Pharmacokinetics:

INSTILL: Peak 0.5-1 hr, duration 1-3 days

Drug interactions of concern to dentistry:

• Avoid concurrent use with pilocarpine

• Increased anticholinergic effects with other anticholinergic drugs (when significant absorption from the eye occurs)

DENTAL CONSIDERATIONS

General:

• Avoid dental light in patient's eyes; offer dark glasses for patient comfort.

• Protect patient's eyes from accidental spatter during dental treatment.

---

hydralazine HCl

(hye-dral'a-zeen)

Apresoline

♣ Novo-Hylazin

Drug class.: Antihypertensive, direct-acting peripheral vasodilator

Action: Vasodilates arteriolar smooth muscle by direct relaxation; reduction in blood pressure with reflex increases cardiac function

Uses: Essential hypertension; parenteral: severe essential hypertension

Dosage and routes:

• *Adult:* PO 10 mg qid 2-4 days, then 25 mg for rest of first wk, then 50 mg qid individualized to desired response, not to exceed 300 mg; IV/IM bol 20-40 mg q4-6h, administer PO as soon as possible; IM 20-40 mg q4-6h

• *Child:* PO 0.75 mg/kg qd 0.75-3 mg/kg/day in 4 divided doses; max 7.5 mg/kg/24 hr; IV bol 0.1-0.2 mg/kg q4-6h; IM 0.1-0.2 mg/kg q4-6h

Available forms include: Inj IV/IM 20 mg/ml; tabs 10, 25, 50, 100 mg

Side effects/adverse reactions:

CNS: Headache, tremors, dizziness, anxiety, peripheral neuritis, depression

*CV: Palpitation, reflex tachycardia, angina, **shock,*** edema, rebound hypertension

GI: Nausea, vomiting, anorexia, diarrhea, constipation

HEMA: ***Leukopenia, agranulocytosis,*** anemia

GU: Impotence, urinary retention, sodium, water retention

INTEG: Rash, pruritus

MISC: Lupuslike symptoms, nasal congestion, muscle cramps

Contraindications: Hypersensitivity to hydralazines, CAD, mitral valvular rheumatic heart disease, rheumatic heart disease

Precautions: Pregnancy category C, CVA, advanced renal disease

Pharmacokinetics:

PO: Onset 20-45 min, peak 1-2 hr, duration 2-4 hr

IV: Onset 5-20 min, peak 10-80 min, duration 2-6 hr, half-life 2-8 hr

Metabolized by liver; less than 10% present in urine

Drug interactions of concern to dentistry:

• Increased tachycardia, angina: IV sympathomimetics (epinephrine, norepinephrine)

• Reduced effects: NSAIDs, indomethacin

DENTAL CONSIDERATIONS

General:

• Monitor vital signs every appointment due to cardiovascular side effects.

• Patients on chronic drug therapy

may rarely have symptoms of blood dyscrasias, which can include infection, bleeding, and poor healing.

• Limit use of sodium-containing products such as saline IV fluids for patients with a dietary salt restriction.

• After supine positioning, have patient sit upright for at least 2 min to avoid orthostatic hypotension.

Consultations:

• In a patient with symptoms of blood dyscrasias, request a medical consult for blood studies and postpone dental treatment until normal values are reestablished.

• Medical consult may be required to assess disease control and patient's ability to tolerate stress.

Teach patient/family:

• Importance of good oral hygiene to prevent soft tissue inflammation

• Caution to prevent injury when using oral hygiene aids

---

hydrochlorothiazide (HTCZ)

(hye-droe-klor-oh-thye′a-zide)

Esidrix, Hydro-Chlor, Hydro-D, HydroDIURIL, Microzide, Oretic

🍁 Apo-Hydro, Diuchlor H, Neo-Codema, Novo-Hydrazide, Urozide

Drug class.: Thiazide diuretic

Action: Acts on distal tubule by increasing excretion of water, sodium, chloride, potassium

Uses: Edema, hypertension, diuresis, CHF

Dosage and routes:

• *Adult:* PO 25-100 mg/day

• *Child >6 mo:* PO 2.2 mg/kg/day in divided doses

• *Child <6 mo:* PO up to 3.3 mg/kg/day in divided doses

Available forms include: Tabs 25, 50, 100 mg; sol 50 mg/5 ml, 100 mg/ml

Side effects/adverse reactions:

▼ *ORAL: Dry mouth, increased thirst,* lichenoid reaction

CNS: Dizziness, fatigue, weakness, drowsiness, paresthesia, anxiety, depression, headache

CV: Irregular pulse, orthostatic hypotension, palpitation, volume depletion

GI: Nausea, vomiting, anorexia, hepatitis, constipation, diarrhea, cramps, pancreatitis, GI irritation

HEMA: ***Aplastic anemia, hemolytic anemia, leukopenia, agranulocytosis, thrombocytopenia, neutropenia***

GU: Frequency, uremia, glucosuria, polyuria

EENT: Blurred vision

INTEG: Rash, urticaria, purpura, photosensitivity, fever

META: Hyperglycemia, hyperuricemia, increased creatinine, BUN

ELECT: Hypokalemia, hypercalcemia, hyponatremia, hypochloremia, hypomagnesemia

Contraindications: Hypersensitivity to thiazides or sulfonamides, anuria, renal decompensation, hypomagnesium

Precautions: Hypokalemia, renal disease, pregnancy category D, hepatic disease, gout, COPD, lupus erythematosus, diabetes mellitus

Pharmacokinetics:

PO: Onset 2 hr, peak 4 hr, duration 6-12 hr; excreted unchanged by kidneys; crosses placenta; enters breast milk

Drug interactions of concern to dentistry:
- Increased photosensitization: tetracycline
- Decreased hypotensive response: NSAIDs, especially indomethacin

DENTAL CONSIDERATIONS

General:
- Monitor vital signs every appointment due to cardiovascular side effects.
- Patients on chronic drug therapy may rarely have symptoms of blood dyscrasias, which can include infection, bleeding, and poor healing.
- After supine positioning, have patient sit upright for at least 2 min before standing to avoid orthostatic hypotension.
- Assess salivary flow as a factor in caries, periodontal disease, and candidiasis.
- Limit use of sodium-containing products such as saline IV fluids for patients with a dietary salt restriction.
- Stress from dental procedures may compromise cardiovascular function; determine patient risk.
- Short appointments and a stress reduction protocol may be required for anxious patients.
- Patients taking diuretics should be monitored for serum K^+ levels.

Consultations:
- In a patient with symptoms of blood dyscrasias, request a medical consult for blood studies and postpone dental treatment until normal values are reestablished.
- Medical consult may be required to assess disease control and patient's ability to tolerate stress.
- Physician should be informed if significant xerostomic side effects occur (increased caries, sore tongue, problems eating or swallowing, difficulty wearing prosthesis) so a medication change can be considered.

Teach patient/family:
- Importance of good oral hygiene to prevent soft tissue inflammation
- Caution to prevent injury when using oral hygiene aids

When chronic dry mouth occurs, advise patient:
- To avoid mouth rinses with high alcohol content due to drying effects
- To use daily home fluoride products for anticaries effect
- To use sugarless gum, frequent sips of water, or saliva substitutes

hydrocodone bitartrate

(hye-droe-koe'done)

Hycodan

Robidone

Drug class.: Narcotic analgesic

Controlled Substance Schedule III, Canada N

Action: Interacts with opioid receptors in the CNS to alter pain perception; acts directly on cough center in medulla to suppress cough

Uses: Hyperactive and nonproductive cough; mild-to-moderate pain; normally used in combination with aspirin or acetaminophen for posttreatment pain control

Dosage and routes:
- *Adult:* PO 5 mg q4h prn or 10 mg q12h (long-acting)
- *Child:* PO 0.15 mg/kg q6h

Available forms include: Caps 5

mg; susp 5 mg/ml; tabs 5, 10 mg (long-acting); some dose forms not available in United States

Side effects/adverse reactions:

▼ *ORAL:* Dry mouth

CNS: ***Convulsions,*** drowsiness, dizziness, light-headedness, confusion, headache, sedation, euphoria, dysphoria, weakness, hallucinations, disorientation

CV: ***Circulatory depression,*** palpitation, tachycardia, bradycardia, change in BP, syncope

GI: Nausea, vomiting, anorexia, constipation, cramps

RESP: ***Respiratory depression***

GU: Increased urinary output, dysuria, urinary retention

EENT: Tinnitus, blurred vision, miosis, diplopia

INTEG: Rash, urticaria, flushing, pruritus

Contraindications: Hypersensitivity, addiction (narcotic)

Precautions: Addictive personality, pregnancy category C, lactation, increased intracranial pressure, MI (acute), severe heart disease, respiratory depression, hepatic disease, renal disease, child <18 yr

Pharmacokinetics: Onset 10-20 min, duration 3-6 hr, half-life 3-4 hr; metabolized in liver; excreted in urine; crosses placenta

Drug interactions of concern to dentistry:

- Increased CNS depression: alcohol, other opioids, phenothiazines, sedative/hypnotics, skeletal muscle relaxants, general anesthetics
- Contraindication: MAO inhibitors
- Increased effects of anticholinergics

DENTAL CONSIDERATIONS

General:

- Monitor vital signs every appointment due to cardiovascular and respiratory side effects.
- After supine positioning, have patient sit upright for at least 2 min to avoid orthostatic hypotension.
- Psychologic and physical dependence may occur with chronic administration.
- Determine why the patient is taking the drug.

Teach patient/family:

- To avoid mouth rinses with high alcohol content due to drying effects

hydrocortisone/ hydrocortisone acetate/hydrocortisone sodium phosphate/ hydrocortisone sodium succinate/ hydrocortisone cypionate

(hye-dro-kor′ti-sone)

Hydrocortisone (tab): Cortef, Hydrocortone

Hydrocortisone cypionate (oral susp): Cortef

Hydrocortisone sodium phosphate (IV/IM/SC): Hydrocortone Phosphate

Hydrocortisone sodium succinate (IV/IM): A-Hydrocort, Solu-Cortef

Hydrocortisone acetate (intraarticular, soft tissue only): Hydrocortone Acetate

Hydrocortisone acetate (rectal): Cortiform

Hydrocortisone (rectal): Cortenema

Drug class.: Corticosteroid

Action: Glucocorticoids have multiple actions that include antiinflammatory and immunosuppressant effects. They inhibit phospholipase A_2, interfering with or reducing the synthesis of prostaglandins and leukotrienes. They also bind to cytoplasmic glucocorticoid receptors (GRs) and enter the cell nucleus to bind with DNA. This results in the synthesis of various enzymes such as collagenase, elastase, and cytokines that play important roles in inflammation and immunosuppression. They also suppress the production of lymphocytes, monocytes, and eosinophils.

Uses: Severe inflammation, shock, adrenal insufficiency, ulcerative colitis, collagen disorders

Dosage and routes:

Adrenal insufficiency/inflammation

• *Adult:* PO 5-30 mg bid-qid; IM/IV 100-250 mg (succinate), then 50-100 mg IM as needed; IM/IV 15-240 mg q12h (phosphate)

Shock

• *Adult:* 500 mg to 2 g q2-6h (succinate)

• *Child:* IM/IV 0.16-1 mg/kg bid-tid (succinate)

Colitis

• *Adult:* Enema 100 mg nightly for 21 days

Available forms include: Retention enema 100 mg/60 ml; tabs 5, 10, 20 mg; inj 25, 50 mg/ml; inj 50 mg/ml; phosphate inj 100, 250, 500, 1000 mg/vial; succinate inj 25, 50 mg/ml

Side effects/adverse reactions:

▼ *ORAL:* Dry mouth, poor wound healing, petechiae, candidiasis

CNS: Depression, flushing, sweating, headache, mood changes

CV: Hypertension, ***circulatory collapse, thrombophlebitis, embolism,*** tachycardia, edema

GI: Diarrhea, nausea, ***pancreatitis, GI hemorrhage,*** increased appetite, abdominal distention

HEMA: ***Thrombocytopenia***

EENT: Fungal infections, increased intraocular pressure, blurred vision

INTEG: Acne, poor wound healing, ecchymosis, petechiae

MS: Fractures, osteoporosis, weakness

Contraindications: Psychosis, hypersensitivity, idiopathic thrombocytopenia, acute glomerulonephritis, amebiasis, fungal infections, nonasthmatic bronchial disease, child <2 yr, AIDS, TB

H

Precautions: Pregnancy category C, diabetes mellitus, glaucoma, osteoporosis, seizure disorders, ulcerative colitis, CHF, myasthenia gravis, renal disease, esophagitis, peptic ulcer, rifampin

Pharmacokinetics:

PO: Onset 1-2 hr, peak 1 hr, duration 1-1.5 days

IM/IV: Onset 20 min, peak 4-8 hr, duration 1-1.5 days

REC: Onset 3-5 days

Metabolized by liver, excreted in urine (17-OHCH, 17-KS), crosses placenta

Drug interactions of concern to dentistry:

• Decreased action: barbiturates, rifabutin, rifampin

• Increased GI side effects: alcohol, salicylates, NSAIDs

• Increased action: ketoconazole, macrolide antibiotics

DENTAL CONSIDERATIONS

General:

• Monitor vital signs every appointment due to cardiovascular side effects.

• Patients on chronic drug therapy may rarely have symptoms of

blood dyscrasias, which can include infection, bleeding, and poor healing.
• Assess salivary flow as a factor in caries, periodontal disease, and candidiasis.
• Place on frequent recall to evaluate healing response.
• Prophylactic antibiotics may be indicated to prevent infection if surgery or deep scaling is planned.
• Avoid prescribing aspirin-containing products.
• Symptoms of oral infections may be masked.
• Determine dose and duration of steroid therapy for each patient to assess the risk for stress tolerance and immunosuppression.
• Patients who have been or are currently on chronic steroid therapy (>2 wk) may require supplemental steroids for dental treatment.
• Determine why the patient is taking the drug.

Consultations:
• In a patient with symptoms of blood dyscrasias, request a medical consult for blood studies and postpone dental treatment until normal values are reestablished.
• Medical consult may be required to assess disease control and patient's ability to tolerate stress.
• Consult may be required to confirm steroid dose and duration of use.

Teach patient/family:
• Importance of good oral hygiene to prevent soft tissue inflammation
• Caution to prevent injury when using oral hygiene aids

When chronic dry mouth occurs, advise patient:
• To avoid mouth rinses with high alcohol content due to drying effects
• To use sugarless gum, frequent sips of water, or saliva substitutes
• To use daily home fluoride products for anticaries effect

---

hydrocortisone/ hydrocortisone acetate/hydrocortisone buteprate/ hydrocortisone butyrate/ hydrocortisone valerate

(hye-droe-kor'ti-sone)

Hydrocortisone: Ala-Cort, Aller-cort, Alphaderm, Cortril, Cort-Dome, Cortifair, Demicort, Dermacort, Dermtex HC, Hydro-Tex, Hytone, Lemoderm, Nutracort, Penecort, Synacort

🍁 Cortef, Lemoderm Cortate, Unicort, Emo-Cort, Prevex-HC

Hydrocortisone acetate: Anusol HC, Corticaine, Cortaid, Carmol-HC, Dermarest, DriCort, Foil-leCort, Gynecort, Lanacort

🍁 Corticreme, Cortacet, Hy-derm, Novohydrocort

Hydrocortisone buteprate: Pandel

Hydrocortisone butyrate: Locoid Cream, Locoid Ointment

Hydrocortisone valerate: Wescort Cream, Westcort Ointment

Drug class.: Topical corticosteroid

Action: Interacts with steroid cytoplasmic receptors to induce antiinflammatory effects; possesses antipruritic, antiinflammatory actions

Uses: Psoriasis, eczema, contact dermatitis, pruritus

Dosage and routes:

• *Adult and child >2 yr:* Apply to affected area qd-qid

Available forms include: Hydrocortisone: oint 0.5%, 1%, 2.5%; cream 0.25%, 0.5%, 1%, 2.5%; lotion 0.25%, 0.5%, 1%, 2%, 2.5%; gel 1%; sol 1%; aerosol/pump spray 0.5%; acetate: oint 0.5%, 1%, 2.5%; cream 0.5%; lotion 0.05%; aerosol 1%; valerate: oint 0.2%; cream 0.2%; buteprate: cream 0.1% in 15 and 45 g; butyrate: oint 0.1%, cream 0.1% (many others)

Side effects/adverse reactions:

▼ *ORAL:* Thinning of mucosa, stinging sensation (oral application site)

INTEG: Burning, dryness, itching, irritation, acne, folliculitis, hypertrichosis, perioral dermatitis, hypopigmentation, atrophy, striae, miliaria, allergic contact dermatitis, secondary infection

Contraindications: Hypersensitivity to corticosteroids, fungal infections, herpetic infections

Precautions: Pregnancy category C, lactation, viral infections, bacterial infections

DENTAL CONSIDERATIONS

General:

• Place on frequent recall to evaluate healing response if used on a chronic basis.

Teach patient/family:

• Importance of good oral hygiene to prevent soft tissue inflammation

• To apply at bedtime or after meals for maximum effect

• That use on oral herpetic ulcerations is contraindicated

• To apply with cotton-tipped applicator by pressing, not rubbing, paste on lesion

• That when used for oral lesions, to return for oral evaluation if response of oral tissues has not occurred in 7-14 days

hydromorphone HCl

(hye-droe-mor′fone)

Dilaudid, Dilaudid HP, Hydrostat IR

♣ PMS-Hydromorphone

Drug class.: Synthetic narcotic analgesic

H

Controlled Substance Schedule II, Canada N

Action: Inhibits ascending pain pathways in CNS, increases pain threshold, alters pain perception

Uses: Moderate-to-severe pain

Dosage and routes:

• *Adult:* PO 1-10 mg q3-6h depending on pain severity and dose form; IM/SC/IV 2-4 mg q4-6h; rec 3 mg hs prn

Available forms include: Inj IM/IV 1, 2, 3, 4, 10 mg/ml; tabs 1, 2, 3, 4 mg; rec supp 3 mg; liquid 5mg/5ml

Side effects/adverse reactions:

▼ *ORAL:* Dry mouth

CNS: Drowsiness, dizziness, confusion, headache, sedation, euphoria

CV: Palpitation, bradycardia, change in BP

GI: Nausea, vomiting, anorexia, constipation, cramps

RESP: ***Respiratory depression***

GU: Increased urinary output, dysuria, urinary retention

EENT: Tinnitus, blurred vision, miosis, diplopia

INTEG: Rash, urticaria, bruising, flushing, diaphoresis, pruritus

Contraindications: Hypersensi-

tivity, addiction (narcotic), MAO inhibitors

Precautions: Addictive personality, pregnancy category C, lactation, increased intracranial pressure, MI (acute), severe heart disease, respiratory depression, hepatic disease, renal disease, child <18 yr

Pharmacokinetics:

PO: Onset 15-30 min, peak 0.5-1.5 hr, duration 4-5 hr; metabolized by liver; excreted by kidneys; crosses placenta; excreted in breast milk

Drug interactions of concern to dentistry:

• Effects may be increased with other CNS depressants: alcohol, narcotics, sedative/hypnotics, skeletal muscle relaxants

• Increased effects of anticholinergic drugs

DENTAL CONSIDERATIONS

General:

• Monitor vital signs every appointment due to cardiovascular and respiratory side effects.

• After supine positioning, have patient sit upright for at least 2 min to avoid orthostatic hypotension.

• Assess salivary flow as a factor in caries, periodontal disease, and candidiasis.

• Psychologic and physical dependence may occur with chronic administration.

• Determine why the patient is taking the drug.

• Avoid in patients with chronic obstructive pulmonary disease.

Teach patient/family:

• To avoid mouth rinses with high alcohol content due to drying effects

hydroxychloroquine sulfate

(hye-drox-ee-klor′oh-kwin)

Plaquenil Sulfate

Drug class.: Antimalarial

Action: Inhibits parasite replications, transcription of DNA to RNA by forming complexes with DNA of parasite

Uses: Malaria caused by *P. vivax, P. malariae, P. ovale, P. falciparum* (some strains); lupus erythematosus; rheumatoid arthritis

Dosage and routes:

Malaria

• *Adult and child:* PO 5 mg/kg/wk on same day of week, not to exceed 400 mg; treatment should begin 2 wk before entering endemic area, continue 8 wk after leaving; if treatment begins after exposure, 800 mg for adult, 10 mg/kg for children in 2 divided doses 6 hr apart

Lupus erythematosus

• *Adult:* PO 400 mg qd-bid, length depends on patient response; maintenance 200-400 mg qd

Rheumatoid arthritis

• *Adult:* PO 400-600 mg qd, then 200-300 mg qd after good response

Available forms include: Tabs 200 mg

Side effects/adverse reactions:

▼ *ORAL:* Discoloration of mucosa, lichenoid lesions

CNS: ***Convulsions,*** headache, stimulation, fatigue, irritability, bad dreams, dizziness, confusion, psychosis, decreased reflexes

CV: ***Asystole with syncope,*** hypotension, heart block

GI: Nausea, vomiting, anorexia, diarrhea, cramps
HEMA: ***Thrombocytopenia, agranulocytosis, hemolytic anemia, leukopenia***
EENT: Blurred vision, corneal changes, retinal changes, difficulty focusing, tinnitus, vertigo, deafness, photophobia, corneal edema
INTEG: ***Exfoliative dermatitis,*** alopecia, pruritus, pigmentation changes, skin eruptions, lichen planus–like eruptions, eczema
Contraindications: Hypersensitivity, retinal field changes, prophyria, children (long-term)
Precautions: Blood dyscrasias, severe GI disease, neurologic disease, alcoholism, hepatic disease, G6PD deficiency, psoriasis, eczema, pregnancy category C
Pharmacokinetics:
PO: Peak 1-2 hr, half-life 3-5 days; metabolized in liver; excreted in urine, feces, breast milk; crosses placenta
Drug interactions of concern to dentistry:
• Hepatotoxicity: alcohol, hepatotoxic drugs

DENTAL CONSIDERATIONS
General:
• Patients on chronic drug therapy may rarely have symptoms of blood dyscrasias, which can include infection, bleeding, and poor healing.
• Avoid dental light in patient's eyes; offer dark glasses for patient comfort.
• Determine why the patient is taking the drug.
Consultations:
• In a patient with symptoms of blood dyscrasias, request a medical consult for blood studies and postpone dental treatment until normal values are reestablished.
Teach patient/family:
• Importance of good oral hygiene to prevent soft tissue inflammation
• To avoid mouth rinses with high alcohol content due to drying effects

---

hydroxyurea

(hye-drox-ee-your-ee'a)
Droxia, Hydrea
Drug class.: Antineoplastic

Action: Acts by inhibiting DNA synthesis without interfering with the synthesis of RNA or protein
Uses: Melanoma, chronic myelocytic leukemia, recurrent or metastatic ovarian cancer, in combination with irradiation therapy for carcinomas of the head and neck (except the lip); sickle-cell anemia
Dosage and routes:
Sickle-cell anemia
• *Child:* PO 15 mg/kg/day single dose, titrated at 12 weeks up to 35 mg/kg/day; monitor CBC q2wk
Solid tumors
• *Adult:* PO 80 mg/kg as a single dose q3d or 20-30 mg/kg as a single dose daily for continuous therapy
With radiation
• *Adult:* PO 80 mg/kg as a single dose q3d
Available forms include: Caps 500 mg
Side effects/adverse reactions:
▼ *ORAL:* Stomatitis, mucositis (with irradiation), lichenoid reaction
CNS: ***Convulsions,*** anorexia, headache, confusion, hallucinations, dizziness

CV: Angina, ischemia
GI: Nausea, vomiting, anorexia, diarrhea, constipation
HEMA: ***Leukopenia, anemia, thrombocytopenia***
GU: Increased BUN, uric acid, creatinine, temporary renal function impairment
INTEG: Rash, urticaria, pruritus, dry skin, facial erythema
Contraindications: Hypersensitivity, leukopenia (<2500/mm^3), thrombocytopenia (<100,000/mm^3),anemia (severe), marked bone marrow depression
Precautions: Pregnancy category D, monitor blood counts and hemoglobin, renal impairment, elderly
Pharmacokinetics:
PO: Readily absorbed with PO use, peak level in 2 hr; 80% excreted in urine
Drug interactions of concern to dentistry:
• None reported
DENTAL CONSIDERATIONS
General:
• Patients receiving chemotherapy may be taking chronic opioids for pain. Consider NSAIDs for dental pain management.
• Patients receiving chemotherapy may require palliative therapy for stomatitis.
• Patients on chronic drug therapy may rarely have symptoms of blood dyscrasias, which can include infection, bleeding, and poor healing.
Consultations:
• Medical consult may be required to assess disease control in the patient.
• In a patient with symptoms of blood dyscrasias, request a medical consult for blood studies and postpone dental treatment until normal values are reestablished.
Teach patient/family:
• That secondary oral infection may occur; must see dentist immediately if infection occurs
When chronic dry mouth occurs, advise patient:
• To avoid mouth rinses with high alcohol content due to drying effects
• To use sugarless gum, frequent sips of water, or saliva substitutes
• To use daily home fluoride products for anticaries effect

hydroxyzine HCl/ hydroxyzine pamoate

(hye-drox′i-zeen)
Atarax, Hyzine, Vistaril, Vistaril IM
Apo-Hydroxyzine, Multipax, Novo-Hydroxyzin
Drug class.: Antianxiety antihistamine

Action: Depresses subcortical levels of CNS, antagonist for histamine H_1-receptors
Uses: Anxiety; preoperatively/ postoperatively to prevent nausea, vomiting; to potentiate narcotic analgesics; sedation; pruritus
Dosage and routes:
• *Adult:* PO 25-100 mg tid-qid
• *Child >6 yr:* 50-100 mg/day in divided doses
• *Child <6 yr:* Up to 50 mg/day in divided doses
Preoperatively/postoperatively
• *Adult:* IM 25-100 mg q4-6h
• *Child:* IM 1.1 mg/kg q4-6h
Available forms include: Tabs 10, 25, 50, 100 mg; caps 25, 50, 100 mg; syrup 10 mg/5 ml; oral susp 25 mg/5 ml; inj IM 25 mg/ml

Side effects/adverse reactions:
▼ *ORAL:* Dry mouth
CNS: Dizziness, drowsiness, confusion, headache, tremors, fatigue, depression, convulsions
Contraindications: Hypersensitivity, pregnancy category not established, avoid in pregnancy
Precautions: Elderly, debilitated, hepatic disease, renal disease
Pharmacokinetics:
PO: Onset 15-30 min, duration 4-6 hr, half-life 3 hr
Drug interactions of concern to dentistry:
- Increased CNS depressant effect: alcohol, all CNS depressants
- Increased anticholinergic effects: other antihistamines, anticholinergics, opioid analgesics

DENTAL CONSIDERATIONS
General:
- Potentiates other CNS depressant drugs. When used in combination, the dose of other CNS depressants should be reduced by one half.
- Assess salivary flow as a factor in caries, periodontal disease, and candidiasis.
- Geriatric patients are more susceptible to drug effects; use lower dose.
- Have someone drive patient to and from dental appointment if the drug is prescribed for dental therapy.

Teach patient/family:
When chronic dry mouth occurs, advise patient:
- To avoid mouth rinses with high alcohol content due to drying effects
- To use sugarless gum, frequent sips of water, or saliva substitutes
- To use daily home fluoride products for anticaries effect

hyoscyamine sulfate
(hye-oh-sye'a-meen)
Anaspaz, Cystospaz-M, Gastrosed, Levbid, Levsin, Levsinex, Neoquess
Drug class.: Anticholinergic

Action: Inhibits muscarinic actions of acetylcholine at postganglionic parasympathetic neuroeffector sites
Uses: Treatment of peptic ulcer disease in combination with other drugs, other GI disorders, other spastic disorders such as parkinsonism, also preoperatively to reduce secretions
Dosage and routes:
- *Adult:* PO/SL 0.125-0.25 mg tid-qid ac, hs; time rel 0.375 q12h; IM/SC/IV 0.25-0.5 mg q6h
- *Child 2-10 yr:* One-half adult dose
- *Child <2 yr:* One-fourth adult dose

Available forms include: Tabs 0.125, 0.13, 0.15 mg; time rel caps 0.375 mg; sol 0.125 mg/ml; elix 0.125 mg/5 ml; inj IM/IV/SC 0.5 mg/ml
Side effects/adverse reactions:
▼ *ORAL: Dry mouth*
CNS: Confusion, stimulation in elderly, headache, insomnia, dizziness, drowsiness, anxiety, weakness, hallucination
CV: Palpitation, tachycardia
GI: Constipation, paralytic ileus, heartburn, nausea, vomiting, dysphagia
GU: Hesitancy, retention, impotence
EENT: Blurred vision, photophobia, mydriasis, cycloplegia, increased ocular tension

H

INTEG: Urticaria, rash, pruritus, anhidrosis, fever, allergic reactions
Contraindications: Hypersensitivity to anticholinergics, narrow-angle glaucoma, GI obstruction, myasthenia gravis, paralytic ileus, GI atony, toxic megacolon, prostatic hypertrophy
Precautions: Hyperthyroidism, CAD, dysrhythmias, CHF, ulcerative colitis, hypertension, hiatal hernia, hepatic disease, renal disease, pregnancy category C, urinary retention
Pharmacokinetics:
PO: Duration 4-6 hr; metabolized by liver, excreted in urine, half-life 3.5 hr
Drug interactions of concern to dentistry:
- Increased anticholinergic effect: other anticholinergics, opioid analgesics
- Decreased effect of phenothiazines, ketoconazole

DENTAL CONSIDERATIONS
General:
- After supine positioning, have patient sit upright for at least 2 min to avoid orthostatic hypotension.
- Assess salivary flow as a factor in caries, periodontal disease, and candidiasis.
- Avoid dental light in patient's eyes; offer dark glasses for patient comfort.

Consultation:
- Physician should be informed if significant xerostomic side effects occur (increased caries, sore tongue, problems eating or swallowing, difficulty wearing prosthesis) so a medication change can be considered.

Teach patient/family:
- Importance of good oral hygiene to prevent soft tissue inflammation

When chronic dry mouth occurs, advise patient:
- To avoid mouth rinses with high alcohol content due to drying effects
- To use sugarless gum, frequent sips of water, or artificial saliva substitutes
- To use daily home fluoride products for anticaries effect

ibuprofen

(eye-byoo-proe'fen)
Bayer Select, Cramp End, Motrin, Rufen, IBU, Ibifon, Ibuprohm
♣ Amersol
OTC: Advil, Dolgesic, Dynafed IB, Excedrin IB, Genpril, Haltran, Ibuprin, Liqui-Gels, Medipren, Menadol, Midol IB, Motrin IB, Nuprin, Pamprin IB, Q-Profen, Trendar
♣ Actiprofen, Apo-Ibuprofen, Novo-Profen, Nu-Ibuprofen
Susp: Children's Advil, Children's Motrin Oral Drops
♣ Children's Apo-Ibuprofen

Drug class.: Nonsteroidal antiinflammatory

Action: Inhibits prostaglandin synthesis by interfering with cyclooxygenase needed for biosynthesis; possesses analgesic, antiinflammatory, antipyretic properties
Uses: Rheumatoid arthritis, osteoarthritis, primary dysmenorrhea, gout, mild-to-moderate pain, fever
Dosage and routes:
- *Adult:* PO 200-800 mg qid, not to exceed 3.2 g/day
- *Child 2-11 yr:* PO oral suspension (OTC) for fever and minor aches and pain, toothache; 7.5 mg/kg up to qid; max daily dose 30 mg/kg

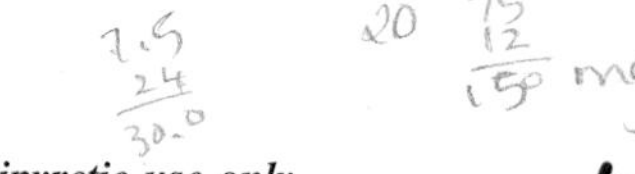

Antipyretic use only
• Child 6 mo-12 yr:
• 5 mg/kg for temperature <102.5° F; 10 mg/kg for higher temperature q4-6h

Available forms include: Tabs 100, 200 (OTC), 300, 400, 600, 800 mg; chew tabs 50, 100 mg; OTC susp 100 mg/5 ml in 60, 120, and 480 ml volumes; caps 100 mg; oral drops 40 mg/ml in 15 ml

Side effects/adverse reactions:

ORAL: Dry mouth, bleeding, stomatitis, lichenoid reaction

CNS: Dizziness, drowsiness, fatigue, tremors, confusion, insomnia, anxiety, depression

CV: Tachycardia, peripheral edema, palpitation, dysrhythmias

GI: ***Cholestatic hepatitis,*** nausea, anorexia, vomiting, diarrhea, jaundice, constipation, flatulence, cramps, peptic ulcer

HEMA: ***Blood dyscrasias***

GU: ***Nephrotoxicity: dysuria, hematuria, oliguria, azotemia***

EENT: Tinnitus, hearing loss, blurred vision

INTEG: Purpura, rash, pruritus, sweating

Contraindications: Hypersensitivity, asthma, severe renal disease, severe hepatic disease, alcohol

Precautions: Pregnancy category not established (use not recommended), lactation, children, bleeding disorders, GI disorders, cardiac disorders, hypersensitivity to other antiinflammatory agents

Pharmacokinetics:

PO: Peak 1-2 hr, half-life 2-4 hr; 90%-99% plasma-protein binding; metabolized in liver (inactive metabolites); excreted in urine (inactive metabolites)

Drug interactions of concern to dentistry:

• GI ulceration, bleeding: aspirin, alcohol, corticosteroids
• Decreased action: salicylates
• Nephrotoxicity: acetaminophen (prolonged use)
• Possible risk of decreased renal function: cyclosporine

When prescribed for dental pain:
• Risk of increased effects: oral anticoagulants, oral antidiabetics, lithium, methotrexate
• Decreased antihypertensive effects of diuretics, β-adrenergic blockers, and ACE inhibitors

DENTAL CONSIDERATIONS

General:

• Patients on chronic drug therapy may rarely have symptoms of blood dyscrasias, which can include infection, bleeding, and poor healing.
• Assess salivary flow as a factor in caries, periodontal disease, and candidiasis.
• Avoid prescribing aspirin-containing products.
• Consider semisupine chair position for patients with arthritic disease.

Consultations:

• In a patient with symptoms of blood dyscrasias, request a medical consult for blood studies and postpone dental treatment until normal values are reestablished.
• Medical consult may be required to assess disease control in the patient.

Teach patient/family:

• To follow labeled directions for OTC products
• Importance of good oral hygiene to prevent soft tissue inflammation
• Caution to prevent injury when using oral hygiene aids

When chronic dry mouth occurs, advise patient:
• To avoid mouth rinses with high alcohol content due to drying effects
• To use sugarless gum, frequent sips of water, or saliva substitutes
• To use daily home fluoride products for anticaries effect

idoxuridine-IDU (ophthalmic)

(eye-dox-yoor'i-deen)
Herplex Liquifilm
Drug class.: Antiviral

Action: Inhibits viral replication by interfering with viral DNA synthesis
Uses: Herpes simplex keratitis, vaccinia virus keratitis, herpes simplex keratoconjunctivitis; unlabeled, has been used for herpes labialis
Dosage and routes:
• *Adult and child:* Instill 1 gtt qh during day and q2h during night; or 1 gtt qmin for 5 min, repeat q4h
Available forms include: Sol 0.1%
Side effects/adverse reactions:
EENT: Poor corneal wound healing, temporary visual haze, overgrowth of nonsusceptible organisms
Contraindications: Hypersensitivity
Precautions: Antibiotic hypersensitivity, pregnancy category C, lactation
Drug interactions of concern to dentistry:
• None reported
DENTAL CONSIDERATIONS
General:
• Avoid dental light in patient's eyes; offer dark glasses for patient comfort.
• Protect patient's eyes from accidental spatter during dental treatment.
• Patient may also have symptomatic oral herpes, which could delay dental treatment. Question patient about any current treatment if oral lesions are present.

imipramine HCl/ imipramine pamoate

(im-ip'ra-meen)
Imipramine HCl: Norfranil, Tipramine, Tofranil
✱ Apo-Imipramine, Impril, Novopramine
Imipramine pamoate: Tofranil-PM Capsules
Drug class.: Antidepressant (tricyclic)

Action: Inhibits both norepinephrine and serotonin (5-HT) uptake in the brain, although the precise antidepressant mechanism remains unclear
Uses: Depression, enuresis in children; unapproved uses include neurogenic pain, panic disorder, migraine headache
Dosage and routes:
• *Adult:* PO/IM 75-100 mg/day in divided doses; may increase by 25-50 mg to 200 mg, not to exceed 300 mg/day; may give daily dose hs
• *Child:* PO 25-75 mg/day
Available forms include: Tabs 10, 25, 50 mg; caps 75, 100, 125 mg
Side effects/adverse reactions:
▼ *ORAL: Dry mouth, unpleasant taste,* stomatitis
CNS: Dizziness, drowsiness, confusion, headache, anxiety, tremors,

stimulation, weakness, insomnia, nightmares, EPS (elderly), increased psychiatric symptoms, paresthesia

CV: Orthostatic hypotension, ECG changes, tachycardia, ***hypertension,*** palpitation

GI: Diarrhea, ***paralytic ileus, hepatitis,*** nausea, vomiting, increased appetite, cramps, epigastric distress, jaundice

HEMA: ***Agranulocytosis, thrombocytopenia, eosinophilia, leukopenia***

GU: Retention, ***acute renal failure***

EENT: Blurred vision, tinnitus, mydriasis

INTEG: Rash, urticaria, sweating, pruritus, photosensitivity

Contraindications: Hypersensitivity to tricyclic antidepressants, recovery phase of MI, convulsive disorders, prostatic hypertrophy

Precautions: Suicidal patients, severe depression, increased intraocular pressure, narrow-angle glaucoma, urinary retention, cardiac disease, hepatic disease, hyperthyroidism, electroshock therapy, elective surgery, elderly, pregnancy category B, MAO inhibitors

Pharmacokinetics:

PO: Steady state 2-5 days, half-life 6-20 hr; metabolized by liver; excreted by kidneys, feces; crosses placenta; excreted in breast milk

Drug interactions of concern to dentistry:

• Increased anticholinergic effects: muscarinic blockers, antihistamines, phenothiazines

• Increased effects of direct-acting sympathomimetics (epinephrine, levonordefrin)

• Potential risk of increased CNS depression: alcohol, barbiturates, benzodiazepines, and other CNS depressants

• Decreased antihypertensive effects: clonidine, guanadrel, guanethidine

DENTAL CONSIDERATIONS

General:

• Monitor vital signs every appointment due to cardiovascular side effects.

• Assess salivary flow as a factor in caries, periodontal disease, and candidiasis.

• Patients on chronic drug therapy may rarely have symptoms of blood dyscrasias, which can include infection, bleeding, and poor healing.

• After supine positioning, have patient sit upright for at least 2 min to avoid orthostatic hypotension.

• Use vasoconstrictors with caution, in low doses, and with careful aspiration. Avoid use of gingival retraction cord with epinephrine.

• Place on frequent recall due to oral side effects.

Consultations:

• In a patient with symptoms of blood dyscrasias, request a medical consult for blood studies and postpone dental treatment until normal values are reestablished.

• Medical consult may be required to assess disease control in the patient.

• Physician should be informed if significant xerostomic side effects occur (increased caries, sore tongue, problems eating or swallowing, difficulty wearing prosthesis) so a medication change can be considered.

Teach patient/family:

• Importance of good oral hygiene to prevent soft tissue inflammation

• Caution to prevent injury when using oral hygiene aids

When chronic dry mouth occurs, advise patient:

• To avoid mouth rinses with high alcohol content due to drying effects

• To use sugarless gum, frequent sips of water, or saliva substitutes

• To use daily home fluoride products for anticaries effect

imiquimod

(i-mi-kwi′mod)

Aldara

Drug class.: Immune response modifier

Action: Mechanism is unknown; imiquimod induces cytokines including interferon-α in animal studies

Uses: External genital and perianal warts, condylomata acuminata

Dosage and routes:

• *Adult:* TOP apply cream 3 days per week at bedtime, leave on the skin for 6-10 hr; remove cream with mild soap and water after treatment; max duration of treatment 16 wk; cream is applied in a thin layer to the wart and rubbed in until no longer visible

Available forms include: Cream 5% in packets containing 250 mg of cream, 12 packets/box

Side effects/adverse reactions:

CNS: Headache, fatigue, fever

GI: Diarrhea

INTEG: Erythema, erosion, flaking, edema, induration, ulceration, scabbing, vesicles

MS: Myalgia

MISC: Fungal infection, flulike symptoms

Contraindications: None listed

Precautions: Has not been evaluated in papilloma viral diseases, cream may weaken condoms and diaphragms, external use only, pregnancy category B, lactation, children <18 yr

Pharmacokinetics:

TOP: Minimal cutaneous absorption

Drug interactions of concern to dentistry:

• None reported

DENTAL CONSIDERATIONS

General:

• Oral manifestations of the disease may occur in the oral mucosa.

• Patient may have history of other STDs.

Consultations:

• Medical consult may be required to assess disease control in the patient.

Teach patient/family:

• To report oral lesions to the dentist

• Importance of updating health and drug history if physician makes any changes in evaluation/drug regimens

indapamide

(in-dap′a-mide)

Lozol

✤ Lozide

Drug class.: Diuretic, thiazide-like

Action: Acts on distal tubule by increasing excretion of water, sodium, chloride, potassium

Uses: Edema, hypertension

Dosage and routes:

• *Adult:* PO 2.5 mg qd in AM, may be increased to 5 mg qd if needed

Available forms include: Tabs 1.25, 2.5 mg

Side effects/adverse reactions:
▼ *ORAL:* Dry mouth
CNS: Headache, dizziness, fatigue, weakness, paresthesia, depression
CV: Orthostatic hypotension, volume depletion, palpitation
GI: Nausea, diarrhea, vomiting, anorexia, cramps, constipation, pancreatitis, abdominal pain, jaundice, hepatitis
HEMA: ***Thrombocytopenia, agranulocytosis, leukopenia, neutropenia, anemia***
GU: Polyuria, dysuria, frequency
EENT: Loss of hearing, tinnitus, blurred vision, nasal congestion, increased intraocular pressure
INTEG: Rash, pruritus, photosensitivity, alopecia, urticaria
MS: Cramps
ELECT: Hypochloremic alkalosis, hypomagnesemia, hyperuricemia, hypercalcemia, hyponatremia, hypokalemia, hyperglycemia

Contraindications: Hypersensitivity, anuria

Precautions: Hypokalemia, dehydration, ascites, hepatic disease, severe renal disease, pregnancy category B

Pharmacokinetics:
PO: Onset 1-2 hr, peak 2 hr, duration up to 36 hr, half-life 14-18 hr; excreted in urine, feces

Drug interactions of concern to dentistry:
• Increased photosensitization: tetracycline
• Decreased hypotensive response: NSAIDs, especially indomethacin

DENTAL CONSIDERATIONS

General:
• Monitor vital signs every appointment due to cardiovascular side effects.
• Patients on chronic drug therapy may rarely have symptoms of blood dyscrasias, which can include infection, bleeding, and poor healing.
• After supine positioning, have patient sit upright for at least 2 min before standing to avoid orthostatic hypotension.
• Assess salivary flow as a factor in caries, periodontal disease, and candidiasis.
• Limit use of sodium-containing products such as saline IV fluids for patients with a dietary salt restriction.
• Stress from dental procedures may compromise cardiovascular function; determine patient risk.
• Short appointments and a stress reduction protocol may be required for anxious patients.
• Patients on diuretic therapy should be monitored for serum K^+ levels.

Consultations:
• In a patient with symptoms of blood dyscrasias, request a medical consult for blood studies and postpone dental treatment until normal values are reestablished.
• Medical consult may be required to assess disease control and patient's ability to tolerate stress.

Teach patient/family:
• Importance of good oral hygiene to prevent soft tissue inflammation
• Caution to prevent injury when using oral hygiene aids

When chronic dry mouth occurs, advise patient:
• To avoid mouth rinses with high alcohol content due to drying effects
• To use sugarless gum, frequent sips of water, or saliva substitutes
• To use daily home fluoride products for anticaries effect

indinavir sulfate

(in-din′a-veer)

Crixivan

Drug class.: Antiviral

Action: Inhibits HIV protease enzyme, preventing cleavage of viral polyproteins and formation of immature noninfectious viral particles

Uses: HIV infection; prophylaxis after needle stick with AZT and lamivudine within 2 hr of needle stick

Dosage and routes:

• *Adult:* PO 800 mg q8h without food, 1 hr before or 2 hr after meal, force fluids; reduce dose to 600 mg q8h with concurrent use of ketoconazole

Available forms include: Caps 200, 400 mg

Side effects/adverse reactions:

▼ *ORAL: Dry mouth, taste alteration,* aphthous stomatitis, gingivitis

CNS: Headache, insomnia, dizziness, somnolence

CV: Palpitation

GI: Abdominal pain, nausea, diarrhea, vomiting, acid regurgitation

RESP: Upper respiratory infection, cough

HEMA: ***Hyperbilirubinemia,*** anemia, lymphadenopathy

GU: Nephrolithiasis, flank pain, hematuria

EENT: Pharyngitis, blurred vision

INTEG: Rash, dry skin, dermatitis

MS: Asthenia, fatigue, back pain

Contraindications: Hypersensitivity; concurrent use with cisapride, triazolam, midazolam, alprazolam, chlordiazepoxide, clonazepam, chlorazepate, diazepam, estazolam, flurazepam, halazepam, quazepam

Precautions: Nephrolithiasis (requires adequate hydration), hyperbilirubinemia, serum transaminase elevation, hepatic impairment, dose reduction of rifabutin required, pregnancy category C, lactation, children

Pharmacokinetics:

PO: Rapid absorption, food reduces absorption, 60% plasma protein bound, peak plasma levels 1 hr, hepatic metabolism, urinary and GI excretion

Drug interactions of interest to dentistry:

• Contraindicated with terfenadine, astemizole, triazolam, midazolam, cisapride

• Reduce dose when given with ketoconazole

• Increased blood levels of: clarithromycin

DENTAL CONSIDERATIONS

General:

• Consider semisupine chair position when GI side effects occur.

• Assess salivary flow as a factor in caries, periodontal disease, candidiasis.

• Monitor vital signs every appointment due to cardiovascular side effects.

• Examine for oral manifestation of opportunistic infection.

• Patients with gastroesophageal reflux may have oral symptoms, including burning mouth, secondary candidiasis, and signs of tooth erosion.

Consultations:

• Medical consult may be required to assess disease control in the patient.

Teach patient/family:

• Importance of good oral hygiene to prevent soft tissue inflammation

• To report oral lesions, soreness, or bleeding to dentist

• Importance of updating health history/drug record if physician makes any changes in evaluations/drug regimens

When chronic dry mouth occurs, advise patient:

• To avoid mouth rinses with high alcohol content due to drying effects

• To use daily home fluoride products for anticaries effect

• To use sugarless gum, frequent sips of water, or saliva substitutes

indomethacin/ indomethacin sodium trihydrate

(in-doe-meth'a-sin)

Indameth, Indocin, Indocin SR

♣ Apo-Indomethacin, Indocid, Indocid SR, Novo-Methacin, Nu-Indo

Drug class.: Nonsteroidal antiinflammatory

Action: Inhibits prostaglandin synthesis by interfering with cyclooxygenase needed for biosynthesis; possesses analgesic, antiinflammatory, antipyretic properties

Uses: Rheumatoid arthritis, osteoarthritis, ankylosing rheumatoid spondylitis, acute gouty arthritis; unapproved uses include closure of patent ductus arteriosus in premature infants

Dosage and routes:

Arthritis

• *Adult:* PO/REC 25 mg bid-tid, may increase by 25 mg/day q1wk, not to exceed 200 mg/day; sus rel 75 mg qd, may increase to 75 mg bid

Acute arthritis

• *Adult:* PO/REC 50 mg tid; use only for acute attack, then reduce dose

Available forms include: Caps 25, 50 mg; ext rel caps 75 mg; susp 25 mg/5 ml; rec supp 50, 100 mg

Side effects/adverse reactions:

▼ *ORAL:* Dry mouth, bleeding, stomatitis, lichenoid reaction

CNS: Dizziness, drowsiness, fatigue, tremors, confusion, insomnia, anxiety, depression

CV: Tachycardia, peripheral edema, palpitation, dysrhythmias

GI: ***Cholestatic hepatitis,*** nausea, anorexia, vomiting, diarrhea, jaundice, constipation, flatulence, cramps, peptic ulcer

HEMA: ***Blood dyscrasias***

GU: ***Nephrotoxicity: dysuria, hematuria, oliguria, azotemia***

EENT: Tinnitus, hearing loss, blurred vision

INTEG: Purpura, rash, pruritus, sweating

Contraindications: Hypersensitivity, asthma, severe renal disease, severe hepatic disease

Precautions: Pregnancy category not listed (use not recommended), lactation, children, bleeding disorders, GI disorders, cardiac disorders, hypersensitivity to other antiinflammatory agents, depression

Pharmacokinetics:

PO: Onset 1-2 hr, peak 3 hr, duration 4-6 hr; 99% plasma-protein binding; metabolized in liver, kidneys; excreted in urine, bile, feces, breast milk; crosses placenta

Drug interactions of concern to dentistry:

• Increased GI bleeding, ulcera-

tion: corticosteroids, alcohol, aspirin, other NSAIDs
• Renal toxicity: acetaminophen (high doses, prolonged use)
• Possible risk of decreased renal function: cyclosporine

When prescribed for dental pain:
• Risk of increased effects: oral anticoagulants, oral antidiabetics, lithium, methotrexate
• Decreased antihypertensive effects of diuretics, β-adrenergic blockers, and ACE inhibitors

DENTAL CONSIDERATIONS

General:
• Avoid prescribing aspirin-containing products.
• Patients on chronic drug therapy may rarely have symptoms of blood dyscrasias, which can include infection, bleeding, and poor healing.
• Assess salivary flow as a factor in caries, periodontal disease, and candidiasis.
• Consider semisupine chair position for patients with arthritic disease.

Consultations:
• In a patient with symptoms of blood dyscrasias, request a medical consult for blood studies and postpone dental treatment until normal values are reestablished.
• Medical consult may be required to assess disease control in the patient.

Teach patient/family:
• Importance of good oral hygiene to prevent soft tissue inflammation
• Caution to prevent injury when using oral hygiene aids

When chronic dry mouth occurs, advise patient:
• To avoid mouth rinses with high alcohol content due to drying effects
• To use sugarless gum, frequent sips of water, or saliva substitutes
• To use daily home fluoride products for anticaries effect

insulin/insulin lispro

(obtained from beef or pork, or human recombinant technology)

(in'su-lin)

Insulin injection USP: Regular Iletin I, Regular Iletin II, U-500, Regular Purified Pork Insulin

✤ Iletin, Iletin II, Novolin ge Toronto

Insulin human injection USP: Humulin-R, Novolin R, Velosulin Human BR

Insulin zinc suspension: Lente Iletin II, Lentel

✤ Iletin, Iletin II, Novolin ge Lente

Insulin zinc suspension, human: Humulin L, Novolin L

Isophane insulin suspension: NPH Iletin I and II, NPH-N

✤ Iletin NPH, Iletin II NPH, Novolin ge NPH

Isophane insulin suspension, human: Humulin N, Novolin N

Isophane insulin and insulin: Humalin 50/50

✤ Novolin ge 50/50

Isophane insulin (human) and insulin (human): Humulin 70/30, Novolin 70/30

✤ Humalin 30/70, Novolin ge 30/70

Human insulin zinc suspension, extended: Ultralente I, Ultralente

Insulin zinc suspension, prompt: Semilente Iletin I

Insulin zinc suspension, extended: Humalin U Ultralente

✤ Humulin_U*, Novolin ge Ultralente*

Insulin analog injection (insulin lispro): Humalog

Drug class.: Exogenous insulin, antidiabetic

Action: Decreases blood glucose; important in the regulation of fat and protein metabolism

Uses: Ketoacidosis, type I (IDDM) and type II (NIDDM) diabetes mellitus, hyperkalemia, hyperalimentation

Dosage and routes:

• *Adult:* SC/IV/IM dosage individualized by blood, urine glucose qd-tid

Available forms include: 100 U/ml and cartridges for NovoPen units

Side effects/adverse reactions: These reactions may reflect either the disease or inappropriate insulin doses.

▼ *ORAL:* Dry mouth (rarely a problem)

CNS: Headache, lethargy, tremors, weakness, fatigue, delirium, sweating

CV: Tachycardia, palpitation

GI: Hunger, nausea

EENT: Blurred vision

INTEG: Flushing, rash, urticaria, warmth, lipodystrophy, lipohypertrophy

META: Hypoglycemia

SYST: ***Anaphylaxis,*** local allergic reactions

Contraindications: Hypersensitivity to protomine

Precautions: Pregnancy category not listed

Pharmacokinetics: Depends on type of insulin used; regular insulin and prompt insulin zinc suspension have rapid onset and short duration; NPH insulin and zinc insulin suspensions are intermediate acting, and protamine zinc insulin and extended zinc insulin are long acting

Drug interactions of concern to dentistry:

• Increased hypoglycemia: salicy-

lates and NSAIDs (large doses and chronic use), alcohol
• Hyperglycemia: corticosteroids, epinephrine

DENTAL CONSIDERATIONS

General:

• Monitor vital signs every appointment due to cardiovascular effects of hypoglycemia.
• Place on frequent recall to evaluate healing response.
• Diabetics may be more susceptible to infection and have delayed wound healing.
• Assess salivary flow as a factor in caries, periodontal disease, and candidiasis.
• Prophylactic antibiotics may be indicated to prevent infection if surgery or deep scaling is planned.
• Ensure that patient is following prescribed diet and regularly takes medication.
• Question patient about self-monitoring of drug's antidiabetic effect, including blood glucose values or finger-stick records.
• Keep a readily available source of sugar or juice in case of insulin overdose.

Consultations:

• Medical consult may be required to assess disease control and patient's tolerance for stress.
• Medical consult may include data from patient's blood glucose monitoring, including glycosylated hemoglobin or HbA_{1c} testing.

Teach patient/family:

• Importance of good oral hygiene to prevent soft tissue inflammation
• Caution to prevent injury when using oral hygiene aids
• To avoid mouth rinses with high alcohol content due to drying effects

interferon alfa-2a/ interferon alfa-2b/ interferon alfa-n1/ interferon alfa-n3/ interferon beta-1a

(in-ter-feer'on)

Interferon alfa-2a: Roferon A
Interferon alfa-2b: Intron A
♣ *Interferon alfa-n1:* Wellferon
Interferon alfa-n3: Alferon N
Interferon beta-1a: Avonex

Drug class.: Biologic response modifier

Action: Antiviral action inhibits viral replication by reprogramming virus; antitumor action suppresses cell proliferation; immunomodulating action phagocytizes target cells

Uses: Hairy cell leukemia in persons >18 yr, condyloma acuminatum, metastatic melanoma, AIDS, Kaposi's sarcoma, bladder carcinoma, lymphomas, malignant myeloma, mycosis fungoides, laryngeal papillomatosis, chronic hepatitis C, chronic hepatitis B in pediatric patients <1 yr

Dosage and routes:

• *Adult:* SC/IM (interferon alfa-2a) 3 million IU × 16-24 wk, then 3 million IU 3 × weekly maintenance; SC/IM (interferon alfa-2b) 2 million IU/m^2 3 × weekly; if severe adverse reactions occur, dose should be reduced by one half; doses will vary to some extent with disease being treated

Condyloma acuminatum (veneral/ genital warts)

• *Adult:* SC/IM (interferon alfa-n3) 0.05 ml (250,000 IU) intralesional, given 2 × weekly × 8 wk; not to exceed 0.5 ml (2.5 million IU); inject into base of wart

Multiple sclerosis

• *Adult:* IM interferon beta-1a 30 μg weekly

Available forms include: Interferon alfa-2a inj 3, 6, 9, 36 million IU/vial; alfa-2b inj 3, 5, 10, 18, 25, 50 million IU/vial; alfa-n3 inj 5 million IU/1 ml vial with 3.3 mg/ml phenol and 1 mg/ml human albumin

Side effects/adverse reactions:

▼ *ORAL: Taste changes,* dry mouth, stomatitis

CNS: Dizziness, confusion, numbness, paresthesia, ***convulsions, coma,*** hallucinations, amnesia, anxiety, mood changes

CV: Edema, hypotension, ***CHF, MI, CVA,*** hypertension, chest pain, palpitation, dysrhythmias

GI: Weight loss

GU: Impotence

INTEG: Rash, dry skin, itching, alopecia, flushing

MISC: Flulike syndrome: fever, fatigue, myalgias, headache, chills

Contraindications: Hypersensitivity

Precautions: Severe hypotension, dysrhythmia, tachycardia, pregnancy category C, lactation, children, severe renal or hepatic disease, convulsion disorder, thrombophlebitis, coagulation disorders, hemophilia

Pharmacokinetics:

SC/IM: Half-life (interferon alfa-2a) 3.7-8.5 hr, peak 3-4 hr; half-life (interferon alfa-2b) 2-7 hr, peak 6-8 hr; alfa-n3: no detectable plasma levels

Drug interactions of concern to dentistry:

• None reported

DENTAL CONSIDERATIONS

General:

• Determine why the patient is taking the drug.
• Monitor vital signs every appointment due to cardiovascular side effects.
• After supine positioning, have patient sit upright for at least 2 min to avoid orthostatic hypotension.
• Palliative medication may be required for oral side effects.
• Assess salivary flow as a factor in caries, periodontal disease, and candidiasis.

Consultations:

• Medical consult may be required to assess disease control in the patient.

Teach patient/family:

• Importance of good oral hygiene to prevent soft tissue inflammation
• To report oral lesions, soreness, or bleeding to dentist

When chronic dry mouth occurs, advise patient:

• To avoid mouth rinses with high alcohol content due to drying effects
• To use sugarless gum, frequent sips of water, or saliva substitutes
• To use daily home fluoride products for anticaries effect
• Importance of updating medical/drug record if physican makes any changes in evaluation or drug regimen

interferon gamma-1b

(in-ter-fer'on)

Actimmune

Drug class.: Biologic response modifier

Action: Species-specific protein synthesized in response to viruses, potent phagocyte-activating effects, stimulates superoxide anion production, enhances oxidative metabolism of macrophages, enhances antibody-dependent cellular cytotoxicity, enhances natural killer cell activity

Uses: Serious infections associated with chronic granulomatous disease

Dosage and routes:

• *Adult:* SC 50 μg/m^2 (1.5 million U/m^2) for patients with a surface area >0.5 m^2; 1.5 μg/kg/dose for patients with a surface area <0.5/m^2; give on Monday, Wednesday, Friday for dosing 3 times weekly

Available forms include: Inj 100 μg (3 million U) single-dose vial

Side effects/adverse reactions:

CNS: Headache, fatigue, fever, chills, depression, confusion, seizures

CV: Hypotension, syncope, tachycardia, heart block

GI: Nausea, anorexia, diarrhea, vomiting, abdominal pain, weight loss, GI bleeding

RESP: Bronchospasm, tachypnea

HEMA: ***Leukopenia, thrombocytopenia,*** deep vein thrombosis

INTEG: Rash, pain at injection site

MS: Myalgia, arthralgia

META: Hyponatremia, hyperglycemia

Contraindications: Hypersensitivity to interferon gamma, *E. coli*–derived products

Precautions: Pregnancy category C, cardiac disease, seizure disorders, CNS disorders, myelosuppression, lactation, children <1 yr; monitor hematologic values q3mo

Pharmacokinetics:

SC: Slow absorption, peak 7 hr, elimination half-life 5.9 hr; dose absorbed 89%

Drug interactions of concern to dentistry:

• None reported

DENTAL CONSIDERATIONS

General:

• Determine why the patient is taking the drug.

• Patients on chronic drug therapy may rarely have symptoms of blood dyscrasias, which can include infection, bleeding, and poor healing.

• Ask patient about side effects associated with drug use (abnormal hematologic values).

• Consider semisupine chair position for patient comfort if GI side effects occur.

• Place on frequent recall to evaluate healing response.

Consultations:

• In a patient with symptoms of blood dyscrasias, request a medical consult for blood studies and postpone dental treatment until normal values are reestablished.

• Medical consult may be required to assess disease control and patient's ability to tolerate stress.

Teach patient/family:

• Importance of good oral hygiene to prevent soft tissue inflammation

• Caution to prevent trauma when using oral hygiene aids

• Importance of updating medical history/drug record if physician makes any changes in evaluation/drug regimens

ipratropium bromide

(i-pra-troe'pee-um)

Atrovent

✦ Apo-Ipravent, Kendral-Ipratropium

Drug class.: Anticholinergic bronchodilator

Action: Inhibits interaction of acetylcholine at receptor sites on the bronchial smooth muscle, resulting in bronchodilation

Uses: Bronchodilation during bronchospasm in those with COPD, bronchitis, emphysema, asthma; not for rapid bronchodilation, maintenance treatment only; rhinorrhea, rhinorrhea associated with allergic and nonallergic perennial rhinitis in children age 6-11 yr

Dosage and routes:

• *Adult and child >5 yr:* 2 inh 4 times daily, not to exceed 12 inh/24 hr

Available forms include: Nasal spray 0.06% (42 μg /spray); aerosol 18 μg /actuation; Canada 20 μg/actuation, 200 inh/container

Side effects/adverse reactions:

▼ *ORAL: Dry mouth,* stomatitis, metallic taste

CNS: Anxiety, dizziness, headache

CV: Palpitation

GI: Nausea, vomiting, cramps

RESP: Cough, worsening of symptoms

EENT: Blurred vision, nasal dryness, nasal bleeding

INTEG: Rash

Contraindications: Hypersensitivity to this drug or atropine

Precautions: Pregnancy category B, lactation, children <12 yr, narrow-angle glaucoma, prostatic hypertrophy, bladder neck obstruction

Pharmacokinetics: Onset 5-15 min, duration 3-4 hr, half-life 2 hr; does not cross blood-brain barrier

Drug interactions of concern to dentistry:

• Increased effects of anticholinergic drugs

DENTAL CONSIDERATIONS

General:

• Monitor vital signs every appointment due to cardiovascular and respiratory side effects.

• Assess salivary flow as a factor in caries, periodontal disease, and candidiasis.

• Acute asthmatic episodes may be precipitated in the dental office. Sympathomimetic inhalants should be available for emergency use.

• Consider semisupine chair position for patients with respiratory disease.

• Place on frequent recall due to oral side effects.

Consultations:

• Medical consult may be required to assess disease control and patient's ability to tolerate stress.

Teach patient/family:

• For inhalation dosage forms, rinse mouth with water after each dose to prevent dryness

When chronic dry mouth occurs, advise patient:

• To avoid mouth rinses with high alcohol content due to drying effects

• To use sugarless gum, frequent sips of water, or saliva substitutes

• To use daily home fluoride products for anticaries effect

irbesartan

(ir-be-sar′tan)

Avapro

Drug class.: Angiotensin II receptor antagonist, antihypertensive

Action: Acts as a competitive antagonist for angiotensin II (AT_1) receptors, inhibiting both vasoconstrictor and aldosterone secreting effects

Uses: Hypertension alone or in combination with other antihypertensive drugs

Dosage and routes:

• *Adult:* PO initial 150 mg qd; some patients may require 300 mg/day; initial dose for volume- or salt-depleted patients is 75 mg/day

Available forms include: Tabs 75, 150, 300 mg

Side effects/adverse reactions:

CNS: Fatigue, headache, dizziness, anxiety

CV: Orthostatic hypotension, increased heart rate

GI: Diarrhea, dyspepsia, heartburn, nausea, vomiting

RESP: URI, pharyngitis

EENT: Rhinitis

INTEG: Rash, urticaria, pruritus

MS: Musculoskeletal trauma, muscle ache

Contraindications: Hypersensitivity, pregnancy (second, third trimester)

Precautions: Hypersensitivity to other angiotensin II receptor antagonists, pregnancy category C, volume- or salt-depleted patients, renal impairment, lactation, children

Pharmacokinetics:

PO: Bioavilaility 60%-80%, rapid absorption, peak serum levels 1.5-2 hr, 90% protein bound, hepatic metabolism, both biliary and renal excretion

Drug interactions of concern to dentistry:

• None reported

DENTAL CONSIDERATIONS

General:

• Monitor vital signs every appointment due to cardiovascular side effects.

• Limit use of sodium-containing products such as saline IV fluids for those patients with a dietary salt restriction.

• Stress from dental procedures may compromise cardiovascular function; determine patient risk.

• Short appointments and a stress reduction protocol may be required for anxious patients.

• Use precaution if sedation or general anesthesia is required; risk of hypotensive episode.

• After supine positioning, have patient sit upright for at least 2 min before standing to avoid orthostatic hypotension.

• Consider semisupine chair position for patient comfort if GI side effects occur.

Consultations:

• Consultation with physician may be needed if sedation or general anesthesia is required.

• Medical consult may be required to assess disease control and patient's ability to tolerate stress; there is risk for a hypotensive episode.

Teach patient/family: Importance

of updating health and drug history if physician makes any changes in evaluation/drug regimens

isocarboxazid

(eye-soe-kar-box'a-zid)

Marplan

Drug class.: Antidepressant—monoamine oxidase inhibitor

Action: Increases concentrations of endogenous norepinephrine, serotonin, and dopamine in CNS storage sites by nonselective inhibition of MAO enzymes; the precise antidepressant mechanism is unknown

Uses: Depression

Dosage and routes:

• *Adult:* PO 10 mg/bid, if tolerated can increase dose 10 mg every 2-4 days to 40 mg by end of first week; max daily dose 60 mg in divided doses

Available forms include: Tabs 10 mg

Side effects/adverse reactions:

▼ *ORAL: Dry mouth*

CNS: Dizziness, sedation, hypomania, headache, mania, insomnia, anxiety, tremors, stimulation, weakness, agitation, convulsions, increased neuromuscular activity

CV: Orthostatic hypotension, syncope, palpitation, tachycardia

GI: Constipation, nausea, diarrhea, abdominal pain

HEMA: ***Agranulocytosis, thrombocytopenia,*** spider telangiectases, anemia (rare)

GU: Sexual dysfunction, urinary retention

EENT: Blurred vision, ocular toxicity

INTEG: Rash

ENDO: ***SIADH-like syndrome,*** hyperprolactinemia

META: Hepatic function abnormalities

MISC: Weight gain

Contraindications: Hypersensitivity to MAO inhibitors, elderly, hypertension, CHF, severe hepatic disease, pheochromocytoma, severe renal disease, severe cardiac disease, foods with high tryptophan or tyramine content, excessive caffeine, sympathomimetics, meperidine

Precautions: Suicidal patients, concurrent use with other antidepressants (patients must stop taking MAO inhibitor 14 days before initiating therapy with other antidepressants), general anesthesia, severe depression, schizophrenia, iabetes mellitus, pregnancy category C, lactation, children <16 yr

Pharmacokinetics:

PO: Good absorption; maximum MAO inhibition 5-10 days, duration up to 2 wk; metabolized by liver, excreted by kidneys

Drug interactions of concern to dentistry:

• Increased pressor effects: indirect-acting sympathomimetics (ephedrine)

• Hyperpyretic crisis, convulsions, hypertensive episode: meperidine, possibly other opioids, carbamazepine

• Increased anticholinergic effects: anticholinergics, antihistamines

• Increased effects of alcohol, barbiturates, benzodiazepines, CNS depressants, SSRIs, tricyclic antidepressants, cyclobenzaprine, bupropion, buspirone, dextromethorphan, antihypertensives

DENTAL CONSIDERATIONS
General:
• Monitor vital signs every appointment due to cardiovascular side effects.
• After supine positioning, have patient sit upright for at least 2 min to avoid orthostatic hypotension.
• Patients on chronic drug therapy may rarely have symptoms of blood dyscrasias, which can include infection, bleeding, and poor healing.
• Consider semisupine chair position for patient comfort if GI side effects occur.
• Assess salivary flow as a factor in caries, periodontal disease, and candidiasis.
• Hypertensive episodes are possible even though there are no specific contraindications to vasoconstrictor use in local anesthetics.
• Short appointments and a stress reduction protocol may be required for anxious patients.
Consultations:
• Medical consult may be required to assess disease control and patient's ability to tolerate stress.
• In a patient with symptoms of blood dyscrasias, request a medical consult for blood studies and postpone treatment until normal values are reestablished.
Teach patient/family:
When chronic dry mouth occurs, advise patient:
• To avoid mouth rinses with high alcohol content due to drying effects
• To use daily home fluoride products for anticaries effect
• To use sugarless gum, frequent sips of water, or saliva substitutes

isoetharine HCl

(eye-soe-eth'a-reen)
Isoetharine
Drug class.: Adrenergic β_2-agonist

Action: Causes bronchodilation by β_2 stimulation, resulting in increased levels of cAMP and causing relaxation of bronchial smooth muscle with little effect on heart rate
Uses: Bronchospasm, asthma
Dosage and routes:
• *Adult:* IPPB 0.5 ml diluted 1:3 with NS
Available forms include: Sol for inh 1%
Side effects/adverse reactions:
▼ *ORAL:* Dry mouth
CNS: Tremors, anxiety, insomnia, headache, dizziness, stimulation
CV: ***Cardiac arrest,*** palpitation, tachycardia, hypertension, dysrhythmias
GI: Nausea
META: Hyperglycemia
Contraindications: Hypersensitivity to sympathomimetics, narrow-angle glaucoma
Precautions: Pregnancy category C, cardiac disorders, hyperthyroidism, diabetes mellitus, prostatic hypertrophy
Pharmacokinetics:
INH: Onset immediate, peak 5-15 min, duration 1-4 hr; metabolized in liver, GI tract, lungs; excreted in urine
Drug interactions of concern to dentistry:
• Increased effects of both drugs: other sympathomimetics
• Increased dysrhythmia: halogenated hydrocarbon anesthetics

DENTAL CONSIDERATIONS

General:

- Assess salivary flow as a factor in caries, periodontal disease, and candidiasis.
- Consider semisupine chair position for patients with respiratory disease.
- Acute asthmatic episodes may be precipitated in the dental office. Sympathomimetic inhalants should be available for emergency use.

Consultations:

- Medical consult may be required to assess disease control and patient's ability to tolerate stress.

Teach patient/family:

- For inhalation dosage forms, rinse mouth with water after each dose to prevent dryness

When chronic dry mouth occurs, advise patient:

- To avoid mouth rinses with high alcohol content due to drying effects
- To use sugarless gum, frequent sips of water, or saliva substitutes
- To use daily home fluoride products for anticaries effect

---

isoniazid (INH)

(eye-soe-nye'a-zid)

Laniazid, Nydrazid

🍁 Isotamine, PMS-Isoniazid

Drug class.: Antitubercular

Action: Bactericidal interference with lipid, nucleic acid biosynthesis

Uses: Treatment/prevention of TB

Dosage and routes:

Treatment

- *Adult:* PO/IM 5 mg/kg qd as single dose for 9 mo-2 yr, not to exceed 300 mg/day
- *Child and infant:* PO/IM 10-20 mg/kg qd as single dose for 18-24 mo, not to exceed 300 mg/day

Prevention

- *Adult:* PO 300 mg qd as single dose for 12 mo
- *Child and infant:* PO/IM 10 mg/kg qd as single dose for 12 mo, not to exceed 300 mg/day

Available forms include: Tabs 50, 100, 300 mg; inj 100 mg/ml; powder, syrup 50 mg/5 ml

Side effects/adverse reactions:

▼ *ORAL:* Lichenoid reaction

CNS: Peripheral neuropathy, ***toxic encephalopathy, convulsions,*** memory impairment, psychosis

GI: ***Jaundice, fatal hepatitis,*** nausea, vomiting, epigastric distress

HEMA: ***Agranulocytosis, hemolytic anemia, aplastic anemia, thrombocytopenia, eosinophilia, methemoglobinemia***

EENT: Blurred vision, optic neuritis

INTEG: Hypersensitivity: fever, skin eruptions, lymphadenopathy, vasculitis

MISC: Dyspnea, B_6 deficiency, pellegra, hyperglycemia, metabolic acidosis, gynecomastia, rheumatic syndrome, SLE-like syndrome

Contraindications: Hypersensitivity, optic neuritis

Precautions: Pregnancy category C; renal disease; diabetic retinopathy cataracts; ocular defects; hepatic disease; fatal hepatitis, especially in Black, Hispanic women; child <13 yr

Pharmacokinetics:

PO: Peak 1-2 hr, duration 6-8 hr

IM: Peak 45-60 min

Metabolized in liver, excreted in urine (metabolites), crosses placenta, excreted in breast milk

Drug interactions of concern to dentistry:
- Increased hepatotoxicity: alcohol, acetaminophen, carbamazepine
- Decreased effectiveness: glucocorticoids, especially prednisolone
- Increased plasma concentration: benzodiazepines, alfentanil
- Decreased effect of ketoconazole, miconazole

DENTAL CONSIDERATIONS
General:
- Patients on chronic drug therapy may rarely have symptoms of blood dyscrasias, which can include infection, bleeding, and poor healing.
- Medical consult may be required to assess disease control in the patient.
- Examine for evidence of oral signs of disease.

Consultations:
- In a patient with symptoms of blood dyscrasias, request a medical consult for blood studies and postpone dental treatment until normal values are reestablished.

Teach patient/family:
- Caution to prevent injury when using oral hygiene aids

---

isoproterenol HCl/ isoproterenol sulfate

(eye-soe-proe-ter′e-nole)

Isuprel, Isuprel Mistometer

Medihaler-Iso

Drug class.: Adrenergic β_1- and β_2-agonist

Action: Has β_1 and β_2 actions; relaxes bronchial smooth muscle and dilates the trachea and main bronchi by increasing levels of cAMP, which relaxes smooth muscles; causes increased contractility and heart rate by acting on β-receptors in heart

Uses: Bronchospasm, asthma, heart block, bradycardia, shock

Dosage and routes:

Asthma, bronchospasm
- *Adult:* SL 10-20 mg q6-8h HCl; inh 1 puff, may repeat in 2-5 min, maintenance 1-2 puffs 4-6 times daily
- *Child:* SL 5-10 mg q6-8h HCl; inh 1 puff, may repeat in 2-5 min, maintenance 1-2 puffs 4-6 times daily

Heart block/bradycardia
- *Adult:* IV 0.02-0.06 mg, then 0.01-0.2 mg or 5 μg/min HCl; IM 0.2 mg, then 0.02-1 mg as needed HCl
- *Child:* IV/IM one-half beginning adult dose

Shock
- *Adult and child:* IV inf 0.5-5 μg/min 1 mg/500 ml D_5W, titrate to BP, CVP, and hourly urine output

Available forms include: Sol for nebuliz 1:400 (0.25%), 1:200 (0.5%), 1:100 (1%); aerosol 0.25%, 0.2%, powd for inh 0.1 mg/cart; inj IV/IM 1:5000 (0.2 mg/ml); glossets (SL) 10 mg

Side effects/adverse reactions:
▼ *ORAL:* Dry mouth, altered taste
CNS: Tremors, anxiety, insomnia, headache, dizziness, stimulation
CV: ***Cardiac arrest,*** palpitation, tachycardia, hypertension
GI: Nausea, vomiting
RESP: Bronchial irritation, edema, dryness of oropharynx
META: Hyperglycemia

Contraindications: Hypersensitivity to sympathomimetics, narrow-angle glaucoma

Precautions: Pregnancy category

C, cardiac disorders, hyperthyroidism, diabetes mellitus, prostatic hypertrophy

Pharmacokinetics:

INH/SL: Onset 1-2 hr

SC: Onset 2 hr

REC: Onset 2-4 hr

Metabolized in liver, lungs, GI tract

Drug interactions of concern to dentistry:

- Hypotension, tachycardia: haloperidol, loxapine, phenothiazines, thioxanthenes
- Increased dysrhythmia: halogenated-hydrocarbon anesthetics

DENTAL CONSIDERATIONS

General:

- Monitor vital signs every appointment due to cardiovascular and respiratory side effects.
- Assess salivary flow as a factor in caries, periodontal disease, and candidiasis.
- Consider semisupine chair position for patients with respiratory disease.
- Short appointments and a stress reduction protocol may be required for anxious patients.
- Acute asthmatic episodes may be precipitated in the dental office. Sympathomimetic inhalants should be available for emergency use.

Teach patient/family:

- For inhalation dosage forms, rinse mouth with water after each dose to prevent dryness

When chronic dry mouth occurs, advise patient:

- To avoid mouth rinses with high alcohol content due to drying effects
- To use sugarless gum, frequent sips of water, or saliva substitutes
- To use daily home fluoride products for anticaries effect

isosorbide dinitrate

(eye'soe-sor-bide)

Cedocard-SR, Dilatrate-SR, Iso-Bid, Isonate, Isordil, Isordil Titradose, Isotrate, Sorbitrate

♣ Apo-ISDN, Coronex, Novosorbide, Sorbitrate SA

Drug class.: Nitrate antianginal

Action: Decreases preload/afterload, which is responsible for decreasing left ventricular end-diastolic pressure, systemic vascular resistance

Uses: Chronic stable angina pectoris, prophylaxis of angina pain

Dosage and routes:

- *Adult:* PO 5-40 mg qid; SL 2.5-10 mg, may repeat q2-3h; chew tabs 5-10 mg prn or q2-3h as prophylaxis; sus rel 40-80 mg q8-12h

Available forms include: Ext rel caps 40 mg; caps 40; tabs 5, 10, 20, 30, 40 mg; chew tabs 5, 10 mg; ext rel tabs 40 mg; SL tabs 2.5, 5, 10 mg

Side effects/adverse reactions:

▼ *ORAL:* Dry mouth, burning sensation to mucosa (SL tabs)

CNS: Vascular headache, flushing, dizziness, weakness, faintness

CV: Postural hypotension, ***collapse,*** tachycardia, syncope

GI: Nausea, vomiting

INTEG: Pallor, sweating, rash

MISC: ***Methemoglobinemia,*** twitching, hemolytic anemia

Contraindications: Hypersensitivity to this drug or nitrites, severe anemia, increased intracranial pressure, cerebral hemorrhage, acute MI

Precautions: Postural hypotension, pregnancy category C, lactation, children

Pharmacokinetics:
SUS ACTION: Duration 6-8 hr
PO: Onset 15-30 min, duration 4-6 hr
SL: Onset 2-5 min, duration 1-4 hr
▼ *ORAL:* Onset 3 min, duration 0.5-3 hr
Metabolized by liver, excreted in urine as metabolites (80%-100%)

Drug interactions of concern to dentistry:
- Increased effects: alcohol and other drugs that can lower blood pressure

DENTAL CONSIDERATIONS
General:
- Monitor vital signs every appointment due to cardiovascular side effects.
- After supine positioning, have patient sit upright for at least 2 min before standing to avoid orthostatic hypotension.
- Assess salivary flow as a factor in caries, periodontal disease, and candidiasis.
- Stress from dental procedures may compromise cardiovascular function; determine patient risk.
- Use vasoconstrictors with caution, in low doses, and with careful aspiration. Avoid use of gingival retraction cord with epinephrine.
- Short appointments and a stress reduction protocol may be required for anxious patients.
- Nitroglycerin should be available in case of acute anginal episode.

Consultations:
- Medical consult may be required to assess disease control and patient's ability to tolerate stress.

Teach patient/family:
- Importance of good oral hygiene to prevent soft tissue inflammation

When chronic dry mouth occurs, advise patient:
- To avoid mouth rinses with high alcohol content due to drying effects
- To use sugarless gum, frequent sips of water, or saliva substitutes
- To use daily home fluoride products for anticaries effect

---

isosorbide mononitrate

(eye'soe-sor-bide)
ISMO, Monoket, IMDUR

Drug class.: Antianginal, organic nitrate

Action: Decreases preload/afterload, which is responsible for decreasing left ventricular end-diastolic pressure, systemic vascular resistance; arterial and venous dilation

Uses: Prevention of angina pectoris due to coronary artery disease

Dosage and routes:
- *Adult:* PO 20 mg bid, 7 hr apart

Available forms include: Tabs 20, 30 mg; ext rel 30, 60, 120 mg

Side effects/adverse reactions:
▼ *ORAL:* Dry mouth
CNS: Vascular headache, flushing, dizziness, weakness, faintness
CV: ***Collapse,*** postural hypotension, tachycardia, syncope
GI: Nausea, vomiting
INTEG: Pallor, sweating, rash
MISC: ***Hemolytic anemia, methemoglobinemia,*** twitching

Contraindications: Hypersensitivity to nitrites, severe anemia, increased intracranial pressure, cerebral hemorrhage, acute MI, closed-angle glaucoma

Precautions: Postural hypotension, pregnancy category C, lactation, children, glaucoma

Pharmacokinetics:
PO: Metabolized by the liver, ex-

creted in urine as metabolites (80%-100%)

Drug interactions of concern to dentistry:

• Increased effects: alcohol and other vasodilator-type drugs

DENTAL CONSIDERATIONS

General:

• Monitor vital signs every appointment due to cardiovascular side effects.

• After supine positioning, have patient sit upright for at least 2 min before standing to avoid orthostatic hypotension.

• Stress from dental procedures may compromise cardiovascular function; determine patient risk.

• Assess salivary flow as a factor in caries, periodontal disease, and candidiasis.

• Short appointments and a stress reduction protocol may be required for anxious patients.

• Consider semisupine chair position for patients with respiratory distress.

• Use vasoconstrictors with caution, in low doses, and with careful aspiration. Avoid use of gingival retraction cord with epinephrine.

• Nitroglycerin should be available in case of an acute anginal episode.

Consultations:

• Medical consult may be required to assess disease control and patient's ability to tolerate stress.

Teach patient/family:

When chronic dry mouth occurs, advise patient:

• To avoid mouth rinses with high alcohol content due to drying effects

• To use sugarless gum, frequent sips of water, or saliva substitutes

• To use daily home fluoride products for anticaries effect

isotretinoin

(eye-soe-tret′i-noyn)

Accutane

♣ Accutane-Roche

Drug class.: Retinoic acid isomer, vitamin A derivative

Action: Decreases sebum secretion; improves cystic acne

Uses: Severe recalcitrant cystic acne

Dosage and routes:

• *Adult:* PO 0.5-2 mg/kg/day in 2 divided doses × 15-20 wk

Available forms include: Caps 10, 20, 40 mg

Side effects/adverse reactions:

▼ *ORAL: Dry lips/mouth, angular cheilosis*

CNS: ***Pseudotumor cerebri,*** lethargy, fatigue, headache, depression

CV: Chest pain

GI: Nausea, vomiting, anorexia, increased liver enzymes, regional ileus, abdominal pain, weight loss

HEMA: ***Thrombocytopenia,*** decreased H & H, WBC, reticulocyte count

GU: ***Hematuria, proteinuria,*** hypouricemia

EENT: Eye irritation, conjunctivitis, epistaxis, dry nose, contact lens intolerance, optic neuritis

INTEG: Dry skin, pruritus, joint/muscle pain, hair loss, photosensitivity, urticaria, bruising, hirsutism, petechiae, hypopigmentation/hyperpigmentation, nail brittleness

MS: Hyperostosis, arthralgia, bone/joint/muscle pain

Contraindications: Hypersensitivity, inflamed skin, pregnancy category X

Precautions: Lactation, diabetes,

I

photosensitivity, hepatic disease, depressive illness

Pharmacokinetics:

PO: Peak 2.9-3.2 hr, half-life 10-20 hr; metabolized in liver; excreted in urine, feces

Drug interactions of concern to dentistry:

- Additive photosensitization: tetracycline
- Pseudotumor cerebri: minocycline or tetracycline
- Increased tissue drying: alcohol

DENTAL CONSIDERATIONS

General:

- Patients on chronic drug therapy may rarely have symptoms of blood dyscrasias, which can include infection, bleeding, and poor healing.
- Assess salivary flow as a factor in caries, periodontal disease, and candidiasis.
- An exaggerated healing response characterized by exuberant granulation tissue has been reported.
- Apply lubricant to dry lips for patient comfort before dental procedures.

Consultations:

- In a patient with symptoms of blood dyscrasias, request a medical consult for blood studies and postpone dental treatment until normal values are reestablished.

Teach patient/family:

- Importance of good oral hygiene to prevent soft tissue inflammation

When chronic dry mouth occurs, advise patient:

- To avoid mouth rinses with high alcohol content due to drying effects
- To use sugarless gum, frequent sips of water, or saliva substitutes
- To use daily home fluoride products for anticaries effect

isoxsuprine HCl

(eye-sox'syoo-preen)

Vasodilan

Drug class.: Peripheral vasodilator

Action: α-adrenoreceptor antagonist with β-adrenoreceptor–stimulating properties; may also act directly on vascular smooth muscle; causes cardiac stimulation, uterine relaxation

Uses: Symptoms of cerebrovascular insufficiency; peripheral vascular disease, including arteriosclerosis obliterans, thromboangiitis obliterans, Raynaud's disease

Dosage and routes:

- *Adult:* PO 10-20 mg tid or qid

Available forms include: Tabs 10, 20 mg

Side effects/adverse reactions:

CNS: Dizziness, weakness, tremors, anxiety

CV: Hypotension, ***tachycardia,*** palpitation, chest pain

GI: Nausea, vomiting, abdominal pain, distention

INTEG: Severe rash, flushing

Contraindications: Hypersensitivity, postpartum, arterial bleeding

Precautions: Pregnancy category C, tachycardia

Pharmacokinetics:

PO: Peak 1 hr, duration 3 hr, half-life 1.25 hr; excreted in urine; crosses placenta

Drug interactions of concern to dentistry:

- Increased effects: alcohol and drugs that also lower blood pressure

DENTAL CONSIDERATIONS

General:

• Monitor vital signs every appointment due to cardiovascular and respiratory side effects.

• After supine positioning, have patient sit upright for at least 2 min before standing to avoid orthostatic hypotension.

• Short appointments and a stress reduction protocol may be required for anxious patients.

• Drugs used for conscious sedation that lower blood pressure may potentiate the hypotensive effects.

• Use vasoconstrictors with caution, in low doses, and with careful aspiration. Avoid use of gingival retraction cord with epinephrine.

Consultations:

• Medical consult may be required to assess disease control and patient's ability to tolerate stress.

---

isradipine

(iz-ra'di-peen)

DynaCirc

Drug class.: Calcium channel blocker

Action: Inhibits calcium ion influx across cell membrane during cardiac depolarization; produces relaxation of coronary vascular smooth muscle, peripheral vascular smooth muscle; dilates coronary vascular arteries; increases myocardial oxygen delivery in patients with vasospastic angina

Uses: Essential hypertension; unapproved use: angina, Raynaud's disease

Dosage and routes:

Hypertension

• *Adult:* PO 2.5 mg bid, increase at 3-4 wk intervals up to 10 mg bid

Angina

• *Adult:* PO 2.5-7.5 mg tid

Available forms include: Caps 2.5, 5 mg

Side effects/adverse reactions:

▼ *ORAL:* Dry mouth (gingival overgrowth has not been documented with this drug)

CNS: Headache, fatigue, dizziness, fainting, sleep disturbances

CV: Peripheral edema, tachycardia, hypotension, chest pain

GI: Nausea, vomiting, diarrhea, gastric upset, constipation, hepatitis

HEMA: ***Thrombocytopenia, leukopenia, anemia***

GU: ***Acute renal failure,*** nocturia, polyuria

INTEG: Rash, pruritus, urticaria, photosensitivity, hair loss

MISC: Flushing

Contraindications: Sick sinus syndrome, second- or third-degree heart block, hypotension <90 mm Hg systolic, hypersensitivity

Precautions: CHF, hypotension, hepatic disease, pregnancy category C, lactation, children, renal disease, elderly

Pharmacokinetics:

PO: Peak plasma levels at 2-3 hr; metabolized in liver; metabolites excreted in urine, feces; excreted in breast milk

Drug interactions of concern to dentistry:

• Decreased effect: indomethacin, possibly other NSAIDs, phenobarbital

• Increased effect: parenteral and inhalational general anesthetics or other drugs with hypotensive actions

• Increased effects of carbamazepine

DENTAL CONSIDERATIONS

General:

• Monitor cardiac status; take vital signs at each appointment because of CV side effects. Consider a stress reduction protocol to prevent stress-induced angina during the dental appointment.

• After supine positioning, have patient sit upright for at least 2 min before standing to avoid orthostatic hypotension.

• Place on frequent recall to monitor gingival condition.

• Limit use of sodium-containing products such as saline IV fluids for patients with a dietary salt restriction.

• Assess salivary flow as a factor in caries, periodontal disease, and candidiasis.

• Use vasoconstrictors with caution, in low doses, and with careful aspiration. Avoid use of gingival retraction cord with epinephrine.

• Patients on chronic drug therapy may rarely have symptoms of blood dyscrasias, which can include infection, bleeding, and poor healing.

Consultations:

• In a patient with symptoms of blood dyscrasias, request a medical consult for blood studies and postpone dental treatment until normal values are reestablished.

• Medical consult may be required to assess disease control and stress tolerance of patient.

Teach patient/family:

• Importance of good oral hygiene to prevent soft tissue inflammation and minimize gingival overgrowth

• Need for frequent oral prophylaxis if overgrowth occurs

When chronic dry mouth occurs, advise patient:

• To avoid mouth rinses with high alcohol content due to drying effects

• To use sugarless gum, frequent sips of water, or saliva substitutes

• To use daily home fluoride products for anticaries effect

---

itraconazole

(i-tra-koe'na-zole)

Sporanox

Drug class.: Antifungal, systemic (triazole)

Action: Inhibits cytochrome P-450 enzymes and blocks synthesis of essential membrane sterols in fungal organism

Uses: Aspergillosis, blastomycosis, histoplasmosis (pulmonary and extrapulmonary); fungal infections of nails (onychomycosis); *Candida* infections of esophagus or mouth (oral sol only)

Dosage and routes:

Blastomycosis and histoplasmosis

• *Adult:* PO 200 mg qd after a full meal, 200 mg bid for immunocompromised; max 400 mg day

Aspergillosis

• *Adult:* PO 200-400 mg qd

Fungal nail infection (tinea unguium)

• *Adult:* PO 200 mg daily for 12 wk

Oral candidiasis

• *Adult:* PO swish and swallow 200 mg/daily for 1-2 wk

Pharyngeal candidiasis

• *Adult:* Swish and swallow 100 mg daily for a minimum of 3 wk

Available forms include: Caps 100 mg; oral sol 10 mg/ml in 150 ml volume; inj 10 mg/ml (IV infusion)

Side effects/adverse reactions:
CNS: Fatigue, headache, dizziness, anorexia, malaise
CV: Hypertension, edema, vertigo
GI: ***Hepatitis,*** *nausea, vomiting, diarrhea, abdominal pain,* hepatic dysfunction
GU: Impotence, albuminuria
INTEG: Rash, pruritus, ***Stevens-Johnson syndrome***
META: Hypokalemia, elevated liver enzymes
MISC: Fever, myalgia, ***anaphylaxis***
Contraindications: Hypersensitivity, cisapride, triazolam, pimozide, quinidine, oral midazolam
Precautions: Pregnancy category C, lactation, liver dysfunction, oral anticoagulants (monitor patient)
Pharmacokinetics:
PO: Peak plasma level 4 hr; highly protein bound (98.5%); take with food; metabolized by liver; 3%-18% excreted in feces, 40% in urine as metabolites
Drug interactions of concern to dentistry:
- Increased risk of rhabdomyolysis: lovastatin and simvastatin
- Increased risk of hypoglycemia: oral antidiabetics
- Increased metabolism: phenobarbital, carbamazepine
- Increased risk of toxicity: cyclosporine
- Contraindicated with triazolam, midazolam, cisapride
- Inhibits metabolism of certain benzodiazepines: alprazolam, chlordiazepoxide, clonazepam, chlorazepate, diazepam, estazolam, flurazepam, halazepam, midazolam, quazepam, triazolam, buspirone, zyloprim, felodipine
- Decreased effects: didanosine
- Increased plasma levels: saquinavir
- Avoid itraconazole use with HMG-CoA reductase inhibitors or lower their dose
- May inhibit the metabolism of warfarin

DENTAL CONSIDERATIONS
General:
- Monitor vital signs every appointment due to cardiovascular side effects.
- Determine why the patient is taking the drug.
- Consider semisupine chair position for patient comfort due to GI effects of drug.

Consultations:
- Medical consult may be required to assess patient's ability to tolerate stress.

K

ketoconazole
(kee-toe-koe'na-zole)
Nizoral, Nizoral Shampoo
Drug class.: Imidazole antifungal

Action: Alters cell membranes and inhibits several fungal enzymes
Uses: Systemic candidiasis, chronic mucocutaneous candidiasis, candiduria, coccidioidomycosis, histoplasmosis, chromomycosis, paracoccidioidomycosis, tinea pedis; unlabeled use: prostate cancer
Dosage and routes:
- *Adult and child >40 kg:* PO 200 mg qd; may increase to 400 mg qd if needed
- *Child >2 yr:* 3.5-6.6 mg/kg/day in a single dose

Cutaneous candidiasis
- *Adult:* TOP apply cream once daily to affected area

Dandruff
- *Adult:* Shampoo twice weekly at 3-day intervals for 4 wk

Available forms include: Tabs 200 mg, cream 2% in 15, 30, and 60 g tubes, shampoo 2% in 120 ml

Side effects/adverse reactions:

▼ *ORAL:* Lichenoid reactions

CNS: Headache, dizziness, lethargy, anxiety, insomnia, dreams, paresthesia

GI: Nausea, vomiting, anorexia, ***hepatotoxicity,*** diarrhea, cramps, abdominal pain, constipation, flatulence, GI bleeding

GU: Gynecomastia, impotence

INTEG: Pruritus, fever, chills, photophobia, rash, dermatitis, purpura, urticaria

SYST: ***Anaphylaxis***

Contraindications: Hypersensitivity, pregnancy category C, lactation, meningitis, loratadine, triazolam, cisapride

Precautions: Renal disease, hepatic disease, achlorhydria (drug-induced)

Pharmacokinetics:

PO: Peak 1-2 hr, half-life 2 hr, terminal 8 hr; highly protein bound; metabolized in liver; excreted in bile, feces; requires acid pH for absorption; distributed poorly to CSF

Drug interactions of concern to dentistry:

• Hepatotoxicity: alcohol, high-dose long-term use, acetaminophen, carbamazepine, sulfonamides

• Increased serum levels: indinavir, saquinavir

• Decreased absorption: antacids (take 2 hr after ketoconazole)

• Contraindicated with triazolam, cisapride, lovastatin

• Inhibits the metabolism of certain benzodiazepines: alprazolam, chlordiazepoxide, clonazepam, clorazepate, diazepam, estazolam, flurazepam, halazepam, midazolam, quazepam, triazolam, zolpidem

• May inhibit metabolism of warfarin

DENTAL CONSIDERATIONS

General:

• To prevent reinoculation of *Candida* infection, dispose of toothbrush or other contaminated oral hygiene devices used during period of infection.

• Determine if medication controls disease.

• Place on frequent recall to evaluate healing response.

• Assess salivary flow as a factor in caries, periodontal disease, and candidiasis.

Teach patient/family:

• To avoid mouth rinses with high alcohol content due to drying effects

---

ketoprofen

(kee-toe-proe'fen)

Orudis, Oruvail, Actron (OTC), Orudis KT (OTC)

✤ Apo-Keto, Apo-Keto-E, Novo-Keto-EC, Orudis-E, Orudis-SR, Rhodis, Rhodis-E

Drug class.: Nonsteroidal antiinflammatory

Action: Inhibits prostaglandin synthesis by interfering with cyclooxygenase needed for biosynthesis; possesses analgesic, antiinflammatory, antipyretic properties

Uses: Osteoarthritis, rheumatoid arthritis, dysmenorrhea; unapproved use includes gouty arthritis, vascular headache

Dosage and routes:

• *Adult:* PO 150-300 mg in divided doses tid-qid, not to exceed 300 mg/day; PO (OTC) 1 or 2 tab q4-6h, limit 6 tabs/day or 75 mg

Available forms include: Tabs (OTC) 12.5 mg; caps 25, 50, 75 mg; sus rel caps 100, 150, 200 mg

Side effects/adverse reactions:

▼ *ORAL:* Stomatitis, bleeding, bitter taste, increased thirst, dry mouth, lichenoid reaction

CNS: Dizziness, drowsiness, fatigue, tremors, confusion, insomnia, anxiety, depression

CV: Tachycardia, peripheral edema, palpitation, dysrhythmias

GI: ***Cholestatic hepatitis,*** nausea, anorexia, vomiting, diarrhea, jaundice, constipation, flatulence, cramps, peptic ulcer

HEMA: ***Blood dyscrasias***

GU: ***Nephrotoxicity: dysuria, hematuria, oliguria, azotemia***

EENT: Tinnitus, hearing loss, blurred vision

INTEG: Purpura, rash, pruritus, sweating

Contraindications: Hypersensitivity, asthma, severe renal disease, severe hepatic disease

Precautions: Pregnancy category B, lactation, children, bleeding disorders, GI disorders, cardiac disorders, hypersensitivity to other antiinflammatory agents, elderly

Pharmacokinetics:

PO: Peak 2 hr, half-life 3-3.5 hr; 99% plasma-protein binding; metabolized in liver; excreted in urine (metabolites), breast milk

Drug interactions of concern to dentistry:

• GI ulceration, bleeding: aspirin, other NSAIDs, alcohol, corticosteroids

• Nephrotoxicity: acetaminophen (prolonged use)

• Possible risk of decreased renal function: cyclosporine

• Increased photosensitizing effect: tetracycline

When prescribed for dental pain:

• Risk of increased effects: oral anticoagulants, oral antidiabetics, lithium, methotrexate

• Decreased effects of diuretics

DENTAL CONSIDERATIONS

General:

• Patients on chronic drug therapy may rarely have symptoms of blood dyscrasias, which can include infection, bleeding, and poor healing.

• Assess salivary flow as a factor in caries, periodontal disease, and candidiasis.

• Avoid prescribing for dental use in first and last trimester of pregnancy.

• Avoid prescribing aspirin-containing products.

• Consider semisupine chair position for patients with arthritic disease.

Consultations:

• In a patient with symptoms of blood dyscrasias, request a medical consult for blood studies and postpone dental treatment until normal values are reestablished.

• Medical consult may be required to assess disease control in the patient.

Teach patient/family:

• Importance of good oral hygiene to prevent soft tissue inflammation

• Caution to prevent injury when using oral hygiene aids

When chronic dry mouth occurs, advise patient:

• To avoid mouth rinses with high alcohol content due to drying effects

K

• To use sugarless gum, frequent sips of water, or saliva substitutes
• To use daily home fluoride products for anticaries effect

ketorolac/ketorolac tromethamine/ ketorolac tromethamine injection

(kee'toe-role-ak)
Toradol

Drug class.: Nonsteroidal antiinflammatory

Action: Inhibits prostaglandin synthesis by interfering with cyclooxygenase needed for biosynthesis; possesses analgesic, antiinflammatory, antipyretic properties

Uses: Acute mild-to-moderate pain, not for chronic pain use

Dosage and routes:

• *Adult <65 yr:* IM one 60 mg dose, or multiple doses of 30 mg q6h (120 mg/day limit); IV one 30 mg dose; PO (oral use is indicated only as continuation therapy to IV/IM doses) 20 mg first dose followed by 10 mg q4-6h (limit 40 mg/day), but only after 60 mg IM as a single dose, 30 mg IV as a single dose, or 30 mg multiple doses IV or IM
• *Adult >65 yr or weight <110 lb or renal impairment:* IM one 30 mg dose, or multiple doses of 15 mg q6h (60 mg/day limit); PO (indicated only as continuation therapy to IV/IM doses) 10 mg first dose followed by 10 mg q4-6h (40 mg/day limit), but only after 30 mg IM single dose, 15 mg IV single dose, or 15 mg multiple dose IV or IM
• *Adult >65 yr:* IV one 15 mg dose

Available forms include: Inj 15, 30 mg (prefilled syringes); tabs 10 mg

Side effects/adverse reactions:

▼ *ORAL:* Dry mouth, lichenoid reaction
CNS: Dizziness, drowsiness, fatigue, tremors, confusion, insomnia, anxiety, depression
CV: Tachycardia, peripheral edema, palpitation, dysrhythmias
GI: ***Cholestatic hepatitis,*** nausea, anorexia, vomiting, diarrhea, jaundice, constipation, flatulence, cramps, peptic ulcer
HEMA: ***Blood dyscrasias***
GU: ***Nephrotoxicity: dysuria, hematuria, oliguria, azotemia***
EENT: Tinnitus, hearing loss, blurred vision
INTEG: Purpura, rash, pruritus, sweating

Contraindications: Hypersensitivity, asthma, severe renal disease, severe hepatic disease, probenecid

Precautions: Pregnancy category B, lactation, children, bleeding disorders, GI disorders, cardiac disorders, hypersensitivity to other antiinflammatory agents

Pharmacokinetics:

IM: Peak 50 min, half-life 6 hr

Drug interactions of concern to dentistry:

• GI ulceration, bleeding: aspirin, alcohol, corticosteroids
• Contraindicated with probenecid
• Possible risk of decreased renal function: cyclosporine

When prescribed for dental pain:

• Risk of increased effects: oral anticoagulants, oral antidiabetics, lithium, methotrexate
• Decreased antihypertensive effects of diuretics, β-blockers, ACE inhibitors

DENTAL CONSIDERATIONS

General:

• Assess salivary flow as a factor in

caries, periodontal disease, and candidiasis.

• Avoid prescribing for dental use in pregnancy.

• Avoid prescribing aspirin-containing products.

• Avoid long-term use for chronic pain syndromes; combined use of IV/IM and oral doses must not exceed 5 days.

Consultations:

• Medical consult may be required to assess disease control in the patient.

Teach patient/family:

• To avoid mouth rinses with high alcohol content due to drying effects

ketotifen fumarate

(kee- toe'ti- fen)

Zaditor

Drug class.: Antihistamine

Action: Noncompetitive antagonist for histamine (H_1) receptors, stabilizes mast cells

Uses: Temporary prevention of itching of the eyes due to allergic conjunctivitis

Dosage and routes:

• *Adult:* Ophth 1 drop in affected eye(s) q8-12h

Available forms include: Ophth sol 5 ml bottle with dropper (0.345 mg of ketotifen fumarate per ml)

Side effects/adverse reactions:

CNS: Headache

EENT: Conjunctival infection, rhinitis, burning, stinging, eye pain, dry eyes, photophobia

INTEG: Rash

Contraindications: Hypersensitivity

Precautions: Prevent contamination of ophthalmic solution by careful use, do not wear contact lens if eyes are red, delay inserting contacts up to 10 min after drops are placed in eyes; pregnancy category C, lactation, children <3 yr

Pharmacokinetics: Limited information

Drug interactions of concern to dentistry:

• None reported

DENTAL CONSIDERATIONS

General:

• Protect patient's eyes from accidental spatter during dental treatment.

• Avoid dental light in patient's eyes; offer dark glasses for patient comfort

labetalol

(la-bet'a-lole)

Normodyne, Trandate

Drug class.: Nonselective adrenergic β-blocker and α-blocker

Action: Produces decreases in BP without reflex tachycardia or significant reduction in heart rate through mixture of α-blocking and β-blocking effects; elevated plasma renins are reduced

Uses: Mild-to-severe hypertension

Dosage and routes:

Hypertension

• *Adult:* PO 100 mg bid; may be given with a diuretic, may increase to 200 mg bid after 2 days, may continue to increase q1-3d; doses may reach 2.4 g/day

Hypertensive crisis

• *Adult:* IV inf 200 mg in 160 ml D_5W, run at 2 ml/min, stop infusion after desired response obtained, repeat q6-8h as needed; IV bol 20 mg over 2 min, may repeat 40-80 mg q10min, not to exceed 300 mg

Available forms include: Tabs 100, 200, 300 mg; inj 5 mg/ml in 20 ml amps

Side effects/adverse reactions:

▼ *ORAL:* Dry mouth, taste changes, lichenoid reaction

CNS: Dizziness, mental changes, drowsiness, fatigue, headache, catatonia, depression, anxiety, nightmares, paresthesias, lethargy

CV: Orthostatic hypotension, bradycardia, ***CHF, ventricular dysrhythmias,*** chest pain, AV block

GI: Nausea, vomiting, diarrhea

RESP: ***Bronchospasm,*** dyspnea, wheezing

HEMA: ***Agranulocytosis, thrombocytopenia***

GU: Impotence, dysuria, ejaculatory failure

EENT: Tinnitus, visual changes, sore throat, double vision, dry/burning eyes

INTEG: Rash, alopecia, urticaria, pruritus, fever

Contraindications: Hypersensitivity to β-blockers, cardiogenic shock, second- or third-degree heart block, sinus bradycardia, CHF, bronchial asthma

Precautions: Major surgery, pregnancy category C, lactation, diabetes mellitus, renal disease, thyroid disease, COPD, well-compensated heart failure, CAD, nonallergic bronchospasm

Pharmacokinetics:

PO: Onset 1-2 hr, peak 2-4 hr, duration 8-12 hr

IV: Peak 5 min

Half-life 6-8 hr; metabolized by liver (metabolites inactive); excreted in urine, bile, breast milk; crosses placenta

Drug interactions of concern to dentistry:

• Decreased metabolism: lidocaine
• Decreased effect: sympathomimetics
• Decreased hypotensive effects: indomethacin and other NSAIDs
• Increased hypotension, myocardial depression: hydrocarbon inhalation anesthetics

DENTAL CONSIDERATIONS

General:

• Monitor vital signs every appointment due to cardiovascular side effects.
• Patients on chronic drug therapy may rarely have symptoms of blood dyscrasias, which can include infection, bleeding, and poor healing.
• Assess salivary flow as a factor in caries, periodontal disease, and candidiasis.
• After supine positioning, have patient sit upright for at least 2 min before standing to avoid orthostatic hypotension.
• Limit use of sodium-containing products, such as saline IV fluids, for patients with a dietary salt restriction.
• Stress from dental procedures may compromise cardiovascular function; determine patient risk.
• Short appointments and a stress reduction protocol may be required for anxious patients.

Consultations:

• Medical consult may be required to assess disease control and patient's ability to tolerate stress.
• In a patient with symptoms of blood dyscrasias, request a medical consult for blood studies and postpone dental treatment until normal values are reestablished.

Teach patient/family:

When chronic dry mouth occurs, advise patient:

- To avoid mouth rinses with high alcohol content due to drying effects
- To use sugarless gum, frequent sips of water, or saliva substitutes
- To use daily home fluoride products for anticaries effect

lamivudine (3TC)

(la-mi′vyoo-deen)

Epivir, Epivir-HBV

Drug class.: Antiviral, nucleoside analog

Action: Inhibition of HIV reverse transcriptase (by active phosphorylated metabolite); also inhibits RNA- and DNA-dependent DNA polymerase

Uses: Used in combination with zidovudine for the treatment of HIV infection and to reduce disease progression and death in AIDS; chronic hepatitis B associated with evidence of hepatitis B viral replication and liver inflammation

Dosage and routes:

HIV infection

- *Adult and child 12-16 yr:* PO 150 mg bid (in combination with zidovudine); for adults with low body weight (<50 kg), the recommended dose is 2 mg/kg bid in combination with zidovudine
- *Child 3 mo-12 yr:* PO 4 mg/kg (limit 150 mg) bid in combination with zidovudine

Chronic hepatitis B

Adult: 100 mg qd (Epivir-HBV dose forms)

Available forms include: Tabs 100, 150 mg; oral sol 5 mg/5ml, 10 mg/ml in 240 ml volume

Side effects/adverse reactions:

CNS: Malaise, fatigue, headache, anorexia, neuropathy, dizziness, insomnia, depression

GI: Nausea, diarrhea, vomiting, abdominal pain, ***pancreatitis***

RESP: Cough, nasal complaints

HEMA: ***Neutropenia,*** anemia

INTEG: Rash

MS: Pain, myalgia

MISC: Fever, chills, peripheral neuropathy, paresthesia

Contraindications: Hypersensitivity, history of pancreatitis as child

Precautions: Reduce dose in renal disease, pregnancy category C, lactation

Pharmacokinetics:

PO: Rapid absorption, wide tissue distribution, low plasma protein binding (36%), eliminated mostly unchanged in urine

Drug interactions of concern to dentistry:

- None reported

DENTAL CONSIDERATIONS

General:

- Patients on chronic drug therapy may rarely have symptoms of blood dyscrasias, which can include infection, bleeding, and poor healing.
- Examine for oral manifestation of opportunistic infections.

Consultations:

- In a patient with symptoms of blood dyscrasias, request a medical consult for blood studies and postpone dental treatment until normal values are reestablished.
- Medical consult may be required to assess disease control and patient's ability to tolerate stress.

Teach patient/family:

• Importance of good oral hygiene to prevent soft tissue inflammation

• Caution patient to prevent trauma when using oral hygiene aids

• That secondary oral infection may occur; must see dentist immediately if infection occurs

---

lamotrigine

(la-moe'tri-jeen)

Lamictal

Drug class.: Antiepileptic

Action: May be due to blockage of voltage-dependent sodium channels with inhibition of excitatory amino acids

Uses: Adjunctive treatment of refractive partial seizures in adults and adjunctive treatment for Lennox-Gastaut syndrome in pediatric and adult patients

Dosage and routes:

• *Adult and child >16 yr:* PO with enzyme-inducing anticonvulsant drugs (but not valproic acid), the initial dose is 50 mg/day × 2 wk, then 50 mg bid × 2 wk; may increase dose 100 mg/wk as needed, limit 500 mg/day

• *Adult and child >16 yr:* PO with enzyme-inducing anticonvulsant drugs and valproic acid, the initial dose is 25 mg qod × 2 wk, then 25 mg/day × 2 wk; may increase dose 25-50 mg/day q1-2wk as needed, limit 150 mg/day

Enzyme-inducing drugs include phenytoin, phenobarbital, and carbamazepine

Available forms include: Tabs 25, 150, 100, 200 mg; chew tabs 5, 25 mg

Side effects/adverse reactions:

▼ *ORAL:* Dry mouth, facial edema (rarely), halitosis, gingival overgrowth, stomatitis

CNS: Dizziness, headache, somnolence, fever, ataxia, insomnia, tremor, depression, anxiety, vertigo

CV: Hot flashes, palpitation, dysrhythmia

GI: Vomiting, nausea, abdominal pain, diarrhea

RESP: Respiratory complaints, cough

HEMA: Anemia, ***leukopenia, leukocytosis***

GU: Dysmenorrhea, vaginitis

EENT: Pharyngitis, rhinitis, blurred vision, diplopia, ear pain

INTEG: Skin rash, ***Stephens-Johnson syndrome, toxic epidermal necrolysis, angioedema,*** pruritus, photosensitivity

MS: Hyperkinesias, neck pain, myasthenia symptoms, arthralgia

Contraindications: Hypersensitivity

Precautions: Pregnancy category C, lactation, elderly, children <16 yr, dose adjustment with other anticonvulsants, seizure risk with drug withdrawal, renal or hepatic impairment; can cause Stevens-Johnson syndrome, toxic epidermal necrolysis

Pharmacokinetics:

PO: Rapid absorption, peak plasma levels 1.3-4.2 hr; 55% plasma protein bound; liver metabolism; renal excretion

Drug interactions of concern to dentistry:

• Increased excretion: high-dose acetaminophen (900 mg tid), but significance is unclear; carbamazepine

• Increased blood levels of carbamazepine

DENTAL CONSIDERATIONS

General:

• Early morning appointments and a stress reduction protocol may be required for anxious patients.

• Determine type of epilepsy, seizure frequency, and quality of seizure control. A stress reduction protocol may be required.

• Evaluate respiration characteristics and rate.

• Assess salivary flow as factor in caries, periodontal disease, and candidiasis.

• Patients on chronic drug therapy may rarely have symptoms of blood dyscrasias, which can include infection, bleeding, and poor healing.

• Place on frequent recall due to oral side effects.

Consultations:

• Medical consult may be required to assess disease control and stress tolerance in the patient.

• In a patient with symptoms of blood dyscrasias, request a medical consult for blood studies and postpone dental treatment until normal values are reestablished.

Teach patient/family:

• Importance of good oral hygiene to prevent soft tissue inflammation

• Use of electric toothbrush if patient has difficulty holding conventional devices

When chronic dry mouth occurs, advise patient:

• To avoid mouth rinses with high alcohol content due to drying effects

• To use daily home fluoride products for anticaries effect

• To use sugarless gum, frequent sips of water, or saliva substitutes

lansoprazole

(lan-soe'pra-zole)

Prevacid

Drug class.: Antisecretory, proton pump inhibitor

Action: Suppresses gastric secretion by inhibiting hydrogen/potassium ATPase enzyme system in gastric parietal cell; characterized as gastric acid pump inhibitor because it blocks final step of acid production

Uses: Short-term treatment for healing and symptomatic relief of active duodenal ulcer and benign gastric ulcer, erosive esophagitis, and GERD; maintenance of healing of duodenal ulcers; long-term treatment of pathologic hypersecretory syndromes

Dosage and routes:

Duodenal ulcers

• *Adult:* PO 15 mg/day ac × 4 wk

Erosive esophagitis

• *Adult:* PO 30 mg/day ac (up to 8 wk)

Hypersecretory syndromes

• *Adult:* PO 60 mg/day (up to 120 mg in divided doses)

H. pylori related

• *Adult:* PO lansoprazole 30 mg along with clarithromycin 500 mg and amoxicillin 1 g bid × 14 days

Gastric ulcer

• *Adult:* PO 30 mg qd × 8 wk

Available forms include: Caps 15, 30 mg

Side effects/adverse reactions:

▼ *ORAL:* Candidiasis, stomatitis, halitosis (all <1%), dry mouth, taste alteration

L

CNS: Headache, dizziness
GI: Abdominal pain, diarrhea, nausea, vomiting
RESP: Cough, asthma, bronchitis, dyspnea
HEMA: Anemia
GU: Abnormal menses, glycosuria, gynecomastia, breast tenderness
EENT: Tinnitus, amblyopia, eye pain
MS: Myalgia, musculoskeletal pain

Contraindications: Hypersensitivity

Precautions: Pregnancy category B, lactation, children <18 yr, elderly (limit doses to 30 mg/day), severe hepatic disease

Pharmacokinetics:
PO: Peak plasma levels 1.7 hr, half-life 1.5 hr; 97% plasma protein bound; extensive liver metabolism; metabolites mainly excreted in feces, less in urine

Drug interactions of concern to dentistry:
- Drug interactions not established but potentially can interfere with absorption of amoxicillin, ketoconazole

DENTAL CONSIDERATIONS
General:
- Consider semisupine chair position for patient comfort due to GI effects of disease.
- Question the patient about tolerance of NSAIDs or aspirin related to GI problem.
- Patients with gastroesophageal reflux may have oral symptoms, including burning mouth, secondary candidiasis, and oral signs of dental erosion.
- Assess salivary flow as factor in caries, periodontal disease, and candidiasis.

Teach patient/family:
- To avoid mouth rinses with high alcohol content due to drying effects

When chronic dry mouth occurs, advise patient:
- To avoid mouth rinses with high alcohol content due to drying effects
- To use daily home fluoride products for anticaries effect
- To use sugarless gum, frequent sips of water, or saliva substitutes

---

latanoprost

(la-ta'noe-prost)
Xalatan

Drug class.: Prostaglandin F_{2a} analogue

Action: A prostanoid F_2 alpha analog believed to reduce intraocular pressure by increasing uveoscleral outflow of aqueous humor

Uses: Open-angle glaucoma and ocular hypertension in patients intolerant to other intraocular pressure–lowering drugs

Dosage and routes:
- *Adult:* Instill 1 drop in affected eye(s) qd in PM

Available forms include: Ophthalmic sol 0.005% (50 μg/ml) in 2.5 ml

Side effects/adverse reactions:
RESP: Upper respiratory infection, cold, flu
EENT: Blurred vision, burning, stinging, itching, foreign body sensation, increased iris pigmentation, dry eye, pain, edema, retinal artery embolus, retinal detachment (rare)
INTEG: Rash
MS: Muscle pain, chest pain, angina pain

Contraindications: Hypersensitivity to lantanoprost or other ingredients in the sterile ophthalmic solution

Precautions: Gradual change in eye color, avoid contamination of sterile solution, renal or hepatic impairment, remove contact lens before using, administer at least 5 min apart if other ophthalmic drug is also used, pregnancy category C, nursing, pediatrics

Pharmacokinetics:

OPHTH: Absorbed through cornea, peak conc 2 hr, hydrolyzed by esterases in cornea to active acid, metabolized in liver, half-life 17 min, renal excretion; onset 3-4 hr, maximum effect 8-12 hr

Drug interactions of concern to dentistry:

• None reported at this time; avoid use of anticholinergic drugs, atropine-like drugs, propanthine, and diazepam (benzodiazepines)

DENTAL CONSIDERATIONS

General:

• Check compliance of patient with prescribed drug regimen for glaucoma.

• Avoid dental light in patient's eyes; offer dark glasses for patient comfort.

• Protect patient's eyes from accidental spatter during dental treatment.

Consultations:

• Medical consult may be required to assess disease control in the patient.

leflunomide

le-flu'no-mide

Arava

Drug class.: Antiarthritic, immunosuppressive

Action: Acts as an immunomodulary agent by blocking dihydroorotate dehydrogenase enzymes, which results in inhibition of pyrimidine synthesis. This results in antiproliferative effects on cells dependent on this pathway.

Uses: To reduce signs and symptoms and to retard structural damage in active rheumatoid arthritis as demonstrated by x-ray erosion and joint space narrowing

Dosage and routes:

• *Adult:* PO loading dose 100 mg × 3 days, maintenance dose 20 mg daily, higher doses not recommended

Available forms include: Tabs 10, 20, 100 mg

Side effects/adverse reactions:

▼ *ORAL:* Mouth ulceration, candidiasis, dry mouth, taste disturbances

CNS: Headache, asthenia, dizziness, paresthesia

CV: Hypertension, palpitation

GI: Diarrhea, abdominal pain, nausea, dyspepsia, colitis

RESP: Cough, URI, bronchitis

HEMA: Anemia

GU: UTI

EENT: Rhinitis, sinusitis

INTEG: Rash, pruritus

META: Elevation of liver enzymes ALT, AST

MS: Synovitis, tenosynovitis, joint discomfort

MISC: Alopecia, allergic reactions

Contraindications: Hypersensi-

L

tivity, pregnancy, woman of childbearing age not using reliable contraception, significant hepatic impairment, hepatitis B or C, lactation

Precautions: Chronic renal or hepatic insufficiency, rifampin, pregnancy category X, child <18 yr

Pharmacokinetics:

PO: Loading dose required, converted to active metabolite, peak levels of metabolite 6-12 hr, half-life of metabolite (2 wk), highly protein bound (99%), metabolites removed by renal (43%) and fecal excretion (48%)

Drug interactions of concern to dentistry:

• None reported

DENTAL CONSIDERATIONS

General:

• Monitor vital signs every appointment due to cardiovascular side effects.

• Consider semisupine chair position for patient if GI side effects occur.

• Examine for oral manifestation of opportunistic infection.

• If acute oral infection occurs, inform physician.

• Assess salivary flow as a factor in caries, periodontal disease, and candidiasis.

Consultations:

• Consult if needed.

Teach patient/family:

• Importance of good oral hygiene to prevent soft tissue inflammation

• Use of electric toothbrush if patient has difficulty holding conventional devices

When chronic dry mouth occurs, advise patient:

• To avoid mouth rinses with high alcohol content due to drying effects

• To use daily home fluoride products for anticaries effect

• To use sugarless gum, frequent sips of water, or saliva substitutes

leucovorin calcium (citrovorum factor/ folinic acid)

(loo-koe-vor′in)

Wellcovorin

Drug class.: Folic acid antagonist antidote, antineoplastic adjunct

Action: Chemically reduced derivative of folic acid; converted to tetrahydrofolate; counteracts folic acid antagonists

Uses: Megaloblastic or macrocytic anemia caused by folic acid deficiency, overdose of folic acid antagonist, methotrexate toxicity, toxicity caused by pyrimethamine or trimethoprim; used with fluorouracil in colorectal cancer

Dosage and routes:

Megaloblastic anemia caused by enzyme deficiency

• *Adult and child:* IM 3-6 mg qd, then 1 mg PO for life

Megaloblastic anemia caused by deficiency of folate

• *Adult and child:* IM 1 mg or less qd, continued until adequate response

Methotrexate toxicity

• *Adult and child:* PO/IM/IV 10 mg/m^2 q6h until methotrexate levels fall

Pyrimethamine toxicity

• *Adult and child:* PO/IM 5 mg qd with each dose of antagonist

Trimethoprim toxicity
• *Adult and child:* PO/IM 400 μg qd
Available forms include: Tabs 5, 10, 15, 25 mg; inj IM 3, 5 mg/ml; powder for inj 50, 100, 350 mg/vial
Side effects/adverse reactions:
RESP: Wheezing
INTEG: Rash, pruritus, erythema
Contraindications: Hypersensitivity, anemias other than megaloblastic not associated with B_{12} deficiency
Precautions: Pregnancy category C
Drug interactions of concern to dentistry:
• None reported
DENTAL CONSIDERATIONS
General:
• Signs of folate deficiency may appear in oral tissues.
• Determine why the patient is taking the drug.
• Patients with severe anemia or cancer or those receiving cancer chemotherapy may have oral complaints. Palliative therapy may be required.
Consultations:
• Medical consult may be required to assess disease control in the patient.
Teach patient/family:
• Importance of good oral hygiene to prevent soft tissue inflammation
• Caution to prevent trauma when using oral hygiene aids
• To report oral lesions, soreness, or bleeding to dentist
• That secondary oral infection may occur; must see dentist immediately if infection occurs
• Importance of updating medical/drug record if physican makes any changes in evaluation/drug regimen

levalbuterol HCl
(lev′al-byoo-ter-ole)
Xopenex
Drug class.: Bronchodilator

Action: Selective β_2-adrenergic agonist; causes relaxation of smooth muscles of all airways
Uses: Treatment or prevention of bronchospasm in adults and children >12 yr with reversible obstructive airway disease
Dosage and routes:
• *Adult and child >12 yr:* Inh 0.63 mg tid by nebulizer
Severe asthma not responding to 0.63 mg
• *Adult and child >12 yr:* Inh 1.25 mg tid by nebulizer
Available forms include: Inh sol 0.63, 1.25 mg in 3 ml vials
Side effects/adverse reactions:
▼ *ORAL:* Dry mouth
CNS: Migraine, dizziness, nervousness, tremor, anxiety, insomnia, paresthesia
CV: Tachycardia, ECG changes
GI: Dyspepsia, diarrhea, nausea, gastroenteritis
RESP: Flulike syndrome, cough
EENT: Rhinitis, sinusitis, turbinate edema, dry throat
META: Increased plasma glucose, decreased serum K^+, eye itch
MS: Back pain, leg cramps
MISC: Pain
Contraindications: Hypersensitivity to this drug or racemic albuterol

Precautions: Paradoxic bronchospasm, cardiovascular disorders, seizures, diabetes, hyperthyroidism, coronary insufficiency, cardiac arrhythmias, hypertension, not to exceed recommended dose, β-adrenergic blockers, MAO inhibitors, tricyclic antidepressants, pregnancy category C, lactation, children <12 yr

Pharmacokinetics:

INH: Relief of bronchoconstriction 20 min, half-life 3-4 hr, low plasma levels

Drug interactions of concern to dentistry:

• Significant reduction of effects: β-adrenergic blockers

• Potentiation of CV effects: MAO inhibitors, tricyclic antidepressants

• No specific dental drug interactions reported

DENTAL CONSIDERATIONS

General:

• Monitor vital signs every appointment due to cardiovascular side effects.

• Assess salivary flow as a factor in caries, periodontal disease, and candidiasis.

• Consider semisupine chair position for patients with respiratory disease.

• Short, midday appointments and a stress reduction protocol may be required for anxious patients.

• Be aware that aspirin or sulfite preservatives in vasoconstrictor-containing products can exacerbate asthma.

• Acute asthmatic episodes may be precipitated in the dental office. Rapid-acting sympathomimetic inhalants should be available for emergency use. A stress reduction protocol may be required.

Consultations:

• Medical consult may be required to assess disease control and patient's ability to tolerate stress.

Teach patient/family:

• For inhalation dosage forms, rinse mouth with water after each dose to prevent dryness

When chronic dry mouth occurs, advise patient:

• To avoid mouth rinses with high alcohol content due to drying effects

• To use daily home fluoride products for anticaries effect

• To use sugarless gum, frequent sips of water, or saliva substitutes

levamisole HCl

(lee-vam'i-sol)

Ergamisol

Drug class.: Immunomodulator

Action: May increase the action of macrophages, monocytes, and T cells, which will restore immune function; complete action is unknown

Uses: Treatment of Dukes' stage C colon cancer, given with fluorouracil after surgical resection

Dosage and routes:

• *Adult:* PO 50 mg q8h × 3 days, begin treatment at least 1 wk but no more than 4 wk after resection, given with fluorouracil 450 mg/m^2/day; IV given daily × 5 days beginning 21-34 days after resection, maintenance is 50 mg q8h × 3 days q2wk × 1 yr, given with fluorouracil 45 mg/m^2/day by IV push qwk starting 28 days after the initial 5-day course × 1 yr

Available forms include: Tab 50 mg (base)

Side effects/adverse reactions:
▼ *ORAL:* Stomatitis, altered taste, lichenoid drug reaction
CNS: Dizziness, headache, paresthesia, somnolence, depression, anxiety, fatigue, fever, mental changes, ataxia, insomnia
CV: Chest pain, edema
GI: Nausea, vomiting, anorexia, diarrhea, constipation, flatulence, dyspepsia, abdominal pain
HEMA: ***Granulocytopenia, leukopenia, thrombocytopenia, agranulocytosis***
EENT: Altered sense of smell, blurred vision, conjunctivitis
INTEG: Rash, pruritus, alopecia, dermatitis, urticaria
META: Hyperbilirubinemia
MISC: Rigors, infection, arthralgia, myalgia

Contraindications: Hypersensitivity

Precautions: Pregnancy category C, lactation, children, blood dyscrasias

Pharmacokinetics:
PO: Peak 1.5-2 hr, elimination half-life 3-4 hr; metabolized by liver

Drug interactions of concern to dentistry:
• Disulfiram-like reaction: alcohol

DENTAL CONSIDERATIONS

General:
• Patients on chronic drug therapy may rarely have symptoms of blood dyscrasias, which can include infection, bleeding, and poor healing.
• Palliative treatment may be required for oral side effects.
• Place on frequent recall to evaluate healing response.
• Consider semisupine chair position when GI side effects occur.

Consultations:
• In a patient with symptoms of blood dyscrasias, request a medical consult for blood studies and postpone dental treatment until normal values are reestablished.
• Medical consult may be required to assess disease control in the patient.

Teach patient/family:
• To call physician if sore throat, swollen lymph nodes, malaise, or fever occur because other infections may exist
• To avoid mouth rinses with high alcohol content
• Importance of good oral hygiene to prevent soft tissue inflammation
• Caution to prevent injury when using oral hygiene aids
• To report oral lesions, soreness, or bleeding to dentist

L

levetiracetam

(lev-tir-a'se-tam)
Keppra
Drug class: Antiepileptic

Action: Mechanism of action is unknown; however, drugs of this type have dopaminergic, cholinergic, and glutamatergic activity; reported to have antiepileptic, anxiolytic, and cognitive enhancing activity; other suggestions include disruption of epileptiform burst firing and seizure propagation.

Uses: Adjunctive therapy in adults with partial onset seizures

Dosage and routes:
• *Adult:* PO initial dose 1000 mg/day given as 500 mg bid; additional doses may be given every 2 wk (1000 mg/day increments); max daily dose 3000 mg; doses must be adjusted with renal impair-

ment; has been used in combination with other antiepileptic drugs
Available forms include: Tabs 250, 500, 750 mg
Side effects/adverse reactions:
Based on limited information
▼ *ORAL:* Ginvitis (unspecified as to cause)
CNS: Drowsiness, somnolence, headache, dizziness, fatigue, amnesia, anxiety, ataxia, depression, emotional lability, hostility, vertigo
GI: Nausea, anorexia, abdominal pain, dyspepsia, diarrhea
RESP: Cough
HEMA: Decrease in mean RBC count, decrease in mean hemoglobin and mean hematocrit, leukopenia
GU: Increase in serum creatinine, UTI
EENT: Pharyngitis, rhinitis, sinusitis, diplopia
INTEG: Rash
MS: Arthralgia
MISC: Asthenia, coordination difficulties, infection
Contraindications: Hypersensitivity
Precautions: Renal impairment, hemodialysis, pregnancy category C, lactation, may increase phenytoin blood levels, risk of seizures on withdrawal, children <16 yr
Pharmacokinetics:
PO: Bioavailability 100%, onset 1 hr, peak plasma levels 20 min-2 hr, half-life 6-8 hr, <10% plasma protein bound, limited hepatic metabolism, renal excretion (66%)
Drug interactions of concern to dentistry:
• None reported
DENTAL CONSIDERATIONS:
General:
• Short appointments and a stress reduction protocol may be required for anxious patients.
• Ask patient about type of epilepsy, seizure frequency, and quality of seizure control.
Consultation:
• Medical consult may be required to assess disease control and the patient's ability to tolerate stress.
• In patients with symptoms of blood dyscrasias, request a medical consult for blood studies and postpone treatment until normal values are reestablished.
Teach patient/family:
• Importance of updating health and drug history if physician makes changes in evaluation/drug regimens

---

levobunolol HCl

(lee-voe-byoo′noe-lole)
AKbeta, Betagan Liquifilm
Drug class.: β-adrenergic blocker

Action: Reduces production of aqueous humor by unknown mechanisms
Uses: Chronic open-angle glaucoma, ocular hypertension
Dosage and routes:
• *Adult:* Instill 1 gtt in affected eye(s) qd or bid
Available forms include: Sol 0.25%, 0.5%
Side effects/adverse reactions:
CNS: Ataxia, dizziness, lethargy
Drug interactions of concern to dentistry:
• Avoid use of anticholinergic drugs, atropine-like drugs, propantheline, and diazepam (benzodiazepines)
DENTAL CONSIDERATIONS
General:
• Check compliance of patient with

prescribed drug regimen for glaucoma.

• Avoid dental light in patient's eyes; offer dark glasses for patient comfort.

Consultations:

• Consultation with physician may be needed if sedation or anesthesia is required.

levocabastine HCl

(lee'voe-kab-as-teen)

Livostin, Livostatin Nasal

Drug class.: Antihistamine, H_1-receptor antagonist

Action: Selective antagonist for histamine at H_1-receptors; little or no systemic absorption; intended for topical effect

Uses: Temporary relief of seasonal allergic conjunctivitis

Dosage and routes:

Ophthalmic

• *Adult and child >12 yr:* Instill 1 gtt in affected eye qid; may continue for up to 2 wk

• *Adult and child >12 yr:* Nasal spray 2 sprays in each nostril bid

Available forms include: Ophth susp 0.05% in 2.5, 5, 10 ml dropper bottles, nasal susp 0.05%

Side effects/adverse reactions:

▼ *ORAL:* Dry mouth

CNS: Headache, fatigue, somnolence

GI: Nausea

RESP: Dyspnea, cough

EENT: Local stinging/burning, red eyes, eyelid edema, lacrimation

INTEG: Rash, erythema

Contraindications: Hypersensitivity; avoid while contact lenses are being used

Precautions: Pregnancy category C, lactation, children <12 yr

Pharmacokinetics:

OPHTH: Systemic absorption low; mean plasma concentration 1-2 ng/ml

Drug interactions of concern to dentistry:

• No documented interactions with dental drugs

DENTAL CONSIDERATIONS

General:

• Question patient about history of allergy to avoid using other potential allergens.

• Avoid dental light in patient's eyes; offer dark glasses for patient comfort.

• Evaluate respiration characteristics and rate.

• Using for less than 2 wk should not present a problem with dry mouth.

Teach patient/family:

When chronic dry mouth occurs, advise patient:

• To avoid mouth rinses with high alcohol content due to drying effects

• To use daily home fluoride products for anticaries effect

• To use sugarless gum, frequent sips of water, or saliva substitutes

levodopa

(lee-voe-doe'pa)

Dopar, Larodopa

Drug class.: Antiparkinson agent

Action: Levodopa is decarboxylated to dopamine, which can interact with dopamine receptors

Uses: Parkinsonism or parkinsonian symptoms

Dosage and routes:

• *Adult:* PO 0.5-1 g qd either bid or qid with food; dose is titrated to

L

tolerated side effects; may be increased by 0.75 g q3-7d, not to exceed 8 g/day

Available forms include: Caps 100, 250, 500 mg; tabs 100, 250, 500 mg

Side effects/adverse reactions:

▼ *ORAL: Dry mouth,* bitter taste

CNS: Involuntary choreiform movements, hand tremors, fatigue, headache, anxiety, twitching, numbness, weakness, confusion, agitation, insomnia, nightmares, psychosis, hallucinations, hypomania, severe depression, dizziness

CV: Orthostatic hypotension, tachycardia, hypertension, palpitation

GI: Nausea, vomiting, anorexia, abdominal distress, flatulence, dysphagia, diarrhea, constipation

HEMA: ***Hemolytic anemia, leukopenia, agranulocytosis***

EENT: Blurred vision, diplopia, dilated pupils

INTEG: Rash, sweating, alopecia

MISC: Urinary retention, incontinence, weight change, dark urine

Contraindications: Hypersensitivity, narrow-angle glaucoma, undiagnosed skin lesions, MAO inhibitors

Precautions: Renal disease, cardiac disease, hepatic disease, respiratory disease, MI with dysrhythmia, convulsions, peptic ulcer, pregnancy category C, asthma, endocrine disease, affective disorders, psychosis, lactation, children <12 yr

Pharmacokinetics:

PO: Peak 1-3 hr, metabolites excreted in urine

Drug interactions of concern to dentistry:

- Decreased absorption: anticholinergics
- Decreased therapeutic effect: benzodiazepines, pyridoxine (vitamin B_6)

DENTAL CONSIDERATIONS

General:

- Patients on chronic drug therapy may rarely have symptoms of blood dyscrasias, which can include infection, bleeding, and poor healing.
- Assess salivary flow as a factor in caries, periodontal disease, and candidiasis.
- After supine positioning, have patient sit upright for at least 2 min before standing to avoid orthostatic hypotension.
- Avoid dental light in patient's eyes; offer dark glasses for patient comfort.

Consultations:

- In a patient with symptoms of blood dyscrasias, request a medical consult for blood studies and postpone dental treatment until normal values are reestablished.
- Take precautions if dental surgery is anticipated and anesthesia is required.
- Medical consult may be required to assess disease control in the patient.

Teach patient/family:

- To use electric toothbrush if patient has difficulty holding conventional devices

When chronic dry mouth occurs, advise patient:

- To avoid mouth rinses with high alcohol content due to drying effects
- To use sugarless gum, frequent sips of water, or saliva substitutes
- To use daily home fluoride products for anticaries effect

levodopa-carbidopa

(lee-voe-doe'pa) (kar-bi-doe'pa)
Sinemet, Sinemet CR

Drug class.: Antiparkinson agent

Action: Decarboxylation of levodopa to periphery is inhibited by carbidopa; more levodopa is made available for transport to brain and conversion to dopamine in the brain

Uses: Treatment of idiopathic, symptomatic, or postencephalitic parkinsonism

Dosage and routes:

• *Adult:* PO 1 tab of 10 mg carbidopa/100 mg levodopa tid or qid in divided doses, not to exceed 8 tabs/day; dose ratio may require adjustments

Available forms include: Tabs 10/100, 25/100, 25/250, 50 mg carbidopa/200 mg levodopa

Side effects/adverse reactions:

▼ *ORAL: Dry mouth,* bitter taste

CNS: Involuntary choreiform movements, hand tremors, fatigue, headache, anxiety, twitching, numbness, weakness, confusion, agitation, insomnia, nightmares, psychosis, hallucinations, hypomania, severe depression, dizziness

CV: Orthostatic hypotension, tachycardia, hypertension, palpitation

GI: Nausea, vomiting, anorexia, abdominal distress, flatulence, dysphagia, diarrhea, constipation

HEMA: ***Hemolytic anemia, leukopenia, agranulocytosis***

EENT: Blurred vision, diplopia, dilated pupils

INTEG: Rash, sweating, alopecia

MISC: Urinary retention, incontinence, weight change, dark urine

Contraindications: Hypersensitivity, narrow-angle glaucoma, undiagnosed skin lesions

Precautions: Renal disease, cardiac disease, hepatic disease, respiratory disease, MI with dysrhythmias, convulsions, peptic ulcer, pregnancy category C

Pharmacokinetics:

PO: Peak 1-3 hr, excreted in urine (metabolites)

Drug interactions of concern to dentistry:

• Decreased absorption: anticholinergics

• Decreased therapeutic effect: benzodiazepines, pyridoxine (vitamin B_6)

DENTAL CONSIDERATIONS

General:

• Patients on chronic drug therapy may rarely have symptoms of blood dyscrasias, which can include infection, bleeding, and poor healing.

• Assess salivary flow as a factor in caries, periodontal disease, and candidiasis.

• After supine positioning, have patient sit upright for at least 2 min before standing to avoid orthostatic hypotension.

• Avoid dental light in patient's eyes; offer dark glasses for patient comfort.

Consultations:

• In a patient with symptoms of blood dyscrasias, request a medical consult for blood studies and postpone dental treatment until normal values are reestablished.

• Take precautions if dental surgery is anticipated and anesthesia is required.

L

• Medical consult may be required to assess disease control in the patient.

Teach patient/family:

• To use electric toothbrush if patient has difficulty holding conventional devices

When chronic dry mouth occurs, advise patient:

• To avoid mouth rinses with high alcohol content due to drying effects

• To use sugarless gum, frequent sips of water, or saliva substitutes

• To use daily home fluoride products for anticaries effect

---

levofloxacin

(lee-voe-flox'a-sin)

Levaquin

Drug class.: Fluoroquinolone antiinfective

Action: A broad-spectrum bactericidal agent that inhibits the enzyme DNA gyrase needed for bacterial DNA replication

Uses: Acute infections due to susceptible bacterial strains causing acute maxillary sinusitis, acute bacterial exacerbation of chronic bronchitis, community-acquired pneumonia, uncomplicated skin and skin structure infections, uncomplicated UTI, and acute pyelonephritis

Dosage and routes:

• *Adult:* PO 250-500 mg q24h for 3-14 days depending on the type of infection

• *Adult:* IV 500 mg by slow infusion over 60 min q24h depending on type of infection

Reduce dose in renal impairment

Available forms include: Tabs 250, 500 mg; vials 500 mg (25 mg/ml); Premix IV bags 250 mg or 500 mg in D_5W (5 mg/ml)

Side effects/adverse reactions:

▼ *ORAL:* Taste alteration, dry mouth (<0.5%)

CNS: Headache, dizziness, insomnia, anorexia, anxiety, tremor

CV: Edema

GI: Abdominal pain, dyspepsia, diarrhea, nausea, flatulence, vomiting

HEMA: Hemolytic anemia

GU: Vaginitis

EENT: Rhinitis, pharyngitis

INTEG: Pruritus, rash, photosensitivity, ***anaphylaxis,*** increased sweating, urticaria, erythema multiforme, Stevens-Johnson syndrome

ENDO: Alteration of blood glucose levels

MS: Tendon rupture

MISC: Chest and back pain

Contraindications: Hypersensitivity to quinolone antiinfectives

Precautions: Children <18 yr; seizure disorders, renal insufficiency, excessive exposure to sunlight, alterations in blood glucose (diabetes), pregnancy category C, lactation, drink fluids liberally; tendon rupture of shoulder, hand, and Achilles tendon

Pharmacokinetics:

PO: Bioavailability 99%, peak plasma levels 1-2 hr; 24%-38% protein bound, limited metabolism, primarily excreted in urine as unchanged drug

IV: After 60 min infusion see peak plasma concentration 6.2 μg/ml; steady state in 48 hr with 500 mg/day

Drug interactions of concern to dentistry:

• Interference with absorption: solutions with multivalent cations (e.g., Mg^{2+})

• Increased seizure risk: NSAIDs

• May increase effects of warfarin

DENTAL CONSIDERATIONS

General:

• Determine why patient is taking the drug.

• If dental drugs prescribed, advise patient of potential for photosensitivity.

Consultations:

• Consult with patient's physician if an acute dental infection occurs and another antiinfective is required.

Teach patient/family:

• To minimize exposure to sunlight and wear sunscreen if sun exposure is planned

• To discontinue treatment and inform dentist immediately if patient experiences pain or inflammation of a tendon, and to rest and refrain from exercise

---

levomethadyl acetate HCl

(lee-voe-meth'a-dil)

Orlaam

Drug class.: Synthetic opioid

Action: Mimics the action of opioid analgesics by interacting with CNS opioid receptors

Uses: Management of opioid dependence

Dosage and routes:

Opioid addiction

• *Adult:* PO initial 20-40 mg 3 × weekly (at 48-72 hr intervals); adjust dose in increments of 5-10 mg over 1 or 2 wk to reach steady state; dose adjustment required for each patient; maintenance 60-90 mg 3 × weekly, limit 140 mg/wk

Available forms include: Sol PO 10 mg/ml in 474 ml; available only from FDA, DEA, or state-approved treatment programs

Side effects/adverse reactions:

ORAL: Dry mouth

CNS: Depression, weakness, postural hypotension, tachycardia

CV: Dysrhythmia

GI: Abdominal pain, constipation, nausea, vomiting

RESP: Coughing

GU: Decreased libido

INTEG: Skin rash, goose flesh

MS: Muscle cramps

MISC: Sweating, flulike symptoms

Contraindications: Hypersensitivity

Precautions: Pregnancy category C, lactation, increased intracranial pressure, MI (acute), severe heart disease, respiratory depression, hepatic disease, renal disease, child <18 yr, addictive personality

Pharmacokinetics:

PO: Onset 2-4 hr, cumulative 22-48 hr; metabolized by liver; excreted by kidneys; crosses placenta; excreted in breast milk

Drug interactions of concern to dentistry:

• Risk of opioid toxicity: opioid analgesics

• Risk of withdrawal symptoms: mixed agonist/antagonist opioids

• Increased CNS effects: alcohol, sedative-hypnotics, other CNS depressants

DENTAL CONSIDERATIONS

General:

• Monitor vital signs every appointment due to cardiovascular side effects.

• Patients using this drug are being treated for opioid dependence; avoid the use of any drug with abuse potential.

• Consider aspirin, acetaminophen, or NSAIDs for the management of dental-related pain.
• Take precautions if dental surgery is anticipated and general anesthesia is required.
• Assess salivary flow as a factor in caries, periodontal disease, and candidiasis.
• If opioid or sedative drugs are required for patient management and comfort, advise current drug abuse care facility or aftercare program as appropriate.

Consultations:
• Consults may be difficult to obtain where treatment confidentiality of drug dependence is followed.
• Medical consult may be required to assess disease control in the patient.

Teach patient/family:
• Importance of good oral hygiene to prevent soft tissue inflammation

When chronic dry mouth occurs, advise patient:
• To avoid mouth rinses with high alcohol content due to drying effects
• To use daily home fluoride products for anticaries effect
• To use sugarless gum, frequent sips of water, or saliva substitutes

levonorgestrel implant

(lee-voe-nor-jes'trel)

Norplant System

Drug class.: Contraceptive system

Action: As a progestin, transforms proliferative endometrium into secretory endometrium; inhibits secretion of pituitary gonadotropins, which prevents follicular maturation and ovulation

Uses: Prevention of pregnancy

Dosage and routes:
• *Adult:* 6 caps subdermally implanted in the upper arm during first 7 days of onset of menses; for long-term use up to 5 yr

Population Council's levonorgestrel
• *Adult:* Two-rod implant system for 3 years of contraception

Available forms include: Kit of 6 caps, 36 mg/cap

Side effects/adverse reactions:
CNS: Dizziness, headache, nervousness
GI: Nausea, abdominal discomfort
GU: Amenorrhea, cervical erosion, breakthrough bleeding, dysmenorrhea, vaginal candidiasis, breast changes, vaginitis
INTEG: Alopecia, dermatitis, hirsutism, acne, hypertrichosis, infection at site, pain/itching at site
MISC: Change in appetite, weight gain

Contraindications: Hypersensitivity, pregnancy category X, thrombophlebitis, undiagnosed genital bleeding, liver tumors, breast carcinoma, liver disease

Precautions: Depression, psychosis, lactation, fluid retention, contact lens wearers

Pharmacokinetics: Max concentration at 24 hr; plasma levels average 0.30 mg/ml over 5 yr as drug is slowly and continuously released

Drug interactions of concern to dentistry:
• Decreased contraception: carbamazepine
• Antibiotics have been shown to decrease effects of oral contraceptives, but no data have been reported on this system

DENTAL CONSIDERATIONS

General:

• Until more data are available, advise patient to use additional contraception when antibiotics are prescribed.

Teach patient/family:

• Importance of good oral hygiene to prevent soft tissue inflammation

---

levothyroxine sodium (T_4, L-thyroxine sodium)

(lee-voe-thye-rox′een)

Euthyrox, Levo-T, Levothroid, Levoxyl, Synthroid

✱ Eltroxin, PMS-Levothyroxine

Drug class.: Thyroid hormone

Action: Increases metabolic rate, with increase in cardiac output, O_2 consumption, body temperature, blood volume, growth/development at cellular level

Uses: Hypothyroidism, myxedema coma, thyroid hormone replacement, cretinism

Dosage and routes:

• *Adult:* PO 0.025-0.1 mg qd, increased by 0.05-0.1 mg q1-4wk until desired response; maintenance 0.1-0.4 mg qd

• *Child:* PO 0.01-0.05 qd; may increase 0.025-0.05 mg q1-4wk until desired response

Cretinism

• *Child:* IV 0.025-0.05 mg qd; may increase by 0.05-0.1 mg PO q2-3wk

Myxedema coma

• *Adult:* IV 0.2-0.5 mg; may increase by 0.1-0.3 mg after 24 hr; place on oral medication as soon as possible

Available forms include: Inj IV 200, 500 µg/vial; tabs 0.025, 0.05, 0.075, 0.088, 0.1, 0.112, 0.125, 0.137, 0.15, 0.175, 0.2, 0.3 mg

Side effects/adverse reactions:

CNS: Anxiety, insomnia, tremors, ***thyroid storm,*** headache

CV: Tachycardia, palpitation, angina, dysrhythmias, ***cardiac arrest,*** hypertension

GI: Nausea, diarrhea, increased or decreased appetite, cramps

MISC: Menstrual irregularities, weight loss, sweating, heat intolerance, fever

Contraindications: Adrenal insufficiency, MI, thyrotoxicosis

Precautions: Elderly, angina pectoris, hypertension, ischemia, cardiac disease, pregnancy category A, lactation

Pharmacokinetics:

IV/PO: Peak 12-48 hr, half-life 6-7 days; distributed throughout body tissues

Drug interactions of concern to dentistry:

• Increased effects of sympathomimetics when thyroid doses are not carefully monitored or in patients with coronary artery disease

DENTAL CONSIDERATIONS

General:

• Uncontrolled hypothyroid patients may be more responsive to CNS depressants.

• Increased nervousness, excitability, sweating, or tachycardia may indicate a patient with uncontrolled hyperthyroidism or a dose of medication that is too high. Uncontrolled patients should be referred for medical treatment.

Consultations:

• Medical consult may be required to assess disease control in the patient.

lidocaine HCl (cardiac)

(lye'doe-kane)

Lidopen Auto-Injector, Xylocaine, Xylocard

Drug class.: Antidysrhythmic (Class IB)

Action: Increases electrical stimulation threshold of ventricle and His-Purkinje system, which stabilizes cardiac membrane and decreases automaticity and excitability of ventricles

Uses: Ventricular tachycardia, ventricular dysrhythmias during cardiac surgery, MI, digitalis toxicity, cardiac catheterization

Dosage and routes:

• *Adult:* IV bol 50-100 mg over 2-3 min, repeat q3-5 min, not to exceed 300 mg in 1 hr, begin IV inf; IV inf 20-50 μg/kg/min; IM 200-300 mg in deltoid muscle

• *Elderly, CHF-reduced liver function:* IV bol give one-half adult dose

• *Child:* IV bol 1 mg/kg, then IV INF 30 μg/kg/min

Available forms include: IV inf 0.2%, 0.4%, 0.8%; IV Ad 4%, 10%, 20%; IV Dir 1%, 2%; IM 300 mg/ml, 10%

Side effects/adverse reactions:

CNS: Headache, dizziness, nervousness, ***convulsions,*** involuntary movement, confusion, tremor, drowsiness, euphoria

CV: Bradycardia, ***hypotension, heart block, cardiovascular collapse, arrest***

GI: Nausea, vomiting, anorexia

RESP: ***Respiratory depression,*** dyspnea

EENT: Blurred vision, tinnitus

INTEG: Rash, urticaria, edema, swelling

MISC: Febrile response, phlebitis at injection site

Contraindications: Hypersensitivity to amides, severe heart block, supraventricular dysrhythmias, Adams-Stokes syndrome, Wolff-Parkinson-White syndrome

Precautions: Pregnancy category B, lactation, children, renal disease, liver disease, CHF, respiratory depression, malignant hyperthermia (questionable), elderly; need to monitor ECG

Pharmacokinetics:

IV: Onset immediate, duration 20 min

IM: Onset 5-15 min, duration 1-1.5 hr

Half-life 1-2 hr; moderate-to-high protein binding; metabolized in liver; excreted in urine; crosses placenta

Drug interactions of concern to dentistry:

• Increased effects: cimetidine, β-blockers, other dysrhythmics

• Increased neuromuscular blockade of neuromuscular blockers, succinylcholine

DENTAL CONSIDERATIONS

General:

• This is an emergency drug used in ICUs, emergency departments, and hospitals. Patients would not be having elective dental treatment.

• Use of lidocaine to control dysrhythmias requires immediate medical consult or removal of patient to emergency care facility.

• Monitor ECG when used; observe for lidocaine toxicity.

• Monitor patient's vital signs and support as required.

lidocaine HCl (local)

(lye'doe-kane)

Dalcaine, Dilocaine, Duo-Trach Kit, L-Caine, Lidoject, Nervocaine, Octocaine, Ultracaine, Xylocaine, Xylocaine-MPF

With vasoconstrictor: Octocaine with Epinephrine, Xylocaine with Epinephrine

Drug class.: Amide local anesthetic

Action: Inhibits ion fluxes across membranes, particularly sodium transport across cell membrane; decreases rise of depolarization phase of action potential; blocks nerve action potential

Uses: Local dental anesthesia; peripheral nerve block; caudal anesthesia; epidural, spinal, surgical anesthesia

Dosage and routes:

Dental injection: infiltration or conduction block

• *Lidocaine 2% without vasoconstrictor:* Max dose 6.6 mg/kg or 300 mg per dental appointment[a] for healthy patients; doses must be adjusted downward for medically compromised, debilitated, or elderly and for each individual patient. **Always use the lowest effective dose, a slow injection rate, and a careful aspiration technique.**

Example calculations illustrating amount of drug administered per dental cartridge(s)

# of cartridges (1.8 ml)	mg of lidocaine (2%)
1	36
2	72
4	144

[a]Maximum dose is cited from *USP-DI,* ed 16, 1996, US Pharmacopeial Convention, Inc., as well as from the manufacturer's package insert. Doses may differ in other published reference resources.

Lidocaine 2% with 1:50,000 epinephrine: Epinephrine 3 μg/kg, with a limit of 0.2 mg/patient.

Manufacturer's package insert indicates that the max dose of lidocaine with vasoconstrictors is 500 mg. Adjust doses for each individual patient as previously indicated.

L

Example calculations illustrating amount of drug administered per dental cartridge(s)

# of cartridges (1.8 ml)	mg of lidocaine (2%)	mg(μg) of vasoconstrictor (1:50,000)
1	36	0.036 (36)
2	72	0.072 (72)
3	108	0.108 (108)
4	144	0.144 (144)
5	180	0.180 (180)
5.5	198	0.198 (198)

Lidocaine 2% with 1:100,000 epinephrine: The same doses and adjustments to doses apply as previously indicated.

Example calculations illustrating amount of drug administered per dental cartridge(s)

# of cartridges (1.8 ml)	mg of lidocaine (2%)	mg(μg) of vasoconstrictor (1:100,000)
1	36	0.018 (18)
2	72	0.036 (36)
3	108	0.054 (54)
6	216	0.108 (108)
8	288	0.144 (144)
10	360	0.180 (180)

Available forms include: Inj 0.5%, 1%, 1.5%, 2%, 4%, 5%; inj with epinephrine 0.5%, 1%, 1.5%, 2%; epinephrine concentrations range from 1:50,000 to 1:200,000; usual dental use is 2% conc with 1:100,000 epinephrine; other % sols are used in medical applications

Side effects/adverse reactions:

▼ *ORAL: Numbness, tingling,* trismus

CNS: ***Convulsions, loss of consciousness,*** drowsiness, disorientation, tremors, shivering, anxiety, restlessness

CV: ***Myocardial depression, cardiac arrest, dysrhythmias,*** bradycardia, hypotension, hypertension, fetal bradycardia

GI: Nausea, vomiting

RESP: ***Status asthmaticus, respiratory arrest, anaphylaxis***

EENT: Blurred vision, tinnitus, pupil constriction

INTEG: Rash, urticaria, allergic reactions, edema, burning, skin discoloration at injection site, tissue necrosis

Contraindications: Hypersensitivity, cross-sensitivity among amides (rare), severe liver disease

Precautions: Elderly, severe drug allergies, pregnancy category B, large doses of local anesthetics in patients with myasthenia gravis

Pharmacokinetics: Onset 2-10 min, duration 20 min to 4 hr; metabolized by liver, metabolites may contribute to toxicity in one dose; excreted in urine (metabolites)

Drug interactions of concern to dentistry:

• CNS depressants: increased risk of CNS depression with all CNS depressants, especially in children and when larger doses are used

• Avoid placing dental cartridges in disinfectant solutions with heavy metals or surface-active agents; may see release of metal ions into local anesthetic solutions with tissue irritation following injection

• Avoid excessive exposure of dental cartridges to light or heat, which hastens deterioration of vasoconstrictor; observe for color change in local anesthetic solution

• Risk of cardiovascular side effects: rapid intravascular administration of local anesthetic containing vasoconstrictor, either alone or in patients taking tricyclic antidepressants, MAO inhibitors, digitalis drugs, cocaine, phenothiazines, β-blockers, and in presence of halogenated hydrocarbon general anesthetics; use smallest effective vasoconstrictor dose and careful aspiration technique

• Avoid use of vasoconstrictors in patients with uncontrolled hyperthyroidism, diabetes, angina, or hypertension; refer these patients for medical treatment before elective dental procedures

DENTAL CONSIDERATIONS

General:

• Monitor vital signs every appointment due to cardiovascular and respiratory side effects.

• Drug is often used with vasoconstrictor for increased duration of action.

• Lubricate dry lips before injection or dental treatment as required.

Teach patient/family:

• To use care to prevent injury while numbness exists and to not chew gum or eat following dental anesthesia

• To report any signs of infection, muscle pain, or fever to dentist when feeling returns

• To report any unusual soft tissue reactions

lidocaine HCl (topical)

(lye'doe-kane)

generic, Xylocaine Viscous

Drug class.: Topically acting local anesthetic, amide

Action: Inhibits nerve impulses from sensory nerves, which produces anesthesia

Uses: Topical anesthesia of inflamed or irritated mucous membranes; to reduce gag reflex in dental radiologic examination or in dental impressions

Dosage and routes:

• *Adult and older child:* Rinse with 5-15 ml q4h, or rinse just before meals to reduce pain of aphthous ulcers; expectorate after rinsing

Available forms include: Top sol 2% in 100, 450 ml bottles

Side effects/adverse reactions:

INTEG: Rash, irritation, sensitization

Contraindications: Hypersensitivity, application to large areas

Precautions: Sepsis, pregnancy category B, denuded skin

DENTAL CONSIDERATIONS

General:

• Do not overuse; use just before eating to reduce pain of aphthous ulcers.

• If affected area is infected, do not apply.

Teach patient/family:

• To report rash, irritation, redness, or swelling to dentist

lidocaine transoral delivery system

(lye'doe-kane)

DentiPatch

Drug class.: Amide local anesthetic

Action: Inhibits nerve impulses from sensory nerves, which produces anesthesia

Uses: Mild topical anesthesia of mucous membranes of the mouth before superficial dental procedures

Dosage and routes:

• *Adult:* TOP apply one patch to area of application after drying with gauze; leave in place until local anesthesia is produced, but *no longer than 15 min*

Available forms include: Patches 2 cm^2 (containing 46.1 mg); carton of 50, 100 patches

Side effects/adverse reactions:

▼ *ORAL: Taste alteration, stomatitis, erythema, mucosa irritation*

CNS: Headache, excitatory or depressor actions, dizziness, nervous-

ness, confusion, tinnitus, twitching, tremors (associated with excessive systemic absorption)
CV: Bradycardia, hypotension, ***cardiovascular collapse*** (with excessive systemic absorption)
GI: Nausea
MISC: Allergic reactions to this agent or to other ingredients in the formulation (rare)
Contraindications: Hypersensitivity to amide-type local anesthetics
Precautions: Local anesthetic toxicity, no pediatric (child <12 yr) or geriatric studies have been made, liver dysfunction, onset longer for maxilla, pregnancy category B, lactation, contains phenylalanine (caution phenylketonurics)
Pharmacokinetics:
TOP: Onset 2.5 min, duration of approximately 30 min after removal; blood levels <0.1 ng/ml limited absorption; hepatic metabolism, urinary excretion
Drug interactions of concern to dentistry:
• None reported with dental drugs

DENTAL CONSIDERATIONS
General:
• Use no more than one patch per area, remove after 15 min to avoid toxicity.
Teach patient/family:
• Advise patient to prevent injury while numbness is present, to not chew gum or eat after dental treatment
• To report unresolved oral lesions to dentist

lincomycin HCl
(lin-koe-mye'sin)
Lincocin, Lincorex
Drug class.: Antibacterial

Action: Binds to 50S subunit of bacterial ribosomes; suppresses protein synthesis
Uses: Infections caused by group A beta-hemolytic streptococci, pneumococci, staphylococci (respiratory tract, skin, soft tissue, urinary tract infections; osteomyelitis; septicemia), and anaerobes
Dosage and routes:
• *Adult:* PO 500 mg q6-8h, not to exceed 8 g/day; IM 600 mg/day or q12h; IV 600 mg-1 g q8-12h, dilute in 100 ml IV sol, infuse over 1 hr, not to exceed 8 g/day
• *Child >1 mo:* PO 30-60 mg/kg/day in divided doses q6-8h; IM 10 mg/kg/day q12h; IV 10-20 mg/kg/day in divided doses q8-12h, dilute to 100 ml IV sol, infuse over 1 hr
Available forms include: Caps 500 mg; caps pediatric 250 mg; inj IM/IV 300 mg/ml
Side effects/adverse reactions:
▼ *ORAL:* Candidiasis
GI: Nausea, vomiting, abdominal pain, diarrhea, ***pseudomembranous colitis***
HEMA: ***Leukopenia, eosinophilia, agranulocytosis, thrombocytopenia***
GU: Vaginitis, increased AST/ALT, bilirubin, alk phosphatase, jaundice, urinary frequency
INTEG: Rash, urticaria, pruritus, erythema, pain, abscess at injection site
Contraindications: Hypersensitivity, ulcerative colitis/enteritis, infants <1 mo

Precautions: Renal disease, liver disease, GI disease, elderly, pregnancy category not listed, lactation

Pharmacokinetics:

PO: Peak 2-4 hr, duration 6 hr

IM: Peak 30 min, duration 8-12 hr

Half-life 4-6 hr; metabolized in liver; excreted in urine, bile, feces as active/inactive metabolites; crosses placenta; excreted in breast milk

Drug interactions of concern to dentistry:

• Decreased action of erythromycin

DENTAL CONSIDERATIONS

General:

• Determine why the patient is taking the drug.

Consultations:

• Medical consult may be required to assess disease control in the patient.

Teach patient/family:

• Importance of good oral hygiene to prevent soft tissue inflammation

• Caution to prevent injury when using oral hygiene aids

• To notify dentist if diarrhea occurs

When used for dental infection, advise patient:

• Taking birth control pill to use additional method of contraception for duration of cycle

• To report sore throat, oral burning sensation, fever, fatigue, any of which could indicate superinfection

• To take at prescribed intervals and complete dosage regimen

• To immediately notify the dentist if signs or symptoms of infection increase

liothyronine sodium (T_3)

(lye-oh-thye′roe-neen)

Cytomel, Triostat

Drug class.: Thyroid hormone

Action: Increases metabolic rate with increase in cardiac output, O_2 consumption, body temperature, blood volume, growth/development at cellular level

Uses: Hypothyroidism, myxedema coma, thyroid hormone replacement, cretinism, nontoxic goiter, T_3 suppression test

Dosage and routes:

• *Adult:* PO 25 μg qd, increased by 12.5-25 μg q1-2wk until desired response; maintenance 25-75 μg qd

Available forms include: Tabs 5, 25, 50 μg

Side effects/adverse reactions:

CNS: Insomnia, tremors, ***thyroid storm (overdose),*** headache

CV: ***Tachycardia, palpitation, angina, dysrhythmias, cardiac arrest,*** hypertension

GI: Nausea, diarrhea, increased or decreased appetite, cramps

MISC: Menstrual irregularities, weight loss, sweating, heat intolerance, fever

Contraindications: Adrenal insufficiency, MI, thyrotoxicosis

Precautions: Elderly, angina pectoris, hypertension, ischemia, cardiac disease, pregnancy category A, lactation

Pharmacokinetics:

PO: Peak 12-48 hr, half-life 0.6-1.4 days

Drug interactions of concern to dentistry:

• Hypertension, tachycardia: ketamine

• Increased effects of sympathomimetics when thyroid doses are not carefully monitored or in patients with coronary artery disease

DENTAL CONSIDERATIONS
General:

• Patients with uncontrolled hypothyroidism may be more responsive to CNS depressants.

• Increased nervousness, excitability, sweating, or tachycardia may indicate a patient with uncontrolled hyperthyroidism or a dose of medication that is too high. Uncontrolled patients should be referred for medical treatment.

Consultations:

• Medical consult may be required to assess disease control in the patient.

liotrix

(lye′oh-trix)
Thyrolar

Drug class.: Thyroid hormone

Action: Increases metabolic rate, cardiac output, O_2 consumption, body temperature, blood volume, growth/development at cellular level

Uses: Hypothyroidism, thyroid hormone replacement

Dosage and routes:

• *Adult and child:* PO 15-30 mg qd, increased by 15-30 mg q1-2wk until desired response, may increase by 15-30 mg q2wk in child

• *Geriatric:* PO 15-30 mg, double dose q6-8wk until desired response

Available forms include: Tabs 15, 30, 60, 120, 180 mg as thyroid equivalent

Side effects/adverse reactions:

CNS: Insomnia, tremors, headache, ***thyroid storm***

CV: Tachycardia, palpitation, angina, dysrhythmias, hypertension, cardiac arrest

GI: Nausea, diarrhea, increased or decreased appetite, cramps

MISC: Menstrual irregularities, weight loss, sweating, heat intolerance, fever

Contraindications: Adrenal insufficiency, MI, thyrotoxicosis

Precautions: Elderly, angina pectoris, hypertension, ischemia, cardiac disease, pregnancy category A, lactation

Pharmacokinetics:

PO: Peak 12-48 hr, half-life 6-7 days

Drug interactions of concern to dentistry:

• Hypertension, tachycardia: ketamine

• Increased effects of sympathomimetics when thyroid doses are not carefully monitored or in patients with coronary artery disease

DENTAL CONSIDERATIONS
General:

• Patients with uncontrolled hypothyroidism may be more responsive to CNS depressants.

• Increased nervousness, excitability, sweating, or tachycardia may indicate a patient with uncontrolled hyperthyroidism or a dose of medication that is too high. Uncontrolled patients should be referred for medical treatment.

Consultations:

• Medical consult may be required to assess disease control in the patient.

Teach patient/family:

• Importance of good oral hygiene to prevent soft tissue inflammation

• To avoid mouth rinses with high alcohol content due to drying effects

lisinopril

(lyse-in'oh-pril)
Prinivil, Zestril

Drug class.: Angiotensin-converting enzyme (ACE) inhibitor

Action: Selectively suppresses renin-angiotensin-aldosterone system; inhibits ACE, which prevents conversion of angiotensin I to angiotensin II

Uses: Mild-to-moderate hypertension, post-MI if hemodynamically stable

Dosage and routes:

• *Adult:* PO 10-40 mg qd; may increase to 80 mg qd if required; PO post-MI initial dose 5 mg, then 5 mg after 24 hr, 10 mg after 48 hr, and 10 mg/day for 6 wk

Available forms include: Tabs 2.5, 5, 10, 20, 40 mg

Side effects/adverse reactions:

▼ *ORAL:* Dry mouth, angioedema

CNS: Vertigo, depression, stroke, insomnia, paresthesia, headache, fatigue, asthenia

CV: Hypotension, chest pain, palpitation, angina, dysrhythmia, syncope

GI: Nausea, vomiting, anorexia, constipation, flatulence, GI irritation

RESP: Cough, dyspnea

HEMA: ***Eosinophilia, leukopenia,*** decreased Hct/Hgb

GU: ***Proteinuria, renal insufficiency,*** sexual dysfunction, impotence

EENT: Blurred vision, nasal congestion

INTEG: Rash, pruritus

Contraindications: Hypersensitivity

Precautions: Pregnancy category C, lactation, renal disease, hyperkalemia

Pharmacokinetics: Peak 6-8 hr; excreted unchanged in urine

Drug interactions of concern to dentistry:

• Increased hypotension: alcohol, phenothiazines

• Decreased hypotensive effects: indomethacin and possibly other NSAIDs, sympathomimetics

DENTAL CONSIDERATIONS

General:

• Monitor vital signs every appointment due to cardiovascular and respiratory side effects.

• After supine positioning, have patient sit upright for at least 2 min before standing to avoid orthostatic hypotension.

• Patients on chronic drug therapy may rarely have symptoms of blood dyscrasias, which can include infection, bleeding, and poor healing.

• Assess salivary flow as a factor in caries, periodontal disease, and candidiasis.

• Limit use of sodium-containing products, such as saline IV fluids, for patients with a dietary salt restriction.

• Use vasoconstrictors with caution, in low doses, and with careful aspiration.

• Short appointments and a stress reduction protocol may be required for anxious patients.

Consultations:

• Medical consult may be required to assess disease control and patient's ability to tolerate stress.

• In a patient with symptoms of blood dyscrasias, request a medical consult for blood studies and postpone dental treatment until normal values are reestablished.

• Take precautions if dental surgery is anticipated and sedation or general anesthesia is required; there is a risk of a hypotensive episode.

Teach patient/family:

• Importance of good oral hygiene to prevent soft tissue inflammation

• Caution to prevent injury when using oral hygiene aids

When chronic dry mouth occurs, advise patient:

• To avoid mouth rinses with high alcohol content due to drying effects

• To use sugarless gum, frequent sips of water, or saliva substitutes

• To use daily home fluoride products for anticaries effect

lithium carbonate/ lithium citrate

(lith'ee-um)

Lithium carbonate: Eskalith, Eskalith CR, Lithane, Lithobid, Lithonate, Lithotabs

🍁 Carbolith, Duralith, Lithizine, PMS-Lithium Carbonate

Lithium citrate: Cibalith-S

🍁 PMS-Lithium Citrate

Drug class.: Antimanic, inorganic salt

Action: May alter sodium and potassium ion transport across cell membrane in nerve, muscle cells; may affect both norepinephrine and serotonin in the CNS

Uses: Manic-depressive illness (manic phase), prevention of bipolar manic depressive psychosis; unapproved use includes depression, vascular headache

Dosage and routes:

• *Adult:* PO 300-600 mg tid, maintenance 300 mg tid or qid; slow rel tabs 300 mg bid, dose should be individualized to maintain blood levels at 0.5-1.5 mEq/L

Available forms include: Caps 150, 300, 600 mg; tabs 300 mg; ext rel tabs 300, 450 mg; oral sol 8 mEq/5 ml

Side effects/adverse reactions:

▼ *ORAL: Increased thirst, dry mouth*

CNS: Headache, drowsiness, dizziness, tremors, twitching, ataxia, seizures, slurred speech, restlessness, confusion, stupor, memory loss, clonic movements

CV: Hypotension, ***circulatory collapse, edema,*** ECG changes, dysrhythmias

GI: Anorexia, nausea, vomiting, diarrhea, incontinence, abdominal pain

HEMA: ***Leukocytosis***

GU: ***Polyuria, glycosuria, proteinuria, albuminuria,*** urinary incontinence, polydipsia, edema

EENT: Tinnitus, blurred vision

INTEG: Drying of hair, alopecia, rash, pruritus, hyperkeratosis

ENDO: Hyponatremia

MS: Muscle weakness

Contraindications: Hepatic disease, renal disease, brain trauma, OBS, pregnancy category D, lactation, children <12 yr, schizophrenia, severe cardiac disease, severe renal disease, severe dehydration

Precautions: Elderly, thyroid disease, seizure disorders, diabetes mellitus, systemic infection, urinary retention

Pharmacokinetics:

PO: Onset rapid, peak 0.5-4 hr, half-life 18-36 hr, depending on age; well absorbed by oral method; 80% of filtered lithium is reabsorbed by the renal tubules; excreted in urine; crosses placenta, blood-brain barrier; excreted in breast milk

Drug interactions of concern to dentistry:

• Increased toxicity: aspirin, indomethacin, other NSAIDs, haloperidol, metronidazole

• Increased effects of neuromuscular blocking agents

DENTAL CONSIDERATIONS

General:

• Assess salivary flow as a factor in caries, periodontal disease, and candidiasis.

• After supine positioning, have patient sit upright for at least 2 min before standing to avoid orthostatic hypotension.

Consultations:

• Medical consult may be required to assess disease control in the patient.

Teach patient/family:

• Importance of good oral hygiene to prevent soft tissue inflammation

• Caution to prevent injury when using oral hygiene aids

When chronic dry mouth occurs, advise patient:

• To avoid mouth rinses with high alcohol content due to drying effects

• To use sugarless gum, frequent sips of water, or saliva substitutes

• To use daily home fluoride products for anticaries effect

lodoxamide tromethamine

(loe-dox'a-mide)

Alomide Ophthalmic

Drug class.: Mast cell stabilizer

Action: Prevents release of mediators of inflammation from mast cells involved with type 1 immediate hypersensitivity reactions

Uses: Vernal keratoconjunctivitis, vernal conjunctivitis, keratitis

Dosage and routes:

Opthalmic

• *Adult and child >2 yr:* 1-2 gtt in each affected eye qid up to 3 mo

Available forms include: Sol 0.1%

Side effects/adverse reactions:

CNS: Headache, dizziness, somnolence

GI: Nausea

RESP: Sneezing

EENT: Burning/stinging eyes, itching, blurred vision, lacrimation, dry nose

INTEG: Rash

Contraindications: Hypersensitivity

Precautions: Pregnancy category B, child <2 yr, lactation, avoid contact lens use

Pharmacokinetics: Elimination half-life 8.5 hr, excreted in urine

Drug interactions of concern to dentistry:

• None reported

DENTAL CONSIDERATIONS

General:

• Question patient about history of allergy to avoid using other potential allergens.

• Avoid dental light in patient's eyes; offer dark glasses for patient comfort.

lomefloxacin HCl

(loe-me-flox'a-sin)

Maxaquin

Drug class.: Fluoroquinolone anti-infective

Action: A broad-spectrum bactericidal agent that inhibits the enzyme

L

DNA gyrase needed for bacterial DNA synthesis

Uses: Treatment of lower respiratory tract infections (pneumonia, bronchitis); genitourinary infections (prostatitis, UTIs); preoperatively to reduce UTIs in transurethral and transrectal surgical procedures due to susceptible gram-negative organisms

Dosage and routes:

• *Adult:* PO 400 mg/day × 7-14 days depending on type of infection

Renal impairment

• *Adult:* PO 200 mg/dose

Prophylaxis of UTI

• *Adult:* PO 400 mg 2-6 hr before surgery

Available forms include: Tabs 400

Side effects/adverse reactions:

▼ *ORAL:* Dry mouth, candidiasis, stomatitis, glossitis

CNS: Dizziness, headache, somnolence, depression, insomnia, nervousness, confusion, agitation

GI: Diarrhea, nausea, vomiting, anorexia, flatulence, heartburn, increased AST/ALT, constipation, abdominal pain, pseudomembranous colitis

EENT: Visual disturbances, phototoxicity

INTEG: Rash, pruritus, urticaria

MS: Tendinitis, tendon rupture

Contraindications: Hypersensitivity to quinolones

Precautions: Pregnancy category C, lactation, children, elderly, renal disease, seizure disorders, excessive sunlight; tendon rupture in shoulder, hand, and Achilles tendons

Pharmacokinetics:

PO: Peak 1-2 hr, half-life 6-8 hr; excreted in urine as active drug, metabolites

Drug interactions of concern to dentistry:

• Decreased effects: antacids

• Increased levels of cyclosporine, caffeine

DENTAL CONSIDERATIONS

General:

• Due to drug interactions, do not use ingestible sodium bicarbonate products such as the air polishing system (Prophy Jet) unless 2 hr have passed since lomefloxacin was taken.

• Use caution in prescribing caffeine-containing analgesics.

• Determine why the patient is taking the drug.

• Avoid dental light in patient's eyes; offer dark glasses for patient comfort.

• Ruptures of the shoulder, hand, and Achilles tendons that required surgical repair or resulted in prolonged disability have been reported with this drug.

Consultations:

• Consult with patient's physician if an acute dental infection occurs and another antiinfective is required.

Teach patient/family:

• Caution to prevent injury when using oral hygiene aids

• To avoid mouth rinses with high alcohol content due to drying effects

• To minimize exposure to sunlight and wear sunscreen if sun exposure is planned

• To discontinue treatment and inform dentist immediately if patient experiences pain or inflammation of a tendon, and to rest and refrain from exercise

lomustine

(loe-mus'teen)

CCNU, CeeNU

Drug class.: Antineoplastic alkylating agent

Action: Interferes with RNA and DNA strands, which leads to cell death

Uses: Hodgkin's disease; lymphomas; melanomas; multiple myeloma; brain, lung, bladder, kidney, colon cancer

Dosage and routes:

• *Adult*: PO 130 mg/m^2 as a single dose q6wk; titrate dose to WBC level; do not give repeat dose unless WBCs are >4000/mm^3, platelet count >100,000/mm^3

Available forms include: Cap 10, 40, 100 mg

Side effects/adverse reactions:

▼ *ORAL: Stomatitis*

GI: Nausea, vomiting, anorexia, ***hepatotoxicity***

RESP: ***Fibrosis, pulmonary infiltrate***

HEMA: ***Thrombocytopenia, leukopenia, myelosuppression, anemia***

GU: ***Azotemia, renal failure***

INTEG: Burning at injection site

Contraindications: Hypersensitivity, leukopenia, thrombocytopenia, pregnancy category D, lactation

Precautions: Radiation therapy, geriatric patient

Pharmacokinetics:

PO: Well absorbed, half-life 16-48 hr; 50% protein bound; metabolized in liver; excreted in urine; crosses blood-brain barrier; excreted in breast milk

Drug interactions of concern to dentistry:

• This drug depresses bone marrow function, which may increase risk of bleeding; avoid drugs that can increase bleeding, such as aspirin, NSAIDs

DENTAL CONSIDERATIONS

General:

• Patients on chronic drug therapy may rarely have symptoms of blood dyscrasias, which can include infection, bleeding, and poor healing.

• Consider semisupine chair position for patient comfort if GI side effects occur.

• Palliative medication may be required for oral side effects.

• Consider local hemostasis measures to prevent excessive bleeding.

• Prophylactic antibiotics may be indicated to prevent infection if surgery or deep scaling is planned.

• Patients taking opioids for acute or chronic pain should be given alternative analgesics for dental pain.

• Avoid prescribing aspirin-containing products.

Consultations:

• In a patient with symptoms of blood dyscrasias, request a medical consult for blood studies and postpone dental treatment until normal values are reestablished.

• Patients on cancer chemotherapy should have an adequate WBC count before completing dental procedures that may produce a wound. Consult to determine blood count before appointment.

Teach patient/family:

• Importance of good oral hygiene to prevent soft tissue inflammation

L

• Caution to prevent trauma when using oral hygiene aids
• That secondary oral infection may occur; must see dentist immediately if infection occurs
• To report oral lesions, soreness, or bleeding to dentist
• To avoid mouth rinses with high alcohol content due to drying and irritating effects
• Importance of updating medical/drug record if physician makes any changes in evaluation/drug regimens

loperamide HCl

(loe-per′a-mide)

Diarr-Eze, Imodium, Imodium A-D, Kaopectate II, Loperacap, Maalox Antidiarrheal, Pepto Diarrhea Control

♣ APO-Loperamide, Nu-Loperamide, PMS-Loperamide Hydrochloride, Rho-Loperamide

Drug class.: Antidiarrheal (opioid)

Action: Direct action on intestinal muscles to decrease GI peristalsis

Uses: Diarrhea (cause undetermined), chronic diarrhea, ileostomy discharge

Dosage and routes:
• *Adult:* PO 4 mg, then 2 mg after each loose stool, not to exceed 16 mg/day
• *Child 2-5 yr:* PO 1 mg, not more than 3 times daily
• *Child 5-8 yr:* PO 2 mg bid on day 1, then 0.1 mg/kg after each loose stool
• *Child 8-12 yr:* PO 2 mg tid on day 1, then 0.1 mg/kg after each loose stool

Available forms include: Tab 2 mg; caps 2 mg; liq 1 mg/5 ml

Side effects/adverse reactions:
▼ *ORAL: Dry mouth*
CNS: Dizziness, drowsiness, fatigue, fever
GI: Nausea, vomiting, constipation, ***toxic megacolon,*** abdominal pain, anorexia
RESP: ***Respiratory depression***
INTEG: Rash

Contraindications: Hypersensitivity, severe ulcerative colitis, pseudomembranous colitis

Precautions: Pregnancy category B, lactation, children <2 yr, liver disease, dehydration, bacterial disease

Pharmacokinetics:
PO: Onset 0.5-1 hr, duration 4-5 hr; metabolized in liver; excreted in feces as unchanged drug; small amount in urine

Drug interactions of concern to dentistry:
• Increased action: opioid analgesics

DENTAL CONSIDERATIONS

General:
• Assess salivary flow as a factor in caries, periodontal disease, and candidiasis.
• Evaluate respiration characteristics and rate.
• Consider semisupine chair position for patient comfort due to GI effects of drug.
• This drug product is normally used only for a few doses for acute problems; however, some patients may have to take it for longer time periods as dictated by contributing disease.

Teach patient/family:
When chronic dry mouth occurs, advise patient:
• To avoid mouth rinses with high

alcohol content due to drying effects
• To use sugarless gum, frequent sips of water, or saliva substitutes
• To use daily home fluoride products for anticaries effect

loracarbef

(loe-ra-kar'bef)
Lorabid

Drug class.: Antibiotic, second-generation cephalosporin

Action: Inhibits bacterial cell wall synthesis, which renders cell wall osmotically unstable
Uses: Gram-negative: *H. influenzae, E. coli, P. mirabilis, Klebsiella;* gram-positive: *S. pneumoniae, S. pyogenes, S. aureus;* upper/lower respiratory tract, urinary tract, skin infections; otitis media; some in vitro activity against anaerobes
Dosage and routes:
UTI
• *Adult:* PO 200-400 mg qd × 14 days
Acute otitis media
• *Child:* PO 15 mg/kg bid × 7 days
Available forms include: Caps 200, 400 mg; susp 100, 200 mg/5 ml
Side effects/adverse reactions:
▼ *ORAL:* Candidiasis, glossitis
CNS: Dizziness, headache, fatigue, paresthesia, fever, chills, confusion
GI: Diarrhea, nausea, vomiting, anorexia, dysgeusia, bleeding, increased AST/ALT, bilirubin, LDH, alk phosphatase, abdominal pain, loose stools, flatulence, heartburn, stomach cramps, colitis, jaundice
RESP: Dyspnea
HEMA: ***Leukopenia, thrombocytopenia, agranulocytosis, neutropenia, lymphocytosis, eosinophilia, pancytopenia, hemolytic anemia, leukocytosis, granulocytopenia,*** anemia
GU: ***Nephrotoxicity, renal failure,*** pyuria, dysuria, reversible interstitial nephritis, vaginitis, pruritus, candidiasis, increased BUN
INTEG: ***Anaphylaxis,*** rash, urticaria, dermatitis
Contraindications: Hypersensitivity to cephalosporins or related antibiotics
Precautions: Pregnancy category B, lactation, children, renal disease
Pharmacokinetics:
PO: Peak 1 hr, half-life 1 hr; excreted in urine as unchanged drug
Drug interactions of concern to dentistry:
• Decreased effects: tetracyclines, erythromycins, lincomycins
When used for dental infection:
• May reduce effect of oral contraceptives

DENTAL CONSIDERATIONS

General:
• Take precautions regarding allergy to medication.
• Determine why the patient is taking the drug.
• Examine for evidence of oral manifestations of blood dyscrasias (infection, bleeding, poor healing).
Consultations:
• Medical consult may be required to assess disease control in the patient.
• Medical consult for blood studies (CBC); leukopenic or thrombocytopenic side effects may result in infection, delayed healing, and ex-

cessive bleeding. Postpone elective dental treatment until normal values are maintained.

Teach patient/family:

• Importance of good oral hygiene to prevent soft tissue inflammation

loratadine

(lor-at'a-deen)

Claritin, Claritin RediTabs

Drug class.: Antihistamine, H_1 histamine antagonist

Action: Acts on blood vessels, GI system, respiratory system by competing with histamine for H_1-receptor site; decreases allergic response by blocking histamine

Uses: Seasonal allergic rhinitis, idiopathic chronic urticaria

Dosage and routes:

• *Adult and child >12 yr:* PO 10 mg qd

Available forms include: Tabs 10 mg

Side effects/adverse reactions:

▼ *ORAL:* Dry mouth

CNS: Dizziness, drowsiness, poor coordination, fatigue, anxiety, euphoria, confusion, paresthesia, neuritis, low incidence of sedation

GI: Nausea, anorexia, diarrhea

RESP: Increased thick secretions, wheezing, chest tightness

GU: Retention, dysuria

EENT: Blurred vision, dilated pupils, tinnitus, nasal stuffiness, dry nose/throat

Contraindications: Hypersensitivity, ketoconazole

Precautions: Pregnancy category B, increased intraocular pressure, bronchial asthma, patients at risk for syncope or drowsiness

Pharmacokinetics:

PO: Peak 1.5 hr; metabolized in liver to active metabolites; excreted in urine

Drug interactions of concern to dentistry:

• Increased CNS depression: all CNS depressants, alcohol

• Increased anticholinergic effect: anticholinergics, antihistamines, antiparkinsonian drugs

• Increased plasma concentration: ketoconazole

DENTAL CONSIDERATIONS

General:

• Assess salivary flow as a factor in caries, periodontal disease, and candidiasis.

• Consider semisupine chair position for patients with respiratory disease.

• Conscious sedation drugs may produce synergistic, sedative action.

Teach patient/family:

• Importance of good oral hygiene to prevent soft tissue inflammation

When chronic dry mouth occurs, advise patient:

• To avoid mouth rinses with high alcohol content due to drying effects

• To use sugarless gum, frequent sips of water, or saliva substitutes

• To use daily home fluoride products for anticaries effect

lorazepam

(lor-a'ze-pam)

Ativan, Lorazepam Intensol

🍁 Apo-Lorazepam, Novo-Lorazem, Nu-Loraz

Drug class.: Benzodiazepine, antianxiety

Controlled Substance Schedule IV

Action: Depresses subcortical levels of CNS, including limbic system and reticular formation
Uses: Anxiety, preoperatively in sedation, acute alcohol withdrawal symptoms, muscle spasm; unapproved use: insomnia
Dosage and routes:
Anxiety
• *Adult:* PO 2-6 mg/day in divided doses, not to exceed 10 mg/day
Insomnia
• *Adult:* PO 2-4 mg hs; only minimally effective after 2 wk continuous therapy
Preoperatively
• *Adult:* IM/IV 2-4 mg; PO 2-4 mg
Available forms include: Tabs 0.5, 1, 2 mg; IM/IV inj 2, 4 mg/ml
Side effects/adverse reactions:
▼ *ORAL:* Dry mouth
CNS: Dizziness, drowsiness, confusion, headache, anxiety, tremors, stimulation, fatigue, depression, insomnia, hallucinations, weakness, unsteadiness, anterograde amnesia
CV: Orthostatic hypotension, ***ECG changes, tachycardia,*** hypotension
GI: Constipation, nausea, vomiting, anorexia, diarrhea
EENT: Blurred vision, tinnitus, mydriasis
INTEG: Rash, dermatitis, itching
Contraindications: Hypersensitivity to benzodiazepines, narrow-angle glaucoma, psychosis, pregnancy category D, child <12 yr, history of drug abuse, COPD
Precautions: Elderly, debilitated, hepatic disease, renal disease
Pharmacokinetics:
PO: Peak 1-3 hr, duration 3-6 hr, half-life 14 hr; metabolized by liver; excreted by kidneys; crosses placenta, excreted in breast milk

Drug interactions of concern to dentistry:
• Increased effects: alcohol, all CNS depressants
• Increased sedation, hallucination: scopolamine

DENTAL CONSIDERATIONS
General:
• After supine positioning, have patient sit upright for at least 2 min before standing to avoid orthostatic hypotension.
• Elderly persons are more prone to orthostatic hypotension and have increased sensitivity to anticholinergic and sedative effects; use lower dose.
• When administered with opioid analgesic, reduce dose of opioid by one third.
• Psychologic and physical dependence may occur with chronic administration.
• Have someone drive patient to and from dental office when used for conscious sedation.
Consultations:
• Medical consult may be required to assess disease control in the patient.
Teach patient/family:
• Importance of good oral hygiene to prevent soft tissue inflammation
• To avoid mouth rinses with high alcohol content due to drying effects

losartan potassium

(loe-sar′tan)
Cozaar

Drug class.: Angiotensin II receptor antagonist

Action: Blocks the vasoconstrictor and aldosterone-releasing effects of angiotensin II

Uses: Hypertension, as a single drug or in combination with other antihypertensives

Dosage and routes:

• *Adult:* PO initial 50 mg/day; can be given once or twice daily in total daily doses ranging from 25-100 mg

Available forms include: Tabs 25, 50 mg

Side effects/adverse reactions:

▼ *ORAL:* Dry mouth (<1%), taste alteration (rare)

CNS: Dizziness, insomnia

CV: Low incidence, including palpitation, hypotension; dysrhythmias

GI: Diarrhea, dyspepsia, nausea

RESP: Cough, infection, dyspnea

GU: Urinary frequency

EENT: Nasal congestion, sinusitis, blurred vision, tinnitus

INTEG: Dry skin, rash, urticaria

MS: Pain, cramps

MISC: Fatigue

Contraindications: Hypersensitivity, second or third trimester of pregnancy

Precautions: Pregnancy category C (first trimester) and D (second or third trimester), lactation, children, sodium- and volume-depleted patients, renal impairment

Pharmacokinetics:

PO: Good oral absorption, peak levels 1 hr, metabolites 3-4 hr; highly bound to plasma proteins; liver metabolism; partially converted to active metabolites (first-pass metabolism); excreted in urine, feces

Drug interactions of concern to dentistry:

• Potential for increased hypotensive effects with other hypotensive drugs and sedatives

• Use ketoconazole with caution because of a potential to inhibit metabolism of losartan

DENTAL CONSIDERATIONS

General:

• Monitor vital signs every appointment due to cardiovascular effects.

• Limit use of sodium-containing products, such as saline IV fluids, for those patients with a dietary salt restriction.

• Stress from dental procedures may compromise cardiovascular function; determine patient risk.

• Assess salivary flow as a factor in caries, periodontal disease, and candidiasis.

• Short appointments and a stress reduction protocol may be required for anxious patients.

• Consider semisupine chair position for patient comfort due to respiratory side effects of drug.

• Use precaution if sedation or general anesthesia is required; risk of hypotensive episode.

Consultations:

• Medical consult may be required to assess disease control and patient's ability to tolerate stress.

Teach patient/family:

• Importance of updating health and drug history if physician makes any changes in evaluation/drug regimens

When chronic dry mouth occurs, advise patient:

• To avoid mouth rinses with high alcohol content due to drying effects

• Of need for daily home fluoride to prevent caries

• To use sugarless gum, frequent sips of water, or saliva substitutes

loteprednol etabonate (optic)

(loe-te-pred′nol)
Lotemax, Alrex
Drug class.: Topical glucocorticoid

Action: Glucocorticoids have multiple actions that include antiinflammatory and immunosuppressant effects. They inhibit phospholipase A_2, interfering with or reducing the synthesis of prostaglandins and leukotrienes. They also bind to cytoplasmic glucocorticoid receptors (GRs) and enter the cell nucleus to bind with DNA. This results in the synthesis of various enzymes such as collagenase, elastase, and cytokines that play important roles in inflammation and immunosuppression. They also suppress the production of lymphocytes, monocytes, and eosinophils.
Uses: For steroid-responsive inflammation of the conjunctiva, cornea, and anterior segments of the globe associated with allergic conjunctivitis, acne rosacea, iritis, superficial punctate keratitis, and so on when topical steroid use is acceptable to reduce inflammation and edema (Lotemax 0.5%); temporary relief of symptoms of seasonal allergic conjunctivitis (Alrex 0.2%)
Dosage and routes:
• *Adult:* TOP instill 1 or 2 gtts into the conjunctival sac of the affected eye qid; during initial treatment (first week) up to 1 gtt qh can be used if necessary; reevaluate if no response in 2 days; also used 24 hr after ocular surgery 1-2 gtts qid for up to 2 wk

Available forms include: Sterile ophthalmic suspension 0.2% and 0.5% in 2.5, 5, 10, 15 ml plastic bottles
Side effects/adverse reactions:
CNS: Headache
RESP: Pharyngitis
EENT: Abnormal vision, blurring, burning, discharge, dry eyes, itching, photophobia, rhinitis.
Contraindications: Hypersensitivity; viral diseases of cornea and conjunctiva, including herpes keratitis, vaccina, and varicella; mycobacteria and fungal eye infections
Precautions: Prolonged use may result in glaucoma, increased risk of secondary ocular infections, delayed healing after cataract surgery; avoid contamination of sterile container; pregnancy category C, lactation, use in children not established
Pharmacokinetics:
INSTILL: Absorbed amounts are believed to be rapidly metabolized, metabolites excreted in urine; systemic effects unknown or not evident
Drug interactions of concern to dentistry:
• None reported
DENTAL CONSIDERATIONS
General:
• Avoid dental light in patient's eyes; offer dark glasses for patient comfort.
• Determine why patient is taking the drug.

L

lovastatin

(loe'va-sta-tin)

Mevacor

Drug class.: Cholesterol-lowering agent

Action: Inhibits HMG-CoA reductase enzyme, which reduces cholesterol synthesis

Uses: As an adjunct in primary hypercholesterolemia (types IIa, IIb), mixed hyperlipidemia; patient should first be placed on a cholesterol-lowering diet; primary prevention of coronary heart disease in patients without symptomatic CV disease who have average to moderately elevated total cholesterol

Dosage and routes:

• *Adult:* PO 20 mg qd with evening meal; may increase to 20-80 mg/day in single or divided doses, not to exceed 80 mg/day; dosage adjustments should be made qmo

Available forms include: Tabs 10, 20, 40 mg

Side effects/adverse reactions:

CNS: Dizziness, headache

GI: Nausea, constipation, diarrhea, dyspepsia, flatus, abdominal pain, heartburn, ***liver dysfunction***

EENT: Blurred vision, dysgeusia, lens opacities

INTEG: Rash, pruritus

MS: Muscle cramps, myalgia, ***myositis, rhabdomyolysis***

Contraindications: Pregnancy category X, lactation, active liver disease, drugs that inhibit the enzyme CYP3A4

Precautions: Past liver disease, alcoholics, severe acute infections, trauma, hypotension, uncontrolled seizure disorders, severe metabolic disorders, electrolyte imbalances

Pharmacokinetics:

PO: Peak 2-4 hr; highly protein bound; metabolized in liver (metabolites); excreted in urine, feces, breast milk; crosses placenta

Drug interactions of concern to dentistry:

• Increased myalgia, myositis: erythromycin, cyclosporine

• Contraindicated with itraconazole, ketoconazole, erythromycin

DENTAL CONSIDERATIONS

General:

• Consider semisupine chair position for patient comfort due to GI side effects.

Teach patient/family:

• To avoid mouth rinses with high alcohol content due to drying effects

loxapine succinate/ loxapine HCl

(lox'a-peen)

Loxitane, Loxitane-C, Loxitane IM

Loxapac

Drug class.: Antipsychotic

Action: Depresses cerebral cortex, hypothalamus, limbic system, all of which control activity and aggression; blocks neurotransmission produced by dopamine at synapse; exhibits strong α-adrenergic, cholinergic-blocking action; mechanism for antipsychotic effects is unclear

Uses: Psychotic disorders

Dosage and routes:

• *Adult:* PO 10 mg bid-qid initially, may be rapidly increased depending on severity of condition, maintenance 60-100 mg/day; IM

12.5-50 mg q4-6h or more until desired response, then start PO form

Available forms include: Caps 5, 10, 25, 50 mg; conc 25 mg/ml; inj IM 50 mg/ml

Side effects/adverse reactions:

▼ *ORAL: Dry mouth*

CNS: Extrapyramidal symptoms: pseudoparkinsonism, akathisia, dystonia, tardive dyskinesia, drowsiness, headache, ***seizures,*** confusion

CV: Orthostatic hypotension, ***cardiac arrest,*** ECG changes, tachycardia

GI: Nausea, vomiting, anorexia, constipation, diarrhea, jaundice, weight gain

RESP: ***Laryngospasm, respiratory depression,*** dyspnea

HEMA: ***Anemia, leukopenia, leukocytosis, agranulocytosis***

GU: Urinary retention, urinary frequency, enuresis, impotence, amenorrhea, gynecomastia

EENT: Blurred vision, glaucoma

INTEG: Rash, photosensitivity, dermatitis

Contraindications: Hypersensitivity, blood dyscrasias, coma, child, brain damage, bone marrow depression, alcohol and barbiturate withdrawal states

Precautions: Pregnancy category C, lactation, seizure disorders, hepatic disease, cardiac disease, prostatic hypertrophy, cardiac conditions, child <16 yr

Pharmacokinetics:

PO: Onset 20-30 min, peak 2-4 hr, duration 12 hr

IM: Onset 15-30 min, peak 15-20 min, duration 12 hr

Initial half-life 5 hr, terminal half-life 19 hr; metabolized by liver; excreted in urine; crosses placenta; excreted in breast milk

Drug interactions of concern to dentistry:

- Increased effects of both drugs: anticholinergics
- Increased CNS depression: alcohol, all CNS depressants
- Decreased effects of sympathomimetics, carbamazepine

DENTAL CONSIDERATIONS

General:

- Patients on chronic drug therapy may rarely have symptoms of blood dyscrasias, which can include infection, bleeding, and poor healing.
- Assess salivary flow as a factor in caries, periodontal disease, and candidiasis.
- Assess for presence of extrapyramidal motor symptoms, such as tardive dyskinesia and akathisia. Extrapyramidal motor activity may complicate dental treatment.
- After supine positioning, have patient sit upright for at least 2 min to avoid orthostatic hypotension.

Consultations:

- In a patient with symptoms of blood dyscrasias, request a medical consult for blood studies and postpone dental treatment until normal values are reestablished.
- If signs of tardive dyskinesia or akathisia are present, refer to physician.
- Physician should be informed if significant xerostomic side effects occur (increased caries, sore tongue, problems eating or swallowing, difficulty wearing prosthesis) so a medication change can be considered.

Teach patient/family:

- Importance of good oral hygiene to prevent soft tissue inflammation
- Caution to prevent injury when using oral hygiene aids
- To use electric toothbrush if patient has difficulty holding conventional devices

When chronic dry mouth occurs, advise patient:

- To avoid mouth rinses with high alcohol content due to drying effects
- To use sugarless gum, frequent sips of water, or saliva substitutes
- To use daily home fluoride products for anticaries effect

---

lypressin

(lye-press'in)

Diapid

Drug class.: Pituitary hormone (8-lysine vasopressin)

Action: Promotes reabsorption of water by action on collecting ducts in kidney; decreases urine excretion

Uses: Nonnephrogenic diabetes insipidus

Dosage and routes:

- *Adult and child >6 wk:* Intranasal 1-2 gtt in each nostril qid; extra dose hs if needed for nocturia

Available forms include: Intranasal 0.185 mg/ml in 8 ml plastic bottle

Side effects/adverse reactions:

CNS: Headache

GI: Nausea, heartburn, cramps

RESP: Cough, shortness of breath, tightness in chest

EENT: Nasal irritation, congestion, rhinitis, conjunctivitis, rhinorrhea

MISC: Chest tightness, cough, dyspnea

Contraindications: Hypersensitivity

Precautions: CAD, pregnancy category C, sensitivity to vasopressin, allergic rhinitis, nasal congestion, hypertension, upper respiratory infection

Pharmacokinetics:

NASAL: Onset 1 hr, duration 3-8 hr, half-life 15 min; metabolized in liver, kidneys; excreted in urine

Drug interactions of concern to dentistry:

- Increased effect: carbamazepine
- Decreased effect: demeclocycline

DENTAL CONSIDERATIONS

General:

- Uncontrolled patients may have excessive loss of body fluids. Ensure that disease is controlled before dental treatment is initiated.

Consultations:

- Medical consult may be required to assess disease control and patient's ability to tolerate stress.

---

magaldrate (aluminum magnesium complex)

(mag'al-drate)

Losopan, Riopan, Riopan Extra Strength

Drug class.: Antacid/aluminum/magnesium hydroxide

Action: Neutralizes gastric acidity

Uses: Antacid for hyperacidity

Dosage and routes:

- *Adult:* PO 480-1080 mg between meals and hs, not to exceed 20 tabs/day; susp 5-10 ml (400-800 mg) with water between meals, hs, not to exceed 100 ml/day

Available forms include: Tabs 480 mg; susp 540 mg/5 ml, 480 mg/5 ml, 1080 mg/5 ml; plus products include simethicone 20 mg

Side effects/adverse reactions:
▼ *ORAL:* Chalky taste
GI: Constipation, diarrhea, nausea, vomiting, thirst, stomach cramps
META: Hypermagnesemia, hypophosphatemia, hypercalcemia
Contraindications: Hypersensitivity to this drug or aluminum products, intestinal obstruction
Precautions: Elderly, fluid restriction, decreased GI motility, GI obstruction, dehydration, renal disease, sodium-restricted diets, pregnancy category C, colitis, gastric outlet obstruction syndrome, colostomy
Pharmacokinetics:
PO: Onset 10-15 min, duration >3 hr
Drug interactions of concern to dentistry:
• Decreased absorption of anticholinergics, corticosteroids, sodium fluoride, tetracycline, ketoconazole, chlordiazepoxide, ciprofloxacin, metronidazole
DENTAL CONSIDERATIONS
General:
• If prescribing oral form of drug in which risk of decreased absorption is reported, advise taking doses at least 2 hr after or before antacid use.
• Avoid drugs that could exacerbate upper GI distress (aspirin and NSAIDs).
• Consider semisupine chair position for patient comfort due to GI effects of disease.

maprotiline HCl

(ma-proe'ti-leen)
Ludiomil
Drug class.: Tetracyclic antidepressant

Action: Blocks reuptake of norepinephrine and serotonin into nerve endings, increasing action of norepinephrine and serotonin at nerve cells
Uses: Depression, depression with anxiety; unapproved use: neurogenic pain, tension headache
Dosage and routes:
• *Adult:* PO 25-75 mg/day in moderate depression; may increase to 150 mg/day, not to exceed 225 mg in hospitalized patients; severely depressed patients who are hospitalized may be given 300 mg/day
• *Elderly:* 50-75 mg/day
Available forms include: Tabs 25, 50, 75 mg
Side effects/adverse reactions:
▼ *ORAL: Dry mouth*
CNS: Dizziness, vertigo, nervousness, drowsiness, ***seizures,*** confusion, headache, anxiety, tremors, stimulation, weakness, insomnia, nightmares, EPS (elderly), increased psychiatric symptoms, sedation, manic hallucinations
CV: Orthostatic hypotension, ECG changes, tachycardia, ***hypertension*** (rare), palpitation
GI: Diarrhea, nausea, vomiting, ***hepatitis, paralytic ileus,*** increased appetite, cramps, epigastric distress, jaundice
HEMA: ***Agranulocytosis, thrombocytopenia, eosinophilia, leukopenia***
GU: Retention, ***acute renal failure***

M

EENT: Blurred vision, tinnitus, mydriasis
INTEG: Rash, urticaria, sweating, pruritus, vasculitis, photosensitivity
Contraindications: Hypersensitivity to tricyclic antidepressants, recovery phase of MI, convulsive disorders, prostatic hypertrophy
Precautions: Suicidal patients, severe depression, increased intraocular pressure, narrow-angle glaucoma, urinary retention, cardiac disease, hepatic or renal disease, hypothyroidism, hyperthyroidism, electroshock therapy, elective surgery, elderly, pregnancy category B, lactation, prostate hypertrophy, schizophrenia, MAO inhibitors
Pharmacokinetics:
PO: Onset 15-30 min, peak 12 hr, duration up to 3 wk, half-life 27-58 hr, steady state 6-10 days; protein binding 80%, metabolized by liver; excreted by kidneys, feces; crosses placenta

Drug interactions of concern to dentistry:

- Increased effects of direct-acting sympathomimetics (epinephrine)
- Potential risk of increased CNS depression: alcohol, and all CNS depressants
- Decreased antihypertensive effect: clonidine, guanadrel, guanethidine

DENTAL CONSIDERATIONS

General:

- Monitor vital signs every appointment due to cardiovascular side effects.
- Patients on chronic drug therapy may rarely have symptoms of blood dyscrasias, which can include infection, bleeding, and poor healing.
- Assess salivary flow as a factor in caries, periodontal disease, and candidiasis.
- After supine positioning, have patient sit upright for at least 2 min before standing to avoid orthostatic hypotension.
- The use of epinephrine in gingival retraction cord is contraindicated. Use vasoconstrictors with caution, in low doses, and with careful aspiration.

Consultations:

- In a patient with symptoms of blood dyscrasias, request a medical consult for blood studies and postpone dental treatment until normal values are reestablished.
- Take precautions if dental surgery is anticipated and anesthesia is required.
- Medical consult may be required to assess disease control in the patient.
- Physician should be informed if significant xerostomic side effects occur (increased caries, sore tongue, problems eating or swallowing, difficulty wearing prosthesis) so a medication change can be considered.

Teach patient/family:

- Importance of good oral hygiene to prevent soft tissue inflammation
- Caution to prevent injury when using oral hygiene aids

When chronic dry mouth occurs, advise patient:

- To avoid mouth rinses with high alcohol content due to drying effects
- To use sugarless gum, frequent sips of water, or saliva substitutes
- To use daily home fluoride products for anticaries effect

masoprocol

(ma-soe'pro-kole)

Actinex

Drug class.: Antineoplastic (topical)

Action: Mechanism is unknown; inhibits lipoxygenase; antiproliferative action against keratinocytes

Uses: Actinic (solar) keratosis

Dosage and routes:

• *Adult:* TOP wash and dry affected area; apply bid

Available forms include: Cream 10% in 30 g tube

Side effects/adverse reactions:

INTEG: Flaking, itching, dryness, edema, burning, tingling, contact dermatitis, erythema

Contraindications: Hypersensitivity to drug or sulfites

Precautions: Avoid occlusive dressings, pregnancy category B, lactation, children, external use only

Pharmacokinetics:

TOP: Absorption <2%

Drug interactions of concern to dentistry:

• None reported

DENTAL CONSIDERATIONS

General:

• If dryness is evident, apply lubricant to dry lips for patient comfort before dental procedures.

mazindol

(may'zin-dole)

Mazanor, Sanorex

Drug class.: Imidazoisoindole anorexiant

Controlled Substance Schedule IV

Action: Exact mechanism of appetite suppression unknown but has amphetamine-like activity and may have an effect on satiety center of hypothalamus

Uses: Exogenous obesity

Dosage and routes:

• *Adult:* PO 1 mg/day 1 hr before first meal of day, then may increase to 1 mg tid 1 hr ac; or 2 mg/day 1 hr before lunch

Available forms include: Tabs 1, 2 mg

Side effects/adverse reactions:

ORAL: Dry mouth, unpleasant taste

CNS: Nervousness, insomnia, restlessness, dizziness, headache, stimulation, irritability, drowsiness, weakness, tremor

CV: Tachycardia, palpitation, edema

GI: Constipation, nausea, anorexia, diarrhea, abdominal discomfort

GU: Impotence, difficulty urinating

EENT: Mydriasis, blurred vision, eye irritation

INTEG: Urticaria, rash, pallor, shivering, sweating

Contraindications: Hypersensitivity, glaucoma, drug abuse, children <12 yr, agitated states, MAO inhibitors

Precautions: Diabetes mellitus, pregnancy category not listed, lactation, caution in operating machinery

Pharmacokinetics:

PO: Onset 0.5-1 hr, duration 8-15 hr; metabolized by liver; excreted by kidneys

Drug interactions of concern to dentistry:

• Hypertensive crisis: MAO inhibitors or within 14 days of MAO inhibitors

• Increased risk of dysrhythmias: hydrocarbon inhalation general anesthetics
• Decreased effects: tricyclics, ascorbic acid, phenothiazines
• Caffeine or caffeine-containing products may increase risk of insomnia
• Increased effects of sympathomimetic amines

DENTAL CONSIDERATIONS

General:

• Monitor vital signs every appointment due to cardiovascular side effects.
• Assess salivary flow as a factor in caries, periodontal disease, and candidiasis.
• Determine why the patient is taking the drug.
• Psychologic and physical dependence may occur with chronic administration.
• Consider semisupine chair position for patient comfort if GI side effects occur.

Consultations:

• Medical consult may be required to assess disease control and patient's ability to tolerate stress.
• Physician should be informed if significant xerostomic side effects occur (increased caries, sore tongue, problems eating or swallowing, difficulty wearing prosthesis) so a medication change can be considered.

Teach patient/family:

When chronic dry mouth occurs, advise patient:

• To avoid mouth rinses with high alcohol content due to drying effects
• To use sugarless gum, frequent sips of water, or saliva substitutes
• To use daily home fluoride products for anticaries effect

mecamylamine HCl

(mek-a-mil'a-meen)

Inversine

Drug class.: Antihypertensive, ganglionic blocker

Action: Occupies receptor site, prevents acetylcholine from attaching to postsynaptic nerve ending in autonomic ganglia

Uses: Moderate-to-severe hypertension, malignant hypertension; unlabeled use: hyperreflexia, smoking cessation

Dosage and routes:

• *Adult:* PO 2.5 mg bid; may increase in increments of 2.5 mg × 2 days until desired response; maintenance 25 mg/day in 3 divided doses

Available forms include: Tabs 2.5 mg

Side effects/adverse reactions:

▼ *ORAL: Dry mouth,* glossitis, bitter taste

CNS: Drowsiness, sedation, dizziness, ***convulsions,*** headache, tremors, weakness, syncope, paresthesia, dizziness

CV: Postural hypotension, ***CHF,*** irregular heart rate

GI: Paralytic ileus, anorexia, nausea, vomiting, constipation

GU: Impotence, urinary retention, decreased libido

EENT: Blurred vision, nasal congestion, dilated pupils

Contraindications: Hypersensitivity, MI, coronary insufficiency, renal disease, glaucoma, organic pyloric stenosis, uremia, uncooperative patients, mild/labile hypertension

Precautions: CVA, prostatic hypertrophy, bladder neck obstruction, urethral stricture, renal dysfunction (elevated BUN), cerebral dysfunction, pregnancy category C, vigorous excercise, stress-related activity

Pharmacokinetics:

PO: Onset 0.5-2 hr, duration 6-12 hr; excreted unchanged in urine, feces, breast milk; crosses placenta

Drug interactions of concern to dentistry:

- Increased vasopressor response: sympathomimetics
- Decreased hypotensive effect: sympathomimetics, NSAIDs, especially indomethacin
- Increased hypotensive response: sedative drugs that may also lower blood pressure

DENTAL CONSIDERATIONS

General:

- Monitor vital signs every appointment due to cardiovascular side effects.
- After supine positioning, have patient sit upright for at least 2 min before standing to avoid orthostatic hypotension.
- Assess salivary flow as a factor in caries, periodontal disease, and candidiasis.
- Consider semisupine chair position for patient comfort due to GI effects of disease.
- Early-morning appointments and a stress reduction protocol may be required for anxious patients.
- Stress from dental procedures may compromise cardiovascular function; determine patient risk.
- Use vasoconstrictors with caution, in low doses, and with careful aspiration.
- Avoid use of gingival retraction cord with epinephrine.
- Limit use of sodium-containing products for patients with a dietary salt restriction (air polishing system and IV fluids).
- Take precautions if dental surgery is anticipated and anesthesia is required.

Consultations:

- Medical consult may be required to assess disease control in the patient.

Teach patient/family:

- Importance of good oral hygiene to prevent soft tissue inflammation

When chronic dry mouth occurs, advise patient:

- To avoid mouth rinses with high alcohol content due to drying effects
- To use daily home fluoride products for anticaries effect
- To use sugarless gum, frequent sips of water, or saliva substitutes

M

---

meclizine HCl

(mek'li-zeen)

Antivert 25, Antivert 50, Bonine, Dramamine II, D-Vert, Meni-D

Bonamine

Drug class.: Antihistamine

Action: A nonspecific CNS depressant with anticholinergic and antihistaminic activity

Uses: Vertigo, motion sickness

Dosage and routes:

- *Adult:* PO 25-100 mg qd in divided doses or 25-50 mg 1 hr before traveling

Available forms include: Tabs 12.5, 25, 50 mg; chew tabs 25 mg; film-coated tabs 25 mg

Side effects/adverse reactions:

ORAL: Dry mouth

CNS: Drowsiness, dizziness, seda-

tion, fatigue, restlessness, headache, insomnia, extrapyramidal symptoms
GI: Nausea, anorexia, vomiting
EENT: Blurred vision
Contraindications: Hypersensitivity to cyclizines
Precautions: Children, narrow-angle glaucoma, urinary retention, lactation, prostatic hypertrophy, elderly, pregnancy category B, asthma
Pharmacokinetics:
PO: Onset 1 hr, duration 8-24 hr, half-life 6 hr
Drug interactions of concern to dentistry:
• Increased effect of alcohol, other CNS depressants, anticholinergics

DENTAL CONSIDERATIONS
General:
• Assess salivary flow as a factor in caries, periodontal disease, and candidiasis.
Teach patient/family:
When chronic dry mouth occurs, advise patient:
• To avoid mouth rinses with high alcohol content due to drying effects
• To use daily home fluoride products for anticaries effect
• To use sugarless gum, frequent sips of water, or saliva substitutes

meclofenamate

(me-kloe-fen-am'ate)
Meclomen
Drug class.: Nonsteroidal antiinflammatory

Action: Inhibits prostaglandin synthesis by interfering with cyclo-oxygenase needed for biosynthesis; possesses analgesic, antiinflammatory, antipyretic properties
Uses: Mild-to-moderate pain, osteoarthritis, rheumatoid arthritis; unapproved use: vascular headache, menorrhagia
Dosage and routes:
Analgesia, antirheumatic
• *Adult:* PO 50-100 mg every 4-6 hr not to exceed 400 mg daily
Available forms include: Caps 50, 100 mg
Side effects/adverse reactions:
▼ *ORAL:* Stomatitis, bitter taste, dry mouth, lichenoid reaction
CNS: Dizziness, drowsiness, fatigue, tremors, confusion, insomnia, anxiety, depression
CV: Tachycardia, peripheral edema, palpitation, dysrhythmias
GI: ***Cholestatic hepatitis,*** *diarrhea,* nausea, anorexia, vomiting, jaundice, constipation, flatulence, cramps, peptic ulcer
HEMA: ***Blood dyscrasias***
GU: ***Nephrotoxicity: dysuria, hematuria, oliguria, azotemia***
EENT: Tinnitus, hearing loss, blurred vision
INTEG: Purpura, rash, pruritus, sweating
Contraindications: Hypersensitivity, asthma induced by aspirin, severe renal disease, severe hepatic disease, allergy to other NSAIDs
Precautions: Pregnancy category not listed, lactation, children, bleeding disorders, upper GI disorders, cardiac disorders, hypersensitivity to other antiinflammatory agents
Pharmacokinetics:
PO: Peak serum levels 30 min, half-life 3-3.5 hr; metabolized in

liver; excreted in urine (metabolites), less in feces and breast milk

Drug interactions of concern to dentistry:

• GI ulceration, bleeding: aspirin, alcohol, corticosteroids

• Nephrotoxicity: acetaminophen (prolonged use)

• Possible risk of decreased renal function: cyclosporine

When prescribed for dental pain:

• Risk of increased effects: oral anticoagulants, oral antidiabetics, lithium, methotrexate

• Decreased effects of diuretics, β-adrenergic blockers

DENTAL CONSIDERATIONS

General:

• Patients on chronic drug therapy may rarely have symptoms of blood dyscrasias, which can include infection, bleeding, and poor healing.

• Assess salivary flow as a factor in caries, periodontal disease, and candidiasis.

• Avoid prescribing for dental use in last trimester of pregnancy.

• Avoid prescribing aspirin-containing products.

• Consider semisupine chair position for patients with rheumatic disease.

Consultations:

• In a patient with symptoms of blood dyscrasias, request a medical consult for blood studies and postpone dental treatment until normal values are reestablished.

• Medical consult may be required to assess disease control in the patient.

Teach patient/family:

• Importance of good oral hygiene to prevent soft tissue inflammation

• Caution to prevent injury when using oral hygiene aids

When chronic dry mouth occurs, advise patient:

• To avoid mouth rinses with high alcohol content due to drying effects

• To use sugarless gum, frequent sips of water, or saliva substitutes

• To use daily home fluoride products for anticaries effect

---

medroxyprogesterone acetate

(me-drox'ee-proe-jes'te-rone)

Amen, Curretab, Cycrin, Depo-Provera, Provera

Drug class.: Progestogen

Action: Inhibits secretion of pituitary gonadotropins, which prevents follicular maturation and ovulation; stimulates growth of mammary tissue; antineoplastic action against endometrial cancer

Uses: Uterine bleeding (abnormal), secondary amenorrhea, endometrial cancer, metastatic renal cancer, contraceptive; with estrogens to reduce incidence of endometrial hyperplasia, cancer

Dosage and routes:

Secondary amenorrhea

• *Adult:* PO 5-10 mg qd × 5-10 days

Endometrial/renal cancer

• *Adult:* IM 400-1000 mg/wk

Uterine bleeding

• *Adult:* PO 5-10 mg qd × 5-10 days starting on 16th day of menstrual cycle

Available forms include: Tabs 2.5, 10 mg; inj susp 100, 400 mg/ml

M

Side effects/adverse reactions:
▼ *ORAL:* Gingival bleeding, gingival overgrowth
CNS: Dizziness, headache, migraines, depression, fatigue
CV: ***Thromboembolism, stroke, pulmonary embolism, MI,*** hypotension, thrombophlebitis, edema
GI: Nausea, ***cholestatic jaundice,*** vomiting, anorexia, cramps, increased weight
GU: Gynecomastia, testicular atrophy, impotence, ***spontaneous abortion,*** endometriosis, amenorrhea, cervical erosion, breakthrough bleeding, dysmenorrhea, vaginal candidiasis, breast changes
EENT: Diplopia
INTEG: Rash, urticaria, acne, hirsutism, alopecia, oily skin, seborrhea, purpura, melasma, photosensitivity
META: Hyperglycemia
Contraindications: Breast cancer, hypersensitivity, thromboembolic disorders, reproductive cancer, genital bleeding (abnormal, undiagnosed), pregnancy category X
Precautions: Lactation, hypertension, asthma, blood dyscrasias, gallbladder disease, CHF, diabetes mellitus, bone disease, depression, migraine headache, convulsive disorders, hepatic disease, renal disease, family history of cancer of breast or reproductive tract
Pharmacokinetics:
PO: Peak levels 2-7 hr, duration 24 hr, depot injection active up to 3 months; metabolized in liver; excreted in urine, feces

DENTAL CONSIDERATIONS
General:
- Place on frequent recall to evaluate inflammatory and healing response.

Teach patient/family:
- Importance of good oral hygiene to prevent soft tissue inflammation

---

mefenamic acid

(me-fe-nam′ik)

Ponstan, Ponstel

Drug class.: Nonsteroidal antiinflammatory

Action: Inhibits prostaglandin synthesis by interfering with cyclooxygenase needed for biosynthesis; possesses analgesic, antiinflammatory, antipyretic properties
Uses: Mild-to-moderate pain, dysmenorrhea, inflammatory disease
Dosage and routes:
- *Adult and child >14 yr:* PO 500 mg, then 250 mg q4h; use not to exceed 1 wk

Available forms include: Caps 250 mg
Side effects/adverse reactions:
▼ *ORAL:* Lichenoid reaction
CNS: Dizziness, drowsiness, fatigue, tremors, confusion, insomnia, anxiety, depression
CV: Tachycardia, peripheral edema, palpitation, dysrhythmias
GI: ***Cholestatic hepatitis,*** nausea, anorexia, vomiting, diarrhea, jaundice, constipation, flatulence, cramps, peptic ulcer
HEMA: ***Blood dyscrasias***
GU: ***Nephrotoxicity: dysuria, hematuria, oliguria, azotemia***
EENT: Tinnitus, hearing loss, blurred vision
INTEG: Purpura, rash, pruritus, sweating
Contraindications: Hypersensitivity, asthma, severe renal disease, severe hepatic disease
Precautions: Pregnancy category C, lactation, children, bleeding dis-

orders, GI disorders, cardiac disorders, hypersensitivity to other anti-inflammatory agents

Pharmacokinetics:

PO: Peak 2 hr, half-life 3-3.5 hr; extensive protein binding; metabolized in liver; excreted in urine (metabolites), breast milk

Drug interactions of concern to dentistry:

- GI bleeding, ulceration: aspirin, alcohol, corticosteroids
- Nephrotoxicity: acetaminophen (prolonged use and high doses)
- Possible risk of decreased renal function: cyclosporine

When prescribed for dental pain:

- Risk of increased effects of oral anticoagulants, oral antidiabetics, lithium, methotrexate
- Decreased effects of diuretics

DENTAL CONSIDERATIONS

General:

- Avoid prescribing for dental use in last trimester of pregnancy.
- Avoid prescribing aspirin-containing products.

Consultations:

- Medical consult may be required to assess disease control in the patient.

---

megestrol acetate

(me-jes'trole)

Megace

Apo-Megestrol

Drug class.: Antineoplastic (progestin)

Action: Affects endometrium by antiluteinizing effect, which is thought to bring about cell death

Uses: Breast, endometrial cancer, renal cell cancer

Dosage and routes:

- *Adult:* PO 40-320 mg/day in divided doses

Available forms include: Tabs 20, 40 mg

Side effects/adverse reactions:

ORAL: Gingival bleeding, gingival overgrowth

CNS: Mood swings

CV: ***Thrombophlebitis***

GI: Nausea, vomiting, anorexia, diarrhea, abdominal cramps

GU: ***Hypercalcemia,*** gynecomastia, fluid retention

INTEG: Alopecia, rash, pruritus, purpura

Contraindications: Hypersensitivity, pregnancy category X

Pharmacokinetics:

PO: Duration 1-3 days, half-life 60 min; metabolized in liver; excreted in feces, breast milk

DENTAL CONSIDERATIONS

General:

- Place on frequent recall to evaluate inflammatory and healing response.
- Patients receiving chemotherapy may require palliative treatment for stomatitis.

Teach patient/family:

- Importance of good oral hygiene to prevent soft tissue inflammation

---

melphalan

(mel'fa-lan)

Alkeran

Drug class.: Antineoplastic

Action: Responsible for cross-linking DNA strands, which leads to cell death

Uses: Palliative treatment of multiple myeloma and nonresectable epithelial carcinoma of the ovary

Dosage and routes:
Multiple myeloma
• *Adult:* PO 6 mg daily for 2-3 wk while evaluating WBC counts; 2 mg maintenance doses may be used depending on blood cell count
Epithelial ovarian cancer
• *Adult:* PO 0.2 mg/kg daily for 5 days as a single course; repeat q4-5wk depending on blood cell count
Available forms include: Tabs 2 mg
Side effects/adverse reactions:
▼ *ORAL:* Stomatitis, oral ulceration
GI: Nausea, vomiting
RESP: ***Fibrosis, dysplasia***
HEMA: ***Thrombocytopenia, neutropenia, myelosuppression,*** anemia
GU: Amenorrhea, hyperuricemia
INTEG: Rash, urticaria
Contraindications: Cancer with prior resistance to drug, lactation, hypersensitivity
Precautions: Pregnancy category D, bone marrow depression, renal impairment
Pharmacokinetics: Half-life 1.5 hr; first-pass hepatic metabolism; plasma levels vary; metabolites excreted in urine
Drug interactions of concern to dentistry:
• Increased toxicity: antineoplastics, radiation
DENTAL CONSIDERATIONS
General:
• Patients receiving chemotherapy may be taking chronic opioids for pain. Consider NSAIDs for dental pain management.
• Patients receiving chemotherapy may require palliative therapy for stomatitis.
• Patients on chronic drug therapy may rarely have symptoms of blood dyscrasias, which can include infection, bleeding, and poor healing.
Consultations:
• Medical consult may be required to assess disease control in the patient.
• In a patient with symptoms of blood dyscrasias, request a medical consult for blood studies and postpone dental treatment until normal values are reestablished.
Teach family/patient:
• About the possibility of secondary oral infection; must see dentist immediately if infection occurs
When chronic dry mouth occurs, advise patient:
• To avoid mouth rinses with high alcohol content due to drying effects
• To use sugarless gum, frequent sips of water, or saliva substitutes
• To use daily home fluoride products for anticaries effect

---

mepenzolate bromide
(me-pen′zoe-late)
Cantil
Drug class.: Gastrointestinal anticholinergic

Action: Inhibits muscarinic actions of acetylcholine at postganglionic parasympathetic neuroeffector sites
Uses: Treatment of peptic ulcer disease, irritable bowel syndrome in combination with other drugs; other GI disorders
Dosage and routes:
• *Adult:* PO 25-50 mg qid with meals, hs; titrate to patient response

Available forms include: Tabs 25 mg

Side effects/adverse reactions:

▼ *ORAL: Dry mouth,* absence of taste

CNS: Confusion, stimulation in elderly, headache, insomnia, dizziness, drowsiness, anxiety, weakness, hallucination

CV: Palpitation, tachycardia

GI: Constipation, ***paralytic ileus,*** heartburn, nausea, vomiting, dysphagia

GU: Hesitancy, retention, impotence

EENT: Blurred vision, photophobia, mydriasis, cycloplegia, increased ocular tension

INTEG: Urticaria, rash, pruritus, anhidrosis, fever, allergic reactions

Contraindications: Hypersensitivity to anticholinergics, narrow-angle glaucoma, GI obstruction, myasthenia gravis, paralytic ileus, GI atony, toxic megacolon

Precautions: Hyperthyroidism, coronary artery disease, dysrhythmias, CHF, ulcerative colitis, hypertension, hiatal hernia, hepatic disease, renal disease, pregnancy category C, elderly, urinary retention, prostatic hypertrophy

Pharmacokinetics:

PO: Onset 1 hr, duration 3-4 hr; metabolized by liver; excreted in urine

Drug interactions of concern to dentistry:

- Increased anticholinergic effect: other anticholinergic drugs
- Constipation, urinary retention: opioid analgesics
- Decreased absorption of ketoconazole; take doses 2 hr apart

DENTAL CONSIDERATIONS

General:

- Monitor vital signs every appointment due to cardiovascular side effects.
- Assess salivary flow as a factor in caries, periodontal disease, and candidiasis.
- Avoid dental light in patient's eyes; offer dark glasses for patient comfort.
- Consider semisupine chair position for patient comfort due to GI effects of disease.

Consultations:

- Physician should be informed if significant xerostomic side effects occur (increased caries, sore tongue, problems eating or swallowing, difficulty wearing prosthesis) so a medication change can be considered.

Teach patient/family:

When chronic dry mouth occurs, advise patient:

- To avoid mouth rinses with high alcohol content due to drying effects
- To use sugarless gum, frequent sips of water, or saliva substitutes
- To use daily home fluoride products for anticaries effect

---

meperidine HCl

(me-per′i-deen)

Demerol

International generic name: pethidine

Drug class.: Synthetic narcotic analgesic

Controlled Substance Schedule II, Canada N

Action: Interacts with opioid receptors in the CNS to alter pain perception

Uses: Moderate-to-severe pain, preoperatively in sedation techniques

Dosage and routes:
Pain
• *Adult:* PO/SC/IM 50-150 mg q3-4h prn; dose should be decreased if given IV
• *Child:* PO/SC/IM 1 mg/kg q4-6h prn, not to exceed 100 mg q4h
Preoperatively
• *Adult:* IM/SC 50-100 mg q30-90 min before surgery; dose should be reduced if given IV
• *Child:* IM/SC 1-2.2 mg/kg 30-90 min before surgery
Available forms include: Inj SC/IM/IV 25, 50, 75, 100 mg/ml; tabs 50, 100 mg; syr 50 mg/5 ml
Side effects/adverse reactions:
ORAL: Dry mouth
CNS: Drowsiness, dizziness, confusion, headache, sedation, euphoria, ***increased intracranial pressure***
CV: Palpitation, bradycardia, change in BP, tachycardia (IV)
GI: Nausea, vomiting, anorexia, constipation, cramps
RESP: ***Respiratory depression***
GU: Increased urinary output, dysuria, urinary retention
EENT: Tinnitus, blurred vision, miosis, diplopia, depressed corneal reflex
INTEG: Rash, urticaria, bruising, flushing, diaphoresis, pruritus
Contraindications: Hypersensitivity, addiction (narcotic), MAO inhibitors, ritonavir, sibutramine
Precautions: Addictive personality, pregnancy category B, lactation, increased intracranial pressure, MI (acute), severe heart disease, respiratory depression, hepatic disease, renal disease, child <18 yr
Pharmacokinetics:
PO: Onset 15 min, peak 1 hr, duration 4-5 hr
SC/IM: Onset 10 min, peak 1 hr, duration 2-4 hr
IV: Onset 5 min, duration 2 hr
Half-life 3-4 hr; metabolized by liver (to active/inactive metabolites); excreted by kidneys; crosses placenta; excreted in breast milk; a toxic metabolite can result from regular use
Drug interactions of concern to dentistry:
• Increased effects with all CNS depressants
• Contraindication: MAO inhibitors, sibutramine
• Increased effects of anticholinergics

DENTAL CONSIDERATIONS
General:
• After supine positioning, have patient sit upright for at least 2 min to avoid orthostatic hypotension.
• Psychologic and physical dependence may occur with chronic administration.
Teach patient/family:
• To avoid mouth rinses with high alcohol content due to drying effects

---

mephenytoin

(me-fen′i-toyn)
Mesantoin
Drug class.: Hydantoin anticonvulsant

Action: Reduces electrical discharges in motor cortex, reducing seizures
Uses: Generalized tonic-clonic seizures, single or complex-partial seizures
Dosage and routes:
• *Adult:* PO 50-100 mg/day, may increase by 50-100 mg q7d, up to

200 mg tid with upper limit 800-1200 mg/day

• *Child:* PO 50-100 mg/day or 100-450 mg/m^2/day in 3 divided doses initially, then increase 50-100 mg q7d, up to 200 mg tid in divided doses q8h; pediatric limit 400 mg/day

Available forms include: Tabs 100 mg

Side effects/adverse reactions:

ORAL: Gingival hyperplasia, oral ulceration (Stevens-Johnson syndrome)

CNS: Drowsiness, dizziness, fatigue, irritability, tremors, insomnia, depression

GI: Nausea, vomiting

RESP: ***Pulmonary fibrosis***

HEMA: ***Agranulocytosis, leukopenia, neutropenia, pancytopenia, eosinophilia, lymphadenopathy***

EENT: Photophobia, conjunctivitis, nystagmus, diplopia

INTEG: Rash, exfoliative dermatitis

Contraindications: Hypersensitivity to hydantoins, sinus bradycardia, heart block, Adams-Stokes syndrome

Precautions: Alcoholism, hepatic disease, renal disease, blood dyscrasias, CHF, elderly, pregnancy category not listed, lactation, respiratory depression, diabetes mellitus

Pharmacokinetics:

PO: Onset 30 min, duration 24-48 hr, half-life (including active metabolite) up to 144 hr; metabolized by liver; excreted by kidneys

Drug interactions of concern to dentistry:

• Decreased effects: chronic alcohol use, barbiturates, antihistamines, CNS depressants, haloperidol, loxapine, xanthines

• Increased effects: benzodiazepines, salicylates, halothane, fluconazole, ketoconazole, metronidazole

• Hepatotoxicity: acetaminophen

• Decreased effects of carbamazepine, acetaminophen, corticosteroids, doxycycline

DENTAL CONSIDERATIONS

General:

• Evaluate respiration characteristics and rate.

• Examine for evidence of oral manifestations of blood dyscrasias (infection, bleeding, poor healing).

• Place on frequent recall to evaluate self-care and healing response.

• Avoid dental light in patient's eyes; offer dark glasses for patient comfort.

• Determine type of epilepsy, seizure frequency, and quality of seizure control. A stress reduction protocol may be required.

• Early-morning appointments and a stress reduction protocol may be required for anxious patients.

Consultations:

• Medical consult for blood studies (CBC); leukopenic or thrombocytopenic side effects may result in infection, delayed healing, and excessive bleeding. Postpone dental treatment until normal values are maintained.

• Take precautions if dental surgery is anticipated and anesthesia is required.

Teach patient/family:

• Importance of good oral hygiene to prevent soft tissue inflammation

• Caution in use of oral hygiene aids to prevent injury

• To avoid mouth rinses with high alcohol content due to drying effects

M

mephobarbital

(me-foe-bar'bi-tal)

Mebaral

✦ Gemonil

Drug class.: Barbiturate anticonvulsant

Controlled Substance Schedule IV, Canada C

Action: A nonspecific depressant of the CNS; may enhance GABA activity in the brain

Uses: Generalized tonic-clonic (grand mal) or absence (petit mal) seizures

Dosage and routes:

- *Adult:* PO 400-600 mg/day or in divided doses
- *Child:* PO 6-12 mg/kg/day in divided doses q6-8h

Available forms include: Tabs 32, 50, 100 mg

Side effects/adverse reactions:

CNS: Dizziness, headache, hangover, paradoxic stimulation, drowsiness, increased pain

CV: Hypotension, bradycardia

GI: Nausea, vomiting, epigastric pain

RESP: Wheezing, hyperpnea

HEMA: ***Thrombocytopenia, agranulocytosis, megaloblastic anemia***

EENT: Tinnitus, hearing loss

INTEG: Rash, urticaria, purpura, erythema multiforme, facial edema

ENDO: Hypoglycemia, hyponatremia, hypokalemia

Contraindications: Hypersensitivity to barbiturates, pregnancy category D

Precautions: Hepatic disease, renal disease, lactation, alcoholism, drug abuse, hyperthyroidism

Pharmacokinetics:

PO: Onset 20-60 min, duration 68 hr

REC: Onset slow, duration 4-6 hr, half-life 34 hr; metabolized by liver; excreted by kidneys

Drug interactions of concern to dentistry:

- Increased effects: alcohol, all CNS depressants
- Decreased effects of corticosteroids, doxycycline, carbamazepine

DENTAL CONSIDERATIONS

General:

- Determine type of epilepsy, seizure frequency, and quality of seizure control. A stress reduction protocol may be required.
- Monitor vital signs every appointment due to cardiovascular and respiratory side effects.
- Patients on chronic drug therapy may rarely have symptoms of blood dyscrasias, which can include infection, bleeding, and poor healing.
- Barbiturates induce liver microsomal enzymes, which alters the metabolism of other drugs.
- Avoid drugs that may lower seizure threshold (phenothiazines).
- Be sure patient is regularly taking medication.

Consultations:

- In a patient with symptoms of blood dyscrasias, request a medical consult for blood studies and postpone dental treatment until normal values are reestablished.
- Medical consult may be required to assess disease control and patient's ability to tolerate stress.

Teach patient/family:

- Importance of good oral hygiene to prevent soft tissue inflammation

• Caution to prevent injury when using oral hygiene aids
• To avoid mouth rinses with high alcohol content due to drying effects

mepivacaine HCl (local)

(me-piv'a-kane)
Carbocaine, Carbocaine with Neo-Cobefrin, Isocaine, Polocaine, Polocaine MPF
With vasoconstrictor: Carbocaine with Neo-Cobefrin, Polocaine/Levonordefrin, Isocaine/Levonordefrin

Drug class.: Amide local anesthetic

Action: Inhibits ion fluxes across membranes, particularly sodium transport across cell membrane; decreases rise of depolarization phase of action potential; blocks nerve action potential

Uses: Local dental anesthesia, nerve block, caudal anesthesia, epidural, pain relief, paracervical block, transvaginal block or infiltration

Dosage and routes:

Dental injection, infiltration, or conduction block

• *Mepivacaine 3% without vasoconstrictor:* Max dose 6.6 mg/kg, or limit of 300 mg per dental appointment[a] for healthy patients; doses must be adjusted downward for medically compromised, debilitated, or elderly and for each individual patient. **Always use lowest effective dose, a slow injection rate, and a careful aspiration technique.**

Example calculations illustrating amount of drug administered per dental cartridge(s)

# of cartridges (1.8 ml)	mg of mepivacaine (3%)
1	54
2	108
4	216

[a]Maximum dose cited from *USP-DI,* ed 16, 1996, US Pharmacopeial Convention, Inc.; drug package inserts indicate max dose of 400 mg. Doses may differ from other published reference resources.

Mepivacaine 2% with levonordefrin 1:20,000: The same considerations for dose adjustment apply as previously indicated. However, the max dose for a single dental appointment is listed at 400 mg.

Example calculations illustrating amount of drug administered per dental cartridge(s)

# of cartridges (1.8 ml)	mg of mepivacaine (2%)	mg (μg) of vasoconstrictor (1:20,000)
1	36	0.090 (90)
2	72	0.180 (180)
3	108	0.270 (270)
5	180	0.450 (450)
8	288	0.720 (720)
10	360	0.900 (900)

Available forms include: Inj 1%, 1.5%, 2%, 3%; inj 2% with levonordefrin 1:20,000

M

Side effects/adverse reactions:
▼ *ORAL:* Numbness, tingling, trismus
CNS: ***Convulsions, loss of consciousness,*** drowsiness, disorientation, tremors, shivering, anxiety, restlessness
CV: ***Myocardial depression, cardiac arrest, dysrhythmias,*** bradycardia, hypotension, hypertension, fetal bradycardia
GI: Nausea, vomiting
RESP: ***Status asthmaticus, respiratory arrest, anaphylaxis***
EENT: Blurred vision, tinnitus, pupil constriction
INTEG: Rash, urticaria, allergic reactions, edema, burning, skin discoloration at injection site, tissue necrosis

Contraindications: Hypersensitivity, cross-sensitivity among amide local anesthetics (rare), elderly, severe liver disease

Precautions: Elderly, severe drug allergies, pregnancy category C

Pharmacokinetics:
INJ: Onset 2-10 min, duration 20 min to 4 hr; metabolized by liver; excreted in urine (metabolites)

Drug interactions of concern to dentistry:

• CNS depressants: may see increased risk of CNS depression with all CNS depressants, especially in children and when larger doses are used
• Avoid placing dental cartridges in disinfectant solutions with heavy metals or surface-active agents; may see release of metal ions into local anesthetic solutions with tissue irritation following injection
• Avoid excessive exposure of dental cartridges to light or heat, which hastens deterioration of vasoconstrictor; observe for color change in local anesthetic solution
• Risk of cardiovascular side effects: rapid intravascular administration of local anesthetic containing vasoconstrictor, either alone or in patients taking tricyclic antidepressants, MAO inhibitors, digitalis drugs, cocaine, phenothiazines, β-blockers, and in the presence of halogenated-hydrocarbon general anesthetics; use smallest effective vasoconstrictor dose and careful aspiration techniques
• Avoid use of vasoconstrictors in patients with uncontrolled hyperthyroidism, diabetes, angina, or hypertension; refer these patients for medical treatment before elective dental procedures

DENTAL CONSIDERATIONS

General:

• Drug is often used with a vasoconstrictor for increased duration of action.
• Monitor vital signs every appointment due to cardiovascular and respiratory side effects.
• Lubricate dry lips before injection.

Teach patient/family:

• To use care to prevent injury while numbness exists and to not chew gum or eat following dental anesthesia
• To report any signs of infection, muscle pain, or fever to dentist when feeling returns
• To report any unusual soft tissue reactions

meprobamate

(me-proe-ba′mate)

Equanil, Meprospan 200/400, Miltown, Probate, Trancot

✦ Apo-Meprobamate

Drug class.: Sedative-hypnotic, anxiolytic

Controlled Substance Schedule IV

Action: Nonspecific CNS depressant; acts in thalamus, limbic system, and spinal cord

Uses: Anxiety disorders

Dosage and routes:

• *Adult:* PO 1.2-1.6 g in 2-3 divided doses, not to exceed 2.4 g/day

• *Child 6-12 yr:* PO 100-200 mg bid-tid

Available forms include: Tabs 200, 400, 600 mg; caps 400 mg; susp rel caps 200, 400 mg

Side effects/adverse reactions:

▼ *ORAL:* Stomatitis, dry mouth

CNS: Dizziness, drowsiness, ***convulsions,*** headache

CV: ***Hyperthermia,*** hypotension, tachycardia, palpitation

GI: Nausea, vomiting, anorexia, diarrhea

HEMA: ***Thrombocytopenia, leukopenia, eosinophilia***

EENT: Blurred vision, tinnitus, mydriasis, slurred speech

INTEG: Urticaria, pruritus, maculopapular rash

Contraindications: Hypersensitivity, renal failure, porphyria, pregnancy category D, history of drug abuse or dependence

Precautions: Suicidal patients, severe depression, renal disease, hepatic disease, elderly

Pharmacokinetics:

PO: Onset 1 hr, half-life 6-16 hr; metabolized by liver; excreted by kidneys, in feces; crosses placenta, excreted in breast milk

Drug interactions of concern to dentistry

• Increased effects: CNS depressants, alcohol

DENTAL CONSIDERATIONS

General:

• Monitor vital signs every appointment due to cardiovascular side effects.

• Patients on chronic drug therapy may rarely have symptoms of blood dyscrasias, which can include infection, bleeding, and poor healing.

• Assess salivary flow as a factor in caries, periodontal disease, and candidiasis.

• Avoid dental light in patient's eyes; offer dark glasses for patient comfort.

• Determine why the patient is taking the drug.

• Psychologic and physical dependence may occur with chronic administration.

Consultations:

• In a patient with symptoms of blood dyscrasias, request a medical consult for blood studies and postpone dental treatment until normal values are reestablished.

• Medical consult may be required to assess disease control in the patient.

Teach patient/family:

• Importance of good oral hygiene to prevent soft tissue inflammation

• Caution to prevent injury when using oral hygiene aids

When chronic dry mouth occurs, advise patient:

• To avoid mouth rinses with high

M

alcohol content due to drying effects
• To use sugarless gum, frequent sips of water, or saliva substitutes
• To use daily home fluoride products for anticaries effect

mercaptopurine (6-MP)

(mer-kap-toe-pyoor'een)
Purinethol

Drug class.: Antineoplastic-antimetabolite

Action: Inhibits purine metabolism at multiple sites, which inhibits DNA and RNA synthesis
Uses: Chronic myelocytic leukemia, acute lymphoblastic leukemia in children, acute myelogenous leukemia
Dosage and routes:
• *Adult and child:* PO 2.5 mg/kg/day, not to exceed 5 mg/kg/day; maintenance 1.5-2.5 mg/kg/day
Available forms include: Tabs 50 mg
Side effects/adverse reactions:
▼ *ORAL:* Gingivitis, stomatitis
CNS: Fever, headache, weakness
GI: Nausea, vomiting, anorexia, diarrhea, ***hepatotoxicity*** (with high doses), jaundice, gastritis
HEMA: ***Thrombocytopenia, leukopenia, myelosuppression, anemia***
GU: ***Renal failure, oliguria, hematuria,*** crystalluria, hyperuricemia
INTEG: Rash, dry skin, urticaria
Contraindications: Patients with prior drug resistance, leukopenia ($<2500/mm^3$), thrombocytopenia ($<100,000/mm^3$), anemia, pregnancy category D
Precautions: Renal disease
Pharmacokinetics:
PO: Incompletely absorbed when taken orally; metabolized in liver; excreted in urine
Drug interactions of concern to dentistry:
• Increased risk of hepatotoxicity: hepatotoxic drugs

DENTAL CONSIDERATIONS
General:
• Patients on chronic drug therapy may rarely have symptoms of blood dyscrasias, which can include infection, bleeding, and poor healing.
• Avoid prescribing aspirin-containing products.
• Prophylactic antibiotics may be indicated to prevent infection if surgery or deep scaling is planned.
• Patients receiving chemotherapy may require palliative treatment for stomatitis.
Consultations:
• In a patient with symptoms of blood dyscrasias, request a medical consult for blood studies and postpone dental treatment until normal values are reestablished.
Teach patient/family:
• Importance of good oral hygiene to prevent soft tissue inflammation
• Caution to prevent injury when using oral hygiene aids
• To avoid mouth rinses with high alcohol content

mesalamine

(me-sal'a-meen)
Asacol, Mesasal, Pentasa, Rowasa
🍁 Salofalk

Drug class.: Antiinflammatory

Action: Unknown, suggested to act

topically in bowel to inhibit prostaglandin synthesis
Uses: Inflammatory bowel disease, ulcerative colitis, maintenance for remission of ulcerative colitis
Dosage and routes:
• *Adult:* PO 800 mg tid for up to 6 wk; rec 500 mg bid for 3-6 wk; retention enema 4 g hs for 3-6 wk
Available forms include: Tabs 400 mg; caps 250 mg; suppos 500 mg; rec susp 4 g/60 ml
Side effects/adverse reactions:
▼ *ORAL:* Lichenoid reactions
CNS: Headache, fever, dizziness, insomnia, asthenia, weakness, fatigue
GI: Cramps, gas, nausea, diarrhea, rectal pain, constipation
EENT: Sore throat
INTEG: Rash, itching, alopecia
SYST: Flu, malaise, back pain, peripheral edema, leg and joint pain, UTI
Contraindications: Hypersensitivity
Precautions: Pregnancy category B, renal disease, lactation, children, sulfite sensitivity
Pharmacokinetics:
REC: Half-life 1 hr, metabolite half-life 5-10 hr; primarily excreted in feces but some in urine as metabolites
DENTAL CONSIDERATIONS
General:
• Consider semisupine chair position for patient comfort due to GI effects of disease.
Consultations
• To reduce any potential risk of antibiotic-associated pseudomembranous colitis, a consult is recommended before selecting an antibiotic for a dental infection.

mesoridazine besylate
(mez-oh-rid'a-zeen)
Serentil, Serentil Concentrate
Drug class.: Phenothiazine antipsychotic

Action: Blocks neurotransmission at dopaminergic synapses in the cerebral cortex, hypothalamus, and limbic system; exhibits strong peripheral α-adrenergic, cholinergic blocking action; mechanism for antipsychotic effects is unclear
Uses: Psychotic disorders, schizophrenia, anxiety, alcoholism, behavioral problems in mental deficiency, chronic brain syndrome
Dosage and routes:
Schizophrenia
• *Adult:* PO 50 mg tid, optimum dose 100-400 mg/day; IM 25 mg, may repeat 0.5-1 hr; dosage range 25-200 mg/day
Behavior problems
• *Adult:* PO 25 mg tid; optimum dose 75-300 mg/day
Alcoholism
• *Adult:* PO 25 mg bid; optimum dose 50-200 mg/day
Schizoaffective disorders
• *Adult:* PO 10 mg tid; optimum dose 30-150 mg/day
Available forms include: Tabs 10, 25, 50, 100 mg; conc 25 mg/ml; inj IM 25 mg/ml
Side effects/adverse reactions:
▼ *ORAL: Dry mouth,* lichenoid reaction
CNS: Extrapyramidal symptoms: pseudoparkinsonism, akathisia, dystonia, tardive dyskinesia, drowsiness, headache
CV: Orthostatic hypotension, ***cardiac arrest,*** hypertension, ECG changes, tachycardia

M

GI: Nausea, vomiting, anorexia, constipation, diarrhea, jaundice, weight gain
RESP: ***Laryngospasm, respiratory depression,*** dyspnea
HEMA: ***Anemia, leukopenia, leukocytosis, agranulocytosis***
GU: Urinary retention, urinary frequency, enuresis, impotence, amenorrhea, gynecomastia
EENT: Blurred vision, glaucoma
INTEG: Rash, photosensitivity, dermatitis

Contraindications: Hypersensitivity, circulatory collapse, liver damage, cerebral arteriosclerosis, coronary disease, severe hypertension/hypotension, blood dyscrasias, coma, brain damage, bone marrow depression, narrow-angle glaucoma

Precautions: Pregnancy category C, lactation, seizure disorders, hypertension, hepatic disease, cardiac disease, prostatic hypertrophy, intestinal obstruction, respiratory conditions

Pharmacokinetics:
PO: Onset erratic, peak 2 hr, duration 4-6 hr
IM: Onset 15-30 min, peak 30 min, duration 6-8 hr
Metabolized by liver, excreted in urine, crosses placenta, excreted in breast milk

Drug interactions of concern to dentistry:

- Increased sedation: other CNS depressants, alcohol, barbiturate anesthetics, opioid analgesics
- Hypotension, tachycardia: epinephrine
- Increased extrapyramidal effects: phenothiazines and related drugs (haloperidol, droperidol), metoclopramide
- Additive photosensitization: tetracyclines
- Increased anticholinergic effects: anticholinergics

DENTAL CONSIDERATIONS

General:

- Monitor vital signs every appointment due to cardiovascular side effects.
- Patients on chronic drug therapy may rarely have symptoms of blood dyscrasias, which can include infection, bleeding, and poor healing.
- After supine positioning, have patient sit upright for at least 2 min before standing to avoid orthostatic hypotension.
- Assess salivary flow as a factor in caries, periodontal disease, and candidiasis.
- Avoid dental light in patient's eyes; offer dark glasses for patient comfort.
- Assess for presence of extrapyramidal motor symptoms, such as tardive dyskinesia and akathisia. Extrapyramidal motor activity may complicate dental treatment.
- Geriatric patients are more susceptible to drug effects; use lower dose.
- Use vasoconstrictors with caution, in low doses, and with careful aspiration. Avoid use of gingival retraction cord with epinephrine.

Consultations:

- In a patient with symptoms of blood dyscrasias, request a medical consult for blood studies and postpone dental treatment until normal values are reestablished.
- Take precautions if dental surgery is anticipated and anesthesia is required.
- Refer to physician if signs of

tardive dyskinesia or akathisia are present.

• Physician should be informed if significant xerostomic side effects occur (increased caries, sore tongue, problems eating or swallowing, difficulty wearing prosthesis) so a medication change can be considered.

Teach patient/family:

• Importance of good oral hygiene to prevent soft tissue inflammation

• Caution to prevent injury when using oral hygiene aids

• To use electric toothbrush if patient has difficulty holding conventional devices

When chronic dry mouth occurs, advise patient:

• To avoid mouth rinses with high alcohol content due to drying effects

• To use sugarless gum, frequent sips of water, or saliva substitutes

• To use daily home fluoride products for anticaries effect

metaproterenol sulfate

(met-a-proe-ter′e-nol)

Alupent

Drug class.: Selective β_2-agonist

Action: Relaxes bronchial smooth muscle by direct action on β_2-adrenergic receptors

Uses: Bronchial asthma, bronchospasm

Dosage and routes:

• *Adult and child >12 yr:* Inh 2-3 puffs; may repeat q3-4h, not to exceed 12 puffs/day

Asthma/bronchospasm

• *Adult:* PO 20 mg q6-8h

• *Child >9 yr or >27 kg:* PO 20 mg q6-8h or 0.4-0.9 mg/kg/dose tid

• *Child 6-9 yr or <27 kg:* PO 10 mg q6-8h or 0.4-0.9 mg/kg/dose tid

Available forms include: Tabs 10, 20 mg; aerosol 0.65 mg/dose; syrup 10 mg/5 ml; sol nebuliz 0.6%, 5%

Side effects/adverse reactions:

▼ *ORAL:* Dry mouth, taste changes

CNS: Tremors, anxiety, insomnia, headache, dizziness, stimulation

CV: ***Cardiac arrest,*** palpitation, tachycardia, hypertension

GI: Nausea

RESP: Cough, throat dryness/irritation, nasal congestion

Contraindications: Hypersensitivity to sympathomimetics, narrow-angle glaucoma

Precautions: Pregnancy category C, cardiac disorders, hyperthyroidism, diabetes mellitus, prostatic hypertrophy

Pharmacokinetics:

PO: Onset 15-30 min, peak 1 hr, duration 4 hr, excreted in urine as metabolites

Drug interactions of concern to dentistry:

• Increased effects of both drugs: other sympathomimetics, CNS stimulants

• Increased dysrhythmias: halogenated hydrocarbon anesthetics

DENTAL CONSIDERATIONS

General:

• Assess salivary flow as a factor in caries, periodontal disease, and candidiasis.

• Consider semisupine chair position for patients with respiratory disease.

• Short appointments and a stress reduction protocol may be required for anxious patients.

• Be aware that aspirin or sulfite

M

preservatives in vasoconstrictor-containing products can exacerbate asthma.

• Acute asthmatic episodes may be precipitated in the dental office. Sympathomimetic inhalants should be available for emergency use.

Consultations:

• Medical consult may be required to assess disease control and patient's ability to tolerate stress.

Teach patient/family:

• For inhalation dosage forms: rinse mouth with water after each dose to prevent dryness

When chronic dry mouth occurs, advise patient:

• To avoid mouth rinses with high alcohol content due to drying effects

• To use sugarless gum, frequent sips of water, or saliva substitutes

• To use daily home fluoride products for anticaries effect

---

metformin HCl

(met-for′min)

🍁 Glucophage, Novo-Metformin

Drug class.: Oral hypoglycemic, biguanide derivative

Action: Exact mechanism unknown, requires insulin secretion to function properly; associated with a decrease in hepatic glucose production and a decrease in intestinal glucose absorption; improves insulin sensitivity through an increase in peripheral glucose uptake and utilization

Uses: Type 2 diabetes mellitus

Dosage and routes:

• *Adult:* Must be individualized; PO initial 500 mg bid with morning and evening meals, increase dose by 500 mg at weekly intervals, daily limit 2500 mg; or 850 mg once daily with morning meal, increase dose in increments of 850 mg every other week, administered in divided doses, max 2550 mg/day

Maintenance dose

• *Adult:* PO 500 or 850 mg bid or tid taken with meals

Available forms include: Tabs 500, 850 mg

Side effects/adverse reactions:

▼ *ORAL:* Unpleasant taste, metallic taste

GI: Diarrhea, nausea, vomiting, abdominal bloating, flatulence

HEMA: ***Megaloblastic anemia,*** lower B_{12} levels

ENDO: Hypoglycemia

MISC: ***Lactic acidosis*** (incidence rare)

Contraindications: Hypersensitivity, renal or hepatic disease, patients receiving radiologic exam with parenteral iodinated contrast media, diabetic ketoacidosis, acute or chronic metabolic acidosis, conditions requiring close blood glucose control; CHF, especially those at risk for hypoperfusion and hypoxemia

Precautions: Elderly, pregnancy category B, lactation, children, interferes with B_{12} absorption

Pharmacokinetics:

PO: Slow absorption, peak concentrations 2-2.5 hr; little or no protein binding; not metabolized; excreted mainly in urine

Drug interactions of concern to dentistry:

• None reported

DENTAL CONSIDERATIONS

General:

• Short appointments and a stress reduction protocol may be required for anxious patients.

• Consider semisupine chair position for patient comfort if GI side effects occur.
• Question patient about self-monitoring of drug's antidiabetic effect, including blood glucose values or finger-stick records.
• Ensure that patient is following prescribed diet and regularly takes medication.
• Patients with diabetes may be more susceptible to infection and have delayed wound healing.
• Place on frequent recall to evaluate healing response.

Consultations:

• Medical consult may be required to assess disease control and patient's ability to tolerate stress.
• Notify physician immediately if symptoms of lactic acidosis are observed (myalgia, respiratory distress, weakness, diarrhea, malaise, muscle cramps, somnolence).
• Medical consult may include data from patient's blood glucose monitoring, including glycosylated hemoglobin or HbA_{1c} testing.
• Oral and maxillofacial surgical procedures associated with significantly restricted food intake require a medical consult and temporary cessation of metformin use.

Teach patient/family:

• Importance of good oral hygiene to prevent soft tissue inflammation
• That alteration of taste may be due to drug side effects

methadone HCl

(meth'a-done)
Dolophine, Methadose
Drug class.: Synthetic narcotic analgesic

Controlled Substance Schedule II, Canada N

Action: Interacts with opioid receptors in the CNS to alter pain perception

Uses: Severe pain, opioid withdrawal program

Dosage and routes:

Pain

• *Adult:* PO/SC/IM 2.5-10 mg q4-12h prn

Narcotic withdrawal

• *Adult:* PO 15-40 mg/day individualized initially, then 20-120 mg/day titrated to patient response

Available forms include: Inj SC/IM 10 mg/ml; tabs 5, 10 mg; oral sol 5, 10 mg/5 ml; dispersible tabs 40 mg

Side effects/adverse reactions:

▼ *ORAL:* Dry mouth

CNS: Drowsiness, dizziness, confusion, headache, sedation, euphoria

CV: Palpitation, bradycardia, change in BP

GI: Nausea, vomiting, anorexia, constipation, cramps, biliary tract spasm

RESP: ***Respiratory depression***

GU: Increased urinary output, dysuria, urinary retention

EENT: Tinnitus, blurred vision, miosis, diplopia

INTEG: Rash, urticaria, bruising, flushing, diaphoresis, pruritus

Contraindications: Hypersensitivity, addiction (narcotic), MAO inhibitors

Precautions: Addictive personality, pregnancy category B, lacta-

M

tion, increased intracranial pressure, MI (acute), severe heart disease, respiratory depression, hepatic disease, renal disease, child <18 yr

Pharmacokinetics:

PO: Onset 30-60 min, duration 6-8 hr, cumulative 22-48 hr

SC/IM: Onset 10-20 min, peak 1 hr, duration 6-8 hr, cumulative 22-48 hr

Half-life 1-1.5 days; 90% bound to plasma proteins; metabolized by liver; excreted by kidneys; crosses placenta; excreted in breast milk

Drug interactions of concern to dentistry:

- Increased CNS depression: alcohol, narcotics, sedative-hypnotics, skeletal muscle relaxants, benzodiazepines, and other CNS depressants
- Increased effects of anticholinergics

DENTAL CONSIDERATIONS

General:

- Assess salivary flow as a factor in caries, periodontal disease, and candidiasis.
- Psychologic and physical dependence may occur with chronic administration.
- Determine why the patient is taking the drug.
- Be aware of the needs of patients who are in recovery from substance abuse.
- In an opioid-dependent patient, NSAIDs are the drugs of choice for posttreatment pain control.

Consultations:

- Patients in the methadone maintenance program should not receive additional opioids or other controlled substances without a consult.

Teach patient/family:

When chronic dry mouth occurs, advise patient:

- To avoid mouth rinses with high alcohol content due to drying effects
- To use sugarless gum, frequent sips of water, or saliva substitutes
- To use daily home fluoride products for anticaries effect

methamphetamine HCl

(meth-am-fet'a-meen)

Desoxyn, Desoxyn Gradumet

Drug class.: Amphetamine

Controlled Substance Schedule II

Action: Increases release of norepinephrine and dopamine in cerebral cortex to reticular activating system

Uses: Exogenous obesity, minimal brain dysfunction, attention deficit disorder with hyperactivity

Dosage and routes:

Attention deficit disorder

- *Child >6 yr:* PO 2.5-5 mg qd or bid increasing by 5 mg/wk

Obesity

- *Adult:* PO 2.5-5 mg, 30 min ac, or 10-15 mg long-acting tab qd in AM

Available forms include: Tabs 5; long-acting tabs 5, 10, 15 mg

Side effects/adverse reactions:

▼ *ORAL:* Dry mouth, unpleasant taste

CNS: Hyperactivity, insomnia, restlessness, talkativeness, dizziness, headache, chills, stimulation, dysphoria, irritability, aggressiveness, tremor

CV: Palpitation, tachycardia, hypertension, decreased heart rate, dysrhythmia
GI: Anorexia, diarrhea, constipation, weight loss, cramps
GU: Impotence, change in libido
INTEG: Urticaria
Contraindications: Hypersensitivity to sympathomimetic amines, hyperthyroidism, hypertension, glaucoma hypertrophy, severe arteriosclerosis, drug abuse, cardiovascular disease, anxiety
Precautions: Gilles de la Tourette's syndrome, pregnancy category C, lactation, child <3 yr
Pharmacokinetics:
PO: Duration 3-6 hr; metabolized by liver; excreted by kidneys; crosses blood-brain barrier
Drug interactions of concern to dentistry:
• Increased effect of methamphetamine: CNS stimulants, sympathomimetics
• Decreased effects of both drugs: haloperidol, sedative-hypnotics
• Ventricular dysrhythmia: inhalation anesthetics

DENTAL CONSIDERATIONS
General:
• Assess salivary flow as a factor in caries, periodontal disease, and candidiasis.
Consultations:
• Physician should be informed if significant xerostomic side effects occur (increased caries, sore tongue, problems eating or swallowing, difficulty wearing prosthesis) so a medication change can be considered.
Teach patient/family:
When chronic dry mouth occurs, advise patient:
• To avoid mouth rinses with high alcohol content due to drying effects
• To use sugarless gum, frequent sips of water, or saliva substitutes
• To use daily home fluoride products for anticaries effect

methantheline bromide

(meth-an′tha-leen)
Banthine
Drug class.: Synthetic anticholinergic

Action: Inhibits muscarinic actions of acetylcholine at postganglionic parasympathetic neuroeffector sites
Uses: Treatment of peptic ulcer disease, irritable bowel syndrome, pancreatitis, gastritis, biliary dyskinesia, pylorospasm, reflex neurogenic bladder in children; unapproved use: reduction in salivation
Dosage and routes:
• *Adult:* PO 50-100 mg q6h
• *Child >1 yr:* PO 12.5-50 mg qid
• *Child <1 yr:* PO 12.5-25 mg qid
Available forms include: Tabs 50 mg
Side effects/adverse reactions:
▼ *ORAL: Dry mouth,* absence of taste
CNS: Confusion, stimulation in elderly, headache, insomnia, dizziness, drowsiness, anxiety, weakness, hallucination
CV: Palpitation, tachycardia
GI: Constipation, paralytic ileus, heartburn, nausea, vomiting, dysphagia
GU: Hesitancy, retention, impotence
EENT: Blurred vision, photophobia, mydriasis, cycloplegia, increased ocular tension, nasal congestion

M

INTEG: Urticaria, rash, pruritus, anhidrosis, fever, allergic reactions

Contraindications: Hypersensitivity to anticholinergics, narrow-angle glaucoma, GI obstruction, myasthenia gravis, paralytic ileus, GI atony, toxic megacolon

Precautions: Hyperthyroidism, CAD, dysrhythmias, CHF, ulcerative colitis, hypertension, hiatal hernia, hepatic disease, renal disease, pregnancy category C, urinary retention, prostatic hypertrophy

Pharmacokinetics:

PO: Onset 30-45 min, duration 4-6 hr; metabolized by liver; excreted in urine, bile

Drug interactions of concern to dentistry:

- Increased anticholinergic effect: H_1 antihistamines, anticholinergics, meperidine
- Decreased absorption of ketoconazole

DENTAL CONSIDERATIONS

General:

- Assess salivary flow as a factor in caries, periodontal disease, and candidiasis.
- Avoid dental light in patient's eyes; offer dark glasses for patient comfort.

Consultations:

- Physician should be informed if significant xerostomic side effects occur (increased caries, sore tongue, problems eating or swallowing, difficulty wearing prosthesis) so a medication change can be considered.

Teach patient/family:

- Importance of good oral hygiene to prevent soft tissue inflammation

When chronic dry mouth occurs, advise patient:

- To avoid mouth rinses with high alcohol content due to drying effects
- To use sugarless gum, frequent sips of water, or saliva substitutes
- To use daily home fluoride products for anticaries effect

methazolamide

(meth-a-zoe'la-mide)

Neptazane

Drug class.: Carbonic anhydrase inhibitor

Action: Decreases production of aqueous humor in eye, which lowers intraocular pressure

Uses: Open-angle glaucoma or preoperatively in narrow-angle glaucoma; can be used with miotic, osmotic agents

Dosage and routes:

- *Adult:* PO 50-100 mg bid or tid

Available forms include: Tabs 25, 50 mg

Side effects/adverse reactions:

▼ *ORAL:* Taste alteration (tingling, burning, numbness has occurred with similar drugs)

CNS: *Drowsiness, paresthesia,* ***convulsions,*** *stimulation, fatigue,* anxiety, depression, headache, dizziness, confusion, sedation, nervousness

GI: *Nausea, vomiting, anorexia,* constipation, diarrhea, melena, weight loss, hepatic insufficiency

HEMA: ***Aplastic anemia, hemolytic anemia, leukopenia, agranulocytosis, thrombocytopenia, purpura, pancytopenia***

GU: *Frequency, hypokalemia,* ***glucosuria, hematuria,*** dysuria, polyuria, uremia

EENT: Myopia, tinnitus

INTEG: *Rash,* ***Stevens-Johnson***

syndrome, pruritus, urticaria, fever, photosensitivity
ENDO: Hyperglycemia
Contraindications: Hypersensitivity to sulfonamides or thiazide diuretics, severe renal disease, severe hepatic disease, electrolyte imbalances (hyponatremia, hypokalemia), hyperchloremic acidosis, Addison's disease, COPD
Precautions: Hypercalciuria, pregnancy category C, lactation, children
Pharmacokinetics:
PO: Slow absorption, onset 2-4 hr, peak 6-8 hr, duration 10-18 hr, half-life 14 hr; excreted in urine; crosses placenta
Drug interactions of concern to dentistry:
• Exacerbation of glaucoma: anticholinergics
• Toxicity: salicylates in large doses

DENTAL CONSIDERATIONS
General:
• Patients on chronic drug therapy may rarely have symptoms of blood dyscrasias, which can include infection, bleeding, and poor healing.
• Avoid prescribing aspirin-containing products.
• Consider semisupine chair position for patient comfort if GI side effects occur.
• Avoid dental light in patient's eyes; offer dark glasses for patient comfort.
• Protect patient's eyes from accidental spatter during dental treatment.
Consultations:
• In a patient with symptoms of blood dyscrasias, request a medical consult for blood studies and postpone dental treatment until normal values are reestablished.
Teach patient/family:
• Importance of good oral hygiene to prevent soft tissue inflammation
• Caution to prevent trauma when using oral hygiene aids

methenamine hippurate/ methenamine mandelamine

(meth-en′a-meen) (hip′yoo-rate)
Methenamine hippurate: Hiprex, Urex
Hip-Rex
Methenamine mandelamine: Mandelamine
Drug class.: Urinary antiinfective

Action: In acid urine, it is hydrolyzed to ammonia and formaldehyde, which are bactericidal
Uses: Prophylaxis and treatment of uncomplicated UTIs
Dosage and routes:
• *Adult and child >12 yr:* PO 1 g q12h, max 4 g/24 hr
• *Child 6-12 yr:* PO 500 mg-1 g q12h
Neurogenic bladder
• *Adult:* PO 1 g qid pc
• *Child 6-12 yr:* PO 500 mg qid pc
• *Child <6 yr:* PO 18 mg/kg in 4 divided doses pc
Available forms include: Tabs 1 g; oral susp 500 mg/5 ml; enteric-coated tabs 500 mg, 1 g
Side effects/adverse reactions:
ORAL: Stomatitis
CNS: Headache
GI: Nausea, vomiting, anorexia, abdominal pain, increased AST/ ALT

M

GU: ***Albuminuria, hematuria,*** dysuria, bladder irritation, crystalluria
EENT: Tinnitus
INTEG: Pruritus, rash, urticaria
Contraindications: Hypersensitivity, severe dehydration, renal insufficiency
Precautions: Renal disease, pregnancy category C, lactation
Pharmacokinetics:
PO: Excreted in urine, half-life 4 hr
Drug interactions of concern to dentistry:
• None

DENTAL CONSIDERATIONS
General:
• Determine why the patient is taking the drug.
• Antibiotics for dental infections are not contraindicated, but a physician notification may be advisable.
• Palliative treatment may be required for oral side effects.
• Consider semisupine chair position for patient comfort due to GI effects of drug.

---

methimazole

(meth-im′a-zole)
Tapazole
Drug class.: Thyroid hormone antagonist

Action: Inhibits synthesis of thyroid hormones by decreasing iodine use in manufacture of thyroglobulin and iodothyronine; does not affect already formed hormones
Uses: Hyperthyroidism, preparation for thyroidectomy, thyrotoxic crisis, thyroid storm
Dosage and routes:
Hyperthyroidism
• *Adult:* PO 15-60 mg per day in divided doses depending on severity of condition; continue until euthyroid; maintenance 5-30 mg qd or in divided doses
• *Child:* PO 0.4 mg/kg/day in divided doses q12h; continue until euthyroid; maintenance dose 0.2 mg/kg/day in one dose or divided doses q12h
Preparation for thyroidectomy
• *Adult and child:* PO same as above; iodine may be added for 10 days before surgery
Thyrotoxic crisis
• *Adult and child:* PO same as hyperthyroidism with iodine and propranolol
Available forms include: Tabs 5, 10 mg
Side effects/adverse reactions:
▼ *ORAL:* Taste alteration
CNS: Drowsiness, headache, vertigo, fever, paresthesias, neuritis
GI: Nausea, diarrhea, vomiting, ***jaundice, hepatitis***
HEMA: ***Agranulocytosis, leukopenia, thrombocytopenia, hypothrombinemia, lymphadenopathy, aplastic anemia,*** bleeding, vasculitis
GU: ***Nephritis***
INTEG: Rash, urticaria, pruritus, alopecia, hyperpigmentation, lupus-like syndrome
ENDO: Enlarged thyroid
MS: Myalgia, arthralgia, nocturnal muscle cramps
Contraindications: Hypersensitivity, pregnancy category D (third trimester), lactation
Precautions: Infection, bone marrow depression, hepatic disease, pregnancy (first, second trimester)

Pharmacokinetics:
PO: Onset 30-40 min, duration 2-4 hr, half-life 1-2 hr; excreted in urine, bile, breast milk; crosses placenta

Drug interactions of concern to dentistry:
• Increased CV side effects in uncontrolled patients: anticholinergics and sympathomimetics
• Patients with uncontrolled hyperthyroidism are at risk when vasoconstrictors are used
• Patients with uncontrolled hypothyroidism may be more responsive to CNS depressants

DENTAL CONSIDERATIONS
General:
• Monitor vital signs every appointment due to cardiovascular effects of disease.
• Patients on chronic drug therapy may rarely have symptoms of blood dyscrasias; examine for evidence of oral manifestations of blood dyscrasias (infection, bleeding, poor healing).
• Evaluate for clotting ability during periodontal instrumentation.
• Evaluate for control of hyperthyroidism. Patients with uncontrolled condition should not be treated in the dental office until thyroid values are normalized.
• Patients with uncontrolled condition should be referred for medical evaluation and treatment.

Consultations:
• Medical consult may be required to assess disease control in the patient.
• Medical consult for blood studies (CBC); leukopenic or thrombocytopenic side effects may result in infection, delayed healing, and excessive bleeding. Postpone elective dental treatment until normal values are maintained.

Teach patient/family:
• Importance of good oral hygiene to prevent soft tissue inflammation
• Caution in use of oral hygiene aids to prevent injury

---

methocarbamol

(meth-oh-kar′ba-mole)
Carbacot, Robaxin, Robaxin 750

Drug class.: Skeletal muscle relaxant

Action: Depresses multisynaptic pathways in the spinal cord

Uses: Adjunct for relief of spasm and pain in musculoskeletal conditions

Dosage and routes:
Pain
• *Adult:* PO 1.5 g × 2-3 days, then 1 g qid; IM 500 mg in each gluteal region, may repeat q8h; IV bol 1-3 g/day at 3 ml/min; IV inf 1 g/250 ml D_5W or NS, not to exceed 3 g/day

Available forms include: Tabs 500, 750 mg; inj IM/IV 100 mg/ml

Side effects/adverse reactions:
▼ *ORAL:* Metallic taste
CNS: Dizziness, weakness, drowsiness, ***seizures,*** headache, tremor, depression, insomnia
CV: Postural hypotension, bradycardia
GI: Nausea, vomiting, hiccups, anorexia
HEMA: Hemolysis, increased hemoglobin (IV only)
GU: Brown, black, or green urine
EENT: Diplopia, temporary loss of vision, blurred vision, nystagmus
INTEG: Rash, pruritus, fever, facial flushing, urticaria

Contraindications: Hypersensitivity, child <12 yr, intermittent porphyria

Precautions: Renal disease, hepatic disease, addictive personalities, pregnancy category C, myasthenia gravis, epilepsy

Pharmacokinetics:

PO: Onset 0.5 hr, peak 1-2 hr, half-life 1-2 hr; metabolized in liver; excreted in urine (unchanged); crosses placenta

Drug interactions of concern to dentistry:

• Increased CNS depression: alcohol, narcotics, sedative-hypnotics

DENTAL CONSIDERATIONS

General:

• Determine why the patient is taking the drug.

• Consider semisupine chair position if back is involved.

Teach patient/family:

• Importance of good oral hygiene to prevent soft tissue inflammation

• Caution to prevent injury when using oral hygiene aids

• To avoid mouth rinses with high alcohol content due to drying effects

---

methotrexate/ methotrexate sodium (amethopterin, mtx)

(meth-oh-trex′ate)

generic, Rheumatrex

Drug class.: Folic acid antagonist, antineoplastic

Action: Inhibits an enzyme that reduces folic acid, which is needed for nucleic acid synthesis in all cells

Uses: Acute lymphocytic leukemia; in combination for breast, lung, head, neck cancer; lymphosarcoma; psoriasis; gestational choriocarcinoma; hydatidiform mole; rheumatoid arthritis

Dosage and routes:

Leukemia

• *Adult and child:* PO 3.3 mg/m^2/day, maintenance 30 mg/m^2/day 2× weekly; IV 2.5 mg/kg q2wk

Choriocarcinoma

• *Adult and child:* PO 15-30 mg/m^2 qd × 5 days, then off 1 wk; may repeat

Available forms include: Tabs 2.5 mg; inj IV 25 mg/ml; powder for inj IV 20, 25, 50, 100, 250 mg; sodium inj IV 2.5, 25 mg/ml

Side effects/adverse reactions:

▼ *ORAL: Ulcerative stomatitis, gingivitis,* bleeding

CNS: ***Convulsions,*** dizziness, headache, confusion, hemiparesis, malaise, fatigue, chills, fever

GI: Nausea, vomiting, anorexia, diarrhea, ***hepatotoxicity, GI hemorrhage,*** abdominal pain, cramps, ulcer, gastritis, hematemesis

HEMA: ***Leukopenia, thrombocytopenia, myelosuppression, anemia***

GU: ***Renal failure, hematuria, azotemia, uric acid nephropathy,*** urinary retention, menstrual irregularities, defective spermatogenesis

INTEG: Rash, alopecia, dry skin, urticaria, photosensitivity, folliculitis, vasculitis, petechiae, ecchymosis, acne, alopecia, painful plaque lesions in psoriasis

MISC: Rare reports of bone and soft tissue necrosis after radiation therapy

Contraindications: Hypersensitivity, leukopenia (<2500/mm^3), thromocytopenia (<100,000/mm^3), anemia, patients with psoriasis and severe renal/hepatic disease, pregnancy category D

Precautions: Renal disease, lactation, other drugs with potential for hepatotoxicity

Pharmacokinetics:

PO: Readily absorbed when taken orally, peak 1-4 hr

IV/IM: Peak 0.5-2 hr

50% plasma protein bound; not metabolized; excreted in urine (unchanged); crosses placenta, blood-brain barrier

Drug interactions of concern to dentistry:

- Increased toxicity: aspirin, alcohol, NSAIDs
- Possible fatal interactions: NSAIDs, high-dose IV methotrexate
- Suspected increase in methotrexate toxicity: amoxicillin

DENTAL CONSIDERATIONS

General:

- Patients on chronic drug therapy may rarely have symptoms of blood dyscrasias, which can include infection, bleeding, and poor healing.
- Avoid prescribing aspirin- or NSAID-containing products.
- Place on frequent recall due to increased risk for infection and to evaluate healing response.
- Determine why the patient is taking the drug.
- Palliative treatment may be needed if stomatitis occurs.

Consultations:

- In a patient with symptoms of blood dyscrasias, request a medical consult for blood studies and postpone dental treatment until normal values are reestablished.
- Medical consult may be required to assess disease control in the patient.

Teach patient/family:

- Importance of good oral hygiene to prevent soft tissue inflammation
- Caution to prevent injury when using oral hygiene aids
- About palliative therapy for sore mouth
- To avoid mouth rinses with high alcohol content due to drying effects

---

methsuximide

(meth-sux'i-mide)

Celontin

Drug class.: Anticonvulsant

Action: Inhibits spike wave formation in absence seizures (petit mal); decreases amplitude, frequency, duration, spread of discharge in minor motor seizures

Uses: Refractory absence seizures (petit mal)

Dosage and routes:

- *Adult and child:* PO 300 mg/day; may increase by 300 mg/wk, not to exceed 1.2 g/day in divided doses

Available forms include: Half-strength caps 150 mg; caps 300 mg

Side effects/adverse reactions:

▼ *ORAL:* Gingival overgrowth, glossitis, ulcers (Stevens-Johnson syndrome)

CNS: Drowsiness, dizziness, fatigue, euphoria, lethargy, irritability, depression, insomnia, anxiety, aggressiveness, ataxia, headache, confusion

GI: Nausea, vomiting, heartburn, anorexia, diarrhea, abdominal pain, cramps, constipation

HEMA: ***Agranulocytosis, aplastic anemia, thrombocytopenia, leuko-***

M

cytosis, eosinophilia, pancytopenia

GU: ***Hematuria, renal damage,*** vaginal bleeding

EENT: Myopia, blurred vision, photophobia

INTEG: ***Stevens-Johnson syndrome,*** urticaria, pruritic erythema, hirsutism

Contraindications: Hypersensitivity to succinimide derivatives

Precautions: Hepatic disease, renal disease, pregnancy category C, lactation

Pharmacokinetics:

PO: Onset 15-30 min, peak 1-2 hr, duration 4-6 hr

REC: Onset slow, duration 4-6 hr

Half-life 2.6-4 hr; metabolized by liver; excreted by kidneys

Drug interactions of concern to dentistry:

• Enhanced CNS depression: alcohol, CNS depressants

• Decreased effects: phenothiazines, thioxanthenes, barbiturates

• Changes in seizure pattern, frequency: haloperidol

DENTAL CONSIDERATIONS

General:

• Patients on chronic drug therapy may rarely have symptoms of blood dyscrasias, which can include infection, bleeding, and poor healing.

• Avoid dental light in patient's eyes; offer dark glasses for patient comfort.

• Determine type of epilepsy, seizure frequency, and quality of seizure control. A stress reduction protocol may be required.

• Place on frequent recall to monitor gingival condition.

Consultations:

• In a patient with symptoms of blood dyscrasias, request a medical consult for blood studies and postpone dental treatment until normal values are reestablished.

• Take precautions if dental surgery is anticipated and anesthesia is required.

• Medical consult may be required to assess disease control in the patient.

Teach patient/family:

• Importance of good oral hygiene to prevent soft tissue inflammation

• Caution to prevent injury when using oral hygiene aids

• To avoid mouth rinses with high alcohol content if oral side effects occur

---

methyldopa/ methyldopate

(meth-il-doe'pa)

Aldomet

♣ Apo-Methyldopa, Dopamet, Novomedopa, Nu-Medopa

Drug class.: Centrally acting antihypertensive

Action: Stimulates central inhibitory α-adrenergic receptors or acts as false transmitter, resulting in reduction of arterial pressure

Uses:

Hypertension

Dosage and routes:

• *Adult:* PO 250 mg bid or tid, then adjusted q2d as needed, 0.5-3 g qd in 2-4 divided doses (maintenance), not to exceed 3 g/day; IV 250-500 mg in 100 ml D_5W q6h, run over 30-60 min, not to exceed 1 g q6h

• *Child:* PO 10 mg/kg/day in 2-4 divided doses, not to exceed 65 mg/kg or 3 g/day, whichever is less; IV 20-40 mg/kg/day in 4 divided doses, not to exceed 65 mg/kg

Available forms include: Tabs 125, 250, 500 mg; oral susp 250 mg/5 ml; inj IV 50 mg/ml

Side effects/adverse reactions:

▼ *ORAL: Dry mouth,* bleeding, lichenoid lesions

CNS: Drowsiness, weakness, dizziness, sedation, headache, depression, psychosis

CV: Bradycardia, myocarditis, orthostatic hypotension, angina, edema, weight gain

GI: Nausea, vomiting, diarrhea, constipation, hepatic dysfunction

HEMA: ***Leukopenia, thrombocytopenia,*** anemia, positive Coombs' test

GU: Impotence, failure to ejaculate

EENT: Nasal congestion, eczema

INTEG: Lupus-like syndrome

Contraindications: Active hepatic disease, hypersensitivity, blood dyscrasias

Precautions: Pregnancy category C, liver disease, eclampsia, severe cardiac disease

Pharmacokinetics:

PO: Peak 4-6 hr, duration 12-24 hr

IV: Peak 2 hr, duration 10-16 hr

Metabolized by liver, excreted in urine

Drug interactions of concern to dentistry:

- Decreased effects: indomethacin and other NSAIDs
- Increased pressor response: epinephrine and other sympathomimetics
- Increased sedation: haloperidol, alcohol, CNS depressants
- Increased hypotensive action of general anesthetics

DENTAL CONSIDERATIONS

General:

- Monitor vital signs every appointment due to cardiovascular side effects.
- Patients on chronic drug therapy may rarely have symptoms of blood dyscrasias, which can include infection, bleeding, and poor healing.
- Assess salivary flow as a factor in caries, periodontal disease, and candidiasis.
- Limit use of sodium-containing products such as saline IV fluids for patients with a dietary salt restriction.
- After supine positioning, have patient sit upright for at least 2 min before standing to avoid orthostatic hypotension.
- Stress from dental procedures may compromise cardiovascular function; determine patient risk.

Consultations:

- In a patient with symptoms of blood dyscrasias, request a medical consult for blood studies and postpone dental treatment until normal values are reestablished.
- Medical consult may be required to assess disease control and stress tolerance in the patient.

Teach patient/family:

- Importance of good oral hygiene to prevent soft tissue inflammation
- Caution to prevent injury when using oral hygiene aids

When chronic dry mouth occurs, advise patient:

- To avoid mouth rinses with high alcohol content due to drying effects
- To use sugarless gum, frequent sips of water, or saliva substitutes

M

• To use daily home fluoride products for anticaries effect

methylphenidate HCl

(meth-il-fen′i-date)

Metadate ER, Methylin, Ritalin, Ritalin SR

♣ PMS-Methylphenidate

Drug class.: CNS stimulant, related to amphetamines

Controlled Substance Schedule II, Canada C

Action: Increases release of norepinephrine, dopamine in cerebral cortex to reticular activating system; exact mode of action not known

Uses: Attention deficit disorder with hyperactivity, narcolepsy

Dosage and routes:

Attention deficit disorder

• *Child >6 yr:* 5 mg before breakfast and lunch, increasing by 5-10 mg/wk, not to exceed 60 mg/day

Narcolepsy

• *Adult:* PO 10 mg bid-tid, 30-45 min before meals; may increase up to 40-50 mg/day

Available forms include: Tabs 5, 10, 20 mg; ext rel tabs 10, 20 mg

Side effects/adverse reactions:

▼ *ORAL:* Dry mouth

CNS: Hyperactivity, insomnia, restlessness, talkativeness, dizziness, headache, akathisia, dyskinesia, Gilles de la Tourette's syndrome

CV: Palpitation, tachycardia, BP changes, angina, dysrhythmias

GI: Nausea, anorexia, diarrhea, constipation, weight loss, abdominal pain

HEMA: ***Thrombocytopenia***

GU: ***Uremia***

INTEG: ***Exfoliative dermatitis,*** urticaria, rash, erythema multiforme

ENDO: Growth retardation

Contraindications: Hypersensitivity, anxiety, history of Gilles de la Tourette's syndrome, history of seizures

Precautions: Hypertension, depression, pregnancy category C, seizures, lactation, drug abuse

Pharmacokinetics:

PO: Onset 0.5-1 hr, duration 4-6 hr; metabolized by liver; excreted by kidneys

Drug interactions of concern to dentistry:

• Increased effects of anticholinergics, CNS stimulants, tricyclic antidepressants, and sympathomimetics

DENTAL CONSIDERATIONS

General:

• Monitor vital signs often due to cardiovascular side effects.

• Patients on chronic drug therapy may rarely have symptoms of blood dyscrasias, which can include infection, bleeding, and poor healing.

• Assess salivary flow as a factor in caries, periodontal disease, and candidiasis.

• Use vasoconstrictors with caution, in low doses, and with careful aspiration.

• Determine why the patient is taking the drug.

Consultations:

• In a patient with symptoms of blood dyscrasias, request a medical consult for blood studies and postpone dental treatment until normal values are reestablished.

• Medical consult may be required to assess disease control in the patient.

Teach patient/family:
• Importance of good oral hygiene to prevent soft tissue inflammation
• Caution to prevent injury when using oral hygiene aids

When chronic dry mouth occurs, advise patient:
• To avoid mouth rinses with high alcohol content due to drying effects
• To use sugarless gum, frequent sips of water, or saliva substitutes
• To use daily home fluoride products for anticaries effect

methylprednisolone/ methylprednisolone acetate/ methylprednisolone sodium succinate

(meth-il-pred-nis'oh-lone)

Methylprednisolone: Medrol, Medrol Dosepak, Meprolone

Methylprednisolone acetate: depMedalone 40, depMedalone 80, Depoject, Depo-Medrol, Depopred 40, Depopred 80, Depo-Prodate, Duralone 40, Duralone 80, Medralone 40, Medralone 80, M-Prednisol 40, M-Prednisol 80, Rep-Pred 40, Rep-Pred 80

Methylprednisolone sodium succinate: A-MethaPred, Solu-Medrol

Drug class.: Glucocorticoid, immediate acting

Action: Glucocorticoids have multiple actions that include antiinflammatory and immunosuppressant effects. They inhibit phospholipase A_2, interfering with or reducing the synthesis of prostaglandins and leukotrienes. They also bind to cytoplasmic glucocorticoid receptors (GRs) and enter the cell nucleus to bind with DNA. This results in the synthesis of various enzymes such as collagenase, elastase, and cytokines that play important roles in inflammation and immunosuppression. They also suppress the production of lymphocytes, monocytes, and eosinophils.

Uses: Severe inflammation, shock, adrenal insufficiency, collagen disorders

Dosage and routes:

Adrenal insufficiency/inflammation
• *Adult:* PO 2-60 mg in 4 divided doses; IM 40-80 mg (acetate); IM/IV 10-250 mg (succinate); intraarticular 4-30 mg (acetate)
• *Child:* IV 117 μg to 1.66 mg/kg in 3-4 divided doses (succinate)

Shock
• *Adult:* IV 100-250 mg q2-6h (succinate)

Available forms include: Tabs 2, 4, 6, 8, 16, 24, 32 mg; inj (acetate) 20, 40, 80 mg/ml

Caution: *Do not administer acetate preparations IV;* inj (succinate) 40, 125, 500, 1000, 2000 mg/vial

Side effects/adverse reactions:
▼ *ORAL:* ***Candidiasis,*** dry mouth, poor wound healing, petechiae
CNS: Depression, flushing, sweating, headache, mood changes
CV: Hypertension, ***circulatory collapse, thrombophlebitis, embolism,*** tachycardia
GI: Diarrhea, nausea, abdominal distention, ***GI hemorrhage, increased appetite, pancreatitis***
HEMA: ***Thrombocytopenia***
EENT: Fungal infections, increased intraocular pressure, blurred vision

M

INTEG: Acne, poor wound healing, ecchymosis, petechiae
MS: Fractures, osteoporosis, weakness
Contraindications: Psychosis, hypersensitivity, idiopathic thrombocytopenia, acute glomerulonephritis, amebiasis, fungal infections, nonasthmatic bronchial disease, child <2 yr, AIDS, TB
Precautions: Pregnancy category C, diabetes mellitus, glaucoma, osteoporosis, seizure disorders, ulcerative colitis, CHF, myasthenia gravis, renal disease, esophagitis, peptic ulcer, rifampin
Pharmacokinetics:
PO: Peak 1-2 hr, duration 1.5 days
IM: Peak 4-8 days, duration 1-4 wk
INTRAARTICULAR: Peak 1 wk
Half-life >3.5 hr

Drug interactions of concern to dentistry:
- Decreased action: barbiturates, rifampin, rifabutin
- Increased GI side effects: alcohol, salicylates, NSAIDs
- Increased action: ketoconazole, macrolide antibiotics
- Hepatotoxicity: acetaminophen (chronic, high doses)

DENTAL CONSIDERATIONS
General:
- Patients on chronic drug therapy may rarely have symptoms of blood dyscrasias, which can include infection, bleeding, and poor healing.
- Assess salivary flow as a factor in caries, periodontal disease, and candidiasis.
- Symptoms of oral infections may be masked.
- Place on frequent recall to evaluate healing response.
- Prophylactic antibiotics may be indicated to prevent infection if surgery or deep scaling is planned.
- Avoid prescribing aspirin-containing products.
- Determine dose and duration of steroid therapy for each patient to assess risk for stress tolerance and immunosuppression.
- Patients who have been or are currently on chronic steroid therapy (>2 wk) may require supplemental steroids for dental treatment.

Consultations:
- In a patient with symptoms of blood dyscrasias, request a medical consult for blood studies and postpone dental treatment until normal values are reestablished.
- Medical consult may be required to assess disease control in the patient.
- Consult may be required to confirm steroid dose and duration of use.

Teach patient/family:
- Importance of good oral hygiene to prevent soft tissue inflammation
- Caution to prevent injury when using oral hygiene aids due to reduced healing response

When chronic dry mouth occurs, advise patient:
- To avoid mouth rinses with high alcohol content due to drying effects
- To use sugarless gum, frequent sips of water, or saliva substitutes
- To use daily home fluoride products for anticaries effect

---

methysergide maleate

(meth-i-ser′jide)
Sansert
Drug class.: Serotonin antagonist

Action: Competitively blocks serotonin HT receptors in CNS and periphery

Uses: Prophylaxis for migraine and other vascular headaches

Dosage and routes:

• *Adult:* PO 4-8 mg daily with meals

Available forms include: Tabs 2 mg

Side effects/adverse reactions:

CNS: Tremors, anxiety, insomnia, headache, dizziness, euphoria, confusion, depersonalization, hallucination, paresthesia, drowsiness

CV: ***Retroperitoneal fibrosis, cardiac fibrosis,*** valvular thickening, palpitation, tachycardia, postural hypertension, angina, thrombophlebitis, ECG changes

GI: Nausea, vomiting, weight gain

HEMA: ***Blood dyscrasias***

INTEG: Flushing, rash, alopecia

MS: Arthralgia, myalgia

Contraindications: Hypersensitivity to ergot, tartrazine, pregnancy category X, occlusion (peripheral, vascular), CAD, hepatic disease, renal or liver disease, peptic ulcer, hypertension, connective tissue disease, fibrotic pulmonary disease, severe atherosclerosis, valvular heart disease

Precautions: Lactation, children

Pharmacokinetics:

PO: Half-life 10 hr; metabolized by liver; excreted in urine (metabolites/unchanged drug)

Drug interactions of concern to dentistry:

• Increased vasoconstriction: systemically administered sympathomimetics

DENTAL CONSIDERATIONS

General:

• Patients on chronic drug therapy may rarely have symptoms of blood dyscrasias, which can include infection, bleeding, and poor healing.

• After supine positioning, have patient sit upright for at least 2 min to avoid orthostatic hypotension.

• Use vasoconstrictors with caution, in low doses, and with careful aspiration.

• Avoid use of gingival retraction cord with epinephrine.

Consultations:

• In a patient with symptoms of blood dyscrasias, request a medical consult for blood studies and postpone dental treatment until normal values are reestablished.

• Medical consult may be required to assess disease control in the patient.

---

metoclopramide HCl

(met-oh-kloe-pra′mide)

Octamide, Reglan

✤ Apo-Metoclop, Maxeran, PMS-Metoclopramide

Drug class.: Central dopamine receptor antagonist

Action: Enhances response to acetylcholine of tissue in upper GI tract, which causes contraction of gastric muscle, relaxes pyloric and duodenal segments, increases peristalsis without stimulating secretions; antiemetic action occurs centrally, possibly by action on chemoreceptor trigger zone

Uses: Prevention of nausea, vomiting induced by chemotherapy, radiation, delayed gastric emptying, gastroesophageal reflux

Dosage and routes:

Nausea/vomiting

• *Adult:* IV 2 mg/kg 30 min before administration of chemotherapy, then q2h × 2 doses, and then q3h × 3 doses

Delayed gastric emptying

• *Adult:* PO 10 mg 30 min ac, hs × 2-8 wk

Gastroesophageal reflux

• *Adult:* PO 10-15 mg qid 30 min ac

Available forms include: Tabs 5, 10 mg; syr 5 mg/5 ml; inj IV 5 mg/ml

Side effects/adverse reactions:

▼ *ORAL:* Dry mouth

CNS: Sedation, fatigue, restlessness, headache, sleeplessness, dystonia, dizziness, drowsiness, tardive dyskinesia, Parkinson-like tremors

CV: Hypotension, supraventricular tachycardia, hypertension (IV)

GI: Constipation, nausea, anorexia, vomiting

HEMA: ***Agranulocytosis, neutropenia, leukopenia***

GU: Decreased libido, prolactin secretion, amenorrhea, galactorrhea

INTEG: Urticaria, rash

Contraindications: Hypersensitivity to this drug or procaine or procainamide, seizure disorder, pheochromocytoma, breast cancer, GI obstruction

Precautions: Pregnancy category B, lactation, GI hemorrhage, CHF, asthma, hypertension, Parkinson's disease, renal failure

Pharmacokinetics:

IV: Onset 1-3 min, duration 1-2 hr

PO: Onset 0.5-1 hr, duration 1-2 hr

IM: Onset 10-15 min, duration 1-2 hr

Half-life 4 hr, metabolized by liver, excreted in urine

Drug interactions of concern to dentistry:

• Decreased GI action: anticholinergics, opioids

• Increased sedation: alcohol, other CNS depressants

• Increased effects of succinylcholine

DENTAL CONSIDERATIONS

General:

• Assess salivary flow as a factor in caries, periodontal disease, and candidiasis.

• Assess for presence of extrapyramidal motor symptoms, such as tardive dyskinesia and akathisia. Extrapyramidal motor activity may complicate dental treatment.

• Determine why the patient is taking the drug.

• Consider semisupine chair position for patient comfort due to GI effects of disease.

Teach patient/family:

When chronic dry mouth occurs, advise patient:

• To avoid mouth rinses with high alcohol content due to drying effects

• To use sugarless gum, frequent sips of water, or saliva substitutes

• To use daily home fluoride products for anticaries effect

---

metolazone

(me-tole'a-zone)

Diulo, Mykrox, Zaroxolyn

Drug class.: Diuretic with thiazide-like effects

Action: Acts on distal tubule by increasing excretion of water, sodium, chloride, and potassium

Uses: Edema, hypertension, CHF

Dosage and routes:

Edema

• *Adult:* PO 5-20 mg/day

Hypertension

• *Adult:* PO 2.5-5 mg/day

Available forms include: Tabs 0.5, 2.5, 5, 10 mg

Side effects/adverse reactions:

▼ *ORAL: Dry mouth, increased thirst*

CNS: Dizziness, fatigue, weakness, drowsiness, paresthesia, anxiety, depression, headache

CV: Irregular pulse, orthostatic hypotension, palpitation, volume depletion

GI: Nausea, vomiting, anorexia, ***hepatitis,*** constipation, diarrhea, cramps, pancreatitis, GI irritation

HEMA: ***Aplastic anemia, hemolytic anemia, leukopenia, agranulocytosis, thrombocytopenia,*** neutropenia

GU: Frequency, ***uremia, glucosuria,*** polyuria

EENT: Blurred vision

INTEG: Rash, urticaria, purpura, photosensitivity, fever

META: Hyperglycemia, hyperuricemia, increased creatinine, BUN

ELECT: Hypokalemia, hypomagnesia, hypercalcemia, hyponatremia, hypochloremia

Contraindications: Hypersensitivity to thiazides or sulfonamides, anuria, pregnancy category D

Precautions: Hypokalemia, renal disease, hepatic disease, gout, COPD, lupus erythematosus, diabetes mellitus

Pharmacokinetics:

PO: Onset 1 hr, peak 2 hr, duration 12-24 hr, half-life 8 hr; excreted unchanged by kidneys; crosses placenta; enters breast milk

Drug interactions of concern to dentistry:

• Increased photosensitization: tetracycline

• Decreased hypotensive response: indomethacin and other NSAIDs

DENTAL CONSIDERATIONS

General:

• Patients on chronic drug therapy may rarely have symptoms of blood dyscrasias, which can include infection, bleeding, and poor healing.

• Assess salivary flow as a factor in caries, periodontal disease, and candidiasis.

• After supine positioning, have patient sit upright for at least 2 min before standing to avoid orthostatic hypotension.

• Short appointments and a stress reduction protocol may be required for anxious patients.

• Limit use of sodium-containing products, such as saline IV fluids, for those patients with a dietary salt restriction.

• Stress from dental procedures may compromise cardiovascular function; determine patient risk.

Consultations:

• In a patient with symptoms of blood dyscrasias, request a medical consult for blood studies and postpone dental treatment until normal values are reestablished.

• Medical consult may be required to assess disease control and patient's ability to tolerate stress.

Teach patient/family:

• Importance of good oral hygiene to prevent soft tissue inflammation

• Caution to prevent injury when using oral hygiene aids

When chronic dry mouth occurs, advise patient:

• To avoid mouth rinses with high alcohol content due to drying effects

• To use sugarless gum, frequent sips of water, or saliva substitutes

• To use daily home fluoride products for anticaries effect

metoprolol tartrate

(met-oh'proe-lol)

Betaloc, Lopressor, Nu-Metop, Toprol XL

♣ Apo-Metoprolol, Lopresor SR, Novometoprol

Drug class.: Antihypertensive, selective β_1-blocker

Action: This is a selective β_1-adrenergic antagonist. At higher doses selectivity may be lost with antagonism of β_2-receptors as well. The antihypertensive mechanism of action is unclear but may include a reduction in cardiac output and inhibition of renin release by the renal juxtaglomerular apparatus. Peripheral resistance decreases with long-term use. The antianginal action (when indicated for this use) may be related to a decrease in myocardial oxygen demand and negative chronotropic and inotropic effects. The antiarrhythmic action (when indicated for this use) has been related to a reduction in spontaneous pacemaker firing and slowing of AV nodal conduction.

Uses: Mild-to-moderate hypertension, acute MI to reduce cardiovascular mortality, angina pectoris

Dosage and routes:

Hypertension

• *Adult:* PO 50 mg bid or 100 mg qd; may give up to 200-450 mg in divided doses

Myocardial infarction

• *Adult:* Early treatment, IV bol 5 mg q2min × 3, then 50 mg PO 15 min after last dose and q6h × 48 hr; late treatment, PO maintenance 100 mg bid × 3 mo

Available forms include: Tabs 50, 100 mg; ext rel 50, 100, 200 mg; inj IV 1 mg/ml

Side effects/adverse reactions:

▼ *ORAL:* Dry mouth

CNS: Insomnia, dizziness, ***depression,*** mental changes, hallucinations, anxiety, headaches, nightmares, confusion, fatigue

CV: Bradycardia, CHF (palpitation), ***cardiac arrest, AV block,*** dysrhythmias, hypotension

GI: Nausea, vomiting, ***diarrhea,*** hiccups, constipation, flatulence, colitis, cramps

RESP: ***Bronchospasm,*** dyspnea, wheezing

HEMA: ***Agranulocytosis, eosinophilia, thrombocytopenic purpura***

GU: Impotence

EENT: Sore throat, dry/burning eyes

INTEG: Rash, purpura, alopecia, dry skin, urticaria, pruritus

Contraindications: Hypersensitivity to β-blockers, cardiogenic shock, second- or third-degree heart block, sinus bradycardia, CHF, bronchial asthma

Precautions: Major surgery, pregnancy category C, lactation, diabetes mellitus, renal disease, thyroid disease, COPD, heart failure, CAD, nonallergic bronchospasm, hepatic disease

Pharmacokinetics:

PO: Peak 2-4 hr, duration 13-19 hr, half-life 3-4 hr; metabolized in liver (metabolites); excreted in urine; crosses placenta; excreted in breast milk

Drug interactions of concern to dentistry:

• Increased hypotension, bradycardia: fentanyl derivatives, inhalation anesthetics

• Decreased antihypertensive ef-

fects: indomethacin and possibly other NSAIDs, sympathomimetics
• May slow metabolism of lidocaine
• Decreased β-blocking effects (or decreased β-adrenergic effects) of epinephrine, levonordefrin, isoproterenol, and other sympathomimetics

DENTAL CONSIDERATIONS

General:

• Monitor vital signs every appointment due to cardiovascular and respiratory side effects.
• After supine positioning, have patient sit upright for at least 2 min before standing to avoid orthostatic hypotension.
• Patients on chronic drug therapy may rarely have symptoms of blood dyscrasias, which can include infection, bleeding, and poor healing.
• Assess salivary flow as a factor in caries, periodontal disease, and candidiasis.
• Stress from dental procedures may compromise cardiovascular function; determine patient risk.
• Short appointments and a stress reduction protocol may be required for anxious patients.
• Use vasoconstrictors with caution, in low doses, and with careful aspiration. Avoid use of gingival retraction cord with epinephrine.

Consultations:

• In a patient with symptoms of blood dyscrasias, request a medical consult for blood studies and postpone dental treatment until normal values are reestablished.
• Medical consult may be required to assess disease control and patient's ability to tolerate stress.
• Take precautions if general anesthesia is required for dental surgery.

Teach patient/family:

• Importance of good oral hygiene to prevent soft tissue inflammation
• Caution to prevent injury when using oral hygiene aids

When chronic dry mouth occurs, advise patient:

• To avoid mouth rinses with high alcohol content due to drying effects
• To use sugarless gum, frequent sips of water, or saliva substitutes
• To use daily home fluoride products for anticaries effect

---

metronidazole/ metronidazole HCl

(me-troe-ni'da-zole)

Flagyl, Flagyl IV RTU, Flagyl 375, Flagyl ER, Helidac, Metric 21, Metro IV, Protostat

🍁 Trikacide, Apo-Metronidazole, Novonidazole

Drug class.: Trichomonacide, amebicide antiinfective

Action: Direct-acting amebicide/ trichomonacide binds, degrades DNA in organism

Uses: Intestinal amebiasis, amebic abscess, trichomoniasis, refractory trichomoniasis, bacterial anaerobic infections, giardiasis; unapproved use: refractory adult periodontitis

Dosage and routes:

Trichomoniasis

• *Adult:* PO 250 mg tid × 7 days, or 2 g in single dose; do not repeat treatment for 2-3 wk

Refractory trichomoniasis

• *Adult:* PO 250 mg bid × 10 days

Amebic abscess

• *Adult:* PO 500-750 mg tid × 5-10 days

• *Child:* PO 35-50 mg/kg/day in 3 divided doses × 10 days

Intestinal amebiasis

• *Adult:* PO 750 mg tid × 5-10 days

• *Child:* PO 35-50 mg/kg/day in 3 divided doses × 10 days; then give oral iodoquinol

Anaerobic bacterial infections

• *Adult:* IV inf 15 mg/kg over 1 hr, then 7.5 mg/kg IV or PO q6h, not to exceed 4 g/day

Periodontitis

• *Adult:* PO 250 mg tid for 7-10 days

Giardiasis

• *Adult:* PO 250 mg tid × 5 days

• *Child:* PO 5 mg/kg tid × 5 days

H. pylori infection

• *Adult:* PO 250 mg 4× daily in combination with 262 mg of bismuth subsalicylate and 500 mg of tetracycline (Helidac), with meals and hs × 14 days, combine with H_2 histamine antagonist

Available forms include: Tabs 250, 375, 500 mg; film-coated tabs 250, 1500 mg; inj IV 5 mg/vial; HCl inj IV 500 mg

Side effects/adverse reactions:

▼ *ORAL:* Dry mouth, furry tongue, bitter taste, metallic taste, glossitis, stomatitis

CNS: Headache, dizziness, ***convulsions,*** confusion, depression, fatigue, drowsiness, insomnia, paresthesia, peripheral neuropathy, incoordination, depression

CV: Flat T waves

GI: Nausea, vomiting, ***pseudomembranous colitis,*** diarrhea, epigastric distress, anorexia, constipation, abdominal cramps

HEMA: ***Leukopenia, bone marrow aplasia***

GU: ***Albuminuria, nephrotoxicity,*** dysuria, cystitis, decreased libido, polyuria, incontinence, dyspareunia

EENT: Blurred vision, sore throat, retinal edema

INTEG: Rash, pruritus, urticaria, flushing

Contraindications: Hypersensitivity to this drug, renal disease, hepatic disease, contracted visual or color fields, blood dyscrasias, pregnancy (first trimester), lactation, CNS disorders

Precautions: *Candida* infections, pregnancy category B (second, third trimesters); avoid unnecessary use because shown to be carcinogenic in rodents

Pharmacokinetics:

IV/PO: Peak 1-2 hr, half-life 6.2-11.5 hr; crosses placenta; excreted in feces

Drug interactions of concern to dentistry:

• Antabuse-like reaction: alcohol, alcohol-containing products

• Decreased action: phenobarbital

DENTAL CONSIDERATIONS

General:

• Patients on chronic drug therapy may rarely have symptoms of blood dyscrasias, which can include infection, bleeding, and poor healing.

• Assess salivary flow as a factor in caries, periodontal disease, and candidiasis.

• Determine why the patient is taking the drug.

Consultations:

• In a patient with symptoms of blood dyscrasias, request a medical consult for blood studies and postpone dental treatment until normal values are reestablished.

• Medical consult may be required to assess disease control in the patient.

Teach patient/family:
• To avoid alcoholic beverages
• That taste alterations may occur
• Importance of good oral hygiene to prevent soft tissue inflammation
• Caution to prevent injury when using oral hygiene aids

When chronic dry mouth occurs, advise patient:
• To avoid mouth rinses with high alcohol content due to drying effects
• To use sugarless gum, frequent sips of water, or saliva substitutes
• To use daily home fluoride products for anticaries effect

mexiletine HCl

(mex'i-le-teen)
Mexitil

Drug class.: Antidysrhythmic (Class IB, lidocaine analog)

Action: Blocks fast sodium channel in His-Purkinje system, which decreases the effective refractory period and shortens the duration of the action potential

Uses: Documented life-threatening ventricular dysrhythmias

Dosage and routes:
• *Adult:* PO 200-400 mg q8h

Available forms include: Caps 150, 200, 250 mg

Side effects/adverse reactions:
▼ *ORAL:* Dry mouth, altered taste, stomatitis

CNS: ***Convulsions,*** headache, dizziness, confusion, tremors, psychosis, nervousness, paresthesia, weakness, fatigue, coordination difficulties, change in sleep habits

CV: ***Heart block, cardiovascular collapse, arrest, left ventricular failure, cardiogenic shock,*** hypotension, bradycardia, angina, PVCs, sinus node slowing, syncope

GI: ***Hepatitis,*** nausea, vomiting, anorexia, diarrhea, abdominal pain, peptic ulcer, GI bleeding

RESP: ***Fibrosis, embolism,*** dyspnea, pneumonia

HEMA: ***Thrombocytopenia, leukopenia, agranulocytosis, hypoplastic anemia,*** SLE syndrome

GU: Urinary hesitancy, decreased libido

EENT: Blurred vision, hearing loss, tinnitus

INTEG: Rash, alopecia, dry skin

MISC: Edema, arthralgia, fever

Contraindications: Hypersensitivity to amides, cardiogenic shock, blood dyscrasias, severe heart block

Precautions: Pregnancy category C, lactation, children, renal disease, liver disease, CHF, respiratory depression, myasthenia gravis

Pharmacokinetics:
PO: Peak 2-3 hr, half-life 12 hr; metabolized by liver; excreted unchanged by kidneys (10%); excreted in breast milk

Drug interactions of concern to dentistry:
• No specific interactions are reported with dental drugs; however, any drug that could affect the cardiac action of mexiletine should be used in the least effective dose, such as other local anesthetics, vasoconstrictors, and anticholinergics

DENTAL CONSIDERATIONS

General:
• Monitor vital signs every appointment due to cardiovascular side effects.
• Patients on chronic drug therapy may rarely have symptoms of blood dyscrasias, which can in-

M

clude infection, bleeding, and poor healing.
- Assess salivary flow as a factor in caries, periodontal disease, and candidiasis.
- Stress from dental procedures may compromise cardiovascular function; determine patient risk.

Consultations:
- In a patient with symptoms of blood dyscrasias, request a medical consult for blood studies and postpone dental treatment until normal values are reestablished.
- Medical consult should be made to assess disease control in the patient.
- Medical consult may be required to assess patient's ability to tolerate stress.

Teach patient/family:
- Importance of good oral hygiene to prevent soft tissue inflammation
- Caution to prevent injury when using oral hygiene aids

When chronic dry mouth occurs, advise patient:
- To avoid mouth rinses with high alcohol content due to drying effects
- To use sugarless gum, frequent sips of water, or saliva substitutes
- To use daily home fluoride products for anticaries effect

miconazole nitrate (topical)

(mi-kon'a-zole)

Micatin, Miconazole-7, Monistat-Derm, Monistat-7, Monistat 3, M-Zole 3

Drug class.: Antifungal

Action: Interferes with fungal cell membrane, which increases permeability, leaking of nutrients

Uses: Tinea pedis, tinea cruris, tinea corporis, tinea versicolor, vaginal or vulvae *Candida albicans*

Dosage and routes:
- *Adult and child:* TOP apply to affected area bid × 2-4 wk
- *Adult:* Intravag give 1 applicator or suppository × 7 days hs; 3-day treatment—intravag insert 200 mg suppository qd with topical cream bid

Available forms include: Cream, lotion, powder, spray 2%; vag cream 2%; vag suppos 100, 200 mg

Side effects/adverse reactions:

GU: Vulvovaginal burning, itching, pelvic cramps

INTEG: Rash, urticaria, stinging, burning, contact dermatitis

Contraindications: Hypersensitivity

Precautions: Child <2 yr, pregnancy category B, lactation

DENTAL CONSIDERATIONS

General:
- Examine oral mucous membranes for signs of fungal infection.
- Broad-spectrum antibiotics may evoke vaginal yeast infections.

Teach patient/family:
- To prevent reinoculation of *Candida* infection, dispose of toothbrush or other contaminated oral hygiene devices used during period of infection

midazolam HCl

(mid'ay-zoe-lam)

Versed

Drug class.: Benzodiazepine general anesthetic, anesthesia adjunct

Controlled Substance Schedule IV

Action: Depresses subcortical levels in CNS; may act on limbic system, reticular formation; may potentiate γ-aminobutyric acid (GABA) by binding to specific benzodiazepine receptors

Uses: Conscious sedation, general anesthesia induction, sedation for diagnostic endoscopic procedures, intubation, preoperative sedation, amnesia

Dosage and routes:

Warning: **Midazolam should be administered by persons trained in the administration of general anesthesia/IV conscious sedation. Patients must be continuously monitored, and facilities for the maintenance of a patent airway, ventilatory support, oxygen supplementation, and circulatory resuscitation must be immediately available.**

ALL DOSES MUST BE INDIVIDUALIZED

Preoperative sedation, ASA I and ASA II <60 yr

• *Adult:* IM 0.07-0.08 mg/kg (usually 5 mg for average adult) 0.5-1 hr before general anesthesia

• *Child:* IM 0.08-0.2 mg/kg 0.5-1 hr before general anesthesia

Induction of general anesthesia

• *Adult <55 yr:* Unpremedicated patients—IV 0.2-0.35 mg/kg over 30 sec, wait 2 min, follow with 25% of initial dose if needed; premedicated patients—0.15-0.35 mg/kg over 20-30 sec, allow 2 min for effect

• *Adult >55 yr:* ASA I or II, unpremedicated—IV 0.15-0.3 mg/kg administered over 20-30 sec; for ASA III or ASA IV, 0.15-0.25 mg/kg over 20-30 sec

Conscious sedation (use 1 mg/ml formulation)

• *Adult <60 yr:* Unpremedicated—IV titrate dose slowly, wait at least 2 min for response, titrate in small increments; doses of more than 5 mg are seldom required; dose may be as low as 1 mg but should not exceed 2.5 mg/min in the average healthy adult; allow at least 2 min to evaluate response; use of the more dilute solution, 1 mg/ml, allows for slower injection control; solutions can be diluted with 0.9% normal saline or dextrose 5% in water; avoid bolus doses; total dose of 5 mg is usually not necessary; patients with narcotic premedication or other CNS depressants: reduce midazolam dose by 30%

• *Adult >60 yr, debilitated:* Unpremedicated—IV (titrate doses) 1 mg or less slowly, wait at least 2 min; total dose of 3.5 mg usually unnecessary; doses must be carefully adjusted for this patient group; patients with other CNS depressant medication: reduce dose by 50%

IV sedation in children

• *Child 6 mo-5 yr:* Caution—IV administer dose over 2-3 min and allow an additional 2-3 min before treatment or giving an additional dose; titrate with small incremental doses; reduce dose if other CNS depressants are used; initial dose 0.05-0.1 mg/kg; do not exceed 6 mg total

• *Child 6-12 yr:* Follow same cautions as for younger children—IV inital dose 0.025-0.05 mg/kg, total dose up to 0.4 mg/kg may be required; do not exceed 10 mg

• *Child 12-16 yr:* IV same as adult dose

Available forms include: Vials 5 mg/ml in 1, 2, 5, 10 ml; 1 mg/ml in 2, 5, 10 ml, syr

Side effects/adverse reactions:

▼ *ORAL:* Increased salivation (be-

cause drugs with anticholinergic action are often used in general anesthesia techniques, salivation is usually not observed), acidic taste
CNS: Retrograde amnesia, headache, oversedation, euphoria, confusion, anxiety, insomnia, slurred speech, paresthesia, weakness, chills, agitation
CV: ***Hypotension, cardiac arrest,*** PVCs, tachycardia, bigeminy, nodal rhythm
GI: Nausea, vomiting, hiccups, increased salivation
RESP: ***Apnea, bronchospasm, respiratory depression, laryngospasm,*** *coughing,* dyspnea
EENT: Blurred vision, nystagmus, diplopia, blocked ears, loss of balance
INTEG: Pain, urticaria, swelling at injection site, rash, pruritus, phlebitis
MS: Involuntary movement, tremor
Contraindications: Hypersensitivity to benzodiazepines, shock, coma, alcohol intoxication, acute narrow-angle glaucoma, ritonavir, nelfinavir, indinavir
Precautions: COPD, CHF, chronic renal failure, chills, elderly, debilitated, pregnancy category D, children <18 yr; to be used only by health care professionals skilled in airway maintenance and ventilation and resuscitation techniques
Pharmacokinetics:
IM: Onset 15 min, peak 0.5-1 hr
IV: Onset 3-5 min, onset of anesthesia 1.5-2.5 min, half-life 1.2-12.3 hr; protein binding 97%; metabolized in liver; metabolites excreted in urine; crosses placenta, blood-brain barrier

Drug interactions of concern to dentistry:
- Prolonged respiratory depression: all CNS depressants, including alcohol, barbiturates, narcotics. *All doses of midazolam must be reduced when used in combination with any CNS depressant. Serious respiratory and cardiovascular depression, including death, has occurred when midazolam is used in combination with other CNS depressants or given too rapidly. Medically compromised and elderly patients are at greater risk.*
- Increased serum levels and prolonged effect of benzodiazepines: erythromycin, ketoconazole, itraconazole, fluconazole, miconazole (systemic), diltiazem
- Contraindicated with nelfinavir, ritonavir, indinavir

DENTAL CONSIDERATIONS
General:
- Monitor vital signs every 5 min during general anesthesia due to cardiovascular and respiratory side effects. Monitor vital signs at regular intervals during recovery.
- Degree of CNS depression is dose dependent; titrate all doses.
- Drug produces amnesia, especially in the elderly patient.
- A longer recovery period could be observed in an obese patient because half-life may be extended.
- Assist patient with ambulation until drowsy period has passed.

Teach patient/family:
- Drug may impair reaction time; avoid driving or potentially hazardous activities until drowsiness or weakness subsides
- That amnesia occurs; events may not be remembered

Treatment of overdose:
- O_2, vasopressors, flumazenil, resuscitation measures as required

miglitol

(mig′li-tol)
Glyset

Drug class.: Oligosaccharide, glucosidase enzyme inhibitor

Action: Inhibits α-glucosidase enzyme in GI tract to slow breakdown of carbohydrates to glucose, which results in reduced plasma glucose levels

Uses: Type 2 diabetes when diet control is ineffective in controlling blood glucose levels, used as single agent or in combination with other oral hypoglycemics

Dosage and routes:

• *Adult:* PO individualize doses; initial dose 25 mg tid with first bite of each meal; maximum recommended dose 100 mg tid; increase initial dose based on side effects and postprandial plasma glucose; usual maintenance dose 50 mg tid

Available forms include: Tabs 25, 50, 100 mg

Side effects/adverse reactions:

GI: Diarrhea, flatulence, abdominal pain, soft stools

INTEG: Rash

MISC: Low serum iron

Contraindications: Hypersensitivity, diabetic ketoacidosis, inflammatory bowel disease, colonic ulceration, partial intestinal obstruction, chronic intestinal diseases associated with disorders of absorption and digestion

Precautions: Renal impairment, hypoglycemia, pregnancy category B, lactation, children

Pharmacokinetics:

PO: Peak plasma levels 2-3 hr; negligible plasma protein binding, not metabolized, urinary excretion

Drug interactions of concern to dentistry:

• None reported with dental drugs; information is lacking at this time

DENTAL CONSIDERATIONS

General:

• Ensure that patient is following prescribed diet and regularly takes medication.

• Type 2 patients may also be using insulin. Should symptomatic hypoglycemia occur while taking this drug, use dextrose rather than sucrose because of interference with sucrose metabolism.

• Place on frequent recall to evaluate healing response.

• Short appointments and a stress reduction protocol may be required for anxious patients.

• Diabetics may be more susceptible to infection and have delayed wound healing.

• Consider semisupine chair position for patient comfort if GI side effects occur.

• Question patient about self-monitoring of drug's antidiabetic effect, including blood glucose values or finger-stick records.

• Examine for oral manifestation of opportunistic infection.

Consultations:

• Medical consult may be required to assess disease control and patient's ability to tolerate stress.

• Medical consult may include data from patient's blood glucose monitoring, including glycosylated hemoglobin or HbA_{1c} testing.

Teach patient/family:

• Importance of updating health and drug history if physician makes any changes in evaluation/drug regimens

• Importance of good oral hygiene to prevent soft tissue inflammation

M

minocycline HCl

(mi-noe-sye'kleen)
Dyancin, Minocin, Vectrin
Drug class.: Tetracycline antiinfective

Action: Inhibits protein synthesis, phosphorylation in microorganisms by binding to 30S ribosomal subunits, reversibly binding to 50S ribosomal subunits; bacteriostatic

Uses: Syphilis, *Chlamydia trachomatis* infection, gonorrhea, lymphogranuloma venereum, rickettsial infections, inflammatory acne, *Mycobacterium marinum, Neisseria* meningitis carriers, actinomycosis, anthrax, ANUG, Aa-induced periodontitis, and other susceptible infections

Dosage and routes:

- *Adult:* PO/IV 200 mg first day, then 100 mg q12h or 50 mg q6h, not to exceed 400 mg/24 hr IV
- *Child >8 yr, <45 kg:* PO/IV 4.4 mg/kg first day, then 2.2 mg/kg/day PO in divided doses q12h

Available forms include: Caps 50, 75, 100 mg; oral susp 25 mg/5 ml; powder for inj IV 100, 200 mg/vial

Side effects/adverse reactions:

▼ *ORAL:* Candidiasis, tooth staining, discolored mucous membranes, discolored tongue, lichenoid reaction

CNS: Dizziness, fever, light-headedness, vertigo

CV: Pericarditis

GI: Nausea, abdominal pain, vomiting, diarrhea, ***hepatotoxicity,*** anorexia, enterocolitis, flatulence, abdominal cramps, epigastric burning

HEMA: ***Eosinophilia, neutropenia, thrombocytopenia, hemolytic anemia***

GU: Increased BUN, ***renal failure, nephrotoxicity,*** polyuria, polydipsia

EENT: Dysphagia

INTEG: Rash, urticaria, photosensitivity, increased pigmentation, ***exfoliative dermatitis,*** pruritus, angioedema, bluish-gray color of skin

Contraindications: Hypersensitivity to tetracyclines, children <8 yr, pregnancy category D

Precautions: Hepatic disease, lactation

Pharmacokinetics:

PO: Peak 2-3 hr, half-life 11-17 hr; 55%-88% protein bound; excreted in urine, feces, breast milk; crosses placenta

Drug interactions of concern to dentistry:

- Decreased effect: antacids, milk, or other calcium- and aluminum-containing products
- Decreased effect of penicillins, oral contraceptives

DENTAL CONSIDERATIONS

General:

- This drug is reported to cause intrinsic staining in erupted permanent teeth not associated with the calcification stage.
- The drug readily distributes to gingival crevicular fluid.
- Do not precribe drug during pregnancy or before age 8 yr due to tooth discoloration.
- Caution patients about driving or performing other tasks requiring alertness.
- Advise patient if dental drugs prescribed have a potential for photosensitivity.
- Do not use ingestible sodium bicarbonate products such as the

air polishing system (Prophy Jet) at the same time dose is taken; take minocycline 2 hr later.

• Determine why the patient is taking the drug.

Consultations:

• Medical consult may be required to assess disease control in the patient.

Teach patient/family:

• Importance of good oral hygiene to prevent soft tissue inflammation
• Caution to prevent injury when using oral hygiene aids
• To avoid mouth rinses with high alcohol content due to drying effects

When used for dental infection, advise patient:

• Taking birth control pill to use additional method of contraception for duration of cycle
• To report sore throat, oral burning sensation, fever, fatigue, any of which could indicate superinfection
• To take at prescribed intervals and complete dosage regimen
• To immediately notify the dentist if signs or symptoms of infection increase

minoxidil

(mi-nox'i-dil)

Systemic: Loniten

Topical: Rogaine for Men, Rogaine for Women

🍁 Apo-gain, Gen-Minoxidil, Minoxigaine

Drug class.: Antihypertensive

Action: Directly relaxes arteriolar smooth muscle, reducing peripheral resistance

Uses: Severe hypertension not responsive to other therapy (used with a diuretic); topically to treat alopecia (mechanism unknown)

Dosage and routes:

• *Adult:* PO 5 mg/day, not to exceed 100 mg daily; usual range 10-40 mg/day in single doses
• *Child <12 yr:* Initial 0.2 mg/kg/day; effective range 0.25-1 mg/kg/day; max 50 mg/day

Alopecia

• *Adult:* Apply topically; rub 1 ml into scalp bid

Available forms include: Tabs 2.5, 10 mg; top 20 mg/ml

Side effects/adverse reactions:

CNS: Drowsiness, dizziness, sedation, headache, depression, fatigue

CV: Severe rebound hypertension on withdrawal, ***CHF, pulmonary edema, pericardial effusion,*** tachycardia, angina, increased T wave, edema, sodium/water retention

GI: Nausea, vomiting

HEMA: Hct, Hgb, erythrocyte count may decrease initially

GU: Gynecomastia, breast tenderness

INTEG: ***Stevens-Johnson syndrome,*** pruritus, rash, hirsutism

Contraindications: Acute MI, dissecting aortic aneurysm, hypersensitivity, pheochromocytoma

Precautions: Pregnancy category C, lactation, children, renal disease, CAD, CHF

Pharmacokinetics:

PO: Onset 30 min, peak 2-3 hr, duration 75 hr, half-life 4.2 hr; metabolized in liver; metabolites excreted in urine, feces

Drug interactions of concern to dentistry:

• Decreased effects: NSAIDs, indomethacin, sympathomimetics

• Increased hypotension: CNS depressant drug used in conscious sedation technique may also lower blood pressure

DENTAL CONSIDERATIONS

General:

• Monitor vital signs every appointment due to cardiovascular side effects.

• Patients on chronic drug therapy may rarely have symptoms of blood dyscrasias, which can include infection, bleeding, and poor healing.

• Limit use of sodium-containing products, such as saline IV fluids, for patients with a dietary salt restriction.

• Short appointments and a stress reduction protocol may be required for anxious patients.

• After supine positioning, have patient sit upright for at least 2 min before standing to avoid orthostatic hypotension.

Consultations:

• In a patient with symptoms of blood dyscrasias, request a medical consult for blood studies and postpone dental treatment until normal values are reestablished.

• Medical consult may be required to assess disease control and stress tolerance in the patient.

mirtazapine

(mir-taz'a-peen)

Remeron

Drug class.: Tetracyclic antidepressant

Action: Mechanism of antidepressant effect is unknown; acts in CNS as an antagonist for presynaptic α_2-adrenergic inhibitory receptors, antagonizes serotonin 5-HT_2 and 5-HT_3 receptors and histamine H_1 receptors

Uses: Depression

Dosage and routes:

• *Adult:* PO initial dose 15 mg qd in PM, effective dose range 15-45 mg/day, allow 1-2 wk between dose changes to evaluate response

Available forms include: Tabs 15, 30, 45 mg

Side effects/adverse reactions:

▼ *ORAL: Dry mouth (25%), thirst,* glossitis, gingival hemorrhage, stomatitis (rare), tongue discoloration, ulcerative stomatitis, salivary gland enlargement, increased salivation, aphthous stomatitis, candidiasis, tongue edema

CNS: Somnolence, dizziness, abnormal dreams, malaise, mania, hypomania, confusion, tremor, migraine

CV: Peripheral edema, hypertension, vasodilation, ***MI,*** angina pectoris, bradycardia, syncope, hypotension

GI: Nausea, constipation, vomiting, abdominal pain, anorexia, increased ALT

RESP: Cough, flulike syndrome, dyspnea

HEMA: ***Agranulocytosis, leukopenia, thrombocytopenia,*** lymphadenopathy, lymphocytosis, pancytopenia, petechia, anemia (all rare)

GU: Urinary frequency

EENT: Sinusitis, eye pain

INTEG: Rash, pruritus, dry skin, herpes simplex, herpes zoster, photosensitivity

MS: Asthenia, arthralgia, back pain, myalgia, neck pain, neck rigidity

MISC: Increased appetite, weight gain, increased cholesterol/triglycerides

Contraindications: Hypersensitivity, MAO inhibitors

Precautions: Hepatic impairment, renal impairment, elderly, pregnancy category C, nursing, pediatric, suicidal ideation, cardiovascular or cerebrovascular disease aggravated by hypotension, avoid alcohol use

Pharmacokinetics:

PO: Rapid absorption, half-life 20-40 hr; peak levels 2 hr, liver metabolism, bioavailability 50%, urinary excretion, 85% plasma protein binding

Drug interactions of concern to dentistry:

- Impairment of cognitive and motor performance with diazepam or other drugs used in conscious sedation
- Use opioid analgesics with caution due to impairment of cognitive or motor performance; NSAIDs may be a more appropriate choice

DENTAL CONSIDERATIONS

General:

- Patients on chronic drug therapy may rarely have symptoms of blood dyscrasias, which can include infection, bleeding, and poor healing.
- Assess salivary flow as a factor in caries, periodontal disease, candidiasis.
- Monitor vital signs every appointment due to cardiovascular side effects.
- Consider semisupine chair position when GI or MS side effects occur.
- Place on frequent recall if oral side effects are a problem.

Consultations:

- In a patient with symptoms of blood dyscrasias, request a medical consult for blood studies and postpone dental treatment until normal values are reestablished.
- Take precaution if dental surgery is anticipated and sedation or general anesthesia is required; there is risk of hypotensive episode.
- Medical consult may be required to assess disease control in the patient.
- Physician should be informed if significant xerostomic side effects occur (increased caries, sore tongue, problems eating or swallowing, difficulty wearing prosthesis) so a medication change can be considered.

Teach patient/family:

- Importance of good oral hygiene to prevent soft tissue inflammation
- Caution to prevent soft tissue trauma when using oral hygiene aids
- Importance of updating health history/drug record if physician makes any changes in evaluations/drug regimens
- Caution about driving or performing other tasks requiring alertness

When chronic dry mouth occurs, advise patient:

- To avoid mouth rinses with high alcohol content due to drying effects
- To use daily home fluoride products for anticaries effect
- To use sugarless gum, frequent sips of water, or saliva substitutes

misoprostol

(mye-soe-prost'ole)

Cytotec

Drug class.: Gastric mucosa protectant

Action: A prostaglandin E_1 analog that inhibits gastric acid secretion, may protect gastric mucosa; can

M

increase bicarbonate, mucus production

Uses: Prevention of onsteroidal antiinflammatory drug–induced gastric ulcers; unapproved use: duodenal ulcers

Dosage and routes:

• *Adult:* PO 200 μg qid with food for duration of NSAID therapy; if 200 μg is not tolerated, 100 μg may be given

Available forms include: Tabs 100, 200 μg

Side effects/adverse reactions:

GI: Diarrhea, nausea, vomiting, flatulence, constipation, dyspepsia, abdominal pain

GU: Spotting, cramps, hypermenorrhea, menstrual disorders

Contraindications: Hypersensitivity, pregnancy category X

Precautions: Lactation, children, elderly, renal disease

Pharmacokinetics:

PO: Peak 12 min; plasma steady state achieved within 2 days; excreted in urine

DENTAL CONSIDERATIONS

General:

• Avoid NSAIDs and salicylates in patients with upper active GI disease; acetaminophen/opioids are more appropriate for pain control in these patients.

Consultations:

• Medical consult may be required to assess disease control in the patient.

---

mitotane

(mye′toe-tane)

Lysodren

Drug class.: Antineoplastic

Action: Acts on adrenal cortex to suppress activity and adrenal steroid production

Uses: Adrenocortical carcinoma; unapproved: Cushing's syndrome

Dosage and routes:

• *Adult:* PO 2-6 g/day in divided doses tid or qid; can increase to 10 g; may need to decrease dose if severe reactions occur

Available forms include: Tabs 500 mg

Side effects/adverse reactions:

CNS: Lethargy, somnolence, vertigo, dizziness, light-headedness, flushing, sedation

GI: Nausea, vomiting, anorexia, diarrhea

GU: ***Proteinuria, hematuria***

EENT: Blurring, retinopathy, double vision

INTEG: Rash

ENDO: ***Adrenal cortical insufficiency***

MS: Muscle ache

Contraindications: Hypersensitivity

Precautions: Lactation, hepatic disease, pregnancy category C, infection

Pharmacokinetics: Adequately absorbed orally (40%), half-life 18-159 days; hepatic metabolism; excreted in urine, bile

Drug interactions of concern to dentistry:

• Increased CNS depression: all CNS depressants

• Decreased effects of corticosteroids; if glucocorticoid replacement is needed, use hydrocortisone

DENTAL CONSIDERATIONS

General:

• Evaluate respiration characteristics and rate.

• Drug may cause adrenal hypofunction, especially under conditions of stress such as surgery, trauma, or acute illness. Patients should be carefully monitored and given hydrocortisone or mineralocorticoid as needed.

- Consider semisupine chair position for patient comfort if GI side effects occur.
- Patients taking opioids for acute or chronic pain should be given alternative analgesics for dental pain.

Consultations:

- Medical consult may be required to assess disease control and patient's ability to tolerate stress.

Teach patient/family:

- That secondary oral infection may occur; must see dentist immediately if infection occurs
- To report oral lesions, soreness, or bleeding to dentist
- Importance of updating medical/drug record if physican makes any changes in evaluation or drug regimen

modafinil

(mo-daf'i-nil)
Provigil

Drug class.: CNS stimulant (orphan drug status)

Action: Mechanism of action remains uncertain; has wake-promoting actions similar to amphetamine and other sympathomimetics; may have CNS α_1-receptor agonist activity; enhancement of dopamine has also been observed in animals

Uses: Improve wakefulness in narcolepsy

Dosage and routes:

- *Adult:* PO 200 mg qd, 400 mg/day doses have been used

Available forms include: Tabs 100, 200 mg

Side effects/adverse reactions:

▼ *ORAL:* Orofacial dyskinesia, dry mouth

CNS: Headache, nervousness, anxiety, insomnia, depression, cataplexy, confusion, amnesia

CV: Hypertension, hypotension

GI: Nausea, diarrhea, anorexia

RESP: Rhinitis, pharyngitis

EENT: Blurred vision

INTEG: Dry skin

META: Abnormal liver function

Contraindications: Hypersensitivity

Precautions: Ischemic heart disease, left ventricular hypertrophy, mitral valve prolapse, recent MI, unstable angina, renal impairment, hepatic impairment, pregnancy category C, lactation, children <16 yr, drug abuse

Pharmacokinetics:

PO: Absorption delayed by food, peak plasma levels 2-4 hr, plasma protein binding (60%), hepatic metabolism, excreted mostly in urine (81%), produces hepatic cytochrome P-450 enzymes (CYP3A4)

Drug interactions of concern to dentistry:

- No documented dental drug interactions reported; however, because it induces cytochrome P-450 enzymes, other P-450 enzyme inducers or inhibitors could result in a drug interaction: antifungal agents, erythromycin

DENTAL CONSIDERATIONS

General:

- Monitor vital signs every appointment due to cardiovascular side effects.
- Assess salivary flow as a factor in caries, periodontal disease, and candidiasis.

M

• Consider semisupine chair position for patient comfort due to GI side effects of drug.
• Short appointments and a stress reduction protocol may be required for anxious patients.

Teach patient/family:
• To prevent trauma when using oral hygiene aids

When chronic dry mouth occurs, advise patient:
• To avoid mouth rinses with high alcohol content due to drying effects
• To use daily home fluoride products for anticaries effect
• To use sugarless gum, frequent sips of water, or saliva substitutes

---

moexipril hydrochloride

(moe′x-i-pril)
Univasc

Drug class.: Angiotensin-converting enzyme (ACE) inhibitor

Action: Selectively suppresses renin-angiotensin-aldosterone system; inhibits ACE; prevents conversion of angiotensin I to angiotensin II; results in dilation of arterial, venous vessels; decreased aldosterone secretion results in diuresis and natriuresis

Uses: Hypertension as a single drug or in combination with a thiazide diuretic

Dosages and routes:

As single drug
• *Adult:* PO 7.5 mg 1 hr ac daily; range 7.5-39 mg/day in 1 or 2 divided doses 1 hr ac

With diuretic
• *Adult:* PO as single drug, but discontinue diuretic 2-3 days to avoid symptomatic hypotension; then restart diuretic carefully, if required; otherwise start with 3.75 mg under medical supervision

Renal impairment
• *Adult:* Dose limited to 15 mg/day

Available forms include: Tabs 7.5, 15 mg

Side effects/adverse reactions:
▼ *ORAL:* ***Angioedema,*** dry mouth (<1%)
CNS: Dizziness, fatigue
CV: Symptomatic hypotension, postural hypotension, hyperkalemia, peripheral edema, chest pain, palpitation
GI: Diarrhea, ***hepatic failure***
RESP: Cough, pharyngitis
HEMA: ***Neutropenia, agranulocytosis***
GU: ***Acute renal failure,*** oliguria, azotemia, urinary frequency
EENT: Tinnitus
INTEG: Flushing, rash, photosensitivity
MS: Myalgia
MISC: ***Anaphylactic reactions***

Contraindications: Hypersensitivity, pregnancy (second or third trimester), angioedema history with other ACE inhibitors

Precautions: Food retards absorption, renal or hepatic impairment, CHF, SLE, scleroderma, renal artery stenosis, lactation, children, pregnancy categories C (first trimester) and D (second and third trimesters)

Pharmacokinetics:
PO: Peak plasma levels 1.5 hr; converted to active metabolite (moexiprilat); 50% plasma protein bound; excreted in urine, feces

Drug interactions of concern to dentistry:
• IV fluids containing potassium: risk of hyperkalemia
• Increased hypotension: other hy-

potensive drugs, alcohol, phenothiazines
• Decreased hypotensive effects: indomethacin, possibly other NSAIDs, sympathomimetics

DENTAL CONSIDERATIONS

General:

• Monitor vital signs every appointment due to cardiovascular side effects.
• After supine positioning, have patient sit upright for at least 2 min before standing to avoid orthostatic hypotension.
• Take precautions if dental surgery is anticipated and general anesthesia is required.
• Patients on chronic drug therapy may rarely have symptoms of blood dyscrasias, which can include infection, bleeding, and poor healing.
• Stress from dental procedures may compromise cardiovascular function; determine patient risk.
• Assess salivary flow as a factor in caries, periodontal disease, and candidiasis.
• Short appointments and a stress reduction protocol may be required for anxious patients.

Consultations:

• Medical consult may be required to assess disease control and patient's ability to tolerate stress.
• In a patient with symptoms of blood dyscrasias, request a medical consult for blood studies and postpone dental treatment until normal values are reestablished.

Teach patient/family:

• Importance of good oral hygiene to prevent soft tissue inflammation
• Caution to prevent trauma when using oral hygiene aids
• To report oral lesions, soreness, or bleeding to dentist

When chronic dry mouth occurs, advise patient:

• To avoid mouth rinses with high alcohol content due to drying effects
• Of need for daily home fluoride to prevent caries
• To use sugarless gum, frequent sips of water, or saliva substitutes

---

molindone HCl

(moe-lin'done)

Moban, Moban Concentrate

Drug class.: Antipsychotic

Action: Depresses cerebral cortex, hypothalamus, limbic system, which control activity, aggression; blocks neurotransmission produced by dopamine at synapse; exhibits strong α-adrenergic, anticholinergic blocking action; mechanism for antipsychotic effects is unclear

Uses: Psychotic disorders

Dosage and routes:

• *Adult:* PO 50-75 mg/day, increasing to 225 mg/day if needed

Available forms include: Tabs 5, 10, 25, 50, 100 mg; conc 20 mg/ml

Side effects/adverse reactions:

▼ *ORAL: Dry mouth*

CNS: Extrapyramidal symptoms: pseudoparkinsonism, akathisia, dystonia, tardive dyskinesia, drowsiness, headache, seizures

CV: Orthostatic hypotension, ***cardiac arrest, tachycardia,*** ECG changes, hypertension

GI: Nausea, vomiting, anorexia, constipation, diarrhea, jaundice, weight gain

RESP: ***Laryngospasm, respiratory depression,*** dyspnea

HEMA: ***Anemia, leukopenia, leukocytosis, agranulocytosis***

M

GU: Urinary retention, urinary frequency, enuresis, impotence, amenorrhea, gynecomastia, menstrual irregularities
EENT: Blurred vision, glaucoma
INTEG: Rash, photosensitivity, dermatitis
Contraindications: Hypersensitivity, coma, child
Precautions: Pregnancy category C, lactation, hypertension, hepatic disease, cardiac disease, Parkinson's disease, brain tumor, glaucoma, urinary retention, diabetes mellitus, respiratory disease, prostatic hypertrophy
Pharmacokinetics:
PO: Onset erratic, peak 1.5 hr, duration 24-36 hr, half-life 1.5 hr; metabolized by liver; excreted in urine, feces; may cross placenta; excreted in breast milk
Drug interactions of concern to dentistry:
• Increased sedation: alcohol, other CNS depressants
• Increased anticholinergic effect: anticholinergics, antihistamines
DENTAL CONSIDERATIONS
General:
• Patients on chronic drug therapy may rarely have symptoms of blood dyscrasias, which can include infection, bleeding, and poor healing.
• Assess salivary flow as a factor in caries, periodontal disease, and candidiasis.
• After supine positioning, have patient sit upright for at least 2 min before standing to avoid orthostatic hypotension.
• Assess for presence of extrapyramidal motor symptoms, such as tardive dyskinesia and akathisia. Extrapyramidal motor activity may complicate dental treatment.
• Geriatric patients are more susceptible to drug effects; use lower dose.
• Use vasoconstrictors with caution, in low doses, and with careful aspiration.
Consultations:
• In a patient with symptoms of blood dyscrasias, request a medical consult for blood studies and postpone dental treatment until normal values are reestablished.
• Medical consult may be required to assess disease control in the patient.
Teach patient/family:
• Importance of good oral hygiene to prevent soft tissue inflammation
• Caution to prevent injury when using oral hygiene aids
When chronic dry mouth occurs, advise patient:
• To avoid mouth rinses with high alcohol content due to drying effects
• To use sugarless gum, frequent sips of water, or saliva substitutes
• To use daily home fluoride products for anticaries effect

montelukast sodium

(mon-te-loo'kast)
Singulair
Drug class.: Selective leukotriene receptor antagonist

Action: Competitive and selective antagonist for cysteinyl leukotriene receptor ($CysLT_1$)
Uses: Prophylaxis and chronic treatment of asthma
Dosage and routes:
• *Adult and child >15 yr:* PO 10 mg hs
• *Child 6-14 yr:* PO 5 mg chewable tab hs

Available forms include: Tabs 5 mg (chewable), 10 mg

Side effects/adverse reactions:

▼ *ORAL: Unspecified dental pain*

CNS: Dizziness, headache

GI: Abdominal pain, dyspepsia, gastroenteritis

RESP: Cough, influenza

EENT: Nasal congestion

META: Increased ALT and AST

MS: Asthenia

MISC: Fatigue

Contraindications: Hypersensitivity

Precautions: Not for acute asthma attacks, not for treatment of exercise-induced bronchospasm or ASA-induced bronchospasm, chewable tablets contain aspartame, pregnancy category B, lactation

Pharmacokinetics:

PO: Rapidly absorbed, peak levels 3-4 hr, bioavailability 73%-64%, highly plasma protein bound (99%), extensive hepatic metabolism, excretion in bile

Drug interactions of concern to dentistry:

• None reported

DENTAL CONSIDERATIONS

General:

• Midday appointments and a stress reduction protocol may be required for anxious patients.

• Avoid prescribing aspirin-containing products.

• Acute asthmatic episodes may be precipitated in the dental office. Rapid-acting sympathomimetic inhalants should be available for emergency use. A stress reduction protocol may be required.

• Be aware that aspirin or sulfite preservatives in vasoconstrictor-containing products can exacerbate asthma.

• Consider semisupine chair position for patients with respiratory disease and when GI side effects are a problem.

Consultations:

• Medical consult may be required to assess disease control in the patient.

Teach patient/family:

• Importance of updating health and drug history if physician makes any changes in evaluation/drug regimens

moricizine

(mor-i'siz-een)

Ethmozine

Drug class.: Antidysrhythmic, type I

Action: Decreased rate of rise of action potential, which prolongs the refractory period and shortens the action potential duration; depression of inward influx if sodium mediates the effects; drug may slow atrial and AV nodal conduction

Uses: Documented life-threatening dysrhythmias

Dosage and routes:

• *Adult:* PO 600-900 mg/day in 3 divided doses

Available forms include: Film-coated tabs 200, 250, 300 mg

Side effects/adverse reactions:

▼ *ORAL:* Dry mouth, altered taste, stomatitis, swelling of lips and tongue

CNS: Dizziness, headache, fatigue, perioral numbness, euphoria, nervousness, sleep disorders, depression, tinnitus, fatigue

*CV: **MI,*** palpitation, chest pain, CHF, hypertension, syncope, dysrhythmias, bradycardia, thrombophlebitis

GI: Nausea, abdominal pain, vomiting, diarrhea
RESP: ***Apnea,*** dyspnea, hyperventilation, asthma, pharyngitis, cough
GU: Sexual dysfunction, difficult urination, dysuria, incontinence
MISC: Sweating, musculoskeletal pain
Contraindications: Second- and third-degree heart block, right bundle branch block, cardiogenic shock, hypersensitivity
Precautions: CHF, hypokalemia, hyperkalemia, sick sinus syndrome, pregnancy category B, lactation, children, impaired hepatic and renal function, cardiac dysfunction
Pharmacokinetics: Peak 0.5-2.2 hr, half-life 1.5-3.5 hr; protein binding >90%; metabolized by the liver; metabolites excreted in feces, urine
Drug interactions of concern to dentistry:
• No specific interactions are reported with dental drugs; however, any drug that could affect the cardiac action of moricizine should be used in the least effective dose (other local anesthetics, vasoconstrictors, anticholinergics)
DENTAL CONSIDERATIONS
General:
• Monitor vital signs every appointment due to cardiovascular side effects.
• Assess salivary flow as a factor in caries, periodontal disease, and candidiasis.
• Stress from dental procedures may compromise cardiovascular function; determine patient risk.
Consultations:
• Medical consult should be made to assess disease control and patient's ability to tolerate stress.
Teach patient/family:
• Importance of good oral hygiene to prevent soft tissue inflammation
• Caution to prevent injury when using oral hygiene aids
When chronic dry mouth occurs, advise patient:
• To avoid mouth rinses with high alcohol content due to drying effects
• To use sugarless gum, frequent sips of water, or saliva substitutes
• To use daily home fluoride products for anticaries effect

---

morphine sulfate
(mor′feen)
Duramorph PF, Kadian, MS Contin, RMS, Roxanol, Roxanol SR
♣ MOS
Drug class.: Narcotic analgesic

Controlled Substance Schedule II, Canada N
Action: Depresses pain impulse transmission at the CNS by interacting with opioid receptors
Uses: Severe pain
Dosage and routes:
• *Adult:* SC/IM 4-15 mg q4h prn; PO 10-30 mg q4h prn; ext rel q12-24h; rec 10-20 mg q4h prn; IV 4-10 mg diluted in 4-5 ml of water for injection, over 5 min
• *Child:* SC 0.1-0.2 mg/kg, not to exceed 15 mg
Available forms include: Inj SC/IM/IV 2, 4, 5, 8, 10, 15 mg/ml; tabs 10, 15, 30 mg; oral sol 10, 20 mg/5 ml, 20 mg/10 ml, 20 mg/ml; oral tabs 15, 30 mg; rec suppos 5, 10, 20 mg; ext rel tabs 30, 60 mg; ext rel caps 20, 50, 100 mg
Side effects/adverse reactions:
▼ *ORAL:* Dry mouth

CNS: Drowsiness, dizziness, confusion, headache, sedation, euphoria
CV: Palpitation, bradycardia, change in BP
GI: Nausea, vomiting, anorexia, constipation, cramps, biliary tract pressure
*RESP: **Respiratory depression***
GU: Increased urinary output, dysuria, urinary retention
EENT: Tinnitus, blurred vision, miosis, diplopia
INTEG: Rash, urticaria, bruising, flushing, diaphoresis, pruritus

Contraindications: Hypersensitivity, addiction (narcotic), hemorrhage, bronchial asthma, increased intracranial pressure, MAO inhibitors

Precautions: Addictive personality, pregnancy category C, lactation, MI (acute), severe heart disease, elderly, respiratory depression, hepatic disease, renal disease, child <18 yr

Pharmacokinetics:
PO: Onset variable, peak variable, duration variable
SC: Onset 15-30 min, peak 50-90 min, duration 3-5 hr
IV: Peak 20 min
Half-life 2.5-3 hr; metabolized by liver; excreted by kidneys; crosses placenta; excreted in breast milk

Drug interactions of concern to dentistry:

- Increased CNS depression: alcohol, all CNS depressants
- Contraindication: MAO inhibitors
- Increased effects of anticholinergics

DENTAL CONSIDERATIONS

General:

- Monitor vital signs every appointment due to cardiovascular and respiratory side effects.
- Assess salivary flow as a factor in caries, periodontal disease, and candidiasis.
- After supine positioning, have patient sit upright for at least 2 min before standing to avoid orthostatic hypotension.
- Psychologic and physical dependence may occur with chronic administration.
- Determine why the patient is taking the drug.
- Consider the use of NSAIDs when additional analgesia is required.

Teach patient/family:

When chronic dry mouth occurs, advise patient:

- To use daily home fluoride products for anticaries effect
- To avoid mouth rinses with high alcohol content due to drying effects
- To use sugarless gum, frequent sips of water, or saliva substitutes

mupirocin/mupirocin calcium

(myoo-peer'o-sin)
Bactroban, Bactroban Nasal 2%
Drug class.: Topical antiinfective, pseudomonic acid A

Action: Inhibits bacterial protein synthesis

Uses: Impetigo caused by *S. aureus,* beta-hemolytic streptococci, *S. pyogenes;* nasal membranes: *S. aureus*

Dosage and routes:

- *TOP:* Apply small amount to affected area tid
- *NASAL:* Divide one half of the ointment from the single-use tube between the nostrils and apply bid for 5 days

M

Available forms include: Oint 2% (20 mg/g), 15, 30 g; nasal oint 2% single-use tube 1 g

Side effects/adverse reactions:

INTEG: Burning, stinging, itching, rash, dry skin, swelling, contact dermatitis, erythema, tenderness, increased exudate

Contraindications: Hypersensitivity

Precautions: Pregnancy category B, lactation

DENTAL CONSIDERATIONS

General:

• The dentist may choose to avoid elective dental treatment if the infected site may be affected by dental treatment.

---

mycophenolate mofetil

(mye-koe-fen′oh-late moe′fe-til)

CellCept

Drug class.: Immunosuppressant

Action: Selective inhibitor of inosine monophosphate dehydrogenase, thereby preventing the synthesis of guanosine nucleotide and resulting in cytostatic effects on T and B lymphocytes

Uses: Prophylaxis of organ rejection in patients receiving allogenic renal transplants, cardiac transplants (in combination with cyclosporine and corticosteroids)

Dosage and routes:

• *Adult:* PO 1 g bid in combination with cortiocosteroids and cyclosporine in renal transplant (within 72 hr of transplant)

Available forms include: Tabs 500 mg; caps 250 mg; powder for inj 500 mg

Side effects/adverse reactions:

▼ *ORAL: Candidiasis*

CNS: Fever, headache, tremor, insomnia, dizziness

CV: Hypertension, chest pain, peripheral edema

GI: Diarrhea, abdominal pain, nausea, dyspepsia, vomiting, GI bleeding

RESP: Infection, dyspnea, cough, pharyngitis

HEMA: ***Leukopenia, sepsis, anemia, thrombocytopenia***

GU: Infection, hematuria, ***renal tubular necrosis***

INTEG: Acne, rash

MS: Back pain, asthenia

Contraindications: Hypersensitivity

Precautions: Active GI diseases, pregnancy category C, lactation, reduce dose in severe chronic renal impairment, increased risk of development of lymphomas or other malignancies and susceptibility to infection

Pharmacokinetics:

PO: Rapidly absorbed; highly plasma bound (97%); metabolized to mycophenolic acid (MPA), the active form of the drug; primary excretion in urine (93%)

Drug interactions of concern to dentistry:

• Increased plasma concentration: acyclovir

• Decreased availability of MPA: drugs that alter the GI flora

DENTAL CONSIDERATIONS

General:

• Determine why the patient is taking the drug.

• Short appointments and a stress reduction protocol may be required for anxious patients.

• Patients who have been or are currently on chronic steroid therapy (>2 wk) may require supplemental steroids for dental treatment.

• Patients on chronic drug therapy may rarely have symptoms of blood dyscrasias, which can include infection, bleeding, and poor healing.

• Place on frequent recall due to oral side effects.

• Determine dose and duration of steroid for patient to assess risk for stress tolerance and immunosuppression.

• Examine for oral manifestation of opportunistic infections.

• Monitor vital signs every appointment due to cardiovascular and respiratory side effects.

• Consider semisupine chair position for patient comfort if GI side effects occur.

• Antibiotic prophylaxis is usually recommended in patients with organ transplants and immunosuppression.

• Monitor time since organ/tissue transplant; note duration of transplant and status of renal function.

• Place on frequent recall due to possible blood dyscrasias and oral side effects.

Consultations:

• Medical consult may be required to assess disease control and patient's ability to tolerate stress.

• In a patient with symptoms of blood dyscrasias, request a medical consult for blood studies and postpone dental treatment until normal values are reestablished.

• Request baseline blood pressure in renal transplant patients for patient evaluation before dental treatment.

Teach patient/family:

• That secondary oral infection may occur; must see dentist immediately if infection occurs

• Importance of good oral hygiene to prevent soft tissue inflammation

• Need for frequent recall due to possible blood dyscrasias and oral side effects

• To report oral lesions, soreness, or bleeding to dentist

nabumetone

(na-byoo′me-tone)

Relafen

Drug class.: Nonsteroidal antiinflammatory

Action: Inhibits prostaglandin synthesis by interfering with cyclooxygenase needed for biosynthesis; possesses analgesic, antiinflammatory, antipyretic properties

Uses: Osteoarthritis, rheumatoid arthritis, acute or chronic treatment

Dosage and routes:

• *Adult:* PO 1000 mg as a single dose; may increase to 1500-2000 mg/day if needed; may give qd or bid

Available forms include: Tabs 500, 750 mg

Side effects/adverse reactions:

▼ *ORAL:* Dry mouth, bleeding, stomatitis, lichenoid reactions

CNS: Dizziness, headache, drowsiness, fatigue, tremors, confusion, insomnia, anxiety, depression, nervousness

CV: Tachycardia, peripheral edema, palpitation, dysrhythmias, CHF

GI: ***Cholestatic hepatitis,*** constipation, flatulence, cramps, peptic ulcer, gastritis, nausea, anorexia, vomiting, diarrhea, jaundice

RESP: ***Bronchospasm,*** dyspnea, pharyngitis

N

HEMA: ***Blood dyscrasias***
GU: ***Nephrotoxicity, dysuria, hematuria, oliguria, azotemia,*** cystitis
EENT: Tinnitus, hearing loss, blurred vision
INTEG: Purpura, rash, pruritus, sweating, photosensitivity

Contraindications: Hypersensitivity to this drug or aspirin, iodides, NSAIDs, asthma, severe renal disease

Precautions: Pregnancy category C, lactation, children, bleeding disorders, GI disorders, cardiac disorders, renal disorders, hepatic dysfunction, elderly

Pharmacokinetics:
PO: Peak 2.5-4 hr, half-life 22-30 hr; plasma protein binding >90%; metabolized in liver to active metabolite; excreted in urine (metabolites), breast milk

Drug interactions of concern to dentistry:
• GI ulceration, bleeding: aspirin, alcohol, corticosteroids
• May decrease effects of nabumetone: salicylates
• Nephrotoxicity: acetaminophen (prolonged use and high doses)
• Possible risk of decreased renal function: cyclosporine

When prescribed for dental pain:
• Risk of increased effects: oral anticoagulants, oral antidiabetics, lithium, methotrexate
• Decreased antihypertensive effects of diuretics, β-adrenergic blockers, and ACE inhibitors

DENTAL CONSIDERATIONS
General:
• Patients on chronic drug therapy may rarely have symptoms of blood dyscrasias, which can include infection, bleeding, and poor healing.
• Assess salivary flow as a factor in caries, periodontal disease, and candidiasis.
• Avoid prescribing for dental use in last trimester of pregnancy.
• Avoid prescribing aspirin-containing products.
• Consider semisupine chair position for patients with arthritic disease.

Consultations:
• In a patient with symptoms of blood dyscrasias, request a medical consult for blood studies and postpone dental treatment until normal values are reestablished.
• Medical consult may be required to assess disease control in the patient.

Teach patient/family:
• Importance of good oral hygiene to prevent soft tissue inflammation
• Caution to prevent injury when using oral hygiene aids

When chronic dry mouth occurs, advise patient:
• To avoid mouth rinses with high alcohol content due to drying effects
• Of need for daily home fluoride
• To use sugarless gum, frequent sips of water, or saliva substitutes

---

nadolol

(nay-doe'lole)
Corgard
♣ Syn-Nadolo

Drug class.: Nonselective β-adrenergic blocker

Action: This is a nonselective β_1- and β_2-adrenergic antagonist. The antihypertensive mechanism of action is unclear, but it may include a reduction in cardiac output and inhibition of renin release by the renal juxtaglomerular apparatus. Peripheral resistance decreases with long-term use. The antianginal action (when indicated for this use) may be related to a decrease in myocardial oxygen demand and negative chronotropic and inotropic effects. The antiarrhythmic action (when indicated for this use) has been related to a reduction in spontaneous pacemaker firing and slowing of AV nodal conduction.

Uses: Chronic stable angina pectoris, mild-to-moderate hypertension; unapproved use: dysrhythmias, MI prophylaxis, vascular headache

Dosage and routes:

• *Adult:* PO 40 mg qd, increase by 40-80 mg q3-7d; maintenance 40-240 mg/day for angina, 40-320 mg/day for hypertension

Available forms include: Oral tabs 20, 40, 80, 120, 160 mg

Side effects/adverse reactions:

▼ *ORAL:* Dry mouth, taste disturbances

CNS: Depression, hallucinations, dizziness, fatigue, lethargy, paresthesia, headache

CV: Bradycardia, hypotension, ***CHF,*** palpitation, AV block

GI: Nausea, vomiting, diarrhea, colitis, constipation, cramps, flatulence, hepatomegaly, pancreatitis

RESP: ***Laryngospasm, bronchospasm,*** dyspnea, respiratory dysfunction, cough, wheezing, nasal stuffiness, pharyngitis

HEMA: ***Agranulocytosis, thrombocytopenia,*** chest pain, peripheral ischemia, flushing, edema, vasodilation, conduction disturbances

EENT: Sore throat

INTEG: Rash, pruritus, fever

Contraindications: Hypersensitivity to this drug, cardiac failure, cardiogenic shock, second- or third-degree heart block, bronchospastic disease, sinus bradycardia, CHF, COPD

Precautions: Diabetes mellitus, pregnancy category C, renal disease, lactation, hyperthyroidism, peripheral vascular disease, myasthenia gravis

Pharmacokinetics:

PO: Onset variable, peak 3-4 hr, duration 17-24 hr, half-life 16-20 hr; not metabolized; excreted in urine (unchanged), bile, breast milk

Drug interactions of concern to dentistry:

• Decreased effects: sympathomimetics (epinephrine, norepinephrine, isoproterenol)

• Slows metabolism of nadolol: lidocaine

• Increased hypotension, myocardial depression: fentanyl derivatives, hydrocarbon inhalation anesthetics

• Decreased hypotensive effect: indomethacin and other NSAIDs

DENTAL CONSIDERATIONS

General:

• Monitor vital signs every appointment due to cardiovascular side effects.

• Patients on chronic drug therapy may rarely have symptoms of blood dyscrasias, which can include infection, bleeding, and poor healing.

• After supine positioning, have patient sit upright for at least 2 min before standing to avoid orthostatic hypotension.

• Limit use of sodium-containing products, such as saline IV fluids, for patients with a dietary salt restriction.

• Assess salivary flow as a factor in

caries, periodontal disease, and candidiasis.

• Stress from dental procedures may compromise cardiovascular function; determine patient risk.

• Short appointments and a stress reduction protocol may be required for anxious patients.

• Consider semisupine chair position for patients with respiratory distress.

Consultations:

• In a patient with symptoms of blood dyscrasias, request a medical consult for blood studies and postpone dental treatment until normal values are reestablished.

• Take precautions if dental surgery is anticipated and anesthesia is required.

• Medical consult may be required to assess disease control and patient's ability to tolerate stress.

Teach patient/family:

• Importance of good oral hygiene to prevent soft tissue inflammation

• Caution to prevent injury when using oral hygiene aids

When chronic dry mouth occurs, advise patient:

• To avoid mouth rinses with high alcohol content due to drying effects

• Of need for daily home fluoride to prevent caries

• To use sugarless gum, frequent sips of water, or saliva substitutes

naftifine HCl

(naf'ti-fin)

Naftin

Drug class.: Topical antifungal

Action: Interferes with cell membrane permeability in fungi such as *T. rubrum, T. mentagrophytes, T. tonsurans, E. floccosum, M. canis, M. audouinii, M. gypseum, Candida,* broad-spectrum antifungal

Uses: Tinea cruris, tinea corporis

Dosage and routes:

• Massage into affected area, surrounding area bid; continue for 7-14 days

Available forms include: Cream 1%

Side effects/adverse reactions:

INTEG: Burning, stinging, dryness, itching, local irritation

Contraindications: Hypersensitivity

Precautions: Pregnancy category B, lactation, children

nalmefene HCl

(nal'me-feen)

Revex

Drug class.: Opioid antagonist

Action: Reverses the effects of opioids by competitive antagonism of opioid receptors

Uses: Management of opioid overdose and complete or partial reversal of opioid drug effects, including respiratory depression

Dosage and routes:

Reversal of opioid depression

• *Adult:* IV use 100 μg/ml strength; initial dose 0.25 μg/kg followed by 0.25 μg/kg, incremental dose at 2-5 min intervals; cumulative doses over 1.0 μg/kg do not provide additional therapeutic effect; titrate all doses

Body weight (kg)	ml of 100 μg/ml solution
50	0.125
60	0.150
70	0.175
80	0.200
90	0.225
100	0.250

Known or suspected opioid overdose

• *Adult:* IV use 1 mg/ml strength; initial 0.5 mg/70 kg; if needed, a second dose of 1.0 mg/70 kg, 2-5 min later; doses over 1.5 mg/70 kg are unlikely to be beneficial

Available forms include: Ampule 100 μg/ml in 1 ml ampule; 1 mg/ml in 2 ml ampule

Side effects/adverse reactions:

▼ *ORAL:* Dry mouth (<1%)

CNS: Dizziness, headache, dysphoria, perception of pain, nervousness

CV: Tachycardia, hypertension, dysrhythmia, hypotension

GI: Nausea, abdominal cramps, vomiting, diarrhea

RESP: Pharyngitis, pulmonary edema

GU: Urinary retention

INTEG: Pruritus

MS: Myalgia, joint pain

MISC: Chills

Contraindications: Hypersensitivity

Precautions: Pregnancy category B, nursing, children, withdrawal symptoms in opioid addicts, renal impairment

Pharmacokinetics:

IV: Onset 2 min, peak plasma conc 1.1-2.3 hr; can also be given IM or SC; hepatic metabolism; excreted in urine

Drug interactions of concern to dentistry:

• None reported

DENTAL CONSIDERATIONS

General:

• This drug is intended for acute use only, but listed side effects can sometimes be seen.

• There is a risk of seizures reported in animal studies; be aware of this as a potential event.

• Serious cardiovascular events have been associated with opioid reversal in postoperative patients; doses should be carefully titrated to reduce these events.

• Buprenorphine depression may not be completely reversed.

• In all cases, the establishment of a patent airway, ventilatory assistance, oxygen administration, and circulatory access should complement or precede opioid antagonist use.

• Significant opioid depression occurring in the dental office may require relocation of the patient to a medical facility for comprehensive management.

• Patients discharged from the office/emergency facility should be carefully observed for the return of opioid-induced depression.

naloxone HCl

(nal-ox′one)

Narcan

Drug class.: Narcotic antagonist

Action: Competes with narcotics at narcotic receptor sites

Uses: Respiratory depression induced by narcotics, to reverse postoperative opioid depression

Dosage and routes:
Narcotic-induced respiratory depression
• *Adult and adolescent:* IV/SC/IM 0.4-2 mg; repeat q2-3 min, if needed
Postoperative respiratory depression
• *Adult:* IV 0.1-0.2 mg q2-3min prn
• *Child:* IV/IM/SC 0.01 mg/kg q2-3min prn
Asphyxia neonatorum
• *Neonates:* IV 0.01 mg/kg given into umbilical vein after delivery; may repeat in q2-3min × 3 doses
Available forms include: Inj IV/IM/SC 0.02, 0.4 mg/ml in 1 ml ampules
Side effects/adverse reactions:
CNS: Drowsiness, nervousness, restlessness, excitement
CV: Rapid pulse, increased or decreased systolic BP high doses
GI: Nausea, vomiting
RESP: Hyperpnea
MISC: Sweating
Contraindications: Hypersensitivity, cardiac irritability
Precautions: Pregnancy category B, opioid dependence
Pharmacokinetics: Onset 1-2 min (IV), 2-5 min (IM), peak effect 5-15 min, duration variable up to 45 min, half-life 60-90 min; metabolized by liver; excreted by kidneys; crosses placenta; excreted in breast milk
Drug interactions of concern to dentistry:
• Antagonizes effects of opioid agonists and mixed agonist/antagonists
DENTAL CONSIDERATIONS
General:
• This drug is intended for acute use only, but listed side effects can sometimes be seen.
• There is a risk of seizures reported in animal studies; be aware of this as a potential event.
• Serious cardiovascular events have been associated with opioid reversal in postoperative patients; doses should be carefully titrated to reduce these events.
• Buprenorphine depression may not be completely reversed.
• In all cases, the establishment of a patent airway, ventilatory assistance, oxygen administration, and circulatory access should complement or precede opioid antagonist use.
• Significant opioid depression occurring in the dental office may require relocation of the patient to a medical facility for comprehensive management.
• Patients discharged from the office/emergency facility should be carefully observed for the return of opioid-induced depression.

naltrexone HCl

(nal-trex′one)
ReVia, Trexan
Drug class.: Narcotic antagonist

Action: Competes with opioids at opioid receptor sites
Uses: Used in treatment of opioid addiction following detoxification
Dosage and routes:
• *Adult:* PO 25 mg, may give 25 mg after 1 hr if there are no withdrawal symptoms; 50-150 mg may be given qd depending on patient need; maintenance 50 mg q24h
Available forms include: Tabs 50 mg
Side effects/adverse reactions:
ORAL: Increased thirst
CNS: Stimulation, drowsiness, diz-

ziness, confusion, convulsion, headache, flushing, hallucinations
CV: Rapid pulse, pulmonary edema, hypertension
GI: Nausea, vomiting, diarrhea, heartburn, ***hepatitis,*** anorexia
RESP: Wheezing, hyperpnea
HEMA: ***Thrombocytopenia, agranulocytosis, leukopenia, neutropenia, hemolytic anemia,*** increased pro-time
EENT: Tinnitus, hearing loss
INTEG: Rash, urticaria, bruising
Contraindications: Hypersensitivity, opioid dependence, hepatic failure, hepatitis
Precautions: Pregnancy category C
Pharmacokinetics:
PO: Onset 15-30 min, peak 1-2 hr, duration is dose dependent, half-life 4 hr; extensive first-pass metabolism; metabolized by liver; excreted by kidneys; crosses placenta; excreted in breast milk
Drug interactions of concern to dentistry:
• Decreased effects of opioid narcotics
DENTAL CONSIDERATIONS
General:
• Monitor vital signs every appointment due to cardiovascular and respiratory side effects.
• Patients on chronic drug therapy may rarely have symptoms of blood dyscrasias, which can include infection, bleeding, and poor healing.
• Patients should not be given opioid analgesics for dental pain management. Substitute with NSAID and long-acting local anesthetics.
• The dental professional must be aware of the patient's disease, and the patient must be active in treatment for chemical dependency.
Consultations:
• In a patient with symptoms of blood dyscrasias, request a medical consult for blood studies and postpone dental treatment until normal values are reestablished.
• Medical consult may be required to assess disease control in the patient.
• Inform aftercare provider or counselor if sedative medications are required for proper management.
Teach patient/family:
• Importance of good oral hygiene to prevent soft tissue inflammation
• Caution to prevent injury when using oral hygiene aids

naphazoline HCl

(naf-az'oh-leen)
AK-Con Ophthalmic, Albalon, Allerest Eye Drops, Allergy Drops, Clear Eyes, Digest 2, Estivin-II, Muro's Opcon, Nafazair, Naphcon, Naphcon Forte, VasoClear, Vasocon
Drug class.: Ophthalmic vasoconstrictor

Action: Vasoconstriction of eye arterioles; decreases eye engorgement by stimulation of α-adrenergic receptors
Uses: Relieves hyperemia, irritation in superficial corneal vascularity
Dosage and routes:
• *Adult:* Instill 1-2 gtt up to tid or qid as needed
Available forms include: Sol 0.01%, 0.012%, 0.02%, 0.025%, 0.03%, 0.05%

Side effects/adverse reactions:
CNS: Headache, dizziness, sedation, anxiety, weakness, sweating (systemic absorption)
CV: ***CV collapse*** (systemic absorption), hypertension, dysrhythmias, tachycardia
EENT: Pupil dilation, increased intraocular pressure, photophobia
Contraindications: Hypersensitivity, glaucoma (narrow-angle)
Precautions: Hypertension, hyperthyroidism, elderly, severe arteriosclerosis, cardiac disease, pregnancy category C
Pharmacokinetics:
INSTILL: Duration 2-3 hr
Drug interactions of concern to dentistry:
• Increased pressor effects: tricyclic antidepressants
DENTAL CONSIDERATIONS
General:
• Monitor vital signs every appointment due to cardiovascular side effects.
• Avoid dental light in patient's eyes; offer dark glasses for patient comfort.
• Protect patient's eyes from accidental spatter during dental treatment.

naproxen/naproxen sodium

(na-prox′en)
Naproxen: EC Naprosyn, Naprosyn, Naprosyn Oral Suspension
♣ Apo-Naproxen, Naprosyn-E, Naprosyn SR, Naxen, Novo-Naprox, Nu-Prox
Naproxen sodium: Anaprox, Anaprox DS, Naprelan, Novo-Naprox Sodium DS; OTC: Aleve
♣ Apo-Napro-Na, Apo-Napro-Na DS, Novo-Naprox Sodium, Synflex, Synflex DS
Drug class.: Nonsteroidal antiinflammatory

Action: Inhibits prostaglandin synthesis by interfering with cyclooxygenase needed for biosynthesis; possesses analgesic, antiinflammatory, antipyretic properties
Uses: Mild-to-moderate pain, osteoarthritis, rheumatoid, juvenile, gouty arthritis, ankylosing spondylitis, primary dysmenorrhea; unapproved use: migraine, PMS, fever
Dosage and routes:
• *Adult:* PO 250-500 mg bid, not to exceed 1 g/day (base); 525 mg, then 275 mg q6-8h prn, not to exceed 1475 mg (sodium); sus rel: 1000 mg once daily
Available forms include: Tabs 200 mg (OTC), 250, 275, 375, 500 mg; sus rel tabs 375, 500 mg; gelcap 220 mg; susp 125 mg/5 ml
Side effects/adverse reactions:
▼ *ORAL:* Stomatitis, bleeding, dry mouth, lichenoid reactions
CNS: Dizziness, drowsiness, fatigue, tremors, confusion, insomnia, anxiety, depression
CV: Tachycardia, peripheral edema, palpitation, dysrhythmias

GI: ***Cholestatic hepatitis,*** nausea, anorexia, vomiting, diarrhea, jaundice, constipation, flatulence, cramps, peptic ulcer
HEMA: ***Blood dyscrasias***
GU: ***Nephrotoxicity: dysuria, hematuria, oliguria, azotemia***
EENT: Tinnitus, hearing loss, blurred vision
INTEG: Purpura, rash, pruritus, sweating

Contraindications: Hypersensitivity, asthma, severe renal disease, severe hepatic disease

Precautions: Pregnancy category B, lactation, children, bleeding disorders, GI disorders, cardiac disorders, hypersensitivity to other antiinflammatory agents, elderly, >2 alcohol drinks daily

Pharmacokinetics:
PO: Peak 2-4 hr, half-life 3-3.5 hr; 99% protein binding; metabolized in liver; excreted in urine (metabolites), breast milk

Drug interactions of concern to dentistry:
- GI ulceration, bleeding: aspirin, alcohol, corticosteroids
- Nephrotoxicity: acetaminophen (chronic use and high doses)
- Possible risk of decreased renal function: cyclosporine
- Increased photosensitization: tetracycline

When prescribed for dental pain:
- Risk of increased effects: oral anticoagulants, oral antidiabetics, lithium, methotrexate
- Decreased antihypertensive effects of diuretics, β-adrenergic blockers, and ACE inhibitors

DENTAL CONSIDERATIONS

General:
- Patients on chronic drug therapy may rarely have symptoms of blood dyscrasias, which can include infection, bleeding, and poor healing.
- Assess salivary flow as a factor in caries, periodontal disease, and candidiasis.
- Avoid prescribing for dental use in last trimester of pregnancy.
- Avoid prescribing aspirin-containing products.
- Consider semisupine chair position for patients with arthritic disease.

Consultations:
- In a patient with symptoms of blood dyscrasias, request a medical consult for blood studies and postpone dental treatment until normal values are reestablished.
- Medical consult may be required to assess disease control in the patient.

Teach patient/family:
- Importance of good oral hygiene to prevent soft tissue inflammation
- Caution to prevent injury when using oral hygiene aids

When chronic dry mouth occurs, advise patient:
- To avoid mouth rinses with high alcohol content due to drying effects
- Of need for daily home fluoride to prevent caries
- To use sugarless gum, frequent sips of water, or saliva substitutes

N

naratriptan HCl

(nar′a-trip-tan)

Amerge

Drug class.: Serotonin agonist

Action: A selective agonist for 5-HT_{1D} and 5-HT_{1B} receptors located on intracranial blood vessels leading to vasoconstriction and possibly inhibition of proinflammatory neuropeptide release

Uses: Acute treatment of migraine attacks with or without aura in adults

Dosage and routes:

• *Adult:* PO 1-2.5 mg with fluids; dose can be repeated once after 4 hr; maximum dose 5 mg/24 hr

Available forms include: Tabs 1, 2.5 mg

Side effects/adverse reactions:

▼ *ORAL:* Dry mouth

CNS: Paresthesias, dizziness, drowsiness, malaise, fatigue

CV: Palpitation, hypertension, tachyarrhythmias

GI: Nausea, vomiting, discomfort, dyspepsia

RESP: Bronchitis, cough

HEMA: Leukocytosis

GU: Bladder inflammation, polyuria

EENT: Throat/neck symptoms, photophobia, sinusitis, tinnitus, blurred vision, vertigo

INTEG: Sweating, rash

ENDO: Polydipsia, thirst

MS: Muscle pain, arthralgia

Contraindications: Hypersensitivity, ischemic heart disease, vasospastic coronary artery disease, cerebrovascular or periperipheral vascular disease, uncontrolled hypertension, severe renal or hepatic impairment, hemiplegic or basilar migraine, ergot-containing drugs

Precautions: Risk of serious cardiovascular events, renal/hepatic dysfunction, SSRI antidepressants, pregnancy category C, lactation, use in children not established, not recommended in elderly

Pharmacokinetics:

PO: Bioavailability 70%, peak levels 2-3 hr, protein binding 28%-31%, metabolized by cytochrome P-450 enzymes; 50% of dose excreted in urine unchanged; 30% as metabolite

Drug interactions of concern to dentistry:

• No specific interactions with dental drugs reported

• Should not be used within 24 hr of another $5HT_1$ agonist

DENTAL CONSIDERATIONS

General:

• This is an acute-use drug, thus it is doubtful that patients will come to the office if acute migraine is present.

• Be aware of patient's disease, its severity, and frequency when known.

• Avoid dental light in patient's eyes; offer dark glasses for patient comfort.

Consultations:

• If treating chronic orofacial pain, consult with physician of record.

• Medical consult may be required to assess disease control and patient's ability to tolerate stress.

Teach patient/family:

• Importance of updating health and drug history if physician makes any changes in evaluation/drug regimens

---

nedocromil sodium

(ne-doe-kroe′mil)

Tilade

Alocril (ophthalmic solution)

Drug class.: Antiasthmatic, mast cell stabilizer

Action: Stabilizes the membrane of the sensitized mast cell, preventing release of chemical mediators after an antigen-IgE interaction

Uses: Prophylaxis only in reversible obstructive airway diseases

(ROADs) such as asthma; ophthalmic solution for allergic conjunctivitis

Dosage and routes:

• *Adult and child >12 yr:* Inh 4 mg bid-qid

Allergic conjunctivitis

• *Adult:* Ophth 1 or 2 drops in each eye bid

Available forms include: Inhaler spray unit, ophthalmic solution

Side effects/adverse reactions:

▼ *ORAL:* Dry/burning mouth, bitter taste (aerosol)

CNS: Headache, dizziness, neuritis

GI: Nausea, vomiting, anorexia

GU: Frequency, dysuria

EENT: Throat irritation, cough, nasal congestion, burning eyes

INTEG: Rash, urticaria, angioedema

MS: Joint pain/swelling

Contraindications: Hypersensitivity to this drug or lactose, status asthmaticus

Precautions: Pregnancy category B, lactation, renal disease, hepatic disease, child <12 yr

Pharmacokinetics:

INH: Peak 15 min, duration 4-6 hr, half-life 80 min; excreted unchanged in feces

DENTAL CONSIDERATIONS

General:

• Assess salivary flow as a factor in caries, periodontal disease, and candidiasis.

• Consider semisupine chair position for patients with respiratory disease.

• Short appointments and a stress reduction protocol may be required for anxious patients.

• Be aware that aspirin or sulfite preservatives in vasoconstrictor-containing products can exacerbate asthma.

Consultations:

• Medical consult may be required to assess disease control in the patient.

Teach patient/family:

• To avoid mouth rinses with high alcohol content due to drying effects

• For inhalation dosage forms, rinse mouth with water after each dose to prevent dryness

nefazodone HCl

(nef-ay'zoe-done)

Serzone

Drug class.: Antidepressant

Action: Inhibits neuronal uptake of serotonin and norepinephrine; the exact mechanism of antidepressant activity remains unknown

Uses: Major depressive disorders

Dosage and routes:

• *Adult:* PO initial dose 200 mg/day in 2 divided doses bid; gradually increase dose in increments of 100-200 mg/day, depending on response and need (all doses are given bid); dose range in clinical trials was 300-600 mg/day; initial doses in elderly should be reduced by one half

Available forms include: Tabs 100, 150, 200, 250 mg

Side effects/adverse reactions:

▼ *ORAL: Dry mouth,* taste alteration, candidiasis (rare), stomatitis

CNS: Somnolence, dizziness, insomnia, confusion, light-headedness, headache, memory impairment, abnormal dreams, mania

CV: Postural hypotension, hypotension, dysrhythmias (rare), peripheral edema

GI: Constipation, nausea, dyspep-

N

sia, diarrhea, increased appetite, gastroenteritis
RESP: Pharyngitis, cough, bronchitis
GU: Urinary frequency, UTI, vaginitis, urinary retention, impotence
EENT: Blurred vision, abnormal vision, visual field defect, eye pain, tinnitus
INTEG: Rash, pruritus, dry skin, urticaria
MS: Neck rigidity
MISC: Flulike syndrome, chills, fever

Contraindications: Hypersensitivity, coadministration of terfenadine or astemizole, MAO inhibitors, cisapride

Precautions: Mania, hypomania, suicidal tendencies, seizures, history of MI or unstable heart conditions, hepatic impairment, pregnancy category C, lactation, child <18 yr, elderly (requires dose adjustment), priapism history, alcohol use

Pharmacokinetics: Bioavailability 20% with PO doses, peak plasma levels 1 hr, half-life 2-4 hr; highly protein bound 99%; extensive hepatic metabolism; metabolites excreted in urine

Drug interactions of concern to dentistry:

- Must *not* be used with terfenadine, astemizole, or MAO inhibitors
- Risk of significant adverse drug interaction with triazolam, alprazolam, alcohol-containing products
- No information available on use of this drug in patients who are candidates for conscious sedation or general anesthesia

DENTAL CONSIDERATIONS

General:

- Assess salivary flow as a factor in caries, periodontal disease, and candidiasis.
- Take vital signs every appointment due to cardiovascular side effects.
- After supine positioning, have patient sit upright for at least 2 min before standing to avoid postural hypotension.
- There is no information concerning the use of vasoconstrictors in patients taking this drug.

Consultations:

- Medical consult may be required to assess disease control in the patient.
- Physician should be informed if significant xerostomic side effects occur (increased caries, sore tongue, problems eating or swallowing, difficulty wearing prosthesis) so a medication change can be considered.
- Because there is no experience with the use of conscious sedation or general anesthesia in patients taking this drug, a medical consult is recommended for risk evaluation.

Teach patient/family:

When chronic dry mouth occurs, advise patient:

- To avoid mouth rinses with high alcohol content due to drying effects
- Of need for daily home fluoride to prevent caries
- To use sugarless gum, frequent sips of water, or saliva substitutes

nelfinavir mesylate

(nel-fin′a-veer)
Viracept
Drug class.: Antiviral

Action: Inhibits HIV-I protease

enzymes leading to the production of immature, noninfectious virus
Uses: HIV infection when indicated by surrogate marker changes in patients receiving nelfinavir in combination with nucleoside analogues or alone for up to 24 wk
Dosage and routes:
• *Adult:* PO tabs 750 mg tid or 1250 mg bid with meals or light snack
• *Child 2-13 yr:* PO 20-30 mg/kg per dose tid with meals or light snack. Oral powder may be used for children unable to take tablets. Oral powder can be mixed with a small amount of water, milk formula, soy formula, soy milk, or dietary supplement. Do not use acidic juices or applesauce.
Available forms include: Tab 250 mg; oral powder 50 mg/g (as free base nelfinavir)
Side effects/adverse reactions:
▼ *ORAL:* Oral ulceration (<2%)
CNS: Anxiety, depression, dizziness, sleep disorder, migraine, insomnia
GI: Diarrhea, nausea, anorexia, dyspepsia, vomiting, hepatitis, pancreatitis, GI bleeding
RESP: Pharyngitis, dyspnea, sinusitis
HEMA: Anemia, leukopenia, thrombocytopenia, abnormal laboratory values
GU: Kidney calculus, sexual dysfunction
EENT: Rhinitis
INTEG: Rash, pruritus, urticaria
META: Increased alkaline phosphatase, creatine phosphokinase, hyperlipidemia, abnormal liver function tests
MS: Arthralgia, asthenia, myalgia, myopathy, cramps
Contraindications: Hypersensitivity, concurrent use with cisapride, triazolam, midazolam, ergot derivatives, rifampin, amiodarone, or quinidine
Precautions: Pediatric use, phenylketonuria (powder contains phenylalanine), diabetes mellitus, hyperglycemia, hepatic impairment, development of resistance, hemophilia, pregnancy category B, lactation, child <2 yr
Pharmacokinetics:
PO: Peak plasma levels 2-4 hr with food; peak plasma levels 3-4 µg/ml, plasma protein bound (98%), hepatic metabolism, active metabolite, excreted mostly in feces (87%), minor urinary excretion (1%-2%)
Drug interactions of concern to dentistry:
• Contraindicated with terfenadine, astemizole, triazolam, midazolam

DENTAL CONSIDERATIONS
General:
• Examine for oral manifestation of opportunistic infection.
• Patient on chronic drug therapy may rarely have symptoms of blood dyscrasias, which can include infection, bleeding, and poor healing.
• Palliative medication may be required for management of oral side effects.
Consultations:
• In a patient with symptoms of blood dyscrasias, request a medical consult for blood studies and postpone treatment until normal values are reestablished.
• Medical consult may be required to assess disease control in the patient.
Teach patient/family:
• Importance of good oral hygiene to prevent soft tissue inflammation

N

Caution to prevent trauma when using oral hygiene aids

• Importance of updating health and drug history if physician makes any changes in evaluation/drug regimens

• That secondary oral infection may occur; must see dentist immediately if infection occurs

neostigmine bromide/ neostigmine methylsulfate

(nee-oh-stig′meen)

Prostigmin Bromide/Prostigmin

Drug class.: Cholinesterase inhibitor

Action: Inhibits destruction of acetylcholine, which increases concentration at sites where acetylcholine is released; this facilitates transmission of impulses across myoneural junction

Uses: Myasthenia gravis, nondepolarizing neuromuscular blocker, antagonist, bladder distention, postoperative ileus

Dosage and routes:

Myasthenia gravis

• *Adult:* PO 15-375 mg/day; IM/IV 0.5-2 mg q1-3h

• *Child:* PO 2 mg/kg/day q3-4h

Tubocurarine antagonist

• *Adult:* IV 0.5-2 mg slowly, may repeat if needed (give 0.6-1.2 mg atropine before this drug)

Abdominal distention/postoperative ileus

• *Adult:* IM/SC 0.25-1 mg q4-6h, depending on condition

Available forms include: Tabs 15 mg; inj IM/SC/IV 1:1000, 1:2000, 1:4000

Side effects/adverse reactions:

ORAL: Increased salivation

CNS: ***Paralysis, convulsions,*** dizziness, headache, sweating, confusion, weakness, incoordination

CV: ***Cardiac arrest,*** tachycardia, dysrhythmias, bradycardia, hypotension, AV block, ECG changes

GI: Nausea, diarrhea, vomiting, cramps, increased secretions

RESP: ***Respiratory depression, bronchospasm, constriction, laryngospasm, respiratory arrest***

GU: Frequency, incontinence

EENT: Miosis, blurred vision, lacrimation

INTEG: Rash, urticaria, flushing

Contraindications: Obstruction of intestine, renal system, pregnancy category C, bromide sensitivity

Precautions: Bradycardia, hypotension, seizure disorders, bronchial asthma, coronary occlusion, hyperthyroidism, dysrhythmias, peptic ulcer, megacolon, poor GI motility, lactation, children

Pharmacokinetics:

PO: Onset 45-75 min, duration 2.5-4 hr

IM/SC: Onset 10-30 min, duration 2.5-4 hr

IV: Onset 4-8 min, duration 2-4 hr

Metabolized in liver, excreted in urine

Drug interactions of concern to dentistry:

• Decreased action: hydrocarbon inhalation anesthetics, corticosteroids

• Decreased action of anticholinergics (may be contraindicated)

• Increased action of succinylcholine

• Increased toxicity of ester-type local anesthetics

DENTAL CONSIDERATIONS

General:

• Monitor vital signs every appointment due to cardiovascular and respiratory side effects.

• Use amide-type local anesthetic agent.

• Early-morning and brief appointments preferred due to effects of disease on oral musculature.

Consultations:

• Take precautions if dental surgery is anticipated and anesthesia is required.

• Medical consult may be required to assess disease control and patient's tolerance for stress.

---

nevirapine (NVP)

(ne-vye'ra-peen)

Viramune

Drug class.: Antiviral

Action: A nonnucleoside reverse transcriptase inhibitor for HIV-1, results in blockade of RNA-dependent and DNA-dependent polymerase

Uses: Used in combination with nucleoside analogs for HIV-1 infection in adults who have demonstrated clinical or immunologic deterioration

Dosage and routes:

• *Adult:* PO 200 mg qd × 14 days; then 200 mg bid in combination with nucleoside analog retroviral agent

Available forms include: Tabs 200 mg

Side effects/adverse reactions:

▼ *ORAL:* Oral ulceration (Stevens-Johnson syndrome)

CNS: Headache, fever, fatigue, somnolence

GI: Nausea, diarrhea

INTEG: ***Rash (Stevens-Johnson syndrome)***

ENDO: Hepatitis

MS: Myalgias, paresthesia

META: Abnormal liver function tests

Contraindications: Hypersensitivity, protease inhibitors

Precautions: Severe life-threatening skin reactions (Stevens-Johnson syndrome), hepatic, renal dysfunction, pregnancy category C, lactation, children

Pharmacokinetics:

PO: Absorption 90%, peak plasma levels 4 hr, plasma protein binding 60%, hepatic metabolism, fecal excretion mainly, urinary excretion also

Drug interactions of concern to dentistry:

• Should not be given with ketoconazole

DENTAL CONSIDERATIONS

General:

• Determine why patient is taking the drug.

• Examine for oral manifestation of opportunistic infection.

Consultations:

• Medical consult may be required to assess disease control in the patient.

Teach patient/family:

• Importance of good oral hygiene to prevent soft tissue inflammation

• To report oral lesions, soreness, or bleeding to dentist

• Importance of updating health history/drug record if physician makes any changes in evaluations/drug regimens

• That secondary oral infection may occur; must see dentist immediately if infection occurs

niacin (vitamin B_3/ nicotinic acid)/ niacinamide (nicotinamide)

(nye'a-sin) (nye-a-sin'a-mide)

Niacin (nicotinic acid): generic, Endur-Acin, Nia-Bid, Niac, Niacels, Niacor, Nicotinex, Nico-400, Nicobid, Niaspan, Nicolar, Slo-Niacin

🍁 Novo-Niacin

Nicotinamide: generic

Drug class.: Vitamin B_3

Action: Needed for conversion of fats, protein, carbohydrates by oxidation-reduction; acts directly on vascular smooth muscle, causing vasodilation; high doses decrease serum lipids

Uses: Pellagra, hyperlipidemias (niacin), peripheral vascular disease (niacin)

Dosage and routes:

Adjunct in hyperlipidemia

• *Adult:* PO 1.5-3 g qd in 3 divided doses after meals, may be increased to 6 g/day; ext rel 500 or 1000 mg for 1 mo, increasing to 1.5 or 2 g hs if inadequate response, daily dose should not be increased >500 mg in 4 wk period

Pellagra

• *Adult:* IM/SC/PO/IV inf 10-20 mg, not to exceed 500 mg total dose

• *Child:* IM/SC/PO/IV inf 300 mg until desired response

Peripheral vascular disease

• *Adult:* PO 250-800 mg qd in divided doses

Available forms include: Nicotinic acid—tabs 20, 25, 50, 100, 500 mg; time rel caps 125, 250, 300, 400, 500 mg; time rel tabs 150 mg; elix 50 mg/5 ml; inj 100 mg/ml; nicotinamide—tabs 50, 100, 500 mg; time rel tabs 1000 mg; inj IV/IM/SC 100 mg/ml

Side effects/adverse reactions:

▼ *ORAL:* Dry mouth

CNS: Paresthesia, headache, dizziness, anxiety

CV: Postural hypotension, vasovagal attacks, dysrhythmias, vasodilation

GI: ***Jaundice,*** nausea, vomiting, anorexia, flatulence, diarrhea, peptic ulcer

RESP: Wheezing

GU: ***Glycosuria, hypoalbuminemia,*** hyperuricemia

EENT: Blurred vision, ptosis

INTEG: Flushing, dry skin, rash, pruritus

Contraindications: Hypersensitivity, peptic ulcer, hepatic disease, lactation, hemorrhage, severe hypotension

Precautions: Glaucoma, cardiovascular disease, CAD, diabetes mellitus, gout, schizophrenia, pregnancy category A

Pharmacokinetics:

PO: Peak 30-70 min, half-life 45 min; metabolized in liver; 30% excreted unchanged in urine

Drug interactions of concern to dentistry:

• None reported

DENTAL CONSIDERATIONS

General:

• Take vital signs every appointment due to cardiovascular side effects.

• After supine positioning, have patient sit upright for at least 2 min before standing to avoid postural hypotension.

• Assess salivary flow as a factor in caries, periodontal disease, and candidiasis.

Teach patient/family:
When chronic dry mouth occurs, advise patient:
• To avoid mouth rinses with high alcohol content due to drying effects
• Of need for daily home fluoride to prevent caries
• To use sugarless gum, frequent sips of water, or saliva substitutes

nicardipine HCl

(nye-kar'de-peen)
Cardene, Cardene IV, Cardene SR
Drug class.: Calcium channel blocker

Action: Inhibits calcium ion influx across cell membrane during cardiac depolarization; produces relaxation of coronary vascular smooth muscle, peripheral vascular smooth muscle; dilates coronary vascular arteries; decreases SA/AV node conduction
Uses: Chronic stable angina pectoris, hypertension
Dosage and routes:
Angina
• *Adult:* PO 20 mg tid initially; may increase after 3 days (range 20-40 mg tid)
Hypertension
• *Adult:* PO 20 mg tid initially, then increase after 3 days (range 20-40 mg tid)
Available forms include: Caps 20, 30 mg; sus rel caps 30, 45, 60 mg; IV 2.5 mg/ml in 10 ml amps
Side effects/adverse reactions:
▼ *ORAL:* Dry mouth, sore throat (gingival overgrowth has been reported with other calcium channel blockers)
CNS: Headache, fatigue, drowsiness, dizziness, anxiety, depression, weakness, insomnia, confusion, paresthesia, somnolence
CV: ***MI, pulmonary edema,*** dysrhythmia, edema, CHF, bradycardia, hypotension, palpitation
GI: ***Hepatitis,*** nausea, vomiting, diarrhea, gastric upset, constipation, abdominal cramps
GU: ***Acute renal failure,*** nocturia, polyuria
INTEG: Rash, pruritus, urticaria, photosensitivity, hair loss
MISC: Blurred vision, flushing, nasal congestion, sweating, shortness of breath, gynecomastia, hyperglycemia, sexual difficulties
Contraindications: Sick sinus syndrome, second- or third-degree heart block, hypotension <90 mm Hg systolic, hypersensitivity
Precautions: CHF, hypotension, hepatic injury, pregnancy category C, lactation, children, renal disease, elderly
Pharmacokinetics:
PO: Onset 10 min, peak 1-2 hr, half-life 2-5 hr; metabolized by liver; excreted in urine (98% as metabolites)
Drug interactions of concern to dentistry:
• Decreased effect: indomethacin, possibly other NSAIDs, phenobarbital
• Increased effect: parenteral and inhalational general anesthetics or other drugs with hypotensive actions
• Increased effects of nondepolarizing muscle relaxants
• Increased effects of carbamazepine

DENTAL CONSIDERATIONS
General:
• Monitor cardiac status; take vital signs at each appointment because of CV side effects. Consider a

stress reduction protocol to prevent stress-induced angina during the dental appointment.

• After supine positioning, have patient sit upright for at least 2 min to avoid orthostatic hypotension.

• Place on frequent recall to monitor gingival condition.

• Limit use of sodium-containing products, such as saline IV fluids, for patients with a dietary salt restriction.

• Assess salivary flow as a factor in caries, periodontal disease, and candidiasis.

• Use vasoconstrictors with caution, in low doses, and with careful aspiration. Avoid use of gingival retraction cord with epinephrine.

Consultations:

• Medical consult may be required to assess disease control and tolerance for stress.

Teach patient/family:

• Importance of good oral hygiene to prevent soft tissue inflammation and minimize gingival overgrowth

• Need for frequent oral prophylaxis if hyperplasia occurs

When chronic dry mouth occurs, advise patient:

• To avoid mouth rinses with high alcohol content due to drying effects

• Of need for daily home fluoride to prevent caries

• To use sugarless gum, frequent sips of water, or saliva substitutes

---

nicotine polacrilex

(nik'o-teen)

Nicorette, Nicorette DS

Drug class.: Smoking deterrent

Action: Agonist at nicotinic receptors in the peripheral and central nervous systems; acts at sympathetic ganglia; on chemoreceptors of the aorta and carotid bodies; also affects adrenal-releasing catecholamines

Uses: Deters cigarette smoking when combined with a program of smoking cessation

Dosage and routes:

• *Adult:* Gum 1 piece chewed for 0.5 hr as needed to abstain from smoking; not to exceed 30/day

Available forms include: Gum 2, 4 mg/piece of gum

Side effects/adverse reactions:

▼ *ORAL:* Burning in mucosa, occlusal stress, unpleasant taste, increased salivation, dry mouth (rare), sore throat

CNS: Dizziness, vertigo, insomnia, headache, confusion, convulsions, depression, euphoria, numbness, tinnitus

CV: Dysrhythmias, tachycardia, palpitation

GI: Nausea, vomiting, anorexia, indigestion, diarrhea, abdominal pain, constipation, eructation

RESP: Breathing difficulty, cough, hoarseness, sneezing, wheezing

Contraindications: Hypersensitivity, immediate post-MI recovery period, severe angina pectoris, pregnancy category X, nicotine patch therapy

Precautions: Vasospastic disease, dysrhythmias, uncontrolled hypertension, diabetes mellitus, pregnancy, children, hyperthyroidism, pheochromocytoma, coronary disease, esophagitis, peptic ulcer, insulin or prescription medications for asthma or depression

Pharmacokinetics:

PO: Onset 15-30 min, half-life 2-3 hr, 30-120 hr (terminal); metabolized in liver; excreted in urine

Drug interactions of concern to dentistry:
• Increased blood levels with cessation of smoking: propoxyphene

DENTAL CONSIDERATIONS

General:
• Take vital signs every appointment due to cardiovascular side effects.
• TMJ disorder may be aggravated by chewing due to heavier viscosity of gum.

Teach patient/family:
• Need for good oral hygiene to prevent periodontal inflammation

When chronic dry mouth occurs, advise patient:
• To avoid mouth rinses with high alcohol content due to drying effects
• Of need for daily home fluoride to prevent caries
• To use sugarless gum, frequent sips of water, or saliva substitutes

When used in conjunction with a smoking cessation program in the dental office, teach:
• All aspects of product use; give package insert to patient and explain
• That gum is to be used only to deter smoking
• To avoid use in pregnancy; birth defects may occur
• To stop smoking when beginning treatment with gum

---

nicotine transdermal system/nicotine spray

(nik′oh-teen)

Habitrol, Nicoderm, NicoDerm CQ, Nicotrol, Nicotrol NS ProStep

Drug class.: Smoking deterrent

Action: Binds to acetylcholine receptors at autonomic ganglia in the adrenal medulla, at neuromuscular junctions, and in the brain

Uses: Cigarette smoking cessation program

Dosage and routes:
• *Adult:* TRANS dose varies with 24 or 16 hr system selected. One example is 21 mg/day for 4-8 wk, then 14 mg/day for 2-4 wk, then 7 mg/day for 2-4 wk; for 22 mg system: 22 mg/day for 4-8 wk, then 11 mg/day for 2-4 wk. For 16 hr system: 15 mg per 16 hr day for 4-6 wk, then 10 mg per 16 hr day for 2-4 wk, then 5 mg per 16 hr day for 2-4 wk.
• *Nasal spray:* One spray in each nostril (1 mg total). Adjust dose to individual of 1 or 2 doses/hr not to exceed 5 doses/hr or 40 doses/day and for no longer than 3 mo.

Available forms include: Transderm patch delivering 7, 11, 14, 21, 22 mg/day for 24 hr system and 5, 10, and 15 mg for 16 hr system; spray pump 0.5 mg of nicotine per actuation

N

Side effects/adverse reactions:
▼ *ORAL:* Dry mouth
CNS: Abnormal dreams, insomnia, nervousness, headache, dizziness, paresthesia
GI: Diarrhea, dyspepsia, constipation, nausea, abdominal pain, vomiting
INTEG: Erythema, pruritus, rash, burning at application site, cutaneous hypersensitivity, sweating
MS: Arthralgia, myalgia

Contraindications: Hypersensitivity, children, pregnancy, lactation, nonsmokers, during immediate post-MI period, life-threatening dysrhythmias, severe or worsening angina pectoris, hypertension

Precautions: Skin disease, angina pectoris, MI, renal or hepatic insufficiency, peptic ulcer, serious cardiac dysrhythmias, hyperthyroidism, pheochromocytoma, insulin-dependent diabetes, elderly, pregnancy category D

Pharmacokinetics:

TRANS: Half-life 3-4 hr; protein binding <5%; 30% is excreted unchanged in urine

Drug interactions of concern to dentistry:

• Decreased dose at cessation of smoking: acetaminophen, caffeine, oxazepam, pentazocine

• Decreased metabolism of propoxyphene

DENTAL CONSIDERATIONS

General:

• Assess salivary flow as a factor in caries, periodontal disease, and candidiasis.

Teach patient/family:

When chronic dry mouth occurs, advise patient:

• To avoid mouth rinses with high alcohol content due to drying effects

• Of need for daily home fluoride to prevent caries

• To use sugarless gum, frequent sips of water, or saliva substitutes

When used in conjunction with a smoking cessation program in the dental office, teach:

• All aspects of product drug; give package insert to patient and explain

• That patch is to be used only to deter smoking

• Not to use during pregnancy; birth defects may occur

• To keep used and unused system out of reach of children and pets; potentially toxic if chewed or swallowed

• To apply once a day to a nonhairy, clean, dry area of skin on upper body or upper outer arm

• To stop smoking immediately when beginning treatment with patch

• To apply promptly after removing from protective patch; system may lose strength

---

nifedipine

(nye-fed′i-peen)

Adalat FT, Procardia, Procardia SL, Procardia XL

♣ Adalat, Adalat CC, Adalat PA, Apo-Nifed, Nu-Nifed, Novo-Nifedin

Drug class.: Calcium channel blocker

Action: Inhibits calcium ion influx across cell membrane during cardiac depolarization; produces relaxation of coronary vascular smooth muscle, dilates coronary arteries; increases myocardial oxygen delivery in patients with vasospastic angina; dilates peripheral arteries

Uses: Chronic stable angina pectoris, vasospastic angina, hypertension (sustained release only)

Dosage and routes:

• *Adult:* PO (immed rel) 10 mg tid, increase in 10 mg increments q4-6h, not to exceed 180 mg or single dose of 30 mg; PO (sus rel) 30-60 mg qd, may increase q7-14 days, doses >120 mg not recommended

Available forms include: Caps 10, 20 mg; sus rel tabs 30, 60, 90 mg

Side effects/adverse reactions:

▼ *ORAL: Gingival overgrowth,* dry mouth

CNS: Giddiness, headache, fatigue, drowsiness, dizziness, anxiety, depression, weakness, insomnia,

light-headedness, paresthesia, tinnitus, blurred vision
CV: Dysrhythmia, edema, CHF, ***MI,*** hypotension, palpitation, pulmonary edema, tachycardia
GI: Nausea, vomiting, diarrhea, gastric upset, constipation, increased liver function studies
GU: Nocturia, polyuria
INTEG: Rash, pruritus, flushing, photosensitivity, hair loss
MISC: Flushing, sexual difficulties, cough, fever, chills
Contraindications: Hypersensitivity
Precautions: CHF, hypotension, sick sinus syndrome, second- or third- degree heart block, hypotension <90 mm Hg systolic, hepatic injury, pregnancy category C, lactation, children, renal disease
Pharmacokinetics:
PO: Onset 20 min, peak 0.5-6 hr, half-life 2-5 hr; metabolized by liver; excreted in urine (98% as metabolites)
Drug interactions of concern to dentistry:
- Decreased effect: indomethacin, possibly other NSAIDs, phenobarbital
- Increased effect: parenteral and inhalational general anesthetics or other drugs with hypotensive actions
- Increased effects of nondepolarizing muscle relaxants
- Increased effects of carbamazepine

DENTAL CONSIDERATIONS
General:
- Monitor cardiac status; take vital signs at each appointment because of CV side effects. Consider a stress reduction protocol to prevent stress-induced angina during the dental appointment.
- After supine positioning, have patient sit upright for at least 2 min before standing to avoid orthostatic hypotension at dismissal.
- Place on frequent recall to monitor gingival condition.
- Limit use of sodium-containing products, such as saline IV fluids, for patients with a dietary salt restriction.
- Assess salivary flow as a factor in caries, periodontal disease, and candidiasis.
- Use vasoconstrictors with caution, in low doses, and with careful aspiration. Avoid use of gingival retraction cord with epinephrine.

Consultations:
- Medical consult may be required to assess disease control and stress tolerance.

Teach patient/family:
- Importance of good oral hygiene to prevent soft tissue inflammation and minimize gingival overgrowth
- Need for frequent oral prophylaxis if hyperplasia occurs

When chronic dry mouth occurs, advise patient:
- To avoid mouth rinses with high alcohol content due to drying effects
- Of need for daily home fluoride to prevent caries
- To use sugarless gum, frequent sips of water, or saliva substitutes

nisoldipine
(nye'sol-di-peen)
Sular

Drug class.: Calcium channel antagonist (dihydropyridine group)

Action: Inhibits calcium ion influx across cell membrane during cardiac depolarization; produces relaxation of coronary vascular smooth muscle; dilates coronary arteries; decreases SA/AV node conduction; dilates peripheral vessels

Uses: Hypertension as a single agent or in combination with other antihypertensive medications

Dosages and routes:

• *Adult <65 yr:* PO initial dose 20 mg daily; can increase dose by 10 mg weekly or at longer intervals depending on patient response and blood pressure control

• *Maintenance dose:* 20-40 mg daily; doses above 60 mg daily are not recommended; do not take with high-fat meals

• *Adult >65 yr or in renal impairment:* PO reduce initial dose to 10 mg daily

Available forms include: Tabs 10, 20, 30, 40 mg

Side effects/adverse reactions:

▼ *ORAL:* Dry mouth, facial edema, gingival overgrowth, glossitis, mouth ulcers

CNS: Headache, dizziness, migraine, abnormal dreams

CV: Peripheral edema, vasodilation, palpitation, CHF, CVA, chest pain, postural hypotension

GI: Anorexia, diarrhea, colitis, dyspepsia, flatulence

HEMA: Anemia, ecchymosis, leukopenia, petechiae

GU: Dysuria, impotence, urinary frequency

EENT: Pharyngitis, sinusitis, abnormal vision, watery eyes

INTEG: Rash, dry skin, pruritus

MS: Arthralgia, leg cramps, myalgia

MISC: Flulike syndrome, malaise

Contraindications: Hypersensitivity

Precautions: Avoid high-fat meals, severe coronary artery disease, monitor blood pressure, CHF, severe hepatic impairment, do not break or crush tablets, pregnancy category C, lactation, geriatric patients

Pharmacokinetics:

PO: Low bioavailability 5%, presystemic metabolism in intestinal wall, peak plasma levels 6-12 hr, highly metabolized, urinary excretion 60%-90%

Drug interactions of concern to dentistry:

• None reported as yet with this drug; however, interactions have been reported with other drugs in this class and include the following:

• Decreased antihypertensive effect: indomethacin, possibly other NSAIDs, phenobarbital

• Increased effect: parenteral and inhalational general anesthetics or other drugs with hypotensive actions

• Increased effects of carbamazepine

DENTAL CONSIDERATIONS:

General:

• Stress from dental procedures may compromise cardiovascular function; determine patient risk.

• Monitor vital signs every appointment due to cardiovascular side effects.

• Short appointments and a stress reduction protocol may be required for anxious patients.

• When taken with grapefruit juice may see increased plasma levels.

• Limit use of sodium-containing products such as saline IV fluids for those patients with a dietary salt restriction.

• After supine positioning, have patient sit upright for at least 2 min before standing to avoid orthostatic hypotension.

• Assess salivary flow as a factor in caries, periodontal disease, and candidiasis.

Consultations:

• Medical consult may be required to assess disease control and patient's ability to tolerate stress.

Teach patient/family:

• Need for frequent oral prophylaxis if gingival overgrowth should occur

When chronic dry mouth occurs, advise patient:

• To avoid mouth rinses with high alcohol content due to drying effects

• To use daily home fluoride products for anticaries effect

• To use sugarless gum, frequent sips of water, or saliva substitutes

---

nitrofurantoin/ nitrofurantoin macrocrystals

(nye-troe-fyoor′an-toyn)

Apo-Nitrofurantoin, Furadantin, Furalan, Furatoin, Macrobid, Macrodantin

Drug class.: Urinary tract antiinfective

Action: Appears to inhibit bacterial enzymes

Uses: UTIs caused by *E. coli, Klebsiella, Pseudomonas, P. vulgaris, P. morganii, Serratia, Citrobacter, S. aureus*

Dosage and routes:

• *Adult and child >12 yr:* PO 50-100 mg qid pc or 50-100 mg hs for long-term treatment

• *Child 1 mo-3 yr:* PO 5-7 mg/kg/day in 4 divided doses; 1-3 mg/kg/day for long-term treatment

Available forms include: Caps 25, 50, 100 mg; tabs 50, 100 mg; susp 25 mg/5 ml

Side effects/adverse reactions:

▼ *ORAL:* Angioedema, brown discoloration of saliva, tooth staining, tingling or burning of mouth

CNS: Dizziness, headache, drowsiness, peripheral neuropathy

GI: Nausea, vomiting, abdominal pain, diarrhea, ***cholestatic jaundice***

INTEG: Pruritus, rash, urticaria, angioedema, alopecia, tooth staining

Contraindications: Hypersensitivity, anuria, severe renal disease

Precautions: Pregnancy category not listed (pregnant women at term), lactation

Pharmacokinetics:

PO: Half-life 20-60 min; crosses blood-brain barrier, placenta; excreted in breast milk; excreted as inactive metabolites in liver

Drug interactions of concern to dentistry:

• Increased effects: anticholinergic drugs

DENTAL CONSIDERATIONS

General:

• Determine why the patient is taking the drug.

Consultations:

• Medical consult may be required to assess disease control in the patient and to select an antiinfective if a dental infection is diagnosed.

N

nitroglycerin

(nye-troe-gli'ser-in)

Nitroglycerin transmucosal tab: Nitrogard

Nitroglycerin lingual aerosol: Nitrolingual

Nitroglycerin extended release cap: Nitrocap T.D., Nitroglyn, Nitrolin, Nitrospan, Nitrocine

Nitroglycerin extended release tab: Nitrong

♣ Nitrong SR

Nitroglycerin injection: Nitro-Bid IV, Tridil

Nitroglycerin sublingual tab: Nitrostat, NitroQuick

Topical dose forms: Nitro-Bid, Nitrol

Nitroglycerin transdermal patch: Deponit, Minitran, Nitro-Dur II, NTS, Transderm-Nitro

Drug class.: Inorganic nitrate, vasodilator

Action: Decreases preload/afterload, which is responsible for decreasing left ventricular end-diastolic pressure, systemic vascular resistance; arterial and venous dilation

Uses: Chronic stable angina pectoris, prophylaxis of angina pain, CHF associated with acute MI, controlled hypotension in surgical procedures

Dosage and routes:

• *Adult:* SL dissolve tablet under tongue when pain begins; may repeat q5min until relief occurs; take no more than 3 tabs/15 min; use 1 tab prophylactically 5-10 min before activities; sus rel cap q6-12h on empty stomach; top 1-2 q8h, increase to 4 q4h as needed; IV 5 μg/min, then increase by 5 μg/min q3-5min, if no response after 20 μg/min, increase by 10-20 μg/min until desired response; trans apply 1 pad qd to a hair-free site

Available forms include: Buccal tabs 1, 2, 3 mg; spray 0.4 mg/meter spray; sus rel caps 2.5, 6.5, 9, 13 mg; sus rel tabs 2.6, 6.5, 9 mg; inj 0.5, 5 mg/ml; SL tabs 0.15, 0.3, 0.4, 0.6 mg; top oint 2%; trans derm syst 0.1, 0.2, 0.3, 0.4, 0.6, 0.8 mg/hr

Side effects/adverse reactions:

▼ *ORAL:* Dry mouth, burning sensation

CNS: Headache, flushing, dizziness

CV: Postural hypotension, ***collapse,*** tachycardia, syncope

GI: Nausea, vomiting

INTEG: Pallor, sweating, rash

Contraindications: Hypersensitivity to this drug or nitrites, severe anemia, increased intracranial pressure, cerebral hemorrhage

Precautions: Postural hypotension, pregnancy category C, lactation

Pharmacokinetics:

SUS REL: Onset 20-45 min, duration 3-8 hr

SL: Onset 1-3 min, duration 30 min

TRANSDERM: Onset 0.5-1 hr, duration 12-24 hr

IV: Onset immediate, duration variable

TRANSMUC: Onset 3 min, duration 10-30 min

AEROSOL: Onset 2 min, duration 30-60 min

TOP OINT: Onset 30-60 min, duration 2-12 hr

Metabolized by liver, excreted in urine

Drug interactions of concern to dentistry:

• Increased hypotensive effects: alcohol, opioids, aspirin in 1 g single doses, benzodiazepines, phenothiazines, and other drugs used in conscious sedation techniques

DENTAL CONSIDERATIONS

General:

• Take vital signs every appointment due to cardiovascular side effects.

• After supine positioning, have patient sit upright for at least 2 min before standing to avoid orthostatic hypotension.

• Assess salivary flow as a factor in caries, periodontal disease, and candidiasis.

• Ensure that patient's drug is easily available if angina occurs.

• A benzodiazepine or nitrous oxide/oxygen may be prescribed to allay anxiety.

• Check expiration date on prescription to ensure drug activity. If bottle has been opened, there is a 3-month shelf life.

• Stress from dental procedures may compromise cardiovascular function; determine patient risk.

• Talk with patient about disease control (frequency of angina episodes).

• Use vasoconstrictors with caution, in low doses, and with careful aspiration. Avoid gingival retraction cord with epinephrine.

• Short appointments and a stress reduction protocol may be required for anxious patients.

• Consider semisupine chair position for patients with cardiovascular disease.

Consultations:

• Medical consult may be required to assess disease control and patient's ability to tolerate stress.

Teach patient/family:

• Importance of good oral hygiene to prevent soft tissue inflammation

• Caution to prevent injury when using oral hygiene aids

When chronic dry mouth occurs, advise patient:

• To avoid mouth rinses with high alcohol content due to drying effects

• Of need for daily home fluoride to prevent caries

• To use sugarless gum, frequent sips of water, or saliva substitutes

---

nizatidine

(ni-za'ti-deen)

Axid, Axid AR

🍁 Apo-Nizatidine

Drug class.: H_2 histamine receptor antagonist

Action: Inhibits histamine at H_2 receptor site in parietal cells, which inhibits gastric acid secretion

Uses: Duodenal ulcer, Zollinger-Ellison syndrome, gastric ulcers, hypersecretory conditions, gastroesophageal reflux disease, stress ulcers; unapproved use includes GI symptoms associated with NSAID use in rheumatoid arthritis

Dosage and routes:

Duodenal ulcer

• *Adult:* PO 300 mg daily hs or 150 mg bid

Maintenance

• *Adult:* PO 150 mg daily hs; gastroesophageal reflux 150 mg bid

Available forms include: Caps 150, 300 mg; tab 75 mg

Side effects/adverse reactions:

CNS: Somnolence, fatigue, insomnia, headache

GI: Nausea, vomiting, abdominal discomfort, diarrhea, constipation

GU: Impotence, decreased libido

INTEG: Pruritus, urticaria, rash, increased sweating

N

Contraindications: Hypersensitivity

Precautions: Pregnancy category C, hepatic disease, renal disease, lactation, children <16 yr

Pharmacokinetics: Peak plasma levels 0.5-3 hr, half-life 2.5-3.5 hr, duration up to 12 hr; primary renal excretion

Drug interactions of concern to dentistry:

- Increased serum salicylate when administered with high doses of aspirin
- Decreased absorption of ketoconazole (take doses 2 hr apart)

DENTAL CONSIDERATIONS

General:

- Avoid prescribing aspirin-containing products in patients with active GI disease.

Teach patient/family:

- To avoid mouth rinses with high alcohol content due to drying effects

---

norethindrone/ norethindrone acetate

(nor-eth-in′drone)

Aygestin, Micronor, Nor-QD

Drug class.: Progesterone derivative

Action: Inhibits secretion of pituitary gonadotropins, which prevents follicular maturation, ovulation

Uses: Uterine bleeding (abnormal), amenorrhea, endometriosis, contraceptive

Dosage and routes:

- *Adult:* PO 5-20 mg qd on days 5-25 of menstrual cycle

Endometriosis

- *Adult:* PO 5 mg qd × 2 wk, then increased by 2.5 mg qd × 2 wk, up to 15 mg qd

Available forms include: Tabs 0.35, 5 mg

Side effects/adverse reactions:

ORAL: Gingival bleeding, gingival overgrowth

CNS: Dizziness, headache, migraines, depression, fatigue

CV: ***Thromboembolism, stroke, pulmonary embolism, MI,*** hypotension, thrombophlebitis, edema

GI: Nausea, ***cholestatic jaundice,*** vomiting, anorexia, cramps, increased weight

GU: Gynecomastia, testicular atrophy, impotence, ***spontaneous abortion,*** amenorrhea, endometriosis, cervical erosion, breakthrough bleeding, dysmenorrhea, vaginal candidiasis, breast changes

EENT: Diplopia

INTEG: Rash, urticaria, acne, hirsutism, alopecia, oily skin, seborrhea, purpura, melasma

META: Hyperglycemia

Contraindications: Breast cancer, hypersensitivity, thromboembolic disorders, reproductive cancer, genital bleeding (abnormal, undiagnosed), cerebral hemorrhage, pregnancy category X

Precautions: Lactation, hypertension, asthma, blood dyscrasias, gallbladder disease, CHF, diabetes mellitus, bone disease, depression, migraine headache, convulsive disorders, hepatic disease, renal disease, family history of breast or reproductive tract cancer

Pharmacokinetics:

PO: Duration 24 hr; metabolized in liver; excreted in urine, feces

Drug interactions of concern to dentistry:

• Decreased effectiveness of oral contraceptives: antibiotics, barbiturates

DENTAL CONSIDERATIONS

General:

• Place on frequent recall to evaluate gingival inflammation if present.

• An increased incidence of dry socket has been reported after extraction.

• Monitor vital signs at each appointment.

Teach patient/family:

• Need for good oral hygiene to prevent periodontal inflammation

• That smoking cessation decreases risk of serious adverse cardiovascular effects

• Need for additional method of birth control while undergoing antibiotic therapy

norfloxacin

(nor-flox′-a-sin)

Noroxin

Drug class.: Fluoroquinolone anti-infective

Action: A broad-spectrum bactericidal agent that inhibits the enzyme DNA gyrase needed for the replication of bacterial DNA

Uses: Adult UTIs (including complicated) caused by *E. coli, E. cloacae, P. mirabilis, K. pneumoniae,* group D strep, indole-positive *Proteus, C. freundii, S. aureus*

Dosage and routes:

Uncomplicated

• *Adult:* PO 400 mg bid × 7-10 days 1 hr before or 2 hr after meals

Complicated

• *Adult:* PO 400 mg bid × 10-21 days; 400 mg qd × 7-10 days in impaired renal function

Available forms include: Tabs 400 mg

Side effects/adverse reactions:

▼ *ORAL:* Dry mouth, stomatitis

CNS: Headache, dizziness, fatigue, somnolence, depression, insomnia

GI: Nausea, constipation, increased ALT/AST, flatulence, heartburn, vomiting, diarrhea

EENT: Visual disturbances, phototoxicity

INTEG: Rash, blue-black discoloration

MS: Tendinitis, tendon rupture

Contraindications: Hypersensitivity to quinolones

Precautions: Pregnancy category C, lactation, children, renal disease, seizure disorders, tendon rupture in shoulder, hand, and Achilles tendons

Pharmacokinetics:

PO: Peak 1 hr, steady state 2 days, half-life 3-4 hr; excreted in urine as active drug, metabolites

Drug interactions of concern to dentistry:

• Decreased absorption: sodium bicarbonate

DENTAL CONSIDERATIONS

General:

• Assess salivary flow as a factor in caries, periodontal disease, and candidiasis.

• Determine why the patient is taking the drug.

• Due to drug interaction, do not use ingestible sodium bicarbonate products such as the air polishing system (Prophy Jet) unless at least 2 hr have passed since norfloxacin was taken.

• Avoid dental light in patient's

N

eyes; offer dark glasses for patient comfort.

• Ruptures of the shoulder, hand, and Achilles tendons that required surgical repair or resulted in prolonged disability have been reported with this drug.

Consultations:

• Consult with patient's physician if an acute dental infection occurs and another antiinfective is required.

Teach patient/family:

• To avoid mouth rinses with high alcohol content due to drying effects

• To discontinue treatment and inform dentist immediately if patient experiences pain or inflammation of a tendon, and to rest and refrain from exercise

---

norgestrel

(nor-jess'trel)
Ovrette

Drug class.: Progesterone derivative

Action: Inhibits secretion of pituitary gonadotropins, which prevents follicular maturation, ovulation

Uses: Oral contraception

Dosage and routes:

• *Adult:* PO 1 tablet qd beginning on day 1 of cycle and continuing

Available forms include: Tabs 0.075 mg

Side effects/adverse reactions:

▼ *ORAL:* Gingival bleeding, dry socket

CNS: Dizziness, headache, migraines, depression, fatigue

CV: ***Thromboembolism, stroke, pulmonary embolism, MI,*** hypotension, thrombophlebitis, edema

GI: Nausea, ***cholestatic jaundice,*** vomiting, anorexia, cramps, increased weight

GU: Gynecomastia, testicular atrophy, impotence, endometriosis, ***spontaneous abortion,*** amenorrhea, cervical erosion, breakthrough bleeding, dysmenorrhea, vaginal candidiasis, breast changes

EENT: Diplopia

INTEG: Rash, urticaria, acne, hirsutism, alopecia, oily skin, seborrhea, purpura, melasma

META: Hyperglycemia

Contraindications: Breast cancer, hypersensitivity, thromboembolic disorders, reproductive cancer, genital bleeding (abnormal, undiagnosed), cerebral hemorrhage, pregnancy category X

Precautions: Lactation, hypertension, asthma, blood dyscrasias, gallbladder disease, CHF, diabetes mellitus, bone disease, depression, migraine headache, convulsive disorders, hepatic disease, renal disease, family history of breast or reproductive tract cancer

Pharmacokinetics:

PO: Duration 24 hr, excreted in urine and feces, metabolized in liver

Drug interactions of concern to dentistry:

• Decreased effectiveness of oral contraceptives: antibiotics, barbiturates

DENTAL CONSIDERATIONS

General:

• Place on frequent recall to evaluate gingival inflammation if present.

• An increased incidence of dry socket has been reported after extraction.

• Monitor vital signs at each appointment.

Teach patient/family:
• Need for good oral hygiene to prevent periodontal inflammation
• That smoking cessation decreases risk of serious and adverse cardiovascular side effects
• Need for additional method of birth control while undergoing antibiotic therapy

nortriptyline HCl

(nor-trip'ti-leen)
Aventyl, Pamelor

Drug class.: Antidepressant—tricyclic

Action: Blocks reuptake of norepinephrine, serotonin into nerve endings, which increases action of norepinephrine, serotonin in nerve cells
Uses: Major depression
Dosage and routes:
• *Adult:* PO 25 mg tid or qid; may increase to 150 mg/day; may give daily dose hs
Available forms include: Caps 10, 25, 75 mg; sol 10 mg/5 ml
Side effects/adverse reactions:
ORAL: Dry mouth, unpleasant taste, bleeding, sublingual adenitis
CNS: Dizziness, drowsiness, confusion, headache, anxiety, tremors, stimulation, weakness, insomnia, nightmares, EPS (elderly), increased psychiatric symptoms
CV: Orthostatic hypotension, ECG changes, tachycardia, ***hypertension,*** palpitation
GI: Constipation, ***hepatitis, paralytic ileus,*** increased appetite, nausea, vomiting, cramps, epigastric distress, jaundice
HEMA: ***Agranulocytosis, thrombocytopenia, eosinophilia, leukopenia***
GU: Retention, ***acute renal failure***
EENT: Blurred vision, tinnitus, mydriasis
INTEG: Rash, urticaria, sweating, pruritus, photosensitivity
Contraindications: Hypersensitivity to tricyclic antidepressants, recovery phase of MI, convulsive disorders, prostatic hypertrophy
Precautions: Suicidal patients, severe depression, increased intraocular pressure, narrow-angle glaucoma, urinary retention, cardiac disease, hepatic disease, hyperthyroidism, electroshock therapy, elective surgery, pregnancy category C, MAO inhibitors
Pharmacokinetics:
PO: Steady state 4-19 days, half-life 18-28 hr; metabolized by liver; excreted by kidneys; crosses placenta; excreted in breast milk
Drug interactions of concern to dentistry:
• Increased anticholinergic effects: muscarinic blockers, antihistamines, phenothiazines
• Increased effects of direct-acting sympathomimetics (epinephrine, levonordefrin)
• Potential risk of increased CNS depression: alcohol, barbiturates, benzodiazepines, and other CNS depressants
• Decreased antihypertensive effect: clonidine, guanadrel, guanethidine

DENTAL CONSIDERATIONS

General:
• Take vital signs every appointment due to cardiovascular side effects.
• Assess salivary flow as a factor in caries, periodontal disease, and candidiasis.
• Patients on chronic drug therapy may rarely have symptoms of

N

blood dyscrasias, which can include infection, bleeding, and poor healing.

• After supine positioning, have patient sit upright for at least 2 min before standing to avoid orthostatic hypotension.

• Use vasoconstrictors with caution, in low doses, and with careful aspiration. Avoid use of gingival retraction cord with epinephrine.

• Place on frequent recall due to oral side effects.

Consultations:

• In a patient with symptoms of blood dyscrasias, request a medical consult for blood studies and postpone dental treatment until normal values are reestablished.

• Medical consult may be required to assess disease control in the patient.

• Physician should be informed if significant xerostomic side effects occur (increased caries, sore tongue, problems eating or swallowing, difficulty wearing prosthesis) so a medication change can be considered.

Teach patient/family:

• Importance of good oral hygiene to prevent soft tissue inflammation

• Caution to prevent injury when using oral hygiene aids

When chronic dry mouth occurs, advise patient:

• To avoid mouth rinses with high alcohol content due to drying effects

• Of need for daily home fluoride to prevent caries

• To use sugarless gum, frequent sips of water, or saliva substitutes

---

nystatin

(nye-sta′tin)

Mycostatin, Nilstat, Nystex

♣ Nadostine, Nyaderm

Drug class.: Antifungal

Action: Interferes with fungal DNA replication; binds sterols in fungal cell membrane, which increases permeability and leaking of cell nutrients

Uses: *Candida* species causing oral, vaginal, intestinal infections

Dosage and routes:

Oral infection

• *Adult:* Susp 400,000-600,000 U qid

• *Adult and child:* TOP apply to affected area bid-tid × 14 days; loz 200,000 up to 400,000 U, dissolve slowly in mouth 4-5 ×/day up to 14 days

• *Child and infant >3 mo:* Susp 250,000-500,000 U qid

• *Newborn and premature infant:* Susp 100,000 U qid

Extemporanous powder: ⅛ teaspoonful powder (500,000 units) in ½ cup of water (120 ml); use as an oral rinse tid or qid

GI infection

• *Adult:* PO 500,000-1,000,000 U tid

Vaginal infection

• *Adult:* Vag tab 100,000 U inserted high into vagina qd-bid × 2 wk

Available forms include: Tabs 500,000 U; vag tabs 100,000 U; powder 50 million, 150 million, 500 million, 1 billion, 2 billion, 5 billion U; susp 100,000 U in 60 ml and 473 ml units; top cream, oint, powder 100,000 U/g in 15 mg and 60 g units; loz 200,000 U

Side effects/adverse reactions:
GI: Nausea, vomiting, anorexia, diarrhea, cramps
INTEG: Rash, urticaria (rare)
Contraindications: Hypersensitivity
Precautions: Pregnancy category not listed
Pharmacokinetics:
PO: Little absorption, excreted in feces

DENTAL CONSIDERATIONS
General:
• Determine why the patient is taking the drug.
• Broad-spectrum antibiotic may contribute to oral *Candida* infections.
Teach patient/family:
• That long-term therapy may be needed to clear infection; to complete entire course of medication
• Not to use commercial mouthwashes for mouth infection unless prescribed by dentist
• To soak full or partial dentures in a suitable antifungal solution nightly
• To prevent reinoculation of *Candida* infection by disposing of toothbrush or other contaminated oral hygiene devices used during period of infection

---

ofloxacin

(oh-flocks'a-sin)
Floxin, Floxin IV
Drug class.: Fluoroquinolone anti-infective

Action: A broad-spectrum bactericidal agent that inhibits the enzyme DNA gyrase needed for the replication of bacterial DNA
Uses: Treatment of lower respiratory tract infections (pneumonia, bronchitis), genitourinary infections (prostatitis, UTIs) caused by *E. coli, K. pneumoniae, C. trachomatis, N. gonorrhoeae;* skin and skin structure infections
Dosage and routes:
Lower respiratory tract infections/ skin and skin structure infections
• *Adult:* PO 400 mg q12h × 10 days
Cervicitis, urethritis
• *Adult:* PO 300 mg q12h × 7 days
Prostatitis
• *Adult:* PO 300 mg q12h × 6 wk
Acute, uncomplicated gonorrhea
• *Adult:* PO 400 mg as a single dose
Pneumonia
• *Adult:* 400 mg by IV infusion given over 60 min q12h × 10 days
Available forms include: Tabs 200, 300, 400 mg; inj 200 mg/50 ml D_5W, 400 mg in 10, 20 ml vials or 100 ml (D_5W) bottles
Side effects/adverse reactions:
▼ *ORAL:* Candidiasis, dry mouth, dysgeusia
CNS: Dizziness, headache, fatigue, somnolence, depression, insomnia, lethargy, malaise, nervousness, anxiety
GI: Diarrhea, nausea, vomiting, anorexia, flatulence, heartburn, increased AST/ALT, abdominal pain/ cramps, constipation, decreased appetite, dyspepsia
EENT: Visual disturbances, phototoxicity
INTEG: Rash, pruritus
MS: Tendinitis, tendon rupture
Contraindications: Hypersensitivity to quinolones
Precautions: Pregnancy category C, lactation, children <18 yr, elderly, renal disease, seizure disorders, excessive sunlight, tendon rupture in shoulder, hand, and Achilles tendons

Pharmacokinetics:
PO: Peak 1-2 hr, steady state 2 days, half-life 9 hr; excreted in urine as active drug, metabolites; 0.9% bioavailability

Drug interactions of concern to dentistry:
• Decreased effects: antacids

DENTAL CONSIDERATIONS
General:
• Due to drug interaction, do not use ingestible sodium bicarbonate products such as the air polishing system (Prophy Jet) unless 2 hr have passed since ofloxacin was taken.
• Examine for oral manifestation of opportunistic infections.
• Avoid dental light in patient's eyes; offer dark glasses for patient comfort.
• Minimize exposure to sunlight and wear sunscreen if sun exposure is planned.
• Ruptures of the shoulder, hand, and Achilles tendons that required surgical repair or resulted in prolonged disability have been reported with this drug.
Consultations:
• Consult with patient's physician if an acute dental infection occurs and another antiinfective is required.
Teach patient/family:
• Importance of good oral hygiene to prevent soft tissue inflammation
• To avoid mouth rinses with high alcohol content due to drying effects
• To discontinue treatment and inform dentist immediately if patient experiences pain or inflammation of a tendon, and to rest and refrain from exercise

ofloxacin (optic)
(oh-flocks'a-sin)
Ocuflox, Ocuflox Opthalmic Solution
Drug class.: Fluroroquinolone antiinfective, topical

Action: A broad-spectrum bactericidal agent that inhibits the enzyme DNA gyrase needed for the replication of DNA
Uses: Treatment of bacterial conjunctivitis caused by susceptible organisms, corneal ulcers
Dosage and routes:
• *Adult and child:* Instill 1 gtt in each eye q2-4h × 2 days; then 1 gtt qid up to 5 days
Available forms include: Sol 3 mg/ml in 5 ml
Side effects/adverse reactions:
CNS: Dizziness
EENT: Burning sensation in eye, photophobia, redness
Contraindications: Hypersensitivity
Precautions: Pregnancy category C, children <1 yr
Pharmacokinetics:
TOP: Low systemic absorption, renal excretion of metabolites

DENTAL CONSIDERATIONS
General:
• Avoid dental light in patient's eyes; offer dark glasses for patient comfort and safety protection during dental treatment.

olanzapine
(oh lan'za-peen)
Zyprexa
Drug class.: Antipsychotic

Action: Antipsychotic mechanism is unknown; acts as an antagonist for serotonin, dopamine, muscarinic, histamine, and α_1-adrenergic receptors

Uses: Psychotic disorders; schizophrenia

Dosage and routes:

• *Adult:* PO initial dose 5-10 mg qd, target dose is 10 mg/day; use 5 mg dose for patients at higher risk for orthostatic hypotension and nonsmoking women >65 yr

Available forms include: Tabs 2.5, 5, 7.5, 10 mg

Side effects/adverse reactions:

▼ *ORAL: Dry mouth (7%)*

CNS: Extrapyramidal events, somnolence, agitation, dizziness, personality disorder, insomnia, nervousness, hostility, headache, anxiety

CV: Orthostatic hypotension, tachycardia

GI: Constipation, increased appetite, abdominal pain

RESP: Rhinitis, cough, pharyngitis

GU: Premenstrual syndrome

INTEG: Vesiculobullous rash

MS: Joint pain, extremity pain, twitching

META: Weight gain, edema, fever

Contraindications: Hypersensitivity

Precautions: Pregnancy category C, lactation, paralytic ileus, elderly; combination of age, smoking, and gender (female) may increase clearance rate; neuroleptic malignant syndrome, CV disease, cerebrovascular disease, seizures, orthostatic hypotension, Alzheimer's dementia, prostate hypertrophy, glaucoma

Pharmacokinetics:

PO: Well absorbed, peak plasma levels 6 hr, hepatic metabolism, half-life 21-54 hr; renal and fecal excretion

Drug interactions of concern to dentistry:

• Potentiation of orthostatic hypotension: diazepam, alcohol

DENTAL CONSIDERATIONS

General:

• Consider semisupine chair position for patient comfort due to GI effects of drug.

• Assess salivary flow as factor in caries, periodontal disease, and candidiasis.

• Monitor vital signs every appointment due to cardiovascular side effects.

• After supine positioning have patient sit upright for at least 2 min to avoid orthostatic hypotension.

• Patients on chronic drug therapy may rarely have symptoms of blood dyscrasias, which can include infection, bleeding, and poor healing.

• Assess for presence of extrapyramidal motor symptoms, such as tardive dyskinesia and akathisia. Extrapyramidal motor activity may complicate dental treatment.

Consultations:

• In a patient with symptoms of blood dyscrasias, request a medical consult for blood studies and postpone dental treatment until normal values are reestablished.

• Medical consult may be required to assess disease control in the patient.

• Physician should be informed if significant xerostomic side effects occur (increased caries, sore tongue, problems eating or swallowing, difficulty wearing prosthesis) so a medication change can be considered.

Teach patient/family:

• Importance of good oral hygiene to prevent soft tissue inflammation

O

• Use of electric toothbrush if patient has difficulty holding conventional devices
• Caution patients about driving or performing other tasks requiring alertness

When chronic dry mouth occurs, advise patient:
• To avoid mouth rinses with high alcohol content due to drying effects
• To use daily home fluoride products for anticaries effect
• To use sugarless gum, frequent sips of water, or saliva substitutes

---

olopatadine HCl

(oh-loe-pa-ta′deen)
Patanol

Drug class.: Opthalmic antihistamine

Action: Selective H_1-receptor antogonist and inhibitor of histamine release from mast cells
Uses: Temporary prevention of itching of eye due to allergic conjunctivitis
Dosage and routes:
• *Adult:* TOP 1 or 2 gtts in each affected eye bid at 6 to 8 hr intervals
Available forms include: Sol 0.1% in 5 ml drop dispenser
Side effects/adverse reactions:
▼ *ORAL: Taste alteration*
EENT: Burning, dry eye, keratitis, lid edema, pruritus, foreign body reaction
MISC: Cold syndrome
Contraindications: Hypersensitivity
Precautions: Topical use only, do not use while wearing contact lenses, pregnancy category C, lactation, children <3 yr
Pharmacokinetics:
TOP: Low to nondetectable plasma levels, peak in 2 hr, renal excretion
Drug interactions of concern to dentistry:
• None reported

DENTAL CONSIDERATIONS
General: Protect patient's eyes from accidental spatter during dental treatment.

---

olsalazine sodium

(ole-sal′a-zeen)
Dipentum

Drug class.: Antiinflammatory, salicylate derivative

Action: Bioconverted to 5-aminosalicylic acid, which decreases inflammation in the colon
Uses: Maintenance of remission of ulcerative colitis in patients intolerant to sulfasalazine
Dosage and routes:
• *Adult:* PO 1 g/day in 2 divided doses with meals
Available forms include: Caps 250 mg
Side effects/adverse reactions:
▼ *ORAL:* Stomatitis
CNS: Headache, insomnia, hallucinations, depression, vertigo, fatigue, drug fever, chills, dizziness, drowsiness, tremors
CV: Allergic myocarditis, second-degree heart block, hypertension, peripheral edema, chest pain, palpitation
GI: Nausea, vomiting, abdominal pain, hepatitis, pancreatitis, diarrhea, bloating
RESP: ***Bronchospasm,*** shortness of breath
HEMA: ***Leukopenia, neutropenia, thrombocytopenia, agranulocytosis, anemia***

GU: Frequency, dysuria, hematuria, impotence
INTEG: ***Stevens-Johnson syndrome,*** erythema, photosensitivity, rash, dermatitis, urticaria, alopecia
SYST: ***Anaphylaxis***
Contraindications: Hypersensitivity to salicylates, child <14 yr
Precautions: Pregnancy category C, lactation, impaired hepatic function, severe allergy, bronchial asthma, renal disease
Pharmacokinetics:
PO: Partially absorbed, peak 1.5 hr, half-life 5-10 hr; excreted in urine as 5-aminosalicylic acid and metabolites; crosses placenta

DENTAL CONSIDERATIONS
General:
• Consider semisupine chair position for patient comfort due to GI effects of disease.
Consultations:
• Avoid drugs that could aggravate an inflammatory colon disease; consult is recommended before selection of an antibiotic.
Teach patient/family:
• Importance of good oral hygiene to prevent soft tissue inflammation
• Caution to prevent injury when using oral hygiene aids
• To avoid mouth rinses with high alcohol content due to drying effects

omeprazole

(oh-me'pray-zol)
Prilosec
♣ Losec
Drug class.: Antisecretory

Action: Suppresses gastric secretion by inhibiting hydrogen/potassium ATPase enzyme system in the gastric parietal cell; characterized as a gastric acid pump inhibitor because it blocks the final step of acid production
Uses: Gastroesophageal reflux disease (GERD), severe erosive esophagitis, poorly responsive systemic GERD, pathologic hypersecretory conditions (Zollinger-Ellison syndrome, systemic mastocytosis, multiple endocrine adenomas), with clarithromycin, short-term treatment of gastric ulcers; not approved for long-term ulcer maintenance therapy
Dosage and routes:
Severe erosive esophagitis/poorly responsive gastroesophageal reflux disease
• *Adult:* PO 20 mg qd × 4-8 wk; take before eating
Gastric ulcers
• *Adult:* PO 40 mg qd × 2 wk, then 20 mg qd × 2 wk
Duodenal ulcer
• *Adult:* PO 40 mg in AM × 14 days with clarithromycin 500 mg tid; on days 15-28, 20 mg daily
Pathologic hypersecretory conditions
• *Adult:* PO 60 mg/day; may increase to 120 mg tid; daily doses >80 mg in divided doses
Available forms include: Cap (delayed release) 10, 20, 40 mg
Side effects/adverse reactions:
▼ *ORAL:* Dry mouth, mucosal atrophy of tongue, taste perversion, candidiasis
CNS: Headache, dizziness, asthenia, nervousness, anxiety disorders
CV: Chest pain, angina, tachycardia, bradycardia, palpitation, peripheral edema
GI: Diarrhea, abdominal pain, vomiting, nausea, constipation, flatulence, acid regurgitation, ab-

O

dominal swelling, anorexia, irritable colon, esophageal candidiasis
RESP: Upper respiratory infections, cough, epistaxis
HEMA: ***Pancytopenia, thrombocytopenia, neutropenia, leukocytosis,*** anemia
GU: ***Proteinuria, hematuria,*** UTI, frequency, increased creatinine, testicular pain, glycosuria
EENT: Tinnitus
INTEG: Rash, dry skin, urticaria, pruritus, alopecia
META: Hypoglycemia, increased hepatic enzymes, weight gain
MISC: Back pain, fever, fatigue, malaise
Contraindications: Hypersensitivity
Precautions: Pregnancy category C, lactation, children
Pharmacokinetics:
PO: Peak 30 min-3.5 hr, half-life 30 min-1 hr; protein binding 95%; eliminated in urine as metabolites and in feces; in the elderly the elimination rate is decreased, bioavailability is increased
Drug interactions of concern to dentistry:
• Increased serum levels: diazepam

DENTAL CONSIDERATIONS
General:
• Question the patient about tolerance of NSAIDs or aspirin related to GI problem.
• Consider semisupine chair position for patient comfort due to GI effects of disease.
• Assess salivary flow as a factor in caries, periodontal disease, and candidiasis.
Teach patient/family:
• Caution to prevent injury when using oral hygiene aids
When chronic dry mouth occurs, advise patient:
• To avoid mouth rinses with high alcohol content due to drying effects
• Of need for daily home fluoride to prevent caries
• To use sugarless gum, frequent sips of water, or saliva substitutes

ondansetron HCl
(on-dan-see'tron)
Zofran, Zofran ODT
Drug class.: Antiemetic

Action: A selective 5-HT_3 antagonist; antiemetic effect may be mediated centrally, peripherally, or both
Uses: Prevention of nausea/vomiting associated with cancer chemotherapy, radiotherapy, and postoperative nausea and vomiting
Dosage and routes:
• *Adult and child >12 yr:* PO 8 mg tid, administer first dose 30 min before chemotherapy and then at 4 and 8 hr intervals, continue 1-2 days after chemotherapy; IV 0.15 mg/kg, give first dose over 15 min and 30 min before chemotherapy and at 4 and 8 hr intervals
Available forms include: Tabs 4, 8 mg; oral disintegrating tab 4, 8 mg; IV 2 mg/ml in 20 ml vials
Side effects/adverse reactions:
▼ *ORAL:* Dry mouth (1%-2%)
CNS: Headache, weakness, possible EPS, grand mal seizures
CV: Hypokalemia, ECG alterations, vascular occlusive events
GI: Constipation, abdominal pain
RESP: ***Bronchospasm***
EENT: Transient blurred vision
INTEG: Rash

MISC: ***Anaphylaxis***
Contraindications: Hypersensitivity
Precautions: Pregnancy category B, lactation, children <12 yr, elderly
Pharmacokinetics:
PO: Well absorbed, peak plasma levels 1.9 hr, food increases absorption; extensive metabolism
IV: Rapid peak levels; protein binding 70%-76%; extensively metabolized
Drug interactions of concern to dentistry:
• None reported
DENTAL CONSIDERATIONS
General:
• Be aware that patient is receiving active chemotherapy.
• Avoid procedures or drugs that could promote nausea/vomiting.
• Patients with cancer may be taking chronic opioids for pain. Consider NSAID for dental pain management.
• Patients receiving chemotherapy may require palliative therapy for stomatitis.
• An increased gag reflex may make dental procedures, such as obtaining radiographs or impressions, difficult.
Consultations:
• Medical consult may be required to assess disease control in the patient.
Teach patient/family:
When chronic dry mouth occurs, advise patient:
• To avoid mouth rinses with high alcohol content due to drying effects
• Of need for daily home fluoride to prevent caries
• To use sugarless gum, frequent sips of water, or saliva substitutes

---

oral contraceptives

Estrogens: ethinyl estradiol, mestranol
Progestins: ethynodiol diacetate, levonorgestrel, norethindrone, norgestimate, norgestrel, desogestrel
Many products are available. Examples:
Monophasic products: Alese, Brevicon, Demulen 1/35, Demulen 1/50, Desogen, Estrostep Fe, Genora 0.5/35, Genora 1/50, Genora 1/35, Levlen, Levite, Levora, Loestrin 21, Loestrin Fe, Lo/Ovral, Modicon, Necon 0.5/35, Nelova 0.5/35E, Necon 1/50, Necon 1/35, Nelova 1/50, Nelova 1/35E, Nordette, Norethin 1/50M, Norethin 1/35E, Norinyl, OrthoCept, Ortho-Cyclen, Ortho-Novum 1/50, Ortho-Novum 1/35, Ovcon-50, Ovral, Brevicon, Modicon, Ovcon 35, Necon, Zovia 1/50E, Zovia 1/35E, others
Biphasic products: Alesse-28, Janest-28, Necon, Nelova 10/11, Ortho-Novum 10/11, Mircette
Triphasic products: Estrostep, Estrostep-21, Tri-Norinyl, Ortho-Novum 7/7/7, Tri-Levlen, Triphasil, Ortho Tri-Cyclen, Trivora, Trivora
Drug class.: Estrogen/progestin combinations

Action: Prevents ovulation by suppressing follicle-stimulating hormone, luteinizing hormone
Uses: To prevent pregnancy, endo-

O

metriosis, hypermenorrhea, hypogonadism; acne (Tri-Cyclen)

Dosage and routes:

• *Adult:* PO 1 qd starting on day 5 of menstrual cycle (day 1 is first day of period)

20/21-tablet packs

• *Adult:* PO 1 qd starting on day 7 of menstrual cycle (day 1 is first day of period); then on for 20 or 21 days, off 7 days

28-tablet packs

• *Adult:* PO 1 qd continuously

Biphasic

• *Adult:* PO 1 qd × 10 days, then next color 1 qd × 11 days

Triphasic

• *Adult:* PO 1 qd; check package insert for each new brand

Endometriosis

• *Adult:* PO 1 qd × 20 days from day 5-24 of cycle

• *Adult:* PO 1 qd; check package insert for specific instructions

Available forms include: Check specific brand

Side effects/adverse reactions:

▼ *ORAL:* Gingival bleeding, dry socket

CNS: Depression, fatigue, dizziness, nervousness, anxiety, headache

CV: Increased BP, thromboembolic conditions, fluid retention, edema

GI: Nausea, vomiting, cramps, diarrhea, bloating, constipation, change in appetite, ***cholestatic jaundice***

HEMA: Increased fibrinogen, clotting factor

GU: Breakthrough bleeding, amenorrhea, spotting, dysmenorrhea, galactorrhea, endocervical hyperplasia, vaginitis, cystitis-like syndrome, breast change

EENT: Optic neuritis, retinal thrombosis, cataracts

INTEG: Melasma, acne, rash, urticaria, erythema multiforme or nodosum, pruritus, hirsutism, alopecia, photosensitivity

ENDO: Decreased glucose tolerance, increased TBG, PBI, T_4, T_3

Contraindications: Pregnancy category X, lactation, reproductive cancer, thrombophlebitis, MI, hepatic tumors, hepatic disease, CAD, women 40 yr and over, CVA

Precautions: Depression, hypertension, renal disease, seizure disorders, lupus erythematosus, rheumatic disease, migraine headache, amenorrhea, irregular menses, breast cancer (fibrocystic), gallbladder disease, diabetes mellitus, heavy smoking, acute mononucleosis, sickle cell disease

Pharmacokinetics:

PO: Excreted in breast milk

Drug interactions of concern to dentistry:

• Decreased effectiveness of oral contraceptives: antibiotics, barbiturates

DENTAL CONSIDERATIONS:

General:

• Monitor vital signs every appointment due to cardiovascular side effects.

• Place on frequent recall to evaluate gingival inflammation, if present.

• An increased incidence of dry socket has been reported after extraction.

• Consider semisupine chair position for patient comfort if GI side effects occur.

Teach patient/family:

• Need for good oral hygiene to prevent periodontal inflammation

• That smoking cessation decreases

risk of serious adverse cardiovascular effects

• Need for additional method of birth control while undergoing antibiotic therapy

orlistat

(or'lih-stat)

Xenical

Drug class.: Antiobesity

Action: A reversible inhibitor of lipases; acts in the intestinal lumen to inhibit both gastric and pancreatic lipases, thereby preventing the metabolism of fats into absorbable fatty acids

Uses: Obesity management, including weight loss and maintenance in conjunction with a reduced-calorie diet; used in patients with a defined body mass index with other risk factors for cardiovascular disease

Dosage and routes:

• *Adult:* PO 120 mg tid with each meal containing fat; give during meal or up to 1 hr after meal

Available forms include: Cap 120 mg

Side effects/adverse reactions:

▼ *ORAL:* Gingiva and tooth disorder (not defined)

CNS: Headache, dizziness, sleep disruption, anxiety

GI: Oily spotting, flatus with discharge, fecal urgency, oily or fatty stool, increased defecation, fecal incontinence, abdominal pain, vomiting

RESP: Influenza, URI, LRI

GU: Menstrual irregularity, UTI

EENT: Otitis

INTEG: Rash, dry skin

MS: Back pain, myalgia, joint discomfort

MISC: Fatigue

Contraindications: Chronic malabsorption syndrome, cholestasis or hypersensitivity reactions to this product, lactation; organic causes of obesity should first be identified

Precautions: Adherence to dietary guidelines, supplemental fat-soluble vitamins may be required along with betacarotene, nephrolithiasis, pregnancy category B, use in children not established

Pharmacokinetics:

PO: Poor oral absorption (minimal), low plasma levels, highly plasma protein bound (99%), metabolized in intestinal wall, majority of dose passes through GI tract for fecal excretion.

Drug interactions of concern to dentistry:

• None reported

DENTAL CONSIDERATIONS

General:

• Although no dental drug interactions are reported, observe expected outcomes of systemically administered drugs.

• Severely obese patients may have type 2 diabetes or cardiovascular diseases.

• Consider semisupine chair position for patient comfort if GI side effects occur.

• Ensure that patient is following prescribed diet and regularly takes medication.

Consultations:

• Medical consult may be required to assess disease control in the patient.

Teach patient/family:

• Importance of updating health and drug history if physician makes any changes in evaluation/ drug regimens

orphenadrine citrate

(or-fen'a-dreen)

Mio-rel, Norflex, Orfo

✤ Antiflex, Banflex, Flexoject, Myolin, Myotrol

Drug class.: Skeletal muscle relaxant, central acting

Action: Acts centrally to depress polysynaptic pathways to relax skeletal muscle, inhibit muscle spasm

Uses: Pain in musculoskeletal conditions

Dosage and routes:

• *Adult:* PO 100 mg bid; IM/IV 60 mg q12h

Available forms include: Tabs 100 mg; sus rel tabs 100 mg; inj IM/IV 30 mg/ml

Side effects/adverse reactions:

▼ *ORAL:* Dry mouth

CNS: Dizziness, weakness, drowsiness, headache, disorientation, insomnia, stimulation, hallucination, agitation, syncope

CV: Tachycardia, palpitation

GI: Nausea, vomiting, constipation

HEMA: ***Aplastic anemia***

GU: Urinary hesitancy, retention

EENT: Pupil dilation, blurred vision, increased intraocular pressure, mydriasis

INTEG: Rash, pruritus, urticaria

Contraindications: Hypersensitivity, narrow-angle glaucoma, GI obstruction, myasthenia gravis, stenosing peptic ulcer, bladder neck obstruction, cardiospasm

Precautions: Pregnancy category not listed, children, cardiac disease, tachycardia, caution in lactation

Pharmacokinetics:

PO: Peak 2 hr, duration 4-6 hr, half-life 14 hr; metabolized in liver; excreted in urine (unchanged)

Drug interactions of concern to dentistry:

• Increased CNS effects: propoxyphene, CNS depressants, alcohol

• Increased anticholinergic effect: other anticholinergics

DENTAL CONSIDERATIONS

General:

• Consider semisupine chair position for patients with back pain.

• Patients on chronic drug therapy may rarely have symptoms of blood dyscrasias, which can include infection, bleeding, and poor healing.

• Assess salivary flow as a factor in caries, periodontal disease, and candidiasis.

Consultations:

• In a patient with symptoms of blood dyscrasias, request a medical consult for blood studies and postpone dental treatment until normal values are reestablished.

• Medical consult may be required to assess disease control in the patient.

Teach patient/family:

• Importance of good oral hygiene to prevent soft tissue inflammation

• Caution to prevent injury when using oral hygiene aids

When chronic dry mouth occurs, advise patient:

• To avoid mouth rinses with high alcohol content due to drying effects

• Of need for daily home fluoride to prevent caries

• To use sugarless gum, frequent sips of water, or saliva substitutes

oseltamivir phosphate

(oh-sel'ta-me-veer)
Tamiflu
Drug class.: Antiviral

Action: Inhibits neuraminidase, which is essential for replication of influenza type A and B viruses
Uses: Uncomplicated acute illness due to influenza infection in adults who have been symptomatic for no more than 2 days; more effective against influenza type A virus
Dosage and routes:
• *Adult:* PO 75 mg bid × 5 days, initiate treatment within 2 days of onset of symptoms
Available forms include: Caps 75 mg
Side effects/adverse reactions:
CNS: Insomnia, vertigo, headache
GI: Nausea, vomiting, abdominal pain
RESP: Bronchitis, cough
MISC: Fatigue
Contraindications: Hypersensitivity
Precautions: Renal impairment, pregnancy category C, lactation, children <18 yr
Pharmacokinetics:
PO: Readily absorbed, hepatic conversion to oseltamivir carboxylate, low plasma protein binding (3%), half-life 1-3 hr, excreted in urine (99%)
Drug interactions of concern to dentistry:
• None reported
DENTAL CONSIDERATIONS
General:
• Acute influenza patients are unlikely to be seen in the dental office except for dental emergencies.
• Consider semisupine chair position for patient comfort due to respiratory effects of disease.

oxacillin sodium

(ox-a-sil'in)
Bactocill, Prostaphlin
Drug class.: Penicillinase-resistant penicillin

Action: Interferes with cell wall replication of susceptible organisms; the cell wall, rendered osmotically unstable, swells and bursts from osmotic pressure
Uses: Effective for gram-positive cocci *(S. aureus, S. pneumoniae)* infections caused by penicillinase-producing *Staphylococcus*
Dosage and routes:
• *Adult and child >40 kg:* PO 500 mg q4-6h (limit 6 g/day); IM/IV 1-2 g q4-6h
• *Child <40 kg:* PO 50-100 mg/kg/day in divided doses q6h
Available forms include: Caps 250, 500 mg; powder for oral susp 250 mg/5 ml; powder for inj IM/IV 250, 500 mg, 1, 2, 4, 10 g
Side effects/adverse reactions:
▼ *ORAL:* Glossitis, candidiasis, black or hairy tongue, stomatitis
CNS: Lethargy, hallucinations, anxiety, depression, twitching, ***coma, convulsions***
GI: Nausea, vomiting, diarrhea, increased AST/ALT, abdominal pain, colitis
HEMA: Thrombocytopenia, transient neutropenia, ***bone marrow depression, granulocytopenia,*** anemia, increased bleeding time
GU: ***Oliguria, proteinuria, hematuria, vaginitis, moniliasis, glomerulonephritis***

O

Contraindications: Hypersensitivity to penicillins

Precautions: Pregnancy category B, hypersensitivity to cephalosporins, neonates, cystic fibrosis

Pharmacokinetics:

PO/IM: Peak 30-60 min, duration 4-6 hr

IV: Peak 5 min, duration 4-6 hr, half-life 30-60 min; metabolized in the liver; excreted in urine, bile, breast milk; crosses placenta

Drug interactions of concern to dentistry:

- Decreased antimicrobial effectiveness: tetracyclines, erythromycins
- Increased concentrations: aspirin, probenecid

DENTAL CONSIDERATIONS

General:

- Consider semisupine chair position for patient comfort if GI side effects occur.
- Examine for oral manifestation of opportunistic infections.
- Take precautions regarding allergy to medication and other drug allergies, such as cephalosporins.
- Determine why the patient is taking the drug.
- The effectiveness of oral contraceptives may be reduced by antibiotics.
- Patients on chronic drug therapy may rarely have symptoms of blood dyscrasias, which can include infection, bleeding, and poor healing.

Consultations:

- In a patient with symptoms of blood dyscrasias, request a medical consult for blood studies and postpone dental treatment until normal values are reestablished.
- Medical consult may be required to assess disease control in the patient.

Teach patient/family:

- Importance of good oral hygiene to prevent soft tissue inflammation
- Caution to prevent injury when using oral hygiene aids

When used for dental infection, advise patient:

- Taking birth control pill to use additional method of contraception for duration of cycle
- To report sore throat, oral burning sensation, fever, fatigue, any of which could indicate superinfection
- To take at prescribed intervals and complete dosage regimen
- To immediately notify the dentist if signs or symptoms of infection increase

---

oxandrolone

(ox-an'droe-lone)

Oxandrin

Drug class.: Androgenic anabolic steroid

Controlled Substance Schedule III

Action: Reverses catabolic tissue processes; promotes buildup of protein; increases erythropoietin production

Uses: Catabolic or tissue wasting processes, such as extensive surgery, burns, infection, or trauma; HIV wasting syndrome; Turner's syndrome

Dosage and routes:

- *Adult:* PO 2.5 mg bid-qid, not to exceed 20 mg qd × 2-3 wk
- *Child:* PO 0.25 mg/kg/day × 2-4 wk, not to exceed 3 mo

Available forms include: Tabs 2.5 mg

Side effects/adverse reactions:
CNS: Dizziness, headache, fatigue, tremors, paresthesia, flushing, sweating, anxiety, lability, insomnia
CV: Increased BP, ***edema*** (in cardiac patients)
GI: ***Cholestatic jaundice, peliosis hepatitis, liver cell tumors,*** nausea, vomiting, constipation, weight gain
HEMA: ***Increased prothrombin time, iron deficiency anemia***
GU: ***Hematuria,*** amenorrhea, vaginitis, decreased libido, decreased breast size, clitoral hypertrophy, testicular atrophy, gynecomastia (males), priapism
EENT: Conjunctional edema, nasal congestion
INTEG: Rash, acneiform lesions, oily hair/skin, flushing, sweating, acne vulgaris, alopecia, hirsutism
ENDO: Abnormal GTT, decreased glucose tolerance, increased LDL
MS: Cramps, spasms
Contraindications: Severe renal disease, severe cardiac disease, severe hepatic disease, hypersensitivity, pregnancy category X, lactation, genital bleeding (abnormal), prostate or breast carcinoma in males, breast cancer in females with hypercalcemia
Precautions: Diabetes mellitus, CV disease, MI, increased risk of prostatic hypertrophy, prostatic carcinoma, virilization (women), increased prothrombin time
Pharmacokinetics:
PO: Metabolized in liver; excreted in urine; crosses placenta; excreted in breast milk
Drug interactions of concern to dentistry:
• Increased risk of bleeding: aspirin
• Edema: ACTH, adrenal steroids

DENTAL CONSIDERATIONS
General:
• Monitor vital signs every appointment due to cardiovascular side effects.
• Determine why the patient is taking the drug.
• Consider local hemostasis measures to prevent excessive bleeding.
• Short appointments and a stress reduction protocol may be required for anxious patients.
• If signs of anemia are observed in oral tissues, physician consult may be required.
• Avoid prescribing aspirin-containing products.
Consultations:
• Medical consult may be required to assess disease control and patient's ability to tolerate stress.
• Medical consult should include partial prothrombin or prothrombin times.
Teach patient/family:
• Importance of good oral hygiene to prevent soft tissue inflammation
• That secondary oral infection may occur; must see dentist immediately if infection occurs

O

oxaprozin

(ox′a-proe-zin)
Daypro
Drug class.: Nonsteroidal antiinflammatory

Action: Inhibits prostaglandin synthesis by interfering with cyclooxygenase needed for biosynthesis; possesses analgesic, antiinflammatory, antipyretic properties
Uses: Rheumatoid arthritis, osteoarthritis, and ankylosing spondylitis

Dosage and routes:

• *Adult:* PO 600 mg once or twice daily; max dose 1800 mg/day

Available forms include: Tabs 600 mg

Side effects/adverse reactions:

▼ *ORAL:* Dry mouth, stomatitis, lichenoid reaction

CNS: Dizziness, drowsiness, fatigue, tremors, confusion, insomnia, anxiety, depression

CV: Tachycardia, peripheral edema, palpitation, dysrhythmias

GI: ***Cholestatic hepatitis,*** nausea, anorexia, vomiting, diarrhea, jaundice, constipation, flatulence, cramps, peptic ulcer

HEMA: ***Blood dyscrasias***

GU: ***Nephrotoxicity: dysuria, hematuria, oliguria, azotemia***

EENT: Tinnitus, hearing loss, blurred vision

INTEG: Purpura, rash, pruritus, sweating, photosensitivity

Contraindications: Hypersensitivity, asthma, severe renal disease, severe hepatic disease

Precautions: Pregnancy category not established, lactation, children, bleeding disorders, GI disorders, cardiac disorders, hypersensitivity to other antiinflammatory agents, diabetes

Pharmacokinetics:

PO: Peak 1-2 hr, half-life 2-4 hr; 90%-99% plasma protein binding; metabolized in liver (inactive metabolites); excreted in urine (inactive metabolites)

Drug interactions of concern to dentistry:

• GI ulceration, bleeding: aspirin, alcohol, corticosteroids

• Decreased action: salicylates

• Nephrotoxicity: acetaminophen (prolonged use and high doses)

• Possible risk of decreased renal function: cyclosporine

When prescribed for dental pain:

• Risk of increased effects: oral anticoagulants, oral antidiabetics, lithium, methotrexate

• Decreased antihypertensive effects of diuretics, β-adrenergic blockers, and ACE inhibitors

DENTAL CONSIDERATIONS

General:

• Patients on chronic drug therapy may rarely have symptoms of blood dyscrasias, which can include infection, bleeding, and poor healing.

• Assess salivary flow as a factor in caries, periodontal disease, and candidiasis.

• Avoid prescribing for dental use in pregnancy.

• Consider semisupine chair position for patients with arthritic disease.

Consultations:

• Medical consult may be required to assess disease control in the patient.

• In a patient with symptoms of blood dyscrasias, request a medical consult for blood studies and postpone dental treatment until normal values are reestablished.

Teach patient/family:

• Importance of good oral hygiene to prevent soft tissue inflammation

• Caution to prevent injury when using oral hygiene aids

When chronic dry mouth occurs, advise patient:

• To avoid mouth rinses with high alcohol content due to drying effects

• Of need for daily home fluoride to prevent caries

• To use sugarless gum, frequent sips of water, or saliva substitutes

oxazepam

(ox-a'ze-pam)

Serax

♣ Apo-Oxazepam, Novoxapam

Drug class.: Benzodiazepine

Controlled Substance Schedule IV

Action: Produces CNS depression by interacting with a benzodiazepine receptor to facilitate the action of the inhibitory neurotransmitter γ-aminobutyric acid (GABA)

Uses: Anxiety, alcohol withdrawal

Dosage and routes:

Anxiety

- *Adult:* PO 10-30 mg tid-qid

Alcohol withdrawal

- *Adult:* PO 15-30 mg tid-qid

Available forms include: Caps 10, 15, 30 mg; tabs 10, 15, 30 mg

Side effects/adverse reactions:

▼ *ORAL:* Dry mouth

CNS: Dizziness, drowsiness, confusion, headache, anxiety, tremors, fatigue, depression, insomnia, hallucinations, paradoxic excitement, transient amnesia, syncope, hangover

CV: Orthostatic hypotension, ***ECG changes, tachycardia,*** hypotension

GI: Nausea, vomiting, anorexia, abdominal discomfort

EENT: Blurred vision, tinnitus, mydriasis

INTEG: Rash, dermatitis, itching

Contraindications: Hypersensitivity to benzodiazepines, narrow-angle glaucoma, psychosis, pregnancy category D, child <12 yr

Precautions: Elderly, debilitated, hepatic disease, renal disease

Pharmacokinetics:

PO: Peak 2-4 hr, half-life 5-15 hr; metabolized by liver; excreted by kidneys

Drug interactions of concern to dentistry:

- Increased effects: CNS depressants, alcohol, and anticonvulsant medications

DENTAL CONSIDERATIONS

General:

- Monitor vital signs every appointment due to cardiovascular side effects.
- Psychologic and physical dependence may occur with chronic administration.
- Geriatric patients are more susceptible to drug effects; use lower dose.
- Assess salivary flow as a factor in caries, periodontal disease, and candidiasis.

Consultations:

- Medical consult may be required to assess disease control in the patient.

Teach patient/family:

- To avoid mouth rinses with high alcohol content due to drying effects

oxidized cellulose

Oxycel, Surgicel

Drug class.: Cellulose hemostatic

Action: Mechanism unclear; may act physically to absorb blood and promote an artificial clot

Uses: Hemostasis in surgery, oral surgery, exodontia

Dosage and routes:

- *Adult and child:* TOP apply using sterile technique as needed; remove after bleeding stops if possible or leave in place if needed

Available forms include: TOP knitted fabric in pads, pledgets, and strips of various sizes

Side effects/adverse reactions:
CNS: Headache in epistaxis
EENT: Sneezing, burning in epistaxis
INTEG: Burning, stinging, encapsulation of fluid, foreign bodies

Contraindications: Hypersensitivity, large artery hemorrhage, oozing surfaces, implantation in bone deficit, placement around optic nerve and optic chiasm

Precautions: Do not autoclave; inactivation of topical thrombin

DENTAL CONSIDERATIONS

General:

• Apply dry; use only amount needed to control bleeding.

• Place loosely and avoid packing; remove excess before closure in surgery; irrigate first, then remove using sterile technique.

• Ensure therapeutic response: decreased bleeding in surgery.

• Can be left in situ when necessary but should be removed once bleeding is controlled.

• Application of topical thrombin solution to the cellulose gauze will inactivate thrombin because of acidity.

---

oxtriphylline

(ox-trye′fi-lin)

Choledyl, Choledyl SA, PMS-Oxtriphylline

✤ Apo-Oxitriphylline

Drug class.: Choline salt of theophylline, bronchodilator

Action: Relaxes smooth muscle of respiratory system by blocking phosphodiesterase, which increases cAMP; 64% theophylline

Uses: Acute bronchial asthma, reversible bronchospasm in chronic bronchitis and COPD

Dosage and routes:

• *Adult and child >12 yr:* PO 200 mg qid

• *Child 2-12 yr:* PO 4 mg/kg q6h; may be increased to desired response, therapeutic level

Available forms include: Elix 100 mg/5 ml; syr 50 mg/5 ml; tabs 100, 200; sus rel tabs 400, 600 mg

Side effects/adverse reactions:
▼ *ORAL:* Bitter taste
CNS: Anxiety, restlessness, insomnia, dizziness, ***convulsions,*** headache, light-headedness, muscle twitching
CV: Palpitation, sinus tachycardia, hypotension
GI: Nausea, vomiting, anorexia, diarrhea, dyspepsia
RESP: Increased rate
INTEG: Flushing, urticaria

Contraindications: Hypersensitivity to xanthines, tachydysrhythmias

Precautions: Elderly, CHF, cor pulmonale, hepatic disease, active peptic ulcer disease, diabetes mellitus, hyperthyroidism, hypertension, children, pregnancy category C, glaucoma, prostatic hypertrophy

Pharmacokinetics:
PO: Peak 1 hr; metabolized in liver; excreted in urine, breast milk; crosses placenta

Drug interactions of concern to dentistry:

• Increased action: erythromycin (macrolides), ephedrine, xanthines, fluoroquinolones

• Decreased therapeutic effects: barbiturates, β-adrenergic blockers, nicotine

DENTAL CONSIDERATIONS

General:

• Evaluate respiration characteristics and rate.

• Consider semisupine chair posi-

tion for patient comfort due to GI effects of disease.

• Short appointments and a stress reduction protocol may be required for anxious patients.

• Be aware that aspirin or sulfite preservatives in vasoconstrictor-containing products can exacerbate asthma.

• Acute asthmatic episodes may be precipitated in the dental office. Sympathomimetic inhalants should be available for emergency use.

• Discuss tobacco cessation for patients using tobacco.

---

oxybutynin chloride

(ox-i-byoo'ti-nin)

Ditropan, Ditropan XL

Drug class.: Antispasmodic

Action: Relaxes smooth muscles in urinary tract

Uses: Antispasmodic for neurogenic bladder, overactive bladder

Dosage and routes:

• *Adult:* PO 5 mg bid-tid, not to exceed 5 mg qid; XL formulation once-daily dosage

• *Child >5 yr:* PO 5 mg bid, not to exceed 5 mg tid

Available forms include: Syr 5 mg/5 ml; tabs 5 mg; ext rel tab 5, 10 mg

Side effects/adverse reactions:

▼ *ORAL: Dry mouth*

CNS: Restlessness, dizziness, drowsiness, ***convulsions,*** confusion, insomnia, weakness, hallucinations

CV: Palpitation, tachycardia, hypotension

GI: Nausea, vomiting, anorexia, abdominal pain, constipation

GU: Dysuria, retention, hesitancy

EENT: Blurred vision, increased intraocular tension

INTEG: Urticaria, dermatitis

Contraindications: Hypersensitivity, GI obstruction, GI hemorrhage, GU obstruction, glaucoma, severe colitis, myasthenia gravis, unstable CV status in acute hemorrhage

Precautions: Pregnancy category C, lactation, suspected glaucoma, children <12 yr, hiatal hernia, esophageal reflux, coronary heart disease, CHF, hypertension

Pharmacokinetics:

PO: Onset 0.5-1 hr, peak 3-4 hr, duration 6-10 hr; metabolized by liver; excreted in urine

Drug interactions of concern to dentistry:

• Increased anticholinergic effect: anticholinergic drugs

• Increased depressant effect of both drugs: CNS depressants, alcohol

DENTAL CONSIDERATIONS

General:

• Assess salivary flow as a factor in caries, periodontal disease, and candidiasis.

• Monitor vital signs every appointment due to cardiovascular side effects.

• Avoid dental light in patient's eyes; offer dark glasses for patient comfort.

• Consider semisupine chair position for patient comfort if GI side effects occur.

Consultations:

• Physician should be informed if significant xerostomic side effects occur (increased caries, sore tongue, problems eating or swallowing, difficulty wearing prosthesis) so a medication change can be considered.

O

Teach patient/family:

- Importance of good oral hygiene to prevent soft tissue inflammation

When chronic dry mouth occurs, advise patient:

- To avoid mouth rinses with high alcohol content due to drying effects
- Of need for daily home fluoride to prevent caries
- To use sugarless gum, frequent sips of water, or saliva substitutes

oxycodone

(ox-i-koe'done)

OxyContin, Percolone, Roxicodone, Roxicodone Intensol, Roxicodone SR

✤ Supeudol

Combinations: Codoxy, Percocet-Demi, Percodan, Tylox

✤ Endodan, Percocet, Roxiprin

Drug class.: Synthetic opioid analgesic

Controlled Substance Schedule II, Canada N

Action: Interacts with opioid receptors in the CNS to alter pain perception

Uses: Moderate-to-severe pain, normally used in combination with aspirin or acetaminophen

Dosage and routes:

- *Adult:* PO 1-2 tab q6h prn (usually in combination with nonopioid analgesics)

Available forms include: Tabs 5 mg; sol 5 mg/5 ml; sus rel tab 10, 30mg; oral sol concentrate 20 mg/ml, con rel tab 10, 20, 40, 80 mg

Side effects/adverse reactions:

▼ *ORAL:* Dry mouth

CNS: Drowsiness, dizziness, confusion, headache, sedation, euphoria

CV: Palpitation, bradycardia, tachycardia

GI: Nausea, vomiting, anorexia, constipation, cramps

RESP: ***Respiratory depression***

GU: Decreased urinary output, oliguria, dysuria, urinary retention

EENT: Tinnitus, blurred vision, miosis, diplopia

INTEG: Rash, urticaria, bruising, flushing, diaphoresis, pruritus

Contraindications: Hypersensitivity, addiction (narcotic)

Precautions: Addictive personality, pregnancy category B, lactation, increased intracranial pressure, MI (acute), severe heart disease, respiratory depression, hepatic disease, renal disease, child <18 yr, physical dependence

Pharmacokinetics:

PO: Onset 10-15 min, peak 0.5-1 hr, duration 4-5 hr; detoxified by liver; excreted in urine, breast milk; crosses placenta

Drug interactions of concern to dentistry:

- Increased effects with other CNS depressants: alcohol, other narcotics, sedative-hypnotics, skeletal muscle relaxants, phenothiazines, benzodiazepines
- Contraindication: MAO inhibitors
- Increased effects of anticholinergics

DENTAL CONSIDERATIONS

General:

- Monitor vital signs every appointment due to cardiovascular and respiratory side effects.
- Assess salivary flow as a factor in caries, periodontal disease, and candidiasis.
- Psychologic and physical dependence may occur with chronic administration.

• Determine why the patient is taking the drug.

Teach patient/family:

• To avoid mouth rinses with high alcohol content due to drying effects

oxymetazoline HCl (nasal)

(ox-i-met-az'oh-leen)

Afrin, Afrin Children's Nose Drops, Allerest 12 Hour Nasal, Dristan 12 Hour, Duramist Plus, Duration, Nasal Decongestant Spray, Nostrilla, NTZ Long-Acting, 12 Hour Sinarest, Sinex Long-Lasting, and many others

Drug class.: Nasal decongestant, sympathomimetic amine

Action: Produces vasoconstriction (rapid, long acting) of arterioles, thereby decreasing fluid exudation, mucosal engorgement

Uses: Nasal congestion

Dosage and routes:

• *Adult and child >6 yr:* Instill 2-3 gtt or sprays to each nostril bid

• *Child 2-6 yr:* Instill 2-3 gtt or sprays 0.025% sol bid, not to exceed 5 days

Available forms include: Sol 0.025%, 0.05%

Side effects/adverse reactions:

CNS: Anxiety, restlessness, tremors, weakness, insomnia, dizziness, fever, headache

GI: Nausea, vomiting, anorexia

EENT: Irritation, burning, sneezing, stinging, dryness, rebound congestion

INTEG: Contact dermatitis

Contraindications: Hypersensitivity to sympathomimetic amines

Precautions: Child <6 yr, elderly, diabetes, cardiovascular disease, hypertension, hyperthyroidism, increased ICP, prostatic hypertrophy, pregnancy category C, glaucoma

Drug interactions of concern to dentistry:

• Increased risk of hypertension: tricyclic antidepressants, but it requires adequate systemic absorption of oxymetazoline

DENTAL CONSIDERATIONS

General:

• Excessive use can lead to rebound congestion and cardiovascular side effects; follow recommended dosing intervals.

• Extensive nasal swelling and congestion could interfere with optimal use of nitrous oxide/oxygen sedation.

oxymetholone

(ox-i-meth'oh-lone)

Anadrol-50

Anapolon 50

Drug class.: Androgenic anabolic steroid

Controlled Substance Schedule III

Action: Reverses catabolic tissue processes; promotes buildup of protein; increases erythropoietin production

Uses: Anemia associated with bone marrow failure and red cell production deficiencies; aplastic anemia, myelofibrosis, and anemia due to myelotoxic drugs

Dosage and routes:

Aplastic anemia

• *Adult and child:* PO 1-5 mg/kg/day, titrated to patient response, with minimum trial period of 3-6 mo

Available forms include: Tabs 50 mg

Side effects/adverse reactions: *CNS:* Dizziness, headache, fatigue, tremors, paresthesia, flushing, sweating, anxiety, lability, insomnia
CV: ***Edema*** (in cardiac patients), increased BP
GI: ***Peliosis hepatitis, liver cell tumors, cholestatic jaundice,*** nausea, vomiting, constipation, weight gain
HEMA: ***Increased prothrombin time, iron deficiency anemia***
GU: ***Hematuria,*** amenorrhea, vaginitis, decreased libido, decreased breast size, clitoral hypertrophy, testicular atrophy, gynecomastia (male), priapism
EENT: Conjunctival edema, nasal congestion
INTEG: Rash, acneiform lesions, oily hair/skin, flushing, sweating, acne vulgaris, alopecia, hirsutism
ENDO: Abnormal GTT, decreased glucose tolerance, increased LDL
MS: Cramps, spasms

Contraindications: Severe renal disease, severe cardiac disease, severe hepatic disease, hypersensitivity, pregnancy category X, lactation, genital bleeding (abnormal), prostate or breast carcinoma (males), breast cancer in females with hypercalcemia

Precautions: Diabetes mellitus, CV disease, MI, increased risk of prostatic hypertrophy, prostatic carcinoma, virilization (women), increased prothrombin time

Pharmacokinetics:
PO: Metabolized in liver, excreted in urine, crosses placenta, excreted in breast milk

Drug interactions of concern to dentistry:
- Increased risk of bleeding: aspirin
- Edema: ACTH, adrenal steroids

DENTAL CONSIDERATIONS

General:
- Monitor vital signs every appointment due to cardiovascular side effects.
- Determine why the patient is taking the drug.
- Consider local hemostasis measures to prevent excessive bleeding.
- Short appointments and a stress reduction protocol may be required for anxious patients.
- Avoid prescribing aspirin-containing products.

Consultations:
- Physician consult may be required if signs of anemia are observed in oral tissues.
- Medical consult may be required to assess disease control and patient's ability to tolerate stress.
- Medical consult should include partial prothrombin or prothrombin times.

Teach patient/family:
- Importance of good oral hygiene to prevent soft tissue inflammation
- That secondary oral infection may occur; must see dentist immediately if infection occurs

---

paclitaxel

(pac-li-tax′el)
Taxol
Drug class.: Antineoplastic

Action: Obtained from Western Yew tree; unique action inhibits microtubule network reorganization essential for cell division

Uses: Metastatic ovarian cancer; second-line treatment for AIDS-related Kaposi's sarcoma; adjuvant treatment of node-positive breast cancer sequential to a course of standard doxorubicin-containing combination chemotherapy

Dosage and routes:

• *Adult:* IV only, after oral premedication with PO dexamethasone, diphenhydramine, and H_2 antagonist, 135 mg/m^2 over 24 hr q3wk, depending on development of neutropenia

Available forms include: Inj 30 mg/5 ml

Side effects/adverse reactions:

▼ *ORAL: Mucositis*

CV: Bradycardia, hypotension, abnormal ECG

GI: Nausea, vomiting, diarrhea, hepatic function impairment

RESP: Allergic dyspnea, infection

HEMA: Bone marrow depression, thrombocytopenia, anemia, bleeding

GU: UTIs

INTEG: Flushing, rash

METAB: Increased bilirubin, increased alkaline phosphatase, AST

MS: Myalgia, arthralgia

MISC: Alopecia, peripheral neuropathy, fever

Contraindications: Hypersensitivity, other products containing polyethylated castor oil, neutropenia $<1500/mm^3$

Precautions: Pregnancy category D, bone marrow depression, AV block, hepatic impairment, lactation, children, recent MI, angina pectoris, CHF history, current use of drug with effect on cardiac conduction system

Pharmacokinetics:

IV: Terminal half-life 5-17 hr; plasma protein binding 88%-98%, hepatic metabolism, excreted in bile

DENTAL CONSIDERATIONS

General:

• Consider semisupine chair position for patient comfort if GI side effects occur.

• Patients receiving chemotherapy may require palliative therapy for stomatitis.

• Patients on chronic drug therapy may rarely have symptoms of blood dyscrasias, which can include infection, bleeding, and poor healing.

Consultations:

• Medical consult may be required to assess disease control in the patient.

Teach patient/family:

• Importance of good oral hygiene to prevent soft tissue inflammation

• Caution to prevent trauma when using oral hygiene aids

---

pancrelipase

(pan-kre-li′pase)

Cotazym, Cotazyme-S, Cotazyme-65B, Enzymase, Ilozyme, Ku-Zyme HP, Pancrease, Pancrease MT 4, Protilase, Ultrase MT, Viokase, Zymase

Drug class.: Digestant

Action: Pancreatic enzyme needed for proper pancreatic functioning in metabolizing lipids, proteins, and carbohydrates

Uses: Exocrine pancreatic secretion insufficiency, cystic fibrosis (digestive aid), steatorrhea, pancreatic enzyme deficiency, chronic pancreatitis

Dosage and routes:

• *Adult and child:* PO 1-3 caps/tabs ac or with meals, or 1 cap/tab with snack or 1-2 pdr pkt ac

Available forms include: Tab 8000, 11,000, 30,000 U; caps 8000,

P

12,000, 30,000 U; enteric-coated caps 4000, 5000, 20,000, 25,000 U; powder 16,800 U

Side effects/adverse reactions:

▼ *ORAL:* Irritation to mucous membranes

GI: Anorexia, nausea, vomiting, diarrhea, cramps

RESP: Asthma attack

GU: Hyperuricuria, hyperuricemia

Contraindications: Allergy to pork

Precautions: Pregnancy category C

DENTAL CONSIDERATIONS

General:

• Consider semisupine chair position for patient comfort due to GI effects of disease.

• To avoid oral irritation, mouth should be rinsed or drug taken with liquid.

---

papaverine HCl

(pa-pav′er-een)

Cerespan, Genabid, Pavabid, Pavacels, Pavacot, Pavagen, Pavarine, Pavased, Pavatine, Pavatym, Paverolan

Drug class.: Peripheral vasodilator

Action: Relaxes all smooth muscle, inhibits cyclic nucleotide phosphodiesterase, which increases intracellular cAMP, causing vasodilation

Uses: Arterial spasm resulting in cerebral and peripheral ischemia; myocardial ischemia associated with vascular spasm or dysrhythmias; angina pectoris; peripheral pulmonary embolism; visceral spasm as in ureteral, biliary, GI colic PVD; unlabeled use: with phentolamine or alprostadil for intracavernous injection for impotence

Dosage and routes:

• *Adult:* PO 100-300 mg 3-5× daily; sus rel 150-300 mg q8-12h; IM/IV 30-120 mg q3h prn

Available forms include: Time rel caps 150; time rel tabs 200 mg; tabs 30, 60, 100, 150, 200, 300 mg; inj IM/IV 30 mg/ml

Side effects/adverse reactions:

CNS: Headache, dizziness, drowsiness, sedation, vertigo, malaise, depression

CV: ***Tachycardia,*** increased BP

GI: ***Hepatotoxicity,*** nausea, anorexia, abdominal pain, constipation, diarrhea, jaundice, altered liver enzymes

RESP: Increased depth of respirations

INTEG: Flushing, sweating, rash, pruritus

Contraindications: Hypersensitivity, complete AV heart block

Precautions: Cardiac dysrhythmias, glaucoma, pregnancy category C, lactation, drug dependency, children, hepatic hyper sensitivity, Parkinson's disease

Pharmacokinetics:

PO: Onset 30 sec, peak 1-2 hr, duration 3-4 hr

SUS REL: Onset erratic; 90% bound to plasma proteins; metabolized in liver; excreted in urine (inactive metabolites)

Drug interactions of concern to dentistry:

• Increased hypotension: alcohol, other drugs that may also lower blood pressure

DENTAL CONSIDERATIONS

General:

• Monitor vital signs every ap-

pointment due to cardiovascular and respiratory side effects.
• Short appointments and a stress reduction protocol may be required for anxious patients.
Consultations:
• Stress from dental procedures may compromise cardiovascular function; determine patient risk.
• Medical consult may be required to assess disease control in the patient.
Teach patient/family:
• To avoid mouth rinses with high alcohol content
• Importance of good oral hygiene to prevent soft tissue inflammation

paroxetine

(pa-rox'e-teen)
Paxil, Paxil CR
Drug class.: Antidepressant

Action: Selectively inhibits the uptake of serotonin in the brain
Uses: Depression, panic disorder, obsessive compulsive disorder, social anxiety disorder; unlabeled use: anxiety
Dosage and routes:
• *Adult:* PO initially 20 mg/day; increase 10 mg weekly to effect; not to exceed 50 mg/day
Panic disorder
• *Adult:* PO 10 mg qd
Available forms include: Tabs 10, 20, 30, 40 mg; caps modified rel 10, 20, 30, 40 mg; con rel tabs 12.5, 25 mg; oral susp 10 mg/5 ml
Side effects/adverse reactions:
▼ *ORAL: Dry mouth,* glossitis, aphthous stomatitis, (<0.1%), salivary gland enlargement (<0.1%), taste perversion
CNS: Somnolence, tremor, sweating, asthenia, insomnia, dizziness
CV: Palpitation, vasodilation, postural hypotension, syncope, tachycardia
GI: Constipation, nausea, diarrhea, anorexia, vomiting, flatulence, weight gain
RESP: Pharyngitis, yawning, respiratory complaints, coughing, rhinitis
GU: Decreased libido, sexual dysfunction, urinary frequency
EENT: Blurred vision, photophobia
SYST: Headache, myopathy, malaise, fever
METAB: Increased serum albumin, blood glucose, alkaline phosphatase
Contraindications: Hypersensitivity, MAO inhibitors
Precautions: Pregnancy category B, lactation, elderly, oral anticoagulants, renal or hepatic impairment, children, other serotonergic drugs
Pharmacokinetics:
PO: Peak plasma levels 5 hr (0.5-11 hr range), half-life 21 hr; highly protein bound; extensive first-pass metabolism; renal excretion
Drug interactions of concern to dentistry:
• Possible increased side effects: highly protein-bound drugs (aspirin), other antidepressants, alcohol
• Increased half-life of diazepam

DENTAL CONSIDERATIONS

General:
• After supine positioning, have patient sit upright for at least 2 min to avoid orthostatic hypotension.
• Assess salivary flow as a factor in caries, periodontal disease, and candidiasis.
• Avoid dental light in patient's eyes; offer dark glasses for patient comfort.

Consultations:

• Medical consult may be required to assess disease control and patient's ability to tolerate stress.

• Physician should be informed if significant xerostomic side effects occur (increased caries, sore tongue, problems eating or swallowing, difficulty wearing prosthesis) so a medication change can be considered.

Teach patient/family:

When chronic dry mouth occurs, advise patient:

• To avoid mouth rinses with high alcohol content due to drying effects

• Of need for daily home fluoride to prevent caries

• To use sugarless gum, frequent sips of water, or saliva substitutes

pemoline

(pem′oh-leen)

Cylert, Cylert Chewable

Drug class.: CNS stimulant

Controlled Substance Schedule IV

Action: Exact mechanism unknown; may act through dopaminergic mechanisms

Uses: Attention deficit disorder with hyperactivity

Dosage and routes:

• *Child >6 yr:* 37.5 mg in AM, increasing by 18.75 mg/wk, not to exceed 112.5 mg/day

Available forms include: Tabs 18.75, 37.5, 75 mg; chew tabs 37.5 mg

Side effects/adverse reactions:

CNS: Hyperactivity, insomnia, restlessness, dizziness, mild depression, headache, stimulation, irritability, aggressiveness, hallucinations, seizures, Tourette's syndrome, drowsiness, dyskinetic movements, fatigue, malaise

GI: Nausea, anorexia, diarrhea, abdominal pain

MISC: Rashes, growth suppression in children, increased liver enzymes, hepatitis, jaundice

Contraindications: Hypersensitivity, hepatic insufficiency

Precautions: Renal disease, pregnancy category B, lactation, drug abuse, child <6 yr; liver function monitoring recommended

Pharmacokinetics:

PO: Peak 2-4 hr, duration 8 hr, half-life 12 hr; metabolized (50%) by liver; excreted (40%) by kidneys

Drug interactions of concern to dentistry:

• Increased irritability, stimulation: caffeine-containing products and food

DENTAL CONSIDERATIONS

General:

• Keep dental appointments short due to effects of disease.

Teach patient/family:

• Use of electric toothbrush for effective plaque control

penbutolol

(pen-byoo′toe-lole)

Levatol

Drug class.: Nonselective β-adrenergic blocker

Action: This is a nonselective β_1- and β_2-adrenergic antagonist. The antihypertensive mechanism of action is unclear, but it may include a reduction in cardiac output and inhibition of renin release by the renal juxtaglomerular apparatus.

Peripheral resistance decreases with long-term use. The antianginal action (when indicated for this use) may be related to a decrease in myocardial oxygen demand and negative chronotropic and inotropic effects. The antiarrhythmic action (when indicated for this use) has been related to a reduction in spontaneous pacemaker firing and slowing of AV nodal conduction.

Uses: Hypertension alone or with thiazide diuretics

Dosage and routes:

• *Adult:* PO 20 mg qd, dose can be increased to 40-80 mg

Available forms include: Tabs 20 mg

Side effects/adverse reactions:

▼ *ORAL:* Dry mouth, taste alteration

CNS: Depression, hallucinations, dizziness, fatigue, lethargy, paresthesia, bizarre dreams, disorientation, syncope, vertigo, headache, sleep disturbances, nervousness, lethargy, behavior change, memory loss

CV: *Bradycardia, hypotension,* ***CHF,*** palpitation, AV block intensification, peripheral vascular insufficiency, vasodilation, chest pain, tachycardia

GI: Nausea, vomiting, diarrhea, colitis, constipation, cramps, hepatomegaly, gastric pain, acute pancreatitis, heartburn, anorexia

RESP: Dyspnea, respiratory dysfunction, *bronchospasm,* laryngospasm

HEMA: ***Agranulocytosis, thrombocytopenia,*** eosinophilia, leukopenia, pulmonary emboli, hyperlipidemia

GU: Impotence, decreased libido, UTIs, renal failure, urinary frequency or retention, dysuria, nocturia

EENT: Sore throat, ***laryngospasm,*** blurred vision, dry eyes

INTEG: Rash, pruritus, fever, photosensitivity

MS: Joint pain, arthralgia, muscle cramps, pain

META: Hyperglycemia, hypoglycemia

MISC: Facial swelling, weight change, Raynaud's phenomenon, lupus syndrome

Contraindications: Hypersensitivity to this drug, cardiac failure, cardiogenic shock, second- or third-degree heart block, bronchospastic disease, sinus bradycardia, CHF

Precautions: Diabetes mellitus, pregnancy category C, renal disease, lactation, hyperthyroidism, COPD, hepatic disease, children, myasthenia gravis, peripheral vascular disease, hypotension

Pharmacokinetics:

PO: Peak levels 1-1.5, half-life 3-5 hr; highly protein bound; hepatic metabolism

Drug interactions of concern to dentistry:

• Decreased hypotensive effect: indomethacin, NSAIDs

• Increased hypotension, myocardial depression: hydrocarbon inhalation anesthetics

• Hypertension, bradycardia: sympathomimetics (epinephrine, ephedrine)

• Slow metabolism of lidocaine

DENTAL CONSIDERATIONS

General:

• Monitor vital signs every appointment due to cardiovascular side effects.

• Patients on chronic drug therapy

P

may rarely have symptoms of blood dyscrasias, which can include infection, bleeding, and poor healing.

• Limit use of sodium-containing products, such as saline IV fluids, for patients with a dietary salt restriction.

• Assess salivary flow as a factor in caries, periodontal disease, and candidiasis.

• After supine positioning, have patient sit upright for at least 2 min before standing to avoid orthostatic hypotension.

• Stress from dental procedures may compromise cardiovascular function; determine patient risk.

• Short appointments and a stress reduction protocol may be required for anxious patients.

• Use vasoconstrictor with caution, in low doses, and with careful aspiration.

• Avoid using gingival retraction cord containing epinephrine.

Consultations:

• In a patient with symptoms of blood dyscrasias, request a medical consult for blood studies and postpone dental treatment until normal values are reestablished.

• Medical consult may be required to assess disease control and patient's ability to tolerate stress.

Teach patient/family:

• Caution to prevent injury when using oral hygiene aids

• Importance of good oral hygiene to prevent soft tissue inflammation

• If taste alterations occur, consider drug effects

When chronic dry mouth occurs, advise patient:

• To avoid mouth rinses with high alcohol content due to drying effects

• Of need for daily home fluoride to prevent caries

• To use sugarless gum, frequent sips of water, or saliva substitutes

penciclovir cream

(pen-sye'kloe-veer)

Denavir

Drug class.: Antiviral

Action: Inhibits viral DNA synthesis needed for viral replication in herpes simplex virus (HSV-1, HSV-2) following cellular kinase conversion to penciclovir triphosphate.

Uses: Recurrent herpes labialis (cold sores)

Dosage and routes:

• *Adult:* TOP apply q2h while awake × 4 days; start treatment early in prodrome or when lesions appear

Available forms include: Cream 1%, 2 g tube

Side effects/adverse reactions:

▼ *ORAL:* Taste alteration

CNS: Headache

INTEG: Hyperthesia, local anesthesia, pruritus, rash

MISC: Allergic reaction, pain

Contraindications: Hypersensitivity

Precautions: Acyclovir-resistant herpes viruses, patients <18 yr, use on mucous membranes not recommended, avoid applications near the eye, pregnancy category B, lactation

Pharmacokinetics:

TOP: Not detected in plasma or urine

DENTAL CONSIDERATIONS

General:

• Use in immunocompromised patients not established.

• Postpone dental treatment when oral herpetic lesions are present.

Teach patient/family:

• To dispose of toothbrush or other contaminated oral hygiene devices used during period of infection to prevent reinoculation of herpetic infection

• To apply with a finger cot or latex glove to prevent herpes infection on fingers

---

penicillin G benzathine

(pen-i-sill'in)

Bicillin L-A, Permapen

✤ Megacillin

Drug class.: Benzathine salt of natural penicillin

Action: Interferes with cell wall replication of susceptible organisms; osmotically unstable cell wall swells and bursts from osmotic pressure

Uses: Respiratory infections, scarlet fever, erysipelas, otitis media, pneumonia, skin and soft tissue infections, bejel, pinta, yaws; effective for gram-positive cocci *(Staphylococcus, S. pyogenes, S. viridans, S. faecalis, S. bovis, S. pneumoniae),* gram-negative cocci *(N. gonorrhoeae),* gram-positive bacilli *(B. anthracis, C. perfringens, C. tetani, C. diphtheriae, L. monocytogenes),* gram-negative bacilli *(E. coli, P. mirabilis, Salmonella, Shigella, Enterobacter, S. moniliformis),* spirochetes *(T. pallidum), Actinomyces*

Dosage and routes:

Early syphilis

• *Adult:* IM 2.4 million U in [illegible] dose

Prophylaxis of rheumatic fever, glomerulonephritis

• *Adult and child >60 lb:* IM 1.2 million U in single dose q2-3wk

• *Child <60 lb:* IM 600,000 U in single dose

Upper respiratory infections (group A streptococcal)

• *Adult:* IM 1.2 million U in single dose

• *Child >27 kg:* IM 900,000 U in single dose

• *Child <27 kg:* IM 50,000 U/kg in single dose

Available forms include: Inj IM 600,000 U/ml; tabs 200,000 U, 1,200,000; 2,400,000, 3,000,000 U/ml

Side effects/adverse reactions:

▼ *ORAL: Candidiasis,* glossitis

CNS: ***Coma, convulsions,*** lethargy, hallucinations, anxiety, depression, twitching

GI: Nausea, vomiting, diarrhea, increased AST/ALT, abdominal pain, colitis

HEMA: ***Bone marrow depression, granulocytopenia,*** anemia, increased bleeding time

GU: ***Oliguria, proteinuria, hematuria, vaginal moniliasis, glomerulonephritis***

INTEG: ***Exfoliative dermatitis,*** rash, urticaria, hives

META: Hyperkalemia, hypokalemia, alkalosis, hypernatremia

MISC: ***Anaphylaxis***

Contraindications: Hypersensitivity to penicillins; neonates

Precautions: Hypersensitivity to cephalosporins, pregnancy category B

P

Pharmacokinetics:
IM: Very slow absorption, hydrolyzed to penicillin G, duration 21-28 days, half-life 30-60 min; excreted in urine, breast milk; crosses placenta

Drug interactions of concern to dentistry:
• Decreased antimicrobial effect of penicillin: tetracyclines, erythromycins, lincomycins
• Increased penicillin concentrations: aspirin, probenecid
• Suspected increased risk of methotrexate toxicity

When used for dental infections:
• Decreased effectiveness of oral contraceptives

DENTAL CONSIDERATIONS

General:
• Take precautions regarding allergy to medication.
• Determine why the patient is taking the drug.
• Place on frequent recall to evaluate healing response.

Consultations:
• Medical consult may be required to assess disease control in the patient.

Teach patient/family:
When used for dental infection, advise patient:
• Taking birth control pill to use additional method of contraception for duration of cycle
• To report sore throat, oral burning sensation, fever, fatigue, any of which could indicate superinfection
• To take at prescribed intervals and complete dosage regimen
• To immediately notify the dentist if signs or symptoms of infection increase

penicillin V potassium/ penicillin V

Beepen-K, Betapen-VK, Ledercillin-VK, V-Cillin K, Veetids
🍁 Apo-Pen-VK, Nadopen-VK, NovoPen-VK, Nu-Pen-VK, Pen-Vee K, PVFK

Drug class.: Semisynthetic penicillin

Action: Interferes with cell wall replication of susceptible organisms; the cell wall, rendered osmotically unstable, swells and bursts from osmotic pressure

Uses: Effective for gram-positive cocci *(S. aureus, S. viridans, S. faecalis, S. bovis, S. pneumoniae),* gram-negative cocci *(N. gonorrhoeae, N. meningitidis),* gram-positive bacilli *(B. anthracis, C. perfringens, C. tetani, C. diphtheriae),* gram-negative bacilli *(S. moniliformis),* spirochetes *(T. pallidum), Actinomyces, Peptococcus,* and *Peptostreptococcus* species

Dosage and routes:

Pneumococcal/staphylococcal infections
• *Adult:* PO 250-500 mg q6h
• *Child <12 yr:* PO 25,000-90,000 U/kg/day in 3-6 divided doses (125 mg = 200,000 U)

Streptococcal infections
• *Adult:* PO 250-500 mg q6-8h × 10 days

Prevention of recurrence of rheumatic fever/chorea
• *Adult:* PO 125-250 mg bid continuously

Vincent's infection of oropharynx
• *Adult:* PO 250-500 mg q6-8h

Available forms include: Tabs 125,

250, 500 mg; caps 250 mg; film-coated tabs 250, 500 mg; powder for oral susp 125, 250 mg/5 ml

Side effects/adverse reactions:

▼ *ORAL:* Candidiasis, glossitis, stomatitis, black hairy tongue, dry mouth, altered taste

CNS: ***Depression, coma, convulsions,*** lethargy, hallucinations, anxiety, twitching

GI: Nausea, vomiting, diarrhea, abdominal pain, colitis, anorexia

HEMA: ***Bone marrow depression, granulocytopenia,*** eosinophilia, anemia, increased bleeding time

GU: ***Oliguria, proteinuria, hematuria, vaginitis, moniliasis, glomerulonephritis***

META: Hyperkalemia, hypokalemia, alkalosis; allergy symptoms: pruritus, urticaria, angioedema, bronchospasm, anaphylaxis

Contraindications: Hypersensitivity to penicillins; neonates

Precautions: Hypersensitivity to cephalosporins, pregnancy category B, lactation

Pharmacokinetics:

PO: Peak 30-60 min, duration 6-8 hr, half-life 30 min; excreted in urine, breast milk

Drug interactions of concern to dentistry:

• Decreased antimicrobial effectiveness of penicillin: tetracyclines, erythromycins, lincomycins

• Increased penicillin concentrations: probenecid

When used for dental infection:

• Decreased effectiveness of oral contraceptives

DENTAL CONSIDERATIONS

General:

• Take precautions regarding allergy to medication.

• Determine why the patient is taking the drug.

• If used for dental infection, place on frequent recall to evaluate healing response.

Consultations:

• Medical consult may be required to assess disease control in the patient.

Teach patient/family:

When used for dental infection, advise patient:

• Taking birth control pill to use additional method of contraception for duration of cycle

• To report sore throat, oral burning sensation, fever, fatigue, any of which could indicate superinfection

• To take at prescribed intervals and complete dosage regimen

• To immediately notify the dentist if signs or symptoms of infection increase

pentamidine/ pentamidine isethionate

(pen-tam'i-deen)

NebuPent, Pentam 300

♣ Pentacarinat, Pneumopent

Drug class.: Antiprotozoal

Action: Interferes with DNA/RNA synthesis in protozoa

Uses: *P. carinii* infections in immunocompromised patients

Dosage and routes:

• *Adult and child:* IV/IM 4 mg/kg/day × 2 wk; nebuliz 600 mg/6 ml NS via specific nebulizer

Available forms include: Inj IV/IM 300 mg/vial; aerosol 300 mg/vial

P

Side effects/adverse reactions:
▼ *ORAL:* Bad taste (metallic), dry mouth, gingivitis, ulcerations or abscess, hypersalivation
CNS: Disorientation, hallucinations, dizziness
CV: Hypotension, ventricular tachycardia, ECG abnormalities
GI: Nausea, vomiting, anorexia, ***acute pancreatitis,*** increased AST/ALT
HEMA: ***Leukopenia, thrombocytopenia,*** anemia
GU: ***Acute renal failure***
INTEG: Sterile abscess, pain at injection site, pruritus, urticaria, rash
META: Hyperkalemia, hypocalcemia, hypoglycemia

Precautions: Blood dyscrasias, hepatic disease, renal disease, diabetes mellitus, cardiac disease, hypocalcemia, pregnancy category C

Pharmacokinetics:
IV/IM: Excreted unchanged in urine (66%)

Drug interactions of concern to dentistry:
- Nephrotoxicity: aminoglycosides, polymyxin B, vancomycin

DENTAL CONSIDERATIONS

General:
- Monitor vital signs every appointment due to cardiovascular side effects.
- Patients on chronic drug therapy may rarely have symptoms of blood dyscrasias, which can include infection, bleeding, and poor healing.
- Place on frequent recall to evaluate healing response.
- Assess salivary flow as a factor in caries, periodontal disease, and candidiasis.
- Consider semisupine chair position for patients with respiratory disease.
- For inhalation dosage forms, rinse mouth with water after each dose to prevent dryness.
- Place on frequent recall due to oral side effects.

Consultations:
- In a patient with symptoms of blood dyscrasias, request a medical consult for blood studies and postpone dental treatment until normal values are reestablished.
- Medical consult may be required to assess disease control in the patient.

Teach patient/family:
- That secondary oral infection may occur; must see dentist immediately if infection occurs
- Importance of good oral hygiene to prevent soft tissue inflammation
- Caution to prevent injury when using oral hygiene aids
- Importance of dietary suggestions to maintain oral and systemic health

When chronic dry mouth occurs, advise patient:
- To avoid mouth rinses with high alcohol content due to drying effects
- Of need for daily home fluoride to prevent caries
- To use sugarless gum, frequent sips of water, or saliva substitutes

---

pentazocine HCl/ pentazocine lactate

(pen-taz'oh-seen)
Talwin, Talwin NX
Drug class.: Synthetic opioid/mixed agonist/antagonist

Controlled Substance Schedule IV

Action: Interacts with opioid receptors in the CNS to alter pain perception

Uses: Moderate-to-severe pain alone or in combination with aspirin or acetaminophen

Dosage and routes:

• *Adult:* PO 50-100 mg q3-4h prn, not to exceed 600 mg/day; IV/IM/SC 30 mg q3-4h prn, not to exceed 360 mg/day

Available forms include: SC/IM/IV 30 mg/ml; tabs (NX) 50 mg in combination with 0.5 mg naloxone

Side effects/adverse reactions:

▼ *ORAL:* Dry mouth

CNS: Drowsiness, dizziness, confusion, headache, sedation, euphoria, hallucinations

CV: Palpitation, bradycardia, tachycardia, decreased BP (high doses)

GI: Nausea, vomiting, anorexia, constipation, cramps

RESP: ***Respiratory depression***

GU: Increased urinary output, dysuria

EENT: Tinnitus, blurred vision, miosis, diplopia

INTEG: Rash, urticaria, bruising, flushing, diaphoresis, pruritus

Contraindications: Hypersensitivity, addiction (narcotic)

Precautions: Addictive personality, pregnancy category B, lactation, increased intracranial pressure, head injury, MI (acute), severe heart disease, respiratory depression, hepatic disease, renal disease, children <18 yr, acute abdominal conditions, Addison's disease, prostatic hypertrophy

Pharmacokinetics:

SC/IM: Onset 15-30 min, peak 1-2 hr, duration 2-4 hr

IV: Onset 2-3 min, duration 4-6 hr

Half-life 2-3 hr; extensive first-pass metabolism with less than 20% entering circulation; metabolized by liver; excreted by kidneys; crosses placenta

Drug interactions of concern to dentistry:

• Increased effects: all CNS depressants, alcohol

• Contraindication: MAO inhibitors

• Do not mix in solutions or syringe with barbiturates

• Additive side effects of opioid agonists

• Increased effects of anticholinergics

• Decreased effects of opioid agonists

DENTAL CONSIDERATIONS

General:

• Monitor vital signs every appointment due to cardiovascular and respiratory side effects.

• Assess salivary flow as a factor in caries, periodontal disease, and candidiasis.

• Consider semisupine chair position for patient comfort if GI side effects occur.

• Psychologic and physical dependence may occur with chronic administration.

Teach patient/family:

When chronic dry mouth occurs, advise patient:

• To avoid mouth rinses with high alcohol content due to drying effects

• Of need for daily home fluoride to prevent caries

• To use sugarless gum, frequent sips of water, or saliva substitutes

P

pentobarbital/ pentobarbital sodium

(pen-toe-bar'bi-tal)
Nembutal Sodium
🍁 Nova-Rectal, Novopentobarb
Drug class.: Sedative-hypnotic barbiturate

Controlled Substance Schedule II, Canada C

Action: Depresses activity in brain cells, primarily in reticular activating system in brainstem; selectively depresses neurons in posterior hypothalamus, limbic structures

Uses: Insomnia, sedation, preoperative medication, increased intracranial pressure, dental anesthetic

Dosage and routes:

- *Adult:* PO 100-200 mg hs; IM 150-200 mg hs; IV 100 mg initially, then up to 500 mg; rec 120-200 mg hs
- *Child:* IM 3-5 mg/kg, not to exceed 100 mg
- *Child 2 mo-1 yr:* Rec 30 mg
- *Child 1-4 yr:* Rec 30-60 mg
- *Child 5-12 yr:* Rec 60 mg
- *Child 12-14 yr:* Rec 60-120 mg

Available forms include: Caps 50, 100 mg; elix 18.2 mg/5 ml; powder, rec supp 30, 60, 120, 200 mg; inj IM/IV 50 mg/ml

Side effects/adverse reactions:

CNS: Lethargy, drowsiness, hangover, ***CNS depression,*** dizziness, paradoxic stimulation in elderly and children, light-headedness, dependence, mental depression, slurred speech

CV: Hypotension, bradycardia, syncope

GI: Nausea, vomiting, diarrhea, constipation, epigastric pain, liver damage (long-term use)

RESP: ***Depression, apnea, laryngospasm, bronchospasm,*** circulatory collapse, hypoventilation

HEMA: ***Agranulocytosis, thrombocytopenia, megaloblastic anemia*** (long-term treatment)

INTEG: Rash, ***Stevens-Johnson syndrome,*** urticaria, pain, abscesses at injection site, angioedema, thrombophlebitis

Contraindications: Hypersensitivity to barbiturates, respiratory depression, addiction to barbiturates, severe liver/renal impairment, porphyria, uncontrolled pain

Precautions: Anemia, pregnancy category D, lactation, hepatic disease, renal disease, hypertension, elderly, acute/chronic pain

Pharmacokinetics:

PO: Onset 15-30 min, duration 4-6 hr

REC: Onset slow, duration 4-6 hr

Half-life 15-48 hr; metabolized by liver; excreted by kidneys (metabolites)

Drug interactions of concern to dentistry:

- Hepatotoxicity: halogenated-hydrocarbon anesthetics
- Increased CNS depression: alcohol, all other CNS depressants
- Increased metabolism of carbamazepine, tricyclic antidepressants, corticosteroids
- Decreased half-life of doxycycline

DENTAL CONSIDERATIONS

General:

- Determine why the patient is taking the drug.
- Monitor vital signs every ap-

pointment due to cardiovascular side effects. Evaluate respiration characteristics and rate.

• Patients on chronic drug therapy may rarely have symptoms of blood dyscrasias, which can include infection, bleeding, and poor healing.

When used for sedation in dentistry:

• Assess vital signs before use and q30min after use as sedative.

• Observe respiratory dysfunction: respiratory depression, character, rate, rhythm; hold drug if respirations <10/min or if pupils dilated.

• After supine positioning, have patient sit upright for at least 2 min before standing to avoid orthostatic hypotension.

• Have someone drive patient to and from dental office when used for conscious sedation.

• Barbiturates induce liver microsomal enzymes, which alters the metabolism of other drugs.

• Geriatric patients are more susceptible to drug effects; use lower dose.

Consultations:

• In a patient with symptoms of blood dyscrasias, request a medical consult for blood studies and postpone dental treatment until normal values are reestablished.

Teach patient/family:

• To avoid driving or other activities requiring alertness

• To avoid alcohol ingestion or CNS depressants; serious CNS depression may result

• To avoid OTC preparations that contain CNS depressants (antihistamines, cold remedies)

pentoxifylline

(pen-tox-i'fi-leen)

Trental

Drug class.: Hemorheologic agent

Action: Decreases blood viscosity, increases blood flow to affected microcirculation, and enhances tissue oxygenation in chronic peripheral arterial disease

Uses: Intermittent claudication related to chronic occlusive arterial disease of the limbs

Dosage and routes:

• *Adult:* PO 400 mg tid with meals

Available forms include: Con rel tabs 400 mg

Side effects/adverse reactions:

▼ *ORAL:* Dry mouth, thirst, bad taste

CNS: Headache, anxiety, tremors, confusion, dizziness, drowsiness, nervousness, agitation, seizures

CV: Angina, dysrhythmias, palpitation, hypotension, chest pain, dyspnea, edema

GI: Nausea, vomiting, anorexia, bloating, belching, constipation, dyspepsia, cholecystitis

EENT: Blurred vision, earache, sore throat, conjunctivitis

INTEG: Rash, pruritus, urticaria, brittle fingernails

MISC: Epistaxis, flulike symptoms: laryngitis, nasal congestion, leukopenia, malaise, weight changes, lymphoedema

Contraindications: Hypersensitivity to this drug or xanthines

Precautions: Pregnancy category C, angina pectoris, cardiac disease, lactation, children, impaired renal function

Pharmacokinetics:

PO: Peak 1 hr, half-life 0.5-1 hr;

P

degradation in liver; excreted in urine

DENTAL CONSIDERATIONS
General:
• Monitor vital signs every appointment due to cardiovascular side effects.
• Assess salivary flow as a factor in caries, periodontal disease, and candidiasis.
• Stress from dental procedures may compromise cardiovascular function; determine patient risk.
• Short appointments and a stress reduction protocol may be required for anxious patients.
• Talk with patient about potential systemic diseases (diabetes, CV disease), which may be associated with claudication.
Consultations:
• Medical consult may be required to assess disease control and patient's ability to tolerate stress.
Teach patient/family:
• Importance of good oral hygiene to prevent soft tissue inflammation
• Caution to prevent injury when using oral hygiene aids
When chronic dry mouth occurs, advise patient:
• To avoid mouth rinses with high alcohol content due to drying effects
• Of need for daily home fluoride to prevent caries
• To use sugarless gum, frequent sips of water, or saliva substitutes

---

pergolide mesylate
(per'go-lide)
Permax
Drug class.: Antiparkinson agent

Action: Dopamine receptor agonist for D_1 and D_2 receptors

Uses: Adjunctive treatment of Parkinson's disease

Dosage and routes:
• *Adult:* PO initial 0.05 mg × 2 days; gradually increase by 0.1-0.15 mg/d q 3rd day over next 12 days. Doses can then be increased by 0.25 mg/d q 3rd day. Average dose 3 mg/day; maximum dose 5 mg/day usually in 3 divided doses/day.

Available forms include: Tabs 0.05, 0.25, 1 mg

Side effects/adverse reactions:
▼ *ORAL: Dry mouth,* sialadenitis, aphthous stomatitis
CNS: Dyskinesia, hallucinations, somnolence, confusion, dizziness, headache, insomnia, tremor, extrapyramidal syndrome, anxiety, psychosis
CV: Postural hypotension, syncope, palpitation, vasodilation
GI: Nausea, constipation, diarrhea, abdominal pain, dyspepsia
RESP: Dyspnea
HEMA: Anemia
GU: Frequency, UTI
EENT: Rhinitis, diplopia
INTEG: Sweating, rash
MS: Back pain, neck pain, myalgia, twitching, arthralgia
MISC: Flulike syndrome, fever, peripheral edema

Contraindications: Hypersensitivity to this drug or ergot derivatives

Precautions: Symptomatic hypotension, cardiac dysrhythmias, dose adjustment for patients on levodopa, discontinue drug slowly, pregnancy category B, lactation, children

Pharmacokinetics:
PO: Plasma protein binding 90%, metabolized, urinary excretion, half-life 27 hr

Drug interactions of concern to dentistry:

• Decreased action: phenothiazines, haloperidol, droperidol, thiothixenes, and metoclopramide

DENTAL CONSIDERATIONS

General:

• Monitor vital signs every appointment due to cardiovascular side effects.

• Short appointments may be required due to disease effects on musculature.

• Use precaution if sedation or general anesthesia is required; risk of hypotensive episode.

• After supine positioning have patient sit upright for at least 2 min before standing to avoid orthostatic hypotension.

• Assess salivary flow as a factor in caries, periodontal disease, candidiasis.

• Assess for presence of extrapyramidal motor symptoms, such as tardive dyskinesia and akathisia. Extrapyramidal motor activity may complicate dental treatment.

• Consider semisupine chair position for patient comfort due to GI effects of drug.

Consultations:

• Medical consult may be required to assess disease control in the patient.

Teach patient/family:

• Use of electric toothbrush if patient has difficulty holding conventional devices

• Importance of updating health history/drug record if physician makes any changes in evaluations/drug regimens

When chronic dry mouth occurs, advise patient:

• To avoid mouth rinses with high alcohol content due to drying effects

• Of need for daily home fluoride to prevent caries

• To use sugarless gum, frequent sips of water, or saliva substitutes

---

perindopril erbumine

(per-in′doe-pril)

Aceon

Drug class.: Angiotensin-converting enzyme (ACE) inhibitor

Action: Selectively suppresses renin-angiotensin-aldosterone system; inhibits ACE; prevents conversion of angiotensin I to angiotensin II; results in dilation of arterial and venous vessels

Uses: Essential hypertension as monotherapy or in combination with other antihypertensive medication

Dosage and routes:

Hypertension

• *Adult:* PO 4 mg qd; can be titrated upward to maximum of 16 mg/day; doses can be given bid if needed

• *Adult >65 yr:* PO daily dose limit 8 mg. NOTE: May have less efficacy in African-American patients

Available forms include: Tabs 2, 4 mg

Side effects/adverse reactions:

▼ *ORAL:* ***Angioedema (lips, tongue, mucous membranes),*** dry mouth, taste disturbances

CNS: Orthostatic hypotension, headache, light-headedness, dizziness, nervousness

CV: Palpitation, edema

GI: Dyspepsia, nausea, diarrhea, abdominal pain, vomiting

RESP: Cough, URI

P

HEMA: ***Agranulocytosis, neutropenia***
GU: Proteinuria, UTI, male sexual dysfunction
EENT: *Sinusitis, ear infection,* rhinitis, pharyngitis, tinnitus
INTEG: Rash
META: *Hyperkalemia,* ALT increase, triglyceride increase
MS: *Asthenia, back pain,* hypertonia, myalgia
MISC: ***Anaphylaxis,*** fever, upper extremity pain

Contraindications: Hypersensitivity to this drug or other ACE inhibitors, patients with a history of angioedema to other ACE inhibitors, pregnancy (second and third trimesters)

Precautions: Renal insufficiency, hypertension with CHF, severe CHF, renal artery stenosis, autoimmune disease, collagen vascular disease, pregnancy category C (first trimester); pregnancy category D (second and third trimesters), lactation

Pharmacokinetics:
PO: Absolute bioavailability 20%-30%, metabolized to active metabolite, perindoprilat, peak plasma levels 1 hr, active metabolite 3-4 hr; protein binding 10%-20%, hepatic metabolism, excreted mostly in urine (75%)

Drug interactions of concern to dentistry:
- Decreased hypotensive effects: NSAIDs, aspirin
- Increased hypotension: caution in use of other drugs that have hypotensive effects

DENTAL CONSIDERATIONS

General:
- Monitor vital signs every appointment due to cardiovascular side effects.
- Limit use of sodium-containing products such as saline IV fluids for those patients with a dietary salt restriction.
- Short appointments and a stress reduction protocol may be required for anxious patients.
- Stress from dental procedures may compromise cardiovascular function; determine patient risk.
- After supine positioning, have patient sit upright for at least 2 min to avoid orthostatic hypotension.
- Use precaution if sedation or general anesthesia is required; risk of hypotensive episode.
- Assess salivary flow as a factor in caries, periodontal disease, and candidiasis.
- Consider semisupine chair position for patient comfort if GI or respiratory side effects occur.
- Patients on chronic drug therapy may rarely have symptoms of blood dyscrasias, which can include infection, bleeding, and poor healing.

Consultations:
- In a patient with symptoms of blood dyscrasias, request a medical consult for blood studies and postpone treatment until normal values are reestablished.
- Medical consult may be required to assess disease control and patient's ability to tolerate stress.

Teach patient/family:
- Importance of updating health and drug history if physician makes any changes in evaluation/drug regimens
- Importance of good oral hygiene to prevent soft tissue inflammation

• To prevent trauma when using oral hygiene aids

When chronic dry mouth occurs, advise patient:

• To avoid mouth rinses with high alcohol content due to drying effects

• To use daily home fluoride products for anticaries effect

• To use sugarless gum, frequent sips of water, or saliva substitutes

---

perphenazine

(per-fen′a-zeen)

Trilafon

♣ PMS Perphenazine, APO-Perphenazine

Drug class.: Phenothiazine antipsychotic

Action: Blocks neurotransmission at dopaminergic synapses in the cerebral cortex, hypothalamus, and limbic system; exhibits strong peripheral α-adrenergic, anticholinergic blocking action; mechanism for antipsychotic effects is unclear

Uses: Psychotic disorders, schizophrenia, alcoholism, nausea, vomiting

Dosage and routes:

Nausea/vomiting/alcoholism/intractable hiccups

• *Adult and child >12 yr:* IM 5-10 mg prn, max 15 mg in ambulatory patients, 30 mg in hospitalized patients; PO 8-16 mg/day in divided doses, up to 24 mg; IV not to exceed 5 mg, give diluted or slow IV drip

Psychiatric use in hospitalized patients

• *Adult:* PO 8-16 mg bid-qid, gradually increased to desired dose, not to exceed 64 mg/day; IM 5 mg q6h, not to exceed 30 mg/day

• *Child >12 yr:* PO 6-12 mg in divided doses

Nonhospitalized patients

• *Adult:* PO 4-8 mg tid or 8-32 mg repeat-action bid; IM 5 mg q6h

Available forms include: Tabs 2, 4, 8, 16 mg; sol 16 mg/5 ml; inj IM 5 mg/ml; sus rel tabs 8 mg

Side effects/adverse reactions:

▼ *ORAL: Dry mouth,* enlarged parotid glands, lichenoid reaction

CNS: Extrapyramidal symptoms: pseudoparkinsonism, akathisia, dystonia, tardive dyskinesia, ***seizures,*** headache

CV: Orthostatic hypotension, ***cardiac arrest, tachycardia,*** ECG changes, syncope

GI: Nausea, vomiting, anorexia, constipation, diarrhea, jaundice, weight gain

RESP: ***Laryngospasm, respiratory depression,*** dyspnea

HEMA: ***Leukopenia, leukocytosis, agranulocytosis,*** anemia

GU: Urinary retention, urinary frequency, enuresis, impotence, amenorrhea, gynecomastia

EENT: Blurred vision, glaucoma

INTEG: Rash, photosensitivity, dermatitis

Contraindications: Hypersensitivity, blood dyscrasias, coma, child <12 yr, brain damage, bone marrow depression

Precautions: Pregnancy category C, lactation, seizure disorders, hypertension, hepatic disease, cardiac disease

Pharmacokinetics:

PO: Onset erratic, peak 2-4 hr

IM: Onset 10 min, peak 1-2 hr,

P

duration 6 hr, occasionally 12-24 hr
Metabolized by liver, excreted in urine, crosses placenta, excreted in breast milk

Drug interactions of concern to dentistry:

- Increased sedation: other CNS depressants, alcohol, barbiturate anesthetics, opioid analgesics
- Hypotension, tachycardia: epinephrine
- Increased extrapyramidal effects: phenothiazines and related drugs (haloperidol, droperidol), metoclopramide
- Additive photosensitization: tetracyclines, fluoroquinolones
- Increased anticholinergic effects: anticholinergics

DENTAL CONSIDERATIONS

General:

- Monitor vital signs every appointment due to cardiovascular side effects.
- Patients on chronic drug therapy may rarely have symptoms of blood dyscrasias, which can include infection, bleeding, and poor healing.
- After supine positioning, have patient sit upright for at least 2 min before standing to avoid orthostatic hypotension.
- Assess salivary flow as a factor in caries, periodontal disease, and candidiasis.
- Avoid dental light in patient's eyes; offer dark glasses for patient comfort.
- Assess for presence of extrapyramidal motor symptoms, such as tardive dyskinesia and akathisia. Extrapyramidal motor activity may complicate dental treatment.
- Geriatric patients are more susceptible to drug effects; use lower dose.
- Use vasoconstrictors with caution, in low doses, and with careful aspiration. Avoid use of gingival retraction cord with epinephrine.

Consultations:

- In a patient with symptoms of blood dyscrasias, request a medical consult for blood studies and postpone dental treatment until normal values are reestablished.
- Take precautions if dental surgery is anticipated and anesthesia is required.
- If signs of tardive dyskinesia or akathisia are present, refer to physician.
- Physician should be informed if significant xerostomic side effects occur (increased caries, sore tongue, problems eating or swallowing, difficulty wearing prosthesis) so a medication change can be considered.

Teach patient/family:

- Importance of good oral hygiene to prevent soft tissue inflammation
- Caution to prevent injury when using oral hygiene aids
- To use electric toothbrush if patient has difficulty holding conventional devices

When chronic dry mouth occurs, advise patient:

- To avoid mouth rinses with high alcohol content due to drying effects
- Of need for daily home fluoride to prevent caries
- To use sugarless gum, frequent sips of water, or saliva substitutes

phenazopyridine HCl

(fen-az-oh-peer'i-deen)

Azo-Standard, Baridium, Eridium, Geridium, Phenazodine, Pyridiate, Pyridium, Urodine, Urogesic, Viridium

🍁 Phenazo

Drug class.: Urinary tract analgesic

Action: Exerts analgesic, anesthetic action on the urinary tract mucosa; exact mechanism of action unknown

Uses: Urinary tract irritation/infection

Dosage and routes:

• *Adult:* PO 100-200 mg tid

• *Child 6-12 yr:* PO 12 mg/kg/24 hr in 3 divided doses

Available forms include: Tabs 95, 100, 200 mg

Side effects/adverse reactions:

CNS: Headache, vertigo

GI: Nausea, vomiting, GI bleeding, diarrhea, heartburn, ***hepatic toxicity***

HEMA: ***Hemolytic anemia, methemoglobinemia*** (with overdose)

GU: ***Renal toxicity, orange-red urine***

INTEG: Rash, urticaria, skin pigmentation

Contraindications: Hypersensitivity, hepatic disease

Precautions: Pregnancy category B, renal disease

Pharmacokinetics:

PO: Metabolized by liver, excreted by kidneys, crosses placenta, duration 6-8 hr

DENTAL CONSIDERATIONS

General:

• Consider semisupine chair position for patient comfort if GI side effects occur.

• Patients on chronic drug therapy may rarely have symptoms of blood dyscrasias, which can include infection, bleeding, and poor healing.

• Be aware that patient might have UTI; question if antiinfectives are also being used.

phendimetrazine tartrate

(fen-dye-me'tra-zeen)

Adipost, Anorex SR, Appecon, Bontril PDM, Obalan, Obezine, Plegine, Prelu-2, Weh-less

Drug class.: Anorexiant, amphetamine-like

Controlled Substance Schedule III

Action: Exact mechanism of action of appetite suppression unknown, but may have an effect on satiety center of hypothalamus

Uses: Exogenous obesity

Dosage and routes:

• *Adult:* PO 35 mg bid-tid 1 hr ac, not to exceed 70 mg tid; sus rel 105 mg qd ac am

Available forms include: Tabs 35 mg; caps 35 mg; sus rel caps 105 mg

Side effects/adverse reactions:

▼ *ORAL:* Dry mouth, unpleasant taste

CNS: Hyperactivity, insomnia, restlessness, dizziness, tremors, headache

CV: Palpitation, tachycardia, hypertension

GI: Nausea, anorexia, diarrhea, constipation, cramps

HEMA: ***Bone marrow depression, leukopenia, agranulocytosis***

P

GU: Dysuria
EENT: Blurred vision
INTEG: Urticaria
Contraindications: Hypersensitivity, hyperthyroidism, hypertension, glaucoma, severe arteriosclerosis, severe cardiovascular disease, children <12 yr, agitated states, MAO inhibitors
Precautions: Drug abuse, anxiety, pregnancy category C, lactation
Pharmacokinetics:
PO: Onset 30 min, peak 1-3 hr, duration 4-20 hr, half-life 2-10 hr; metabolized by liver; excreted by kidneys; crosses placenta; excreted in breast milk
Drug interactions of concern to dentistry:
• Hypertensive crisis: MAO inhibitors or within 14 days of MAO inhibitors
• Increased risk of dysrhythmia: hydrocarbon inhalation general anesthetics
• Decreased effect: tricyclic antidepressants, ascorbic acid, phenothiazines
• Caffeine or caffeine-containing products: may increase risk of insomnia and dry mouth

DENTAL CONSIDERATIONS
General:
• Monitor vital signs every appointment due to cardiovascular side effects.
• Assess salivary flow as a factor in caries, periodontal disease, and candidiasis.
• Determine why the patient is taking the drug.
• Psychologic and physical dependence may occur with chronic administration.
• Patients on chronic drug therapy may rarely have symptoms of blood dyscrasias, which can include infection, bleeding, and poor healing.
Consultations:
• In a patient with symptoms of blood dyscrasias, request a medical consult for blood studies and postpone dental treatment until normal values are reestablished.
Teach patient/family:
• Importance of good oral hygiene to prevent soft tissue inflammation
• To report oral lesions, soreness, or bleeding to dentist
• Caution to prevent injury when using oral hygiene aids
When chronic dry mouth occurs, advise patient:
• To avoid mouth rinses with high alcohol content due to drying effects
• Of need for daily home fluoride to prevent caries
• To use sugarless gum, frequent sips of water, or saliva substitutes

---

phenelzine sulfate
(fen′el-zeen)
Nardil
Drug class.: Antidepressant, MAO inhibitor

Action: Increases concentrations of endogenous epinephrine, norepinephrine, serotonin, dopamine in storage sites in CNS by inhibition of MAO; antidepressant mechanism uncertain
Uses: Depression when uncontrolled by other means
Dosage and routes:
• *Adult:* PO 45 mg/day in 3 divided doses; may increase to 60 mg/day;

dose should be reduced to 15 mg/day for maintenance; not to exceed 90 mg/day

Available forms include: Tabs 15 mg

Side effects/adverse reactions:

▼ *ORAL:* Dry mouth

CNS: Dizziness, drowsiness, confusion, headache, anxiety, tremors, stimulation, weakness, hyperreflexia, mania, insomnia, fatigue, weight gain

CV: Orthostatic hypotension, hypertension, dysrhythmias, hypertensive crisis, peripheral edema

GI: Constipation, nausea, vomiting, *anorexia,* diarrhea, weight changes, abdominal pain

HEMA: Anemia

GU: Change in libido, frequency

EENT: Blurred vision

INTEG: Rash, flushing, increased perspiration

*ENDO: **SIADH-like syndrome***

Contraindications: Hypersensitivity to MAO inhibitors, elderly, hypertension, CHF, severe hepatic disease, pheochromocytoma, severe renal disease, severe cardiac disease, fluoxetine, meperidine

Precautions: Suicidal patients, convulsive disorders, severe depression, schizophrenia, hyperactivity, diabetes mellitus, pregnancy category C

Pharmacokinetics: Metabolized by liver, excreted by kidneys

Drug interactions of concern to dentistry:

• Increased anticholinergic effect: anticholinergics, haloperidol, phenothiazines, antihistamines

• Hyperpyretic crisis, convulsions, hypertensive episode: meperidine, carbamazepine, cyclobenzapine

• Cardiac dysrhythmia: caffeine-containing medications

• Increased risk of serotonin syndrome: tricyclic antidepressants, other serotonin reuptake inhibitors

• Increased sedative effects of alcohol, barbiturates, benzodiazepines, CNS depressants

• Increased pressor effects: indirect-acting sympathomimetics such as ephedrine, amphetamine

DENTAL CONSIDERATIONS

General:

• Monitor vital signs every appointment due to cardiovascular side effects.

• Assess salivary flow as a factor in caries, periodontal disease, and candidiasis.

• After supine positioning, have patient sit upright for at least 2 min before standing to avoid orthostatic hypotension.

• Hypertensive episodes are possible even though there are no specific contraindications to vasoconstrictor use in local anesthetics.

• Avoid prescribing caffeine-containing products.

• Take precautions if dental surgery is anticipated and general anesthesia is required.

Consultations:

• Medical consult may be required to assess disease control and patient's ability to tolerate stress.

Teach patient/family:

• To use electric toothbrush if patient has difficulty holding conventional devices

When chronic dry mouth occurs, advise patient:

• To avoid mouth rinses with high alcohol content due to drying effects

P

• Of need for daily home fluoride to prevent caries
• To use sugarless gum, frequent sips of water, or saliva substitutes

phenobarbital/ phenobarbital sodium

(fee-noe-bar'bi-tal)

Ancalixir, Barbita, Luminal Sodium, Solfoton

Drug class.: Barbiturate anticonvulsant

Controlled Substance Schedule IV

Action: A nonspecific depressant of the CNS; may enhance GABA activity in the brain

Uses: All forms of epilepsy, status epilepticus, febrile seizures in children, sedation, insomnia; unapproved uses: hyperbilirubinemia, chronic cholestasis

Dosage and routes:

Seizures

• *Adult:* PO 100-200 mg/day in divided doses tid or total dose hs
• *Child:* PO 4-6 mg/kg/day in divided doses q12h; may be given as single dose hs

Status epilepticus

• *Adult:* IV inf 10 mg/kg; run no faster than 50 mg/min; may give up to 20 mg/kg
• *Child:* IV inf 5-10 mg/kg; may repeat q10-15 min, up to 20 mg/kg; run no faster than 50 mg/min

Sedation

• *Adult:* PO 30-120 mg/day in 2-3 divided doses
• *Child:* PO 6 mg/kg/day in 3 divided doses

Preoperative sedation

• *Adult:* IM 100-200 mg 1-1.5 hr before surgery
• *Child:* IM 16-100 mg 1-1.5 hr before surgery

Hyperbilirubinemia

• *Neonate:* PO 7 mg/kg/day from days 1-5 after birth; IM 5 mg/kg/day on day 1, then PO on days 2-7 after birth

Chronic cholestasis

• *Adult:* PO 90-180 mg/day in 2-3 divided doses
• *Child <12 yr:* PO 3-12 mg/kg/day in 2-3 divided doses

Available forms include: Caps 16 mg; elix 15, 20 mg/5 ml; tabs 8, 15, 16, 30, 32, 60, 65, 100 mg; inj 30, 60, 65, 130 mg/ml; powder for inj 120 mg/ampule

Side effects/adverse reactions:

CNS: Drowsiness, somnolence, paradoxic excitement (elderly), lethargy, hangover headache, flushing, hallucinations, coma, agitation, confusion, vertigo, insomnia, fever

CV: Bradycardia, hypotension, syncope

GI: Nausea, vomiting, diarrhea, constipation, liver damage (with chronic use)

RESP: Hypoventilation, apnea, respiratory depression, laryngospasm, bronchospasm, circulatory collapse

INTEG: ***Stevens-Johnson syndrome, angioedema,*** rash, urticaria, local pain, swelling, necrosis, thrombophlebitis, pemphigus-like reaction

Contraindications: Hypersensitivity to barbiturates, porphyria, hepatic disease, respiratory disease, nephritis, hyperthyroidism, diabetes mellitus, elderly, lactation, pregnancy category D

Precautions: Anemia

Pharmacokinetics:
PO: Onset 2-60 min, peak 8-12 hr, duration 6-10 hr, half-life 53-118 hr; metabolized by liver; excreted by kidneys; crosses placenta; excreted in breast milk

Drug interactions of concern to dentistry:
• Increased effects: alcohol, all CNS depressants, saquinavir
• Decreased effects of corticosteroids, doxycycline, carbamazepine

DENTAL CONSIDERATIONS

General:
• Determine why the patient is taking the drug.
• Monitor vital signs every appointment due to cardiovascular side effects. Evaluate respiration characteristics and rate.
• Patients on chronic drug therapy may rarely have symptoms of blood dyscrasias, which can include infection, bleeding, and poor healing.

When used for sedation in dentistry:
• Assess vital signs before use and q30min after use as sedative.
• Observe respiratory dysfunction: respiratory depression, character, rate, rhythm; hold drug if respirations <10/min or if pupils are dilated.
• After supine positioning, have patient sit upright for at least 2 min to avoid orthostatic hypotension.
• Have someone drive patient to and from dental office when used for conscious sedation.
• Barbiturates induce liver microsomal enzymes, which alters the metabolism of other drugs.
• Geriatric patients are more susceptible to drug effects; use lower dose.

Consultations:
• In a patient with symptoms of blood dyscrasias, request a medical consult for blood studies and postpone dental treatment until normal values are reestablished.

Teach patient/family:
• To avoid driving or other activities requiring alertness
• To avoid alcohol ingestion or CNS depressants; serious CNS depression may result
• To use OTC preparations with caution because they may contain other CNS depressants (antihistamines, cold remedies)

phenoxybenzamine HCl

(fen-ox-ee-ben'za-meen)
Dibenzyline

Drug class.: Antihypertensive

Action: α-adrenergic blocker that binds to α-adrenergic receptors, dilating peripheral blood vessels; lowers peripheral resistance; lowers blood pressure

Uses: Hypertensive episodes associated with pheochromocytoma; unapproved use: benign prostatic hypertrophy

Dosage and routes:
• *Adult:* PO 10 mg bid; increase by 10 mg qod, not to exceed 60 mg/day; usual range: 20-40 mg bid-tid

Available forms include: Caps 10 mg

Side effects/adverse reactions:
ORAL: Dry mouth
CNS: Dizziness, flushing, drowsiness, sedation, weakness, confusion, headache, malaise, fatigue, lassitude

CV: Postural hypotension, tachycardia, palpitation
GI: Nausea, vomiting, diarrhea
GU: Inhibition of ejaculation
EENT: Nasal congestion, miosis
INTEG: Allergic contact dermatitis

Contraindications: Hypersensitivity, CHF, angina, cerebral vascular insufficiency, coronary arteriosclerosis

Precautions: Severe renal disease, severe pulmonary disease, pregnancy category C, lactation

Pharmacokinetics:
PO: Onset 2 hr, peak 4-6 hr, duration 3-4 days, half-life 24 hr; metabolized in liver; excreted in urine, bile

Drug interactions of concern to dentistry:
- Decreased pressor response of ephedrine, phenylephrine, and epinephrine

DENTAL CONSIDERATIONS

General:
- Assess salivary flow as a factor in caries, periodontal disease, and candidiasis.
- After supine positioning, have patient sit upright for at least 2 min before standing to avoid orthostatic hypotension.
- Monitor vital signs every appointment due to cardiovascular side effects.
- Stress from dental procedures may compromise cardiovascular function; determine patient risk.
- Short appointments and a stress reduction protocol may be required for anxious patients.
- Avoid use of gingival retraction cord with epinephrine.

Consultations:
- Medical consult may be required before any dental treatment to assess disease control and patient's ability to tolerate stress.

Teach patient/family:
When chronic dry mouth occurs, advise patient:
- To avoid mouth rinses with high alcohol content due to drying effects
- Of need for daily home fluoride to prevent caries
- To use sugarless gum, frequent sips of water, or saliva substitutes

phensuximide

(fen-sux'i-mide)
Milontin

Drug class.: Anticonvulsant, succinimide

Action: Suppresses spike, wave formation in absence seizures (petit mal); decreases amplitude, frequency, duration, spread of discharge in minor motor seizures

Uses: Absence (petit mal) seizures; unapproved use: complex partial seizures

Dosage and routes:
- *Adult and child:* PO 500 mg-1 g bid or tid

Available forms include: Caps 500 mg

Side effects/adverse reactions:
▼ *ORAL:* Gingival bleeding, ulcerations (Stevens-Johnson syndrome); swelling of tongue and gingival enlargement (rare)
CNS: Drowsiness, dizziness, fatigue, euphoria, lethargy, anxiety, depression, irritability, insomnia, aggressiveness, weakness, headache
GI: Nausea, vomiting, heartburn, anorexia, diarrhea, abdominal pain, cramps, constipation

HEMA: ***Agranulocytosis, aplastic anemia, thrombocytopenia, leukocytosis, eosinophilia, pancytopenia***
GU: ***Hematuria, renal damage,*** urinary frequency, vaginal bleeding
EENT: Myopia, blurred vision
INTEG: ***Stevens-Johnson syndrome,*** urticaria, pruritic erythema, hirsutism
Contraindications: Hypersensitivity to succinimide derivatives
Precautions: Lactation, hepatic disease, pregnancy category D, renal disease, intermittent porphyria
Pharmacokinetics:
PO: Peak 1-4 hr, half-life 5-12 hr; metabolized by liver; excreted by kidneys
Drug interactions of concern to dentistry:
• Enhanced CNS depression: CNS depressants, alcohol
• Decreased effects: phenothiazines, thioxanthenes, bartiturates
DENTAL CONSIDERATIONS
General:
• Patients on chronic drug therapy may rarely have symptoms of blood dyscrasias, which can include infection, bleeding, and poor healing.
• Ask about type of epilepsy, seizure frequency, and quality of seizure control.
• A stress reduction protocol may be required for anxious patients.
• Consider semisupine chair position if GI side effects occur.
Consultations:
• In a patient with symptoms of blood dyscrasias, request a medical consult for blood studies and postpone dental treatment until normal values are reestablished.
• Medical consult may be required to assess disease control and patient's ability to tolerate stress.
Teach patient/family:
• Importance of good oral hygiene to prevent gingival inflammation
• To avoid mouth rinses with high alcohol content due to drying effects
• To prevent injury when using oral hygiene aids
• To report oral lesions, soreness, or bleeding to dentist

phentermine HCl/ phentermine resin

(fen′ter-meen)
Adipex-P, Fastin, Ionamin, Obe-Nix, Obestine-30, Oby-Cap, Panshapem, Phentercot, Phentride, Teramine, T-Diet, Zantryl
Drug class.: Sympathomimetic, anorexant

Controlled Substance Schedule IV
Action: Exact mechanism of action of appetite suppression unknown, but may have an effect on satiety center of hypothalamus
Uses: Exogenous obesity
Dosage and routes:
• *Adult:* PO 8 mg tid 30 min before meals or 15-37.5 mg qd
Available forms include: Tabs 8, 30, 37.5 mg; caps 15, 18.75, 30, 37.5 mg; time rel caps 30 mg
Side effects/adverse reactions:
ORAL: Dry mouth, unpleasant taste
CNS: Insomnia, restlessness, agitation, hyperactivity, dizziness, tremor, headache, anxiety, agitation, euphoria, dyskensia
CV: Palpitation, tachycardia, hypertension, ECG changes, dysrhythmias

P

GI: Nausea, anorexia, constipation, diarrhea
HEMA: ***Bone marrow depression, agranulocytosis, leukopenia***
GU: Impotence, change in libido, dysuria, urinary frequency
EENT: Blurred vision, mydriasis
INTEG: Urticaria, rash
Contraindications: Hypersensitivity, hyperthyroidism, hypertension, glaucoma, severe arteriosclerosis, angina pectoris, cardiovascular disease, child <12 yr, MAO inhibitor–type medications
Precautions: Pregnancy category C, lactation, drug abuse, anxiety, tolerance
Pharmacokinetics:
SUS REL: Duration 10-14 hr; metabolized by liver; excreted by kidneys
PO (NOT CON REL DOSE FORMS): Rapid onset, duration 4 hr
Drug interactions of concern to dentistry:
- Hypertensive crisis: MAO inhibitors or within 14 days of MAO inhibitors
- Increased risk of dysrhythmia: hydrocarbon inhalation general anesthetics
- Decreased effect: tricyclic antidepressants, ascorbic acid, phenothiazines
- Caffeine or caffeine-containing products may increase risk of insomnia

DENTAL CONSIDERATIONS
General:
- Monitor vital signs every appointment due to cardiovascular side effects.
- Assess salivary flow as a factor in caries, periodontal disease, and candidiasis.
- Determine why the patient is taking the drug.
- Psychologic and physical dependence may occur with chronic administration.
- Patients on chronic drug therapy may rarely have symptoms of blood dyscrasias, which can include infection, bleeding, and poor healing.

Consultations:
- In a patient with symptoms of blood dyscrasias, request a medical consult for blood studies and postpone dental treatment until normal values are reestablished.

Teach patient/family:
- Importance of good oral hygiene to prevent soft tissue inflammation
- To prevent injury when using oral hygiene aids
- To report oral lesions, soreness, or bleeding to dentist

When chronic dry mouth occurs, advise patient:
- To avoid mouth rinses with high alcohol content due to drying effects
- Of need for daily home fluoride to prevent caries
- To use sugarless gum, frequent sips of water, or saliva substitutes

---

phentolamine mesylate
(fen-tole'a-meen)
Regitine
Rogitine
Drug class.: Antihypertensive

Action: α-adrenergic blocker; binds to α-adrenergic receptors, dilating peripheral blood vessels, lowering peripheral resistances, lowering blood pressure
Uses: Hypertension, pheochromocytoma, prevention and treatment of dermal necrosis following extravasation of norepinephrine or

dopamine; unlabeled use: with papaverine for intracavernous injection for impotence

Dosage and routes:

Treatment of hypertensive episodes in pheochromocytoma

• *Adult:* IV/IM 5 mg 1-2 hr before surgery; repeat if necessary

• *Child:* IV/IM 1 mg 1-2 hr before surgery; repeat if necessary

Prevention/treatment of necrosis

• *Adult:* 5-10 mg/10 ml NS injected into area of norepinephrine extravasation within 12 hr; preventive dose 10 mg to each 1000 ml norepinephrine solution

Available forms include: Inj IM/IV 5 mg/ml

Side effects/adverse reactions:

▼ *ORAL: Dry mouth*

CNS: Dizziness, flushing, weakness

CV: Hypotension, tachycardia, angina, dysrhythmias, ***MI***

GI: Nausea, vomiting, diarrhea, abdominal pain

EENT: Nasal congestion

Contraindications: Hypersensitivity, MI, coronary insufficiency, angina, peptic ulcer

Precautions: Pregnancy category C, lactation

Pharmacokinetics:

IV: Peak 2 min, duration 10-15 min

IM: Peak 15-20 min, duration 3-4 hr

Metabolized in liver, excreted in urine

Drug interactions of concern to dentistry:

• Hypotension, tachycardia: epinephrine

• Decreased pressor effects of epinephrine, ephedrine

DENTAL CONSIDERATIONS

General:

• This is an acute-use drug; hypertension and pheochromocytoma are the immediate concerns in the patient.

• Patients with untreated pheochromocytoma or with extreme hypertension requiring the use of this drug and who are not controlled are not candidates for elective dental treatment. Physican consult is required.

• Short appointments and a stress reduction protocol may be required for anxious patients.

• Stress from dental procedures may compromise cardiovascular function; determine patient risk.

• Use vasoconstrictors with caution, in low doses, and with careful aspiration. Avoid use of gingival retraction cord with epinephrine.

• Assess vital signs at each appointment due to nature of disease.

Consultations:

• Medical consult may be required to assess disease control and patient's ablilty to tolerate stress.

phenylephrine HCl (nasal)

(fen-ill-ef′rin)

Alconefrin, Neo-Synephrine, Doktors, Duration, Rhinall, Nostril, Sinex

Drug class.: Nasal decongestant, sympathomimetic

Action: Produces rapid and long-acting vasoconstriction of arterioles, thereby decreasing fluid exudation, mucosal engorgement

Uses: Nasal congestion (temporary relief)

Dosage and routes:

• *Adult:* Instill 2-3 gtt or sprays to nasal mucosa bid (0.25%-1%) q3-4h

• *Child 6-12 yr:* Instill 1-2 gtt or sprays (0.25%) q3-4h
• *Child <6 yr:* Instill 2-3 gtt or sprays (0.125%) q3-4h
Available forms include: Sol 0.125%, 0.16%, 0.25%, 0.5%, 1%
Side effects/adverse reactions:
▼ *ORAL: Dry mouth,* bitter taste
CNS: Anxiety, restlessness, tremors, weakness, insomnia, dizziness, fever, headache
GI: Nausea, vomiting, anorexia
EENT: Irritation, burning, sneezing, stinging, dryness, rebound congestion
INTEG: Contact dermatitis
Contraindications: Hypersensitivity to sympathomimetic amines, MAO inhibitors
Precautions: Child <6 yr, elderly, diabetes, cardiovascular disease, hypertension, hyperthyroidism, increased IOP, prostatic hypertrophy, pregnancy category C, glaucoma, ischemic heart disease, excessive use
Drug interactions of concern to dentistry:
• None reported with normal topical use
With systemic absorption, see risk of:
• Bradycardia: β-adrenergic blockers
• Increased dysrhythmias and hypertension: tricyclic antidepressants
DENTAL CONSIDERATIONS
General:
• Consider semisupine chair position for patient comfort due to respiratory effects of disease.
• Assess salivary flow as a factor in caries, periodontal disease, and candidiasis.
• Patients with significant nasal congestion may complicate nasal administration of nitrous oxide/oxygen sedation.
Teach patient/family:
That this product is not indicated for prolonged use because of congestion rebound; however, this may not always be the case

---

phenytoin sodium/ phenytoin sodium extended/phenytoin sodium prompt

(fen′i-toyn)

Dilantin, Dilantin Infatabs, Dilantin Kapseals, Diphenylan, Phenytex

Drug class.: Hydantoin anticonvulsant

Action: Inhibits spread of seizure activity in motor cortex
Uses: Generalized tonic-clonic (grand mal) seizures, status epilepticus, nonepileptic seizures, trigeminal neuralgia, cardiac dysrhythmias (Class Ib) caused by digitalis-type drugs
Dosage and routes:
Seizures
• *Adult:* IV loading dose 900 mg-1.5 g run at 50 mg/min; if patient has received phenytoin, 100-300 mg run at 50 mg/min; PO loading dose 900 mg-1.5 g divided tid, then 300 mg/day (extended) or divided tid (extended/prompt)
• *Child:* IV loading dose 15 mg/kg run at 50 mg/min; if patient has received phenytoin, 5-7 mg/kg run at 50 mg/min, may repeat in 30 min; PO loading dose 15 mg/kg divided q8-12h, then 5-7 mg/kg in divided doses q12h

Ventricular dysrhythmias

• *Adult:* PO loading dose 1 g divided over 24 hr, then 500 mg/day for 2 days, maintenance 300 mg PO daily; IV 250 mg given over 5 min until dysrhythmias subside or 1 g is given, or 100 mg q15min until dysrhythmias subside or 1 g is given

• *Child:* PO 3-8 mg/kg or 250 mg/m²/day as single dose or divided in 2 doses; IV 3-8 mg/kg given over several min, or 250 mg/m²/day as single dose or divided in 2 doses

Available forms include: Susp 30, 125 mg/5 ml; chew tabs 50 mg; inj 50 mg/ml; ext rel caps 30, 100 mg; caps prompt 30, 100 mg

Side effects/adverse reactions:

▼ *ORAL: Gingival overgrowth,* oral ulceration (Stevens-Johnson syndrome), taste loss

CNS: Drowsiness, dizziness, insomnia, paresthesia, depression, headache, confusion, slurred speech, ataxia, numbness

CV: Hypotension, ventricular fibrillation

GI: Nausea, vomiting, constipation, ***hepatitis,*** anorexia, weight loss, jaundice, epigastric pain

HEMA: ***Agranulocytosis, leukopenia, aplastic anemia, thrombocytopenia, megaloblastic anemia***

GU: Nephritis, albuminuria

EENT: Nystagmus, diplopia, blurred vision

INTEG: Rash, ***Stevens-Johnson syndrome,*** lupus erythematosus, hirsutism

MISC: Lymphadenopathy, hyperglycemia

Contraindications: Hypersensitivity, psychiatric condition, pregnancy category D, bradycardia, SA and AV block, Stokes-Adams syndrome

Precautions: Allergies, hepatic disease, renal disease

Pharmacokinetics:

PO: Duration 5 hr; metabolized by liver; excreted by kidneys

Drug interactions of concern to dentistry:

• Increased serum levels by: ketaconazole, fluconazole, fluoxetine, metronidazole

• Decreased effects: barbiturates, carbamazepine, chloral hydrate

• Hepatotoxicity: acetaminophen (chronic use and high doses only)

• Decreased effects of corticosteroids, doxycycline

DENTAL CONSIDERATIONS

General:

• Patients on chronic drug therapy may rarely have symptoms of blood dyscrasias, which can include infection, bleeding, and poor healing.

• Place on frequent recall to evaluate gingival condition and self-care.

• Short appointments and a stress reduction protocol may be required for anxious patients.

• Ask about type of epilepsy, seizure frequency, and quality of seizure control.

Consultations:

• In a patient with symptoms of blood dyscrasias, request a medical consult for blood studies and postpone dental treatment until normal values are reestablished.

• Medical consult may be required to assess disease control and the patient's ability to tolerate stress.

Teach patient/family:

• Importance of good oral hygiene

to prevent soft tissue inflammation and minimize gingival overgrowth
• Caution to prevent injury when using oral hygiene aids

phytonadione (vitamin k_1)

(fye-toe-na-dye'one)

AquaMEPHYTON, Konakion, Mephyton

Drug class.: Vitamin K_1, fat-soluble vitamin

Action: Needed for adequate blood clotting (factors II, VII, IX, X)

Uses: Vitamin K malabsorption, hypoprothrombinemia, prevention of hypoprothrombinemia caused by oral anticoagulants

Dosage and routes:

Hypoprothrombinemia caused by vitamin K malabsorption

• *Adult:* PO/IM 2-25 mg; may repeat or increase to 50 mg
• *Child:* PO/IM 5-10 mg
• *Infants:* PO/IM 2 mg

Prevention of hemorrhagic disease of the newborn

• *Neonate:* SC/IM 0.5-1 mg after birth; repeat in 6-8 hr if required

Hypoprothrombinemia caused by oral anticoagulants

• *Adult:* PO/SC/IM 2.5-10 mg; may repeat 12-48 hr after PO dose or 6-8 hr after SC/IM dose, based on PT

Available forms include: Tabs 5 mg; inj aqueous colloidal IM/IV; inj aqueous dispersion 2, 10 mg/ml (IM only)

Side effects/adverse reactions:

▼ *ORAL:* Unusual taste

CNS: Headache, ***brain damage*** (large doses)

CV: Cardiac irregularities

GI: Nausea, vomiting

HEMA: ***Hemolytic anemia, hemoglobinuria, hyperbilirubinemia***

INTEG: Rash, urticaria, flushing, erythema, sweating

MISC: Bronchospasms, dyspnea, cramplike pain

Contraindications: Hypersensitivity, severe hepatic disease, last few weeks of pregnancy

Precautions: Pregnancy category C

Pharmacokinetics:

PO/INJ: Readily absorbed from duodenum and requires bile salts, rapid hepatic metabolism, onset of action 6-12 hr, normal PT in 12-24 hr, crosses placenta, renal and biliary excretion

Drug interactions of concern to dentistry:

• Decreased action: broad-spectrum antibiotics, salicylates (high doses)
• Antagonist to oral anticoagulants

DENTAL CONSIDERATIONS

General:

• Determine why the patient is taking this drug. Medical consult should be made before dental treatment.
• Patients on chronic drug therapy may rarely have symptoms of blood dyscrasias, which can include infection, bleeding, and poor healing.

Consultations:

• Medical consultation to determine coagulation stability.

pilocarpine HCl/ pilocarpine nitrate (optic)

(pye-loe-kar′peen)

Adsorbocarpine, Akarpine, Isopto Carpine, Ocu-Carpine, Pilocar, Pilagan, Piloptic, Pilostat

♣ Miocarpine

Drug class.: Miotic, cholinergic agonist

Action: Acts directly on cholinergic receptor sites; induces miosis, spasm of accommodation, fall in intraocular pressure, caused by stimulation of ciliary, pupillary sphincter muscles, which leads to pulling of iris from filtration angle, resulting in increased outflow of aqueous humor

Uses: Primary glaucoma, early stages of wide-angle glaucoma (less useful in advanced stages), chronic open-angle glaucoma, acute narrow-angle glaucoma before emergency surgery; also used to neutralize mydriatics used during eye exam; may be used alternately with mydriatics to break adhesions between iris and lens

Dosage and routes:

- *Adult and child:* Instill sol 1-2 gtt of 1% or 2% solution in eye q6-8h; instill 20-40 μg/hr (Ocusert Pilo) in cul-de-sac of eye

Available forms include: Sol 0.25%-10%

Side effects/adverse reactions:

▼ *ORAL:* Excessive salivation

CV: Hypotension, tachycardia

GI: Nausea, vomiting, abdominal cramps, diarrhea

RESP: ***Bronchospasm***

EENT: Blurred vision, browache, twitching of eyelids, eye pain with change in focus

Contraindications: Bradycardia, hyperthyroidism, coronary artery disease, hypertension, obstruction of GI/urinary tracts, epilepsy, parkinsonism, asthma

Precautions: Bronchial asthma, hypertension, pregnancy category C

DENTAL CONSIDERATIONS

General:

- Avoid drugs with anticholinergic activity, such as antihistamines, opioids, benzodiazepines, propantheline, atropine, and scopolamine.
- Avoid dental light in patient's eyes; offer dark glasses for patient comfort.
- Monitor vital signs every appointment due to cardiovascular and respiratory side effects.

Consultations:

- Medical consult may be required to assess disease control in the patient.

P

pilocarpine HCl (oral)

(pye-loe-kar′peen)

Salagen

Drug class.: Cholinergic agonist (parasympathomimetic)

Action: Mimics the action of acetylcholine on muscarinic receptors

Uses: Treatment of symptoms of xerostomia from salivary gland hypofunction caused by radiotherapy for cancer of the head and neck and Sjögren's syndrome

Dosage and routes:

- *Adult:* PO initially 5 mg tid; 10 mg tid may be considered for patients who are not responding adequately and who can tolerate the lower doses

Available forms include: Tabs 5 mg

Side effects/adverse reactions:

▼ *ORAL:* Taste alteration

CNS: Dizziness, headache, nervousness, anxiety

CV: Flushing, edema, tachycardia, palpitation, hypotension, hypertension, bradycardia

GI: Nausea, dyspepsia, diarrhea, abdominal pain, vomiting, diarrhea

HEMA: Leukopenia, lymphadenopathy

GU: Urinary frequency

EENT: Rhinitis, lacrimation, pharyngitis, amblyopia, conjunctivitis, sinusitis

INTEG: Rash

MS: Asthenia

MISC: Sweating (high doses)

Contraindications: Uncontrolled asthma, hypersensitivity, when miosis is undesirable (acute iritis, narrow-angle glaucoma)

Precautions: Pregnancy category C, children, lactation, cardiovascular disease, retinal diseases, pulmonary diseases (asthma, chronic bronchitis, COPD), biliary tract disease, history of renal colic, psychiatric disorders

Pharmacokinetics:

PO: Onset 20 min, peak effect 1 hr, duration 3-5 hr; renal excretion

Drug interactions of concern to dentistry

• With β-adrenergic agonists: use with caution; possibility of conduction disturbances

• Reduced effect: anticholinergic drugs

• Enhanced effects: other cholinergic agonists

DENTAL CONSIDERATIONS

General:

• Patients receiving chemotherapy may require palliative treatment for stomatitis.

• Assess salivary flow as a factor in caries, periodontal disease, and candidiasis.

• Monitor vital signs every appointment due to cardiovascular side effects.

• Place on frequent recall due to oral effects of head and neck radiation.

Consultations:

• Medical consult may be required to assess disease control in the patient.

• Medical consult may be necessary before prescribing for those patients with cardiovascular, retinal, or respiratory disease.

Teach patient/family:

• To use caution when driving at night or performing hazardous activities in reduced lighting (visual blurring)

• That sweating can become extensive with high dose; have patient take plenty of fluids, observe for dehydration, or discontinue drug

When chronic dry mouth occurs, advise patient:

• To avoid mouth rinses with high alcohol content due to drying effects

• Of need for daily home fluoride to prevent caries

• To use sugarless gum, frequent sips of water, or saliva substitutes

pimozide

(pi′moe-zide)

Orap

Drug class.: Antipsychotic, antidyskinetic

Action: Blocks dopamine effects in the CNS

Uses: Motor and phonic tics in Gilles de la Tourette's syndrome; unapproved use: psychotic disorders

Dosage and routes:

• *Adult and child >12 yr:* PO 1-2 mg qd in divided doses, usual dose 10 mg/day

Available forms include: Tabs 2 mg

🍁 Tabs 4 mg

Side effects/adverse reactions:

▼ *ORAL: Dry mouth,* thirst, altered taste

CNS: Extrapyramidal symptoms: pseudoparkinsonism, akathisia, dystonia, tardive dyskinesia, drowsiness, headache, neuroleptic malignant syndrome, seizures, lethargy, sedation, muscle tightness

CV: Orthostatic hypotension, ***cardiac arrest, tachycardia,*** hypertension, ECG changes

GI: Nausea, vomiting, anorexia, constipation, diarrhea, jaundice, weight gain

GU: Urinary retention, urinary frequency, enuresis, impotence, amenorrhea, gynecomastia

EENT: Blurred vision, cataracts

INTEG: Rash, photosensitivity, dermatitis, hyperpyrexia

Contraindications: Hypersensitivity, CNS depression/coma, parkinsonism, liver disease, blood dyscrasias, renal disease, tics other than syndrome, cardiac dysrhythmias, macrolide antiinfectives, itraconazole

Precautions: Child <12 yr, pregnancy category C, lactation, hypertension, hepatic disease, cardiac disease, renal disease, breast cancer, hypokalemia

Pharmacokinetics:

PO: Onset erratic, peak 6-8 hr, half-life 50-55 hr; metabolized by liver; excreted in urine, feces

Drug interactions of concern to dentistry:

• Increased CNS depression: alcohol, CNS depressants

• Increased effects of both drugs: phenothiazines

• Increased effects of anticholinergic drugs

• Prolonged QT interval, fatal cardiac arrhythmia, contraindicated: clarithromycin, erythromycin, azithromycin, dirithromycin, itraconazole

DENTAL CONSIDERATIONS

General:

• Assess salivary flow as a factor in caries, periodontal disease, and candidiasis.

• Monitor vital signs every appointment due to cardiovascular side effects.

• Assess for presence of extrapyramidal motor symptoms, such as tardive dyskinesia and akathisia. Extrapyramidal motor activity may complicate dental treatment.

• After supine positioning, have patient sit upright for at least 2 min to avoid orthostatic hypotension.

• Consider action of drug in assessment of altered taste.

Consultations:

• Medical consult may be required to assess disease control in the patient.

P

• If signs of tardive dyskinesia or akathisia are present, refer to physician.

Teach patient/family:

• Importance of good oral hygiene to prevent soft tissue inflammation
• Caution to prevent injury when using oral hygiene aids

When chronic dry mouth occurs, advise patient:

• To avoid mouth rinses with high alcohol content due to drying effects
• Of need for daily home fluoride to prevent caries
• To use sugarless gum, frequent sips of water, or saliva substitutes

---

pindolol

(pin′doe-lole)

Visken

✤ Syn-Pindolol, Novo-Pindol

Drug class.: Nonselective β-adrenergic blocker

Action: This is a nonselective β_1- and β_2-adrenergic antagonist. The antihypertensive mechanism of action is unclear, but it may include a reduction in cardiac output and inhibition of renin release by the renal juxtaglomerular apparatus. Peripheral resistance decreases with long-term use. The antianginal action (when indicated for this use) may be related to a decrease in myocardial oxygen demand and negative chronotropic and inotropic effects. The antiarrhythmic action (when indicated for this use) has been related to a reduction in spontaneous pacemaker firing and slowing of AV nodal conduction.

Uses: Mild-to-moderate hypertension

Dosage and routes:

• *Adult:* PO 5 mg bid, usual dose 15 mg/day (5 mg tid); may increase by 10 mg/day q3-4wk to a max of 60 mg/day

Available forms include: Tabs 5, 10 mg

Side effects/adverse reactions:

▼ *ORAL:* Dry mouth, taste changes

CNS: Insomnia, dizziness, hallucinations, anxiety, fatigue

CV: ***CHF, AV block,*** edema, chest pain, palpitation, claudication, tachycardia, ***cardiac arrest,*** hypertension, syncope

GI: Nausea, abdominal pain, ***mesenteric arterial thrombosis, ischemic colitis,*** vomiting, diarrhea

RESP: Dyspnea, ***bronchospasm,*** cough, rales

HEMA: ***Agranulocytosis, thrombocytopenia, purpura***

GU: Impotence, pollakiuria

EENT: Visual changes, double vision, sore throat, dry burning eyes

INTEG: Rash, alopecia, pruritus, fever

MISC: Joint pain, muscle pain, hypoglycemia

Contraindications: Hypersensitivity to β-blockers, cardiogenic shock, heart block (second or third degree), sinus bradycardia, CHF, cardiac failure, bronchial asthma, lactation

Precautions: Major surgery, pregnancy category B, diabetes mellitus, renal disease, thyroid disease, COPD, well-compensated heart failure, CAD, nonallergic bronchospasm, impaired hepatic function, children

Pharmacokinetics:

PO: Peak 1-2 hr, half-life 3-4 hr; 60%-65% is metabolized by liver;

excreted 35%-50% unchanged; excreted in breast milk

Drug interactions of concern to dentistry:

- Increased hypotension, bradycardia: anticholinergics, hydrocarbon inhalation anesthetics, fentanyl derivatives
- Decreased antihypertensive effects: indomethacin, sympathomimetics
- Increased effect of both drugs: phenothiazines, xanthines
- Decreased bronchodilation: theophyllines
- Hypertension, bradycardia: epinephrine, ephedrine
- Slow metabolism of drug: lidocaine

DENTAL CONSIDERATIONS

General:

- Monitor vital signs every appointment due to cardiovascular side effects.
- Patients on chronic drug therapy may rarely have symptoms of blood dyscrasias, which can include infection, bleeding, and poor healing.
- Stress from dental procedures may compromise cardiovascular function; determine patient risk.
- Use vasoconstrictors with caution, in low doses, and with careful aspiration. Avoid use of gingival retraction cord with epinephrine.
- Consider semisupine chair position for patient comfort if GI side effects occur.
- Assess salivary flow as a factor in caries, periodontal disease, and candidiasis.
- Consider drug effects if taste alteration occurs.

Consultations:

- In a patient with symptoms of blood dyscrasias, request a medical consult for blood studies and postpone dental treatment until normal values are reestablished.
- Medical consult may be required to assess disease control and patient's ability to tolerate stress.

Teach patient/family:

- Need for good oral hygiene to prevent soft tissue inflammation
- Caution to prevent injury when using oral hygiene aids

When chronic dry mouth occurs, advise patient:

- To avoid mouth rinses with high alcohol content due to drying effects
- Of need for daily home fluoride to prevent caries
- To use sugarless gum, frequent sips of water, or saliva substitutes

pioglitazone

(pi-oh-glit′a-zone)

Actos

Drug class.: Antidiabetic, oral

Note: This drug was marketed in late 1999 and limited information was available at publication time.

Action: An agonist for peroxisome proliferator-activated receptor gamma (PPAR-γ); improves target cell response to insulin without increasing insulin secretion; insulin must be present for this drug to act

Uses: Monotherapy, as an adjunct to diet and exercise in patients with type 2 diabetes mellitus; may also be used with metformin when metformin, diet, and exercise are not adequate for control

Dosage and routes:

- *Adult:* PO 15-45 mg qd

Available forms include: Tabs 15, 30, 45 mg

Side effects/adverse reactions:
CNS: Paresthesias
CV: Edema
GI: Abdominal pain
HEMA: Anemia
ENDO: Hypoglycemia, ↑LDL cholesterol, ↑CPK
MISC: Weight gain

Contraindications: Hypersensitivity or hypersensitivity to other glitazone oral antidiabetics

Precautions: Hepatic dysfunction, renal impairment (?), pregnancy, lactation, children

Pharmacokinetics:
PO: Data lacking; some metabolism by cytochrome P-450 3A4 enzymes; highly plasma protein bound (98%), hepatic metabolism, some renal excretion

Drug interactions of concern to dentistry:
- None reported

DENTAL CONSIDERATIONS
General:
- Ensure that patient is following prescribed diet and regularly takes medication.
- Place on frequent recall to evaluate healing response.
- Short appointments and a stress reduction protocol may be required for anxious patients.
- Diabetics may be more susceptible to infection and have delayed wound healing.
- Question patient about self-monitoring of drug's antidiabetic effect, including blood glucose values or finger-stick records.
- Consider semisupine chair position for patient comfort if GI side effects occur.

Consultations:
- Medical consult may be required to assess disease control and patient's ability to tolerate stress.
- Medical consult may include data from patient's blood glucose monitoring, including glycosylated hemoglobin or HbA_{1c} testing.

Teach patient/family:
- To prevent trauma when using oral hygiene aids
- Importance of updating health and drug history if physician makes any changes in evaluation/drug regimens

pirbuterol acetate

(perr-byoo′ter-ole)
Maxair

Drug class.: Bronchodilator

Action: Causes bronchodilation with little effect on heart rate by acting on β-receptors, causing increased cAMP and relaxation of smooth muscle

Uses: Reversible bronchospasm (prevention, treatment), including asthma; may be given with theophylline or steroids

Dosage and routes:
- *Adult and child >12 yr:* Aerosol 1-2 inh (0.4 mg) q4-6h; do not exceed 12 inh/day

Available forms include: Aerosol delivers 0.2 mg pirbuterol/actuation

Side effects/adverse reactions:
▼ *ORAL:* Taste changes, dry mouth
CNS: Tremors, anxiety, insomnia, headache, dizziness, stimulation, restlessness, hallucinations, drowsiness, irritability
CV: Palpitation, tachycardia, hypertension, angina, hypotension, dysrhythmias
GI: Heartburn, nausea, vomiting, anorexia

RESP: ***Bronchospasm,*** dyspnea, coughing
EENT: Dry nose, irritation of nose/throat
MS: Muscle cramps
Contraindications: Hypersensitivity to sympathomimetics, tachycardia
Precautions: Lactation, pregnancy category C, cardiac disorders, hyperthyroidism, diabetes mellitus, prostatic hypertrophy
Pharmacokinetics:
INH: Onset 3 min, peak 0.5-1 hr, duration 5 hr

DENTAL CONSIDERATIONS
General:
- Acute asthmatic episodes may be precipitated in the dental office. Sympathomimetic inhalants should be available for emergency use.
- Be aware that aspirin or sulfite preservatives in vasoconstrictor-containing products can exacerbate asthma.
- Monitor vital signs every appointment due to cardiovascular and respiratory side effects.
- Assess salivary flow as a factor in caries, periodontal disease, and candidiasis.
- Consider semisupine chair position for patients with respiratory disease.
- Short appointments and a stress reduction protocol may be required for anxious patients.

Consultations:
- Medical consult may be required to assess disease control and patient's ability to tolerate stress.

Teach patient/family:
- For inhalation dosage forms: rinse mouth with water after each dose to prevent dryness

When chronic dry mouth occurs, advise patient:
- To avoid mouth rinses with high alcohol content due to drying effects
- Of need for daily home fluoride to prevent caries
- To use sugarless gum, frequent sips of water, or saliva substitutes

---

piroxicam

(peer-ox'i-kam)
Feldene
✦ Apo-Piroxicam, Novo-Pirocam, Nu-Pirox, PMS-Piroxicam
Drug class.: Nonsteroidal antiinflammatory

Action: Inhibits prostaglandin synthesis by interfering with cyclooxygenase needed for biosynthesis; possesses analgesic, antiinflammatory, antipyretic properties
Uses: Osteoarthritis, rheumatoid arthritis; unapproved use: gouty arthritis
Dosage and routes:
- *Adult:* PO 20 mg qd or 10 mg bid

Available forms include: Caps 10, 20 mg
✦ Suppositories 10, 20 mg
Side effects/adverse reactions:
▼ *ORAL:* Stomatitis, bleeding, dry mouth, lichenoid reaction
CNS: Dizziness, drowsiness, headache, insomnia, depression, malaise, somnolence, nervousness, vertigo
CV: Peripheral edema
GI: Nausea, anorexia, vomiting, diarrhea, ***cholestatic hepatitis,*** jaundice, constipation, flatulence, cramps, peptic ulcer, epigastric distress, bleeding
HEMA: ***Blood dyscrasias***

P

GU: ***Nephrotoxicity: hematuria, oliguria, azotemia***
EENT: Tinnitus, hearing loss, blurred vision
INTEG: Purpura, rash, pruritus, sweating, photosensitivity, pemphigus-like reaction
META: Elevated ALT/AST, hypoglycemia
Contraindications: Hypersensitivity, asthma, severe renal disease, severe hepatic disease, ritonavir
Precautions: Pregnancy category C, lactation, children, bleeding disorders, GI disorders, cardiac disorders, hypersensitivity to other antiinflammatory agents, hypertension
Pharmacokinetics:
PO: Peak 2 hr, half-life 3-3.5 hr; 99% protein binding; metabolized in liver; excreted in urine (metabolites), breast milk

Drug interactions of concern to dentistry:
- GI ulceration, bleeding: aspirin, alcohol, corticosteroids
- Nephrotoxicity: acetaminophen (prolonged use and high doses)
- Possible risk of decreased renal function: cyclosporine
- Decreased action: salicylates

When prescribed for dental pain:
- Risk of increased effects of oral anticoagulants, oral antidiabetics, lithium, methotrexate
- Decreased antihypertensive effects of diuretics, β-adrenergic blockers, ACE inhibitors

DENTAL CONSIDERATIONS
General:
- Patients on chronic drug therapy may rarely have symptoms of blood dyscrasias, which can include infection, bleeding, and poor healing.
- Assess salivary flow as a factor in caries, periodontal disease, and candidiasis.
- Avoid prescribing for dental use during pregnancy.
- Minimize use of aspirin-containing products.
- Consider semisupine chair position for patients with arthritic disease or if GI side effects occur.

Consultations:
- In a patient with symptoms of blood dyscrasias, request a medical consult for blood studies and postpone dental treatment until normal values are reestablished.
- Medical consult may be required to assess disease control in the patient.

Teach patient/family:
- Importance of good oral hygiene to prevent soft tissue inflammation
- Caution to prevent injury when using oral hygiene aids
- To report oral lesions, soreness, or bleeding to dentist

When chronic dry mouth occurs, advise patient:
- To avoid mouth rinses with high alcohol content due to drying effects
- Of need for daily home fluoride to prevent caries
- To use sugarless gum, frequent sips of water, or saliva substitutes

---

polymyxin B sulfate (ophthalmic)

(pol-i-mix'in)
Aerosporin
Drug class.: Antiinfective (ophthalmic)

Action: Inhibits cell wall permeability in susceptible organism

Uses: Superficial external ocular infections

Dosage and routes:

• *Adult and child:* Instill 1-2 gtt of 0.1%-0.25% sol bid-qid × 7-10 days

Available forms include: Powder for sol 500,000 U

Side effects/adverse reactions:

EENT: Poor corneal wound healing, temporary visual haze, overgrowth of nonsusceptible organisms, photosensitivity

Contraindications: Hypersensitivity; viral, mycobacterial, or fungal ocular infection

Precautions: Antibiotic hypersensitivity, pregnancy category B

DENTAL CONSIDERATIONS

General:

• Avoid dental light in patient's eyes; offer dark glasses for patient comfort and safety during dental treatment.

polythiazide

(pol-i-thye'azide)

Renese

Drug class.: Thiazide diuretic

Action: Acts on distal tubule by increasing excretion of water, sodium, chloride, potassium

Uses: Edema, hypertension, diuresis

Dosage and routes:

• *Adult:* PO 1-4 mg/day

Available forms include: Tabs 1, 2, 4 mg

Side effects/adverse reactions:

▼ *ORAL:* Dry mouth, increased thirst, bitter taste, lichenoid reaction

CNS: Drowsiness, paresthesia, anxiety, depression, headache, dizziness, fatigue, weakness, restlessness, syncope

CV: Irregular pulse, orthostatic hypotension, palpitation, volume depletion, dehydration

GI: Nausea, vomiting, anorexia, constipation, diarrhea, cramps, pancreatitis, GI irritation, hepatitis

HEMA: ***Aplastic anemia, hemolytic anemia, leukopenia, agranulocytosis, thrombocytopenia,*** neutropenia

GU: Frequency, polyuria, uremia, glucosuria, impotence, reduced libido

EENT: Blurred vision

INTEG: Rash, urticaria, purpura, photosensitivity, fever

META: Hyperglycemia, hyperuricemia, increased creatinine, BUN

ELECT: Hypokalemia, hypercalcemia, hyponatremia, hypochloremia

Contraindications: Hypersensitivity to thiazides or sulfonamides, anuria, renal decompensation, pregnancy category D

Precautions: Hypokalemia, renal disease, hepatic disease, gout, COPD, lupus erythematosus, diabetes mellitus

Pharmacokinetics:

PO: Onset 2 hr, peak 6 hr, duration 24-48 hr, half-life 26 hr; excreted unchanged by kidneys; crosses placenta; excreted in breast milk

Drug interactions of concern to dentistry:

• Decreased hypotensive response: indomethacin, NSAIDs, sympathomimetics

• Increased toxicity of nondepolarizing skeletal muscle relaxants

DENTAL CONSIDERATIONS

General:

• Take vital signs every appointment due to cardiovascular side effects.

P

• Patients on chronic drug therapy may rarely have symptoms of blood dyscrasias, which can include infection, bleeding, and poor healing.
• After supine positioning, have patient sit upright for at least 2 min before standing to avoid orthostatic hypotension.
• Assess salivary flow as a factor in caries, periodontal disease, and candidiasis.

Consultations:

• In a patient with symptoms of blood dyscrasias, request a medical consult for blood studies and postpone dental treatment until normal values are reestablished.
• Medical consult may be required to assess disease control in the patient.

Teach patient/family:

• Need for good oral hygiene to prevent periodontal inflammation
• Caution to prevent injury when using oral hygiene aids

When chronic dry mouth occurs, advise patient:

• To avoid mouth rinses with high alcohol content due to drying effects
• Of need for daily home fluoride to prevent caries
• To use sugarless gum, frequent sips of water, or saliva substitutes

potassium bicarbonate/ potassium acetate/ potassium chloride/ potassium gluconate/ potassium phosphate

Potassium bicarbonate effervescent: K^+ Care ET, K-Electrolyte, K-Ide, Klor-Con/EF, K-Lyte, Vesant
Potassium chloride: Cena-K, K^+ 10, Kaochlor, Kaon-Cl, KayCiel, K-Dur, K-Lease, K-Lor, Klor-Con 8, Klor-Con 10, Klotrix, K-Norm, K-Tab, Micro-K, Slow-K, Ten-K
🍁 Apo-K, Kalium, Novolente-K
Potassium gluconate: Glu-K, Kaon, Kayelixir

Drug class.: Potassium electrolyte

Action: Needed for adequate transmission of nerve impulses and cardiac contraction, renal function, intracellular ion maintenance

Uses: Prevention and treatment of hypokalemia

Dosage and routes:

Potassium bicarbonate

• *Adult:* PO dissolve 25-50 mEq in water qd-qid

Potassium acetate—hypokalemia

• *Adult and child:* PO 40-100 mEq/day in divided doses 2-4 days

Hypokalemia (prevention)

• *Adult and child:* PO 20 mEq/day in 2-4 divided doses

Potassium chloride

• *Adult:* PO 40-100 mEq in divided doses tid-qid; IV 20 mEq/hr when diluted as 40 mEq/1000 ml, not to exceed 150 mEq/day

Potassium gluconate

• *Adult:* PO 40-100 mEq in divided doses tid-qid

Potassium phosphate

• *Adult:* IV 1 mEq/hr in sol of 60 mEq/L, not to exceed 150 mEq/

day; PO 40-100 mEq/day in divided doses
Available forms include: Liq 20, 30, 40, 45 mEq per 15 ml; powder 15, 20, 25 mEq per packet; effervescent tabs 20, 25, 50 mEq per tablet; con rel tabs 6.7, 8.0, 10 mEq per tab; ext rel tabs 10, 20 mEq per tab; con rel caps 8, 10 mEq per capsule; IV preps 10 mEq/g, 40 mEq/ml in 10, 20 ml vials
Side effects/adverse reactions:
CNS: Confusion, hyperkalemia
CV: ***Cardiac depression, dysrhythmias, arrest, peaking T waves, lowered R and depressed RST, prolonged P-R interval, widened QRS complex,*** bradycardia
GI: Nausea, vomiting, cramps, pain, diarrhea, ulceration of small bowel
GU: Oliguria
INTEG: Cold extremities, rash
Contraindications: Renal disease (severe), severe hemolytic disease, Addison's disease, hyperkalemia, acute dehydration, extensive tissue breakdown
Precautions: Cardiac disease, potassium-sparing diuretic therapy, systemic acidosis, pregnancy category A, renal impairment
Pharmacokinetics:
PO: Excreted by kidneys and in feces
IV: Immediate onset of action
Drug interactions of concern to dentistry:
• Decreased potassium requirement: corticosteroids
• Increased GI side effects: anticholinergic drugs, NSAIDs
• Increased serum potassium: NSAIDs, cyclosporine
DENTAL CONSIDERATIONS
General:
• Patients taking potassium supplements will normally be taking a diuretic. Compliance with potassium supplements can be a problem. Verify serum potassium levels as required.
• Consider semisupine chair position for patient comfort if GI side effects occur.

povidone iodine

(poe'vi-done)
ACU-dyne, Aerodine, Betadine, Biodine, Efodine, Iodex-P, Mallisol, Minidyne, Polydine
✤ Proviodine
Drug class.: Iodophor disinfectant

Action: Destroys a wide variety of microorganisms by local irritation, germicidal action
Uses: Cleansing wounds, disinfection, preoperative skin preparation removal
Dosage and routes:
• *Adult and child:* Sol use as needed, topical only
Available forms include: Top—a variety of solutions, ointments, aerosols, foams, creams, gels, and pads
Side effects/adverse reactions:
GU: ***Renal damage***
META: Metabolic acidosis
INTEG: Irritation
Contraindications: Hypersensitivity to iodine, pregnancy category D (vaginal antiseptic)
Precautions: Extensive burns
Drug interactions of concern to dentistry:
• Do not use with alcohol or hydrogen peroxide
DENTAL CONSIDERATIONS
General:
• Assess for allergies to seafood; if present, drug should not be used.

P

• Store in tight, light-resistant container.
• Evaluate area of the body involved for irritation, rash, breaks, dryness, and scales.

Teach patient/family:
• To discontinue use if rash, irritation, or redness occurs

pramipexole dihydrochloride

(pra-mi-pex'ole)
Mirapex

Drug class.: Antiparkinson agent

Action: Acts as a dopamine agonist at D_2 receptor sites

Uses: Idiopathic Parkinson's disease

Dosage and routes:
• *Adult:* PO all doses should be titrated gradually beginning with an initial dose of 0.125 mg tid for 5-7 days; doses can be increased by increments each week to a tolerated range of 1.5-4.5 mg/day in 3 divided doses; dose must be reduced in renal impairment

Available forms include: Tabs 0.125, 0.25, 1, 1.5 mg

Side effects/adverse reactions:
▼ *ORAL:* Dry mouth, taste perversion
CNS: Hallucinations, dizziness, somnolence, insomnia, headache, malaise
CV: Postural hypotension, edema
GI: Nausea, constipation, dyspepsia, anorexia
GU: Impotence, urinary frequency
EENT: Vision abnormalities
INTEG: Rash
MS: Extrapyramidal syndrome
MISC: Asthenia, accidental injury

Contraindications: Hypersensitivity

Precautions: Orthostatic hypotension, hallucination risk higher >65 yr, renal insufficiency, caution in driving a car (somnolence), risk of falling asleep while performing daily activities, pregnancy category C, lactation, use not established in children

Pharmacokinetics:
PO: Rapid absorption, peak levels in 2 hr, bioavailability 90%, low plasma protein binding (15%), 90% of dose excreted unchanged in urine

Drug interactions of concern to dentistry:
• Increased CNS depression: all CNS depressants
• Possible decreased effects: dopamine antagonists (phenothiazines, butyrophenones, or thiothanxenes) and metoclopramide

DENTAL CONSIDERATIONS

General:
• Monitor vital signs every appointment due to cardiovascular side effects.
• Assess salivary flow as factor in caries, periodontal disease, and candidiasis.
• Consider semisupine chair position for patient comfort if GI side effects occur.
• After supine positioning, have patient sit upright for at least 2 min to avoid orthostatic hypotension.

Consultations:
• Medical consult may be required to assess disease control and patient's ability to tolerate stress.

Teach patient/family:
• Importance of good oral hygiene to prevent soft tissue inflammation
• Caution to prevent trauma when using oral hygiene aids

• Use of electric toothbrush if patient has difficulty holding conventional devices
• Importance of updating health and drug history if physician makes any changes in evaluation/drug regimens

When chronic dry mouth occurs, advise patient:

• To avoid mouth rinses with high alcohol content due to drying effects
• To use daily home fluoride products for anticaries effect
• To use sugarless gum, frequent sips of water, or saliva substitutes

pravastatin sodium

(pra'va-sta-tin)
Pravachol

Drug class.: Antihyperlipidemic

Action: Inhibits HMG-CoA reductase enzyme, which reduces cholesterol synthesis

Uses: As an adjunct in primary hypercholesterolemia (types IIa, IIb) and mixed dyslipidemia, reduction in apolipoprotein B, prevention of first heart attack, cardiovascular disease, may reduce rate of nonfatal and fatal MI, reduce risk of stroke or TIA in post-MI patient with normal cholesterol levels

Dosage and routes:

• *Adult:* PO 10-20 mg qd at hs (range 10-40 mg qd)

Available forms include: Tabs 10, 20 mg

Side effects/adverse reactions:

CNS: Headache, dizziness, psychic disturbances, fatigue
CV: Chest pain
GI: ***Liver dysfunction, hepatitis,*** pancreatitis, nausea, constipation, diarrhea, dyspepsia, flatus, abdominal pain, heartburn, vomiting
GU: Gynecomastia, libido loss
EENT: Lens opacities, common cold, rhinitis, cough, cataracts
INTEG: Rash, pruritus
MS: ***Myositis, rhabdomyolysis,*** muscle cramps, myalgia
MISC: Alopecia, edema

Contraindications: Hypersensitivity, pregnancy category X, lactation, active liver disease

Precautions: Past liver disease, alcoholics, severe acute infections, trauma, hypotension, uncontrolled seizure disorders, severe metabolic disorders, electrolyte imbalances

Pharmacokinetics:

PO: Peak 1-1.5 hr; highly protein bound; metabolized by liver; excreted in urine, feces, breast milk; crosses placenta

Drug interactions of concern to dentistry:

• Increased risk of myopathy or rhabdomyolysis: erythromycin, itraconazole

DENTAL CONSIDERATIONS

General:

• Monitor vital signs every appointment due to possible cardiovascular disease.
• Consider semisupine chair position for patient comfort if GI side effects occur.

prazosin HCl

(pra'zoe-sin)
Minipress

Drug class.: Antihypertensive, α-adrenergic antagonist

Action: Reduction in blood pressure results from blockage of α-adrenergic receptors and reduced peripheral resistance

Uses: Hypertension; unapproved use: CHF, urinary retention in prostatic hypertrophy, pheochromocytoma

Dosage and routes:

• *Adult:* PO 1 mg bid or tid, increasing to 20 mg qd in divided doses if required; usual range 6-15 mg/day, not to exceed 1 mg initially

Available forms include: Caps 1, 2, 5 mg

🍁 Tabs 1, 2, 5 mg

Side effects/adverse reactions:

▼ *ORAL:* Dry mouth, lichenoid drug reaction

CNS: Dizziness, headache, drowsiness, anxiety, depression, vertigo, weakness, fatigue, light-headedness, lethargy, syncope

CV: Palpitation, orthostatic hypotension, tachycardia, edema, dyspnea, angina

GI: Nausea, vomiting, diarrhea, constipation, abdominal pain

GU: Urinary frequency, incontinence, impotence, priapism

EENT: Blurred vision, epistaxis, tinnitus, red sclera

Contraindications: Hypersensitivity, severe CHF

Precautions: Pregnancy category C, children

Pharmacokinetics:

PO: Onset 2 hr, peak 1-3 hr, duration 6-12 hr, half-life 2-4 hr; metabolized in liver; excreted via bile, feces (>90%), in urine (<10%)

Drug interactions of concern to dentistry:

• Increased effects: epinephrine

• Decreased effect: indomethacin, NSAIDs

DENTAL CONSIDERATIONS

General:

• Monitor vital signs every appointment due to cardiovascular side effects.

• After supine positioning, have patient sit upright for at least 2 min before standing to avoid orthostatic hypotension.

• Assess salivary flow as a factor in caries, periodontal disease, and candidiasis.

• Limit use of sodium-containing products, such as saline IV fluids, for patients with a dietary salt restriction.

• Stress from dental procedures may compromise cardiovascular function; determine patient risk.

• Short appointments and a stress reduction protocol may be required for anxious patients.

Consultations:

• Medical consult may be required to assess disease control in the patient.

Teach patient/family:

When chronic dry mouth occurs, advise patient:

• To avoid mouth rinses with high alcohol content due to drying effects

• Of need for daily home fluoride to prevent caries

• To use sugarless gum, frequent sips of water, or saliva substitutes

---

prednicarbate

(pred′ni-kar-bate)

Dermatop Emollient Cream

Drug class.: Topical corticosteroid, group III potency

Action: Glucocorticoids have multiple actions that include antiinflammatory and immunosuppressant effects. They inhibit phospholipase A_2, interfering with or reducing the synthesis of prosta-

glandins and leukotrienes. They also bind to cytoplasmic glucocorticoid receptors (GRs) and enter the cell nucleus to bind with DNA. This results in the synthesis of various enzymes such as collagenase, elastase, and cytokines that play important roles in inflammation and immunosuppression. They also suppress the production of lymphocytes, monocytes, and eosinophils.
Uses: Relief of inflammatory and pruritic manifestations of corticosteroid-responsive dermatoses
Dosage and routes:
• *Adult:* Top apply a thin film to affected area bid
Available forms include: Cream 0.1% in 15, 60 g
Side effects/adverse reactions:
INTEG: ***Skin atrophy,*** pruritus, burning, urticaria, edema, rash
Contraindications: Hypersensitivity
Precautions: Pregnancy category C, lactation, children <18 yr, occlusive dressings; bacterial, viral, or fungal skin infections
Drug interactions of concern to dentistry:
• None reported

DENTAL CONSIDERATIONS
General:
• Determine why the patient is taking the drug.
• Use on oral herpetic ulcerations is contraindicated.

prednisolone/ prednisolone acetate/ prednisolone phosphate/ prednisolone tebutate

(pred-niss'oh-lone)
Prednisolone: Delta-Cortef, Prelone
Prednisolone acetate (not for IV use): Articulose-50, Key-Pred 25 and 50, Pedaject-50, Predalone-50, Predcor-25 and 50, Predicort-50
Prednisolone tebutate: Hydeltra TBA, Nor-Pred TBA, Pedalone TBA, Predcor-TBA, Prednisol TBA
Prednisolone sodium phosphate: Hydeltrasol, Key-Pred-SP, Pediapred, Predate S, Pedicort-RP
Drug class.: Glucocorticoid, immediate acting

Action: Glucocorticoids have multiple actions that include antiinflammatory and immunosuppressant effects. They inhibit phospholipase A_2, interfering with or reducing the synthesis of prostaglandins and leukotrienes. They also bind to cytoplasmic glucocorticoid receptors (GRs) and enter the cell nucleus to bind with DNA. This results in the synthesis of various enzymes such as collagenase, elastase, and cytokines that play important roles in inflammation and immunosuppression. They also suppress the production of lymphocytes, monocytes, and eosinophils.
Uses: Severe inflammation, immunosuppression, neoplasms, adrenal insufficiency
Dosage and routes:
• *Adult:* PO 5-60 mg/day; IM 4-60 mg/day (acetate, phosphate); IV

P

4-60 mg (phosphate); 4-5 mg in small joints, 10-20 mg in large joints (phosphate); 8-20 mg in joint lesion (tebutate); 40 mg intralesional (acetate); 10-30 mg soft tissue (phosphate); syr 15 mg/5 ml

Available forms include: Tabs 5 mg; inj 25, 50 mg/ml (acetate); inj 20 mg/ml (terbutate); inj 20 mg/ml (phosphate); PO liq 5 mg/5 ml

Side effects/adverse reactions:

▼ *ORAL: Candidiasis,* dry mouth, delayed wound healing, petechiae

CNS: Depression, flushing, sweating, headache, mood changes

CV: Hypertension, ***circulatory collapse, thrombophlebitis, embolism,*** tachycardia

GI: Diarrhea, nausea, abdominal distention, ***GI hemorrhage, pancreatitis,*** increased appetite

HEMA: ***Thrombocytopenia***

EENT: Fungal infections, increased intraocular pressure, blurred vision

INTEG: Acne, delayed wound healing, ecchymosis, petechiae, striae

MS: Fractures, osteoporosis, muscle weakness

Contraindications: Psychosis, hypersensitivity, idiopathic thrombocytopenia, acute glomerulonephritis, amebiasis, fungal infections, nonasthmatic bronchial disease, child <2 yr

Precautions: Pregnancy category C, diabetes mellitus, glaucoma, osteoporosis, seizure disorders, ulcerative colitis, CHF, myasthenia gravis, ulcerative GI disease, rifampin

Pharmacokinetics:

PO: Peak 1-2 hr, duration 2 days

IM: Peak 3-45 hr

Drug interactions of concern to dentistry:

- Decreased action: barbiturates, rifampin, rifabutin
- Increased side effects: alcohol, salicylates, NSAIDs
- Increased action: ketoconazole, macrolide antibiotics (erythromycin, clarithromycin, azithromycin)
- Hepatotoxicity: acetaminophen (chronic use, high doses)

DENTAL CONSIDERATIONS

General:

- Take vital signs every appointment due to cardiovascular side effects.
- Patients on chronic drug therapy may rarely have symptoms of blood dyscrasias, which can include infection, bleeding, and poor healing.
- Assess salivary flow as a factor in caries, periodontal disease, and candidiasis.
- Avoid prescribing aspirin-containing products.
- Place on frequent recall to evaluate healing response.
- Prophylactic antibiotics may be indicated to prevent infection if surgery or deep scaling is planned.
- Symptoms of oral infections may be masked.
- Determine dose and duration of steroid therapy for each patient to assess risk for stress tolerance and immunosuppression.
- Patients who have been or are currently on chronic steroid therapy (>2 wk) require supplemental steroids for dental treatment.
- Determine why the patient is taking the drug.

Consultations:

- In a patient with symptoms of blood dyscrasias, request a medical consult for blood studies and postpone dental treatment until normal values are reestablished.
- Medical consult may be required

to assess disease control in the patient.

• Consult may be required to confirm steroid dose and duration of use.

Teach patient/family:

• Importance of good oral hygiene to prevent soft tissue inflammation

• Caution to prevent injury when using oral hygiene aids

When chronic dry mouth occurs, advise patient:

• To avoid mouth rinses with high alcohol content due to drying effects

• Of need for daily home fluoride to prevent caries

• To use sugarless gum, frequent sips of water, or saliva substitutes

---

prednisone

(pred′ni-sone)

Deltasone, Liquid Pred, Meticorten, Orasone, Prednicen-M, Prednisone Intensol, Sterapred

🍁 Apo-Prednisone, Winpred

Drug class.: Glucocorticoid, intermediate acting

Action: Glucocorticoids have multiple actions that include antiinflammatory and immunosuppressant effects. They inhibit phospholipase A_2, interfering with or reducing the synthesis of prostaglandins and leukotrienes. They also bind to cytoplasmic glucocorticoid receptors (GRs) and enter the cell nucleus to bind with DNA. This results in the synthesis of various enzymes such as collagenase, elastase, and cytokines that play important roles in inflammation and immunosuppression. They also suppress the production of lymphocytes, monocytes, and eosinophils.

Uses: Severe inflammation, immunosuppression, neoplasms, multiple sclerosis, collagen disorders, dermatologic disorders

Dosage and routes:

• *Adult:* PO 2.5-15 mg bid-qid, then qd or qod; maintenance up to 250 mg/day

Available forms include: Tabs 1, 2.5, 5, 10, 20, 25, 50 mg; oral sol 5 mg/5 ml; syr 5 mg/5 ml

Side effects/adverse reactions:

▼ *ORAL: Candidiasis,* dry mouth, poor wound healing, petechiae

CNS: Depression, flushing, sweating, headache, mood changes

CV: Hypertension, ***circulatory collapse, thrombophlebitis, embolism,*** tachycardia

GI: Diarrhea, nausea, abdominal distention, ***GI hemorrhage, pancreatitis,*** increased appetite

HEMA: ***Thrombocytopenia***

EENT: Fungal infections, increased intraocular pressure, blurred vision

INTEG: Acne, poor wound healing, ecchymosis, petechiae

MS: Fractures, osteoporosis, weakness

Contraindications: Psychosis, hypersensitivity, idiopathic thrombocytopenia, acute glomerulonephritis, amebiasis, fungal infections, nonasthmatic bronchial disease, child <2 yr, AIDS, TB

Precautions: Pregnancy category C, diabetes mellitus, glaucoma, osteoporosis, seizure disorders, ulcerative colitis, CHF, myasthenia gravis, renal disease, esophagitis, peptic ulcer, rifampin

Pharmacokinetics:

PO: Peak 1-2 hr, duration 1-1.5 days, half-life 3.5-4 hr

P

Drug interactions of concern to dentistry:

- Decreased action: barbiturates, rifampin, rifabutin
- Increased side effects: alcohol, salicylates, NSAIDs
- Increased action: ketoconazole, macrolide antibiotics
- Hepatotoxicity: acetaminophen (chronic, high doses)

DENTAL CONSIDERATIONS

General:

- Monitor vital signs every appointment due to cardiovascular side effects.
- Patients on chronic drug therapy may rarely have symptoms of blood dyscrasias, which can include infection, bleeding, and poor healing.
- Avoid aspirin-containing products.
- Assess salivary flow as a factor in caries, periodontal disease, and candidiasis.
- Symptoms of oral infections may be masked.
- Place on frequent recall to evaluate healing response.
- Prophylactic antibiotics may be indicated to prevent infection if surgery or deep scaling is planned.
- Determine dose and duration of steroid therapy for each patient to assess risk for stress tolerance and immunosuppression.
- Patients who have been or are currently on chronic steroid therapy (>2 wk) may require supplemental steroids for dental treatment.
- Determine why the patient is taking the drug.

Consultations:

- In a patient with symptoms of blood dyscrasias, request a medical consult for blood studies and postpone dental treatment until normal values are reestablished.
- Medical consult may be required to assess disease control in the patient.
- Consult may be required to confirm steroid dose and duration of use.

Teach patient/family:

- Importance of good oral hygiene to prevent soft tissue inflammation
- Caution to prevent injury when using oral hygiene aids

When chronic dry mouth occurs, advise patient:

- To avoid mouth rinses with high alcohol content due to drying effects
- Of need for daily home fluoride to prevent caries
- To use sugarless gum, frequent sips of water, or saliva substitutes

prilocaine hydrochloride (local)

(pry'lo-kane)

Citanest

With vasoconstrictor: Citanest Forte with epinephrine

Drug class.: Amide local anesthetic

Action: Inhibits ion fluxes across membranes, particularly sodium transport across cell membrane; decreases rise of depolarization phase of action potential; blocks nerve action potential

Uses: Local dental anesthesia

Dosage and routes:

Dental injection: infiltration or conduction block

- *Prilocaine 4% without vasoconstrictor:* Max dose of 400 mg over a 2 hr period per dental appointment for healthy adult patient[a]; doses must be adjusted for medically compromised, debilitated, or elderly and for each individual patient. Doses in excess of 400 mg have caused methemoglobinemia. **Always use the lowest effective dose, a slow injection rate, and a careful aspiration technique.**

Example calculations illustrating amount of drug administered per dental cartridge(s)

# of dental cartridges (1.8 ml)	mg of prilocaine (4%)
1	72
2	144
3	216
4	288

[a]Max dose cited from *USP-DI,* ed 16, 1996, US Pharmacopeial Convention, Inc, as well as manufacturer package insert. Doses may differ in other published reference resources.

• *Prilocaine 4% with epinephrine 1:200,000:* Recommended doses are the same; adjust doses for each individual as previously indicated

Example calculations illustrating amount of drug administered per dental cartridge(s)

# of cartridges (1.8 ml)	mg of prilocaine (4%)	mg (μg) vasoconstrictor (1:200,000)
1	72	0.009 (9)
2	144	0.018 (18)
4	288 mg	0.036 mg (36)

Available forms include: 4% sol, 4% sol with epinephrine 1:200,000

Side effects/adverse reactions:
▼ *ORAL: Numbness, tingling,* trismus
CNS: ***Convulsions, loss of consciousness,*** drowsiness, disorientation, tremors, shivering, anxiety, restlessness
CV: ***Myocardial depression, cardiac arrest, dysrhythmias,*** bradycardia, hypotension, hypertension
GI: Nausea, vomiting
RESP: ***Status asthmaticus, respiratory arrest, anaphylaxis***
HEMA: ***Methemoglobinemia***
INTEG: Rash, urticaria, allergic reactions

Contraindications: Hypersensitivity, cross-sensitivity among amides (rare), severe liver disease

Precautions: Elderly, pregnancy category B, large doses of local anesthetic in myasthenia gravis, risk of methemoglobinemia

Pharmacokinetics:
INJ: Onset 2-10 min, duration 2-4 hr; metabolized in liver; excreted in urine

Drug interactions of concern to dentistry:

• CNS depressants: increased risk of CNS depression with all CNS depressants, especially in children and when larger doses are used

• Avoid placing dental cartridges in disinfection solutions with heavy metals or surface-active agents; may see release of ions into local anesthetic solutions with tissue irritation following injection

• Avoid excessive exposure of dental cartridges to light or heat; hastens deterioration of vasoconstrictor; observe for color change in local anesthetic solution

• Risk of cardiovascular side effects; rapid intravascular administration of local anesthetic contain-

P

ing vasoconstrictor, either alone or in patients taking tricyclic antidepressants, MAO inhibitors, digitalis drugs, cocaine, phenothiazines, β-blockers, and in the presence of halogenated-hydrocarbon general anesthetics; use smallest effective vasoconstrictor dose and careful aspiration technique
• Avoid use of vasoconstrictors in patients with uncontrolled hyperthyroidism, diabetes, angina, or hypertension; refer these patients for medical treatment before elective dental treatment

DENTAL CONSIDERATIONS

General:
• Monitor vital signs every appointment due to cardiovascular side effects.
• Often used with vasoconstrictor for increased duration of action.
• Lubricate dry lips before injection or dental treatment as required.

Teach patient/family:
• To use care to prevent injury while numbness exists and to not chew gum or eat following dental anesthesia
• To report any signs of infection, muscle pain, or fever to dentist when feeling returns
• To report any unusual soft tissue reactions

primaquine phosphate

(prim'a-kween)

generic

Drug class.: Antiprotozoal

Action: Action is unknown; thought to destroy exoerythrocytic forms by gametocidal action

Uses: Malaria caused by *P. vivax;* unapproved use: with clindamycin in the treatment of *P. carinii* in AIDS

Dosage and routes:
• *Adult:* PO 15 mg base qd × 2 wk
• *Child:* PO 0.9 mg/kg base daily × 2 wk

Available forms include: Tabs 26.3 mg (equivalent to 15 mg base)

Side effects/adverse reactions:
CNS: Headache
CV: Hypertension
GI: Nausea, vomiting, anorexia, cramps
HEMA: ***Agranulocytosis, granulocytopenia, leukopenia, hemolytic anemia, leukocytosis,*** mild anemia, ***methemoglobinemia***
EENT: Blurred vision, difficulty focusing
INTEG: Pruritus, skin eruptions

Contraindications: Hypersensitivity, anemia, lupus erythematosus, methemoglobinemia, porphyria, rheumatoid arthritis, methemoglobin reductase deficiency, G6PD deficiency

Precautions: Pregnancy category C

Pharmacokinetics:
PO: Half-life 3.7-9.6 hr; metabolized by liver (metabolites)

Drug interactions of concern to dentistry:
• None

DENTAL CONSIDERATIONS

General:
• Patients on chronic drug therapy may rarely have symptoms of blood dyscrasias, which can include infection, bleeding, and poor healing.
• Avoid dental light in patient's eyes; offer dark glasses for patient comfort.

Consultations:
• In a patient with symptoms of

blood dyscrasias, request a medical consult for blood studies and postpone dental treatment until normal values are reestablished.

Teach patient/family:

• Importance of good oral hygiene to prevent soft tissue inflammation

• Caution to prevent injury when using oral hygiene aids

---

primidone

(pri'mi-done)

Myidone, Mysoline

✱ APO-Primidone, PMS-Primidone, Sertan

Drug class.: Anticonvulsant, barbiturate derivative

Action: Raises seizure threshold by unknown mechanism; may be related to facilitation of GABA; metabolized to phenobarbital

Uses: Generalized tonic-clonic (grand mal), complex-partial psychomotor seizures

Dosage and routes:

• *Adult and child >8 yr:* PO 250 mg/day; may increase by 250 mg/wk, not to exceed 2 g/day in divided doses qid

• *Child <8 yr:* PO 125 mg/day; may increase by 125 mg/wk, not to exceed 1 g/day in divided doses qid

Available forms include: Tabs 50, 250 mg; susp 250 mg/5 ml

Side effects/adverse reactions:

CNS: Stimulation, drowsiness, dizziness, confusion, sedation, headache, flushing, hallucinations, coma, psychosis, ataxia, vertigo

GI: Nausea, vomiting, anorexia

HEMA: ***Thrombocytopenia, leukopenia, neutropenia, eosinophilia, megaloblastic anemia,*** reduces serum folate level, lymphadenopathy

GU: Impotence, polyuria

EENT: Diplopia, nystagmus, edema of eyelids

INTEG: Rash, edema, alopecia, lupus-like syndrome

Contraindications: Hypersensitivity, porphyria, pregnancy category D

Precautions: COPD, hepatic disease, renal disease, hyperactive children

Pharmacokinetics:

PO: Peak 4 hr, half-life 3-24 hr; excreted by kidneys, in breast milk

Drug interactions of concern to dentistry:

• Increased CNS depression: alcohol, other CNS depressants

• Increased metabolism/hepatotoxicity: halothane, halogenated-hydrocarbon inhalation anesthetics

• Increased seizure threshold: haloperidol, phenothiazines

• Decreased effects of acetaminophen, corticosteroids, doxycycline, fenoprofen

DENTAL CONSIDERATIONS

General:

• Ask about type of epilepsy, seizure frequency, and quality of seizure control.

• After supine positioning, have patient sit upright for at least 2 min before standing to avoid orthostatic hypotension.

• Patients on chronic drug therapy may rarely have symptoms of blood dyscrasias, which can include infection, bleeding, and poor healing.

• Short appointments and a stress reduction protocol may be required for anxious patients.

Consultations:

• Medical consult may be required to assess disease control and patient's ability to tolerate stress.

P

• In a patient with symptoms of blood dyscrasias, request a medical consult for blood studies and postpone dental treatment until normal values are reestablished.

Teach patient/family:

• Importance of good oral hygiene to prevent soft tissue inflammation

• Caution to prevent injury when using oral hygiene aids

• To avoid mouth rinses with high alcohol content due to drying effects

probenecid

(proe-ben′e-sid)

Benemid, Probalan

🍁 Benuryl

Drug class.: Uricosuric

Action: Inhibits tubular reabsorption of urates, with increased excretion of uric acids

Uses: Hyperuricemia in gout, gouty arthritis, adjunct to cephalosporin or penicillin treatment by reducing excretion and maintaining high blood levels

Dosage and routes:

Gout/gouty arthritis

• *Adult:* PO 250 mg bid for 1 wk, then 500 mg bid, not to exceed 2 g/day; maintenance 500 mg/day for 6 mo

Adjunct in penicillin/cephalosporin treatment

• *Adult and child >50 kg:* PO 500 mg qid with antibiotic

• *Child <50 kg:* PO 25 mg/kg, then 40 mg/kg in divided doses qid

Available forms include: Tabs 500 mg

Side effects/adverse reactions:

▼ *ORAL:* Painful gingivae, increased thirst

CNS: Drowsiness, headache

CV: Bradycardia

GI: Gastric irritation, nausea, vomiting, anorexia, ***hepatic necrosis***

RESP: ***Apnea,*** irregular respirations

GU: ***Nephrotic syndrome,*** glycosuria, frequency

INTEG: Rash, dermatitis, pruritus, fever

META: Acidosis, hypokalemia, hyperchloremia, hyperglycemia

Contraindications: Hypersensitivity, severe hepatic disease, blood dyscrasias, severe renal disease, CrCl <50 mg/min, history of uric acid calculus, ketorolac

Precautions: Pregnancy category B, severe respiratory disease, lactation, cardiac edema, child <2 yr

Pharmacokinetics:

PO: Peak 2-4 hr, duration 8 hr, half-life 8-10 hr; metabolized by liver; excreted in urine; crosses placenta

Drug interactions of concern to dentistry:

• Increased toxicity: dapsone, indomethacin, other NSAIDs, acyclovir

• Increased sedation: benzodiazepines

• Decreased action: alcohol, salicylates

• Increased duration of action: penicillins, cephalosporins

• Contraindicated: ketorolac

DENTAL CONSIDERATIONS

General:

• Avoid prescribing aspirin-containing products.

Teach patient/family:

• Importance of good oral hygiene to prevent soft tissue inflammation

• Caution to prevent injury when using oral hygiene aids

• To avoid mouth rinses with high alcohol content due to drying effects

procainamide HCl

(proe-kane-a'mide)

Procan SR, Procanbid, Promine, Pronestyl, Pronestyl SR

Drug class.: Antidysrhythmic (Class IA)

Action: Depresses excitability of cardiac muscle to electrical stimulation and slows conduction in atrium, bundle of His, and ventricle

Uses: PVCs, atrial fibrillation, PAT, atrial dysrhythmias, ventricular tachycardia

Dosage and routes:

Atrial fibrillation/PAT

• *Adult:* PO 1-1.25 g, may give another 750 mg if needed; if no response then 500 mg-1 g q2h until desired response; maintenance 50 mg/kg in divided doses q6h

Ventricular tachycardia

• *Adult:* PO 1 g; maintenance 50 mg/kg/day given in 3 hr intervals; sus rel tabs 500 mg-1.25 g q6h

Other dysrhythmias

• *Adult:* IV bol 100 mg q5min, given 25-50 mg/min, not to exceed 500 mg; then IV inf 2-6 mg/min

Available forms include: Caps 250, 375, 500 mg; tabs 250, 375, 500 mg; sus rel tabs 250, 500, 750, 1000 mg; inj IV 100, 500 mg/ml

Side effects/adverse reactions:

▼ *ORAL:* Dry mouth

CNS: Headache, dizziness, confusion, psychosis, restlessness, irritability, weakness

CV: Hypotension, ***heart block, cardiovascular collapse, arrest***

GI: Nausea, vomiting, anorexia, diarrhea, hepatomegaly

HEMA: ***Agranulocytosis, thrombocytopenia, neutropenia, hemolytic anemia,*** SLE syndrome

INTEG: Rash, urticaria, edema, swelling, pruritus

Contraindications: Hypersensitivity, myasthenia gravis, severe heart block

Precautions: Pregnancy category C, lactation, children, renal disease, liver disease, CHF, respiratory depression, elderly

Pharmacokinetics:

PO: Peak 1-2 hr, duration 3 hr (8 hr extended)

IM: Peak 10-60 min, duration 3 hr Half-life 3 hr; metabolized in liver to active metabolites; excreted unchanged by kidneys (60%)

Drug interactions of concern to dentistry:

• Decreased effects: barbiturates

• Increased effects of neuromuscular blockers, anticholinergics

DENTAL CONSIDERATIONS

General:

• Monitor vital signs every appointment due to cardiovascular side effects.

• Patients on chronic drug therapy may rarely have symptoms of blood dyscrasias, which can include infection, bleeding, and poor healing.

• After supine positioning, have patient sit upright for at least 2 min before standing to avoid orthostatic hypotension.

• Assess salivary flow as a factor in caries, periodontal disease, and candidiasis.

• Stress from dental procedures may compromise cardiovascular function; determine patient risk.

Consultations:

• In a patient with symptoms of blood dyscrasias, request a medical

P

consult for blood studies and postpone dental treatment until normal values are reestablished.

• Medical consult may be required to assess disease control and patient's ability to tolerate stress.

Teach patient/family:

• Importance of good oral hygiene to prevent soft tissue inflammation

• Caution to prevent injury when using oral hygiene aids

When chronic dry mouth occurs, advise patient:

• To avoid mouth rinses with high alcohol content due to drying effects

• Of need for daily home fluoride to prevent caries

• To use sugarless gum, frequent sips of water, or saliva substitutes

---

procarbazine HCl

(proe-kar'ba-zeen)

Matulane

✤ Natulan

Drug class.: Antineoplastic, miscellaneous

Action: Inhibits DNA, RNA, protein synthesis; has multiple sites of action; a nonvesicant, also inhibits monoamine oxidase enzymes

Uses: Lymphoma, Hodgkin's disease, cancers resistant to other therapy

Dosage and routes:

• *Adult:* PO 2-4 mg/kg/day for first wk; maintain dosage of 4-6 mg/kg/day until platelets and WBC count fall; after recovery: 1-2 mg/kg/day

• *Child:* PO 50 mg/day for 7 days, then 100 mg/m^2 until desired response, leukopenia, or thrombocytopenia occurs; 50 mg/day is maintenance after bone marrow recovery

Available forms include: Caps 50 mg

Side effects/adverse reactions:

▼ *ORAL:* Petechiae, bleeding, dry mouth, stomatitis

CNS: Headache, dizziness, insomnia, hallucinations, confusion, coma, pain, chills, fever, sweating, paresthesia

CV: Orthostatic hypotension, fast or slow heartbeat

GI: Nausea, vomiting, anorexia, diarrhea, constipation

RESP: Cough, pneumonitis

HEMA: ***Thrombocytopenia, anemia, leukopenia, myelosuppression, bleeding tendencies,*** purpura, petechiae, epistaxis

GU: Azospermia, cessation of menses

EENT: Retinal hemorrhage, nystagmus, photophobia, diplopia

INTEG: Rash, pruritus, dermatitis, alopecia, herpes, hyperpigmentation

Contraindications: Hypersensitivity, thrombocytopenia, bone marrow depression

Precautions: Renal disease, hepatic disease, pregnancy category D, radiation therapy

Pharmacokinetics:

PO: Peak levels 1 hr; concentrates in liver, kidney, skin; metabolized in liver, excreted in urine

Drug interactions of concern to dentistry:

• Increased CNS depression: barbiturates, antihistamines, narcotics

• Disulfiram-like reaction: ethyl alcohol

• Hypertension: indirect-acting sympathomimetics

• Increased anticholinergic effect: anticholinergic drugs, antihistamines

• Increased risk of severe toxic

reactions: tricyclic antidepressants, meperidine and other opioids, tyramine-containing foods and other MAO inhibitors; may also include cyclobenzaprine and carbamazepine

DENTAL CONSIDERATIONS

General:

• Patients on chronic drug therapy may rarely have symptoms of blood dyscrasias, which can include infection, bleeding, and poor healing.

• Monitor vital signs every appointment due to cardiovascular side effects.

• Consider semisupine chair position when GI side effects occur.

• Assess salivary flow as a factor in caries, periodontal disease, and candidiasis.

• After supine positioning, have patient sit upright for at least 2 min before standing to avoid orthostatic hypotension.

• Avoid dental light in patient's eyes; offer dark glasses for patient comfort.

• Avoid aspirin-containing products because of bleeding risk.

• Avoid use of gingival retraction cord with epinephrine.

• Patients receiving chemotherapy may require palliative treatment for stomatitis.

Consultations:

• In a patient with symptoms of blood dyscrasias, request a medical consult for blood studies and postpone dental treatment until normal values are reestablished.

• Take precautions if dental surgery is anticipated and sedation or general anesthesia is required; there is risk of hypotensive episode.

Teach patient/family:

• Importance of good oral hygiene to prevent soft tissue inflammation

• Caution to prevent injury when using oral hygiene aids

• To report oral lesions, soreness, or bleeding to dentist

When chronic dry mouth occurs, advise patient:

• To avoid mouth rinses with high alcohol content due to drying effects

• Of need for daily home fluoride to prevent caries

• To use sugarless gum, frequent sips of water, or saliva substitutes

---

prochlorperazine edisylate/ prochlorperazine maleate

(proe-klor-per′a-zeen)

Compazine

🍁 PMS Prochlorperazine, Prorazin, Stemetil

Drug class.: Phenothiazine antipsychotic

Action: Blocks neurotransmission at dopaminergic synapses in the cerebral cortex, hypothalamus, and limbic system; exhibits strong peripheral α-adrenergic, anticholinergic blocking action; mechanism for antipsychotic effects is unclear

Uses: Antipsychotic; for nausea, vomiting

Dosage and routes:

Psychiatry

• *PO:* 5-10 mg tid-qid, increasing dosage every 2-3 days; more severe cases start 10 mg tid-qid; patients may tolerate 100-150 mg/day

Postoperative nausea/vomiting

• *Adult:* IM 5-10 mg 1-2 hr before

anesthesia, may repeat in 30 min; IV 5-10 mg 15-30 min before anesthesia; IV inf 20 mg/L D_5W or NS 15-30 min before anesthesia, not to exceed 40 mg/day

Severe nausea/vomiting

- *Adult:* PO 5-10 mg tid-qid; sus rel 15 mg qd in AM or 10 mg q12h; rec 25 mg/bid; IM 5-10 mg; may repeat q4h, not to exceed 40 mg/day
- *Child 18-39 kg:* PO 2.5 mg tid or 5 mg bid, not to exceed 15 mg/day; IM 0.132 mg/kg
- *Child 14-17 kg:* PO/rec 2.5 mg bid-tid, not to exceed 10 mg/day; IM 0.132 mg/kg
- *Child 9-13 kg:* PO/rec 2.5 mg qd-bid, not to exceed 7.5 mg/day; IM 0.132 mg/kg

Available forms include: Oral syr 5 mg/ml; inj 5 mg/ml; tabs 5, 10, 25 mg; ext rel caps 10, 15, 30 mg; suppos 2.5, 5, 25 mg

Side effects/adverse reactions:

ORAL: Dry mouth, metallic taste, lichenoid reaction

*CNS: Euphoria, **depression, extrapyramidal symptoms,*** restlessness, tremor, dizziness

*CV: **Circulatory failure, tachycardia***

GI: Nausea, vomiting, anorexia, diarrhea, constipation, weight loss, cramps

*RESP: **Respiratory depression***

Contraindications: Hypersensitivity to phenothiazines, coma, seizure, encephalopathy, bone marrow depression

Precautions: Children <2 yr, pregnancy category C, elderly

Pharmacokinetics:

PO: Onset 30-40 min, duration 3-4 hr

SUS REL: Onset 30-40 min, duration 10-12 hr

REC: Onset 60 min, duration 3-4 hr

IM: Onset 10-20 min, duration 12 hr

Metabolized by liver, excreted by kidneys, crosses placenta, excreted in breast milk

Drug interactions of concern to dentistry:

- Increased sedation: other CNS depressants, alcohol, barbiturate anesthetics, opioid analgesics
- Hypotension, tachycardia: epinephrine
- Increased extrapyramidal effects: phenothiazines and related drugs (haloperidol, droperidol), metoclopramide
- Additive photosensitization: tetracyclines
- Increased anticholinergic effects: anticholinergics

DENTAL CONSIDERATIONS

General:

- Monitor vital signs every appointment due to cardiovascular side effects.
- Patients on chronic drug therapy may rarely have symptoms of blood dyscrasias, which can include infection, bleeding, and poor healing.
- After supine positioning, have patient sit upright for at least 2 min before standing to avoid orthostatic hypotension.
- Assess salivary flow as a factor in caries, periodontal disease, and candidiasis.
- Avoid dental light in patient's eyes; offer dark glasses for patient comfort.
- Assess for presence of extrapyramidal motor symptoms, such as tardive dyskinesia and akathisia. Extrapyramidal motor activity may complicate dental treatment.

• Geriatric patients are more susceptible to drug effects; use lower dose.
• Use vasoconstrictors with caution, in low doses, and with careful aspiration.

Consultations:
• In a patient with symptoms of blood dyscrasias, request a medical consult for blood studies and postpone dental treatment until normal values are reestablished.
• Take precautions if dental surgery is anticipated and anesthesia is required.
• If signs of tardive dyskinesia or akathisia are present, refer to physician.

Teach patient/family:
• Importance of good oral hygiene to prevent soft tissue inflammation
• Caution to prevent injury when using oral hygiene aids
• To use electric toothbrush if patient has difficulty holding conventional devices

When chronic dry mouth occurs, advise patient:
• To avoid mouth rinses with high alcohol content due to drying effects
• Of need for daily home fluoride to prevent caries
• To use sugarless gum, frequent sips of water, or saliva substitutes

---

procyclidine HCl

(proe-sye'kli-deen)
Kemadrin
🍁 PMS-Procyclidine, Procyclid

Drug class.: Anticholingergic, antidyskinetic

Action: Blockade of central acetylcholine receptors

Uses: Parkinson symptoms, extrapyramidal symptoms associated with neuroleptic drugs

Dosage and routes:
• *Adult:* PO 2.5 mg tid pc, titrated to patient response up to 5 mg tid

Available forms include: Tabs 2.5, 5 mg; elixir 2.5 mg/5 ml

Side effects/adverse reactions:
▼ *ORAL: Dry mouth,* glossitis
CNS: Confusion, anxiety, restlessness, irritability, delusions, hallucinations, headache, sedation, depression, incoherence, dizziness, light-headedness, memory loss
CV: Palpitation, tachycardia, postural hypotension, bradycardia
GI: Constipation, nausea, vomiting, abdominal distress, paralytic ileus, ***epigastric distress***
GU: Hesitancy, retention
EENT: Blurred vision, photophobia, dilated pupils, difficulty swallowing, mydriasis
INTEG: Rash, urticaria, dermatoses
MS: Weakness, cramping
MISC: Increased temperature, flushing, decreased sweating, hyperthermia, heatstroke, numbness of fingers

Contraindications: Hypersensitivity, narrow-angle glaucoma, myasthenia gravis, GI/GU obstruction, child <3 yr, megacolon, stenosing peptic ulcer

Precautions: Pregnancy category C, elderly, lactation, tachycardia, prostatic hypertrophy, children, kidney or liver disease, drug abuse, hypotension, hypertension, psychiatric patients

Pharmacokinetics:
PO: Onset 30-45 min, duration 4-6 hr

Drug interactions of concern to dentistry:
• Increased anticholinergic effect:

antihistamines, anticholingergics, meperidine
• Increased CNS depression: alcohol, CNS depressants

DENTAL CONSIDERATIONS
General:
• Monitor vital signs every appointment due to cardiovascular side effects.
• Assess salivary flow as a factor in caries, periodontal disease, and candidiasis.
• After supine positioning, have patient sit upright for at least 2 min before standing to avoid orthostatic hypotension.
• Avoid dental light in patient's eyes; offer dark glasses for patient comfort.
• Do not ingest sodium bicarbonate products, such as the air polishing system (Prophy Jet), within 1 hr of taking procyclidine.
• Place on frequent recall due to oral side effects.
Consultations:
• Medical consult may be required to assess disease control in the patient.
• Medical consult may be required to assess patient's ability to tolerate stress.
Teach patient/family:
• Use of electric toothbrush if patient has difficulty holding conventional devices
• Importance of good oral hygiene to prevent soft tissue inflammation
• Caution to prevent injury when using oral hygiene aids
When chronic dry mouth occurs, advise patient:
• To avoid mouth rinses with high alcohol content due to drying effects
• To use daily home fluoride products for anticaries effect
• To use sugarless gum, frequent sips of water, or saliva substitutes

---

promazine HCl

(proe'ma-zeen)
Sparine

Drug class.: Phenothiazine antipsychotic

Action: Blocks neurotransmission at dopaminergic synapses in the cerebral cortex, hypothalamus, and limbic system; exhibits strong peripheral α-adrenergic, anticholinergic blocking action; mechanism for antipsychotic effects is unclear
Uses: Psychotic disorders, schizophrenia, nausea, vomiting, alcohol withdrawal
Dosage and routes:
Psychosis
• *Adult:* PO 10-200 mg q4-6h, max dose 1000 mg/day; IM 50-150 mg, followed in 30 min with additional dose up to a total dose of 300 mg
• *Child >12 yr:* PO 10-25 mg q4-6h
Nausea/vomiting
• *Adult:* PO 25-50 mg q4-6h; IM 50 mg; IV not recommended but may use in concentrations of <25 mg/ml
Available forms include: Tabs 25, 50, 100 mg; inj IV/IM 25, 50 mg/ml
Side effects/adverse reactions:
▼ *ORAL: Dry mouth,* candidiasis, lichenoid reaction
CNS: Extrapyramidal symptoms: pseudoparkinsonism, akathisia, dystonia, tardive dyskinesia, drowsiness, headache, ***seizures***
CV: Orthostatic hypotension, ***car-***

diac arrest, tachycardia, ECG changes

GI: Nausea, vomiting, anorexia, constipation, diarrhea, jaundice, weight gain

RESP: ***Laryngospasm, respiratory depression,*** dyspnea

HEMA: ***Leukopenia, leukocytosis, agranulocytosis,*** anemia

GU: Urinary retention, urinary frequency, enuresis, impotence, amenorrhea, gynecomastia

EENT: Blurred vision, glaucoma, dry eyes

INTEG: Rash, photosensitivity, dermatitis

Contraindications: Hypersensitivity, blood dyscrasias, coma, child <12 yr, brain damage, bone marrow depression, glaucoma

Precautions: Pregnancy category C, lactation, seizure disorders, hypertension, hepatic disease, cardiac disease

Pharmacokinetics:

PO: Onset erratic, peak 2-4 hr

IM: Onset 15 min, peak 1 hr

Duration 4-6 hr; metabolized by liver; excreted in urine; crosses placenta; excreted in breast milk

Drug interactions of concern to dentistry:

- Increased sedation: other CNS depressants, alcohol, barbiturate anesthetics, opioid analgesics
- Hypotension, tachycardia: epinephrine
- Increased extrapyramidal effects: phenothiazines and related drugs (haloperidol, droperidol), metoclopramide
- Additive photosensitization: tetracyclines
- Increased anticholinergic effects: anticholinergics

DENTAL CONSIDERATIONS

General:

- Patients on chronic drug therapy may rarely have symptoms of blood dyscrasias, which can include infection, bleeding, and poor healing.
- After supine positioning, have patient sit upright for at least 2 min before standing to avoid orthostatic hypotension.
- Assess salivary flow as a factor in caries, periodontal disease, and candidiasis.
- Avoid dental light in patient's eyes; offer dark glasses for patient comfort.
- Assess for presence of extrapyramidal motor symptoms, such as tardive dyskinesia and akathisia. Extrapyramidal motor activity may complicate dental treatment.
- Geriatric patients are more susceptible to drug effects; use lower dose.
- Use vasoconstrictors with caution, in low doses, and with careful aspiration.
- Examine for oral manifestation of opportunistic infections.

Consultations:

- In a patient with symptoms of blood dyscrasias, request a medical consult for blood studies and postpone dental treatment until normal values are reestablished.
- Take precautions if dental surgery is anticipated and anesthesia is required.
- If signs of tardive dyskinesia or akathisia are present, refer to physician.
- Physician should be informed if significant xerostomic side effects occur (increased caries, sore tongue, problems eating or swal-

P

lowing, difficulty wearing prosthesis) so a medication change can be considered.

Teach patient/family:

• Importance of good oral hygiene to prevent soft tissue inflammation

• Caution to prevent injury when using oral hygiene aids

• To use electric toothbrush if patient has difficulty holding conventional devices

When chronic dry mouth occurs, advise patient:

• To avoid mouth rinses with high alcohol content due to drying effects

• Of need for daily home fluoride to prevent caries

• To use sugarless gum, frequent sips of water, or saliva substitutes

---

promethazine HCl

(proe-meth'a-zeen)

Phenameth, Phenazine, Phenergan, Phenergan Fortis, Phenergan Plain, Shogan

♣ Anergan, Histanil, Pentazine, Phencen-50, Prorex, V-Gan

Drug class.: Antihistamine, H_1-receptor antagonist

Action: Acts on blood vessels, GI, respiratory system by competing with histamine for H_1-receptor site; decreases allergic response by blocking histamine

Uses: Motion sickness, rhinitis, allergy symptoms, sedation, nausea, preoperative or postoperative sedation

Dosage and routes:

Nausea

• *Adult:* PO/IM 25 mg, may repeat 12.5-25 mg q4-6h; rec 12.5-25 mg q4-6h

• *Child:* PO/IM/rec 0.5 mg/lb q4-6h

Motion sickness

• *Adult:* PO 25 mg bid

• *Child:* PO/IM/rec 12.5-25 mg bid

Allergy/rhinitis

• *Adult:* PO 12.5 mg qid or 25 mg hs

• *Child:* PO 6.25-12.5 mg tid or 25 mg hs

Sedation

• *Adult:* PO/IM 25-50 mg hs

• *Child:* PO/IM/rec 12.5-25 mg hs

Sedation (preoperative/postoperative)

• *Adult:* PO/IM/IV 25-50 mg

• *Child:* PO/IM/IV 12.5-25 mg

Available forms include: Tabs 12.5, 25, 50 mg; syr 6.25, 25 mg/5 ml; supp 12.5, 25, 50 mg; inj 25, 50 mg/ml

Side effects/adverse reactions:

▼ *ORAL:* Dry mouth

CNS: Dizziness, drowsiness, poor coordination, fatigue, anxiety, euphoria, confusion, paresthesia, neuritis

CV: Hypotension, palpitation, tachycardia

GI: Constipation, nausea, vomiting, anorexia, diarrhea

RESP: Increased thick secretions, wheezing, chest tightness

HEMA: ***Thrombocytopenia, agranulocytosis, hemolytic anemia***

GU: Retention, dysuria, frequency

EENT: Blurred vision, dilated pupils, tinnitus, nasal stuffiness, dry nose/throat, photosensitivity

INTEG: Rash, urticaria, photosensitivity

Contraindications: Hypersensitivity to H_1-receptor antagonist, acute asthma attack, lower respiratory tract disease

Precautions: Increased intraocular

pressure, renal disease, cardiac disease, hypertension, bronchial asthma, seizure disorder, stenosed peptic ulcers, hyperthyroidism, prostatic hypertrophy, bladder neck obstruction, pregnancy category C

Pharmacokinetics:

PO: Onset 20 min, duration 4-6 hr; metabolized in liver; excreted by kidneys, GI tract (inactive metabolites)

Drug interactions of concern to dentistry:

- Increased CNS depression: alcohol, all CNS depressants
- Hypotension: general anesthetics
- Increased effect of anticholinergic drugs

DENTAL CONSIDERATIONS

General:

- Determine why the patient is taking the drug.
- Patients on chronic drug therapy may rarely have symptoms of blood dyscrasias, which can include infection, bleeding, and poor healing.
- Monitor vital signs every appointment due to cardiovascular side effects.
- Assess salivary flow as a factor in caries, periodontal disease, and candidiasis.
- Assess vital signs q30min after use as sedative.

Teach patient/family:

When chronic dry mouth occurs, advise patient:

- To avoid mouth rinses with high alcohol content due to drying effects
- Of need for daily home fluoride to prevent caries
- To use sugarless gum, frequent sips of water, or saliva substitutes

propafenone

(proe-pa-fen′one)

Rythmol

Drug class.: Antidysrhythmic (Class IC)

Action: Able to slow conduction velocity; reduces cardiac muscle membrane responsiveness; inhibits automaticity; increases ratio of effective refractory period to action potential duration; β-blocking activity

Uses: Documented life-threatening dysrhythmias; unapproved use: sustained ventricular tachycardia

Dosage and routes:

- *Adult:* PO initial doses 150 mg q8h; allow a 3-4 day interval before increasing dose; 900 mg max daily dose

Available forms include: Tabs 150, 300 mg

Side effects/adverse reactions:

▼ *ORAL:* Dry mouth, altered taste, stomatitis

CNS: ***Seizures,*** headache, dizziness, abnormal dreams, syncope, confusion

CV: ***Sudden death,*** dysrhythmias, palpitation, AV block, intraventricular conduction delay, AV dissociation, CHF, atrial flutter

GI: Nausea, vomiting, ***hepatitis,*** constipation, dyspepsia, cholestasis, abnormal liver function studies

RESP: Dyspnea

HEMA: ***Leukopenia, agranulocytosis, granulocytopenia, thrombocytopenia,*** anemia

EENT: Blurred vision, tinnitus

INTEG: Rash

Contraindications: Second- and third-degree heart block, right bun-

P

dle branch block, cardiogenic shock, hypersensitivity, bradycardia, uncontrolled CHF, sick sinus node syndrome, marked hypotension, bronchospastic disorders

Precautions: CHF, hypokalemia, hyperkalemia, recent MI, nonallergic bronchospasm, pregnancy category C, lactation, children, hepatic or renal disease

Pharmacokinetics: Peak 3-5 hr, half-life 2-10 hr; metabolized in liver; excreted in urine (metabolite)

Drug interactions of concern to dentistry:

- No specific interactions are reported; however, any drug that could affect the cardiac action of propafenone (other local anesthetics, vasoconstrictors, anticholinergics) should be used in the least effective dose

DENTAL CONSIDERATIONS

General:

- Monitor vital signs every appointment due to cardiovascular side effects.
- Patients on chronic drug therapy may rarely have symptoms of blood dyscrasias, which can include infection, bleeding, and poor healing.
- Assess salivary flow as a factor in caries, periodontal disease, and candidiasis.
- Stress from dental procedures may compromise cardiovascular function; determine patient risk.
- Consider semisupine chair position for patients with respiratory distress.

Consultations:

- In a patient with symptoms of blood dyscrasias, request a medical consult for blood studies and postpone dental treatment until normal values are reestablished.
- Medical consult may be required to assess disease control and patient's ability to tolerate stress.

Teach patient/family:

- Importance of good oral hygiene to prevent soft tissue inflammation
- Caution to prevent injury when using oral hygiene aids

When chronic dry mouth occurs, advise patient:

- To avoid mouth rinses with high alcohol content due to drying effects
- Of need for daily home fluoride to prevent caries
- To use sugarless gum, frequent sips of water, or saliva substitutes

---

propantheline bromide

(proe-pan'the-leen)

Pro-Banthine

✦ Propanthel

Drug class.: Anticholinergic

Action: Inhibits muscarinic actions of acetylcholine at postganglionic parasympathetic neuroeffector sites

Uses: Treatment of peptic ulcer disease, irritable bowel syndrome, duodenography, urinary incontinence; unapproved use: reduction in salivary flow

Dosage and routes:

- *Adult:* PO 15 mg tid ac, 30 mg hs
- *Elderly:* PO 7.5 mg tid ac

Antisialagogue

- *Adult:* 7.5-15 mg 45-60 min before dental appointment

Available forms include: Tabs 7.5, 15 mg

Side effects/adverse reactions:

▼ *ORAL: Dry mouth,* absence of taste

CNS: Confusion, stimulation in elderly, headache, insomnia, dizzi-

ness, drowsiness, anxiety, weakness, hallucinations
CV: Palpitation, tachycardia
*GI: Constipation, **paralytic ileus,*** heartburn, nausea, vomiting, dysphagia
GU: Hesitancy, retention, impotence
EENT: Blurred vision, photophobia, mydriasis, cycloplegia, increased ocular tension
INTEG: Urticaria, rash, pruritus, anhidrosis, fever, allergic reactions
Contraindications: Hypersensitivity to anticholinergics, narrow-angle glaucoma, GI obstruction, myasthenia gravis, paralytic ileus, GI atony, toxic megacolon
Precautions: Hyperthyroidism, CAD, dysrhythmias, CHF, ulcerative colitis, hypertension, hiatal hernia, hepatic disease, renal disease, pregnancy category C, urinary retention, prostatic hypertrophy
Pharmacokinetics:
PO: Onset 30-45 min, duration 6 hr; metabolized by liver, GI system; excreted in urine, bile
Drug interactions of concern to dentistry:
• Increased anticholinergic effect: other anticholinergic drugs
• Constipation, urinary retention: opioid analgesics
• Decreased absorption of ketoconazole; take doses 2 hr apart
DENTAL CONSIDERATIONS
General:
• Assess salivary flow as a factor in caries, periodontal disease, and candidiasis.
• Avoid dental light in patient's eyes; offer dark glasses for patient comfort.
• Place on frequent recall due to oral side effects.
• Avoid prescribing aspirin-containing products.
• Consider semisupine chair position for patient comfort due to GI effects of disease.
Consultations:
• Physician should be informed if significant xerostomic side effects occur (increased caries, sore tongue, problems eating or swallowing, difficulty wearing prosthesis) so a medication change can be considered.
Teach patient/family:
When chronic dry mouth occurs, advise patient:
• To avoid mouth rinses with high alcohol content due to drying effects
• Of need for daily home fluoride to prevent caries
• To use sugarless gum, frequent sips of water, or saliva substitutes

---

propofol
(proe-po'fole)
Diprivan
Drug class.: General anesthetic

Action: Produces dose-dependent CNS depression; mechanism of action is unknown
Uses: Induction or maintenance of anesthesia as part of balanced anesthetic technique
Dosage and routes:
Warning: **Propofol should be administered by persons trained in the administration of general anesthesia. Patients must be continuously monitored, and facilities for maintenance of a patent airway, ventilatory support, oxygen supplementation, and circulatory resuscitation must be immediately available. Strict aseptic**

P

technique must be followed in handling propofol.

Induction of general anesthesia

• *Adult <55 yr:* IV 2-2.5 mg/kg, approximately 40 mg q10sec until induction onset

• *Child >3 yr:* IV 2.5-3.5 mg/kg over 20-30 sec

• *Elderly or ASA III or IV patients:* IV: 1-1.5 mg/kg, approximately 20 mg q10sec until induction onset

Maintenance

• *Adult <55 yr:* IV 0.1-0.2 mg/kg/min (6-12 mg/kg/hr)

• *Child >3 yr:* IV 125-300 μg/kg/min (7.5-18 mg/kg/hr)

• *Elderly or ASAIII or IV patients:* IV 0.05-0.1 mg/kg/min (3-6 mg/kg/hr)

Intermittent bolus (maintenance)

• *Adult:* IV increments of 25-50 mg as needed

• *Only general dose information is listed because all doses should be individualized and carefully adjusted for each patient.*

Available forms include: Inj 10 mg/ml in 20 ml amp, 50, 100 ml infusion vials

Side effects/adverse reactions:

▼ *ORAL:* Dry mouth, strange taste

CNS: Movement, headache, jerking, fever, dizziness, shivering, tremor, confusion, somnolence, paresthesia, agitation, abnormal dreams, euphoria, fatigue, dystonia

CV: Bradycardia, hypotension, hypertension, PVC, PAC, tachycardia, abnormal ECG, ST segment depression

GI: Nausea, vomiting, abdominal cramping, swallowing

RESP: ***Apnea, cough, hiccups,*** dyspnea, hypoventilation, sneezing, wheezing, tachypnea, hypoxia

GU: Urine retention, green urine

EENT: Blurred vision, tinnitus, eye pain

INTEG: Flushing, phlebitis, hives, burning/stinging at injection site

MS: Myalgia

META: Hyperlipidemia

MISC: Anaphylaxis

Contraindications: Hypersensitivity

Precautions: Elderly, debilitated, respiratory depression, severe respiratory disorders, cardiac dysrhythmias, pregnancy category B, labor and delivery, lactation, children <3 yr, epilepsy

Pharmacokinetics:

IV: Onset 40 sec, rapid distribution, half-life 1-8 min, terminal elimination half-life 5-10 hr; metabolized in liver by conjugation to inactivate metabolites; 70% excreted in urine

Drug interactions of concern to dentistry:

• Increased CNS depression: alcohol, narcotics, sedative-hypnotics, antipsychotics, skeletal muscle relaxants, inhalational anesthetics

DENTAL CONSIDERATIONS

General:

• Monitor vital signs at regular intervals during recovery after use as anesthetic.

• Have someone drive patient to and from dental office if used for general anesthesia.

• Geriatric patients more susceptible to drug effects; use lower dose.

• Use only with resuscitative equipment available and only by qualified persons trained in anesthesia.

Monitor:

• Injection site: phlebitis, burning/stinging.

• ECG for changes: PVC, PAC, ST segment changes.

• Allergic reactions: hives.

Administer:

• After diluting with D_5W, use only glass containers when mixing; not stable in plastic.

• By injection (IV only).

• Alone; do not mix with other agents before using.

Perform/provide:

• Storage in light-resistant area at room temperature.

• Coughing, turning, deep breathing for postoperative patients.

• Safety measures: siderails, night light, call bell within reach.

Evaluate:

• CNS changes: movement, jerking, tremors, dizziness, LOC, pupil reaction.

• Respiratory dysfunction: respiratory depression, character, rate, rhythm; notify physician if respirations are <10/min.

Treatment of overdose:

• Discontinue drug, artificial ventilation, administer vasopressor agents or anticholinergics.

---

propoxyphene napsylate/ propoxyphene HCl

(proe-pox′i-feen)

Cotanal-65, Darvon, Darvon-N, PP-Cap

Drug class.: Synthetic opioid narcotic analgesic

Controlled Substance Schedule IV

Action: Depresses pain impulse transmission in the CNS by interacting with opioid receptors

Uses: Mild-to-moderate pain

Dosage and routes:

• *Adult:* PO 65 mg q4h prn (HCl); PO 100 mg q4h prn (napsylate)

Available forms include: HCl—tabs 32, 65 mg; napsylate—tabs 100 mg; susp 10 mg/ml

Side effects/adverse reactions:

▼ *ORAL:* Dry mouth

CNS: Drowsiness, dizziness, confusion, headache, sedation, ***convulsions, hyperthermia,*** euphoria

CV: ***Dysrhythmias,*** palpitation, bradycardia, change in BP

GI: Nausea, vomiting, anorexia, constipation, cramps

RESP: ***Respiratory depression***

GU: Increased urinary output, dysuria

EENT: Tinnitus, blurred vision, miosis, diplopia

INTEG: ***Rash,*** urticaria, bruising, flushing, diaphoresis, pruritus

Contraindications: Hypersensitivity to ASA products (some preparations), addiction (narcotic), ritonavir

Precautions: Addictive personality, pregnancy category C, lactation, increased intracranial pressure, MI (acute), severe heart disease, respiratory depression, hepatic disease, renal disease, child <18 yr, alcoholism

Pharmacokinetics:

PO: Onset 15-30 min, peak 2-3 hr, duration 4-6 hr; metabolized by liver; half-life 6-12 hr; excreted by kidneys (as metabolites); equimolar doses of HCl or napsylate provide similar plasma levels

Drug interactions of concern to dentistry:

• Increased effects with other CNS depressants: alcohol, narcotics, sedative-hypnotics, skeletal muscle relaxants

• Contraindication: MAO inhibitors

P

• Increased effects of anticholinergics, antihypertensives, carbamazepine

DENTAL CONSIDERATIONS

General:

• Monitor vital signs due to cardiovascular and respiratory side effects.

• Consider semisupine chair position for patient comfort if GI side effects occur.

• Assess salivary flow as a factor in caries, periodontal disease, and candidiasis.

• Psychologic and physical dependence may occur with chronic administration.

• When combined with nonopioid analgesics (aspirin, NSAIDS, acetaminophen), permits better-quality pain relief.

Teach patient/family:

When chronic dry mouth occurs, advise patient:

• To avoid mouth rinses with high alcohol content due to drying effects

• Of need for daily home fluoride to prevent caries

• To use sugarless gum, frequent sips of water, or artificial saliva substitutes

propranolol HCl

(proe-pran'oh-lole)

Inderal, Inderal LA

🍁 Apo-Propranolol, Detensol, Novo-Pranol, PMS-Propranolol

Drug class.: Nonselective β-adrenergic blocker

Action: This is a nonselective β_1- and β_2-adrenergic antagonist. The antihypertensive mechanism of action is unclear, but it may include a reduction in cardiac output and inhibition of renin release by the renal juxtaglomerular apparatus. Peripheral resistance decreases with long-term use. The antianginal action (when indicated for this use) may be related to a decrease in myocardial oxygen demand and negative chronotropic and inotropic effects. The antiarrhythmic action (when indicated for this use) has been related to a reduction in spontaneous pacemaker firing and slowing of AV nodal conduction.

Uses: Chronic stable angina pectoris, hypertension, supraventricular dysrhythmias (class II), migraine, MI prophylaxis, pheochromocytoma, essential tremor, hypertrophic cardiomyopathy, anxiety

Dosage and routes:

Dysrhythmias

• *Adult:* PO 10-30 mg tid-qid; IV bol 0.5-3 mg over 1 mg/min; may repeat in 2 min

Hypertension

• *Adult:* PO sus rel 40 mg bid or 80 mg qd initially; usual dose 120-240 mg/day bid-tid or 120-160 mg qd

Angina

• *Adult:* PO sus rel 80-320 mg in divided doses bid-qid or 80 mg qd; usual dose 160 mg qd

MI

• *Adult:* PO 180-240 mg/day tid-qid

Migraine

• *Adult:* PO sus rel 80 mg/day or in divided doses; may increase to 160-240 mg/day in divided doses

Available forms include: Sus rel caps 80, 120, 160 mg; tabs 10, 20, 40, 60, 80, 90 mg; inj 1 mg/ml, oral sol 4 mg, 8 mg/ml, conc oral sol 80 mg/ml; sus rel cap 60 mg

Side effects/adverse reactions:

▼ *ORAL:* Dry mouth, lichenoid reaction

CNS: Depression, hallucinations, dizziness, fatigue, lethargy, paresthesias, bizarre dreams, disorientation
CV: Bradycardia, hypotension, ***CHF,*** palpitation, AV block, peripheral vascular insufficiency, vasodilation
GI: Nausea, vomiting, diarrhea, colitis, constipation, cramps, hepatomegaly, gastric pain, acute pancreatitis
RESP: Bronchospasm, dyspnea, respiratory dysfunction
HEMA: ***Agranulocytosis, thrombocytopenia***
GU: Impotence, decreased libido, UTIs
EENT: ***Laryngospasm,*** blurred vision, sore throat, dry eyes
INTEG: Rash, pruritus, fever
MS: Joint pain, arthralgia, muscle cramps, pain
META: Hypoglycemia
MISC: Facial swelling, weight change, Raynaud's disease

Contraindications: Hypersensitivity to this drug, cardiac failure, cardiogenic shock, second- and third-degree heart block, bronchospastic disease, sinus bradycardia, CHF

Precautions: Diabetes mellitus, pregnancy category C, renal disease, lactation, hyperthyroidism, COPD, hepatic disease, children, myasthenia gravis, peripheral vascular disease, hypotension

Pharmacokinetics:
PO: Onset 30 min, peak 1-1.5 hr
IV: Onset 2 min, peak 15 min, duration 3-6 hr, half-life 3-5 hr (immed rel), 8-11 hr (sus rel); metabolized by liver; crosses placenta, blood-brain barrier; excreted in breast milk

Drug interactions of concern to dentistry:
- Decreased hypotensive effect: indomethacin, NSAIDs
- Increased hypotension, myocardial depression: hydrocarbon inhalation anesthetics
- Hypertension, bradycardia: sympathomimetics (epinephrine, ephedrine)
- Slow metabolism of lidocaine

DENTAL CONSIDERATIONS

General:
- Monitor vital signs every appointment due to cardiovascular side effects.
- Patients on chronic drug therapy may rarely have symptoms of blood dyscrasias, which can include infection, bleeding, and poor healing.
- Limit use of sodium-containing products, such as saline IV fluids, for patients with a dietary salt restriction.
- Assess salivary flow as a factor in caries, periodontal disease, and candidiasis.
- After supine positioning, have patient sit upright for at least 2 min before standing to avoid orthostatic hypotension.
- Stress from dental procedures may compromise cardiovascular function; determine patient risk.
- Short appointments and a stress reduction protocol may be required for anxious patients.
- Consider semisupine chair position for patients with respiratory distress.
- Use vasoconstrictors with caution, in low doses, and with careful aspiration. Avoid use of gingival retraction cord with epinephrine.

Consultations:
- In a patient with symptoms of

blood dyscrasias, request a medical consult for blood studies and postpone dental treatment until normal values are reestablished.

- Medical consult may be required to assess disease control and patient's ability to tolerate stress.

Teach patient/family:

- Caution to prevent injury when using oral hygiene aids
- Importance of good oral hygiene to prevent soft tissue inflammation

When chronic dry mouth occurs, advise patient:

- To avoid mouth rinses with high alcohol content due to drying effects
- Of need for daily home fluoride to prevent caries
- To use sugarless gum, frequent sips of water, or saliva substitutes

---

propylthiouracil (PTU)

(proe-pil-thye-oh-yoor'a-sil)

generic

Propyl-Thyracil

Drug class.: Thyroid hormone antagonist

Action: Blocks synthesis of thyroid hormones T_3, T_4 (triiodothyronine), and T_4 (thyroxine)

Uses: Preparation for thyroidectomy, thyrotoxic crisis, hyperthyroidism, thyroid storm

Dosage and routes:

Hyperthyroidism

- *Adult:* PO 100 mg tid, increasing to 300 mg q8h if condition is severe; continue to euthyroid state, then 100 mg qd-tid
- *Child >10 yr:* PO 100 mg tid; continue to euthyroid state, then 25 mg tid to 100 mg bid
- *Child 6-10 yr:* PO 50-150 mg in divided doses q8h

Available forms include: Tabs 50 mg

Side effects/adverse reactions:

ORAL: Loss of taste, bleeding (rare)

CNS: Drowsiness, headache, vertigo, fever, paresthesias, neuritis

GI: Nausea, diarrhea, vomiting, ***jaundice, hepatitis***

HEMA: ***Agranulocytosis, leukopenia, thrombocytopenia, hypothrombinemia, lymphadenopathy,*** bleeding, vasculitis, periarteritis

GU: ***Nephritis***

INTEG: Rash, urticaria, pruritus, alopecia, hyperpigmentation, lupus-like syndrome

MS: Myalgia, arthralgia, nocturnal muscle cramps

Contraindications: Hypersensitivity, pregnancy category D, lactation

Precautions: Infection, bone marrow depression, hepatic disease

Pharmacokinetics:

PO: Onset 30-40 min, duration 2-4 hr, half-life 1-2 hr; excreted in urine, bile, breast milk; crosses placenta

Drug interactions of concern to dentistry:

- Increased CV side effects in uncontrolled patients: anticholinergics and sympathomimetics
- Patients with uncontrolled hyperthyroidism are at risk when vasoconstrictors are used
- Patients with uncontrolled hypothyroidism may be more responsive to CNS depressants

DENTAL CONSIDERATIONS

General:

- Patients on chronic drug therapy may rarely have symptoms of blood dyscrasias, which can include infection, bleeding, and poor healing.

• Patients with uncontrolled hyperthyroidism should not be treated in the dental office until thyroid values are normalized.
• Uncontrolled patients should be referred for medical evaluation and treatment.
• Monitor vital signs every appointment due to cardiovascular side effects.
• Consider semisupine chair position for patient comfort if GI side effects occur.

Consultations:
• Medical consult may be required to assess disease control and patient's ability to tolerate stress.

---

protriptyline HCl

(proe-trip'te-leen)
Vivactil
Triptil

Drug class.: Tricyclic antidepressant

Action: Inhibits both norepinephrine and serotonin (5-HT) uptake in the brain, although the precise antidepressant mechanism remains unclear

Uses: Depression; unapproved use: adjunctive use in narcolepsy and attention-deficit disorders

Dosage and routes:
• *Adult:* PO 15-40 mg/day in divided doses; may increase to 60 mg/day
• *Adolescent and elderly:* PO 5 mg tid

Available forms include: Tabs 5, 10 mg

Side effects/adverse reactions:
ORAL: Dry mouth, unpleasant taste, bleeding, stomatitis
CNS: Dizziness, drowsiness, confusion, headache, anxiety, tremors, stimulation, weakness, insomnia, nightmares, EPS (elderly), increased psychiatric symptoms, paresthesia
CV: Orthostatic hypotension, ECG changes, tachycardia, ***hypertension,*** palpitation
GI: Diarrhea, ***paralytic ileus, hepatitis,*** increased appetite, nausea, vomiting, cramps, epigastric distress, jaundice
HEMA: ***Agranulocytosis, thrombocytopenia, eosinophilia, leukopenia***
GU: Retention, ***acute renal failure***
EENT: Blurred vision, tinnitus, mydriasis
INTEG: Rash, urticaria, sweating, pruritus, photosensitivity

Contraindications: Hypersensitivity to tricyclic antidepressants, recovery phase of MI, convulsive disorders, prostatic hypertrophy

Precautions: Suicidal patients, severe depression, increased intraocular pressure, narrow-angle glaucoma, urinary retention, cardiac disease, hepatic disease, hyperthyroidism, electroshock therapy, elective surgery, pregnancy category not established, MAO inhibitors

Pharmacokinetics:
PO: Onset 15-30 min, peak 24-30 hr, duration 4-6 hr, therapeutic effect 2-3 wk, half-life 67-89 hr; metabolized by liver; excreted by kidneys; crosses placenta

Drug interactions of concern to dentistry:
• Increased anticholinergic effects: muscarinic blockers, antihistamines, phenothiazines
• Increased effects of direct-acting sympathomimetics (epinephrine, levonordefrin)
• Possible risk of increased CNS

P

depression: alcohol, barbiturates, benzodiazepines, and other CNS depressants

• Decreased antihypertensive effects of: clonidine, guanadrel, guanethidine

DENTAL CONSIDERATIONS

General:

• Take vital signs every appointment due to cardiovascular side effects.

• Assess salivary flow as a factor in caries, periodontal disease, and candidiasis.

• Patients on chronic drug therapy may rarely have symptoms of blood dyscrasias, which can include infection, bleeding, and poor healing.

• After supine positioning, have patient sit upright for at least 2 min before standing to avoid orthostatic hypotension.

• Use vasoconstrictors with caution, in low doses, and with careful aspiration. Avoid use of gingival retraction cord with epinephrine.

• Place on frequent recall due to oral side effects.

Consultations:

• In a patient with symptoms of blood dyscrasias, request a medical consult for blood studies and postpone dental treatment until normal values are reestablished.

• Medical consult may be required to assess disease control in the patient.

• Physician should be informed if significant xerostomic side effects occur (increased caries, sore tongue, problems eating or swallowing, difficulty wearing prosthesis) so a medication change can be considered.

Teach patient/family:

• Importance of good oral hygiene to prevent soft tissue inflammation

• Caution to prevent injury when using oral hygiene aids

When chronic dry mouth occurs, advise patient:

• To avoid mouth rinses with high alcohol content due to drying effects

• Of need for daily home fluoride to prevent caries

• To use sugarless gum, frequent sips of water, or saliva substitutes

---

pseudoephedrine HCl/ pseudoephedrine sulfate

(soo-doe-e-fed′rin)

Balminil, Benylin Decongestant, Cenafed, Children's Sufedrin, Dorcol, Effidac24, Genaphed, Halofed, Novafed, PediaCare Infant's, Pseudogest, Sudafed, Sudafed 12 Hour, Sudafed Liquid

♣ Eltor 120, Robidrine

Drug class.: α-adrenergic agonist

Action: Acts primarily on α-receptors, causing vasoconstriction in blood vessels; has some beta activity and to a lesser degree CNS stimulant effects

Uses: Decongestant, nasal congestion

Dosage and routes:

• *Adult:* PO 60 mg q6h; ext rel 60-120 mg q12h

• *Child 6-12 yr:* PO 30 mg q6h, not to exceed 120 mg/day

• *Child 2-6 yr:* PO 15 mg q6h, not to exceed 60 mg/day

Available forms include: Ext rel caps 120 mg; sol 15 mg, 30 mg/5 ml drops; 7.5 mg/0.8 ml drops; tabs 30, 60 mg; ext rel tabs 120 mg

Side effects/adverse reactions:

▼ *ORAL:* Dry mouth

CNS: Tremors, anxiety, ***seizures,*** insomnia, headache, dizziness, anxiety, hallucinations

CV: ***Dysrhythmias,*** palpitation, tachycardia, hypertension, chest pain

GI: Anorexia, nausea, vomiting

GU: Dysuria

EENT: Dry nose, irritation of nose and throat

Contraindications: Hypersensitivity to sympathomimetics, narrow-angle glaucoma, lactation

Precautions: Pregnancy category B, cardiac disorders, hyperthyroidism, diabetes mellitus, prostatic hypertrophy

Pharmacokinetics:

PO: Onset 15-30 min, duration 4-6 hr, 8-12 hr (ext rel); metabolized in liver; excreted in feces, breast milk

Drug interactions of concern to dentistry:

- Dysrhythmia: hydrocarbon inhalation anesthetics
- Increased CNS, CV effects: sympathomimetics

DENTAL CONSIDERATIONS

General:

- Assess salivary flow as a factor in caries, periodontal disease, and candidiasis.
- Monitor vital signs every appointment due to cardiovascular side effects.
- Consider semisupine chair position for patient comfort if GI side effects occur.

Teach patient/family:

- Use of electric toothbrush if patient has difficulty holding conventional devices

When chronic dry mouth occurs, advise patient:

- To avoid mouth rinses with high alcohol content due to drying effects
- Of need for daily home fluoride to prevent caries
- To use sugarless gum, frequent sips of water, or saliva substitutes

pyrazinamide

(peer-a-zin'a-mide)

generic

✤ PMS-Pyrazinamide, Tebrazid

Drug class.: Antitubercular

Action: Bactericidal interference with lipid, nucleic acid biosynthesis

Uses: TB, as an adjunct with other drugs

Dosage and routes:

- *Adult:* PO 20-35 mg/kg/day in 3-4 divided doses, not to exceed 3 g/day

Available forms include: Tabs 500 mg

Side effects/adverse reactions:

CNS: Headache

GI: ***Hepatotoxicity,*** abnormal liver function tests, peptic ulcer

HEMA: ***Hemolytic anemia***

GU: Urinary difficulty, increased uric acid

INTEG: Photosensitivity, urticaria

Contraindications: Hypersensitivity

Precautions: Pregnancy category C, child <13 yr

Pharmacokinetics:

PO: Peak 2 hr, half-life 9-10 hr; metabolized in liver, excreted in urine (metabolites/unchanged drug)

P

DENTAL CONSIDERATIONS

General:

• Determine why the patient is taking the drug (for prophylaxis or active therapy).

• Determine that noninfectious status exists by ensuring that (1) anti-TB drugs have been taken >3 wk, (2) culture has confirmed TB susceptibility to antiinfectives, (3) patient has had three consecutive negative sputum smears, and (4) patient is not in the coughing stage.

Consultations:

• Medical consult may be required to assess disease control in the patient.

Teach patient/family:

• Importance of taking medications for full length of regimen to ensure effectiveness of treatment and to prevent the emergence of resistant strains

---

pyridostigmine bromide

(peer-id-oh-stig′meen)

Mestinon, Mestinon SR, Regonol

Drug class.: Cholinergic

Action: Inhibits destruction of acetylcholine, which increases concentration at sites where acetylcholine is released; this facilitates transmission of impulses across myoneural junction

Uses: Nondepolarizing muscle relaxant antagonist, myasthenia gravis

Dosage and routes:

Myasthenia gravis

• *Adult:* PO initial 30-60 mg q3-4h, titrate as required, not to exceed 1.5 g/day; IM/IV 1/30 of PO dose q2-3h; sus rel 180-540 mg 1-2 × daily at intervals of at least 6 hr

Tubocurarine antagonist

• *Adult:* 0.6-1.2 mg IV atropine, then 10-20 mg

Available forms include: Tabs 60 mg; sus rel tabs 180 mg; syr 60 mg/5 ml; inj IM/IV 5 mg/ml

Side effects/adverse reactions:

▼ *ORAL: Salivation, tongue weakness*

CNS: ***Convulsions,*** dizziness, headache, sweating, confusion, incoordination, paralysis

CV: Bradycardia, ***cardiac arrest,*** tachycardia, dysrhythmias, AV block, hypotension, ECG changes

GI: Nausea, diarrhea, vomiting, cramps

RESP: Increased bronchial secretions, ***respiratory depression, bronchospasm, constriction, laryngospasm, respiratory arrest,*** SOB

GU: Frequency, incontinence

EENT: Miosis, blurred vision, lacrimation

INTEG: Rash, urticaria, flushing

MS: Weakness (arms, neck), cramps, twitching

Contraindications: Bradycardia, hypotension, obstruction of intestine, renal system, sensitivity to bromides

Precautions: Seizure disorders, bronchial asthma, coronary occlusion, hyperthyroidism, dysrhythmias, peptic ulcer, megacolon, poor GI motility, pregnancy category C, elderly, lactation

Pharmacokinetics:

PO: Onset 20-30 min, duration 3-6 hr

IM/IV/SC: Onset 2-15 min, duration 2.5-4 hr; metabolized in liver, excreted in urine

Drug interactions of concern to dentistry:

• Decreased effects: atropine, scopolamine, and other anticholinergic drugs; methocarbamol

• Reduced rate of metabolism of ester local anesthetics

• Avoid anticholinergic drugs to control excessive salivation

DENTAL CONSIDERATIONS

General:

• Monitor vital signs every appointment due to cardiovascular and respiratory side effects.

• After supine positioning, have patient sit upright for at least 2 min before standing to avoid orthostatic hypotension.

• Schedule short appointments due to effects of disease on oral musculature.

• Avoid dental light in patient's eyes; offer dark glasses for patient comfort.

• Place on frequent recall due to oral side effects.

• Consider semisupine chair position if GI side effects occur.

Consultations:

• Medical consult may be required to assess disease control in the patient.

• Consult with physician about adjusting dose if excessive salivation becomes a problem.

Teach patient/family:

• Use of electric toothbrush or other oral hygiene aids if patient has difficulty in maintaining oral hygiene

• Importance of good oral hygiene to prevent soft tissue inflammation

• To prevent injury when using oral hygiene aids

pyridoxine HCl/ vitamin B_6

(peer-i-dox'een)

Nestrex

Drug class.: Vitamin B_6, water soluble

Action: Needed for fat, protein, and carbohydrate metabolism as a coenzyme

Uses: Vitamin B_6 deficiency associated with inborn errors of metabolism, inadequate diet; unapproved use: drug-induced deficiencies

Dosage and routes:

Vitamin B_6 deficiency (dietary deficiency)

• *Adult:* PO 10-20 mg qd × 3 wk, then 2-5 mg qd (large doses ranging from 50-200 mg daily are usually required for drug-induced deficiency)

• *Child:* PO 2-10 mg qd × 3 wk, then 2-5 mg qd

Available forms include: Tabs 25, 50, 100 mg; time rel tabs 100 mg; inj IM/IV 100 mg/ml

Side effects/adverse reactions:

CNS: Paresthesia, flushing, warmth, lethargy ataxia (rare with normal renal function)

INTEG: Pain at injection site

Contraindications: Hypersensitivity

Precautions: Pregnancy category A, lactation, children, Parkinson's disease

Pharmacokinetics:

PO/INJ: Half-life 2-3 wk; metabolized in liver; excreted in urine

Drug interactions of concern to dentistry:

• Decreased effectiveness: levodopa

• Decreased serum levels of phenytoin, phenobarbital

DENTAL CONSIDERATIONS

General:

• Vitamin B deficiency and peripheral neuropathy may manifest with oral symptoms of glossitis and cheilosis.

---

quazepam

(kway'ze-pam)

Doral

Drug class.: Benzodiazepine, sedative-hypnotic

Controlled Substance Schedule IV

Action: Produces CNS depression by interacting with a benzodiazepine receptor to facilitate the action of the inhibitory neurotransmitter γ-aminobutyric acid (GABA)

Uses: Insomnia

Dosage and routes:

• *Adult:* PO 15 mg hs; may decrease if needed

Available forms include: Tabs 7.5, 15 mg

Side effects/adverse reactions:

▼ *ORAL:* Dry mouth, taste alteration

CNS: Lethargy, drowsiness, daytime sedation, dizziness, confusion, light-headedness, headache, anxiety, irritability, weakness, tremor, depression

CV: Chest pain, pulse changes, palpitation, tachycardia

GI: Nausea, vomiting, diarrhea, heartburn, abdominal pain, constipation, anorexia

HEMA: ***Leukopenia, granulocytopenia*** (rare)

MISC: Joint pain, congestion, dermatitis, sweating

Contraindications: Hypersensitivity to benzodiazepines, pregnancy category X, lactation, ritonavir

Precautions: Hepatic disease, renal disease, suicidal individuals, drug abuse, elderly, psychosis, child <18 yr, lactation, depression, pulmonary insufficiency

Pharmacokinetics:

PO: Onset 15-45 min, duration 7-8 hr; metabolized by liver; excreted by kidneys (inactive/active metabolites); crosses placenta; excreted in breast milk

Drug interactions of concern to dentistry:

• Increased effects of diazepam: CNS depressants, alcohol

• Delayed elimination: erythromycin

DENTAL CONSIDERATIONS

General:

• Assess salivary flow as a factor in caries, periodontal disease, and candidiasis.

• Psychologic and physical dependence may occur with chronic administration.

• Geriatric patients are more susceptible to drug effects; use a lower dose.

• Avoid using this drug in a patient with a history of drug abuse or alcoholism.

• Increased serum levels and prolonged effect of benzodiazepines: erythromycin, ketoconazole, itraconazole, fluconazole, miconazole (systemic).

Consultations:

• Medical consult may be required to assess disease control in the patient.

Teach patient/family:

When chronic dry mouth occurs, advise patient:

• To avoid mouth rinses with high

alcohol content due to drying effects
• Of need for daily home fluoride to prevent caries
• To use sugarless gum, frequent sips of water, or saliva substitutes

quetiapine fumarate

(kwe-tye'a-peen)
Seroquel
Drug class.: Antipsychotic, atypical

Action: Acts as an agonist at serotonin ($5HT_2$) receptors and to a lesser extent at dopamine (DA_2) receptors
Uses: Schizophrenia
Dosage and routes:
• *Adult:* PO initial dose 25 mg bid, on second day increase dose by 25 mg bid or tid, as tolerated, to target range of 300-400 mg daily by the fourth day; doses of 75 mg daily have been used
Available forms include: Tabs 25, 200, 200 mg
Side effects/adverse reactions:
▼ *ORAL: Dry mouth* (8%-17%), taste perversion
CNS: Somnolence, headache, agitation, insomnia, dizziness, extrapyramidal symptoms, anorexia
CV: Orthostatic hypotension, tachycardia, palpitation, peripheral edema
GI: Abdominal pain, constipation, dyspepsia
RESP: Cough, dyspnea
HEMA: Leukopenia
EENT: Rhinitis, ear pain, pharyngitis, dry eyes, conjunctivitis
INTEG: Rash, sweating, pruritus
META: Elevation of liver enzymes, cholesterol, triglycerides
MS: Asthenia, dysorthia, hypertonia
MISC: Weight gain, flulike syndrome
Contraindications: Hypersensitivity, severe CNS depression
Precautions: Renal impairment, hepatic impairment, CV disease, thyroid disease, hyperprolactinemia, neuromalignant syndrome, tardive dyskinesia, seizure disorders, cataracts, dementia, suicide tendency, pregnancy category C, lactation
Pharmacokinetics:
PO: Peak serum levels 1.5 hr; hepatic metabolism, renal excretion (70% as unchanged drug)
Drug interactions of concern to dentistry:
• Risk of increased CNS depression: CNS depressants

DENTAL CONSIDERATIONS
General:
• Monitor vital signs every appointment due to cardiovascular and respiratory side effects.
• Assess salivary flow as factor in caries, periodontal disease, and candidiasis.
• Assess for presence of extrapyramidal motor symptoms, such as tardive dyskinesia and akathisia. Extrapyramidal motor activity may complicate dental treatment.
• After supine positioning, have patient sit upright for at least 2 min before standing to avoid orthostatic hypotension.
• Consider semisupine chair position for patient comfort if GI side effects occur.
• Patients on chronic drug therapy may rarely have symptoms of blood dyscrasias, which can include infection, bleeding, and poor healing.
• Place on frequent recall due to oral side effects.

Q

Consultations:

- In a patient with symptoms of blood dyscrasias, request a medical consult for blood studies and postpone treatment until normal values are reestablished.
- Medical consult may be required to assess disease control and patient's ability to tolerate stress.
- If signs of tardive dyskinesia or akathisia are present, refer to physician.
- Consultation with physician may be needed if sedation or general anesthesia is required.
- Physician should be informed if significant xerostomic side effects occur (increased caries, sore tongue, problems eating or swallowing, difficulty wearing prosthesis) so a medication change can be considered.

Teach patient/family:

- Caution to prevent trauma when using oral hygiene aids
- Use of electric toothbrush if patient has difficulty holding conventional devices
- Importance of good oral hygiene to prevent soft tissue inflammation
- Importance of updating health and drug history if physician makes any changes in evaluation/ drug regimens
- To be aware of oral side effects and potential sequelae

When chronic dry mouth occurs, advise patient:

- To avoid mouth rinses with high alcohol content due to drying effects
- To use daily home fluoride products for anticaries effect
- To use sugarless gum, frequent sips of water, or saliva substitutes

quinapril

(kwyn'a-pril)

Accupril

Drug class.: Angiotension-converting enzyme (ACE) inhibitor

Action: Selectively suppresses renin-angiotensin-aldosterone system; inhibits ACE; prevents conversion of angiotensin I to angiotensin II; results in dilation of arterial, venous vessels

Uses: Hypertension, alone or in combination with thiazide diuretics

Dosage and routes:

- *Adult:* PO 10 mg qd initially, then 20-80 mg/day divided bid or qd

Available forms include: Tabs 5, 10, 20, 40 mg

Side effects/adverse reactions:

▼ *ORAL:* Dry mouth

CNS: Headache, dizziness, fatigue, somnolence, depression, malaise, nervousness, vertigo

CV: Hypotension, postural hypotension, syncope, palpitation, angina pectoris, MI, tachycardia, vasodilation

GI: Nausea, constipation, vomiting, gastritis, GI hemorrhage

RESP: Cough, bronchitis

HEMA: ***Thrombocytopenia, agranulocytosis***

GU: Increased BUN, creatinine, decreased libido, impotence

INTEG: ***Angioedema,*** rash, sweating, photosensitivity, pruritus

MS: Arthralgia, arthritis, myalgia, back pain

META: Hyperkalemia

MISC: Amblyopia

Contraindications: Hypersensitivity, children

Precautions: Pregnancy category D, impaired renal/liver function, dialysis patients, hypovolemia, blood dyscrasias, CHF, COPD, asthma, elderly, lactation

Pharmacokinetics:

PO: Peak 0.5-1 hr, half-life 2 hr; serum protein binding 97%; metabolized by liver (metabolites); metabolites excreted in urine

Drug interactions of concern to dentistry:

• Increased hypotension: alcohol, phenothiazines

• Decreased hypotensive effects: indomethacin and possibly other NSAIDs, sympathomimetics

DENTAL CONSIDERATIONS

General:

• Monitor vital signs every appointment due to cardiovascular side effects.

• After supine positioning, have patient sit upright for at least 2 min before standing to avoid orthostatic hypotension.

• Patients on chronic drug therapy may rarely have symptoms of blood dyscrasias, which can include infection, bleeding, and poor healing.

• Assess salivary flow as a factor in caries, periodontal disease, and candidiasis.

• Limit use of sodium-containing products, such as saline IV fluids, for patients with a dietary salt restriction.

• Use vasoconstrictors with caution, in low doses, and with careful aspiration.

• Stress from dental procedures may compromise cardiovascular function; determine patient risk.

• Short appointments and a stress reduction protocol may be required for anxious patients.

Consultations:

• Medical consult may be required to assess disease control and patient's ability to tolerate stress.

• In a patient with symptoms of blood dyscrasias, request a medical consult for blood studies and postpone dental treatment until normal values are reestablished.

• Take precautions if dental surgery is anticipated and sedation or general anesthesia is required; there is risk of a hypotensive episode.

Teach patient/family:

• Importance of good oral hygiene to prevent soft tissue inflammation

• Caution to prevent injury when using oral hygiene aids

When chronic dry mouth occurs, advise patient:

• To avoid mouth rinses with high alcohol content due to drying effects

• Of need for daily home fluoride to prevent caries

• To use sugarless gum, frequent sips of water, or saliva substitutes

---

Q

quinidine gluconate/ quinidine polygalacturonate/ quinidine sulfate

(kwin'i-deen)

Cardioquin, Cin-Quin, Duraquin, Quinaglute, Quinalan, Quinidex Extentabs, Quinora

♣ Apo-Quinidine, Novoquindin, Quinate

Drug class.: Antidysrhythmic (Class IA)

Action: Prolongs effective refractory period; decreases myocardial excitability, conduction velocity, and contractility; indirect anticholinergic properties

Uses: PVCs, atrial flutter and fibrillation, PAT, ventricular tachycardia

Dosage and routes:

Atrial fibrillation/flutter

• *Adult:* PO 200 mg q2-3h × 5-8 doses; may increase qd until sinus rhythm is restored; max 4 g/day given only after digitalization

Paroxysmal supraventricular tachycardia

• *Adult:* PO 400-600 mg q2-3h

All other dysrhythmias

• *Adult:* PO 50-200 mg as a test dose, then 200-400 mg q4-6h

Available forms include: Gluconate—sus rel tabs 324 mg; inj 80 mg/ml in 10 ml vials; sulfate—tabs 100, 200 mg; caps 200, 300 mg; sus rel tabs 300 mg; polygalacturonate—tabs 275 mg

Side effects/adverse reactions:

▼ *ORAL: Bitter taste, lichenoid drug reaction*

CNS: Headache, dizziness, involuntary movement, confusion, psychosis, restlessness, irritability, syncope, excitement

CV: Hypotension, bradycardia, ***heart block, cardiovascular collapse, arrest,*** PVCs

GI: Diarrhea, ***hepatotoxicity,*** nausea, vomiting, anorexia

RESP: Dyspnea, ***respiratory depression***

HEMA: ***Thrombocytopenia,*** hemolytic anemia, agranulocytosis, hypoprothrombinemia

EENT: Cinchonism: tinnitus, blurred vision, hearing loss, mydriasis, disturbed color vision

INTEG: Rash, urticaria, angioedema, swelling, photosensitivity

Contraindications: Hypersensitivity, blood dyscrasias, severe heart block, myasthenia gravis, itraconazole

Precautions: Pregnancy category C, lactation, children, renal disease, potassium imbalance, liver disease, CHF, respiratory depression

Pharmacokinetics:

PO: Peak 0.5-6 hr (depending on form given), duration 6-8 hr, half-life 6-7 hr; metabolized in liver; excreted unchanged by kidneys

Drug interactions of concern to dentistry:

• May decrease effects of quinidine: barbiturates

• Increased anticholinergic effect: anticholinergic drugs

• Increased effects of neuromuscular blockers

• Contraindicated with: itraconazole

DENTAL CONSIDERATIONS

General:

• Monitor vital signs every appointment due to cardiovascular and respiratory side effects.

• Patients on chronic drug therapy may rarely have symptoms of blood dyscrasias, which can include infection, bleeding, and poor healing.

• After supine positioning, have patient sit upright for at least 2 min before standing to avoid orthostatic hypotension.

• Use vasoconstrictors with caution, in low doses, and with careful aspiration. Avoid use of gingival retraction cord with epinephrine.

• Consider semisupine chair position for patient comfort if GI side effects occur.

Consultations:

• In a patient with symptoms of blood dyscrasias, request a medical

consult for blood studies and postpone dental treatment until normal values are reestablished.
• Medical consult may be required to assess patient's ability to tolerate stress.

Teach patient/family:
• Importance of good oral hygiene to prevent soft tissue inflammation

quinine sulfate

(kwye'nine)
generic
Drug class.: Antimalarial

Action: Schizonticidal, but mechanism is unclear; increases refractory period in skeletal muscle

Uses: *P. falciparum* malaria, nocturnal leg cramps

Dosage and routes:
• *Adult:* PO 650 mg q8h over 3-7 days, given with concurrent antiinfective drugs

Available forms include: Caps 65, 162.5, 200, 300, 325 mg; tabs 260

Side effects/adverse reactions:
▼ *ORAL:* Lichenoid drug reaction
CNS: ***Convulsion,*** headache, stimulation, fatigue, irritability, bad dreams, dizziness, fever, confusion, anxiety
CV: ***Acute circulatory failure,*** angina, dysrhythmias, tachycardia, hypotension
GI: Nausea, vomiting, anorexia, diarrhea, epigastric pain
HEMA: ***Thrombocytopenia, purpura, hypothrombinemia, hemolysis***
GU: Dysuria
EENT: Blurred vision, corneal changes, retinal changes, difficulty focusing, tinnitus, vertigo, deafness, photophobia, diplopia, night blindness
INTEG: Pruritus, pigment changes, skin eruptions, lichen planus–like eruptions, flushing, facial edema, sweating
ENDO: Hypoglycemia

Contraindications: Hypersensitivity, G6PD deficiency, retinal field changes, pregnancy category X

Precautions: Blood dyscrasias, severe GI disease, neurologic disease, severe hepatic disease, psoriasis, cardiac dysrhythmias, tinnitus

Pharmacokinetics:
PO: Peak 1-3 hr, half-life 4-5 hr; metabolized in liver; excreted in urine

Drug interactions of concern to dentistry:
• Decreased absorption: magnesium or aluminum salts
• Prolonged duration of neuromuscular blocking drugs

DENTAL CONSIDERATIONS

General:
• Patients on chronic drug therapy may rarely have symptoms of blood dyscrasias, which can include infection, bleeding, and poor healing.
• Avoid dental light in patient's eyes; offer dark glasses for patient comfort.
• Monitor vital signs every appointment due to cardiovascular side effects.
• Consider semisupine chair position for patient comfort if GI side effects occur.

Consultations:
• Medical consult may be required to assess disease control in the patient.
• In a patient with symptoms of blood dyscrasias, request a medical

Q

consult for blood studies and postpone dental treatment until normal values are reestablished.

Teach patient/family:

• Importance of good oral hygiene to prevent soft tissue inflammation

quinupristin/ dalfopristin

(qwen'yoo-pris-ten) (dal'fo-pris-ten)

Synercid I.V.

Drug class.: Antiinfective, streptogramin

Action: Combination of quinupristin (30%) with dalfopristin (70%); inhibition of the synthesis of bacterial protein by irreversible binding to 50S ribosomal subunits

Uses: Serious or life-threatening infections due to vancomycin-resistant *Enterococcus faecium*; skin and skin structure infections caused by *Streptococcus pyogenes* or methicillin-resistant *Staphylococcus aureus*

Dosage and routes:

• *Adult:* IV infusion in D_5W over 60 min; for vancomycin-resistant *E. faecium,* 7.5 mg/kg q8h; for complicated skin and skin structure infections, 7.5 mg/kg q12h with minimum dose duration of 7 days

• *Child <16 yr:* Limited data available; no dose adjustment required

Available forms include: Single-dose vial: quinupristin 150 mg and dalfopristin 350 mg in each vial

Side effects/adverse reactions:

▼ *ORAL:* Candidiasis

CNS: Headache, chest pain

CV: Infusion site reactions (pain, inflammation), peripheral edema

GI: Nausea, vomiting, ***pseudomembranous colitis,*** diarrhea, abdominal pain, dyspepsia, pancreatitis

GU: UTI

INTEG: Rash, pruritus

META: Hyperbilirubenemia, elevation of ALT, AST

MS: Arthralgia, myalgia, leg cramps

MISC: Asthenia, allergic reaction

Contraindications: Known hypersensitivity or prior hypersensitivity to other streptogramins, heparin flush

Precautions: Venous irritation, inhibits cytochrome P-450 3A4 enzymes, pregnancy category B, lactation

Pharmacokinetics:

IV: Both constituents are converted to active metabolites, short half-life but prolonged postantibiotic effect on *S. aureus* and *S. pneumoniae,* peak concentration 1 hr, protein binding quinupristin (55%-78%), dalfopristin (11%-26%), extensive metabolism in liver and blood, renal excretion 20%, mostly fecal excretion

Drug interactions of concern to dentistry:

• Patients with serious, life-threatening systemic infections will not be candidates for dental care except for extreme emergencies

DENTAL CONSIDERATIONS

General:

• Examine for oral manifestation of opportunistic candida infection.

rabeprazole sodium

(ra-bee'pry-zole)

Aciphex

Drug class.: Antisecretory

Action: Suppresses gastric acid

secretion by inhibiting hydrogen/potassium ATPase enzyme system in the gastric parietal cell; characterized as a gastric acid pump inhibitor because it blocks the final step in acid production.

Uses: Gastroesophageal reflux disease (GERD), duodenal ulcers, and hypersecretory conditions (Zollinger-Ellison disease)

Dosage and routes:

GERD and duodenal ulcer

- *Adult:* PO 20 mg qd × 4-8 wk; if healing is not evident can continue 8 wk more

Hypersecretory conditions

- *Adult:* PO 60 mg qd; higher dose of 60 mg bid has been used

Available forms include: Del rel tabs 20 mg

Side effects/adverse reactions:

▼ *ORAL:* Dry mouth, mouth ulceration

CNS: Headache, insomnia, anxiety, abnormal dreams

CV: Hypertension, ECG abnormalities, syncope, palpitation, bundle branch block

GI: Diarrhea, nausea, abdominal pain

RESP: Dyspnea, asthma, hiccups

HEMA: Anemia, abnormal blood cell counts

EENT: Dry eyes, eye pain

INTEG: Photosensitivity, rash, pruritus, sweating

ENDO: Alteration in thyroid function

META: Weight gain, gout, abnormal liver function tests

MS: Asthenia, chest pain, neck rigidity, myalgia

MISC: Fever

Contraindications: Hypersensitivity

Precautions: Do not break, crush, or chew tablets, pregnancy category B, avoid nursing, pediatric use not studied

Pharmacokinetics:

PO: Delayed release tablets: bioavailability 52%, peak plasma levels 2-5 hr, half-life 1-2 hr, highly plasma protein bound (96.3%), extensive hepatic metabolism (CYP450 3A), about 90% excreted in urine

Drug interactions of concern to dentistry:

- None documented

DENTAL CONSIDERATIONS

General:

- Assess salivary flow as a factor in caries, periodontal disease, and candidiasis.
- Consider semisupine chair position for patient comfort due to GI side effects of disease.
- Question the patient about tolerance of NSAIDs or aspirin related to GI problems.

Teach patient/family:

- To prevent trauma when using oral hygiene aids

When chronic dry mouth occurs, advise patient:

- To avoid mouth rinses with high alcohol content due to drying effects
- To use daily home fluoride products for anticaries effect
- To use sugarless gum, frequent sips of water, or saliva substitutes

R

raloxifene hydrochloride

(ral-ox′i-feen)

Evista

Drug class.: Synthetic estrogen

Action: Acts as a selective estrogen receptor modulator (SERM) to reduce resorption of bone and decrease overall bone turnover; may act as an estrogen antagonist in uterine and breast tissues

Uses: Prevention and treatment of osteoporosis in postmenopausal women, supplemented with calcium as based on need

Dosages and routes:

• *Adult:* PO 60 mg daily was used in clinical trials

Available forms include: Tabs 60 mg

Side effects/adverse reactions:

CNS: Insomnia, depression

CV: Chest pain, *hot flashes*

GI: Nausea, vomiting, dyspepsia, flatulence

RESP: Cough

GU: Vaginitis, UTI, cystitis, leukorrhea, vaginal bleeding

EENT: Sinusitis, pharyngitis

INTEG: Rash, sweating

ENDO: Weight gain

MS: Leg cramps, arthralgia, myalgia

MISC: Flulike syndrome, infection

Contraindications: Hypersensitivity, pregnancy, prior history of venous thromboembolic events, premenopausal use, lactation, children

Precautions: Hepatic impairment, risk of thromboembolitic events, pregnancy category X, lactation

Pharmacokinetics:

PO: Rapidly absorbed, bioavailability 2%, plasma levels depend on systemic interconversion and enterohepatic cycling, highly bound to plasma proteins, extensive first-pass metabolism, glucuronide metabolites, mainly excreted in feces, urinary excretion is minor

Drug interactions of concern to dentistry:

• Reduced absorption: ampicillin

• Risk of potential drug interactions with other highly plasma protein–bound drugs is unknown, such as NSAIDS, aspirin, and diazepam

DENTAL CONSIDERATIONS:

General:

• This drug should be discontinued 72 hr before prolonged immobilization such as hospitalization, postsurgical recovery, and bed rest.

• Consider short appointments and dental chair position if needed for patient comfort.

Consultations:

• Medical consult may be required to assess disease control and patient's ability to tolerate stress.

ramipril

(ra-mi′pril)

Altace

Drug class.: Angiotensin-converting enzyme (ACE) inhibitor

Action: Selectively suppresses renin-angiotensin-aldosterone system; inhibits ACE; prevents conversion of angiotensin I to angiotensin II; results in dilation of arterial, venous vessels

Uses: Hypertension; alone or in combination with thiazide diuretics; CHF immediately after MI

Dosage and routes:

• *Adult:* PO 2.5 mg qd initially, then 2.5-20 mg/day divided bid or qd; renal impairment: 1.25 mg qd with CrCl <40 ml/min/1.73 m^2, increase as needed to max of 5 mg/day

Available forms include: Caps 1.25, 2.5, 5, 10 mg

Side effects/adverse reactions:

▼ *ORAL:* Angioedema (lips, tongue, mucous membranes), dry mouth

CNS: Headache, dizziness, ***convulsions,*** anxiety, insomnia, paresthesia, fatigue, depression, malaise, vertigo, hearing loss

CV: Hypotension, chest pain, palpitation, angina, syncope, dysrhythmia

GI: Nausea, constipation, vomiting, dyspepsia, dysphagia, anorexia, diarrhea, abdominal pain

RESP: Cough, dyspnea

HEMA: ***Eosinophilia, leukopenia,*** decreased Hct/Hgb

GU: ***Proteinuria,*** increased BUN, creatinine, impotence

INTEG: ***Angioedema,*** rash, sweating, photosensitivity, pruritus

MS: Arthralgia, arthritis, myalgia

META: Hyperkalemia

Contraindications: Hypersensitivity to ACE inhibitors, pregnancy category D, lactation, children

Precautions: Impaired renal/liver function, dialysis patients, hypovolemia, blood dyscrasias, CHF, COPD, asthma, elderly

Pharmacokinetics:

PO: Peak 1 hr, half-life 5 hr, duration 24 hr; high serum protein binding; metabolized by liver; metabolites excreted in urine, feces

Drug interactions of concern to dentistry:

- Increased hypotension: alcohol, phenothiazines
- Decreased hypotensive effects: indomethacin and possibly other NSAIDs, sympathomimetics

DENTAL CONSIDERATIONS

General:

- Monitor vital signs every appointment due to cardiovascular and respiratory side effects.
- After supine positioning, have patient sit upright for at least 2 min before standing to avoid orthostatic hypotension.
- Patients on chronic drug therapy may rarely have symptoms of blood dyscrasias, which can include infection, bleeding, and poor healing.
- Assess salivary flow as a factor in caries, periodontal disease, and candidiasis.
- Limit use of sodium-containing products, such as saline IV fluids, for patients with a dietary salt restriction.
- Use vasoconstrictors with caution, in low doses, and with careful aspiration.
- Stress from dental procedures may compromise cardiovascular function; determine patient risk.
- Short appointments and a stress reduction protocol may be required for anxious patients.

Consultations:

- Medical consult may be required to assess patient's ability to tolerate stress.
- In a patient with symptoms of blood dyscrasias, request a medical consult for blood studies and postpone dental treatment until normal values are reestablished.
- Take precautions if dental surgery is anticipated and sedation or general anesthesia is required; there is risk of a hypotensive episode.

Teach patient/family:

- Importance of good oral hygiene to prevent soft tissue inflammation

R

• Caution to prevent injury when using oral hygiene aids

When chronic dry mouth occurs, advise patient:

• To avoid mouth rinses with high alcohol content due to drying effects

• Of need for daily home fluoride to prevent caries

• To use sugarless gum, frequent sips of water, or saliva substitutes

---

ranitidine

(ra-nye'te-deen)

Zantac, Zantac EFFERdose, Zantac 150 GELdose; OTC: Zantac 75, Zantac 75 EFFERdose

🍁 Apo-Ranitidine, Gen-Ranitidine, Novo-Ranitidine, Nu-Ranit, Zantac-C

Drug class.: H_2 histamine receptor antagonist

Action: Inhibits histamine at H_2-receptor site in parietal cells, which inhibits gastric acid secretion

Uses: Duodenal ulcer, Zollinger-Ellison syndrome, gastric ulcers, hypersecretory conditions, gastroesophageal reflux disease, stress ulcers; unapproved use: GI symptoms associated with NSAID use in rheumatoid arthritis

Dosage and routes:

• *Adult:* PO 150 mg bid or 300 mg hs; IM 50 mg q6-8h; IV bol 50 mg diluted to 20 ml over 5 min q6-8h; IV int inf 50 mg/100 ml D_5 over 15-20 min q6-8h; PO (OTC dose) 75 mg qd-bid

Available forms include: Tabs (OTC) 75 mg; tabs 150, 300 mg; syrup 15 mg/ml; inj IM/IV 0.5, 25 mg/ml; effervesent tabs 75, 150 mg; effervesent granules 150 mg

Side effects/adverse reactions:

CNS: Headache, sleeplessness, dizziness, confusion, agitation, depression, hallucination

CV: Tachycardia, bradycardia, PVCs

GI: ***Hepatotoxicity,*** constipation, abdominal pain, diarrhea, nausea, vomiting

GU: Impotence, gynecomastia

EENT: Blurred vision, increased intraocular pressure

INTEG: Urticaria, rash, fever

Contraindications: Hypersensitivity

Precautions: Pregnancy category B, lactation, child <12 yr, hepatic disease, renal disease

Pharmacokinetics:

PO: Peak 2-3 hr, duration 8-12 hr, half-life 2-3 hr; less than 10% metabolized by liver; excreted in urine, breast milk

Drug interactions of concern to dentistry:

• Decreased absorption of diazepam, ketoconazole (take doses 2 hr apart)

DENTAL CONSIDERATIONS

General:

• Avoid prescribing aspirin-containing products in patients with active GI disease.

• Consider semisupine chair position for patient comfort due to GI effects of disease.

---

repaglinide

(re-pag'lin-ide)

Prandin

Drug class.: Oral antidiabetic, meglitinide class

Action: Lowers blood glucose by stimulation of insulin release from the pancreatic β-cells; binds to ATP-dependent potassium channels in functioning β-cells with opening of calcium channels and subsequent insulin release

Uses: Type 2 diabetes mellitus when hyperglycemia cannot be controlled by diet and exercise. May also be used in combination with metformin.

Dosage and routes:

Adult not previously treated or whose HbA_{1c} is <8%

• *Adult:* PO initial dose 0.5 mg before meals; doses can be given 2, 3, or 4 times/day depending on blood glucose control; dose range 0.5-4.0 mg with limit of 16 mg/day

Adult previously treated with blood glucose–lowering drugs and whose HbA_{1c} is ≥8%

• *Adult:* PO initial dose 1 or 2 mg before meals

Available forms include: Tabs 0.5, 1, 2 mg

Side effects/adverse reactions:

CNS: Headache, paresthesia

CV: Chest pain, angina, palpitation, hypertension, ECG changes

GI: Diarrhea, nausea, vomiting, constipation, dyspepsia

RESP: URI, bronchitis

EENT: Sinusitis, rhinitis

META: Hypoglycemia

MS: Arthralgia, back pain

Contraindications: Hypersensitivity, diabetic ketoacidosis, type 1 diabetes

Precautions: Increased cardiac mortality, hypoglycemia, hypoglycemia in patients taking β-adrenergic blockers, monitor laboratory values, pregnancy category C, lactation, pediatric patients

Pharmacokinetics:

PO: Rapid absorption, bioavailability 56%, peak plasma levels 1 hr; half-life 1 hr; plasma protein binding 98%, hepatic metabolism, metabolites excreted mainly in feces, small amount in urine

Drug interactions of concern to dentistry:

• Clinical studies have not been completed; metabolism may be inhibited by ketoconazole, miconazole, erythromycin

• Risk of increased hypoglycemia: NSAIDs, salicylates

DENTAL CONSIDERATIONS

General:

• If dentist prescribes any of the drugs listed in the drug interactions section, monitor patient blood sugar levels.

• Consider semisupine chair position for patient comfort due to GI side effects of drug.

• Ensure that patient is following prescribed diet and regularly takes medication.

• Place on frequent recall to evaluate healing response.

• Short appointments and a stress reduction protocol may be required.

• Diabetics may be more susceptible to infection and have delayed wound healing.

Consultations:

• Medical consult may include data from patient's blood glucose monitoring, including glycosylated hemoglobin or HbA_{1c} testing.

• Medical consult may be required to assess disease control and patient's ability to tolerate stress.

Teach patient/family:

• To prevent trauma when using oral hygiene aids

R

• Importance of updating health and drug history if physician makes any changes in evaluation/drug regimens

reserpine

(re-ser'peen)

♣ Novoreserpine, Reserfia

Drug class.: Antiadrenergic agent; antihypertensive

Action: Depletes catecholamine stores in CNS and in adrenergic nerve endings

Uses: Hypertension

Dosage and routes:

Hypertension

• *Adult:* PO 0.25-0.5 mg qd for 1-2 wk, then 0.1-0.25 mg qd maintenance

Available forms include: Tabs 0.1, 0.25, 1 mg

Side effects/adverse reactions:

▼ *ORAL: Dry mouth,* bleeding

CNS: Drowsiness, fatigue, lethargy, dizziness, depression, anxiety, headache, increased dreaming, nightmares, convulsions, Parkinsonism, EPS (high doses)

CV: ***Thrombocytopenic purpura,*** bradycardia, chest pain, dysrhythmias, prolonged bleeding time

GI: Nausea, vomiting, cramps, peptic ulcer, increased appetite, anorexia

RESP: Bronchospasm, dyspnea, cough, rales

GU: Impotence, dysuria, nocturia, sodium, water retention, edema, breast engorgement, galactorrhea, gynecomastia

EENT: Lacrimation, miosis, blurred vision, ptosis, epistaxis

INTEG: Rash, purpura, alopecia, flushing, warm feeling, pruritus, ecchymosis

Contraindications: Hypersensitivity, depression, suicidal patients, active peptic ulcer disease, ulcerative colitis, pregnancy category C

Precautions: Pregnancy, lactation, seizure disorders, renal disease

Pharmacokinetics:

PO: Peak 4 hr, duration 2-6 wk, half-life 50-100 hr; metabolized by liver; excreted in urine, feces, breast milk; crosses placenta, blood-brain barrier

Drug interactions of concern to dentistry:

• Increased CNS depression: barbiturates, alcohol, opioids

• Increased pressor effects: epinephrine

• Decreased pressor effects: ephedrine

• Decreased hypotensive effect: indomethacin and possibly other NSAIDs

DENTAL CONSIDERATIONS

General:

• Monitor vital signs every appointment due to cardiovascular side effects.

• Patients on chronic drug therapy may rarely have symptoms of blood dyscrasias, which can include infection, bleeding, and poor healing.

• Assess salivary flow as a factor in caries, periodontal disease, and candidiasis.

• After supine positioning, have patient sit upright for at least 2 min before standing to avoid orthostatic hypotension.

• Limit use of sodium-containing products, such as saline IV fluids, for patients with a dietary salt restriction.

Consultations:

• Medical consult may be required

to assess disease control in the patient.

Teach patient/family:

• Importance of good oral hygiene to prevent soft tissue inflammation

When chronic dry mouth occurs, advise patient:

• To avoid mouth rinses with high alcohol content due to drying effects

• Of need for daily home fluoride to prevent caries

• To use sugarless gum, frequent sips of water, or saliva substitutes

riboflavin (vitamin B_2)

(rey'boo-flay-vin)

Various generic sources

Drug class.: Vitamin B_2, water soluble

Action: Needed for normal tissue respiratory reactions; functions as a coenzyme

Uses: Vitamin B_2 deficiency

Dosage and routes:

• *Adult and child >12 yr:* PO 5-50 mg qd

• *Child <12 yr:* PO 2-10 mg qd

Available forms include: Tabs 5, 10, 25, 50, 100 mg

Side effects/adverse reactions:

GU: Yellow discoloration of urine (large doses)

Contraindications: Child <12 yr

Precautions: Pregnancy category A, lactation

Pharmacokinetics:

PO: Readily absorbed, half-life 65-85 min; 60% protein bound; unused amounts excreted in urine (unchanged)

Drug interactions of concern to dentistry:

• Chronic alcohol use impairs absorption

• Patients taking tricyclic antidepressants or phenothiazines may require supplement

DENTAL CONSIDERATIONS

General:

• Patients deficient in B vitamins, including riboflavin, may have cheilosis, bald tongue, beefy red-colored tongue, glossitis, or anemia.

• Determine why the patient is taking the drug.

Teach patient/family:

• About addition of needed foods that are rich in riboflavin

rifabutin

(rif'a-byoo-ten)

Mycobutin

Drug class.: Antimycobacterial agent

Action: Inhibits DNA-dependent RNA polymerase synthesis of bacterial RNA

Uses: Prevention of disseminated *M. avium* complex (MAC) disease with advanced HIV infection

Dosage and routes:

• *Adult:* PO 300 mg qd

Available forms include: Cap 150 mg

Side effects/adverse reactions:

▼ *ORAL:* Altered taste, colored saliva (brownish-orange)

CNS: Asthenia, headache, anorexia, insomnia

GI: Abdominal pain, flatulence, nausea, vomiting, diarrhea

HEMA: ***Leukopenia, neutropenia, thrombocytopenia***

GU: Discolored urine

INTEG: Rash

MS: Myalgia

MISC: Fever

R

Contraindications: Hypersensitivity, active TB

Precautions: Pregnancy category B, lactation, concurrent corticosteroid therapy

Pharmacokinetics:

PO: Peak 2-4 hr, terminal half-life average 45 hr; moderately protein bound; hepatic metabolism; both renal and fecal excretion

Drug interactions of concern to dentistry:

• Decreases plasma concentrations of corticosteriods; may be significant

DENTAL CONSIDERATIONS

General:

• Examine for evidence of oral signs of opportunistic disease.

• Determine why the patient is taking the drug.

• Patients on chronic drug therapy may rarely have symptoms of blood dyscrasias, which can include infection, bleeding, and poor healing.

Consultations:

• Medical consult may be required to assess patient's ability to tolerate stress.

• In a patient with symptoms of blood dyscrasias, request a medical consult for blood studies and postpone dental treatment until normal values are reestablished.

Teach patient/family:

• To avoid mouth rinses with high alcohol content due to drying effects

• Importance of good oral hygiene to prevent soft tissue inflammation

---

rifampin

(rif'am-pin)

Rifadin, Rifadin IV, Rimactane

🍁 Rofact

Drug class.: Antitubercular antiinfective

Action: Inhibits DNA-dependent RNA polymerase synthesis of bacterial RNA

Uses: Pulmonary TB, meningococcal carriers (prevention); unapproved uses: leprosy and atypical mycobacterial infections

Dosage and routes:

• *Adult:* PO 600 mg/day as single dose 1 hr ac or 2 hr pc

• *Child >5 yr:* PO 10-20 mg/kg/day as single dose 1 hr ac or 2 hr pc; not to exceed 600 mg/day, with other antituberculars

Meningococcal carriers

• *Adult:* PO 600 mg bid × 2 days

• *Child >5 yr:* PO 10 mg/kg bid × 2 days, not to exceed 600 mg/dose

Available forms include: Caps 150, 300 mg

Side effects/adverse reactions:

▼ *ORAL:* Stomatitis, glossitis, candidiasis, bleeding, discolored saliva

CNS: Headache, fatigue, anxiety, drowsiness, confusion

GI: ***Pseudomembranous colitis,*** nausea, vomiting, anorexia, diarrhea, heartburn, pancreatitis

HEMA: ***Hemolytic anemia, eosinophilia, thrombocytopenia, leukopenia***

GU: ***Hematuria, acute renal failure, hemoglobinuria***

EENT: Visual disturbances

INTEG: Rash, pruritus, urticaria, pemphigus-like reaction

MS: Ataxia, weakness

MISC: Flulike symptoms, menstrual disturbances, edema, shortness of breath

Contraindications: Hypersensitivity

Precautions: Pregnancy category C, lactation, hepatic disease, blood dyscrasias, concurrent therapy with corticosteroids

Pharmacokinetics:

PO: Peak 2-3 hr, duration >24 hr, half-life 3 hr; metabolized in liver (active/inactive metabolites); excreted in urine as free drug (30% crosses placenta); excreted in breast milk

Drug interactions of concern to dentistry:

- Increased risk of hepatotoxicity: acetaminophen (chronic use and high doses), alcohol, hydrocarbon inhalation anesthetics (except isoflurane)
- Decreased effects of corticosteroids, dapsone, diazepam, ketoconazole, fluconazole, itraconazole

DENTAL CONSIDERATIONS

General:

- Examine for oral manifestation of opportunistic infections.
- Patients on chronic drug therapy may rarely have symptoms of blood dyscrasias, which can include infection, bleeding, and poor healing.
- Determine why the patient is taking the drug (prophylaxis or active therapy).
- Determine that noninfectious status exists by ensuring that (1) anti-TB drugs have been taken >3 wk, (2) culture has confirmed TB susceptibility to antiinfectives, (3) patient has had three consecutive sputum smears, and (4) patient is not in the coughing stage.

Consultations:

- Medical consult may be required to assess patient's ability to tolerate stress.
- In a patient with symptoms of blood dyscrasias, request a medical consult for blood studies and postpone dental treatment until normal values are reestablished.

Teach patient/family:

- To avoid mouth rinses with high alcohol content due to drying effects
- Importance of good oral hygiene to prevent soft tissue inflammation
- Importance of taking medications for full length of regimen to ensure effectiveness of treatment and to prevent the emergence of resistant strains

---

rifapentine

(rif'a-pen-teen)

Priftin

Drug class.: Antimycobacterial agent

Action: Inhibits DNA-dependent RNA polymerase; bactericidal for *Mycobacterium tuberculosis*

Uses: Pulmonary tuberculosis in combination with other antituberculosis drugs; unlabeled use includes prophylaxis of *Mycobacterium avium* complex in patients with AIDS

Dosage and routes:

- *Adult:* PO in combination with other anti-TB drugs; intensive phase 600 mg twice weekly at an interval of not less than 3 days for 2 mo, then continue once weekly for 4 mo in combination with another anti-TB drug; concomitant use of pyridoxine (B_6) is recommended for malnourished patients,

R

patients predisposed to neuropathy, and adolescents; can give with food

Available forms include: Tabs 150 mg

Side effects/adverse reactions:

NOTE: Adverse effects are reported for combination drug therapy only and may or may not be due solely to rifapentine.

▼ *ORAL:* Reddish discoloration of saliva

CNS: Anorexia, headache, dizziness

CV: Hypertension

GI: Nausea, vomiting, dyspepsia, diarrhea, ***pseudomembranous colitis,*** hyperbilirubinemia

HEMA: Anemia, lymphopenia, thrombocytosis, ***leukopenia, neutropenia***

GU: Hyperuricemia, pyuria, proteinuria, hematuria

EENT: Hemoptysis

INTEG: Rash, pruritus, acne, urticaria

META: Increased ALT, AST

MS: Arthralgia, gout

MISC: Fatigue, reddish discoloration of urine, sweat, tears

Contraindications: Hypersensitivity to rifampin, rifabuten

Precautions: Significant hepatic dysfunction, induces hepatic microsomal enzymes, pregnancy category C, lactation, children <12 yr

Pharmacokinetics:

PO: Slow absorption, peak levels 5-6 hr, highly plasma protein bound (97%-93%), hepatic metabolism, 25-desacetylrifapentine is active metabolite, hepatic metabolism, excreted in feces (70%) and urine (17%)

Drug interactions of concern to dentistry:

• May accelerate metabolism of clarithromycin, doxycycline, ciprofloxacin, fluconazole, ketoconazole, itraconazole, diazepam, barbiturates, corticosteroids, methadone, sildenafil, tricyclic antidepressants

DENTAL CONSIDERATIONS

General:

• Determine why patient is taking the drug (prophylaxis or active therapy).

• Examine for oral manifestation of opportunistic infections.

• Patients on chronic drug therapy may rarely have symptoms of blood dyscrasias, which can include infection, bleeding, and poor healing.

• Determine that noninfectious status exists by ensuring that (1) anti-TB drugs have been taken >3 wk, (2) culture has confirmed TB susceptibility to antiinfectives, (3) patient has had three consecutive negative sputum smears, and (4) patient is not in the coughing stage.

• Consider semisupine chair position for patient comfort due to GI side effects of drug.

Consultations:

• Medical consult may be required to assess disease control and patient's ability to tolerate stress.

• In a patient with symptoms of blood dyscrasias, request a medical consult for blood studies and postpone treatment until normal values are reestablished.

Teach patient/family:

• To avoid mouth rinses with high alcohol content due to drying effects

• To prevent trauma when using oral hygiene aids

• Importance of good oral hygiene to prevent soft tissue inflammation

• Importance of taking medication for full length of regimen to ensure effectiveness of treatment and prevent emergence of resistant strains
• Of potential for extrinsic oral staining side effect

riluzole

(ril′yoo-zole)
Rilutek

Drug class.: Glutamate antagonist

Action: Inhibits presynaptic release of glutamate in CNS; may also interfere with effects of excitatory amino acids and inactivation of voltage-dependent sodium channels

Uses: Treatment of amyotrophic lateral sclerosis (Lou Gehrig's disease)

Dosage and routes:

• *Adult:* PO 50 mg bid 1 hr before morning and evening meals or 2 hr after meals

Available forms include: Tabs 50 mg

Side effects/adverse reactions:

▼ *ORAL: Dry mouth* (3%), stomatitis (1%), candidiasis (0.5%), circumoral paresthesia (1.3%), glossitis

CNS: Asthenia, dizziness, depression, headache, hypertonia, insomnia, incoordination, anorexia

CV: Hypertension, peripheral edema, tachycardia, palpitation, postural hypotension

GI: Nausea, vomiting, dyspepsia, anorexia, diarrhea, flatulence

RESP: Cough, sinusitis

HEMA: ***Neutropenia***

GU: UTI

EENT: Rhinitis

INTEG: Pruritus, eczema

META: Weight loss, liver enzyme abnormalities

MS: Stiffness, worsening of spasticity, fasciculation

Contraindications: Hypersensitivity

Precautions: Hepatic impairment, renal impairment, hypertension, other CNS disorders, pregnancy category C, lactation, children

Pharmacokinetics:

PO: Well absorbed, extensively metabolized by liver, excreted in urine/feces

Drug interactions of concern to dentistry:

• Unknown

DENTAL CONSIDERATIONS

General:

• Short appointments may be required due to nature of disease process.
• Monitor vital signs every appointment due to cardiovascular and respiratory side effects.
• Consider semisupine chair position for patient comfort.
• Assess salivary flow as factor in caries, periodontal disease, and candidiasis.
• Examine for oral manifestation of opportunistic infection.
• Patients on chronic drug therapy may rarely have symptoms of blood dyscrasias, which can include infection, bleeding, and poor healing.
• After supine positioning, have patient sit upright for at least 2 min before standing to avoid orthostatic hypotension.

Consultations:

• Medical consult may be required to assess disease control in the patient.
• In a patient with symptoms of

blood dyscrasias, request a medical consult for blood studies and postpone treatment until normal values are reestablished.

Teach patient/family:

• Instructions for management of oral hygiene, including use of electric toothbrush or directions to caregiver

• That professional oral hygiene home care may be needed

• Caution to prevent trauma when using oral hygiene aids

When chronic dry mouth occurs, advise patient:

• To avoid mouth rinses with high alcohol content due to drying effects

• To use daily home fluoride products for anticaries effect

• To use sugarless gum, frequent sips of water, or saliva substitutes

rimantadine HCl

(ri-man′ta-deen)

Flumadine

Drug class.: Antiviral

Action: May inhibit viral uncoating

Uses: Adult—prophylaxis and treatment of illnesses caused by strains of influenza A virus; child—prophylaxis against influenza A virus

Dosage and routes

Prophylaxis

• *Adult:* PO 100 mg bid; patients with severe hepatic dysfunction, renal failure, and elderly nursing home patients 100 mg/day

• *Child >10 year:* PO use adult dose

• *Child <10 yr:* PO 5 mg/kg once daily, not to exceed 150 mg

Treatment

• *Adult:* PO 100 mg bid; 100 mg/day recommended for patients with severe hepatic dysfunction, patients with renal failure, and elderly nursing home patients; continue therapy for 7 days from initial onset of symptoms

Available forms include: Tabs 100 mg; syrup 50 mg/5 ml in 60, 240, 480 ml

Side effects/adverse reactions:

▼ *ORAL: Dry mouth,* stomatitis, altered taste

CNS: Insomnia, dizziness, headache, fatigue, nervousness, anorexia, depression

CV: Palpitation, hypertension, tachycardia, syncope

GI: Nausea, vomiting, diarrhea, dyspepsia

RESP: Dyspnea

EENT: Tinnitus, eye pain

INTEG: Rash

MS: Asthenia

Contraindications: Hypersensitivity, hypersensitivity to amantadine, nursing mothers, children <1 yr

Precautions: Pregnancy category C, elderly, epilepsy, hepatic or renal impairment, emergence of resistant viral strains

Pharmacokinetics:

PO: Peak plasma levels 6 hr; 40% plasma protein binding; hepatic metabolism; renal excretion

Drug interactions of concern to dentistry:

• Reduced peak plasma levels: aspirin, acetaminophen

DENTAL CONSIDERATIONS

General:

• Monitor vital signs at each appointment due to cardiovascular side effects.

• Determine why the patient is

taking the drug (will probably be used only during peak seasons for influenza).

• Assess salivary flow as a factor in caries, periodontal disease, and candidiasis.

Teach patient/family:

• Importance of good oral hygiene to prevent soft tissue inflammation

When chronic dry mouth occurs, advise patient:

• To avoid mouth rinses with high alcohol content due to drying effects

• Of need for daily home fluoride to prevent caries

• To use sugarless gum, frequent sips of water, or saliva substitutes

rimexolone

(re-mex′oh-lone)

Vexol

Drug class.: Corticosteroid

Action: Glucocorticoids have multiple actions that include antiinflammatory and immunosuppressant effects. They inhibit phospholipase A_2, interfering with or reducing the synthesis of prostaglandins and leukotrienes. They also bind to cytoplasmic glucocorticoid receptors (GRs) and enter the cell nucleus to bind with DNA. This results in the synthesis of various enzymes such as collagenase, elastase, and cytokines that play important roles in inflammation and immunosuppression. They also suppress the production of lymphocytes, monocytes, and eosinophils.

Uses: Inflammation of the eye associated with ocular surgery and uveitis

Dosage and routes:

Ocular surgery

• *Adult:* Opth top after postoperative inflammation, instill 1 or 2 gtt qid beginning 24 hr after surgery; continue up to 2 wk

Uveitis

• *Adult:* Ophth top use 1 or 2 gtt in affected eye qh while awake × 1 wk; then 1 or 2 gtt q2h while awake × 1 week; then reduce dose according to need

Available forms include: Susp 1% in 5, 10 ml droptainers

Side effects/adverse reactions:

▼ *ORAL:* Alteration of taste (rare)

CNS: Headache (rare)

CV: Hypotension (rare)

EENT: Blurred vision, ocular pain, corneal edema, ulceration, increased ocular pressure

INTEG: Pruritus

Contraindications: Hypersensitivity, fungal or herpetic infections of eye

Precautions: Increased intraocular pressure, pregnancy category C, lactation, children, secondary ocular infections

Pharmacokinetics:

OPHTH TOP: Immediate onset, systemic absorption, extensive metabolism, excretion in feces

Drug interactions of concern to dentistry:

• None reported

DENTAL CONSIDERATIONS

General:

• Determine why the patient is taking the drug.

• Protect patient's eyes from accidental spatter during dental treatment.

• Avoid dental light in patient's eyes; offer dark glasses for patient comfort.

risedronate sodium

(ris-ed′roe-nate)
Actonel
Drug class.: Bisphosphonate

Action: Binds to bone hydroxyapatite, inhibits osteoclast-mediated bone resorption, and modulates bone metabolism
Uses: Paget's disease of bone
Dosage and routes:
• *Adult:* PO 30 mg daily × 2 mo, take at least 30 min before first food or drink of the day (other than water), take in upright position with 6-8 oz water, avoid lying down for 30 min after dose is taken; patient should also take supplemental calcium and vitamin D if dietary intake is inadequate
Available forms include: Tabs 30 mg
Side effects/adverse reactions:
CNS: Headache, dizziness
CV: Chest pain, peripheral edema
GI: Diarrhea, abdominal pain, nausea, constipation, belching, colic
RESP: Bronchitis, sinusitis
EENT: Amblyopia, tinnitus, dryness
INTEG: Rash
MS: Asthenia, arthralgia, bone pain, leg cramps, myasthenia
MISC: Flulike symptoms
Contraindications: Hypersensitivity, hypocalcemia
Precautions: Upper GI disease, avoid use in significant renal impairment, pregnancy category C, lactation, pediatric patients
Pharmacokinetics:
PO: Rapid oral absorption, food decreases bioavailability, bisphosphonates are not metabolized, renal excretion, unabsorbed drug excreted in feces

Drug interactions of concern to dentistry:
• Retarded absorption: calcium, antacids, medications with divalent cations
• Increased GI side effects: NSAIDs, aspirin

DENTAL CONSIDERATIONS
General:
• Be aware of the oral manifestations of Paget's disease (macrognathia, alveolar pain).
• Consider semisupine chair position for patient comfort due to GI side effects of drug.
• Short appointments may be required for patient comfort.
Consultations:
• Medical consult may be required to assess disease control in the patient.
Teach patient/family:
• Use of electric toothbrush if patient has difficulty holding conventional devices

risperidone

(ris-per′i-done)
Risperdal
Drug class: Antipsychotic (benzisoxazole derivative)

Action: Unclear, but may be related to antagonism for dopamine(D_2) and serotonin (5-HT_2) receptors; also has affinity for alpha receptors and histamine (H_1) receptors
Uses: Psychotic disorders
Dosage and routes:
• *Adult:* PO initial 1 mg bid; increase by 1 mg bid on second and third day to 3 mg bid (target dose); further dose increase at 1 wk intervals; dose range 4-16 mg/day; re-

duce doses for elderly or debilitated patients or for those with severe renal or hepatic impairment (limit 3 mg/day)
Available forms include: Tabs 0.25, 0.5, 1, 2, 3, 4 mg; oral sol 1 mg/ml

Side effects/adverse reactions:
▼ *ORAL: Dry mouth,* stomatitis, taste alteration (rare)
CNS: Anxiety, ***neuromalignant syndrome,*** *EPS, dystonia, somnolence, hyperkinesia, dizziness,* tardive dyskinesia, syncope, motor impairment, insomnia
CV: Dysrhythmias, orthostatic hypotension, *tachycardia*
GI: Nausea, constipation, dyspepsia
RESP: Cough, dyspnea
HEMA: ***Thrombocytopenia,*** purpura, anemia, leukocytosis, leukopenia (all rare)
GU: Decreased libido, sexual dysfunction (male), menorrhagia, priapism, amenorrhea
EENT: Rhinitis, sinusitis, visual changes
INTEG: Rash, dry skin, photosensitivity
MS: Arthralgia
MISC: Hyperprolactinemia, akathisia

Contraindications: Hypersensitivity

Precautions: Pregnancy category C, lactation, seizures, suicidal patients, cardiac diseases, renal or hepatic impairment, elderly

Pharmacokinetics:
PO: Good absorption, peak plasma levels 1-2 hr; high plasma protein binding; extensive hepatic metabolism (active metabolite); renal excretion

Drug interactions of concern to dentistry:
- Increased excretion: chronic use of carbamazepine
- Increased sedation: other CNS depressants, alcohol, barbiturate anesthesia, opioid analgesics
- Increased extrapyramidal effects: phenothiazines and related drugs (haloperidol, droperidol), metoclopramide
- Additive photosensitization: tetracyclines
- Increased anticholinergic effects: anticholinergics such as atropine and scopolamine

DENTAL CONSIDERATIONS

General:
- Monitor vital signs every appointment due to cardiovascular side effects.
- Patients on chronic drug therapy may rarely have symptoms of blood dyscrasias, which can include infection, bleeding, and poor healing.
- After supine positioning, have patient sit upright for at least 2 min before standing to avoid orthostatic hypotension.
- Assess salivary flow as a factor in caries, periodontal disease, and candidiasis.
- Consider semisupine chair position for patient comfort due to GI effects of drug.
- Assess for presence of extrapyramidal motor symptoms, such as tardive dyskinesia and akathisia. Extrapyramidal motor activity may complicate dental treatment.
- Use vasoconstrictors with caution, in low doses, and with careful aspiration; avoid use of gingival retraction cord with epinephrine.

Consultations:
- In a patient with symptoms of

blood dyscrasias, request a medical consult for blood studies and postpone dental treatment until normal values are reestablished.

• Take precautions if dental surgery is anticipated and anesthesia is required.

• If signs of tardive dyskinesia or other extrapyramidal symptoms are present, refer to physician.

• Physician should be informed if significant xerostomic side effects occur (increased caries, sore tongue, problems eating or swallowing, difficulty wearing prosthesis) so a medication change can be considered.

Teach patient/family:

• Importance of good oral hygiene to prevent soft tissue inflammation

• Caution to prevent injury when using oral hygiene aids

• Use of electric toothbrush if patient has difficulty holding conventional devices

When chronic dry mouth occurs, advise patient:

• To avoid mouth rinses with high alcohol content due to drying effects

• To use daily home fluoride products for anticaries effect

• To use sugarless gum, frequent sips of water, or saliva substitutes

---

ritonavir

(ri-toe′na-veer)

Norvir

Drug class.: Antiviral protease inhibitor

Action: Inhibits HIV-1 and HIV-2 proteases essential for production of HIV virion particles

Uses: Treatment of HIV infection in adults and children as single-drug therapy or in combination with nucleoside analogues

Dosage and routes:

• *Adult:* PO 600 mg bid with food; start with lower doses if nausea is a problem at outset

Available forms include: Caps 100 mg; oral sol 80 mg/ml in 240 ml

Side effects/adverse reactions:

▼ *ORAL: Circumoral paresthesia,* taste alteration, dry mouth

CNS: Headache, dizziness, somnolence, insomnia, anorexia

CV: Hypotension, palpitation, syncope

GI: Nausea, vomiting, abdominal pain, diarrhea

RESP: Cough, asthma, hiccough

HEMA: Anemia

GU: Dysuria

EENT: Pharyngitis

INTEG: Rash, urticaria, acne

MS: Asthenia, arthralgia, weakness

MISC: Peripheral paresthesia, weight loss

Contraindications: Hypersensitivity; **note multiple drug interactions with potential adverse effects**

Precautions: Hepatic impairment, pregnancy category B, lactation, children <12 yr, alters lab chemistry values (triglycerides, ALT, AST, GGT, CPK, uric acid)

Pharmacokinetics:

PO: Peak plasma levels with food 2 hr, hepatic metabolism, active metabolite excreted in feces, highly plasma protein bound (98%), half-life 3-5 hr

Drug interactions of concern to dentistry:

• Contraindicated with alprazolam, clorazepate, diazepam, cisapride, bupropion, estazolam, flurazepam, midazolam, triazolam, zolpidem, meperidine, piroxicam, propoxyphene, chlordiazepoxide, halazepam, quazepam

• Increased plasma levels: clarithromycin, fluconazole, fluoxetine, desipramine, theophylline

• Possible alcohol-disulfiram reaction: metronidazole, disulfiram

• Decreased plasma levels with carbamazepine, dexamethasone, phenobarbital

Multiple drug interactions are reported; check before prescribing dental drugs.

DENTAL CONSIDERATIONS

General:

• Monitor vital signs every appointment due to cardiovascular side effects.

• Examine for oral manifestation of opportunistic infection.

• Place on frequent recall to evaluate healing response.

• Assess salivary flow as a factor in caries, periodontal disease, and candidiasis.

• Consider semisupine chair position for patient comfort due to GI effects of drug.

Consultations:

• Medical consult may be required to assess disease control in the patient.

Teach patient/family:

• Importance of good oral hygiene to prevent soft tissue inflammation

• That secondary oral infection may occur; must see dentist immediately if infection occurs

When chronic dry mouth occurs, advise patient:

• To avoid mouth rinses with high alcohol content due to drying effects

• To use daily home fluoride products for anticaries effect

• To use sugarless gum, frequent sips of water, or saliva substitutes

rizatriptan benzoate

(rye-za-trip'tan)

Maxalt, Maxalt-MLT

Drug class.: Serotonin agonist

Action: A selective agonist for 5-HT_{1D} and 5-HT_{1B} receptors on intracranial vessels leading to vasoconstriction and possibly inhibition of proinflammatory neuropeptide release

Uses: Acute treatment of migraine attacks with or without aura

Dosage and routes:

• *Adult:* PO initial dose 5-10 mg, can repeat dose in 2 hr, limit 30 mg/24 hr

Orally disintegrating tablet (MLT)

• *Adult:* PO remove tablet from sealed pouch immediately before use; place tablet on tongue, allow it to dissolve, and swallow with saliva; 5-10 mg initial dose, can repeat in 2 hr, limit 30 mg/24 hr

Available forms include: Tabs 5, 10 mg; orally disintegrating tab 5, 10 mg

Side effects/adverse reactions:

▼ *ORAL:* Dry mouth

CNS: Fatigue, somnolence, dizziness, paresthesia, euphoria

CV: Palpitation, syncope, orthostatic hypotension

GI: Nausea, diarrhea, vomiting

RESP: Dyspnea, URI

GU: Hot flashes

EENT: Dry throat, nasal congestion, blurred vision, eye dryness

INTEG: Flushing

MS: Muscle weakness, arthralgia

MISC: Asthenia, pain or pressure (chest, neck, throat)

Contraindications: Hypersensi-

tivity, MAO inhibitors, uncontrolled hypertension, ischemic heart disease, cerebrovascular or peripheral vascular disease, ergot-type drugs

Precautions: Risk of serious cardiovascular events, renal/hepatic impairment, SSRI antidepressants, pregnancy category C, lactation, use in children not established

Pharmacokinetics:

PO: Bioavailability 45%, mean peak plasma levels 1-1.5 hr for oral tablet, MLT tablets slower rate of absorption, peak levels 1.6-2.5 hr, metabolized by MAO type A metabolites excreted in urine (82%) and feces (12%), plasma protein binding (14%)

Drug interactions of concern to dentistry:

- Increased plasma levels: propranolol
- No specific interactions with dental drugs reported
- Should not be used within 24 hr of another 5-HT agonist

DENTAL CONSIDERATIONS

General:

- This is an acute-use drug, thus it is doubtful that patients will be treated in the office if acute migraine is present.
- Be aware of patient's disease, its severity, and frequency when known.
- Avoid dental light in patient's eyes; offer dark glasses for patient comfort.
- Short appointments and a stress reduction protocol may be required for anxious patients.
- After supine positioning, have patient sit upright for at least 2 min to avoid orthostatic hypotension.

Consultations:

- If treating chronic orofacial pain, consult with physician of record.
- Medical consult may be required to assess disease control and patient's ability to tolerate stress.

Teach patient/family:

- Importance of updating health and drug history if physician makes any changes in evaluation/drug regimens

rofecoxib

(ro-fa-cox'ib)

Vioxx

Drug class.: Nonsteroidal antiinflammatory analgesic

Action: A selective inhibitor of cyclooxygenase 2 (COX 2) enzymes, thereby preventing the synthesis of prostaglandins

Uses: Relief of signs and symptoms of osteoarthritis; acute pain in adults, including dental pain; and primary dysmenorrhea

Dosage and routes:

Osteoarthritis

- *Adult:* PO initial dose 12.5 mg daily; max recommended dose 25 mg daily

Acute pain and primary dysmenorrhea

- *Adult:* PO 50 mg qd; use for more than 5 days for acute pain has not been studied

Available forms include: Tabs 12.5, 25 mg; oral susp 12.5 mg/5 ml and 25 mg/5 ml in 150 ml volumes

Side effects/adverse reactions:

▼ *ORAL:* Dry mouth, aphthous stomatitis (low incidence)

CNS: Dizziness, fatigue, headache

CV: Hypertension (high dose), edema, PVC, tachycardia, palpitation
GI: Abdominal pain, diarrhea, dyspepsia, heartburn, epigastric discomfort, nausea
RESP: URI, bronchitis
HEMA: Anemia
GU: UTI
EENT: Sinusitis
INTEG: Rash, urticaria
MS: Back pain
MISC: Asthenia, influenza-like disease

Contraindications: Hypersensitivity; patients who have experienced asthma, urticaria, or allergic-type reactions to aspirin or other NSAIDs

Precautions: Serious GI toxicity including ulceration and bleeding; prior history of GI disease (ulcer or bleeding); preexisting asthma, severe renal impairment, severe hepatic impairment, dehydrated patients, fluid retention, CHF, hypertension, pregnancy category C, lactation, children <18 yr; patients should be made aware of potential GI and hepatic side effects

Pharmacokinetics:
PO: Bioavailability 93%, peak plasma levels 2-3 hr; high-fat meal delays peak plasma time; highly plasma protein bound (87%), hepatic metabolism, renal excretion (72%), minor fecal excretion

Drug interactions of concern to dentistry:
- Possible increased GI symptoms: aspirin
- As with other NSAIDs: reduced effectiveness of diuretics, ACE inhibitors
- Decreased plasma levels: rifampin
- Increased plasma levels of lithium, methotrexate, warfarin

DENTAL CONSIDERATIONS
General:
- Assess salivary flow as a factor in caries, periodontal disease, and candidiasis.
- Update health and drug history if physician makes changes in evaluation/drug regimens.
- Monitor vital signs every appointment due to cardiovascular side effects.
- Consider semisupine chair position for patient comfort if GI side effects occur.

Teach patient/family:
- Importance of good oral hygiene to prevent soft tissue inflammation
- Use of electric toothbrush if patient has difficulty holding conventional devices

When chronic dry mouth occurs, advise patient:
- To avoid mouth rinses with high alcohol content due to drying effects
- To use daily home fluoride products for anticaries effect
- To use sugarless gum, frequent sips of water, or saliva substitutes

R

ropinirole HCl

(roe-pin'i-role)
ReQuip
Drug class.: Antiparkinson agent

Action: Acts as a dopamine (D_2 and D_3) receptor agonist in the caudate-putamen region of the brain

Uses: Parkinson's disease

Dosage and routes:
- *Adult:* PO initial 0.25 mg tid with weekly incremental dose increase based on patient response

Dose schedule

Week	Dose	Total daily dose
1	0.25 mg tid	0.75 mg
2	0.5 mg tid	1.5 mg
3	0.75 mg tid	2.25 mg
4	1.0 mg tid	3.0 mg

Available forms include: Tabs 0.25, 0.5, 1, 2, 5 mg

Side effects/adverse reactions:

▼ *ORAL: Dry mouth*

CNS: Confusion, hallucination, drowsiness, somnolence, euphoria, dyskinesia, dizziness, headache

CV: Supraventricular ectopy, postural hypotension, syncope, fatigue, bradycardia

GI: Nausea, vomiting, dyspepsia, constipation

RESP: Bronchitis, URI

HEMA: ***Thrombocytopenia*** (rare), B_{12} deficiency, hypochromic anemia

GU: UTI

EENT: Pharyngitis, blurred vision, rhinitis

INTEG: Sweating

ENDO: Decrease in prolactin levels

META: Increased alkaline phosphotase, increased BUN

MS: Asthenia, leg cramps

MISC: Viral infection

Contraindications: Hypersensitivity

Precautions: Cardiovascular disease, severely impaired renal or hepatic function, lactation, pregnancy category C, syncope, hypotension

Pharmacokinetics:

PO: Peak plasma levels 1-2 hr, good oral absorption, bioavailability 55%, hepatic metabolism, 40% plasma protein binding, urinary excretion of metabolites

Drug interactions of concern to dentistry:

• Possible increase in sedation with all CNS depressants

• Possible diminished effects: dopamine antagonists, phenothiazines, haloperidol, droperidol, and metoclopramide

DENTAL CONSIDERATIONS

General:

• Monitor vital signs every appointment due to cardiovascular side effects.

• Assess salivary flow as factor in caries, periodontal disease, and candidiasis.

• After supine positioning, have patient sit upright for at least 2 min before standing to avoid orthostatic hypotension.

• Patients on chronic drug therapy may rarely have symptoms of blood dyscrasias, which can include infection, bleeding, and poor healing.

• Consider semisupine chair position for patient comfort if GI side effects occur.

Consultations:

• In a patient with symptoms of blood dyscrasias, request a medical consult for blood studies and postpone treatment until normal values are reestablished.

• Medical consult may be required to assess disease control and patient's ability to tolerate stress.

Teach patient/family:

• Caution to prevent trauma when using oral hygiene aids

• Use of electric toothbrush if patient has difficulty holding conventional devices

• Importance of good oral hygiene to prevent soft tissue inflammation

• Importance of updating health

and drug history if physician makes any changes in evaluation/drug regimens

When chronic dry mouth occurs, advise patient:

- To avoid mouth rinses with high alcohol content due to drying effects
- To use daily home fluoride products for anticaries effect
- To use sugarless gum, frequent sips of water, or saliva substitutes

rosiglitazone maleate

(ros-i-gli'ta-zone)

Avandia

Drug class.: Oral antidiabetic

Action: An agonist for peroxisome proliferator-activated receptor gamma (PPAR-γ); improves target cell response to insulin without increasing insulin secretion; insulin must be present for this drug to act

Uses: Monotherapy, as an adjunct to diet and exercise in patients with type 2 diabetes mellitus; may also be used with metformin when metformin, diet, and exercise are not adequate for control

Dosage and routes:

- *Adult:* PO initial dose 4 mg in a single dose or 2 equal doses daily; after evaluation (12 wk) can increase to 8 mg daily

With metformin

- *Adult:* PO 4 mg daily as a single dose or 2 equal doses; after evaluation (12 wk) can increase dose to 8 mg daily

Available forms include: Tabs 2, 4, 8 mg

Side effects/adverse reactions:

CNS: Headache
CV: Edema
GI: Diarrhea
RESP: URI
HEMA: Anemia, decrease hemoglobin/hematocrit
EENT: Sinusitis
META: Hyperglycemia, hypoglycemia, hyperbilirubinemia
MISC: Fatigue

Contraindications: Hypersensitivity, patients with jaundice associated with use of troglitazone, type 1 diabetes

Precautions: May cause resumption of ovulation in premenopausal anovulatory women (risk of pregnancy), patients with edema, advanced heart failure, hepatic impairment, monitor liver enzymes, pregnancy category C, lactation

Pharmacokinetics:

PO: Absolute bioavailability 99%, peak plasma levels approximately 1 hr, half-life 3-4 hr; highly bound to plasma proteins (99.8%), extensive metabolism (CYP450 2C8), excreted mostly in urine (64%)

Drug interactions of concern to dentistry:

- None reported

DENTAL CONSIDERATIONS

General:

- Ensure that patient is following prescribed diet and regularly takes medication.
- Place on frequent recall to evaluate healing response.
- Short appointments and a stress reduction protocol may be required for anxious patients.
- Diabetics may be more susceptible to infection and have delayed wound healing.
- Question patient about self-monitoring of drug's antidiabetic effect, including blood glucose values or finger-stick records.

Consultations:

- Medical consult may include data

from patient's blood glucose monitoring, including glycosylated hemoglobin or HbA_{1c} testing.
• Medical consult may be required to assess disease control and patient's ability to tolerate stress.

Teach patient/family:
• To prevent trauma when using oral hygiene aids
• Importance of updating health and drug history if physician makes any changes in evaluation/drug regimens

salmeterol xinafoate

(sal-me'te-role)

Serevent, Serevent Diskus

Drug class.: Long-acting selective β_2-agonist

Action: Relaxes bronchial smooth muscle by directly acting on β_2-adrenergic receptors; also inhibits release of mast cell mediators

Uses: Bronchospasm associated with COPD, maintenance treatment of asthma and exercise-induced bronchospasm

Dosage and routes:

Bronchospasm and asthma
• *Adult and child >12 yr:* PO inh 2 puffs bid (12 hr apart); avoid higher doses and more frequent use; inh (powder) 1 inhalation of 50 μg bid

Exercise-induced bronchospasm (prevention)
• *Adult and child >12 yr:* 2 puffs 30-60 min before exercise, not more than once q12h and not in patients using the drug on a regular basis

Available forms include: Canisters 13 g containing 120 actuations, 6.5 g containing 60 actuations; inh powder 50 μg/disk

Side effects/adverse reactions:
▼ *ORAL: Dry throat,* dental pain (1%-3%, type or origin not defined)
CNS: Headache, tremors, anxiety, dizziness, vertigo, nervousness, fatigue
CV: Tachycardia, palpitation
GI: Stomachache, nausea, vomiting, diarrhea
RESP: Upper/lower respiratory infections, cough, ***bronchospasm***
GU: Dysmenorrhea
EENT: Ear/nose/throat infections, nasopharyngitis, sinus headache
INTEG: Rash, urticaria
MS: Tremor, joint pain, muscular soreness, myalgia, back pain, muscle cramps, myositis
MISC: Immediate hypersensitivity reactions

Contraindications: Hypersensitivity

Precautions: Pregnancy category C, lactation, children <12 yr, hepatic impairment, coronary insufficiency, dysrhythmias, hypertension, convulsive disorders; **not for acute symptoms,** not to exceed recommended dose, paradoxic bronchospasm may occur with use; not recommended for use with a spacer or other aerosol device

Pharmacokinetics:
PO/INH: Rapid onset 5-15 min, peak 4 hr, duration 12 hr; plasma levels are not used to predict local effects in the lung; 94%-98% plasma protein bound; metabolized in liver; excreted mainly in feces, to a lesser degree in urine

Drug interactions of concern to dentistry:
• Increased cardiovascular effects: tricyclic antidepressants

DENTAL CONSIDERATIONS

General:

• Monitor vital signs every appointment due to cardiovascular and respiratory side effects.

• Be aware that aspirin or sulfite preservatives in vasoconstrictor-containing products can exacerbate asthma.

• Acute asthmatic episodes may be precipitated in the dental office. Rapid-acting sympathomimetic inhalants should be available for emergency use. Salmeterol is not a rapid-acting drug and is not intended for use in acute asthmatic attacks.

• Consider semisupine chair position for patients with respiratory disease.

• Midmorning appointments and a stress reduction protocol may be required for anxious patients.

Consultations:

• Medical consult may be required to assess disease control and stress tolerance in the patient.

Teach patient/family:

• Importance of good oral hygiene to prevent soft tissue inflammation

---

salsalate

(sal'sa-late)

Amigesic, Anaflex 750, Disalcid, Marthritic, Mono-Gesic, Salflex, Salsitab

Drug class.: Salicylate, nonnarcotic analgesic

Action: Blocks formation of peripheral prostaglandins, which cause pain and inflammation; antipyretic action results from inhibition of hypothalamic heat-regulating center; does not inhibit platelet aggregation

Uses: Mild-to-moderate pain or fever, including arthritis, juvenile rheumatoid arthritis

Dosage and routes:

• *Adult:* PO 500-1000 mg in 2 or 3 doses/day

Available forms include: Caps 500 mg; tabs 500, 750 mg

Side effects/adverse reactions:

CNS: Stimulation, drowsiness, dizziness, confusion, ***convulsions,*** headache, flushing, hallucinations, coma

CV: Rapid pulse, ***pulmonary edema***

GI: Nausea, vomiting, GI bleeding, diarrhea, heartburn, anorexia, ***hepatotoxicity***

RESP: Wheezing, hyperpnea

HEMA: ***Thrombocytopenia, agranulocytosis, leukopenia, neutropenia, hemolytic anemia,*** increased prothrombin time

EENT: Tinnitus, hearing loss

INTEG: Rash, urticaria, bruising

ENDO: Hypoglycemia, hyponatremia, hypokalemia, alteration in acid-base balance

Contraindications: Hypersensitivity to salicylates, NSAIDs, GI bleeding, bleeding disorders, children <3 yr, vitamin K deficiency

Precautions: Anemia, hepatic disease, renal disease, Hodgkin's disease, pregnancy category C, lactation

Pharmacokinetics:

PO: Half-life 1 hr; highly protein bound; metabolized by liver; excreted by kidneys; slowly crosses blood-brain barrier and placenta

Drug interactions of concern to dentistry:

• Increased risk of GI complaints

S

and occult blood loss: alcohol, NSAIDs, corticosteroids
• Increased risk of bleeding: oral anticoagulants, valproic acid, dipyridamole
• Avoid prolonged or concurrent use with NSAIDs, corticosteroids, acetaminophen
• Increased risk of hypoglycemia: oral antidiabetics
• Increased risk of toxicity: methotrexate, lithium, zidovudine
• Decreased effects of probenecid, sulfinpyrazone

DENTAL CONSIDERATIONS

General:

• Patients on chronic drug therapy rarely have symptoms of blood dyscrasias, which can include infection, bleeding, and poor healing.
• Potential cross-allergies with other salicylates such as aspirin.
• Consider semisupine chair position for patients with inflammatory joint diseases.
• Avoid prescribing aspirin-containing products because this drug is a salicylate.
• If used for dental patients, take with food or milk to decrease GI complaints; give 30 min before meals or 2 hr after meals; take with a full glass of water.

Consultations:

• In a patient with symptoms of blood dyscrasias, request a medical consult for blood studies and postpone dental treatment until normal values are reestablished.
• Medical consult may be required to assess disease control in the patient.

Teach patient/family:

• That salicylates should not be placed directly on a tooth or oral mucosa due to risk of chemical burns
• Not to exceed recommended dosage; acute toxicity may result
• To read label on other OTC drugs; many contain aspirin
• To avoid alcohol ingestion; GI bleeding may occur
• Importance of good oral hygiene to prevent soft tissue inflammation
• Caution to prevent injury when using oral hygiene aids

saquinavir mesylate

(sa-kwin'a-veer)

Invirase, Fotovase

Drug class.: Antiviral

Action: Inhibits HIV protease important for viral replication

Uses: Used in combination with nucleoside analogs, zidovudine, or zalcitabine in the treatment of AIDS

Dosage and routes:

Invirase

• *Adult:* PO 600 mg tid; take within 2 hr after eating with a nucleoside analog

Fotovase

• *Adult:* PO 1200 mg tid; take within 2 hr after eating with a nucleoside analog

Available forms include: Caps 200 mg

Side effects/adverse reactions:

▼ *ORAL:* Buccal mucosal ulceration (<2%), dry mouth, taste alteration, stomatitis

CNS: Headache, paresthesia, extremity numbness, dizziness, peripheral neuropathy

CV: Hypotension, syncope (infrequent)

GI: Diarrhea, abdominal discomfort, nausea, dyspepsia

RESP: Cough, dyspnea, pharyngitis, rhinitis, sinusitis

HEMA: Anemia, ***thrombocytopenia, pancytopenia***
GU: UTI
EENT: Blepharitis, earache, eye irritation, tinnitus
INTEG: Rash, pruritus, photosensitivity
ENDO: Dry eyes
MS: Musculoskeletal pain, myalgia

Contraindications: Hypersensitivity, rifampin

Precautions: Hepatic impairment, child <16 yr, pregnancy category B, lactation (unknown), bone marrow suppression, renal impairment

Pharmacokinetics:
PO: Peak serum levels 3 hr, serum levels decrease by 8 hr; hepatic metabolism; renal excretion

Drug interactions of concern to dentistry:
- Increased plasma levels of terfenadine, astemizole, clindamycin, troleandomycin, ketoconazole, itraconazole
- Increased metabolism of carbamazepine, dexamethasone, phenobarbital

DENTAL CONSIDERATIONS

General:
- Examine for oral manifestations of opportunistic infections.
- Patients on chronic drug therapy may rarely have symptoms of blood dyscrasias, which can include infection, bleeding, and poor healing.
- Palliative medication may be required for management of oral side effects.

Consultations:
- Medical consult may be required to assess disease control in the patient.
- In a patient with symptoms of blood dyscrasias, request a medical consult for blood studies and postpone dental treatment until normal values are reestablished.

Teach patient/family:
- Importance of good oral hygiene to prevent soft tissue inflammation
- Caution to prevent trauma when using oral hygiene aids
- That secondary oral infection may occur; must see dentist immediately if infection occurs
- Importance of updating medical/drug history if physician makes any changes in evaluation or drug regimen

---

scopolamine (transdermal)

(skoe-pol'a-meen)
Transderm Scop
Transderm-V

Drug class.: Anticholinergic

Action: Competitive antagonism of acetylcholine at receptor sites in the eye, smooth muscle, cardiac muscle, glandular cells; inhibition of vestibular input to the CNS, resulting in inhibition of vomiting reflex

Uses: Prevention of motion sickness; prevent nausea, vomiting associated with anesthesia or opiate analgesia

Dosage and routes:
- *Adult:* Patch 1 placed behind ear 4-5 hr before travel

Not recommended for children

Available forms include: Patch 0.5, 1.5 mg

Side effects/adverse reactions:
ORAL: Dry mouth
CNS: Dizziness, drowsiness, confusion, disorientation, memory disturbances, hallucinations

GU: Difficult urination
EENT: Blurred vision, dilated pupils, altered depth perception, photophobia, dry/itchy/red eyes, acute narrow-angle glaucoma
INTEG: Rash, erythema
Contraindications: Hypersensitivity, glaucoma
Precautions: Children, elderly, pregnancy category C; pyloric, urinary, bladder neck, intestinal obstruction; liver, kidney disease
Pharmacokinetics:
PATCH: Onset 4-5 hr, duration 72 hr

Drug interactions of concern to dentistry:
- Increased anticholinergic effects: propantheline and other anticholinergic drugs
- Increased risk of CNS depression: alcohol, all CNS depressants

DENTAL CONSIDERATIONS
General:
- Avoid dental light in patient's eyes; offer dark glasses for patient comfort.

Teach patient/family:
- To avoid mouth rinses with high alcohol content due to drying effects

---

secobarbital/ secobarbital sodium

(see-koe-bar′bi-tal)
Seconal
Novosecobarb

Drug class.: Sedative-hypnotic barbiturate

Controlled Substance Schedule II, Canada G
Action: Nonselective depression of the CNS, ranging from sedation to hypnosis to anesthesia to coma depending on the dose administered
Uses: Insomnia, sedation, preoperative medication, status epilepticus, acute tetanus convulsions
Dosage and routes:
Insomnia
- *Adult:* PO/IM 100-200 mg hs

Sedation (preoperatively)
- *Adult:* PO 100-200 mg 1-2 hr preoperatively
- *Child:* PO 2-6 mg/kg 1-2 hr preoperatively; rectal up to a max of 100 mg

Status epilepticus
- *Adult and child:* IM/IV 250-350 mg

Available forms include: Caps 50, 100 mg; tabs 100 mg; inj IM/IV 50 mg/ml
Side effects/adverse reactions:
ORAL: Oral ulcerations (rare), bleeding (rare)
CNS: Lethargy, drowsiness, hangover, dizziness, paradoxic stimulation in the elderly and children, light-headedness, dependence, CNS depression, mental depression, slurred speech
CV: Hypotension, bradycardia
GI: Nausea, vomiting, diarrhea, constipation
RESP: ***Apnea, laryngospasm, bronchospasm,*** depression
HEMA: ***Agranulocytosis, thrombocytopenia, megaloblastic anemia*** (long-term treatment)
INTEG: Rash, ***Stevens-Johnson syndrome,*** urticaria, pain, abscesses at injection site, angioedema, thrombophlebitis
Contraindications: Hypersensitivity to barbiturates, respiratory depression, addiction to barbiturates, severe liver impairment, porphyria, uncontrolled severe pain

Precautions: Anemia, pregnancy category D, lactation, hepatic disease, renal disease, hypertension, elderly, acute/chronic pain

Pharmacokinetics:

IM: Onset 10-15 min, duration 3-6 hr

REC: Onset slow, duration 3-6 hr

Half-life 15-40 hr; metabolized by liver; excreted by kidneys (metabolites)

Drug interactions of concern to dentistry:

- Hepatotoxicity: halogenated hydrocarbon anesthetics
- Increased CNS depression: alcohol, all CNS depressants
- Increased metabolism of carbamazepine, tricyclic antidepressants, corticosteroids
- Decreased half-life of doxycycline

DENTAL CONSIDERATIONS

General:

- Determine why the patient is taking the drug.
- Monitor vital signs every appointment due to cardiovascular side effects. Evaluate respiration characteristics and rate.
- Patients on chronic drug therapy may rarely have symptoms of blood dyscrasias, which can include infection, bleeding, and poor healing.

When used for sedation in dentistry:

- Assess vital signs before use and q30min after use as sedative.
- Observe respiratory dysfunction: respiratory depression, character, rate, rhythm; hold drug if respirations <10/min or if pupils are dilated.
- After supine positioning, have patient sit upright for at least 2 min before standing to avoid orthostatic hypotension.
- Have someone drive patient to and from dental office when used for conscious sedation.
- Barbiturates induce liver microsomal enzymes, which alter the metabolism of other drugs.
- Geriatric patients are more susceptible to drug effects; use a lower dose.

Consultations:

- In a patient with symptoms of blood dyscrasias, request a medical consult for blood studies and postpone dental treatment until normal values are reestablished.

Teach patient/family:

- To avoid driving or other activities requiring alertness
- To avoid alcohol ingestion and CNS depressants; serious CNS depression may result
- Caution when using OTC preparations that contain CNS depressants (antihistamines, cold remedies)

selegiline HCl (l-deprenyl)

(se-le'ji-leen)

Carbex, Eldepryl

Apo-Selegiline, Gen-Selegiline, Novo-Selegiline, Nu-Selegiline, SD Deprenyl

Drug class.: Antiparkinson agent

Action: Increased dopaminergic activity by inhibiting MAO type B activity

Uses: Adjunct management of Parkinson's disease in patients being treated with levodopa/carbidopa

S

Dosage and routes:

• *Adult:* PO 10 mg/day in divided doses of 5 mg at breakfast and lunch; doses of 20 mg/day increase the risk of side effects/drug interactions

Available forms include: Tabs 5 mg

Side effects/adverse reactions:

▼ *ORAL:* Dry mouth

CNS: Increased tremors, chorea, restlessness, blepharospasm, increased bradykinesia, grimacing, tardive dyskinesia, dystonic symptoms, involuntary movements, increased apraxia, hallucinations, dizziness, mood changes, nightmares, delusions, lethargy, apathy, overstimulation, sleep disturbances, headache, migraine, numbness, muscle cramps, confusion, anxiety, tiredness, vertigo, personality change, back/leg pain

CV: Orthostatic hypotension, hypertension, dysrhythmia, palpitation, angina pectoris, hypotension, tachycardia, edema, sinus bradycardia, syncope

GI: Nausea, vomiting, constipation, weight loss, anorexia, diarrhea, heartburn, rectal bleeding, poor appetite, dysphagia

RESP: Asthma, shortness of breath

GU: Slow urination, nocturia, prostatic hypertrophy, hesitation, retention, frequency, sexual dysfunction

EENT: Diplopia, blurred vision, tinnitus

INTEG: Increased sweating, alopecia, hematoma, rash, photosensitivity, facial hair

Contraindications: Hypersensitivity; fluoxetine, meperidine

Precautions: Pregnancy category C, lactation, children

Pharmacokinetics:

PO: Rapidly absorbed, peak 0.5-2 hr; rapidly metabolized (active metabolites: *N*-desmethyldeprenyl, l-amphetamine, l-methamphetamine); metabolites excreted in urine

Drug interactions of concern to dentistry:

• ***Fatal interaction:*** opioids (especially meperidine); do not administer together

• Risk of serotonin syndrome: serotonin uptake inhibitors (fluoxetine, sertraline, paroxetine)

DENTAL CONSIDERATIONS

General:

• Monitor vital signs every appointment due to cardiovascular side effects.

• After supine positioning, have patient sit upright for at least 2 min before standing to avoid orthostatic hypotension.

• Assess for presence of extrapyramidal motor symptoms, such as tardive dyskinesia and akathisia. Extrapyramidal motor activity may complicate dental treatment.

• Assess salivary flow as a factor in caries, periodontal disease, and candidiasis.

Consultations:

• Medical consult may be required to assess disease control and patient's ability to tolerate stress.

• If signs of tardive dyskinesia or akathisia are present, refer to physician.

Teach patient/family:

• To use electric toothbrush if patient has difficulty holding conventional devices

When chronic dry mouth occurs, advise patient:

• To avoid mouth rinses with high

alcohol content due to drying effects
• Of need for daily home fluoride to prevent caries
• To use sugarless gum, frequent sips of water, or saliva substitutes

sertraline

(ser'tra-leen)
Zoloft
Drug class.: Antidepressant

Action: Selectively inhibits the uptake of serotonin in the brain
Uses: Major depression, obsessive-compulsive disorder, panic disorder; posttraumatic stress disorder
Dosage and routes:
• *Adult:* PO 50 mg qd; may increase to a max of 200 mg/day; do not change dose at intervals of <1 wk; administer qd in AM or PM
Available forms include: Tabs 50, 100 mg
✤ Caps 25, 50, 100, 150, 200 mg
Side effects/adverse reactions:
▼ *ORAL: Dry mouth,* aphthous stomatitis (<0.1%), taste alteration, lichenoid reaction
CNS: Insomnia, headache, dizziness, somnolence, tremor, fatigue, twitching, confusion
CV: Palpitation, chest pain, postural hypotension, syncope
GI: Diarrhea, nausea, dyspepsia, constipation, anorexia, vomiting, flatulence
RESP: Rhinitis, pharyngitis, coughing
GU: Male sexual dysfunction, micturition disorder
EENT: Vision abnormalities, tinnitus
INTEG: Sweating, rash
MS: Myalgia

Contraindications: Hypersensitivity, MAOIs
Precautions: Pregnancy category B, lactation, elderly, hepatic/renal disease, epilepsy
Pharmacokinetics:
PO: Peak 6-10 hr, elimination half-life 25 hr; plasma protein binding 99%; extensively metabolized; metabolites excreted in urine
Drug interactions of concern to dentistry:
• Increased CNS depression: alcohol, CNS depressants
• Increased side effects: highly protein-bound drugs (aspirin)
• Increased half-life of diazepam

DENTAL CONSIDERATIONS
General:
• Monitor vital signs every appointment due to cardiovascular side effects.
• After supine positioning, have patient sit upright for at least 2 min to avoid orthostatic hypotension.
• Assess salivary flow as a factor in caries, periodontal disease, and candidiasis.
• Avoid dental light in patient's eyes; offer dark glasses for patient comfort.
• Consider semisupine chair position for patient comfort if GI side effects occur.
Consultations:
• Medical consult may be required to assess patient's ability to tolerate stress.
• Physician should be informed if significant xerostomic side effects occur (increased caries, sore tongue, problems eating or swallowing, difficulty wearing prosthesis) so a medication change can be considered.

S

Teach patient/family:
- To use electric toothbrush if patient has difficulty holding conventional devices

When chronic dry mouth occurs, advise patient:
- To avoid mouth rinses with high alcohol content due to drying effects
- Of need for daily home fluoride to prevent caries
- To use sugarless gum, frequent sips of water, or saliva substitutes

---

sibutramine

(si-byoo'tra-meen)

Meridia

Drug class.: Amphetamine analog anorexiant

Controlled Substance Schedule IV

Action: Anoretic action unclear, blocks the reuptake of norepinephrine, serotonin, and dopamine; action depends on formation of two active metabolites, M_1 and M_2

Uses: Obesity

Dosage and routes:
- *Adult:* PO initial dose 10 mg/day; after 4 wk can titrate dose to 15 mg/day; doses >15 mg/day are not recommended

Available forms include: Caps 5, 10, 15 mg

Side effects/adverse reactions:

▼ *ORAL: Dry mouth,* taste prevention

CNS: Headache, insomnia, irritability, asthenia, migraine

CV: Tachycardia, hypertension, palpitation

GI: Abdominal pain, dyspepsia, nausea

GU: Dysmenorrhea, UTI

EENT: Rhinitis, pharyngitis

MS: Back pain, arthralgia

MISC: Flu syndrome

INTEG: Skin rash, dry skin

META: Elevated ALT, AST, alkaline phosphatase

Contraindications: Hypersensitivity, MAO inhibitor, anorexia nervosa, severe hepatic or renal impairment, CAD, CHF, arrhythmias, stroke, other CNS appetite suppressants, meperidine

Precautions: Requires monitoring of BP, risk of serotonin syndrome with other serotonin reuptake inhibitors, glaucoma, pregnancy category C, lactation, children <16 yr, elderly, seizures

Pharmacokinetics:

PO: Rapid absorption, extensive first-pass metabolism, two active metabolites (M_1 and M_2), highly protein bound (94%-97%), hepatic metabolism; excreted mostly in urine, less in feces

Drug interactions of concern to dentistry:
- Avoid use of meperidine: risk of serotonin syndrome

DENTAL CONSIDERATIONS

General:
- Monitor vital signs every appointment due to cardiovascular side effects.
- Assess salivary flow as factor in caries, periodontal disease, and candidiasis.
- Information on any abuse liability is unknown.
- Determine why patient is taking the drug.

Teach patient/family:

When chronic dry mouth occurs, advise patient:
- To avoid mouth rinses with high alcohol content due to drying effects

• Of need for daily home fluoride to prevent caries
• To use sugarless gum, frequent sips of water, or saliva substitutes

sildenafil citrate

(sil-den'a-fil)
Viagra
Drug class.: Impotence therapy

Action: A selective inhibitor of cyclic guanosine monophosphate (cGMP)–specific phosphodiesterase type 5 (PDE5). It enhances the effect of nitric oxide (produced by sexual stimulation) that is involved in increased production of cGMP, all of which are involved in the physiologic processes leading to penile erection. cGMP is required for smooth muscle relaxation in the corpus cavernosum that allows inflow of blood.
Uses: Male erectile dysfunction
Dosage and routes:
• *Adult:* PO (male only) 50 mg taken as needed approximately 1 hr before sexual activity with once-a-day dosing at a maximum. The dosage range is 25-100 mg based on tolerance and effectiveness. It can be taken anywhere from 0.5-4 hr before sexual activity. Sexual activity is required for effective response.
Available forms include: Tabs 25, 50, 100 mg
Side effects/adverse reactions:
▼ *ORAL:* Dry mouth, glossitis (very low incidence)
CNS: Headache, dizziness, insomnia, somnolence, abnormal dreams
CV: Flushing, syncope, palpitation
GI: Dyspepsia, diarrhea, vomiting, dysphagia, gastritis
RESP: Dyspnea, increased cough, asthma
GU: UTI, cystitis, nocturia, urinary frequency, abnormal ejaculation
EENT: Nasal congestion, sinusitis
INTEG: Rash, urticaria, pruritus, contact dermatitis
MS: Musculoskeletal pain, synovitis
Contraindications: Hypersensitivity, patients who are currently using organic nitrates
Precautions: Complete medical and physical exam to determine cause of erectile dysfunction; because of cardiac risk associated with sexual activity, cardiovascular status should be evaluated; anatomic deformation of penis, conditions predisposing to priapism (sickle cell anemia, anemia, multiple myeloma, leukemia), retinitis pigmentosa, not indicated for women, children, or newborns, pregnancy category B; hepatic or renal impairment, men >65 yr
Pharmacokinetics:
PO: Rapid oral absorption, bioavailability 40%, peak plasma levels 30 min-2 hr, hepatic metabolism by cytochrome P-450 enzymes, active metabolite, highly plasma protein bound (96%), major excretion route in feces, lesser route in urine
Drug interactions of concern to dentistry:
• Avoid use of nitroglycerin within 24 hr
• Increased plasma levels due to interference with metabolism: cimetidine, erythromycin, ketoconazole, itraconazole

DENTAL CONSIDERATIONS
General:
• This is an acute-use drug intended to be taken just before

S

sexual activity, and the reported incidence of oral side effects did not differ from a placebo. However, the potential interacting drugs should be avoided.

simvastatin

(sim'va-sta-tin)

Zocor

Drug class.: Antihyperlipidemic

Action: Inhibits HMG-CoA reductase enzyme, which reduces cholesterol synthesis

Uses: As an adjunct in primary hypercholesterolemia and mixed dyslipidemia (types IIa, IIb), treatment of hypertriglyceridemia (Frederickson type IV) and type III hyperlipoproteinemia, to reduce risk of stroke or TIA

Dosage and routes:

• *Adult:* PO 5-10 mg qd with evening meal; may increase to 5-40 mg/day in single or divided doses; not to exceed 40 mg/day; dosage adjustments should be made qmo

Available forms include: Tabs 5, 10, 20, 40, 80 mg

Side effects/adverse reactions:

CNS: Dizziness, headache

GI: Nausea, constipation, diarrhea, dyspepsia, flatulence, abdominal pain, heartburn, ***liver dysfunction***

EENT: Blurred vision, dysgeusia, lens opacities

INTEG: Rash, pruritus

MS: Muscle cramps, myalgia, ***myositis, rhabdomyolysis***

Contraindications: Pregnancy category X, lactation, active liver disease

Precautions: Past liver disease, alcoholics, severe acute infections, trauma, hypotension, uncontrolled seizure disorders, severe metabolic disorders, electrolyte imbalances

Pharmacokinetics:

PO: Peak 1-2.5 hr; highly protein bound; metabolized in liver (active metabolites); excreted in bile, feces

Drug interactions of concern to dentistry:

• Increased myalgia, myositis: erythromycin, cyclosporin, itraconazole

DENTAL CONSIDERATIONS

General:

• Consider semisupine chair position for patient comfort due to GI side effects.

sodium fluoride

Fluoritabs, Flura-Drops, Flurodex Karidium, Luride Lozi-Tabs, Pediaflor, Pedi-Dent, Solu-Flur; also found in pediatric vitamin formulas

Fluor-A-Day, Fluotic

Drug class.: Fluoride ion

Action: Interacts with tooth structure to increase resistance to acid dissolution; promotes enamel remineralization and inhibits dental plaque microorganisms

Uses: Prevention of dental caries, osteoporosis

Dosage and routes:

• *Adult and child >12 yr:* TOP 10 ml 0.2% sol qd after brushing teeth; rinse mouth for >1 min with sol

• *Child 6-12 yr:* TOP 5 ml 0.2% sol

Revised fluoride supplement schedules (infants and children—ADA, American Academy of Pediatric Dentistry, American Academy of Pediatrics)

• Must ascertain fluoride concentration in patient's drinking water before prescribing, as shown in the following tables:

USA—fluoride supplementation schedule

Child's age	<0.3 ppm	0.3-0.6 ppm	>0.6 ppm
birth-6 mo	0.0	0.0	0.0
6 mo-3 yr	0.25 mg/day	0.0	0.0
3-6 yr	0.50 mg/day	0.25 mg/day	0.0
6-16 yr	1.0 mg/day	0.50mg/ day	0.0

Canada—fluoride supplementation schedule

Age	Canadian Paediatric Society (applies to all children)	Canadian Dental Association (Applies to children with high risk of caries)
6 mo-2 yr	0.25 mg/day	0
3-5 yr	0.50 mg/day	0.25 mg/day (0.5 mg/day if fluoridated toothpaste is not used regularly)
6-12 yr	Not applicable	1.00 mg/day
6-16 yr	1.0 mg/day	Not applicable

Reference: Kowalchuk I: New guidelines on fluoride supplementation for children, *CMAJ* 154(7):1007-1008, 1996.

Available forms include: Chew tabs 0.25 mg; tabs 0.5, 1 mg, effervescent tabs 10 mg; drops 0.125, 0.25, 0.5 mg/ml; rinse supplements 0.2 mg/ml; rinse 0.01%, 0.02%, 0.09%; gel 0.1%, 0.5%, 1.23%

Side effects/adverse reactions:

▼ *ORAL:* Mottled enamel (chronic use), stomatitis

ACUTE OVERDOSE: ***Black tarry stools, bloody vomit, diarrhea, decreased respiration, increased salivation, watery eyes***

CHRONIC OVERDOSE: ***Hypocalcemia, tetany, respiratory arrest, constipation, loss of appetite, nausea, vomiting, weight loss***

Contraindications: Hypersensitivity, renal insufficiency, GI ulcerations

Precautions: Child <6 yr (must evaluate total fluoride ingestion), pregnancy category not established

Pharmacokinetics:

PO: Efficient oral absorption; distributed to calcified tissues (bones and teeth); excreted in urine, feces; crosses placenta, excreted in breast milk

Drug interactions of concern to dentistry:

• Avoid use with dairy products and gastric alkalinizers

DENTAL CONSIDERATIONS

General:

• Determine fluoride concentration in water supply, then calculate dosage.

• In the United states, the use of fluoride supplements is not recommended when community drinking water contains at least 0.6 ppm fluoride or after age 16.

• Recommended dose should not be exceeded or dental fluorosis and osseous changes may occur.

• To reduce risk of accidental ingestion and overdosage, ADA recommends that a limit of 264 mg sodium fluoride be dispensed in prepackaged containers.

- Give drops after meals with fluids or undiluted tablets; may be chewed; do not swallow whole; may be given with water or juice; avoid milk.
- Systemic fluoride use during pregnancy has not been shown to prevent tooth decay in children.

Teach patient/family:

- To monitor children using gel or rinse; not to be swallowed
- Not to drink, eat, or rinse mouth for at least 0.5 hr after topical use
- To apply after brushing and flossing hs
- To store out of children's reach

Treatment of acute overdose:

- Gastric lavage with calcium chloride or calcium hydroxide solution to precipitate fluoride
- Maintenance of high urine output
- Refer to hospital emergency facility

sodium fluoride (topical)

Sodium fluoride (topical) nonabrasive: Karigel, Neutracare, Prevident

Sodium fluoride (topical) without abrasive: Prevident 5000 Plus

Drug class.: Fluoride ion

Action: Interacts with enamel surface to increase resistance to acid dissolution; promotes enamel remineralization and inhibits dental plaque microorganisms

Uses: Prevention of dental caries, hypersensitive root surfaces

Dosage and routes:

- *Adult and child >6 yr:* Nonabrasive gels—use daily; apply thin ribbon to toothbrush for at least 1 min after regular brushing, preferably at bedtime; adults expectorate and refrain from eating, drinking, and rinsing; pediatric patients 6-16 yr expectorate and rinse after use; abrasive gels—use as above instead of toothpaste

Available forms include: Gel or cream 2 oz (56 g) squeeze tube 0.5% (as 1.1% sodium fluoride) with and without mild abrasive

Other fluoride topical products include the following daily-use gels: 1.1% APF (Thera-Flur); 0.4% SnF_2 (Control, Easy-Gel, Flocare, Flo-Gel, Florentine, Gel-Kam, Gel-Pro, Gel-Tin, Perfect Choice, Quick-Gel, Stan-Gard, Stop Gel)

Rinses: 0.05% APF daily use (NaF-rinse, Phos-Flur) and 0.2% NaF weekly use (NaFrinse, Point-Two, Preventive, Prevident)

Product strength	Percent F^- ion	ppm F equivalence
1.1% NaF	0.5	4950
0.4% SnF_2	0.10	970
0.2% NaF	0.10	910
0.05% NaF	0.02	230

Contraindications: Hypersensitivity; may be used in areas of fluoridated drinking water

Precautions: Child <6 yr (repeated swallowing of agent could cause dental fluorosis); do not use in pediatric patients <6 yr, infants. Supervise children <6 yr. A 2 oz tube of 1.1% NaF contains 250 mg fluoride, more than twice the amount that the ADA recommends to be dispensed in 1 container. Ingestion of as little as 0.29 oz could cause acute toxicity in a 1-year-old child. Repeated swallowing could cause fluorosis.

DENTAL CONSIDERATIONS
General:
• Neutral sodium fluoride preparations are recommended for patients with exposed root surfaces, which may be hypersensitive.
Teach patient/family:
• To apply daily a thin ribbon of dental cream or gel to toothbrush and brush thoroughly for 2 min, preferably at bedtime
• That adults should expectorate after use and should not eat, drink, or rinse for 30 min
• That children ages 6-16 yr should expectorate after use and rinse mouth thoroughly to avoid swallowing fluoride

---

sotalol HCl

(soe'ta-lole)
Betapace
♣ Sotacor

Drug class.: Nonselective β-adrenergic blocker

Action: This is a nonselective β_1- and β_2-adrenergic antagonist. The antihypertensive mechanism of action is unclear, but it may include a reduction in cardiac output and inhibition of renin release by the renal juxtaglomerular apparatus. Peripheral resistance decreases with long-term use. The antianginal action (when indicated for this use) may be related to a decrease in myocardial oxygen demand and negative chronotropic and inotropic effects. The antiarrhythmic action (when indicated for this use) has been related to a reduction in spontaneous pacemaker firing and slowing of AV nodal conduction.
Uses: Life-threatening ventricular dysrhythmias (class II)

Dosage and routes:
• *Adult:* PO initial 80 mg bid; may be increased gradually to 240 or 320 mg/day; some patients may require 480-640 mg/day
Available forms include: Tabs 80, 160, 240
Side effects/adverse reactions:
CNS: Fatigue, dizziness, asthenia, light-headedness, headache, insomnia, sedation
CV: ***Bradycardia, dysrhythmia, hypotension, CHF, syncope,*** chest pain, palpitation
GI: Nausea, vomiting, dyspepsia
RESP: ***Asthma, dyspnea***
GU: Sexual dysfunction
EENT: Visual problems
INTEG: Rash
Contraindications: Hypersensitivity to this drug, cardiac failure, cardiogenic shock, second- or third-degree heart block, bronchospastic disease, sinus bradycardia, CHF
Precautions: Pregnancy category B, lactation, diabetes mellitus, renal disease
Pharmacokinetics:
PO: Peak plasma levels 2.5-4 hr, half-life 12 hr; low protein binding; excreted in urine unchanged
Drug interactions of concern to dentistry:
• Decreased hypotensive effect: NSAIDs, indomethacin
• Increased hypotension, myocardial depression: hydrocarbon inhalation anesthetics
• Hypertension, bradycardia: sympathomimetics
• Slow metabolism of lidocaine
DENTAL CONSIDERATIONS
General:
• Monitor vital signs every appointment due to cardiovascular side effects.

S

• After supine positioning, have patient sit upright for at least 2 min before standing to avoid orthostatic hypotension.
• Stress from dental procedures may compromise cardiovascular function; determine patient risk.
• Use vasoconstrictors with caution, in low doses, and with careful aspiration. Avoid use of gingival retraction cord with epinephrine.
• Short appointments and a stress reduction protocol may be required for anxious patients.

Consultations:

• Medical consult should be made to assess disease control and patient's ability to tolerate stress.

sparfloxacin

(spar-flox'a-sin)

Zagam

Drug class.: Fluoroquinolone anti-infective

Action: A broad-spectrum bactericidal agent that inhibits the enzyme DNA gyrase needed for bacterial DNA replication

Uses: Community-acquired pneumonia and acute bacterial exacerbations of chronic bronchitis chaused by susceptible microorganisms *(C. pneumoniae, H. influenza, M. pneumonia, S. pneumoniae, K. pneumoniae, M. catarrhalis, S. aureus, E. cloacae)*

Dosage and routes:

• *Adult >18 yr:* PO 400 mg first day, then 200 mg qd for total of 10 days therapy (total 11 tabs)

Renal impairment

• *Adult >18 yr:* PO 400 mg first day; then 200 mg q48h for total of 9 days therapy (6 tabs)

Available forms include: Tabs 200 mg

Side effects/adverse reactions:

▼ *ORAL: Taste alteration,* dry mouth

CNS: Headache, insomnia, convulsions, toxic psychoses, dizziness, light-headedness

CV: Prolonged QT interval, vasodilation, palpitation, postural hypotension

GI: Diarrhea, nausea, dyspepsia, abdominal pain, vomiting, flatulence, ***pseudomembranous colitis***

RESP: Pharyngitis, epistaxis, cough, sinusitis

HEMA: Cyanosis, ecchymosis

GU: Vaginitis, dysuria

EENT: Ear pain, tinnitus, diplopia, eye pain

INTEG: Photosensitization, pruritus

MS: Rupture of Achilles tendon, tendons in shoulder or hand

MISC: ***Anaphylaxis***

Contraindications: Hypersensitivity, photosensitivity, disopyramide, amiodarone, and class Ia and III antiarrhythmics, cisapride, bepridil; patients with prolonged QT_c interval, hypokalemia, significant bradycardia

Precautions: Antacids retard absorption, renal impairment, avoid exposure to sun, artificial ultraviolet light, patients <18 yr, seizures, CV arrhythmics, MI, congestive heart failure, pregnancy category C, lactation

Pharmacokinetics:

PO: Oral bioavailability 92%, peak plasma levels 3-6 hr, hepatic metabolism, equally excreted in urine and feces

Drug interactions of concern to dentistry:

• Avoid concurrent use with erythromycin, cisapride, pentamidine, tricyclic antidepressants, phenothiazines

• Concurrent administration with antacids greatly reduces oral absorption, can increase warfarin levels

DENTAL CONSIDERATIONS

General:

• Contraindicated for patients whose lifestyle or employment will not permit compliance with photosensitivity precautions.

• Determine why patient is taking the drug.

• Assess salivary flow as factor in caries, periodontal disease, and candidiasis.

• Consider semisupine chair position for patient comfort if GI side effects occur.

• Avoid dental light in patient's eyes; offer dark glasses for patient comfort.

Consultations:

• Consult with patient's physician if an acute dental infection occurs and another antiinfective is required.

Teach patient/family:

• To avoid exposure to sunlight and wear sunscreen if sun exposure is planned during treatment and for 5 days after treatment is stopped

spironolactone

(speer-on-oh-lak'tone)

Aldactone

♣ Novospiroton

Drug class.: Potassium-sparing diuretic

Action: Competes with aldosterone at receptor sites in distal tubule, resulting in excretion of sodium chloride, water, retention of potassium and phosphate

Uses: Edema, hypertension, diuretic-induced hypokalemia, primary hyperaldosteronism (diagnosis, short-term treatment, long-term treatment), nephrotic syndrome, cirrhosis of the liver with ascites

Dosage and routes:

Edema/hypertension

• *Adult:* PO 25-200 mg qd in single or divided doses

• *Child:* PO 3.3 mg/kg/day in single or divided doses

Hypokalemia

• *Adult:* PO 25-100 mg/day; if PO, K supplements must not be used

Primary hyperaldosteronism diagnosis

• *Adult:* PO 400 mg/day for 4 days or 4 wk depending on test, then 100-400 mg/day maintenance

Available forms include: Tab 25, 50, 100 mg

Side effects/adverse reactions:

▼ *ORAL:* Gingival bleeding (rare); dry mouth may be a symptom of hyponatremia, lichenoid drug reaction

CNS: Headache, confusion, drowsiness, lethargy, ataxia

GI: Diarrhea, ***bleeding*** (rare), gastritis, cramps, vomiting

HEMA: Decreased WBCs, platelets

INTEG: Rash, pruritus, urticaria

ENDO: Impotence, gynecomastia, irregular menses, amenorrhea, postmenopausal bleeding, hirsutism, deepening voice

ELECT: ***Hyperkalemia,*** hyperchloremic metabolic acidosis, hyponatremia

Contraindications: Hypersensi-

S

tivity, anuria, severe renal disease, hyperkalemia, pregnancy category not established

Precautions: Dehydration, hepatic disease, lactation

Pharmacokinetics:

PO: Onset 24-48 hr, peak 48-72 hr; metabolized in liver; excreted in urine; crosses placenta

Drug interactions of concern to dentistry:

• Nephrotoxicity: indomethacin and possibly other NSAIDs

• Decreased antihypertensive effect: indomethacin and possibly other NSAIDs

DENTAL CONSIDERATIONS

General:

• Monitor vital signs every appointment due to cardiovascular side effects.

• Assess salivary flow as a factor in caries, periodontal disease, and candidiasis.

• If dry mouth occurs, follow usual preventive and palliative measures, but consider hyponatremia as a contributing factor.

• Consider semisupine chair position for patient comfort if GI side effects occur.

Consultations:

• Medical consult may be required to assess disease control and patient's ability to tolerate stress.

Teach patient/family:

When chronic dry mouth occurs, advise patient:

• To avoid mouth rinses with high alcohol content due to drying effects

• Of need for daily home fluoride to prevent caries

• To use sugarless gum, frequent sips of water, or saliva substitutes

stanozolol

(stan-oh'zoe-lole)

Winstrol

Drug class.: Androgenic anabolic steroid

Controlled Substance Schedule III

Action: Reverses catabolic tissue processes; promotes buildup of protein; increases erythropoietin production

Uses: Hereditary angioedema prophylaxis

Dosage and routes:

Angioedema

• *Adult:* PO 2 mg tid, then decrease q1-3mo, down to 2 mg qd or q2d

• *Child 6-12 yr:* PO up to 2 mg/day only during the attack

• *Child <6 yr:* PO 1 mg/day only during the attack

Available forms include: Tabs 2 mg

Side effects/adverse reactions:

CNS: Dizziness, headache, fatigue, tremors, paresthesia, flushing, sweating, anxiety, lability, insomnia

CV: ***Edema*** (in cardiac patients), increased BP

GI: ***Peliosis hepatitis, liver cell tumors, cholestatic jaundice,*** nausea, vomiting, constipation, weight gain

HEMA: Increased prothrombin time, iron deficiency anemia

GU: ***Hematuria,*** amenorrhea, vaginitis, decreased libido, decreased breast size, clitoral hypertrophy, testicular atrophy, gynecomastia (males), priapism

EENT: Conjunctival edema, nasal congestion

INTEG: Rash, acneiform lesions,

oily hair/skin, flushing, sweating, acne vulgaris, alopecia, hirsutism
ENDO: Abnormal GTT, decreased glucose tolerance, increased LDL
MS: Cramps, spasms

Contraindications: Severe renal disease, severe cardiac disease, severe hepatic disease, hypersensitivity, pregnancy category X, lactation, genital bleeding (abnormal), prostate or breast carcinoma in males, breast cancer in females with hypercalcemia, nephrosis

Precautions: Diabetes mellitus, CV disease, MI, increased risk of prostatic hypertrophy, prostatic carcinoma, virilization (women), increased prothrombin time

Pharmacokinetics:
PO: Metabolized in liver, excreted in urine, crosses placenta, excreted in breast milk

Drug interactions of concern to dentistry:

- Increased risk of bleeding: aspirin
- Edema: ACTH, adrenal steroids

DENTAL CONSIDERATIONS

General:

- Determine why the patient is taking the drug.
- Consider local hemostasis measures to prevent excessive bleeding.
- Psychologic and physical dependence may occur with chronic administration.
- Short appointments and a stress reduction protocol may be required for anxious patients.
- Monitor vital signs every appointment due to cardiovascular side effects.
- Avoid prescribing aspirin-containing products.

Consultations:

- If signs of anemia are observed in oral tissues, physician consult may be required.
- Medical consult may be required to assess disease control and patient's ability to tolerate stress.
- Medical consult should include partial prothrombin time, prothrombin time, or INR.

Teach patient/family:

- Importance of good oral hygiene to prevent soft tissue inflammation
- That secondary oral infection may occur; must see dentist immediately if infection occurs

stavudine (d4t)

(stav'yoo-deen)
Zerit

Drug class.: Antiviral, nucleoside analog

Action: A nucleoside analog that undergoes phosphorylation by cellular enzymes and inhibits HIV replication by termination of DNA elongation and inhibition of HIV reverse transcriptase

Uses: Treatment of advanced HIV infection when intolerant of other therapies or if significant deterioration occurs while receiving other therapies

Dosage and routes:

- *Adult:* PO 40 mg bid for patients >60 kg; 30 mg bid for patients <60 kg; dose interval 12 hr apart; doses must be adjusted to creatinine clearance and appearance of peripheral neuropathy
- *Child:* Approved dose information not yet available

Available forms include: Caps 15, 20, 30, 40 mg; powder after reconstitution 1 mg/ml solution in 202 ml

S

Side effects/adverse reactions:
▼ *ORAL:* Ulcerative stomatitis, aphthous stomatitis
CNS: Headache, asthenia, malaise, anorexia, neuropathy, insomnia, anxiety, depression, nervousness
CV: Chest pain
GI: Abdominal pain, diarrhea, nausea, vomiting, ***pancreatitis***
RESP: Dyspnea
HEMA: ***Neutropenia, thrombocytopenia,*** lymphadenopathy
GU: Dysuria
EENT: Conjunctivitis, abnormal vision
INTEG: Rash, pruritus
MS: Myalgia, arthralgia
MISC: Chills, fever, peripheral neurologic symptoms, sweating
Contraindications: Hypersensitivity
Precautions: Pregnancy category C, lactation, children, alcoholism, hepatic or renal impairment; monitor for peripheral neuropathy
Pharmacokinetics:
PO: Rapid absorption, peak plasma levels <1 hr; renal excretion
Drug interactions of concern to dentistry:
• None reported at this time

DENTAL CONSIDERATIONS
General:
• Examine for oral disease.
• Palliative treatment of oral ulcers may be required if they occur.
• Patients on chronic drug therapy may rarely have symptoms of blood dyscrasias, which can include infection, bleeding, and poor healing.
• Consider semisupine chair position for patient comfort due to GI effects of drug.
• Place on frequent recall due to oral side effects and immunocompromised condition.

Consultations:
• Refer to physician if signs of peripheral neuropathy occur.
• In a patient with symptoms of blood dyscrasias, request a medical consult for blood studies and postpone dental treatment until normal values are reestablished.
• Medical consult may be required to assess disease control in the patient.

Teach patient/family:
• Importance of good oral hygiene to prevent soft tissue inflammation
• To prevent injury when using oral hygiene aids
• To see dentist if secondary oral infection occurs
• To report oral lesions, soreness, or bleeding to dentist

---

sucralfate

(soo-kral′fate)
Carafate
Apo-Sucralfate, Sulcrate
Drug class.: Protectant, aluminum salt of a sulfated sucrose

Action: Forms an ulcer-adherent complex that covers and protects the ulcer site
Uses: Duodenal ulcer
Dosage and routes:
• *Adult:* PO 1 g qid 1 hr ac, hs
Available forms include: Tabs 1 g
Side effects/adverse reactions:
▼ *ORAL:* Metallic taste, dry mouth
CNS: Drowsiness, dizziness
GI: Constipation, nausea, gastric pain, vomiting
INTEG: Urticaria, rash, pruritus
Contraindications: Hypersensitivity
Precautions: Pregnancy category B, lactation, children

Pharmacokinetics:
PO: Duration up to 5 hr

Drug interactions of concern to dentistry:

- Gastric irritation: chloral hydrate
- Decreased absorption of tetracyclines, fluoroquinolones

DENTAL CONSIDERATIONS
General:

- Prescribe acetaminophen for analgesia if needed. ASA and NSAIDs are contraindicated in active upper GI disease.
- Consider semisupine chair position for patient comfort due to GI effects of disease.
- Tetracycline doses should be given 2 hr before or after the sucralfate dose.

Teach patient/family:

- To avoid mouth rinses with high alcohol content due to drying effects

---

sulconazole nitrate

(sul-kon'a-zole)
Exelderm
Drug class.: Topical antifungal

Action: Interferes with fungal cell membrane, which increases permeability and leaking of nutrients
Uses: Treatment of tinea pedis, tinea corporis, tinea cruris, tinea versicolor; unapproved use: cutaneous candidiasis
Dosage and routes:

- *Adult:* TOP apply once or twice daily × 3 wk, except tinea pedis use × 4 wk

Available forms include: Cream 1%; sol 1%
Side effects/adverse reactions:
INTEG: Stinging, burning, itching, redness
Contraindications: Hypersensitivity
Precautions: Pregnancy category C
DENTAL CONSIDERATIONS
General:

- There are no significant dental considerations. One possible concern will be those few patients with topical candidiasis, in whom broad-spectrum antiinfectives could potentially contribute to a superinfection.

---

sulfacetamide sodium (ophthalmic)

(sul-fa-see'ta-mide)
AK-Sulf, Bleph-10, Cetamide, Isopto Cetamide, Ocu-Sul, Sodium Sulamyd, Sulfare-Forte, Sulfair, and others
♣ Sulfex
Drug class.: Antibacterial sulfonamide

Action: Inhibits folic acid synthesis by preventing PABA use, which is necessary for bacterial growth
Uses: Conjunctivitis, superficial eye infections, corneal ulcers
Dosage and routes:

- *Adult and child:* Instill 1-2 gtt q2-3h; top apply 0.5-1 inch oint into conjunctival sac qid-tid and hs

Available forms include: Sterile ophth sol 10%, 15%, 30%; sterile ophth oint 10%
Side effects/adverse reactions:
EENT: Burning, stinging, swelling
Contraindications: Hypersensitivity
Precautions: Cross-sensitivity with other sulfas; pregnancy category C

S

Drug interactions of concern to dentistry:
• No specific interactions listed

DENTAL CONSIDERATIONS
General:
• Protect patient's eye from accidental spatter during dental treatment.
• Avoid dental light in patient's eyes; offer dark glasses for patient comfort.

---

sulfamethizole

(sul-fa-meth'i-zole)
Thiosulfil Forte
Drug class.: Sulfonamide, short acting

Action: Interferes with bacterial biosynthesis of proteins by competitive antagonism of PABA
Uses: UTIs
Dosage and routes:
• *Adult:* PO 0.5-1 g tid-qid
• *Child >2 mo:* PO 30-45 mg/kg/day in divided doses q6h
Available forms include: Tabs 500 mg
Side effects/adverse reactions:
▼ *ORAL:* Stomatitis, glossitis
CNS: ***Convulsions,*** headache, confusion, insomnia, hallucinations, depression, vertigo, fatigue, anxiety, drug fever, chills
CV: ***Allergic myocarditis***
GI: Nausea, vomiting, abdominal pain, ***hepatitis, enterocolitis,*** pancreatitis, diarrhea
HEMA: ***Leukopenia, neutropenia, thrombocytopenia, agranulocytosis, hemolytic anemia***
GU: ***Renal failure, toxic nephrosis,*** increased BUN, creatinine, crystalluria
INTEG: ***Stevens-Johnson syndrome,*** erythema, photosensitivity, rash, dermatitis, urticaria
SYST: ***Anaphylaxis***
Contraindications: Hypersensitivity to sulfonamides, pregnancy at term
Precautions: Pregnancy category C, lactation, impaired hepatic function, severe allergy, bronchial asthma
Pharmacokinetics:
PO: Rapidly absorbed, peak 2 hr; 90% bound to plasma proteins; excreted in urine, breast milk; crosses placenta

Drug interactions of concern to dentistry:
• Increased photosensitizing effects: tetracyclines
• Decreased effect of penicillin

DENTAL CONSIDERATIONS
General:
• Determine why the patient is taking the drug.
• Patients on chronic drug therapy may rarely have symptoms of blood dyscrasias, which can include infection, bleeding, and poor healing.
• Consider semisupine chair position for patient comfort if GI side effects occur.

Consultations:
• In a patient with symptoms of blood dyscrasias, request a medical consult for blood studies and postpone dental treatment until normal values are reestablished.
• Medical consult may be required to assess disease control in the patient.

Teach patient/family:
• Importance of good oral hygiene to prevent soft tissue inflammation
• Caution to prevent trauma when using oral hygiene aids

• To report oral lesions, soreness, or bleeding to dentist
• If taking birth control pill, to use additional method of contraception for duration of cycle

sulfamethoxazole

(sul-fa-meth-ox′a-zole)
Gantanol
♣ Apo-Sulfamethoxazole
Drug class.: Sulfonamide

Action: Interferes with bacterial biosynthesis of proteins by competitive antagonism of PABA
Uses: UTIs, lymphogranuloma venereum, systemic infections
Dosage and routes:
• *Adult:* PO 2 g, then 1 g bid or tid for 7-10 days
• *Child >2 mo:* PO 50-60 mg/kg, then 25-30 mg/kg bid, not to exceed 75 mg/kg day
Lymphogranuloma venereum
• *Adult:* PO 1 g bid for 14 days
Available forms include: Tabs 500 mg; oral susp 500 mg/5 ml
Side effects/adverse reactions:
▼ *ORAL:* Stomatitis, glossitis, gingival bleeding
CNS: Headache, insomnia, hallucinations, depression, vertigo, fatigue, anxiety, convulsions, drug fever, chills, drowsiness
CV: ***Allergic myocarditis***
GI: Nausea, vomiting, abdominal pain, ***hepatitis, enterocolitis,*** pancreatitis, diarrhea, anorexia
HEMA: ***Leukopenia, thrombocytopenia, agranulocytosis, hemolytic anemia, aplastic anemia***
GU: ***Renal failure, toxic nephrosis,*** increased BUN, creatinine, crystalluria, hematuria, proteinuria
INTEG: ***Stevens-Johnson syndrome,*** rash, dermatitis, urticaria, erythema, photosensitivity, alopecia
SYST: ***Anaphylaxis***
Contraindications: Hypersensitivity to sulfonamides, sulfonylureas, thiazide, loop diuretics, salicylates, pregnancy at term
Precautions: Pregnancy category C, lactation, impaired hepatic function, severe allergy, bronchial asthma
Pharmacokinetics:
PO: Poorly absorbed, peak 3-4 hr, 50%-70% bound to plasma proteins, half-life 7-12 hr; excreted in urine (unchanged 90%), breast milk; crosses placenta
Drug interactions of concern to dentistry:
• Decreased effect: ester-type local anesthetics (procaine, tetracaine)
• Increased photosensitizing effect: tetracycline
• Decreased effect of penicillins

DENTAL CONSIDERATIONS
General:
• Determine why the patient is taking the drug.
• Patients on chronic drug therapy may rarely have symptoms of blood dyscrasias, which can include infection, bleeding, and poor healing.
• Consider semisupine chair position for patient comfort if GI side effects occur.
• Palliative medication may be required for management of oral side effects.
Consultations:
• Medical consult may be required to assess disease control in the patient.
• In a patient with symptoms of sulfamethoxazole/trimethoprim blood dyscrasias, request a medical

S

consult for blood studies and postpone dental treatment until normal values are reestablished.

Teach patient/family:

• Importance of good oral hygiene to prevent soft tissue inflammation

sulfamethoxazole/trimethoprim (SMZ/TMP) (co-trimazole)

(sulf-a-meth-ox'a-zole)/(tri-meth'o-prim)

Bactrim, Cofatrim Forte, Cotarim, Septra, Sulfatrim (also all DS brands)

♣ Apo-Sulfatrim, Novo-Trimel, Nu-Cotrimox, Roubac

Drug class.: Sulfonamide and folic acid antagonist

Action: Sulfamethoxazole interferes with bacterial biosynthesis of proteins by competitive antagonism of PABA when adequate levels are maintained; trimethoprim blocks synthesis of tetrahydrofolic acid; this combination blocks two consecutive steps in bacterial synthesis of essential nucleic acids/protein

Uses: UTIs, otitis media, acute and chronic prostatitis, shigellosis, *P. carinii* pneumonitis, chronic bronchitis, chancroid

Dosage and routes:

Urinary tract infections

• *Adult:* PO 160 mg TMP/800 mg SMZ q12h × 10-14 days

• *Child:* PO 8 mg/kg TMP/40 mg/kg SMZ qd in 2 divided doses q12h

Otitis media

• *Child:* PO 8 mg/kg TMP/40 mg/kg SMZ qd in 2 divided doses q12h × 10 days

Chronic bronchitis

• *Adult:* PO 160 mg TMP/800 mg SMZ q12h × 14 days

Pneumocystis carinii pneumonitis

• *Adult and child:* PO 20 mg/kg TMP/100 mg/kg SMZ qd in 4 divided doses q6h × 14 days; IV 15-20 mg/kg/day (based on TMP) in 3-4 divided doses for up to 14 days

Dosage reduction necessary in moderate-to-severe renal impairment (CrCl <30 ml/min)

Available forms include: Tabs 80 mg TMP/400 mg SMZ; DS (double strength): 160 mg TMP/800 mg SMZ; susp 40 mg/200 mg/5 ml; IV inj 16 mg/80 mg/ml

Side effects/adverse reactions:

▼ *ORAL:* Candidiasis, glossitis, stomatitis (Stevens-Johnson syndrome), salivary gland pain

CNS: Headache, insomnia, hallucinations, depression, vertigo, fatigue, anxiety, convulsions, drug fever, chills, aseptic meningitis

CV: ***Allergic myocarditis***

GI: Nausea, vomiting, abdominal pain, ***hepatitis, enterocolitis,*** pancreatitis, diarrhea, anorexia

RESP: Cough, shortness of breath

HEMA: ***Leukopenia, neutropenia, thrombocytopenia, agranulocytosis, hemolytic anemia, hypoprothrombinemia, Henoch-Schönlein purpura, methemoglobinemia, eosinophilia***

GU: ***Renal failure, toxic nephrosis,*** increased BUN, creatinine, crystalluria

INTEG: ***Stevens-Johnson syndrome,*** rash, dermatitis, urticaria, erythema, photosensitivity, pain, inflammation at injection site

SYST: ***Anaphylaxis, SLE***

Contraindications: Hypersensitivity to trimethoprim or sulfonamides, pregnancy at term, megaloblastic anemia, infants <2 mo, CrCl <15 ml/min, lactation

Precautions: Pregnancy category C, renal disease, elderly, G6PD deficiency, impaired hepatic function, possible folate deficiency, severe allergy, bronchial asthma

Pharmacokinetics:

PO: Rapidly absorbed, peak 1-4 hr, half-life 8-13 hr; highly bound to plasma proteins; excreted in urine (metabolites and unchanged), breast milk; crosses placenta; TMP achieves high levels in prostatic tissue and fluid

Drug interactions of concern to dentistry:

• None identified

DENTAL CONSIDERATIONS

General:

• Determine why the patient is taking the drug.

• Patients on chronic drug therapy may rarely have symptoms of blood dyscrasias, which can include infection, bleeding, and poor healing.

• Ensure that dental therapy does not interfere with fluid intake.

Consultations:

• In a patient with symptoms of blood dyscrasias, request a medical consult for blood studies and postpone dental treatment until normal values are reestablished.

• Inform physician if antibiotics are required for dental infection.

Teach patient/family:

• Importance of good oral hygiene to prevent soft tissue inflammation

• Caution to prevent injury when using oral hygiene aids

sulfasalazine

(sul-fa-sal'a-zeen)

Asulfidine-En-Tabs, Azulfidine

♣ PMS-Sulfasalazine, Salazopyrin EN-Tab, SAS-500

Drug class.: Sulfonamide derivative with antiinflammatory action

Action: Acts as pro-drug to deliver sulfapyridine and mesalamine (5-aminosalicylic acid) to the colon

Uses: Ulcerative colitis, Crohn's disease, rheumatoid arthritis

Dosage and routes:

• *Adult:* PO 3-4 g/day in divided doses; maintenance 1.5-2 g/day in divided doses q6h

• *Child >2 yr:* PO 40-60 mg/kg/day in 4-6 divided doses, then 20-30 mg/kg/day in 4 doses; max 2 g/day

Available forms include: Tabs 500 mg; oral susp 250 mg/5 ml; enteric-coated tabs 500 mg

Side effects/adverse reactions:

▼ *ORAL:* Stomatitis, glossitis, ulcers (Stevens-Johnson syndrome), bleeding, lichenoid reaction

CNS: Headache, ***convulsions,*** confusion, insomnia, hallucinations, depression, vertigo, fatigue, anxiety, drug fever, chills

CV: ***Allergic myocarditis***

GI: Nausea, vomiting, abdominal pain, anorexia, ***hepatitis,*** pancreatitis, diarrhea

HEMA: ***Leukopenia, neutropenia, thrombocytopenia, agranulocytosis, hemolytic anemia***

GU: Reversible low sperm count, ***renal failure, toxic nephrosis,*** increased BUN, creatinine, crystalluria

INTEG: ***Stevens-Johnson syn-***

S

drome, rash, dermatitis, urticaria, erythema, photosensitivity
SYST: ***Anaphylaxis***
Contraindications: Hypersensitivity to sulfonamides or salicylates, pregnancy at term, child <2 yr, intestinal or urinary obstruction
Precautions: Pregnancy category B, lactation, impaired hepatic function, severe allergy, bronchial asthma, impaired renal function, intolerance to aspirin
Pharmacokinetics:
PO: Partially absorbed, peak 1.5-6 hr, half-life 5-10 hr; excreted in urine as sulfasalazine (15%), sulfapyridine (60%), 5-aminosalicylic acid, and metabolites (20%-33%); excreted in breast milk; crosses placenta
Drug interactions of concern to dentistry:
• Increased photosensitizing effects: tetracycline
• Decreased absorption: folic acid
DENTAL CONSIDERATIONS
General:
• Patients on chronic drug therapy may rarely have symptoms of blood dyscrasias, which can include infection, bleeding, and poor healing.
• Question patient about response to antibiotics to avoid responses that might provoke pseudomembranous colitis.
• Palliative medication may be required for management of oral side effects.
• Consider semisupine chair position for patient comfort due to GI effects of disease.
Consultations:
• Medical consult may be required to assess disease control and patient's ability to tolerate stress.
• In a patient with symptoms of blood dyscrasias, request a medical consult for blood studies and postpone dental treatment until normal values are reestablished.
Teach patient/family:
• Caution to prevent injury when using oral hygiene aids

---

sulfinpyrazone

(sul-fin-peer'a-zone)
Anturane
Anturan, Apo-Sulfinpyrazone, Novopyrazone
Drug class.: Uricosuric

Action: Inhibits tubular reabsorption of urates, with increased excretion of uric acid; inhibits prostaglandin synthesis, which decreases platelet aggregation
Uses: Chronic gouty arthritis
Dosage and routes:
Gout/gouty arthritis
• *Adult:* PO 100-200 mg bid for 1 wk, then 200-400 mg bid, not to exceed 800 mg/day
Available forms include: Tabs 100 mg; caps 200 mg
Side effects/adverse reactions:
ORAL: Bleeding (rare)
CNS: ***Convulsions, coma,*** dizziness
GI: Gastric irritation, nausea, vomiting, anorexia, ***hepatic necrosis,*** GI bleeding
RESP: ***Apnea,*** irregular respirations
HEMA: ***Agranulocytosis*** (rare)
GU: Renal calculi, hypoglycemia
EENT: Tinnitus
INTEG: Rash, dermatitis, pruritus, fever, photosensitivity
Contraindications: Hypersensitivity to pyrazolone derivatives, severe hepatic disease, blood dys-

crasias, severe renal disease, CrCl <50 mg/min, active peptic ulcer, GI inflammation, renal calculi

Precautions: Pregnancy category C, lactation

Pharmacokinetics:

PO: Peak 1-2 hr, duration 4-6 hr, half-life 3 hr; metabolized by liver, excreted in urine

Drug interactions of concern to dentistry:

• Increased bleeding: NSAIDs, aspirin

• Decreased effects of salicylates

DENTAL CONSIDERATIONS

General:

• Consider local hemostasis measures to prevent excessive bleeding.

• Avoid prescribing aspirin-containing products.

• Patients on chronic drug therapy may rarely have symptoms of blood dyscrasias, which can include infection, bleeding, and poor healing.

• Consider semisupine chair position for patient comfort if GI side effects occur.

• Evaluate respiration characteristics and rate.

Consultations:

• In a patient with symptoms of blood dyscrasias, request a medical consult for blood studies and postpone dental treatment until normal values are reestablished.

Teach patient/family:

• Caution to prevent injury when using oral hygiene aids

sulfisoxazole

(sul-fi-sox'a-zole)

Apo-Sulfisoxazole, Novo-Soxazole, Sulfizole

Drug class.: Sulfonamide, short acting; antiinfective

Action: Interferes with bacterial biosynthesis of proteins by competitive antagonism of PABA

Uses: Urinary tract, systemic infections; chancroid; trachoma; toxoplasmosis; acute otitis media; lymphogranuloma venereum; eye infections

Dosage and routes:

• *Adult:* PO 2-4 g loading dose, then 1-2 g qid × 7-10 days

• *Child >2 mo:* PO 75 mg/kg or 2 g/m^2 loading dose, then 120-150 mg/kg/day or 4 g/m^2/day in divided doses q6h, not to exceed 6 g/day

Available forms include: Tabs 500 mg; syr/pediatric susp 500 mg/5 ml

Side effects/adverse reactions:

▼ *ORAL:* Stomatitis, ulcers (Stevens-Johnson syndrome)

CNS: ***Convulsions,*** headache, insomnia, hallucinations, depression, vertigo, fatigue, anxiety, drug fever, chills, drowsiness

CV: ***Allergic myocarditis***

GI: Nausea, vomiting, abdominal pain, ***hepatitis, enterocolitis,*** pancreatitis, diarrhea, anorexia

HEMA: ***Leukopenia, thrombocytopenia, agranulocytosis, hemolytic anemia, aplastic anemia***

GU: ***Renal failure, toxic nephrosis,*** increased BUN, creatinine, crystalluria, hematuria, proteinuria

INTEG: ***Stevens-Johnson syndrome,*** rash, dermatitis, urticaria, erythema, photosensitivity, alopecia

SYST: ***Anaphylaxis***

Contraindications: Hypersensitivity to sulfonamides, sulfonylureas, thiazide, loop diuretics, salicylates, pregnancy at term

Precautions: Pregnancy category C, lactation, impaired hepatic function, severe allergy, bronchial asthma

Pharmacokinetics:

PO: Rapidly absorbed, peak 2-4 hr, half-life 4-7 hr; 85% protein bound; excreted in urine; crosses placenta

Drug interactions of concern to dentistry:

- Decreased effect: ester-type local anesthetics (procaine, tetracaine)
- Increased photosensitizing effect: tetracycline
- Decreased effect of penicillins, cephalosporins

DENTAL CONSIDERATIONS

General:

- Patients on chronic drug therapy may rarely have symptoms of blood dyscrasias, which can include infection, bleeding, and poor healing.
- Determine why the patient is taking the drug.
- Palliative medication may be required for management of oral side effects.
- Consider semisupine chair position for patient comfort if GI side effects occur.

Consultations:

- Medical consult may be required to assess disease control in the patient.
- In a patient with symptoms of blood dyscrasias, request a medical consult for blood studies and postpone dental treatment until normal values are reestablished.

Teach patient/family:

- Importance of good oral hygiene to prevent soft tissue inflammation

---

sulindac

(sul-in'dak)

Clinoril

Apo-Sulin, Novo-Sundac

Drug class.: Nonsteroidal antiinflammatory

Action: Inhibits prostaglandin synthesis by interfering with cyclooxygenase, an enzyme needed for biosynthesis; possesses analgesic, antiinflammatory, antipyretic properties

Uses: Osteoarthritis, rheumatoid arthritis, acute gouty arthritis, tendinitis, bursitis, ankylosing spondylitis

Dosage and routes:

Arthritis

- *Adult:* PO 150 mg bid with food, may increase to 200 mg bid; max dose 400 mg day

Bursitis/acute arthritis

- *Adult:* PO 200 mg bid × 1-2 wk, then reduce dose

Available forms include: Tabs 150, 200 mg

Side effects/adverse reactions:

ORAL: Dry mouth, gingival bleeding, mucosal ulceration and soreness, white spots in mouth or lips, aphthous stomatitis, bitter taste, glossitis, lichenoid reaction

CNS: Dizziness, drowsiness, fatigue, tremors, confusion, insomnia, anxiety, depression

CV: Tachycardia, peripheral edema, palpitations, dysrhythmias

GI: ***Cholestatic hepatitis,*** constipa-

tion, flatulence, cramps, peptic ulcer, nausea, anorexia, vomiting, diarrhea, jaundice
HEMA: ***Blood dyscrasias***
GU: ***Nephrotoxicity: dysuria, hematuria, oliguria, azotemia***
EENT: Tinnitus, hearing loss, blurred vision
INTEG: Purpura, rash, pruritus, sweating
Contraindications: Hypersensitivity, asthma (provoked by aspirin or NSAIDs), severe renal disease, severe hepatic disease, systemic lupus erythematosus
Precautions: Pregnancy category not established, lactation, children, bleeding disorders, GI disorders, cardiac disorders, hypersensitivity to other NSAIDs, geriatric patients
Pharmacokinetics:
PO: Peak 2 hr, half-life 3-3.5 hr; 93% protein binding; metabolized in liver; excreted in urine (metabolites), breast milk
Drug interactions of concern to dentistry:
• Increased bleeding, GI effects: alcohol, aspirin, steroids, other NSAIDs
• Renal toxicity: acetaminophen (prolonged use)
• Possible risk of decreased renal function: cyclosporine
• Increased photosensitizing effect: tetracycline
• Increased toxicity of methotrexate, cyclosporine
• Decreased plasma levels: diflunisal
DENTAL CONSIDERATIONS
General:
• Patients on chronic drug therapy may rarely have symptoms of blood dyscrasias, which can include infection, bleeding, and poor healing.
• Assess salivary flow as a factor in caries, periodontal disease, and candidiasis.
• Avoid prescribing in last trimester of pregnancy.
• Should oral inflammation or lesions occur, refer to physican and consider palliative treatment for the lesions.
• Consider semisupine chair position due to GI side effects, if present.
Consultations:
• Medical consult may be required to assess disease control in the patient.
• In a patient with symptoms of blood dyscrasias, request a medical consult for blood studies and postpone dental treatment until normal values are reestablished.
Teach patient/family:
• To report oral lesions, soreness, or bleeding to dentist
• Caution to prevent injury in use of oral hygiene aids
• Importance of good oral hygiene to prevent soft tissue inflammation
When chronic dry mouth occurs, advise patient:
• To avoid mouth rinses with high alcohol content due to drying effects
• Of need for daily home fluoride to prevent caries
• To use sugarless gum, frequent sips of water, or saliva substitutes

sumatriptan succinate

(soo-ma-trip′tan)
Imitrex
Drug class.: Serotonin agonist

Action: Selective agonist for the vascular 5-HT (serotonin) receptor in cranial arteries, causing vasodilation with little or no effect on peripheral pressure

Uses: Migraine headaches; cluster headaches

Dosage and routes:

• *Adult:* SC 6 mg; max 2 injections/24 hr; side effects may limit dose

• *Adult:* PO 25-100 mg as a single dose; then, if required, 100 mg q2h, not to exceed 300 mg/day. If migraine returns after injection, 1 tab q2h, not to exceed 200 mg/day

• *Adult:* Intranasal 5, 10, or 20 mg as a single dose given in one nostril; dose may be repeated once after 2 hr with a daily limit of 40 mg

Available forms include: Tabs 25, 50, 100 mg; inj 12 mg/ml self-use syringes/vial; nasal spray 5 and 20 mg in 100 μl nasal spray device

Side effects/adverse reactions:

▼ *ORAL:* Discomfort in jaw/mouth/tongue

CNS: Dizziness, vertigo, drowsiness, sedation, headache, anxiety, fatigue

CV: Hypertension, hypotension, bradycardia, palpitation, dysrhythmias, coronary vasospasm

GI: Abdominal discomfort, dysphagia, diarrhea, reflux

RESP: Chest tightness, pressure in chest, dyspnea

GU: Dysuria

EENT: Discomfort in throat/sinuses/nasal cavity, photophobia

INTEG: Redness at injection site, sweating, rashes

MS: Weakness, neck pain, cramps, myalgia

MISC: Tingling, hot or burning sensation, numbness

Contraindications: IV use, ischemic heart disease, MI, uncontrolled hypertension and ergot-containing drugs

Precautions: Pregnancy category C, hepatic and renal impairment, elderly, lactation, children

Pharmacokinetics:

PO: Rapid onset, peak serum levels 5-20 min, terminal half-life 115 min

Drug interactions of concern to dentistry:

• None reported; avoid ergot-containing medications

DENTAL CONSIDERATIONS

General:

• Be aware of the patient's disease, its severity, and frequency when known.

• Monitor vital signs every appointment due to cardiovascular side effects.

• Avoid dental light in patient's eyes; offer dark glasses for patient comfort.

Consultations:

• If treating chronic orofacial pain, consult with physician of record.

Teach patient/family:

• That oral symptoms uncommonly occur and will disappear when drug is discontinued

---

tacrine HCl

(tak'reen)

Cognex

Drug class.: Cholinesterase inhibitor

Action: A centrally acting, reversible inhibitor of cholinesterase enzyme

Uses: Treatment of mild-to-moderate cognitive defects associated with Alzheimer's disease

Dosage and routes:

• *Adult:* PO initially 10 mg qid × 4

wk min; after 4 wk titrate dose to 20 mg qid; higher doses up to 120-160 mg/day in 4 equal doses; monitored every 4 wk, all doses depend on transaminase levels and patient responses

Available forms include: Caps 10, 20, 30, 40 mg

Side effects/adverse reactions:

▼ *ORAL:* Glossitis, dry mouth, stomatitis, increased salivation (variable, low incidence)

CNS: Dizziness, confusion, ataxia, agitation, headache, paresthesia, nervousness, EPS, Bell's palsy (rare)

CV: Hypertension, peripheral edema, bradycardia, hypotension

GI: Increase in serum transaminase levels, nausea, vomiting, diarrhea, ***hepatotoxicity***

RESP: Dyspnea, upper respiratory infection, coughing

HEMA: ***Leukopenia, thrombocytopenia,*** lymphadenopathy, anemia

GU: Urinary frequency or incontinence, infection

EENT: Rhinitis, sinusitis

INTEG: ***Rash,*** flushing of skin

MS: Arthralgia, muscle hypertonia

Contraindications: Hypersensitivity; previously treated patients with jaundice associated with elevated total bilirubin >3 mg/dl

Precautions: Pregnancy category C, cardiovascular disease, GI ulcers, general anesthesia, smokers, liver disease, seizures, asthma, lactation, children, decrease in absolute neutrophil count; liver enzyme monitoring required

Pharmacokinetics:

PO: Peak plasma levels 1-2 hr; plasma levels are higher in females; hepatic metabolism; renal excretion

Drug interactions of concern to dentistry:

• Potential increase in GI complaints: NSAIDs

• Action inhibited by anticholinergic drugs

• Increased effects with succinylcholine and other cholinergic agonists

DENTAL CONSIDERATIONS

General:

• Patients on chronic drug therapy may rarely have symptoms of blood dyscrasias, which can include infection, bleeding, and poor healing.

• Monitor vital signs every appointment due to cardiovascular and respiratory side effects.

• After supine positioning, have patient sit upright for at least 2 min before standing to avoid orthostatic hypotension.

• Assess salivary flow as a factor in caries, periodontal disease, and candidiasis.

• Take precautions if dental surgery is anticipated and anesthesia is required.

• Consider semisupine chair position for patient comfort due to GI effects of drug.

• Place on frequent recall because early attention to dental health is important for Alzheimer's patients.

Consultations:

• Medical consult may be required to assess disease control in the patient.

• In a patient with symptoms of blood dyscrasias, request a medical consult for blood studies and postpone dental treatment until normal values are reestablished.

Teach patient/family:

• Importance of good oral hygiene to prevent soft tissue inflammation

• To prevent injury when using oral hygiene aids
• Use of electric toothbrush if patient has difficulty holding conventional devices

When chronic dry mouth occurs, advise patient:

• To avoid mouth rinses with high alcohol content due to drying effects
• Of need for daily home fluoride to prevent caries
• To use sugarless gum, frequent sips of water, or saliva substitutes

---

tacrolimus (FK506)

(ta-kroe'li-mus)

Prograf

Drug class.: Immunosuppressant

Action: Inhibits T-lymphocyte activation, leading to immunosuppression

Uses: Prophylaxis of organ rejection in patients receiving allogeneic liver or kidney transplants; used in conjunction with steroids; unapproved uses: other transplant tissues, including bone marrow, pancreas, small bowel, also severe recalcitrant psoriasis

Dosage and routes:

• *Adult:* PO initial 0.15-0.30 mg/kg/day in 2 divided doses 12 hr apart no sooner than 6 hr after transplant and 8-12 hr after discontinuing IV infusion dose; IV (if patient cannot take PO) initial 0.05-0.10 mg/kg/day by infusion no sooner than 6 hr after graft
• *Pediatric:* 0.1 mg/kg/day IV and 0.3 mg/kg/day PO; show increased tolerance for doses at high end of adult schedules

Available forms include: Caps 1, 5 mg; inj 5 mg/ml in 1 mg ampule

Side effects/adverse reactions:

▼ *ORAL:* Candidiasis

CNS: Tremors, headache, insomnia, paresthesia, anorexia, neurotoxicity, seizures

CV: Hyperkalemia, hypertension

GI: Diarrhea, nausea, vomiting, constipation

RESP: Pleural effusion, dyspnea

HEMA: Anemia, leukocytosis, thrombocytopenia, lymphoproliferative disorders, lymphoma

GU: ***Nephrotoxicity,*** hyperuricemia, oliguria, UTI

INTEG: Rash, pruritus

MISC: Anaphylaxis, *hyperglycemia*

Contraindications: Hypersensitivity, simultaneous use with cyclosporine, castor oil derivative allergy, potassium-sparing diuretics, lactation

Precautions: Pregnancy category C, renal impairment, hepatic impairment; discontinue cyclosporine doses 24 hr before using this drug

Pharmacokinetics:

PO: Peak levels 1.5-3.5 hr; highly bound to plasma proteins, erythrocytes; liver metabolism; urinary excretion of metabolites

Drug interactions of concern to dentistry:

• No confirmed studies to date: avoid drugs with potential for renal impairment
• Risk of increased blood levels with clotrimazole, fluconazole, ketoconazole, clarithromycin, erythromycin, and methylprednisolone
• Risk of decreased blood levels with carbamazepine, phenobarbital

DENTAL CONSIDERATIONS

General:

• Patients on immunosuppressant therapy have an increased susceptibility to infection.
• Patients on chronic drug therapy

may rarely have symptoms of blood dyscrasias, which can include infection, bleeding, and poor healing.

• Monitor vital signs every appointment due to cardiovascular side effects.

• Prophylactic antibiotics may be indicated to prevent infection if surgery or deep scaling is planned.

• Examine for evidence of oral candidiasis. Topically acting antifungals may be preferred.

Consultations:

• Medical consult may be required to assess disease control in the patient.

• In a patient with symptoms of blood dyscrasias, request a medical consult for blood studies and postpone dental treatment until normal values are reestablished.

• Consult with patient's physician for recommendations for possible antibiotic prophylaxis before dental treatment or when considering the use of systemic antifungals.

Teach patient/family:

• Importance of good oral hygiene to prevent soft tissue inflammation

• Caution to prevent injury when using oral hygiene aids

• Use of electric toothbrush if patient has difficulty holding conventional devices

• That secondary oral infection may occur; must see dentist immediately if infection occurs

• To report oral lesions, soreness, or bleeding to dentist

tamoxifen citrate

(ta-mox'i-fen)

Med Tamoxifen, Nolvadex

🍁 Apo-Tamoxifen, Gen-Tamoxifen, Novo-Tamoxifen, Tamofen, Tamone, Tamoplex

Drug class.: Antineoplastic, antiestrogen hormone

Action: Inhibits cell division by binding to cytoplasmic receptors (estrogen receptors); resembles normal cell complex but inhibits DNA synthesis

Uses: Advanced breast carcinoma that has not responded to other therapy in estrogen receptor–positive patients (usually postmenopausal), to reduce the incidence of breast cancer in healthy women with high risk of developing the disease

Dosage and routes:

• *Adult:* PO 10-20 mg bid or 20 mg daily

Available forms include: Tabs 10, 20 mg

Side effects/adverse reactions:

▼ *ORAL:* Altered taste

CNS: Hot flashes, headache, lightheadedness, depression

CV: Chest pain

GI: Nausea, vomiting

HEMA: ***Thrombocytopenia, leukopenia***

GU: Vaginal bleeding, pruritus vulvae

EENT: Ocular lesions, retinopathy, corneal opacity, blurred vision (high doses)

INTEG: Rash, alopecia

META: Hypercalcemia

Contraindications: Hypersensitivity, pregnancy category D

Precautions: Leukopenia, thrombocytopenia, lactation, cataracts
Pharmacokinetics:
PO: Peak 4-7 hr, half-life 7 days (1 wk terminal); excreted primarily in feces

DENTAL CONSIDERATIONS
General:
• Patients on chronic drug therapy may rarely have symptoms of blood dyscrasias, which can include infection, bleeding, and poor healing.
• Consider semisupine chair position for patient comfort if GI side effects occur.
Consultations:
• Medical consult may be required to assess disease control in the patient.
• In a patient with symptoms of blood dyscrasias, request a medical consult for blood studies and postpone dental treatment until normal values are reestablished.
Teach patient/family:
• Importance of good oral hygiene to prevent soft tissue inflammation

---

tamsulosin HCl

(tam-soo'loe-sin)
Flomax

Drug class.: Adrenoreceptor antagonist

Action: Acts as an antagonist for α-adrenoreceptors in the prostate
Uses: Benign prostatic hyperplasia (BPH)
Dosage and routes:
• *Adult:* PO 0.4 mg given 30 min after the same meal each day; patients failing to respond after 2-4 wk can be increased to 0.8 mg daily

Available forms include: Tabs 0.4 mg
Side effects/adverse reactions:
▼ *ORAL:* Tooth disorder (not defined)
CNS: Dizziness, vertigo, headache, somnolence, insomnia
CV: Orthostatic hypotension
GI: Nausea, diarrhea
RESP: Cough, pharyngitis
GU: Decreased libido, abnormal ejaculation
EENT: Rhinitis, amblyopia
MS: Asthenia, back pain, chest pain
MISC: Infection
Contraindications: Hypersensitivity
Precautions: Potential syncope risk due to hypotension, vertigo, dizziness, carcinoma of prostate, avoid use with other α-adrenoreceptor antagonists, not for use in women, pregnancy category B, lactation, children (not for use)
Pharmacokinetics:
PO: Good oral absorption, maximum plasma levels 4.5 hr (fasting), highly bound to plasma proteins (94%-99%), extensive liver metabolism, renal excretion
Drug interactions of concern to dentistry:
• No interactions reported with usual dental drugs. It is possible but not known that risk of orthostatic hypotension could be increased with conscious sedation techniques.
• Opioids and anticholinergic drugs may enhance urinary retention; use alternative analgesics (NSAIDs)
• Caution in use or avoid concurrent use with other adrenergic antagonists

DENTAL CONSIDERATIONS
General:
• Monitor vital signs every appointment due to cardiovascular and respiratory side effects.
• Consider semisupine chair position for patient comfort when GI side effects occur.
• After supine positioning, have patient sit upright for at least 2 min before standing to avoid orthostatic hypotension.

---

tazarotene topical

(taz-ar′oh-teen)
Tazorac
Drug class.: Topical retinoid

Action: Unclear; binds to retinoid receptors and inhibits mouse ornithine decarboxynase activity associated with cell proliferation and hyperplasia; also inhibits corneocyte accumulation in rhino mouse skin
Uses: Topical treatment in stable plaque psoriasis, mild to moderate facial acne vulgaris
Dosage and routes:
Psoriasis
• *Adult:* TOP apply a thin film once daily in evening to psoriatic lesions to no more than 20% of body surface area; skin should be clean and dry before applying; avoid application to unaffected skin
Acne vulgaris
• *Adult:* TOP apply a thin film once daily in evening to skin area where acne lesions appear; skin should be dry and clean (0.1% gel only)
Available forms include: Topical gel 0.05% and 0.1% in 30 g and 100 g sizes
Side effects/adverse reactions:
INTEG: Pruritus, burning, stinging, erythema, worsening of psoriasis, rash, dermatitis, fissuring, dry skin, bleeding, desquamations
Contraindications: Pregnancy, hypersensitivity, eczematous skin
Precautions: Pregnancy category X, use birth control measures in women of childbearing age, avoid contact with eyes, eyelids, mouth; exposure to tanning (sun, sun lamps) or drugs that cause photosensitivity, lactation, children <12 yr
Pharmacokinetics:
TOP: After application converted to active metabolite by esterase hydrolysis, metabolite highly plasma protein bound (99%); half-life 18 hr; renal and fecal excretion; systemic absorption less than 1%, 4.5% found in stratum corneum layers of epidermis
Drug interactions of concern to dentistry:
• Increased risk of photosensitivity: tetracyclines, fluoroquinolones, phenothiazines
• Caution in use with systemic vitamin A
DENTAL CONSIDERATIONS
General:
• Apply lubricant to dry lips for patient comfort before dental procedures.
• Advise patient if dental drugs are prescribed that have a potential for photosensitivity.
Teach patient/family:
• Should not be used if pregnant
• Avoid application to oral mucous membranes or lips

T

telmisartan

(tel-mi-sar'tan)
Micardis

Drug class.: Angiotensin II (AT_1) receptor antagonist

Action: Blocks the vasoconstrictor and aldosterone releasing effects of angiotensin II

Uses: Hypertension, as a single drug or in combination with other antihypertensives

Dosage and routes:

• *Adult:* PO initial dose 40 mg qd, daily dosage range 20-80 mg

Available forms include: Tabs 40, 80 mg

Side effects/adverse reactions:

CNS: Headache, dizziness, fatigue
CV: Peripheral edema
GI: Diarrhea, dyspepsia, abdominal pain, nausea
RESP: URI, coughing
GU: UTI
EENT: Sinusitis, pharyngitis
MS: Myalgia
MISC: Back pain

Contraindications: Hypersensitivity

Precautions: Discontinue if pregnancy occurs, risk of fetal and neonatal injury, correct volume depletion if present, hepatic impairment, impaired renal function; pregnancy category C (first trimester) and D (second, third trimesters), lactation

Pharmacokinetics:

PO: Peak levels 0.5-1 hr, bioavailability is dose dependent at 40 mg (42%), excreted in feces (97%), some hepatic metabolism, highly plasma protein bound.

Drug interactions of concern to dentistry:

• None reported

DENTAL CONSIDERATIONS

General:

• Monitor vital signs every appointment due to cardiovascular side effects.
• Stress from dental procedures may compromise cardiovascular function; determine patient risk.
• Use precaution if sedation or general anesthesia is required; risk of hypotensive episode.
• Short appointments and a stress reduction protocol may be required for anxious patients.
• Limit use of sodium-containing products such as saline IV fluids for those patients with a dietary salt restriction.

Consultations:

• Medical consult may be required to assess disease control and patient's ability to tolerate stress.

temazepam

(te-maz'e-pam)
Restoril

Drug class.: Benzodiazepine, sedative-hypnotic

Controlled Substance Schedule IV, Canada F

Action: Produces CNS depression at limbic, thalamic, hypothalamic levels of the CNS; interacts with benzodiazepine receptors to facilitate action of the inhibitory neurotransmitter γ-aminobutyric acid (GABA)

Uses: Sedative and hypnotic for insomnia

Dosage and routes:

• *Adult:* PO 15-30 mg hs

Available forms include: Caps 15, 30 mg

Side effects/adverse reactions:
CNS: Lethargy, drowsiness, daytime sedation, dizziness, confusion, light-headedness, headache, anxiety, irritability
CV: Chest pain, pulse changes
GI: Nausea, vomiting, diarrhea, heartburn, abdominal pain, constipation, anorexia
HEMA: ***Leukopenia, granulocytopenia*** (rare)
Contraindications: Hypersensitivity to benzodiazepines, pregnancy category X, lactation, intermittent porphyria
Precautions: Anemia, hepatic disease, renal disease, suicidal individuals, drug abuse, elderly, psychosis, child <18 yr, acute narrow-angle glaucoma
Pharmacokinetics:
PO: Onset 30-45 min, duration 6-8 hr, half-life 8-14 hr; metabolized by liver; excreted by kidneys; crosses placenta; excreted in breast milk

Drug interactions of concern to dentistry:
• Increased action of both drugs: alcohol, all CNS depressants

DENTAL CONSIDERATIONS
General:
• Psychologic and physical dependence may occur with chronic administration.
• Geriatric patients are more susceptible to drug effects; use lower dose.

Teach patient/family:
• Importance of good oral hygiene to prevent soft tissue inflammation

terazosin HCl

(ter-ay′zoe-sin)
Hytrin
Drug class.: Antihypertensive, antiadrenergic

Action: Decreases total vascular resistance, which is responsible for a decrease in BP; this occurs by blockade of α_1-adrenoreceptor
Uses: Hypertension as a single agent or in combination with diuretics or β-blockers; benign prostatic hypertrophy
Dosage and routes:
• *Adult:* PO 1 mg hs; usual dose range 1-5 mg daily; may increase dose slowly to desired response; not to exceed 20 mg/day
Benign prostatic hypertrophy
• *Adult:* PO initial dose 1 mg hs; increase dose by increasing daily to achieve the desired response; 10 mg/day may be required
Available forms include: Tabs 1, 2, 5, 10 mg
Side effects/adverse reactions:
▼ *ORAL:* Dry mouth
CNS: Dizziness, headache, drowsiness, anxiety, depression, vertigo, weakness, fatigue
CV: Orthostatic hypotension, palpitation, tachycardia, edema, rebound hypertension
GI: Nausea, vomiting, diarrhea, constipation, abdominal pain
RESP: Dyspnea, pharyngitis, rhinitis
GU: Urinary urgency, incontinence, impotence
EENT: Epistaxis, tinnitus, red sclera, nasal congestion, sinusitis
Contraindications: Hypersensitivity
Precautions: Pregnancy category C, children, lactation

T

Pharmacokinetics:
PO: Peak 1 hr, half-life 9-12 hr; highly bound to plasma proteins; metabolized in liver; excreted in urine, feces

Drug interactions of concern to dentistry:
• Decreased effects: NSAIDs, indomethacin

DENTAL CONSIDERATIONS
General:
• Monitor vital signs every appointment due to cardiovascular side effects.
• After supine positioning, have patient sit upright for at least 2 min before standing to avoid orthostatic hypotension.
• Assess salivary flow as a factor in caries, periodontal disease, and candidiasis.
• Limit use of sodium-containing products, such as saline IV fluids, for patients with a dietary salt restriction.
• Consider semisupine chair position for patient comfort if GI side effects occur.

Teach patient/family:
When chronic dry mouth occurs, advise patient:
• To avoid mouth rinses with high alcohol content due to drying effects
• Of need for daily home fluoride to prevent caries
• To use sugarless gum, frequent sips of water, or saliva substitutes

terbinafine HCl

(ter-bin'a-feen)
Lamisil

Drug class.: Antifungal, systemic

Action: Inhibits key enzyme, squalene epoxidase, involved with sterol synthesis with resultant fungal cell death

Uses: Treatment of onychomycosis of the toenail or fingernail caused by dermatophytes (tinea unguium)

Dosage and routes:
Fingernail onychomycosis
• *Adult:* PO 250 mg qd × 6 wk
Toenail onychomycosis
• *Adult:* PO 250 mg qd × 12 wk

Available forms include: Tabs 250 mg

Side effects/adverse reactions:
▼ *ORAL: Taste disturbances*
GI: Diarrhea, dyspepsia, abdominal pain, nausea, flatulence, cholestatic hepatitis (rare)
HEMA: ***Severe neutropenia*** (rare), transient decrease in absolute lymphocyte counts
INTEG: Rash, urticaria, pruritus
META: Abnormal liver tests
MS: Arthralgia, myalgia
MISC: Malaise, fatigue

Contraindications: Hypersensitivity

Precautions: Preexisting liver or renal disease, pregnancy category B, use not recommended during nursing, pediatric patients

Pharmacokinetics:
PO: Bioavailability 40%, peak plasma levels approximately 2 hr; highly plasma protein bound (99%), extensive metabolism, excreted in urine (70%)

Drug interactions of concern to dentistry:
• None reported

DENTAL CONSIDERATIONS
General:
• Determine why patient is taking the drug.
• Consider semisupine chair position for patient comfort if GI side effects occur.

• Patients on chronic drug therapy may rarely have symptoms of blood dyscrasias, which can include infection, bleeding, and poor healing.

Consultations:

• In a patient with symptoms of blood dyscrasias, request a medical consult for blood studies and postpone treatment until normal values are reestablished.

Teach patient/family:

• Importance of good oral hygiene to prevent soft tissue inflammation

• To prevent trauma when using oral hygiene aids

terbinafine HCl (topical)

(ter-bin′a-feen)

Lamisil, Lamisil AT, Lamisil Derma-Gel

Drug class.: Antifungal

Action: Inhibits key enzyme, squalene epoxidase, involved with sterol synthesis with resultant fungal cell death

Uses: Tinea pedis, tinea cruris, tinea corporis; unapproved uses: cutaneous candidiasis, tinea versicolor

Dosage and routes:

• *Adult:* TOP apply to affected area bid until symptoms show significant improvement, usually 7-14 days; duration usually 7 days, but should not exceed 4 wk

Available forms include: Cream 1% in 15, 30 g containers

Side effects/adverse reactions:

INTEG: Irritation, burning, drying, itching

Contraindications: Hypersensitivity

Precautions: Pregnancy category B, lactation, children <12 yr

Drug interactions of concern to dentistry:

• None reported

terbutaline sulfate

(ter-byoo′ta-leen)

Brethaire, Brethine, Bricanyl

Drug class.: Selective β_2-agonist

Action: Relaxes bronchial smooth muscle by direct action on β_2-adrenergic receptors

Uses: Bronchospasm, asthma prophylaxis, premature labor inhibitor

Dosage and routes:

Bronchospasm

• *Adult and child >6 yr:* Inh 2 puffs qmin, then q4-6h; PO 2.5-5 mg q8h; SC 0.25 mg q8h

Premature labor

• *Adult:* IV inf 0.01 mg/min, increased by 0.005 mg q10min, not to exceed 0.025 mg/min; SC 0.25 mg qh; PO 5 mg q4h × 48 hr, then 5 mg q6h as maintenance for above doses

Available forms include: Tabs 2.5, 5 mg; aerosol 0.2 mg/actuation; inj 1 mg/ml in 2 ml ampules

Side effects/adverse reactions:

▼ *ORAL:* Dry mouth, unusual taste

CNS: Tremors, anxiety, insomnia, headache, dizziness, stimulation

CV: Palpitation, tachycardia, hypertension, ***cardiac arrest***

GI: Nausea, vomiting

Contraindications: Hypersensitivity to sympathomimetics, narrow-angle glaucoma, tachydysrhythmias

Precautions: Pregnancy category B, cardiac disorders, hyperthyroidism, diabetes mellitus, prostatic hy-

T

pertrophy, lactation, elderly, hypertension, glaucoma

Pharmacokinetics:

PO: Onset 0.5 hr, duration 4-8 hr

SC: Onset 6-15 min, duration 1.5-hr

INH: Onset 5-30 min, duration 3-6 hr

Drug interactions of concern to dentistry:

• Increased CNS side effects: other sympathomimetics

• Risk of dysrhythmias with halogenated-hydrocarbon anesthetics

• Increased vascular side effects: tricyclic antidepressants

DENTAL CONSIDERATIONS

General:

• Consider semisupine chair position for patients with respiratory disease.

• Monitor vital signs every appointment due to cardiovascular side effects.

• Assess salivary flow as a factor in caries, periodontal disease, and candidiasis.

• Be aware that aspirin or sulfite preservatives in vasoconstrictor-containing products can exacerbate asthma.

• Acute asthmatic episodes may be precipitated in the dental office. Sympathomimetic inhalants should be available for emergency use.

• Midday appointments and a stress reduction protocol may be required for anxious patients.

Teach patient/family:

• For inhalation dosage forms: to rinse mouth with water after each dose to help prevent dryness

• Use of electric toothbrush if patient has difficulty holding conventional devices

When chronic dry mouth occurs, advise patient:

• To avoid mouth rinses with high alcohol content due to drying effects

• Of need for daily home fluoride to prevent caries

• To use sugarless gum, frequent sips of water, or saliva substitutes

terconazole

(ter-kone'a-zole)

Terazol 3, Terazol 7

Drug class.: Local antifungal

Action: Interferes with fungal DNA replication; binds sterols in fungal cell membranes, which increases permeability, leaking of nutrients

Uses: Vaginal, vulval, vulvovaginal candidiasis (moniliasis)

Dosage and routes:

• *Adult:* Vag 5 g (1 applicator) hs × 3-7 days depending on dose form selected for use; suppos 1 hs × 3 days

Available forms include: Vag cream 0.4%; vag suppos 80 mg

Side effects/adverse reactions:

GU: Vulvovaginal burning, itching, pelvic cramps

INTEG: Rash, urticaria, stinging, burning

MISC: Headache, body pain

Contraindications: Hypersensitivity

Precautions: Children <2 yr, pregnancy, lactation

DENTAL CONSIDERATIONS

General:

• Be aware that broad-spectrum antibiotics can exacerbate vaginal candidiasis.

testosterone/ testosterone cypionate/ testosterone enanthate/testosterone propionate

(tess-toss'ter-one)

Testosterone (IM use only): Andro-100, Histerone-50, Histerone-100, Testamone-100, Testaqua, Testoject-50

♣ Malogen

Testosterone cypionate (IM use only): Andro-Cyp, Andronate, depAndro, Depotest, Duratest, Testoject, Testred Cypionate, Virilon IM

♣ Depo-Testosterone

Testosterone enanthate (IM use only): Andro LA, Andropository, Andryl 200, Delalest, Test-PA, Testone LA

♣ Delatestryl, Malogex

Testosterone propionate (IM use only): Testex

♣ Malogen

Testosterone transdermal: Testaderm

Drug class.: Androgen, anabolic steroid

Controlled Substance Schedule III

Action: In many tissues testosterone is converted to dihydrotestosterone, which interacts with cytoplasmic protein receptors to increase protein production; natural hormone that functions to regulate spermatogenesis and male secondary sex characteristics; also functions as an anabolic steroid

Uses: Treatment of androgen deficiency, delayed puberty, female breast cancer, certain anemias, gender changes, cryptorchidism

Dosage and routes:

Replacement therapy

- *Adult (male):* IM 50-400 mg q2-4wk (cypionate or enanthate)
- *Adult (male):* IM 25-50 mg 2-3 × weekly (testosterone or propionate)
- *Adult (male):* Scrotal patch 1 patch (4 or 6 mg) q22-24h

Breast cancer

- *Adult (female):* IM 200-400 mg q2-4 wk (cypionate or enanthate)
- *Adult (female):* IM 50-100 mg 3 × weekly (testosterone or propionate)

Delayed puberty

- *Child (male):* M 100 mg (max) per mo up to 4-6 mo (all forms)

Available forms include: Propionate inj IM 100 mg/ml; enanthate inj IM 100, 200 mg/ml; cypionate inj IM 50, 100, 200 mg/ml; testosterone IM 25, 50, 100 mg/ml; scrotal patch 4, 6 mg

Side effects/adverse reactions:

CNS: Dizziness, headache, fatigue, tremors, paresthesias, flushing, sweating, anxiety, lability, insomnia

CV: ***Edema*** (in cardiac patients), increased BP

GI: ***Hepatic necrosis*** (rare), ***cholestatic jaundice,*** nausea, vomiting, constipation, weight gain

HEMA: Increased prothrombin time, iron deficiency anemia

GU: Amenorrhea, gynecomastia (males), hematuria, priapism, vaginitis, decreased libido, decreased breast size, clitoral hypertrophy, testicular atrophy

EENT: Conjunctional edema, nasal congestion

INTEG: Rash, acneiform lesions,

T

oily hair/skin, flushing, sweating, acne vulgaris, alopecia, hirsutism
ENDO: Abnormal GTT
MS: Cramps, spasms, hypercalcification in breast
Contraindications: Severe renal disease, severe cardiac disease, severe hepatic disease, hypersensitivity, pregnancy category X, lactation, genital bleeding (abnormal), prostate or breast carcinoma (males), breast cancer in females with hypercalcemia
Precautions: Diabetes mellitus, CV disease, MI, increased risk of prostatic hypertrophy, prostatic carcinoma, virilization (women), increased prothrombin time
Pharmacokinetics:
IM: Highly protein bound, metabolized in liver, half-life 10-20 min; excreted in urine, breast milk; crosses placenta
PATCH: Absorption from scrotal skin much higher than other skin sites, half-life 10-100 min, peak levels 2-4 hr

Drug interactions of concern to dentistry:
- Increased risk of bleeding: aspirin
- Edema: ACTH, adrenal steroids

DENTAL CONSIDERATIONS
General:
- Avoid prescribing aspirin-containing products.
- Determine why the patient is taking the drug.
- Consider local hemostasis measures to prevent excessive bleeding.
- Short appointments and a stress reduction protocol may be required for anxious patients.
- Prophylactic antibiotics may be indicated to prevent infection if surgery or deep scaling is planned.
- Physician consult may be required if signs of anemia are observed in oral tissues.

Consultations:
- Medical consult may be required to assess disease control and patient's ability to tolerate stress.
- Medical consult should include partial prothrombin or prothrombin times.

Teach patient/family:
- Importance of good oral hygiene to prevent soft tissue inflammation
- Alert the patient to the possibility of secondary oral infection and the need to see dentist immediately if infection occurs

tetracaine/tetracaine HCl (topical)

(tet′ra-cane)
Pontocaine, Pontocaine Cream
Drug class.: Topical anesthetic (ester group)

Action: Inhibits nerve impulses from sensory nerves, which produces anesthesia
Uses: Local anesthesia of mucous membranes, pruritus, sunburn, sore throat, cold sores, oral pain, rectal pain and irritation, control of gagging
Dosage and routes:
- *Adult:* TOP apply to affected area using smallest effective amount at point of needle insertion
- *Adult and adolescent:* Aerosol spray 2 metered sprays (1.4 mg); adult limit 20 mg

Available forms include: Oint 0.5%; cream 1%; metered spray 0.7 mg/spray
Side effects/adverse reactions:
INTEG: Rash, irritation, sensitization, dermatitis

MISC: Hypersensitivity reactions (systemic), angioedema
More severe systemic reactions can be observed if excessive absorption leads to toxic doses
Contraindications: Hypersensitivity, infants <1 yr, application to large areas, PABA allergies
Precautions: Child <12 yr, sepsis, pregnancy category C, lactation, local infection, geriatric, debilitated patient
Pharmacokinetics:
TOP: Onset 3-10 min, duration up to 60 min; metabolized in plasma when absorbed; excreted in urine
Drug interactions of concern to dentistry:
- Specific drug interactions are not listed; it would be wise to use with caution in patients taking tocainide, mexiletine; significant systemic absorption could lead to synergistic and potentially toxic effects

DENTAL CONSIDERATIONS
General:
- Apply smallest effective dose; apply to small area because significant absorption can occur, especially from denuded areas.
- Absorption of excessive amounts of drug may lead to signs of local anesthetic toxicity; with correct use, toxicity is a rare event.
- Use aerosol with caution; advise patient not to inhale spray.
- Use for topical anesthesia or temporary relief of symptoms; reevaluate if symptoms persist.
- Toxic amounts can be absorbed from denuded mucosa or skin.
- Apply with cotton-tipped applicator by pressing, not rubbing, paste on lesion.

Teach patient/family:
- How to apply
- Not to chew gum or eat while numbness is present after dental treatment

Symptoms of systemic toxicity could include:
- Nervousness, nausea, excitement followed by drowsiness, convulsions, cardiac and respiratory depression
- Symptoms may vary because they depend on the amount of drug actually absorbed

---

tetracycline/tetracycline HCl

(tet-ra-sye'kleen)
Achromycin, Helidac Therapy, Panmycin, Robitet, Sumycin, Tetracyn
♣ Apo-Tetra, Novotetra, Nu-Tetra
Drug class.: Tetracycline, broad-spectrum antibiotic

Action: Inhibits protein synthesis and phosphorylation in microorganisms; bacteriostatic
Uses: Syphilis, *C. trachomatis,* gonorrhea, lymphogranuloma venereum, *M. pneumoniae,* rickettsial infections, acne, actinomycosis, anthrax, bronchitis, GU infections, sinusitis, and many other infections produced by susceptible organisms; *H. pylori*–associated duodenal ulcer
Dosage and routes:
- *Adult:* PO 250-500 mg q6h 1 hr before or 2 hr after meals; IM 250 mg/day or 150 mg q12h; IV 250-500 mg q8-12h
- *Child >8 yr:* PO 25-50 mg/kg/day in divided doses q6h 1 hr before or 2 hr after meals; IM 15-25 mg/kg/day in divided doses q8-12h; IV 10-20 mg/kg/day in divided doses q12h

T

Gonorrhea
• *Adult:* PO 1.5 g, then 500 mg qid for a total of 9 g over 7 days
Chlamydia trachomatis
• *Adult:* PO 500 mg qid × 7 days
Syphilis
• *Adult:* PO 2-3 g in divided doses × 10-15 days; must treat 30 days if syphilis duration >1 yr
Urethral syndrome in women
• *Adult:* PO 500 mg qid × 7 days
Acne
• *Adult:* 1 g/day in divided doses; maintenance 125-500 mg/day
Available forms include: Oral susp 125 mg/5 ml; caps 100, 200, 500 mg; tabs 100, 250, 500 mg
Side effects/adverse reactions:
▼ *ORAL: Tooth discoloration in children <8 yr, candidiasis, tongue discoloration and hypertrophy of papilla,* enamel hypoplasia, bleeding (long-term use), stomatitis, lichenoid drug reaction, erythema multiforme
CNS: Fever, headache, paresthesia
CV: Pericarditis
GI: Nausea, abdominal pain, vomiting, diarrhea, anorexia, ***hepatotoxicity,*** enterocolitis, flatulence, abdominal cramps, epigastric burning
HEMA: ***Eosinophilia, neutropenia, thrombocytopenia, leukocytosis, hemolytic anemia***
GU: Increased BUN
EENT: Dysphagia
INTEG: Rash, urticaria, photosensitivity, increased pigmentation, ***exfoliative dermatitis, angioedema,*** pruritus
Contraindications: Hypersensitivity to tetracyclines, children <8 yr, pregnancy category D, lactation
Precautions: Renal disease, hepatic disease

Pharmacokinetics:
PO: Peak 2-3 hr, duration 6 hr, half-life 6-10 hr; 20%-60% protein bound; excreted in urine; crosses placenta; excreted in breast milk
Drug interactions of concern to dentistry:
• Decreased absorption: $NaHCO_3$, other antacids
• Decreased effect of penicillins, cephalosporins

DENTAL CONSIDERATIONS
General:
• Determine why the patient is taking tetracycline.
• Broad-spectrum antibiotics may be a factor in oral or vaginal *Candida* infections.
• Advise patient if dental drugs prescribed have a potential for photosensitivity.
Consultations:
• Medical consult may be required to assess disease control in the patient.
Teach patient/family:
• Importance of good oral hygiene to prevent soft tissue inflammation
• Caution to prevent injury when using oral hygiene aids
• To avoid milk products; to take with a full glass of water
• To take tetracycline doses 1 hr before or 2 hr after air polishing device (Prophy Jet), if used
When used for dental infection, advise patient:
• Taking birth control pill to use additional method of contraception for duration of cycle
• To report sore throat, oral burning sensation, fever, fatigue, any of which could indicate superinfection
• To take at prescribed intervals and complete dosage regimen

• To immediately notify the dentist if signs or symptoms of infection increase

tetracycline periodontal fiber

(tet-ra-sye'kleen)

Actisite

Drug class.: Tetracycline, broad-spectrum antiinfective

Action: Antimicrobial effect related to inhibition of protein synthesis; decreases incidence of postsurgical inflammation and edema; suppresses bacteria and acts as a barrier to bacterial entry; acts on cementum or fibroblasts to enhance periodontal ligament regeneration

Uses: Adjunctive treatment in adult periodontitis

Dosage and routes:

• *Fiber:* Adjust length to fit pocket depth and contour of teeth treated; fiber should contact base of pocket; apply cyanoacrylate adhesive to secure fiber for 10 days; replace if lost before 7 days; up to 11 teeth can be treated

Available forms include: Topical supplied in boxes of 10 fibers, each 23 cm long and each with 12.7 mg tetracycline

Side effects/adverse reactions:

▼ *ORAL: Gingival inflammation and pain, glossitis,* local erythema, candidiasis, staining of tongue

EENT: Minor throat irritation

INTEG: Photosensitivity

Contraindications: Hypersensitivity, children <8 yr, acutely abscessed periodontal pocket

Precautions: Pregnancy category C, lactation, children, superinfection, patients with predisposition to candidiasis; must remove fibers after 10 days

Pharmacokinetics:

TOP: In vitro release rate 2 μg/cm/hr; gingival concentration maintained over 10 days; plasma levels below detectable limits

Drug interactions of concern to dentistry:

• It is not known if the tetracycline fiber will decrease the effectiveness of oral contraceptives; however, manufacturer recommends suggesting the use of an alternative form of contraception during the remaining cycle to female patients taking oral contraceptives

DENTAL CONSIDERATIONS

General:

• Take precautions regarding allergy to tetracyclines.

• Examine oral mucosa for candidiasis before placing fiber.

Teach patient/family:

• Do not chew hard, crusty, or sticky foods

• Do not brush or floss near treated area, but clean other teeth

• Avoid other oral hygienic practices that could dislodge fibers, such as the use of toothpicks

• Do not probe or pick at the treated area

• Notify dentist if fiber dislodges or falls out

• Notify dentist if pain, swelling, or other symptoms occur

theophylline/ theophylline sodium glycinate

(thee-off'i-lin)

Aerolate Sr, Asmalix, Elixophyllin, Quibron-T, Lanophyllin, Respbid, Slo-Bid, Slo-Phyllin, Theobid, Theo-clear, Theo-Dur, Theo-Dur Sprinkle, Theolair, Theo-24, Theovent, Uni-Dur, Uniphyl

♣ Apo-Theo-LA, PMS-Theophylline

Drug class.: Xanthine

Action: Relaxes smooth muscle of respiratory system by blocking phosphodiesterase, which increases cAMP

Uses: Bronchial asthma, bronchospasm of COPD, chronic bronchitis; unapproved use: apnea in the neonate

Dosage and routes:

Bronchospasm, bronchial asthma

• *Adult:* PO 100-200 mg q6h, dosage must be individualized; rec 250-500 mg q8-12h

• *Child:* PO 50-100 mg q6h, not to exceed 12 mg/kg/24 hr

COPD, chronic bronchitis

• *Adult:* PO 330-660 mg q6-8h pc (sodium glycinate)

• *Child >12 yr:* PO 220-330 mg q6-8h pc (sodium glycinate)

• *Child 6-12 yr:* PO 330 mg q6-8h pc (sodium glycinate)

• *Child 3-6 yr:* PO 110-165 mg q6-8h pc (sodium glycinate)

• *Child 1-3 yr:* PO 55-110 mg q6-8h pc (sodium glycinate)

Available forms include: Caps 50, 100, 200, 250 mg; tabs 100, 125, 200, 225, 250, 300 mg; time rel tabs 100, 200, 250, 300, 400, 500 mg; time rel caps 50, 65, 100, 125 mg; thiamine HCl (vitamin B_1) 130, 200, 250, 260, 300, 400, 500 mg; elix 80, 11.25 mg/15 ml; sol 80 mg/15 ml; liq 80, 150, 160 mg/15 ml; susp 300 mg/15 ml

Side effects/adverse reactions:

▼ *ORAL:* Bitter taste, dry mouth

CNS: Anxiety, restlessness, insomnia, dizziness, convulsions, headache, light-headedness, muscle twitching

CV: Palpitation, sinus tachycardia, hypotension, other dysrhythmias

GI: Nausea, vomiting, anorexia, diarrhea, dyspepsia, gastric distress

RESP: Increased rate

INTEG: Flushing, urticaria

Contraindications: Hypersensitivity to xanthines, tachydysrhythmias

Precautions: Elderly, CHF, cor pulmonale, hepatic disease, active peptic ulcer disease, diabetes mellitus, hyperthyroidism, hypertension, children, pregnancy category C

Pharmacokinetics:

PO: Peak 1 hr; metabolized in liver; excreted in urine, breast milk; crosses placenta

Drug interactions of concern to dentistry:

• Increased action: erythromycin, ciprofloxacin

• Increased risk of cardiac dysrhythmia: halothane inhalation anesthesia, CNS stimulants

• Decreased effect: barbiturates, carbamazepine, ketoconazole

• May decrease sedative effects of benzodiazepines

DENTAL CONSIDERATIONS

General:

• Consider semisupine chair posi-

tion for patients with respiratory disease.

• Monitor vital signs every appointment due to cardiovascular side effects.

• Assess salivary flow as a factor in caries, periodontal disease, and candidiasis.

• Be aware that aspirin or sulfite preservatives in vasoconstrictor-containing products can exacerbate asthma.

• Acute asthmatic episodes may be precipitated in the dental office. Sympathomimetic inhalants should be available for emergency use.

• Midday appointments and a stress reduction protocol may be required for anxious patients.

Consultations:

• Medical consult may be required to assess disease control in the patient.

Teach patient/family:

When chronic dry mouth occurs, advise patient:

• To avoid mouth rinses with high alcohol content due to drying effects

• Of need for daily home fluoride to prevent caries

• To use sugarless gum, frequent sips of water, or saliva substitutes

---

thiamine HCl (vitamin B_1)

(thye'a-min)

Bewon, Biamine

♣ Betaxin

Drug class.: Vitamin B_1, water soluble

Action: Needed for carbohydrate metabolism

Uses: Vitamin B_1 deficiency or prophylaxis, beriberi, Wernicke-Korsakoff syndrome

Dosage and routes:

Recommended dietary allowance (RDA)

• *Adult:* PO men 1.2-1.5 mg; women 1.0-1.1 mg; pregnant women 1.5 mg; lactating women 1.6 mg

• *Child:* PO ages 1-3, 0.7 mg; ages 4-6, 0.9 mg; ages 7-10, 1 mg

Beriberi

• *Adult (critical):* IM or slow IV 5-100 mg tid; use injection only when necessary

• *Adult:* PO 5-10 mg tid with multivitamin, then RDA (dose recommendations are highly variable)

• *Infant (mild):* PO 10 mg qd

Alcohol-induced deficiency:

• *Adult:* PO 40 mg qd

Available forms include: Tabs 10, 25, 50, 100, 250, 500 mg; enteric-coated tabs 20 mg; inj IM/IV 100, 200 mg/ml

Side effects/adverse reactions:

NOTE: Parenteral doses are more likely to cause severe adverse reactions

▼ *ORAL:* ***Angioedema***

CNS: Weakness, restlessness

CV: ***Collapse, pulmonary edema,*** hypotension

GI: Nausea, diarrhea, hemorrhage

EENT: Tightness of throat

INTEG: Cyanosis, sweating, warmth

SYST: ***Anaphylaxis*** (after parenteral doses)

Contraindications: None known

Precautions: Pregnancy category A, sensitivity to thiamine, Wernicke's encephalopathy

Pharmacokinetics:

PO/INJ: Unused amounts excreted in urine (unchanged)

DENTAL CONSIDERATIONS
General:
• Determine why the patient is taking this vitamin.
Teach patient/family:
• Food sources to be included in diet: yeast, whole grain, beef, liver, legumes

---

thiethylperazine maleate

(thye-eth-il-per'a-zeen)
Torecan
Drug class.: Phenothiazine-type, antiemetic

Action: Acts centrally by blocking chemoreceptor trigger zone, which in turn acts on vomiting center
Uses: Nausea, vomiting
Dosage and routes:
• *Adult:* PO/IM/rec 10 mg qd-tid
Available forms include: Tabs 10 mg; supp 10 mg; inj 5 mg/ml
Side effects/adverse reactions:
▼ *ORAL:* Dry mouth, metallic taste
CNS: Euphoria, depression, ***convulsions,*** restlessness, tremor, EPS, drowsiness
CV: ***Circulatory failure, tachycardia,*** postural hypotension, ECG changes
GI: Nausea, vomiting, anorexia, diarrhea, constipation, weight loss, cramps
RESP: ***Respiratory depression***
GU: Urinary retention, dark urine
Contraindications: Hypersensitivity to phenothiazines, coma, seizure, encephalopathy, bone marrow depression
Precautions: Children <2 yr, pregnancy category C, elderly
Pharmacokinetics:
PO: Onset 45-60 min
REC: Onset 45-60 min
Metabolized by liver; excreted by kidneys; crosses placenta; excreted in breast milk
Drug interactions of concern to dentistry:
• Increased anticholinergic action: anticholinergics
• Increased CNS depression, hypotension: alcohol, CNS depressants
DENTAL CONSIDERATIONS
General:
• Defer elective dental treatment when symptoms are present.
Consultations:
• Medical consult may be required to assess disease control in the patient.

---

thioridazine HCl

(thye-oh-rid'a-zeen)
Mellaril
♣ Apo-Thioridazine, Novo-Ridazine
Drug class.: Phenothiazine antipsychotic

Action: Blocks neurotransmission at dopaminergic synapses in the cerebral cortex, hypothalamus, and limbic system; exhibits strong peripheral α-adrenergic, anticholinergic blocking action; mechanism for antipsychotic effects is unclear
Uses: Psychotic disorders, schizophrenia, behavioral problems in children, alcohol withdrawal as adjunct, anxiety, major depressive disorders, organic brain syndrome
Dosage and routes:
Psychosis
• *Adult:* PO 25-100 mg tid; max dose 800 mg/day; dose is gradually increased to desired response, then reduced to minimum maintenance

Depression/behavioral problems/ organic brain syndrome
• *Adult:* PO 25 tid; range from 10 mg bid-qid to 50 mg tid-qid
• *Child 2-12 yr:* PO 0.5-3 mg/kg/day in divided doses
Available forms include: Tabs 10, 15, 25, 50, 100, 150, 200, 300 mg; conc 30, 100 mg/ml; susp 25, 100 mg/5 ml
Side effects/adverse reactions:
▼ *ORAL: Dry mouth,* movements of lips and tongue (tardive dyskinesia), erythema multiforme, lichenoid reaction
CNS: Extrapyramidal symptoms: pseudoparkinsonism, akathisia, dystonia, tardive dyskinesia, ***seizures, headache,*** confusion
CV: Orthostatic hypotension, ***cardiac arrest,*** ECG changes, ***tachycardia***
GI: Nausea, vomiting, anorexia, constipation, diarrhea, jaundice, weight gain
RESP: ***Laryngospasm,*** dyspnea, ***respiratory depression***
HEMA: Anemia, ***leukopenia, leukocytosis, agranulocytosis***
GU: Urinary retention, enuresis, impotence, amenorrhea, gynecomastia
EENT: Blurred vision, glaucoma, dry eyes
INTEG: Rash, photosensitivity, dermatitis
Contraindications: Hypersensitivity, blood dyscrasias, coma, child <2 yr, brain damage, bone marrow depression
Precautions: Pregnancy category C, lactation, seizure disorders, hypertension, hepatic disease, cardiac disease
Pharmacokinetics:
PO: Onset erratic, peak 2-4 hr, half-life 26-36 hr; metabolized by liver; excreted in urine; crosses placenta; excreted in breast milk
Drug interactions of concern to dentistry:
• Increased sedation: other CNS depressants, alcohol, barbiturate anesthetics, opioid analgesics
• Hypotension, tachycardia: epinephrine (systemic)
• Increased extrapyramidal effects: phenothiazines and related drugs (haloperidol, droperidol), metoclopramide
• Additive photosensitization: tetracyclines
• Increased anticholinergic effects: anticholinergics

DENTAL CONSIDERATIONS

General:
• Monitor vital signs every appointment due to cardiovascular side effects.
• Patients on chronic drug therapy may rarely have symptoms of blood dyscrasias, which can include infection, bleeding, and poor healing.
• After supine positioning, have patient sit upright for at least 2 min before standing to avoid orthostatic hypotension.
• Assess salivary flow as a factor in caries, periodontal disease, and candidiasis.
• Avoid dental light in patient's eyes; offer dark glasses for patient comfort.
• Assess for presence of extrapyramidal motor symptoms, such as tardive dyskinesia and akathisia. Extrapyramidal motor activity may complicate dental treatment.
• Geriatric patients are more susceptible to drug effects; use lower dose.
• Use vasoconstrictors with cau-

T

tion, in low doses, and with careful aspiration.

Consultations:

• In a patient with symptoms of blood dyscrasias, request a medical consult for blood studies and postpone dental treatment until normal values are reestablished.

• Take precautions if dental surgery is anticipated and anesthesia is required.

• Refer to physician if signs of tardive dyskinesia or akathisia are present.

• Physician should be informed if significant xerostomic side effects occur (increased caries, sore tongue, problems eating or swallowing, difficulty wearing prosthesis) so a medication change can be considered.

Teach patient/family:

• Importance of good oral hygiene to prevent soft tissue inflammation

• Caution to prevent injury when using oral hygiene aids

• To use electric toothbrush if patient has difficulty holding conventional devices

When chronic dry mouth occurs, advise patient:

• To avoid mouth rinses with high alcohol content due to drying effects

• Of need for daily home fluoride to prevent caries

• To use sugarless gum, frequent sips of water, or saliva substitutes

---

thiothixene

(thye-oh-thix'een)

Navane

Drug class.: Thioxanthene/antipsychotic

Action: Depresses cerebral cortex, hypothalamus, limbic system, which control activity, aggression; blocks neurotransmission produced by dopamine at the synapse; exhibits strong peripheral α-adrenergic blocking action; mechanism for antipsychotic effects is unclear

Uses: Psychotic disorders, schizophrenia, acute agitation

Dosage and routes:

• *Adult:* PO 2-5 mg bid-qid depending on severity of condition; dose is gradually increased to 15-30 mg/day if needed; IM 4 mg bid-qid, max dose 30 mg qd; administer PO dose as soon as possible

Available forms include: Caps 1, 2, 5, 10, 20 mg; conc 5 mg/ml; inj IM 2 mg/ml; powder for inj 5 mg/ml

Side effects/adverse reactions:

▼ *ORAL: Dry mouth,* uncontrolled tongue and lip movements

CNS: Extrapyramidal symptoms: pseudoparkinsonism, akathisia, dystonia, tardive dyskinesia, headache, seizures

CV: Orthostatic hypotension, ***cardiac arrest, tachycardia,*** hypertension, ECG changes

GI: Nausea, vomiting, anorexia, constipation, diarrhea, jaundice, weight gain

RESP: ***Laryngospasm, respiratory depression,*** dyspnea

HEMA: ***Leukopenia, leukocytosis, agranulocytosis,*** anemia

GU: Urinary retention, enuresis, impotence, amenorrhea, gynecomastia

EENT: Blurred vision, glaucoma

INTEG: Rash, photosensitivity, dermatitis

Contraindications: Hypersensitivity, blood dyscrasias, child <12 yr, bone marrow depression, circulatory collapse, CNS depression, coma, alcoholism, CV disease, hepatic disease, Reye's syndrome, narrow-angle glaucoma

Precautions: Pregnancy category C, lactation, seizure disorders, hypertension, hepatic disease

Pharmacokinetics:

PO: Onset slow, peak 2-8 hr, duration up to 12 hr

IM: Onset 15-30 min, peak 1-6 hr, duration up to 12 hr

Half-life 34 hr; metabolized by liver; excreted in urine; crosses placenta; excreted in breast milk

Drug interactions of concern to dentistry:

• Increased sedation: other CNS depressants, alcohol, barbiturate anesthetics, opioid analgesics

• Hypotension, tachycardia: epinephrine (systemic)

• Increased extrapyramidal effects: phenothiazines and related drugs (haloperidol, droperidol), metoclopramide

• Additive photosensitization: tetracyclines

• Increased anticholinergic effects: anticholinergics

DENTAL CONSIDERATIONS

General:

• Monitor vital signs every appointment due to cardiovascular side effects.

• Patients on chronic drug therapy may rarely have symptoms of blood dyscrasias, which can include infection, bleeding, and poor healing.

• After supine positioning, have patient sit upright for at least 2 min before standing to avoid orthostatic hypotension.

• Assess salivary flow as a factor in caries, periodontal disease, and candidiasis.

• Assess for presence of extrapyramidal motor symptoms, such as tardive dyskinesia and akathisia. Extrapyramidal motor activity may complicate dental treatment.

• Use vasoconstrictors with caution, in low doses, and with careful aspiration.

• Avoid dental light in patient's eyes; offer dark glasses for patient comfort.

• Geriatric patients are more susceptible to drug effects; use lower dose.

Consultations:

• In a patient with symptoms of blood dyscrasias, request a medical consult for blood studies and postpone dental treatment until normal values are reestablished.

• Take precautions if dental surgery is anticipated and anesthesia is required.

• If signs of tardive dyskinesia or akathisia are present, refer to physician.

Teach patient/family:

• Importance of good oral hygiene to prevent soft tissue inflammation

• Caution to prevent injury when using oral hygiene aids

• To use electric toothbrush if patient has difficulty holding conventional devices

When chronic dry mouth occurs, advise patient:

• To avoid mouth rinses with high alcohol content due to drying effects

• Of need for daily home fluoride to prevent caries

• To use sugarless gum, frequent sips of water, or saliva substitutes

T

thyroid USP (desiccated)

(thye'roid)

Armour Thyroid, S-P-T, Thyrar, Thyroid Strong, Westroid

🍁 Cholaxin

Drug class.: Thyroid hormone

Action: Increases metabolic rates; increases cardiac output, O_2 consumption, body temperature, blood volume, growth/development at cellular level

Uses: Hypothyroidism, cretinism, myxedema

Dosage and routes:

Hypothyroidism

- *Adult:* PO 65 mg qd, increased by 65 mg q30d until desired response; maintenance dose 65-195 mg qd
- *Geriatric:* PO 7.5-15 mg qd, double dose q6-8wk until desired response

Creatinism/juvenile hypothyroidism

- *Child >1 yr:* PO up to 180 mg qd titrated to response
- *Child 4-12 mo:* PO 3-60 mg qd
- *Child 1-4 mo:* PO 15-30 mg qd, may increase q2wk, titrated to response; maintenance dose 30-45 mg qd

Myxedema

- *Adult:* PO 16 mg qd, double dose q2wk; maintenance 65-195 mg/day

Available forms include: Tabs 16, 32, 65, 98, 130, 195, 260, 325 mg; enteric-coated tabs 32, 65, 130 mg; sugar-coated tabs 32, 65, 130, 195 mg; caps 65, 130, 195, 325 mg

Side effects/adverse reactions:

CNS: Insomnia, tremors, headache, thyroid storm

CV: ***Cardiac arrest,*** tachycardia, palpitation, angina, dysrhythmias, hypertension

GI: Nausea, diarrhea, increased or decreased appetite, cramps

MISC: Menstrual irregularities, weight loss, sweating, heat intolerance, fever

Contraindications: Adrenal insufficiency, MI, thyrotoxicosis

Precautions: Elderly, angina pectoris, hypertension, ischemia, cardiac disease, pregnancy category A, lactation

Pharmacokinetics:

PO: Peak 12-48 hr, half-life 6-7 days

Drug interactions of concern to dentistry:

- Increased effects of sympathomimetics in those patients when thyroid doses are not carefully monitored or with coronary artery disease

DENTAL CONSIDERATIONS

General:

- Increased nervousness, excitability, sweating, or tachycardia may indicate uncontrolled hyperthyroidism or a dose of medication that is too high. Uncontrolled patients should be referred for medical treatment.

Consultations:

- Medical consult may be required to assess disease control in the patient.

tiagabine HCl

(tye-ag'a-been)

Gabitril

Drug class.: Anticonvulsant

Action: Antiseizure mechanism unknown; acts as an antagonist for γ-aminobytric acid (GABA) uptake and may enhance the activity of GABA

Uses: Adjunctive therapy for partial seizures

Dosage and routes:

• *Adult:* PO initial dose 4 mg; increase dose by 4-8 mg increments at weekly intervals until response or up to 32 mg/day

• *Child 12-18 yr:* PO initial dose 4 mg/day; after 1 wk can increase dose 2-8 mg/day; thereafter can be increased by 4-8 mg at weekly intervals up to total dose of 32 mg/day

Available forms include: Tabs 4, 12, 16, 20 mg

Side effects/adverse reactions:

▼ *ORAL:* Dry mouth (1%), gingivitis, stomatitis, gingival hyperplasia (uncommon)

CNS: Sedation, dizziness, headache, memory impairment, emotional state, nervousness, tremor, depression, confusion

CV: Hypertension, palpitation, tachycardia, edema

GI: Abdominal pain, nausea, diarrhea, vomiting, constipation, dyspepsia

RESP: Cough, bronchitis, dyspnea

HEMA: Lymphadenopathy

GU: UTI

EENT: Pharyngitis, amblyopia, ear pain

INTEG: Pruritus, rash, dry skin

MS: Asthenia, myalgia

MISC: Flulike syndrome, pain

Contraindications: Hypersensitivity

Precautions: Hepatic disease, Alzheimer's disease, dementia, organic brain disease, stroke

Pharmacokinetics:

PO: Rapid absorption, peak plasma levels 0.5-1 hr; highly plasma protein bound (95%), hepatic metabolism, some enterohepatic circulation

Drug interactions of concern to dentistry:

• Increased tiagabine clearance: carbamazepine, phenobarbital

• Use CNS depressants with caution because possible additional effects may occur

DENTAL CONSIDERATIONS

General:

• Monitor vital signs every appointment due to cardiovascular and respiratory side effects.

• Consider semisupine chair position for patient comfort when GI side effects occur.

• Short appointments and a stress reduction protocol may be required for anxious patients.

• Determine type of epilepsy, seizure frequency, and quality of seizure control.

• Assess salivary flow as factor in caries, periodontal disease, and candidiasis.

• Place on frequent recall if oral side effects occur.

Consultations:

• Consultation with physician may be needed if sedation or general anesthesia is required.

Teach patient/family:

• Caution to prevent trauma when using oral hygiene aids

• Use of electric toothbrush if patient has difficulty holding conventional devices

• Importance of good oral hygiene to prevent soft tissue inflammation

• Importance of updating health and drug history if physician makes any changes in evaluation/drug regimens

• To be aware of oral side effects and potential sequelae

When chronic dry mouth occurs, advise patient:

- To avoid mouth rinses with high alcohol content due to drying effects
- To use daily home fluoride products for anticaries effect
- To use sugarless gum, frequent sips of water, or saliva substitutes

---

ticlopidine

(tye-chloe′pi-deen)

Ticlid

Drug class.: Platelet aggregation inhibitor

Action: Inhibits first and second phases of ADP-induced effects in platelet aggregation

Uses: Reducing the risk of stroke in high-risk patients

Dosage and routes:

- *Adult:* PO 250 mg bid with food

Available forms include: Tabs 250 mg

Side effects/adverse reactions:

GI: ***Cholestatic jaundice, hepatitis,*** increased cholesterol, LDL, VLDL, nausea, vomiting, diarrhea, GI discomfort

HEMA: ***Bleeding (epistaxis, hematuria, conjunctival hemorrhage, GI bleeding), agranulocytosis, neutropenia, thrombocytopenia, erythroleukemia, thrombotic thrombocytopenic purpura***

INTEG: Rash, pruritus

Contraindications: Hypersensitivity, active liver disease, blood dyscrasias

Precautions: Past liver disease, renal disease, elderly, pregnancy category B, lactation, children; increased bleeding risk requires hematologic monitoring every 2 wk for the first 3 mo of therapy

Pharmacokinetics: Peak 1-3 hr, half-life increases with repeated dosing; metabolized by the liver; excreted in urine, feces

Drug interactions of concern to dentistry:

- Increased bleeding tendencies: aspirin, NSAIDs

DENTAL CONSIDERATIONS

General:

- Patients on chronic drug therapy may rarely have symptoms of blood dyscrasias, which can include infection, bleeding, and poor healing.
- Consider local hemostatic measures to prevent excessive bleeding.

Consultations:

- Medical consult may be required to assess disease control and patient's ability to tolerate stress. Consult should include data on hematologic profile.

Teach patient/family:

- Caution to prevent injury when using oral hygiene aids

---

tiludronate disodium

(tye-loo′droe-nate)

Skelid

Drug class.: Biphosphonate derivative

Action: Acts to inhibit bone resorption by a mechanism that involves inhibition of osteoclastic activity

Uses: Paget's disease of bone in patients with twice normal upper limit values for serum alkaline phosphatase (SAP) and who are symptomatic and at risk for future complications

Dosage and routes:
• *Adult:* PO 400 mg/day taken with 6-8 oz of plain water only for 3 mo; do not take with other beverages; do not eat for 2 hr after dosing
Available forms include: Tabs 200 mg
Side effects/adverse reactions:
▼ *ORAL:* Tooth disorder (not specified), dry mouth (<1%)
CNS: Headache, dizziness, paresthesia, nervousness, anxiety
CV: Peripheral edema, hypertension
GI: Nausea, diarrhea, dyspepsia, vomiting
RESP: URI, cough, pharyngitis
EENT: Rhinitis, sinusitis, cataract, conjunctivitis, glaucoma
INTEG: Rash, pruritus
ENDO: Hyperparathyroidism
META: Vitamin D deficiency
MS: Back pain, chest pain, arthralgia
MISC: Flulike symptoms
Contraindications: Hypersensitivity, severe renal failure
Precautions: Pregnancy category C, lactation, safety in children <18 yr not established
Pharmacokinetics:
PO: Rapid but incomplete absorption, bioavailability 6% (fasted), peak plasma levels 2 hr, little or no metabolism, excreted in urine
Drug interactions of concern to dentistry:
• Bioavailability decreased by calcium, food, aluminum or magnesium antacids
• Do not take indomethacin, aspirin, or calcium supplements 2 hr before or after tilundronate
DENTAL CONSIDERATIONS
General:
• Be aware of oral manifestations of Paget's disease (macrognathia, alveolar pain).
• Consider semisupine chair position for patient comfort when GI side effects occur.
• Consider short appointments for patient comfort.
• Assess salivary flow as a factor in caries, periodontal disease, candidiasis.
Consultations:
• Medical consult may be required to assess disease control in the patient.
Teach patient/family:
• Caution to prevent trauma when using oral hygiene aids
• Importance of good oral hygiene to prevent soft tissue inflammation
• Importance of updating health and drug history if physician makes any changes in evaluation/drug regimens
When chronic dry mouth occurs, advise patient:
• To avoid mouth rinses with high alcohol content due to drying effects
• To use daily home fluoride products for anticaries effect
• To use sugarless gum, frequent sips of water, or saliva substitutes

timolol maleate
(tye'moe-lole)
Blocadren
Apo-Timol, Novo-Timol
Drug class.: Nonselective β-adrenergic blocker

Action: This is a nonselective β_1- and β_2-adrenergic antagonist. The antihypertensive mechanism of action is unclear, but it may include a reduction in cardiac output and inhibition of renin release by the renal juxtaglomerular apparatus. Peripheral resistance decreases with long-term use. The antianginal action (when indicated for this use) may be related to a decrease in myocardial oxygen demand and negative chronotropic and inotropic effects. The antiarrhythmic action (when indicated for this use) has been related to a reduction in spontaneous pacemaker firing and slowing of AV nodal conduction.

Uses: Mild-to-moderate hypertension, reduction of mortality risk after MI, migraine prophylaxis; unapproved uses: essential tremors, angina, cardiac dysrhythmias, anxiety

Dosage and routes:

Hypertension

• *Adult:* PO 10 mg bid, may increase by 10 mg q2-3d, not to exceed 60 mg/day

Myocardial infarction

• *Adult:* 10 mg bid

Available forms include: Tabs 5, 10, 20 mg

Side effects/adverse reactions:

▼ *ORAL:* Dry mouth

CNS: Insomnia, dizziness, hallucinations, anxiety

CV: ***CHF,*** hypotension, bradycardia, edema, chest pain, claudication

GI: Nausea, vomiting, abdominal pain, ***mesenteric arterial thrombosis, ischemic colitis,*** diarrhea

RESP: ***Bronchospasm, dyspnea,*** cough, rales

HEMA: ***Agranulocytosis, thrombocytopenia***

GU: Impotence, frequency

EENT: Visual changes, double vision, sore throat, dry/burning eyes

INTEG: Rash, alopecia, pruritus, fever

META: Hypoglycemia

MISC: Joint pain, muscle pain

Contraindications: Hypersensitivity to β-blockers, cardiogenic shock, second- or third-degree heart block, sinus bradycardia, CHF, cardiac failure

Precautions: Major surgery, pregnancy category C, lactation, diabetes mellitus, renal disease, thyroid disease, COPD, well-compensated heart failure, CAD, nonallergic bronchospasm

Pharmacokinetics:

PO: Peak 2-4 hr, half-life 3-4 hr; excreted 30%-45% unchanged; 60%-65% is metabolized by liver; excreted in breast milk

Drug interactions of concern to dentistry:

• Increased hypotension, bradycardia: anticholinergics, sympathomimetics (epinephrine)

• Decreased antihypertensive effects: indomethacin and other NSAIDs

• May slow metabolism of lidocaine

DENTAL CONSIDERATIONS

General:

• Monitor vital signs every appointment due to cardiovascular side effects.

• Patients on chronic drug therapy may rarely have symptoms of blood dyscrasias, which can include infection, bleeding, and poor healing.

• Assess salivary flow as a factor in caries, periodontal disease, and candidiasis.

• Limit use of sodium-containing products, such as saline IV fluids, for patients with a dietary salt restriction.

• After supine positioning, have patient sit upright for at least 2 min before standing to avoid orthostatic hypotension.

• Stress from dental procedures may compromise cardiovascular function; determine patient risk.
• Short appointments and a stress reduction protocol may be required for anxious patients.
• Consider semisupine chair position for patients with nausea or respiratory distress.

Consultations:
• In a patient with symptoms of blood dyscrasias, request a medical consult for blood studies and postpone dental treatment until normal values are reestablished.
• Medical consult may be required to assess disease control and patient's ability to tolerate stress.

Teach patient/family:
• Importance of good oral hygiene to prevent soft tissue inflammation
• Caution to prevent injury when using oral hygiene aids

When chronic dry mouth occurs, advise patient:
• To avoid mouth rinses with high alcohol content due to drying effects
• Of need for daily home fluoride to prevent caries
• To use sugarless gum, frequent sips of water, or saliva substitutes

---

timolol maleate (optic)

(tye'moe-lole)

Beta-Tim, Betimol, Med Timolol, Timoptic Solution, Timodal, Timoptic-XE

♣ Apo-Timop, Gen-Timolol, Novo-Timolol, Nu-Timol

Drug class.: β-adrenergic blocker

Action: Reduces production of aqueous humor by unknown mechanism

Uses: Ocular hypertension, chronic open-angle glaucoma, secondary glaucoma, aphakic glaucoma

Dosage and routes:
• *Adult:* Instill 1 gtt of 0.25% sol in affected eye(s) bid, then 1 gtt for maintenance; may increase to 1 gtt of 0.5% sol bid if needed

Available forms include: Sol 0.25%, 0.5%, in 2.5, 5, 10, 15 ml; also unit dose container (Ocudose)

Side effects/adverse reactions:
CNS: Weakness, fatigue, depression, anxiety, headache, confusion
CV: Bradycardia, hypotension, dysrhythmias
GI: Nausea
RESP: ***Bronchospasm***
EENT: Eye irritation, conjunctivitis, keratitis
INTEG: Rash, urticaria

Contraindications: Hypersensitivity, asthma, second- or third-degree heart block, right ventricular failure, congenital glaucoma (infants), COPD

Precautions: May be absorbed systemically, can mask hypoglycemia in patients with diabetes, pregnancy category C, lactation, children

Pharmacokinetics:
INSTILL: Onset 15-30 min, peak 1-2 hr, duration 24 hr

Drug interactions of concern to dentistry:
• Avoid use of anticholinergic drugs, atropine-like drugs, propantheline, and diazepam (benzodiazepines)

DENTAL CONSIDERATIONS

General:
• Check compliance of patient with prescribed drug regimen for glaucoma.
• Avoid dental light in patient's eyes; offer dark glasses for patient comfort.

Consultations:

- Consultation with physician may be needed if sedation or anesthesia is required.

tizanidine HCl

(tye-zan'i-deen)

Zanaflex

Drug class.: Centrally acting α_2-adrenergic agonist

Action: Acts as an agonist at α_2-adrenoreceptor sites; believed to reduce spasticity by increasing presynaptic inhibition on motor neurons

Uses: Treatment of acute and intermittent management of increased muscle tone due to spasticity (multiple sclerosis, spinal cord injury)

Dosage and routes:

- *Adult:* PO initial 4 mg at 6-8 hr intervals; increase dose by 2-4 mg steps to satisfactory reduction of muscle tone; daily dose limit 36 mg

Available forms include: Tabs 4 mg

Side effects/adverse reactions:

▼ *ORAL: Dry mouth (3-10%)*

CNS: Light-headedness, dizziness, sedation, hallucination, drowsiness, psychosis, nervousness

CV: Hypotension, bradycardia, orthostatic hypotension, syncope

GI: Abdominal pain, diarrhea, dyspepsia, constipation

GU: UTI, candidiasis

EENT: Blurred vision, rhinitis, pharyngitis, ear pain

INTEG: Skin rash

META: Liver injury, liver enzymes elevated

MS: Asthenia, increased spasm, myasthenia

Contraindications: Hypersensitivity

Precautions: Long-term use, concurrent hypotensive drugs, renal impairment, oral contraceptives, pregnancy category C, lactation, elderly, children

Pharmacokinetics:

PO: Half-life 2.5 hr, peak levels 1.5 hr, first-pass metabolism, extensively metabolized, 30% plasma protein bound, excretion in urine and feces

Drug interactions of concern to dentistry:

- Additive CNS side effects: ethanol and other CNS depressants
- Orthostatic hypotension: drugs that lower blood pressure

DENTAL CONSIDERATIONS

General:

- Monitor vital signs every appointment due to cardiovascular side effects.
- Short appointments may be required due to effects of disease on musculature.
- Use precaution if sedation or general anesthesia is required; risk of hypotensive episode.
- Assess salivary flow as factor in caries, periodontal disease, and candidiasis.
- After supine positioning, have patient sit upright for at least 2 min before standing to avoid orthostatic hypotension.

Consultations:

- Medical consult may be required to assess disease control and patient's ability to tolerate stress.

Teach patient/family:

- Not to drive or perform other tasks requiring alertness

• Use of electric toothbrush if patient has difficulty holding conventional devices

When chronic dry mouth occurs, advise patient:

• To avoid mouth rinses with high alcohol content due to drying effects

• To use daily home fluoride products for anticaries effect

• To use sugarless gum, frequent sips of water, or saliva substitutes

tobramycin (ophthalmic)

(toe-bra-mye'sin)

Tobrex

♣ AK-Tob

Drug class.: Antiinfective

Action: Inhibits bacterial protein synthesis

Uses: Infection of eye

Dosage and routes:

• *Adult and child:* Instill 1-2 gtt q1-4h depending on infection; oint 1 cm bid-tid

Available forms include: Oint 0.3%; sol 0.3%

Side effects/adverse reactions:

EENT: Poor corneal wound healing, visual haze (temporary), overgrowth of nonsusceptible organisms

Contraindications: Hypersensitivity

Precautions: Antibiotic hypersensitivity, pregnancy category D

DENTAL CONSIDERATIONS

General:

• Avoid directing dental light into patient's eyes; provide dark glasses during treatment to avoid irritation.

• Protect patient's eyes from accidental spatter during dental treatment.

tocainide HCl

(toe-kay'nide)

Tonocard

Drug class.: Antidysrhythmic (Class IB), lidocaine analog

Action: Decreases sodium and potassium conductance, which decreases myocardial excitability

Uses: Documented life-threatening ventricular dysrhythmias

Dosage and routes:

• *Adult:* PO 400 mg q8h; range 1200-1800 mg/day

Available forms include: Tabs 400, 600 mg

Side effects/adverse reactions:

▼ *ORAL:* Dry mouth, oral ulcerations, erythema multiforme (rare)

CNS: *Headache, dizziness,* ***seizures,*** involuntary movement, confusion, psychosis, restlessness, irritability, paresthesia, tremors

CV: *Hypotension, bradycardia,* ***heart block, cardiovascular collapse, arrest, CHF,*** chest pain, angina, PVCs, tachycardia

GI: Nausea, vomiting, anorexia, diarrhea, hepatitis

RESP: ***Respiratory depression, pulmonary fibrosis,*** dyspnea

HEMA: ***Blood dyscrasias: leukopenia, agranulocytosis, hypoplastic anemia, thrombocytopenia***

EENT: Tinnitus, blurred vision, hearing loss

INTEG: Rash, urticaria, edema, swelling

Contraindications: Hypersensitivity to amides, severe heart block

Precautions: Pregnancy category C, lactation, children, renal dis-

T

ease, liver disease, CHF, respiratory depression, myasthenia gravis, blood dyscrasias

Pharmacokinetics:

PO: Peak 0.5-3 hr; half-life 10-17 hr; metabolized by liver; excreted in urine

Drug interactions of concern to dentistry:

• No specific interactions are reported with dental drugs; however, any drug that could affect the cardiac action of tocainide (local anesthetics, vasoconstrictors, and anticholinergics) should be used in the least effective dose

DENTAL CONSIDERATIONS

General:

• Monitor vital signs every appointment due to cardiovascular and respiratory side effects.

• After supine positioning, have patient sit upright for at least 2 min before standing to avoid orthostatic hypotension.

• Patients on chronic drug therapy may rarely have symptoms of blood dyscrasias, which can include infection, bleeding, and poor healing.

• Assess salivary flow as a factor in caries, periodontal disease, and candidiasis.

• Stress from dental procedures may compromise cardiovascular function; determine patient risk.

Consultations:

• In a patient with symptoms of blood dyscrasias, request a medical consult for blood studies and postpone dental treatment until normal values are reestablished.

• Medical consult may be required to assess disease control and patient's ability to tolerate stress.

Teach patient/family:

• Importance of good oral hygiene to prevent soft tissue inflammation

• Caution to prevent injury when using oral hygiene aids

When chronic dry mouth occurs, advise patient:

• To avoid mouth rinses with high alcohol content due to drying effects

• Of need for daily home fluoride to prevent caries

• To use sugarless gum, frequent sips of water, or saliva substitutes

tolazamide

(tole-az'a-mide)

Tolinase

Drug class.: Sulfonylurea (first-generation) oral antidiabetic

Action: Causes functioning β-cells in pancreas to release insulin, leading to drop in blood glucose levels; may improve binding to insulin receptors or increase the number of insulin receptors; this drug is not effective if patient lacks functioning β-cells

Uses: Type II (NIDDM) diabetes mellitus

Dosage and routes:

• *Adult:* PO 100 mg/day for FBS <200 mg/dl or 250 mg/day for FBS >200 mg/dl; dose should be titrated to patient response (1 g or less/day)

Available forms include: Tabs 100, 250, 500 mg

Side effects/adverse reactions:

▼ *ORAL:* Lichenoid reaction

CNS: Headache, weakness, fatigue, lethargy, dizziness, vertigo, tinnitus

GI: ***Hepatotoxicity, jaundice,*** heartburn, nausea, vomiting, diarrhea, constipation, gas

HEMA: ***Leukopenia, thrombocyto-***

penia, agranulocytosis, aplastic anemia, pancytopenia, hemolytic anemia

INTEG: Rash, (rare) allergic reactions, pruritus, urticaria, eczema, photosensitivity, erythema

ENDO: ***Hypoglycemia***

Contraindications: Hypersensitivity to sulfonylureas, juvenile or brittle diabetes

Precautions: Pregnancy category C, elderly, cardiac disease, thyroid disease, severe hypoglycemic reactions, renal disease, hepatic disease

Pharmacokinetics:

PO: Completely absorbed by GI route; onset 4-6 hr, peak 4-8 hr, duration 12-24 hr, half-life 7 hr; highly protein bound; metabolized in liver; excreted in urine (metabolites), breast milk

Drug interactions of concern to dentistry:

• Increased hypoglycemic reaction: NSAIDs, salicylates, ketoconazole, miconazole

• Decreased action of tolazamide: corticosteroids, sympathomimetics (epinephrine)

DENTAL CONSIDERATIONS

General:

• Patients on chronic drug therapy may rarely have symptoms of blood dyscrasias, which can include infection, bleeding, and poor healing.

• Place on frequent recall to evaluate healing response.

• Short appointments and a stress reduction protocol may be required for anxious patients.

• Patients with diabetes may be more susceptible to infection and have delayed wound healing.

• Ensure that patient is following prescribed diet and regularly takes medication.

• Question patient about self-monitoring of drug's antidiabetic effect.

• Avoid prescribing aspirin-containing products.

Consultations:

• In a patient with symptoms of blood dyscrasias, request a medical consult for blood studies and postpone dental treatment until normal values are reestablished.

• Medical consult may be required to assess disease control in the patient.

Teach patient/family:

• Importance of good oral hygiene to prevent soft tissue inflammation

• To avoid mouth rinses with high alcohol content due to drying effects

tolbutamide

(tole-byoo'ta-mide)

Orinase, Tol-Tab

Apo-Tolbutamide, Mobenol, Novo-Butamide

Drug class.: Sulfonylurea (first-generation) oral antidiabetic

Action: Causes functioning β-cells in pancreas to release insulin, leading to drop in blood glucose levels; may improve binding to insulin receptors or increase the number of insulin receptors; this drug is not effective if patient lacks functioning β-cells

Uses: Type II diabetes mellitus

Dosage and routes:

• *Adult:* PO 1-2 g/day in divided doses, titrated to patient response

Available forms include: Tabs 250, 500 mg

Side effects/adverse reactions:

ORAL: Changes in taste sensation, lichenoid reaction

CNS: Headache, weakness, pares-

thesia, tinnitus, dizziness, vertigo
GI: ***Hepatotoxicity, cholestatic jaundice,*** nausea, fullness, heartburn, diarrhea
HEMA: ***Leukopenia, thrombocytopenia, agranulocytosis, aplastic anemia,*** increased AST/ALT, alk phosphatase
INTEG: Rash, allergic reactions, pruritus, urticaria, eczema, photosensitivity, erythema
ENDO: ***Hypoglycemia***
MS: Joint pain

Contraindications: Hypersensitivity to sulfonylureas, juvenile or brittle diabetes

Precautions: Pregnancy category C, elderly, cardiac disease, thyroid disease, severe hypoglycemic reactions, renal disease, hepatic disease

Pharmacokinetics:
PO: Completely absorbed by GI route, onset 30-60 min, peak 3-5 hr, duration 6-12 hr, half-life 4-5 hr; 90%-95% is plasma protein bound; metabolized in liver; excreted in urine (metabolites), breast milk

Drug interactions of concern to dentistry:
• Increased hypoglycemic reactions: NSAIDs, salicylates, ketoconazole, miconazole
• Decreased effects: corticosteroids, sympathomimetics

DENTAL CONSIDERATIONS
General:
• Patients on chronic drug therapy may rarely have symptoms of blood dyscrasias, which can include infection, bleeding, and poor healing.
• Ensure that patient is following prescribed diet and regularly takes medication.
• Question patient about self-monitoring of drug's antidiabetic effect, including blood glucose values or finger-stick records.
• Place on frequent recall to evaluate healing response.
• Short appointments and a stress reduction protocol may be required for anxious patients.
• Patients with diabetes may be more susceptible to infection and have delayed wound healing.
• Avoid prescribing aspirin-containing products.

Consultations:
• In a patient with symptoms of blood dyscrasias, request a medical consult for blood studies and postpone dental treatment until normal values are reestablished.
• Medical consult may be required to assess disease control in the patient.
• Medical consult may include data from patient's blood glucose monitoring, including glycosylated hemoglobin or HbA_{1c} testing.

Teach patient/family:
• Importance of good oral hygiene to prevent soft tissue inflammation
• To avoid mouth rinses with high alcohol content due to drying effects

tolcapone

(tole'ka-pone)
Tasmar

Drug class.: Antiparkinsonian

Action: Reversibly and selectively inhibits catechol-*O*-methyltransferase (COMT) and may alter the plasma pharmacokinetics of levodopa; levodopa (with carbidopa) plasma levels are more sustained

Uses: Adjunct to levodopa and carbidopa in the treatment of Parkinson's disease

Dosage and routes:

• *Adult:* PO initial 100 mg or 200 mg tid as an adjunct to levodopa/carbidopa therapy; max daily dose 600 mg

Available forms include: Tabs 100, 200 mg

Side effects/adverse reactions:

▼ *ORAL: Xerostomia (5%-6%)*

CNS: Hallucinations, dyskinesia, sleep disorders, dystonia, anorexia, headache, dizziness, confusion, somnolence, excessive dreaming

CV: Orthostatic hypotension, chest pain

GI: ***Hepatocellular injury,*** diarrhea, nausea, anorexia, abdominal pain, constipation, vomiting

RESP: Pulmonary effusion, URI

GU: Hematuria, UTI, discolored urine

EENT: Sinus congestion

META: Elevation of SGT and AST

MS: Muscle cramps

MISC: Sweating, fatigue

Contraindications: Hypersensitivity, patients with SGPT/ALT and SGOT/AST exceeding upper limit of normal or other signs of hepatic impairment; informed consent required; history of nontraumatic rhabdomyolysis, hyperpyrexia, and confusion related to medication

Precautions: Discontinue drug with signs of hepatocellular injury, MAO inhibitors, hypotension, dyskinesia, pregnancy category C, lactation

Pharmacokinetics:

PO: Rapidly absorbed, bioavailability 65%, highly plasma protein bound (99.9%), hepatic metabolism, 60% excreted in urine, 40% in feces

Drug interactions of concern to dentistry:

• Increased sedation: alcohol and all CNS depressants

• No other data for dental drugs reported

DENTAL CONSIDERATIONS

General:

• Notify physician immediately if symptoms of liver failure are observed (bleeding, jaundice, etc.).

• Assess salivary flow as a factor in caries, periodontal disease, and candidiasis.

• After supine positioning, have patient sit upright for at least 2 min to avoid orthostatic hypotension.

• Consider semisupine chair position for patient comfort due to GI side effects of drug.

Consultations:

• Medical consult may be required to assess disease control in the patient.

• Take precaution if dental surgery is anticipated; general anesthesia is required.

Teach patient/family:

• Use of electric toothbrush if patient has difficulty holding conventional devices

When chronic dry mouth occurs, advise patient:

• To avoid mouth rinses with high alcohol content due to drying effects

• To use daily home fluoride products for anticaries effect

• To use sugarless gum, frequent sips of water, or saliva substitutes

T

tolmetin sodium

(tole'met-in)
Tolectin, Tolectin DS
♣ Novo-Tolmetin

Drug class.: Nonsteroidal antiinflammatory

Action: Inhibits prostaglandin synthesis by interfering with cyclooxygenase needed for biosynthesis
Uses: Osteoarthritis, rheumatoid arthritis, juvenile rheumatoid arthritis
Dosage and routes:
• *Adult:* PO 400 mg tid, not to exceed 2 g/day
• *Child >2 yr:* PO 15-30 mg/kg/day in 3 or 4 divided doses
Available forms include: Tabs 200, 600 mg; caps 400 mg
Side effects/adverse reactions:
▼ *ORAL:* Dry mouth, gingival bleeding, mucosal ulceration, lichenoid reaction
CNS: Dizziness, drowsiness, fatigue, tremors, confusion, insomnia, anxiety, depression
CV: Tachycardia, peripheral edema, palpitation, dysrhythmias
GI: ***Cholestatic hepatitis,*** nausea, anorexia, vomiting, diarrhea, jaundice, constipation, flatulence, cramps, peptic ulcer
HEMA: ***Blood dyscrasias***
GU: ***Nephrotoxicity: dysuria, hematuria, oliguria, azotemia***
EENT: Tinnitus, hearing loss, blurred vision
INTEG: Purpura, rash, pruritus, sweating
Contraindications: Hypersensitivity, asthma, severe renal disease, severe hepatic disease
Precautions: Pregnancy category C, lactation, children, bleeding disorders, GI disorders, cardiac disorders, hypersensitivity to aspirin, NSAIDs, peptic ulcer disease, geriatric patients
Pharmacokinetics:
PO: Peak 2 hr, half-life 3-3.5 hr; 99% protein binding; metabolized in liver; excreted in urine (metabolites), breast milk
Drug interactions of concern to dentistry:
• Increased risk of GI side effects: ASA, NSAIDs, ethanol (alcohol)
• Nephrotoxicity: acetaminophen (prolonged use and high doses)
• Possible risk of decreased renal function: cyclosporine
• Decreased antihypertensive effect of diuretics, β-adrenergic blockers, and ACE inhibitors

DENTAL CONSIDERATIONS

General:
• Patients on chronic drug therapy may rarely have symptoms of blood dyscrasias, which can include infection, bleeding, and poor healing.
• Monitor vital signs every appointment due to cardiovascular side effects.
• Assess salivary flow as a factor in caries, periodontal disease, and candidiasis.
• Avoid prescribing for dental use in last trimester of pregnancy.
• Possibility of cross-allergenicity when patient is allergic to aspirin.
Consultations:
• Medical consult may be required to assess disease control in the patient.
• In a patient with symptoms of blood dyscrasias, request a medical consult for blood studies and postpone dental treatment until normal values are reestablished.

Teach patient/family:

- Importance of good oral hygiene to prevent soft tissue inflammation
- Caution to prevent injury when using oral hygiene aids

When chronic dry mouth occurs, advise patient:

- To avoid mouth rinses with high alcohol content due to drying effects
- Of need for daily home fluoride to prevent caries
- To use sugarless gum, frequent sips of water, or saliva substitutes

tolnaftate (topical)

(tole-naf'tate)

Aftate, Genaspor, NP-27, Tinactin, Ting, Zeasorb-AF

♣ Pitrex

Drug class.: Antifungal, topical

Action: Interferes with fungal cell membrane, which increases permeability, leaking of cell nutrients

Uses: Tinea pedis, tinea cruris, tinea corporis, tinea capitis, tinea unguium, versicolor

Dosage and routes:

- *Adult and child:* TOP apply to affected area bid for 2-6 wk, rub in

Available forms include: Cream, powder, aerosol powder, aerosol liq, gel, pump spray, liq 1% sol

Side effects/adverse reactions:

INTEG: Rash, urticaria, stinging

Contraindications: Hypersensitivity, nail infections

Precautions: Pregnancy category C, lactation

tolterodine tartrate

(tole-ter'o-deen)

Detrol

Drug class.: Antispasmodic

Action: Inhibits muscarinic actions of acetylcholine at postganglionic receptors

Uses: Overactive bladder, with symptoms of urinary frequency or incontinence

Dosage and routes:

- *Adult:* PO initial dose 2 mg bid; may be reduced to 1 mg bid based on individual response

With hepatic dysfunction or concurrent use with inhibitors of cytochrome P-450 3A4

- *Adult:* PO 1 mg bid

Available forms include: Tabs 1, 2 mg

Side effects/adverse reactions:

▼ *ORAL: Dry mouth (39.5%)*

CNS: Headache, dizziness, fatigue, vertigo, somnolence, paresthesia, nervousness

GI: Dyspepsia, constipation, abdominal pain, nausea, diarrhea

RESP: URI, bronchitis, coughing

GU: Urinary retention, dysuria, UTI

EENT: Xerophthalmia, blurred vision, rhinitis

INTEG: Rash, erythema, pruritus, dry skin

MS: Arthralgia, back pain

MISC: Weight gain, flulike symptoms

Contraindications: Hypersensitivity, urinary retention, gastric retention, uncontrolled narrow-angle glaucoma

Precautions: Bladder obstruction, pyloric stenosis, GI obstructive disorders, treated narrow-angle glau-

T

coma, significant hepatic dysfunction, renal impairment, pregnancy category C, lactation, pediatric use
Pharmacokinetics:
PO: Onset 1 hr, peak serum levels 1-2 hr, highly plasma protein bound (96%), hepatic metabolism, active metabolite, urinary excretion (77%)
Drug interactions of concern to dentistry:
• Studies not available; however, drugs that inhibit cytochrome P-450 3A4 enzymes, such as erythromycin, clarithromycin, ketoconazole, itraconazole, and fluoxetine, require a dose reduction to 1 mg bid
• Increased anticholinergic effects: possibly with other anticholinergic drugs

DENTAL CONSIDERATIONS
General:
• Assess salivary flow as a factor in caries, periodontal disease, and candidiasis.
• Consider semisupine chair position for patient comfort due to GI side effects of drug.
• Avoid dental light in patient's eyes; offer dark glasses for patient comfort.
• Avoid drugs with anticholinergic activity, such as antihistamines, opioids, benzodiazepines, propantheline, atropine, and scopolamine.
Consultations:
• Physician should be informed if significant xerostomic side effects occur (e.g., increased caries, sore tongue, problems eating or swallowing, difficulty wearing prosthesis) so a medication change can be considered.
Teach patient/family:
• Importance of good oral hygiene to prevent soft tissue inflammation

When chronic dry mouth occurs, advise patient:
• To avoid mouth rinses with high alcohol content due to drying effects
• To use daily home fluoride products for anticaries effect
• To use sugarless gum, frequent sips of water, or saliva substitutes

---

topiramate
(toe-pyre'a-mate)
Topamax
Drug class.: Anticonvulsant

Action: Anticonvulsant action is unclear; blocks repetitively elicited action potentials and enhances GABA activity along with antagonism of kainate activity on non-NMDA receptors
Uses: Adjunctive therapy for adult patients with partial-onset seizures or for primary generalized tonic-clonic seizures; Lennox-Gastaut syndrome
Dosage and routes:
• *Adult and child 2-16 yr:* PO 400 mg/day in 2 divided doses; initiate therapy at 50 mg/day and titrate to effective dose level
Available forms include: Tabs 25, 100, 200 mg
Side effects/adverse reactions:
▼ *ORAL:* Dry mouth (1.1%), gingival overgrowth (rare), taste alteration
CNS: Psychomotor slowing, somnolence, fatigue, ataxia, confusion, dizziness, memory problems, irritability, depression
CV: Palpitation, bradycardia
GI: Nausea, dyspepsia, abdominal pain
RESP: Coughing, bronchitis

HEMA: Epistaxis, ***leukopenia, purpura, thrombycytopenia***
GU: Hematuria, UTI
EENT: Decreased hearing, eye pain, photophobia
INTEG: Dermatitis, acne
MS: Back pain, asthenia, leg pain, myalgia
MISC: Paresthesia

Contraindications: Hypersensitivity

Precautions: Renal impairment, hepatic impairment, rapid drug withdrawal, kidney stones, pregnancy category C, lactation, children

Pharmacokinetics:
PO: Rapid oral absorption, peak plasma levels 2 hr, low protein binding (13%-17%), 70% excreted in urine unchanged, little metabolism

Drug interactions of concern to dentistry:
• Increased CNS depression: opioids, sedatives, ethanol, and other CNS depressants

DENTAL CONSIDERATIONS

General:
• Patients on chronic drug therapy may rarely have symptoms of blood dyscrasias, which can include infection, bleeding, and poor healing.
• Short appointments and a stress reduction protocol may be required for anxious patients.
• Assess salivary flow as factor in caries, periodontal disease, and candidiasis.
• Avoid dental light in patient's eyes; offer dark glasses for patient comfort.
• Determine type of epilepsy, seizure frequency, and quality of seizure control. A stress reduction protocol may be required.

Consultations:
• In a patient with symptoms of blood dyscrasias, request a medical consult for blood studies and postpone dental treatment until normal values are reestablished.
• Medical consult may be required to assess disease control in the patient.

Teach patient/family:
• Importance of good oral hygiene to prevent soft tissue inflammation
• Caution to prevent trauma when using oral hygiene aids
• Use of electric toothbrush if patient has difficulty holding conventional devices
• Importance of updating health and drug history if physician makes any changes in evaluation/drug regimens

When chronic dry mouth occurs, advise patient:
• To avoid mouth rinses with high alcohol content due to drying effects
• To use daily home fluoride products for anticaries effect
• To use sugarless gum, frequent sips of water, or saliva substitutes

toremifene citrate

(tore'em-i-feen)
Fareston

Drug class.: Antineoplastic, antiestrogen agent

Action: Inhibits cell division by binding to cytoplasmic receptors (estrogen receptors); resembles normal cell complex but inhibits DNA synthesis

Uses: Metastatic breast cancer in postmenopausal women with estrogen receptor–positive or unknown tumors

Dosage and routes:
• *Adult:* PO 60 mg qd continued until disease progression is observed
Available forms include: Tabs 60 mg
Side effects/adverse reactions:
CNS: Dizziness
CV: Edema
GI: Nausea, vomiting
HEMA: Thrombophlebitis, thrombosis
GU: Vaginal discharge, vaginal bleeding
EENT: Cataracts, dry eyes, abnormal visual fields, glaucoma
INTEG: Sweating
ENDO: Hot flashes
META: Elevated SGOT, alkaline phosphatase, bilirubin, hypercalcemia
Contraindications: Hypersensitivity
Precautions: Thromboembolic diseases, endometrial hyperplasia, hypercalcemia with bone metastases, monitor leukocyte and platelet counts, pregnancy category D, tumor flare
Pharmacokinetics:
PO: Well absorbed, peak levels average 3 hr, extensive metabolism with active metabolite, enterohepatic circulation, highly protein bound (99.5%), excreted mainly in feces, 10% in urine
Drug interactions of concern to dentistry:
• None reported
DENTAL CONSIDERATIONS
General:
• Patients on chronic drug therapy may rarely have symptoms of blood dyscrasias, which can include infection, bleeding, and poor healing.
• Consider semisupine chair position for patient comfort due to GI side effects of drug.
Consultations:
• Medical consult may be required to assess disease control in the patient.
Teach patient/family:
• Importance of good oral hygiene to prevent soft tissue inflammation

---

torsemide
(tore'se-mide)
Demadex
Drug class.: Loop diuretic

Action: Acts on loop of Henle to decrease the reabsorption of chloride, sodium, and potassium with resultant diuresis
Uses: Hypertension and edema associated with CHF, liver disease, chronic renal failure
Dosage and routes:
Hypertension
• *Adult:* PO 5 mg/day; may increase to 10 mg after 4-6 wk if required
CHF, chronic renal failure
• *Adult:* PO or IV, 10-20 mg/day; may increase if inadequate response; no data for doses >200 mg
Hepatic cirrhosis
• *Adult:* PO or IV 5-10 mg/day
Available forms include: Tabs 5, 10, 20, 100 mg; inj IV 10 mg/ml in 2, 5 ml amps
Side effects/adverse reactions:
CNS: Dizziness, headache, fatigue, insomnia, nervousness, syncope
CV: Orthostatic hypotension, ECG abnormalities, chest pain, edema, dysrhythmias
GI: Diarrhea, nausea, dyspepsia, irritation, GI bleeding
RESP: Cough

GU: Excessive urination
EENT: Sore throat, rhinitis
INTEG: Rash, photosensitvity
MS: *Asthenia,* muscle cramps, arthralgia
Contraindications: Hypersensitivity, anuria, severe electrolyte depletion, hypersensitivity to sulfonylureas, hepatic coma, cisapride
Precautions: Pregnancy category B, lactation, children <18 yr, dehydration, systemic lupus erythematosus, ototoxicity, electrolyte imbalance
Pharmacokinetics:
PO: Onset 1 hr, peak effects 1-2 hr, duration 6-8 hr; liver metabolism; renal excretion
IV: Onset 10 min, peak effect 1 hr, duration 6-8 hr
Drug interactions of concern to dentistry:
• Increased electrolyte imbalance: systemic corticosteroids
• Masked ototoxicity: phenothiazines
• Decreased antihypertensive effects: NSAIDs, especially indomethacin
• Increased sweating, hot flashes, weakness, CV symptoms: chloral hydrate (rare)

DENTAL CONSIDERATIONS
General:
• Monitor vital signs every appointment due to cardiovascular side effects.
• After supine positioning, have patient sit upright for at least 2 min before standing to avoid orthostatic hypotension.
• Patients on high-potency loop diuretics should be questioned about serum potassium levels or potassium supplement use.
• Short appointments and a stress reduction protocol may be required for anxious patients.
• Consider semisupine chair position if GI side effects occur.
Consultations:
• Medical consult may be required to assess disease control and stress tolerance in the patient.
Teach patient/family:
• Importance of updating health history/drug record if physician makes any changes in evaluation/drug regimen

---

tramadol HCl
(tra′ma-dole)
Ultram
Drug class.: Synthetic opioid analgesic

Action: Unknown, but it has been shown to bind to opioid receptors and inhibit the reuptake of norepinephrine and serotonin
Uses: Moderate-to-severe pain
Dosage and routes:
• *Adult:* PO 50-100 mg q4-6h, limit 400 mg/day (do not exceed limit); for moderately severe pain, 100 mg initial dose may be required
Moderate chronic pain not requiring rapid analgesic onset
• *Adult:* PO initial 25 mg/day, then titrate doses by 25 mg as separate doses q3d to maximum dose of 100 mg, then titrate doses by 50 mg q3d to max of 200 mg daily; max daily dose 400 mg
Renal/hepatic impairment or elderly 65 yr or older
• *Adult:* PO limit dose to 300 mg/day

T

Cirrhosis

• *Adult:* PO limit dose to 50 mg q12h

Available forms include: Tabs 50 mg

Side effects/adverse reactions:

▼ *ORAL:* Dry mouth (<5%), stomatitis

CNS: Dizziness, vertigo, headache, somnolence, seizures, anxiety, confusion, drug abuse risk

CV: Vasodilation, palpitation

GI: Constipation, vomiting, dyspepsia, diarrhea, flatulence

GU: Urinary retention, frequency

EENT: Visual disturbances

INTEG: Pruritus, sweating, rash

MS: Hypertonia

MISC: Malaise

Contraindications: Hypersensitivity to tramadol, codeine, or other opioids; acute alcohol, hypnotic, other opioid, or psychotropic drug intoxication, opioid addicts; pregnancy category C; lactation; child <16 yr; elderly; renal or hepatic impairment; risk of seizures in patients taking MAO inhibitors, tricyclic antidepressants, or other drugs that reduce the seizure threshold; increased intracranial pressure due to head injury

Precautions: Not a controlled substance, but dependence and abuse are possible

Pharmacokinetics:

PO: Rapid oral absorption, can be given with food, peak levels 2 hr, half-life 6-7 hr; hepatic metabolism; excreted in urine

Drug interactions of concern to dentistry:

• Increased risk of respiratory depression: anesthetics, alcohol

• Significant increase in metabolism: carbamazepine

• Increased serum concentrations: quinidine

• Increased risk of seizures: MAO inhibitors, tricyclic antidepressants, selective serotonin reuptake inhibitors

• Increased risk of sedation: other CNS depressant drugs, alcohol

DENTAL CONSIDERATIONS

General:

• Determine why the patient is taking the drug.

• Patients taking opioids for acute or chronic pain should be given alternative analgesics for dental pain.

• Geriatric patients are more susceptible to drug effects; use lower dose.

• Assess salivary flow as a factor in caries, periodontal disease, and candidiasis.

• Take precautions if dental surgery is anticipated and general anesthesia is required.

• Risk of cross-hypersensitivity to other opioid analgesics.

Teach patient/family:

• Caution to prevent trauma when using oral hygiene aids

• That opioid drugs may alter reaction time; caution patient about driving or operating complex equipment

When chronic dry mouth occurs, advise patient:

• To avoid mouth rinses with high alcohol content due to drying effects

• To use daily home fluoride products for anticaries effect

• To use sugarless gum, frequent sips of water, or saliva substitutes

trandolapril

(tran'dole-a-pril)
Mavik

Drug class.: Angiotensin-converting enzyme (ACE) inhibitor

Action: Selectively suppresses renin-angiotensin-aldosterone system; inhibits ACE; prevents conversion of angiotension I to angiotensin II; results in reduced peripheral resistance, decreased aldosterone secretion, and increase in plasma renin

Uses: Hypertension alone or in combination with other antihypertensive medications; maintenance therapy to prevent CHF after MI; ventricular dysfunction after MI

Dosage and routes:

Not taking diuretic

• *Adult:* PO initial dose 1 mg (non–African-American patient) and 2 mg (African-American patient) daily; adjust dose to BP response; usual dose 2-4 mg daily

Taking diuretic

• *Adult:* Discontinue diuretic for 2-3 days before initiating trandolapril therapy, add diuretic if BP is not controlled

When diuretic cannot be discontinued

• *Adult:* Initial dose is 0.5 mg with caution and medical supervision until BP is stabilized

Available forms include: Tabs 1 mg, 2 mg, and 4 mg

Side effects/adverse reactions:

▼ *ORAL:* ***Angioedema (lips, tongue, mucous membranes)***

CNS: Dizziness, drowsiness, insomnia, vertigo, headache, fatigue

CV: Hypotension, syncope, bradycardia, chest pain, palpitation, AV first-degree block, bradycardia, hyperkalemia

GI: Diarrhea, ***pancreatitis,*** cholestatic jaundice

RESP: Cough, URI, dyspnea

HEMA: ***Neutropenia, leukopenia***

GU: Impotence, decreased libido

EENT: Throat inflammation, epistaxis

INTEG: Pruritus, rash, pemphigus

MS: Cramps, gout, extremity pain

MISC: ***Anaphylactoid reactions***

Contraindications: Hypersensitivity or angioedema with prior use of ACE inhibitors, second or third trimester of pregnancy, lactation

Precautions: Angioedema (higher rate in African-American patients), congestive heart failure, ischemic heart disease, aortic stenosis, cerebrovascular disease, monitor WBC in SLE or scleroderma, impaired renal function, hyperkalemia, pregnancy category C (first trimester), pregnancy category D (second, third trimester), pediatric patients, potassium-sparing diuretics

Pharmacokinetics:

PO: Active metabolite trandolaprilat, peak levels trandolapril 1 hr, trandolaprilat 4-10 hr, excreted 66% in feces, 33% in urine, protein binding 80%

Drug interactions of concern to dentistry:

• Decreased absorption of tetracycline

• Drugs that lower blood pressure could possibly exaggerate hypotensive effects

DENTAL CONSIDERATIONS

General:

• Monitor vital signs every appointment due to cardiovascular disease.

• Limit use of sodium-containing

products such as saline IV fluids for those patients with a dietary salt restriction.

• Stress from dental procedures may compromise cardiovascular function; determine patient risk.

• Short appointments and a stress reduction protocol may be required for anxious patients.

• Use precaution if sedation or general anesthesia is required; risk of hypotensive episode.

• After supine positioning, have patient sit upright for at least 2 min before standing to avoid orthostatic hypotension.

• Consider semisupine chair position for patient comfort due to respiratory side effects of drug.

• Patients on chronic drug therapy may rarely have symptoms of blood dyscrasias, which can include infection, bleeding, and poor healing.

• Importance of updating health and drug history if physician makes any changes in evaluation/drug regimens.

Consultations:

• Medical consult may be required to assess disease control and patient's ability to tolerate stress.

Teach patient/family:

• Importance of good oral hygiene to prevent soft tissue inflammation

• Caution to prevent trauma when using oral hygiene aids

---

tranexamic acid

(tran-ex-am′ik)

Cyklokapron

Drug class.: Hemostatic, antithrombolytic

Action: Competitive inhibitor of plasminogen activation, decreases the conversion of plasminogen to plasmin; a much higher dose acts as a noncompetitive inhibitor of plasmin

Uses: Prophylaxis and treatment of hemophilia patients to reduce or prevent hemorrhage during and after extractions; unapproved uses: in hyperfibrinolysis-induced hemorrhage, angioedema; oral rinse (with systemic therapy) to reduce bleeding in oral surgery patients who are also taking anticoagulants

Dosage and routes:

Dental extraction in hemophilia patient

• *Adult and adolescent:* IV immediately before surgery, 10 mg/kg; after surgery give 25 mg/kg tid or qid for 2-8 days

• *Adult and adolescent:* PO beginning day before surgery, 25 mg/kg tid or qid; after surgery give 25 mg/kg tid or qid for 2-8 days; patients unable to take PO meds—IV, 10 mg/kg tid-qid

NOTE: Reduce dose with moderate to severe renal impairment

Unlabled use: Dental procedures producing bleeding in patients taking oral anticoagulants (rinse)

Some reports suggest the use of tranexamic oral rinse for use in patients who cannot reduce their use of oral anticoagulants. One report (Ramstrom et al: *J Oral Maxillofac Surg* 51:1211-1216, 1963) used the following procedure:

• *Adult:* Before suturing, the area is irrigated with 10 ml of 4.8% tranexamic acid solution. Patients rinse for 2 min 4 times daily for the next 7 days. No food or drink is to be consumed within 1 hr of using mouthwash. Tranexamic acid mouthwash is not commercially

available in Canada or the USA. It could be extemporaneously prepared using the commercial tablets or injection. Because stability data for aqueous solutions are lacking, extemporaneous solutions should be freshly prepared.
In another report (Souto et al: *J Oral Maxillofac Surg* 54:27-32, 1996) a mouth rinse of 1 ampule of the antifibrinolytic agent for 2 min q6h for 2 days was used.
Available forms include: Tabs 500 mg; amps 100 mg/ml in 10 ml size
Side effects/adverse reactions:
CNS: Giddiness
CV: Hypotension (IV doses)
GI: Nausea, vomiting, diarrhea
EENT: Blurred vision
Contraindications: Patients with acquired defective color vision, subarachnoid hemorrhage
Precautions: Pregnancy category B, lactation, reduce dose in renal impairment, limited use experience in children
Pharmacokinetics:
PO: Bioavailability 30%-50%, low protein binding (<3%), peak plasma levels 3 hr, little metabolism, renal excretion
Drug interactions of concern to dentistry:
• Increased risk of bleeding: drugs that affect coagulation
• Factor IX complex: increased risk of thrombotic complications when used concurrently
DENTAL CONSIDERATIONS
General:
• Has been used as an antifibrinolytic mouthwash following oral surgery to prevent hemorrhage in patients taking oral anticoagulants.
Consultations:
• Hematologist consult is strongly recommended.
Teach patient/family:
• Importance of updating health and drug history if physician makes any changes in evaluation/drug regimens
• To report hemorrhage or bleeding not responding to postsurgical hemostasis
• Caution to prevent trauma when using oral hygiene aids

---

tranylcypromine sulfate

(tran-il-sip′roe-meen)
Parnate

Drug class.: Antidepressant, MAO inhibitor

Action: Increases concentrations of endogenous norepinephrine, serotonin, and dopamine in CNS storage sites by inhibiting MAO; the precise antidepressant mechanism is unknown
Uses: Depression (when uncontrolled by other means)
Dosage and routes:
• *Adult:* PO 10 mg bid; may increase to 30 mg/day after 2 wk; max 60 mg/day
Available forms include: Tabs 10 mg
Side effects/adverse reactions:
▼ *ORAL:* Dry mouth
CNS: Dizziness, drowsiness, confusion, headache, anxiety, tremors, stimulation, weakness, hyperreflexia, mania, insomnia, fatigue, weight gain
CV: Orthostatic hypotension, hypertension, dysrhythmias, hypertensive crisis
GI: Anorexia, constipation, nausea, vomiting, diarrhea, weight gain
HEMA: Anemia
GU: Change in libido, urinary retention

T

EENT: Blurred vision
INTEG: Rash, flushing, increased perspiration
ENDO: ***SIADH-like syndrome***
Contraindications: Hypersensitivity to MAO inhibitors, elderly, hypertension, CHF, severe hepatic disease, pheochromocytoma, severe renal disease, severe cardiac disease
Precautions: Suicidal patients, convulsive disorders, severe depression, schizophrenia, hyperactivity, diabetes mellitus, pregnancy category C
Pharmacokinetics:
PO: Metabolized in liver, excreted by kidneys, crosses placenta, excreted in breast milk
Drug interactions of concern to dentistry:
• Increased pressor effects: indirect-acting sympathomimetics (ephedrine)
• Hyperpyretic crisis, convulsions, hypertensive episode, and death: carbamazepine, meperidine, and possibly other opioids
• Increased anticholinergic effects: anticholinergics and antihistamines
• Increased effects of alcohol, barbiturates, benzodiazepines, CNS depressants, fluoxetine, tricyclic antidepressants

DENTAL CONSIDERATIONS
General:
• After supine positioning, have patient sit upright for at least 2 min before standing to avoid orthostatic hypotension.
• Take vital signs every appointment due to cardiovascular side effects.
• Assess salivary flow as a factor in caries, periodontal disease, and candidiasis.
• Hypertensive episodes are possible even though there are no specific contraindications to vasoconstrictor use in local anesthetics.
Consultations:
• Medical consult may be required to assess patient's ability to tolerate stress.
Teach patient/family:
• To use electric toothbrush if patient has difficulty holding conventional devices
When chronic dry mouth occurs, advise patient:
• To avoid mouth rinses with high alcohol content due to drying effects
• Of need for daily home fluoride to prevent caries
• To use sugarless gum, frequent sips of water, or saliva substitutes

---

trazodone HCl

(traz′oh-done)
Desyrel, Trazon, Trialodine
Drug class.: Antidepressant

Action: Selectively inhibits serotonin-specific reuptake in the brain
Uses: Depression; unapproved use: chronic pain, diabetes-associated painful neuropathy, burning mouth syndrome
Dosage and routes:
• *Adult:* PO 150 mg/day in divided doses; may be increased by 50 mg/day q3-4d, not to exceed 600 mg/day
Available forms include: Tabs 50, 100, 150, 300 mg
Side effects/adverse reactions:
▼ *ORAL: Dry mouth,* stomatitis
CNS: Dizziness, drowsiness, confusion, headache, anxiety, tremors, stimulation, weakness, insomnia, nightmares, EPS (elderly), increase in psychiatric symptoms

CV: Orthostatic hypotension, ECG changes, tachycardia, ***hypertension,*** palpitations
GI: Diarrhea, ***paralytic ileus, hepatitis,*** increased appetite, nausea, vomiting, cramps, epigastric distress, jaundice
HEMA: ***Agranulocytosis, thrombocytopenia, eosinophilia, leukopenia***
GU: Retention, ***acute renal failure, priapism***
EENT: Blurred vision, tinnitus, mydriasis
INTEG: Rash, urticaria, sweating, pruritus, photosensitivity

Contraindications: Hypersensitivity to tricyclic antidepressants, recovery phase of myocardial infarction, convulsive disorders, prostatic hypertrophy

Precautions: Suicidal patients, severe depression, increased intraocular pressure, narrow-angle glaucoma, urinary retention, cardiac disease, hepatic disease, hyperthyroidism, electroshock therapy, elective surgery, pregnancy category C

Pharmacokinetics:
PO: Half-life 4.4-7.5 hr; metabolized by liver; excreted by kidneys, feces

Drug interactions of concern to dentistry:
• Increased anticholinergic effects: anticholinergic drugs
• Increased CNS depression: alcohol, all other CNS depressants

DENTAL CONSIDERATIONS
General:
• Take vital signs every appointment due to cardiovascular side effects.
• Patients on chronic drug therapy may rarely have symptoms of blood dyscrasias, which can include infection, bleeding, and poor healing.
• Assess salivary flow as a factor in caries, periodontal disease, and candidiasis.
• After supine positioning, have patient sit upright for at least 2 min before standing to avoid orthostatic hypotension.

Consultations:
• In a patient with symptoms of blood dyscrasias, request a medical consult for blood studies and postpone dental treatment until normal values are reestablished.
• Medical consult may be required to assess disease control in the patient.
• Physician should be informed if significant xerostomic side effects occur (increased caries, sore tongue, problems eating or swallowing, difficulty wearing prosthesis) so a medication change can be considered.

Teach patient/family:
• To report oral lesions, soreness, or bleeding to dentist
When chronic dry mouth occurs, advise patient:
• To avoid mouth rinses with high alcohol content due to drying effects
• Of need for daily home fluoride to prevent caries
• To use sugarless gum, frequent sips of water, or saliva substitutes

T

tretinoin (vitamin A acid, retinoic acid)

(tre'ti-noyn)

Avita, Retin-A, Retin-A Regimen Kit, Renova

🍁 Stieva-A, Stieva-A Forte

Drug class.: Vitamin A acid

Action: Decreases cohesiveness of follicular epithelium, decreases microcomedone formation

Uses: Acne vulgaris; unlabeled uses: skin cancer, lichen planus

Dosage and routes:

• *Adult and child:* Topical; cleanse area, apply hs, cover lightly

Available forms include: Topical; cream 0.1%, 0.05%; gel 0.025%, 0.01%; liq 0.05%

Side effects/adverse reactions:

INTEG: Rash, stinging, warmth, redness, erythema, blistering, crusting, peeling, contact dermatitis, hypopigmentation, hyperpigmentation

Contraindications: Hypersensitivity

Precautions: Pregnancy category C, lactation, eczema, sunburn

Pharmacokinetics:

TOP: Poor absorption, excreted in urine

Drug interactions of concern to dentistry:

• Increased peeling: medication-containing agents such as alcohol or astringents

• Avoid concurrent use with photosensitizing drugs: tetracycline, fluoroquinolones, sulfonamides

DENTAL CONSIDERATIONS

General:

• May cause dry, peeling skin if used around lips; provide lip lubricant for patient comfort during dental treatment.

• Advise patient if dental drugs prescribed have a potential for photosensitivity.

Teach patient/family:

• To avoid application on normal skin or getting cream in eyes, mouth, or other mucous membranes

triamcinolone acetonide

(trye-am-sin'oh-lone)

Azmacort Oral Inhaler, Nasacort AQ Nasal Spray

Drug class.: Glucocorticoid, intermediate acting

Action: Glucocorticoids have multiple actions that include antiinflammatory and immunosuppressant effects. They inhibit phospholipase A_2, interfering with or reducing the synthesis of prostaglandins and leukotrienes. They also bind to cytoplasmic glucocorticoid receptors (GRs) and enter the cell nucleus to bind with DNA. This results in the synthesis of various enzymes such as collagenase, elastase, and cytokines that play important roles in inflammation and immunosuppression. They also suppress the production of lymphocytes, monocytes, and eosinophils.

Uses: Maintenance treatment of chronic asthma (Azmacort); seasonal and perennial allergic rhinitis (Nasacort)

Dosage and routes:

• *Adult:* Oral inh 2 inhalations tid or qid or 4 inhalations bid

• *Adult and child >12 yr:* Nasal spray initial 2 sprays in each nostril daily; may increase to bid after 4-7 days and patient response; maintenance dose 1 spray in each nostril daily

• *Child 6-12 yr:* Oral inh 1 or 2 inhalations tid or qid or 2-4 inhalations bid; max 12 inh/day

Available forms include: Oral inh 20 g inhaler 100 μg per actuation/ 240 metered dose container; nasal spray 15 g container 55 μg per actuation/100 metered dose spray container

Side effects/adverse reactions:

▼ *ORAL: Candidiasis*

EENT: Dry throat, hoarseness, irritation

Contraindications: Acute asthma, status asthmaticus, nonasthmatic bronchitis, hypersensitivity

Precautions: TB; untreated fungal, bacterial, or viral infections of respiratory tract; pregnancy category C, lactation, children <6 yr; different doses may be required for patients on systemic glucocorticoids or patients with chickenpox, measles

Pharmacokinetics:

INH ORAL: Little systemic absorption from lungs, hepatic metabolism

NASAL SPRAY: Little systemic absorption, peak plasma levels 1.5 hr

Drug interactions of concern to dentistry:

• None reported

DENTAL CONSIDERATIONS

General:

• Place on frequent recall due to oral side effects.

• Evaluate respiration characteristics, rate.

• Midday appointments and a stress reduction protocol may be required for anxious patients.

• Acute asthmatic episodes may be precipitated in the dental office. Rapid-acting sympathomimetic inhalants should be available for emergency use. Triamcinolone is not a rapid-acting drug and is not intended for use in acute asthmatic attacks.

• Be aware that aspirin or sulfite preservatives in vasoconstrictor-containing products can exacerbate asthma.

• Examine for oral manifestation of opportunistic infection.

Consultations:

• Medical consult may be required to assess disease control in the patient.

Teach patient/family:

• Importance of good oral hygiene to prevent soft tissue inflammation

• Importance of gargling, rinsing mouth with water, and expectorating after each aerosol dose

triamcinolone/ triamcinolone acetonide/ triamcinolone diacetate/triamcinolone hexacetonide

(trye-am-sin'oh-lone)

Triamcinolone (oral): Aristocort, Kenacort

Triamcinolone acetonide: Cenocort A-40, Cinonide 40 Kenaject-40, Kenalog-10, Kenalog-40, Tac-3, Triam-A, Triamonide 40, Tri-Kort, Trilog

Triamcinolone diacetate (not for IV use): Amcort, Aristocort forte, Aristocort Intralesional, Articulose LA, Cenocort Forte, Cinalone 40, Kenacort Diacetate, Triam Forte, Triamolone 40, Trilone

🍁 Tristoject

Triamcinolone diacetate syrup: Aristocort

Triamcinolone hexacetonide (not for IV use): Aristocort Intraarticular, Aristospan Intralesional

Drug class.: Glucocorticoid, intermediate-acting

Action: Glucocorticoids have multiple actions that include antiinflammatory and immunosuppressant effects. They inhibit phospholipase A_2, interfering with or reducing the synthesis of prostaglandins and leukotrienes. They also bind to cytoplasmic glucocorticoid receptors (GRs) and enter the cell nucleus to bind with DNA. This results in the synthesis of various enzymes such as collagenase, elastase, and cytokines that play important roles in inflammation and immunosuppression. They also suppress the production of lymphocytes, monocytes, and eosinophils.

Uses: Severe inflammation; immunosuppression; neoplasms; asthma (steroid dependent); collagen, respiratory, dermatologic disorders; seasonal and perennial allergic rhinitis

Dosage and routes:

• *Adult:* PO dose depends on disease to be treated with a range of 4-48 mg per day as a single dose or divided dose

• *Child:* PO dose depends on disease to be treated; suggested dose is 1.7 mg/kg as a single dose or divided dose

Parenteral doses

• *Adult:* Triamcinolone acetonide—IM, 40-80 mg at 4 wk intervals; intraarticular, 2.5-15 mg; intralesional, up to 1 mg per injection site; triamcinolone diacetate—IM, 40 mg once weekly; intraarticular, intralesional, or soft tissue 3-48 mg repeated at 1-8 wk intervals; triamcinolone hexacetonide—intraarticular, 2-20 mg at 3-4 wk intervals; intralesional up to 0.5 mg per square inch of skin, repeat as needed

Available forms include: Tabs 1, 2, 4, 8, 16 mg; syr 2 mg/5 ml, 4.85 mg/5 ml; inj 25, 40 mg/ml diacetate; inj 3, 10, 40 mg/ml acetonide; inj 20, 5 mg/ml hexacetonide

Side effects/adverse reactions:

▼ *ORAL: Candidiasis,* poor wound healing, petechiae, dry mouth

CNS: Depression, flushing, sweating, headache, mood changes

CV: Hypertension, circulatory collapse, thrombophlebitis, embolism, tachycardia, edema

*GI: Diarrhea, nausea, abdominal distention, **GI hemorrhage, pancreatitis,*** increased appetite
*HEMA: **Thrombocytopenia***
EENT: Fungal infections, increased intraocular pressure, blurred vision
INTEG: Acne, poor wound healing, ecchymosis, petechiae
MS: Fractures, osteoporosis, weakness

Contraindications: Psychosis, hypersensitivity, idiopathic thrombocytopenia, acute glomerulonephritis, amebiasis, fungal and viral infections, nonasthmatic bronchial disease, child <2 yr, AIDS, TB

Precautions: Pregnancy category D, diabetes mellitus, glaucoma, osteoporosis, seizure disorders, ulcerative colitis, CHF, myasthenia gravis, renal disease, esophagitis, peptic ulcer, herpetic infections, rifampin

Pharmacokinetics:
PO/IM: Peak 1-2 hr, 2 days, 1-6 wk (IM), half-life 2-5 hr

Drug interactions of concern to dentistry:
- Decreased action: barbiturates, rifampin, rifabutin
- Increased GI side effects: alcohol, salicylates, NSAIDs
- Increased action: ketoconazole, macrolide antibiotics

DENTAL CONSIDERATIONS
General:
- Symptoms of oral infections may be masked.
- Examine for oral manifestation of opportunistic infections.
- Oral side effects may be more common with inhalation products; significant steroid side effects are more likely to occur with chronic systemic doses.
- Acute asthmatic episodes may be precipitated in the dental office. Rapid-acting sympathomimetic inhalants should be available for emergency use. A stress reduction protocol may be required.
- Monitor vital signs every appointment due to cardiovascular side effects.
- Assess salivary flow as a factor in caries, periodontal disease, and candidiasis.
- Prophylactic antibiotics may be indicated to prevent infection.
- Place on frequent recall to monitor healing response.
- Determine dose and duration of steroid therapy for each patient to assess risk for stress tolerance and immunosuppression.
- Be aware that aspirin or sulfite preservatives in vasoconstrictor-containing products can exacerbate asthma.
- Patients who have been or are currently on chronic steroid therapy (>2 wk) may require supplemental steroids for dental treatment.

Consultations:
- Medical consult may be required to assess disease control in the patient.
- Consult may be required to confirm steroid dose and duration of use.

Teach patient/family:
- Importance of good oral hygiene to prevent soft tissue inflammation
- To report oral lesions, soreness, or bleeding to dentist

When chronic dry mouth occurs, advise patient:
- To avoid mouth rinses with high alcohol content due to drying effects
- To use daily home fluoride products for anticaries effect

• To use sugarless gum, frequent sips of water, or saliva substitutes

triamcinolone acetonide (topical)

(trye-am-sin'oh-lone)

Aristocort, Aristicort A, Aristocort C, Aristocort D, Aristocort R, Delta-Tritex, Flutex, Kenalog, Kenalog-H, Kenalog in Orabase, Kenonel, Oracort, Oralone, Triacet, Tri-derm, Trianide, Triaderm

Drug class.: Topical corticosteroid, synthetic fluorinated agent, group II potency (0.5%), group III potency (0.1%), group IV potency (0.025%)

Action: Interacts with steroid cytoplasmic receptors to induce antiinflammatory effects; possesses antipruritic, antiinflammatory actions

Uses: Psoriasis, eczema, contact dermatitis, pruritus; topical dental paste used to treat nonviral inflammatory oral lesions, including aphthous stomatitis, lichen planus, and cicatricial pemphigoid

Dosage and routes:

• *Adult and child:* Apply to affected area bid-qid

Available forms include: Oint 0.025%, 0.1%, 0.5%; cream 0.025%, 0.1%, 0.5%; lotion 0.025%, 0.1%; aerosol 0.2 mg/2 sec; paste 0.1%

Side effects/adverse reactions:

▼ *ORAL:* Mucosal thinning and petechial hemorrhage (rare), stinging sensation (oral application)

INTEG: Burning, dryness, itching, irritation, acne, folliculitis, hypertrichosis, perioral dermatitis, hypopigmentation, atrophy, striae, allergic contact dermatitis, secondary infection

Contraindications: Hypersensitivity to corticosteroids, fungal or viral (herpetic) infections

Precautions: Pregnancy category C, lactation, viral infections, bacterial infections, diabetes mellitus, TB

DENTAL CONSIDERATIONS

General:

• Apply approximately 0.25 inch; measure with cotton-tipped applicator; press on lesion, do not rub. Use after brushing and eating and at bedtime for optimal effect.

• When used for oral lesions, return for oral evaluation if response of oral tissues has not occurred in 7-14 days.

Teach patient/family:

• To avoid sunlight on affected area; burns may occur

• Not to use on herpetic lesions

triamterene

(trye-am'ter-een)

Dyrenium

Drug class.: Potassium-sparing diuretic

Action: Acts on distal tubule to inhibit reabsorption of sodium and chloride; increases potassium retention

Uses: Edema; hypertension; more commonly used in combination with a thiazide diuretic

Dosage and routes:

• *Adult:* PO 100 mg bid pc, not to exceed 300 mg

Available forms include: Cap 50, 100 mg; tab 50, 100 mg

Side effects/adverse reactions:

▼ *ORAL:* Dry mouth

CNS: Confusion, nervousness, numbness in hands or feet, weakness, headache, dizziness

GI: Nausea, diarrhea, vomiting, jaundice, liver disease
HEMA: ***Thrombocytopenia, megaloblastic anemia,*** low folic acid levels
GU: ***Azotemia, interstitial nephritis,*** increased BUN, creatinine, renal stones
INTEG: Photosensitivity, rash
ELECT: Hyperkalemia, hyponatremia, hypochloremia

Contraindications: Hypersensitivity, anuria, severe renal disease, severe hepatic disease, hyperkalemia, pregnancy category D

Precautions: Dehydration, hepatic disease, lactation, CHF, renal disease, cirrhosis

Pharmacokinetics:

PO: Onset 2 hr, peak 6-8 hr, duration 12-16 hr, half-life 3 hr; metabolized in liver; excreted in bile, urine

Drug interactions of concern to dentistry:

- Nephrotoxicity: possible risk with indomethacin, NSAIDs
- Decreased antihypertensive effect: possible risk with NSAIDs, indomethacin
- Decreased effect of folic acid

DENTAL CONSIDERATIONS

General:

- Limit use of sodium-containing products, such as saline IV fluids, for those patients with a dietary salt restriction.
- Assess salivary flow as a factor in caries, periodontal disease, and candidiasis.
- Take vital signs every appointment due to cardiovascular effects and possible hyperkalemia.
- Patients on chronic drug therapy may rarely have symptoms of blood dyscrasias, which can include infection, bleeding, and poor healing.

Consultations:

- In a patient with symptoms of blood dyscrasias, request a medical consult for blood studies and postpone dental treatment until normal values are reestablished.
- Medical consult may be required to assess disease control in the patient.

Teach patient/family:

- Importance of good oral hygiene to prevent soft tissue inflammation
- Caution to prevent injury when using oral hygiene aids
- To report oral lesions, soreness, or bleeding to dentist

When chronic dry mouth occurs, advise patient:

- To avoid mouth rinses with high alcohol content due to drying effects
- Of need for daily home fluoride to prevent caries
- To use sugarless gum, frequent sips of water, or saliva substitutes

---

triazolam

(trye-ay'zoe-lam)

Halcion

♣ Apo-Triazo, Gen-Triazolam, Novo-Triolam, Nu-Triazo

Drug class.: Benzodiazepine, sedative-hypnotic

Controlled Substance Schedule IV, Canada F

Action: Produces CNS depression by interacting with a benzodiazepine receptor to facilitate the action of the inhibitory neurotransmitter γ-aminobutyric acid (GABA)

T

Uses: Insomnia; unlabeled use: oral sedation of anxious dental patients

Dosage and routes:

• *Adult:* PO 0.125-0.5 mg hs

• *Elderly:* PO 0.125-0.25 mg hs

Available forms include: Tabs 0.125, 0.25, 0.5 mg

Side effects/adverse reactions:

▼ *ORAL:* Dry mouth

CNS: Headache, lethargy, drowsiness, daytime sedation, dizziness, confusion, light-headedness, anxiety, irritability, amnesia, poor coordination

CV: Chest pain, pulse changes

GI: Nausea, vomiting, diarrhea, heartburn, abdominal pain, constipation

HEMA: ***Leukopenia, granulocytopenia*** (rare)

Contraindications: Hypersensitivity to benzodiazepines, pregnancy category X, lactation, intermittent porphyria, ketoconazole, itraconazole, cisipride, ritonavir, indinavir, nelfinavir

Precautions: Anemia, hepatic disease, renal disease, suicidal individuals, drug abuse, elderly, psychosis, child <15 yr, acute narrow-angle glaucoma, seizure disorders

Pharmacokinetics:

PO: Onset 30-45 min, duration 6-8 hr, half-life 2-3 hr; metabolized by liver; excreted by kidneys (inactive metabolites); crosses placenta; excreted in breast milk

Drug interactions of concern to dentistry:

• Increased effects: erythromycin

• Increased sedation: alcohol, CNS depressants, opioid analgesics, diltiazem, anesthetics

• Avoid use with ketoconazole, itraconazole, cisapride, ritonavir, indinavir, nelfinavir

• Caution if used with fluvoxamine, reduce dose by 50%

DENTAL CONSIDERATIONS

General:

• Assess salivary flow as a factor in caries, periodontal disease, and candidiasis.

• If dizziness occurs, provide assistance when escorting patient to and from dental chair.

• When used for conscious sedation, have someone drive patient to and from dental office.

• Avoid the use of this drug in a patient with a history of drug abuse or alcoholism.

• Geriatric patients are more susceptible to drug effects; use a lower dose.

• Psychologic and physical dependence may occur with chronic administration.

• Determine why the patient is taking the drug.

• Patients on chronic drug therapy may rarely have symptoms of blood dyscrasias, which can include infection, bleeding, and poor healing.

Teach patient/family:

When chronic dry mouth occurs, advise patient:

• To avoid mouth rinses with high alcohol content due to drying effects

• Of need for daily home fluoride to prevent caries

• To use sugarless gum, frequent sips of water, or saliva substitutes

trifluoperazine HCl

(trye-floo-oh-per′a-zeen)

Stelazine

✤ Apo-Trifluoperazine, Novo-Flurazine, PMS-Trifluoperazine, Solazine, Terfluzine

Drug class.: Phenothiazine antipsychotic

Action: Blocks neurotransmission at dopaminergic synapses in the cerebral cortex, hypothalamus, and limbic system; exhibits strong peripheral α-adrenergic, anticholinergic blocking action; mechanism for antipsychotic effects is unclear

Uses: Psychotic disorders, nonpsychotic anxiety, schizophrenia

Dosage and routes:

Psychotic disorders

• *Adult:* PO 2-5 mg bid, usual range 15-20 mg/day, may require 40 mg/day or more; IM 1-2 mg q4-6h

• *Child >6 yr:* PO 1 mg qd or bid; IM not recommended for children, but 1 mg may be given qd or bid

Nonpsychotic anxiety

• *Adult:* PO 1-2 mg bid, not to exceed 5 mg/day; do not give longer than 12 wk

Available forms include: Tabs 1, 2, 5, 10, 20 mg; conc 10 mg/ml; inj IM 2 mg/ml

Side effects/adverse reactions:

▼ *ORAL: Dry mouth*

CNS: Extrapyramidal symptoms: pseudoparkinsonism, akathisia, dystonia, tardive dyskinesia, seizures, headache, lichenoid reaction

CV: Orthostatic hypotension, hypertension, ***cardiac arrest,*** ECG changes, ***tachycardia***

GI: Nausea, vomiting, anorexia, constipation, diarrhea, jaundice, weight gain

RESP: ***Laryngospasm,*** dyspnea, ***respiratory depression***

HEMA: Anemia, ***leukopenia, leukocytosis, agranulocytosis***

GU: Urinary retention, enuresis, impotence, amenorrhea, gynecomastia

EENT: Blurred vision, glaucoma, dry eyes

INTEG: Rash, photosensitivity, dermatitis

Contraindications: Hypersensitivity, cardiovascular disease, coma, blood dyscrasias, severe hepatic disease, child <6 yr, glaucoma

Precautions: Breast cancer, seizure disorders, pregnancy category C, lactation, diabetes mellitus, respiratory conditions, prostatic hypertrophy

Pharmacokinetics:

PO: Onset rapid, peak 2-3 hr, duration 12 hr

IM: Onset immediate, peak 1 hr, duration 12 hr

Metabolized by liver, excreted in urine, crosses placenta, excreted in breast milk

Drug interactions of concern to dentistry:

• Increased sedation: other CNS depressants, alcohol, barbiturate anesthetics, opioid analgesics

• Hypotension, tachycardia: epinephrine

• Increased extrapyramidal effects: phenothiazines and related drugs (haloperidol, droperidol), metoclopramide

• Additive photosensitization: tetracyclines

• Increased anticholinergic effects: anticholinergics

T

DENTAL CONSIDERATIONS

General:

• Monitor vital signs every appointment due to cardiovascular side effects.

• Patients on chronic drug therapy may rarely have symptoms of blood dyscrasias, which can include infection, bleeding, and poor healing.

• After supine positioning, have patient sit upright for at least 2 min before standing to avoid orthostatic hypotension.

• Assess salivary flow as a factor in caries, periodontal disease, and candidiasis.

• Avoid dental light in patient's eyes; offer dark glasses for patient comfort.

• Assess for presence of extrapyramidal motor symptoms, such as tardive dyskinesia and akathisia. Extrapyramidal motor activity may complicate dental treatment.

• Geriatric patients are more susceptible to drug effects; use lower dose.

• Use vasoconstrictors with caution, in low doses, and with careful aspiration.

Consultations:

• In a patient with symptoms of blood dyscrasias, request a medical consult for blood studies and postpone dental treatment until normal values are reestablished.

• Take precautions if dental surgery is anticipated and anesthesia is required.

• Physician should be informed if significant xerostomic side effects occur (increased caries, sore tongue, problems eating or swallowing, difficulty wearing prosthesis) so a medication change can be considered.

• If signs of tardive dyskinesia or akathisia are present, refer to physician.

Teach patient/family:

• Importance of good oral hygiene to prevent soft tissue inflammation

• Caution to prevent injury when using oral hygiene aids

• To use electric toothbrush if patient has difficulty holding conventional devices

When chronic dry mouth occurs, advise patient:

• To use daily home fluoride products for anticaries effect

• To avoid mouth rinses with high alcohol content due to drying effects

• To use sugarless gum, frequent sips of water, or saliva substitutes

---

triflupromazine HCl

(trye-floo-proe'ma-zeen)

Vesprin

Drug class.: Phenothiazine, antipsychotic

Action: Blocks neurotransmission at dopaminergic synapses in the cerebral cortex, hypothalamus, and limbic system; exhibits strong peripheral α-adrenergic, anticholinergic blocking action; mechanism for antipsychotic effects is unclear

Uses: Psychotic disorders, schizophrenia, acute agitation, nausea, vomiting

Dosage and routes:

Psychosis

• *Adult:* IM 60 mg; not to exceed 150 mg/day

• *Child >2.5 yr:* IM 0.2-0.25 mg/kg to max total dose of 10 mg/day

Nausea/vomiting

• *Adult:* IM 5-15 mg q4h, max 60 mg qd; IV 1 mg, max 3 mg/day

• *Child >2.5 yr:* IM 0.2 mg/kg, max 10 mg qd; do not give IV to child

Available forms include: Inj IM/IV 10, 20 mg/ml

Side effects/adverse reactions:

▼ *ORAL:* Dry mouth, metallic taste, lichenoid reaction

CNS: Extrapyramidal symptoms: pseudoparkinsonism, akathisia, dystonia, tardive dyskinesia, drowsiness, headache, ***seizures***

CV: Orthostatic hypotension, hypertension, ***cardiac arrest,*** ECG changes, ***tachycardia***

GI: Nausea, vomiting, anorexia, constipation, diarrhea, jaundice, weight gain

RESP: ***Laryngospasm,*** dyspnea, ***respiratory depression***

HEMA: Anemia, ***leukopenia, leukocytosis, agranulocytosis***

GU: Urinary retention, urinary frequency, enuresis, impotence, amenorrhea, gynecomastia

EENT: Blurred vision, glaucoma

INTEG: Rash, photosensitivity, dermatitis

Contraindications: Hypersensitivity, blood dyscrasias, coma, child <2.5 yr, brain damage, bone marrow depression

Precautions: Pregnancy category C, lactation, seizure disorders, hepatic disease, cardiac disease

Pharmacokinetics:

IV/IM: Onset erratic, peak 2-4 hr, duration 4-6 hr

IM: Onset 15-30 min, peak 15-20 min, duration 4-6 hr

Metabolized by liver; excreted in urine, feces; crosses placenta; excreted in breast milk

Drug interactions of concern to dentistry:

• Oversedation: other CNS depressants, opioid analgesics, alcohol, barbiturate anesthetics

• Hypotension, tachycardia: epinephrine

• Increased anticholinergic effects: anticholinergics

• Increased photosensitivity: tetracyclines

• Increased extrapyramidal effects: phenothiazines and related drugs (haloperidol, droperidol), metoclopramide

DENTAL CONSIDERATIONS

General:

• The primary use of this drug is to control nausea/vomiting, which may preclude elective dental therapy.

• Assess salivary flow as a factor in caries, periodontal disease, and candidiasis.

• Examine for evidence of blood dyscrasias (infection, bleeding, poor healing).

• After supine positioning, have patient sit upright for at least 2 min before standing to avoid orthostatic hypotension.

• Assess for the presence of extrapyramidal motor symptoms such as tardive dyskinesia and akathisia. Extrapyramidal motor activity may complicate dental treatment.

• Avoid dental light in patient's eyes; offer dark glasses for patient comfort.

• Monitor vital signs every appointment due to cardiovascular side effects.

• Geriatric patients are more susceptible to drug effects; use a lower dose.

• Use vasoconstrictors with caution, in low doses, and with careful aspiration.

• Take precautions if dental surgery is anticipated and anesthesia is required.

Consultations:

• Medical consult for blood studies (CBC); leukopenic and thrombocytopenic side effects may result in infection, delayed healing, and excessive bleeding. Postpone dental treatment until normal values are maintained.

• If signs of tardive dyskinesia or akathisia are present, refer to physician.

Teach patient/family:

• Importance of good oral hygiene to prevent soft tissue inflammation

• Use of electric toothbrush if patient has difficulty holding conventional devices

• Caution in use of oral hygiene aids to prevent injury

This drug will not be used chronically; however, *when chronic dry mouth occurs, advise patient:*

• To avoid mouth rinses with high alcohol content due to drying effects

• Of need for daily home fluoride to prevent caries

• To use sugarless gum, frequent sips of water, or saliva substitutes

trifluridine (ophthalmic)

(trye-flure'i-deen)

Viroptic Ophthalmic Solution

Drug class.: Antiviral

Action: Inhibits viral DNA synthesis and replication

Uses: Primary keratoconjunctivitis, recurring epithelial keratitis, keratitis associated with herpes simplex virus types 1 and 2, and vicciniavirus

Dosage and routes:

• *Adult and child:* Instill 1 gtt q2h while awake, not to exceed 9 gtt/day, until corneal epithelium is regrown; then 1 gtt q4h × 1 wk

Available forms include: Sol 1% in 7.5 ml container

Side effects/adverse reactions:

EENT: Burning, stinging, swelling, photophobia

Contraindications: Hypersensitivity

Precautions: Antibiotic hypersensitivity, pregnancy category C

Drug interactions of concern to dentistry:

• None reported

DENTAL CONSIDERATIONS

General:

• Protect patient's eyes from accidental spatter during dental treatment.

• Avoid dental light in patient's eyes; offer dark glasses for patient comfort.

Evaluate:

• Therapeutic response: absence of redness, inflammation, tearing

• Allergy: itching, lacrimation, redness, swelling

trihexyphenidyl HCl

(trye-hex-ee-fen'i-dil)

Trihexane, Trihexy

♣ Apo-Trihex, Artane, PMS-Trihexyphenidyl

Drug class.: Antiparkinsonian, anticholinergic

Action: Blocks central muscarinic receptors, which decreases the severity of involuntary movements

Uses: Parkinson symptoms

Dosage and routes:
Parkinson symptoms
• *Adult:* PO 1 mg, increased by 2 mg q3-5d to a total of 6-10 mg/day
Drug-induced extrapyramidal symptoms
• *Adult:* PO 1 mg/day; usual dose 5-15 mg/day
Available forms include: Tabs 2, 5 mg; sus rel caps 5 mg; elix 2 mg/5 ml
Side effects/adverse reactions:
ORAL: Dry mouth, soreness of mouth or tongue
CNS: Confusion, anxiety, restlessness, irritability, delusions, hallucinations, headache, sedation, depression, incoherence, dizziness, flushing, weakness
CV: Palpitation, tachycardia, postural hypotension
GI: Constipation, ***paralytic ileus,*** nausea, vomiting, abdominal distress
GU: Hesitancy, retention
EENT: Blurred vision, photophobia, dilated pupils, difficulty swallowing
INTEG: Urticaria, rash
MS: Weakness, cramping
MISC: Suppression of lactation, nasal congestion, decreased sweating, increased temperature
Contraindications: Hypersensitivity, narrow-angle glaucoma, myasthenia gravis, GI/GU obstruction, tachycardia, myocardial ischemia, unstable CV disease
Precautions: Pregnancy category C, children, gastric ulcer
Pharmacokinetics:
PO: Onset 1 hr, peak 2-3 hr, duration 6-12 hr; excreted in urine
Drug interactions of concern to dentistry:
• Increased anticholinergic effects: scopolamine, atropine, phenothiazines, antihistamines, and other anticholinergics
• Increased CNS depression: alcohol, CNS depressants
• Decreased effects of phenothiazines

DENTAL CONSIDERATIONS
General:
• Assess salivary flow as a factor in caries, periodontal disease, and candidiasis.
• Place on frequent recall due to oral side effects.
• After supine positioning, have patient sit upright for at least 2 min before standing to avoid orthostatic hypotension.
• Avoid dental light in patient's eyes; offer dark glasses for patient comfort.
Teach patient/family:
• Importance of good oral hygiene to prevent soft tissue inflammation
• To use electric toothbrush if patient has difficulty holding conventional devices
When chronic dry mouth occurs, advise patient:
• To avoid mouth rinses with high alcohol content due to drying effects
• Of need for daily home fluoride to prevent caries
• To use sugarless gum, frequent sips of water, or saliva substitutes

T

trimethadione
(trye-meth-a-dye'one)
Tridione
Drug class.: Anticonvulsant

Action: Increases the threshold for

seizures initiated in the cortex, decreases CNS synaptic stimulation to low-frequency impulses

Uses: Refractory absence (petit mal) seizures

Dosage and routes:

• *Adult:* PO 300 mg tid; may increase by 300 mg/wk, not to exceed 600 mg qid

• *Child >6 yr:* PO 0.9 g/day in divided doses tid or qid

• *Child 2-6 yr:* PO 0.6 g/day in divided doses tid or qid

• *Child <2 yr:* PO 0.3 g/day in divided doses tid or qid

Available forms include: Caps 300 mg; chew tabs 150 mg

Side effects/adverse reactions:

▼ *ORAL: Bleeding gums*

CNS: Drowsiness, dizziness, fatigue, paresthesia, irritability, headache, insomnia, myasthenia gravis syndrome

CV: Hypertension, hypotension

GI: Nausea, vomiting, abnormal liver function tests

HEMA: ***Thrombocytopenia, agranulocytosis, leukopenia, neutropenia, hemolytic anemia, eosinophilia, aplastic anemia,*** increased pro-time

GU: ***Fatal nephrosis,*** vaginal bleeding, albuminuria, nephrosis, abdominal pain, weight loss

EENT: Photophobia, diplopia, epistaxis, retinal hemorrhage, scotomata, hemeralopia

INTEG: ***Exfoliative dermatitis,*** rash, alopecia, petechiae, erythema

Contraindications: Hypersensitivity, blood dyscrasias, pregnancy category D

Precautions: Hepatic disease, renal disease, retinal disease, porphyria, lactation, systemic lupus erythematosus

Pharmacokinetics:

PO: Peak 30 min-2 hr, half-life 10 days; excreted by kidneys

Drug interactions of concern to dentistry:

• Increased CNS depression: all CNS depressants

DENTAL CONSIDERATIONS

General:

• Short appointments and a stress reduction protocol may be required for anxious patients.

• Determine type of epilepsy, seizure frequency, and quality of seizure control. A stress reduction protocol may be required.

• Patients on chronic drug therapy may rarely have symptoms of blood dyscrasias, which can include infection, bleeding, and poor healing.

• Avoid dental light in patient's eyes; offer dark glasses for patient comfort.

• Place on frequent recall due to oral side effects.

• Monitor vital signs every appointment due to cardiovascular side effects.

Consultations:

• Obtain a medical consult for blood studies (CBC) because leukopenic and thrombocytopenic effects of drug may result in infection, delayed healing, and excessive bleeding. Dental treatment should be postponed until normal values are maintained.

• Medical consult may be required to assess disease control and patient's ability to tolerate stress.

Teach patient/family:

• Importance of good oral hygiene to prevent soft tissue inflammation

• To prevent trauma when using oral hygiene aids

trimethobenzamide

(trye-meth-oh-ben'za-mide)

Arrestin, Benzacot, Bio-Gan, Stemetic, Tebamide, Ticon, Tigan, T-Gen, Tegamide, Triban, Tribenzagan

Drug class.: Antiemetic

Action: Acts centrally by blocking chemoreceptor trigger zone, which in turn acts on vomiting center

Uses: Nausea, vomiting, prevention of postoperative vomiting

Dosage and routes:

Postoperative vomiting

• *Adult:* IM/rec 200 mg before or during surgery; may repeat 3 hr after

Discontinuing anesthesia

• *Child 13-40 kg:* PO/rec 100-200 mg tid-qid

• *Child <13 kg:* PO/rec 100 mg tid-qid

Nausea/vomiting

• *Adult:* PO 250 mg tid-qid; IM/rec 200 mg tid-qid

Available forms include: Caps 100, 250 mg; supp 100, 200 mg; inj IM 100 mg/ml

Side effects/adverse reactions:

▼ *ORAL:* Dry mouth

CNS: *Drowsiness,* restlessness, headache, dizziness, insomnia, confusion, nervousness, tingling, *vertigo,* extrapyramidal symptoms

CV: Hypertension, hypotension, palpitation

GI: Nausea, anorexia, diarrhea, vomiting, constipation

EENT: Blurred vision, diplopia, nasal congestion, photosensitivity

INTEG: Rash, urticaria, fever, chills, flushing

Contraindications: Hypersensitivity, shock, children (parenterally)

Precautions: Children, cardiac dysrhythmias, elderly, asthma, pregnancy category C, prostatic hypertrophy, bladder neck obstruction, narrow-angle glaucoma, stenosing peptic ulcer, pyloroduodenal obstruction

Pharmacokinetics:

PO: Onset 20-40 min, duration 3-4 hr

IM: Onset 15 min, duration 2-3 hr

Metabolized by liver, excreted by kidneys

Drug interactions of concern to dentistry:

• Increased effect: CNS depressants

• May mask ototoxic symptoms associated with antibiotics or large doses of salicylates

DENTAL CONSIDERATIONS

General:

• Nausea and vomiting may be accompanied by dehydration and electrolyte imbalance and should be corrected as part of treatment.

• Defer elective dental treatment when symptoms are present.

trimetrexate glucuronate

(tri-me-trex'ate)

Neutrexin

Drug class.: Folate antagonist

Action: Inhibits the enzyme dihydrofolate reductase, which leads to interference with DNA, RNA, and protein synthesis in the *P. carinii* organism

Uses: Alternative therapy for *P. carinii* pneumonia in immunocompromised patients, including patients with AIDS; unapproved uses: lung, prostate, colon cancer

T

Dosage and routes:
Must be given concurrently with leucovorin
• *Adult:* IV infusion 45 mg/m^2 once daily over 60-90 min; leucovorin is given IV 20 mg/m^2 over 5-10 min q6h for total dose of 80 mg/m^2; course of treatment is 21 days with trimetrexate and 24 days with leucovorin
Available forms include: IV 25 mg/5 ml vials with or without 50 mg leucovorin
Side effects/adverse reactions:
▼ *ORAL:* Oral ulceration if leucovorin is not used
GI: Nausea, vomiting, ***hepatotoxicity,*** mucosal ulceration
HEMA: ***Neutropenia (<1000/mm^3), thrombocytopenia (<75,000/mm^3),*** *anemia (Hgb <8 g/dl)*
GU: Renal toxicity
INTEG: Rash, pruritus
MISC: Hyponatremia, hypocalcemia
Contraindications: Hypersensitivity to trimetrexate, methotrexate, or leucovorin
Precautions: Pregnancy category D, lactation, child <18 yr; impaired hematologic, renal, or hepatic function; serious bone marrow depression can occur if leucovorin is not used concurrently
Pharmacokinetics:
IV: Extended plasma levels up to 72 hr; highly plasma protein bound 95%-98%; hepatic metabolism; renal excretion
Drug interactions of concern to dentistry:
• Alteration of plasma levels: concurrent use with erythromycin, ketoconazole, and fluconazole
• Alteration in trimetrexate metabolites: acetaminophen

DENTAL CONSIDERATIONS
General:
• Examine for evidence of oral manifestations of blood dyscrasia (infection, bleeding, poor healing).
• Place on frequent recall due to oral side effects.
• Determine why the patient is taking the drug.
• Examine for oral manifestations of opportunistic infections.
• Consider local hemostasis measures to prevent excessive bleeding.
• Palliative treatment may be required for stomatitis.
• Refer to physician if oral ulcerative lesions occur.
• Consider semisupine chair position for patient comfort due to GI effects of disease.
Consultations:
• Obtain a medical consult for blood studies (CBC) because leukopenic or thrombocytopenic side effects may result in infection, delayed healing, and excessive bleeding. Postpone elective dental treatment until normal values are maintained.
• Medical consult may be required to assess disease control in the patient.
Teach patient/family:
• Importance of good oral hygiene to prevent soft tissue inflammation
• Caution to prevent injury when using oral hygiene aids
• That secondary oral infection may occur; must see dentist immediately if infection occurs

trimipramine maleate

(tri-mi′pra-meen)

Surmontil

♣ Apo-Trimip, Novo-Trimipramine, Rhotrimine

Drug class.: Antidepressant—tricyclic

Action: Inhibits both norepinephrine and serotonin (5-HT) uptake in the brain, although the precise antidepressant mechanism remains unclear

Uses: Depression, enuresis in children; unlabeled uses: chronic pain, burning mouth syndrome

Dosage and routes:

• *Adult:* PO 75 mg/day in divided doses; may be increased to 200 mg/day

• *Child >6 yr:* PO 25 mg hs; may increase to 50 mg in children <12 yr or 75 mg in children >12 yr

Available forms include: Caps 25, 50, 100 mg

Side effects/adverse reactions:

▼ *ORAL: Dry mouth,* unpleasant taste

CNS: Dizziness, drowsiness, confusion, headache, anxiety, tremors, stimulation, weakness, insomnia, nightmares, EPS (elderly), increase in psychiatric symptoms

CV: Orthostatic hypotension, ECG changes, tachycardia, ***hypertension,*** palpitation

GI: Diarrhea, ***paralytic ileus, hepatitis,*** increased appetite, nausea, vomiting, cramps, epigastric distress, jaundice

HEMA: ***Agranulocytosis, thrombocytopenia, eosinophilia, leukopenia***

GU: Retention, ***acute renal failure***

EENT: Blurred vision, tinnitus, mydriasis

INTEG: Rash, urticaria, sweating, pruritus, photosensitivity

Contraindications: Hypersensitivity to tricyclic antidepressants, recovery phase of MI, convulsive disorders, prostatic hypertrophy

Precautions: Suicidal patients, severe depression, increased intraocular pressure, narrow-angle glaucoma, urinary retention, cardiac disease, hepatic disease, hyperthyroidism, electroshock therapy, elective surgery, pregnancy category C, MAO inhibitors

Pharmacokinetics:

PO: Steady state 2-6 days, half-life 7-30 hr; metabolized by liver; excreted by kidneys

Drug interactions of concern to dentistry:

• Increased anticholinergic effects: muscarinic blockers, antihistamines, phenothiazines

• Increased effects of direct-acting sympathomimetics (epinephrine, levonordefrin)

• Possible risk of increased CNS depression: alcohol, barbiturates, benzodiazepines, and other CNS depressants

• Decreased antihypertensive effects: clonidine, guamadrel, guanethidine

DENTAL CONSIDERATIONS

General:

• Take vital signs every appointment due to cardiovascular side effects.

• Assess salivary flow as a factor in caries, periodontal disease, and candidiasis.

• Patients on chronic drug therapy may rarely have symptoms of

blood dyscrasias, which can include infection, bleeding, and poor healing.
• After supine positioning, have patient sit upright for at least 2 min to avoid orthostatic hypotension.
• Use vasoconstrictors with caution, in low doses, and with careful aspiration. Avoid use of gingival retraction cord with epinephrine.
• Place on frequent recall due to oral side effects.

Consultations:
• In a patient with symptoms of blood dyscrasias, request a medical consult for blood studies and postpone dental treatment until normal values are reestablished.
• Medical consult may be required to assess disease control in the patient.
• Physician should be informed if significant xerostomic side effects occur (increased caries, sore tongue, problems eating or swallowing, difficulty wearing prosthesis) so a medication change can be considered.

Teach patient/family:
• Importance of good oral hygiene to prevent soft tissue inflammation
• Caution to prevent injury when using oral hygiene aids

When chronic dry mouth occurs, advise patient:
• To avoid mouth rinses with high alcohol content due to drying effects
• Of need for daily home fluoride to prevent caries
• To use sugarless gum, frequent sips of water, or saliva substitutes

tripelennamine HCl

(tri-pel-en′a-meen)

PBZ, PBZ-SR

Drug class.: Antihistamine, H_1-receptor antagonist

Action: Acts by competing with histamine for H_1-receptor sites; decreases allergic response by blocking histamine effects

Uses: Rhinitis, allergy symptoms

Dosage and routes:
• *Adult:* PO 25-50 mg q4-6h, not to exceed 600 mg/day; time rel 100 mg bid-tid, not to exceed 600 mg/day
• *Child >5 yr:* Time rel 50 mg q8-12h, not to exceed 300 mg/day
• *Child <5 yr:* PO 5 mg/kg/day in 4-6 divided doses, not to exceed 300 mg/day

Available forms include: Tabs 25, 50 mg; time rel tabs 100 mg

Side effects/adverse reactions:

▼ *ORAL:* Dry mouth

CNS: Dizziness, drowsiness, poor coordination, fatigue, anxiety, euphoria, confusion, paresthesia, neuritis

CV: Hypotension, palpitation, tachycardia

GI: Constipation, nausea, vomiting, anorexia, diarrhea

RESP: Increased thick secretions, wheezing, chest tightness

HEMA: ***Thrombocytopenia, agranulocytosis, hemolytic anemia***

GU: Retention, dysuria, frequency

EENT: Blurred vision, dilated pupils, tinnitus, nasal stuffiness, dry nose/throat

INTEG: Rash, urticaria, photosensitivity

Contraindications: Hypersensi-

tivity to H_1-receptor antagonist, acute asthma attack, lower respiratory tract disease

Precautions: Dental patients with chronic dry mouth, increased intraocular pressure, renal disease, cardiac disease, hypertension, bronchial asthma, seizure disorder, stenosed peptic ulcers, hyperthyroidism, prostatic hypertrophy, bladder neck obstruction, pregnancy category C

Pharmacokinetics:

PO: Onset 15-30 min, duration 4-6 hr; detoxified in liver; excreted by kidneys

Drug interactions of concern to dentistry:

- Increased CNS depression: CNS depressants, barbiturates, narcotics, hypnotics, tricyclic antidepressants, alcohol
- Increased photosensitization: tetracyclines
- Increased anticholinergic effects: muscarinic blockers

DENTAL CONSIDERATIONS

General:

- Assess salivary flow as a factor in caries, periodontal disease, and candidiasis.
- Patients on chronic drug therapy may rarely have symptoms of blood dyscrasias, which can include infection, bleeding, and poor healing.
- Consider semisupine chair position for patients with respiratory disease.
- Monitor vital signs every appointment due to cardiovascular side effects.

Teach patient/family:

When chronic dry mouth occurs, advise patient:

- To avoid mouth rinses with high alcohol content due to drying effects
- Of need for daily home fluoride to prevent caries
- To use sugarless gum, frequent sips of water, or saliva substitutes

troglitazone

(troe′gli-ta-zone)

Rezulin

Drug class.: Oral antidiabetic

Action: Improves target cell response to insulin without increasing pancreatic insulin secretion; insulin must be present for this drug to act

Uses: Type 2 diabetes for patients currently on insulin whose hyperglycemia is inadequately controlled despite 30 U of insulin/day; combination therapy with sulfonylureas or metformin

Dosage and routes:

- *Adult:* PO initial 200 mg/day in patients on insulin therapy; patients not responding—increase dose after 2-4 wk; combination with sulfonylureas—200 mg qd

Available forms include: Tabs 200, 300, 400 mg

Side effects/adverse reactions:

CNS: Headache, dizziness

CV: Peripheral edema

GI: Nausea, diarrhea

HEMA: Small increases in hemoglobin, hematocrit, neutrophils

GU: UTI

EENT: Rhinitis, pharyngitis

MS: Asthenia, back pain

META: Elevation of AST, ALT, ***severe idiosyncratic hepatocellular injury***, liver function monitoring is required

MISC: Infection, pain

T

Contraindications: Hypersensitivity

Precautions: Hepatic disease, ALT levels >1.5 times upper limit of normal, monitor liver enzymes, pregnancy category B, lactation, children

Pharmacokinetics:

PO: Rapid absorption, peak plasma levels 2-3 hr, plasma protein binding 99%, liver metabolism (P-450 enzymes), excreted in urine

Drug interactions of concern to dentistry: None reported

DENTAL CONSIDERATIONS

General:

• Ensure that patient is following prescribed diet and regularly takes medication.

• Place on frequent recall to evaluate healing response.

• Short appointments and a stress reduction protocol may be required for anxious patients.

• Diabetics may be more susceptible to infection and have delayed wound healing.

• Question patient about self-monitoring of drug's antidiabetic effect, including blood glucose values or finger-stick records.

• Consider semisupine chair position for patient comfort if GI side effects occur.

Consultations:

• Medical consult may be required to assess disease control and patient's ability to tolerate stress.

• Medical consult may include data from patient's blood glucose monitoring, including glycosylated hemoglobin or HbA_{1c} testing.

Teach patient/family:

• Caution to prevent trauma when using oral hygiene aids

• Importance of updating health and drug history if physician makes any changes in evaluation/drug regimens

trovafloxacin mesylate/ alatrofloxacin mesylate

(troe'va-flox-a-sin)

(ala-troe'flox-a-sin)

Trovafloxacin mesylate oral: Trovan

Alatrofloxacin mesylate injection: Trovan I.V.

Drug class.: A fluoronaphthyridone antiinfective (related to the fluoroquinolones)

Action: A broad-spectrum, bactericidal antiinfective that inhibits the enzymes DNA gyrase and topoisomerase IV; both enzymes are essential for proper DNA activity leading to bacterial cell division

Uses: For infections caused by susceptible microorganisms in nosocomial pneumonia, community-acquired pneumonia, acute bacterial exacerbated chronic bronchitis, acute sinusitis, abdominal infections, gynecologic infections, UTI, bacterial prostatitis, skin and skin structure infections, and selected STDs

Dosage and routes:

• *Adults >18 yr:* PO dose depends on type of infection; range 100-200 mg daily for 1-14 days

• *Adults >18 yr:* IV dose depends on type of infection; range 200-300 mg daily; single IV doses can be followed by appropriate oral doses for 10-14 days

Available forms include: Tabs 100 and 200 mg; vials IV (alatrofloxacin for injection) 5 mg/ml in 40 and 60 ml

Side effects/adverse reactions:

▼ *ORAL:* Dry mouth, stomatitis, angular cheilitis

CNS: Dizziness, headache, lightheadedness, confusion, anxiety, hallucinations

CV: Hypotension, palpitation, flushing, peripheral edema, chest pain

GI: Vomiting, nausea, diarrhea, abdominal pain, flatulence, ***antibiotic-associated pseudomembranous colitis***

RESP: Dyspnea, bronchospasm, coughing

HEMA: Anemia, leukopenia, thrombocytopenia

GU: Vaginitis, frequency of urination, abnormal renal function

EENT: Rhinitis, sinusitis

INTEG: Pruritus, rash, photosensitization

META: Increased liver enzymes

MS: Arthralgia, myalgia, muscle cramps

MISC: Pain on injection, increased sweating, fatigue, fever, ***anaphylaxis***

Contraindications: Hypersensitivity and allergy to the fluoroquinolones

Precautions: Children <18 yr, mild to moderate cirrhosis, potential for liver damage, exposure to sunlight, visible or ultraviolet radiation, seizure disorders, cerebral atherosclerosis, pregnancy category C, lactation

Pharmacokinetics:

PO: Good oral absorption, bioavailability 88%, can be administered with food, peak serum levels 1.7 hr, plasma protein binding 76%, wide tissue distribution, excreted in breast milk, hepatic metabolism, excretion in feces and urine, 50% of dose is excreted unchanged in feces

IV: Alatrofloxacin is a prodrug converted to trovafloxacin

Drug interactions of concern to dentistry:

• Reduction in absorption: magnesium or aluminum antacid products, iron salts, sucralfate, and morphine within 30 min of oral trovafloxacin; separate doses by at least 2 hr

• Increases serum levels of caffeine

DENTAL CONSIDERATIONS:

General:

• Determine why patient is taking the drug; specific infection.

• Do not use ingestible sodium bicarbonate products, such as the air polishing system (Prophy Jet), within 2 hours of drug use.

• Examine for oral manifestation of opportunistic infection.

• Avoid dental light in patient's eyes; offer dark glasses for patient comfort.

• Use caution in prescribing caffeine-containing analgesics.

Consultations:

• Medical consult may be required to assess disease control in the patient.

• Consult with patient's physician if an acute dental infection occurs and another antiinfective is required.

Teach patient/family:

• To prevent trauma when using oral hygiene aids

• Importance of good oral hygiene to prevent soft tissue inflammation

• To avoid mouth rinses with high alcohol content due to drying effects

T

ursodiol

(er'soe-dye-ole)

Actigall, Ursofalk

Drug class.: Gallstone solubilizing agent

Action: Suppresses hepatic synthesis, secretion of cholesterol; inhibits intestinal absorption of cholesterol

Uses: Dissolution of radiolucent, noncalcified gallbladder stones (<20 mm in diameter) in which surgery is not indicated; prevent gallstones in obese patients experiencing rapid weight loss

Dosage and routes:

• *Adult:* PO 8-10 mg/kg/day in 2-3 divided doses using gallbladder ultrasound q6mo; determine if stones have dissolved; if so, continue therapy and repeat ultrasound within 1-3 mo

Gallstone prevention

• *Adult:* PO 300 mg bid for 4-6 mo

Available forms include: Caps 300 mg

Side effects/adverse reactions:

▼ *ORAL:* Metallic taste, stomatitis

CNS: Headache, anxiety, depression, insomnia, fatigue

GI: Diarrhea, nausea, vomiting, abdominal pain, constipation, flatulence, dyspepsia, biliary pain

RESP: Cough, rhinitis

INTEG: Pruritus, rash, urticaria, dry skin, sweating, alopecia

MS: Arthralgia, myalgia, back pain

Contraindications: Calcified cholesterol stones, radiopaque stones, radiolucent bile pigment stones, chronic liver disease, hypersensitivity

Precautions: Pregnancy category B, lactation, children

Pharmacokinetics:

PO: 80% excreted in feces, 20% metabolized, excreted into bile, lost in feces

Drug interactions of concern to dentistry:

• Reduced action: aluminum-based antacids

DENTAL CONSIDERATIONS

General:

• Consider semisupine chair position for patient comfort due to GI effects of disease.

• Some opioids can cause spasm of bile duct leading to epigastric distress. Use caution in use for sedation or pain control. NSAIDs may be better choice.

• Consider drug as a factor in the diagnosis of altered taste.

valacyclovir HCl

(val-ay-sye'kloe-veer)

Valtrex, Zelitrex (Europe)

Drug class.: Antiviral

Action: Converted to acyclovir, which interferes with DNA synthesis required for viral replication

Uses: Herpes zoster in immunocompetent patients, genital herpes, recurrent genital herpes

Dosage and routes:

Initial herpes infection

• *Adult:* PO 1 g tid × 7 days with or without meals

Recurrent genital herpes treatment

• *Adult:* PO 500 mg bid × 5 days

Available forms include: Caps 500 mg, 1 g

Side effects/adverse reactions:

▼ *ORAL:* Glossitis, medication taste; although unknown for this drug, lichenoid drug reactions are reported with acyclovir

CNS: *Headache,* ***convulsions,*** tremors, confusion, lethargy, hallucinations, dizziness
GI: *Nausea,* vomiting, diarrhea, increased ALT/AST, abdominal pain, colitis
HEMA: ***Bone marrow depression, granulocytopenia, thrombocytopenia, leukopenia, megaloblastic anemia,*** anemia, increased bleeding time
GU: *Vaginitis, candidiasis,* ***glomerulonephritis, acute renal failure,*** oliguria, proteinuria, hematuria, changes in menses
INTEG: Rash, urticaria, pruritus
MS: Asthenia

Contraindications: Hypersensitivity to valacyclovir or acyclovir, avoid with patients with HIV or bone marrow or renal transplants due to risk of hemolytic uremic syndrome

Precautions: Pregnancy category B, renal impairment, lactation, children; reduce dose in renal impairment

Pharmacokinetics:
PO: Rapid absorption and conversion to acyclovir, renal excretion, extensive tissue distribution

Drug interactions of concern to dentistry:
• None reported in otherwise uncompromised patients

DENTAL CONSIDERATIONS

General:
• Determine why the patient is taking the drug.
• Be aware of general discomfort associated with shingles; acute symptoms may preclude patient's routine dental visit or mandate short appointments.
• Patients on chronic drug therapy may rarely have symptoms of blood dyscrasias, which can include infection, bleeding, and poor healing.

Consultations:
• Medical consult may be required to assess disease control in the patient.
• In a patient with symptoms of blood dyscrasias, request a medical consult for blood studies and postpone dental treatment until normal values are reestablished.

Teach patient/family:
• Importance of good oral hygiene to prevent soft tissue inflammation
• Caution to prevent trauma when using oral hygiene aids

---

valproic acid/valproate sodium/divalproex sodium

(val-proe'ate)
Divalproex sodium: Depakote, Depakote Sprinkle
♣ Epival
Valproate sodium: Depacon
Valproic acid: Depakene
♣ Alti-Valproic, Dom-Valproic, MedValproic, Novo-Valproic, Nu-Valproic, Penta-Valproic, PMS-Valproic Acid
Drug class.: Anticonvulsant

Action: Increased levels of γ-aminobutyric acid (GABA) in the brain

Uses: Simple, complex (petit mal) absence, mixed seizures; divalproex for manic episodes in bipolar disorder, complex partial seizures, migraine prophylaxis; unlabled use: tonic-clonic (grand mal) seizures

Dosage and routes:
• *Adult and child:* PO 15 mg/kg/day divided in 2-3 doses; may increase by 5-10 mg/kg/day qwk,

V

not to exceed 30 mg/kg/day in 2-3 divided doses

Manic episodes in bipolar disorder

• *Adult:* PO initially 75 mg in divided doses; increase dose to desired effect with max dose 60 mg/kg/day

Migraine prophylaxis

• *Adult and child >16 yr:* PO ext rel 250 mg bid, up to 1000 mg/day

Available forms include: Caps 250 mg; caps sprinkles 125 mg; delayed rel tabs 125, 250, 500 mg; syr 250 mg/5 ml; inj single dose vial 5 ml

Side effects/adverse reactions:

▼ *ORAL:* Prolonged bleeding, delayed healing, gingival enlargement (rare)

CNS: Sedation, drowsiness, dizziness, headache, incoordination, paresthesia, depression, hallucinations, behavioral changes, tremors, aggression, weakness

GI: Nausea, vomiting, abdominal pain, ***hepatic failure, pancreatitis, toxic hepatitis,*** anorexia, cramps, constipation, diarrhea, dyspepsia

HEMA: ***Thrombocytopenia, leukopenia, lymphocytosis,*** increased prothrombin time

GU: Enuresis, irregular menses

INTEG: Rash, alopecia, bruising

MISC: Asthenia

Contraindications: Hypersensitivity, hepatic disease or significant hepatic dysfunction

Precautions: MI (recovery phase), hepatic disease, renal disease, Addison's disease, pregnancy category D, lactation

Pharmacokinetics:

PO: Onset 15-30 min, peak 1-4 hr, duration 4-6 hr

REC: Absorption of enteric coated divalproex is delayed 1 hr

Drug interactions of concern to dentistry:

• Increased effects: CNS depressants; carbamazepine, phenobarbital levels may be increased; phenothiazines can lower the seizure threshold

• Increased bleeding and toxicity: salicylates, NSAIDs

• Increased serum levels of amitriptyline, nortriptyline (start with low dose and monitor)

DENTAL CONSIDERATIONS

General:

• Patients on chronic drug therapy may rarely have symptoms of blood dyscrasias, which can include infection, bleeding, and poor healing.

• Evaluate for clotting ability during gingival instrumentation because inhibition of platelet aggregation may occur.

• Consider semisupine chair position for patient comfort if GI side effects occur.

• Place on frequent recall if gingival overgrowth occurs.

• Ask about type of epilepsy, seizure frequency, and quality of seizure control.

Consultations:

• In a patient with symptoms of blood dyscrasias, request a medical consult for blood studies and postpone dental treatment until normal values are reestablished.

• Medical consult may be required to assess disease control in the patient.

Teach patient/family:

• Importance of good oral hygiene to prevent soft tissue inflammation and minimize gingival overgrowth

• Caution to prevent injury when using oral hygiene aids

• To use electric toothbrush if pa-

tient has difficulty holding conventional devices
• Need for frequent oral prophylaxis if gingival overgrowth occurs
• To report oral lesions, soreness, or bleeding to dentist

valsartan

(val-sar'tan)

Diovan

Drug class.: Angiotensin II receptor (AT_1) antagonist

Action: Acts as a competitive antagonist for angiotensin II receptors, inhibiting both vasoconstrictor and aldosterone secreting effects

Uses: Hypertension as a single drug or in combination with other antihypertensive medications

Dosage and routes:
• *Adult:* PO initial dose 80 mg/day; adjust initial dose upward or add a diuretic; dose range 80-320 mg qd

Available forms include: Caps 80, 160 mg

Side effects/adverse reactions:

▼ *ORAL:* Taste alterations

CNS: Insomnia, dizziness, fatigue, vertigo

CV: Edema, palpitation

RESP: Cough, URI

GI: Diarrhea, dyspepsia, nausea

GU: Impotence

MS: Arthralgia, back pain, leg pain, muscle cramp

Contraindications: Hypersensitivity, second and third trimesters of pregnancy

Precautions: Pregnancy category C (first trimester), D (second and third trimesters), volume depletion, less effect in African-Americans, liver impairment, lactation, children <18 yr, elevated labs for liver function, BUN, and potassium

Pharmacokinetics:

PO: Bioavailability 25%, highly plasma protein bound (95%), peak plasma levels 2-4 hr, limited metabolism; excreted in feces 83%, urine 13%

Drug interactions of concern to dentistry:
• Possible reduction in effect: ketoconazole

DENTAL CONSIDERATIONS

General:
• Monitor vital signs every appointment due to cardiovascular side effects.
• Limit use of sodium-containing products such as saline IV fluids for those patients with a dietary salt restriction.
• Stress from dental procedures may compromise cardiovascular function; determine patient risk.
• Short appointments and a stress reduction protocol may be required for anxious patients.
• Use precaution if sedation or general anesthesia is required; risk of hypotensive episode.

Consultations:
• Medical consult may be required to assess disease control and patient's ability to tolerate stress.

vancomycin HCl

(van-koe-mye'sin)

Vancocin

Drug class.: Glucopeptide-type antiinfective

Action: Inhibits bacterial cell wall synthesis

Uses: Resistant staphylococcal infections, pseudomembranous colitis, staphylococcal enterocolitis, endocarditis prophylaxis for dental procedures

Dosage and routes:

Serious staphylococcal infections

• *Adult:* IV 500 mg q6h or 1 g q12h

• *Child:* IV 40 mg/kg/day divided q6h

• *Neonate:* IV 15 mg/kg initially followed by 10 mg/kg q8-12h

Pseudomembranous colitis/staphylococcal enterocolitis

• *Adult:* PO 500 mg-2 g/day in 3-4 divided doses for 7-10 days

• *Child:* PO 40 mg/kg/day divided q6h, not to exceed 2 g/day

Available forms include: Pulvules 125, 250 mg; powder for oral sol 1, 10 g; powder for inj IV 500 mg

Side effects/adverse reactions:

▼ *ORAL:* Bitter taste sensation

CV: ***Cardiac arrest, vascular collapse***

GI: Nausea

RESP: Wheezing, dyspnea

HEMA: ***Leukopenia, eosinophilia, neutropenia***

GU: ***Nephrotoxicity, fatal uremia,*** increased BUN, creatinine, albumin

EENT: ***Ototoxicity, permanent deafness,*** tinnitus

INTEG: Chills, fever, rash, thrombophlebitis at injection site, urticaria, pruritus, necrosis

SYST: ***Anaphylaxis***

Contraindications: Hypersensitivity, decreased hearing

Precautions: Renal disease, pregnancy category C, lactation, elderly, neonates

Pharmacokinetics:

PO/IV: Oral absorption poor; rapid peak plasma levels with IV infusion of repeated doses; little metabolism because most of drug is excreted by kidney; delayed clearance occurs with renal dysfunction

Drug interactions of concern to dentistry:

• Ototoxicity or nephrotoxicity: aminoglycosides and high-dose salicylates

• Increased effects of nondepolarizing muscle relaxants

DENTAL CONSIDERATIONS

General:

• Monitor vital signs every appointment due to cardiovascular side effects.

• Administer IV slowly over 1 hr; an administration that is too rapid can lead to a fall in blood pressure (monitor) and a red rash on the face, neck, and chest due to local histamine release. No specific treatment is required for this reaction; evaluate recovery progress.

• Determine why the patient is taking the drug.

Consultations:

• Medical consult may be required to assess disease control in the patient.

---

venlafaxine HCl

(ven′la-fax-een)

Effexor, Effexor XR

Drug class.: Bicyclic antidepressant

Action: Inhibits both norepinephrine and serotonin (5-HT) uptake and to a lesser extent dopamine, but the precise antidepressant mechanism remains unclear

Uses: Depression

Dosage and routes:

• *Adult:* PO 75 mg/day in 2 or 3 divided doses; can increase dose 75 mg/day at no less than 4-day intervals; max dose 375 mg/day in 3 divided doses

Available forms include: Tabs 25, 37.5, 50, 75, 100 mg; ext rel caps 37.5, 75, 150 mg

Side effects/adverse reactions:

▼ *ORAL: Dry mouth,* glossitis (rare), cheilitis, gingivitis, candidiasis

CNS: Somnolence, dizziness, migrane, nervousness, anxiety, headache, anorexia, mania, hypomania

CV: Hypertension, tachycardia, vasodilation, postural hypotension

GI: Nausea, constipation, vomiting, dyspepsia

RESP: Dyspnea, bronchitis, yawning

HEMA: Ecchymosis, anemia, thrombocytopenia, leukopenia

GU: Abnormal ejaculation (male), male impotence, painful urination, decreased libido

EENT: Blurred vision, ear pain

INTEG: Sweating, rash, pruritus

MS: Asthenia, tremor, trismus

MISC: General body discomfort, asthenia

Contraindications: Hypersensitivity, concurrent use with an MAO inhibitor–type drug presents risk of severe reaction

Precautions: Pregnancy category C, lactation, children <18 yr, sustained hypertension with use, renal or hepatic impairment, elderly, long-term use (>4-6 wk), history of seizures, suicidal patients, mania

Pharmacokinetics:

PO: Good bioavailability (92%), metabolized in liver, active metabolite, renal excretion, plasma protein binding is low (27%)

Drug interactions of concern to dentistry:

- None currently reported; however, because this drug is similar in action to other antidepressants, it would be wise to avoid excessive amounts of vasoconstrictors, especially in gingival retraction cords
- Increased CNS depression: all CNS depressants

DENTAL CONSIDERATIONS

General:

- Monitor vital signs every appointment due to cardiovascular side effects.
- After supine positioning, have patient sit upright for at least 2 min before standing to avoid orthostatic hypotension.
- Assess salivary flow as a factor in caries, periodontal disease, and candidiasis.
- Examine for evidence of oral manifestations of blood dyscrasias (infection, bleeding, poor healing).
- Place on frequent recall to evaluate healing response.
- Consider semisupine chair position for patient comfort due to GI effects of disease.

Consultations:

- Medical consult may be required to assess disease control in the patient.
- Physician should be informed if significant xerostomic side effects occur (increased caries, sore tongue, problems eating or swallowing, difficulty wearing prosthesis) so a medication change can be considered.
- Obtain a medical consult for blood studies (CBC) because leukopenic or thrombocytopenic side effects may result in infection, delayed healing, and excessive bleeding. Postpone elective dental treatment until normal values are maintained.

Teach patient/family:

- Importance of good oral hygiene to prevent soft tissue inflammation

• Caution to prevent injury when using oral hygiene aids

When chronic dry mouth occurs, advise patient:

• To avoid mouth rinses with high alcohol content due to drying effects

• Of need for daily home fluoride to prevent caries

• To use sugarless gum, frequent sips of water, or saliva substitutes

---

verapamil/verapamil HCl

(ver-ap'a-mil)

Calan, Calan SR, Isoptin, Isoptin SR, Verelan

✤ Apo-Verap, Novo-Veramil, Nu-Verap

Drug class.: Calcium-channel blocker

Action: Inhibits calcium ion influx across cell membrane during cardiac depolarization; produces relaxation of coronary vascular smooth muscle; dilates coronary arteries; decreases SA/AV node conduction; dilates peripheral arteries

Uses: Chronic stable angina pectoris, vasospastic angina, dysrhythmias (class IV), hypertension; unlabeled uses: migraine headache, cardiomyopathy

Dosage and routes:

• *Adult:* PO 80 mg tid or qid, increase qwk; ext rel PO 120-240 mg qd; IV bol 5-10 mg over >2 min, repeat if necessary in 30 min

• *Child 1-15 yr:* IV bol 0.1-0.3 mg/kg over >2 min, repeat in 30 min, not to exceed 10 mg in a single dose

• *Child 0-1 yr:* IV bol 0.1-0.2 mg/kg over >2 min with ECG monitoring, repeat if necessary in 30 min

Available forms include: Tabs 40, 80, 120; sus rel tabs 120, 180, 240 mg; ext rel caps 120, 180, 240, 360 mg; inj 2.5 mg/ml

Side effects/adverse reactions:

▼ *ORAL: Gingival enlargement,* dry mouth, ulcers

CNS: Headache, drowsiness, dizziness, anxiety, depression, weakness, insomnia, confusion, lightheadedness

CV: Edema, ***CHF,*** bradycardia, hypotension, palpitation, AV block

GI: Nausea, diarrhea, gastric upset, constipation, increased liver function studies

GU: Nocturia, polyuria

Contraindications: Sick sinus syndrome, second- or third-degree heart block, hypotension <90 mm Hg systolic, cardiogenic shock, severe CHF

Precautions: CHF, hypotension, hepatic injury, pregnancy category C, lactation, children, renal disease, concomitant β-blocker therapy

Pharmacokinetics:

IV: Onset 3 min, peak 3-5 min, duration 10-20 min

PO: Onset variable, peak 3-4 hr, duration 17-24 hr

Half-life 4 min (biphasic), 3-7 hr (terminal); metabolized by liver; excreted in urine (96% as metabolites)

Drug interactions of concern to dentistry:

• Decreased effect: indomethacin, possibly other NSAIDs, phenobarbital

• Increased effect: parenteral and inhalation general anesthetics or other drugs with hypotensive actions

• Increased effects of nondepolarizing muscle relaxants
• Increased effects of carbamazepine

DENTAL CONSIDERATIONS
General:
• Monitor cardiac status; take vital signs at each appointment because of CV side effects. Consider a stress reduction protocol to prevent stress-induced angina during the dental appointment.
• After supine positioning, have patient sit upright for at least 2 min before standing to avoid orthostatic hypotension at dismissal.
• Place on frequent recall to monitor gingival condition.
• Limit use of sodium-containing products, such as saline IV fluids, for patients with a dietary salt restriction.
• Assess salivary flow as a factor in caries, periodontal disease, and candidiasis.
• Use vasoconstrictors with caution, in low doses, and with careful aspiration. Avoid use of gingival retraction cord with epinephrine.
Consultations:
• In a patient with symptoms of blood dyscrasias, request a medical consult for blood studies and postpone dental treatment until normal values are reestablished.
• Medical consult may be required to assess disease control and patient's tolerance for stress.
Teach patient/family:
• Importance of good oral hygiene to prevent soft tissue inflammation and minimize gingival overgrowth
• Need for frequent oral prophylaxis if gingival overgrowth occurs
When chronic dry mouth occurs, advise patient:
• To avoid mouth rinses with high alcohol content due to drying effects
• Of need for daily home fluoride to prevent caries
• To use sugarless gum, frequent sips of water, or saliva substitutes

---

vidarabine (ophthalmic)

(vye-dare'a-been)
Vira-A Ophthalmic
Drug class.: Antiviral

Action: Inhibits viral DNA synthesis by blocking DNA polymerase
Uses: Keratoconjunctivitis due to herpes simplex virus
Dosage and routes:
• *Adult and child:* TOP 0.5 inch oint into conjunctival sac q3h 5 × daily
Available forms include: Oint 3%
Side effects/adverse reactions:
EENT: Burning, stinging, photophobia, pain, temporary visual haze
Contraindications: Hypersensitivity
Precautions: Antibiotic hypersensitivity, pregnancy category C
DENTAL CONSIDERATIONS
General:
• Protect patient's eyes from spatter during dental procedures.
• Avoid dental light in patient's eyes; offer dark glasses for patient comfort.

---

vitamin A

Aquasol A
Drug class.: Fat-soluble vitamin

Action: Vitamin A (retinol) combines with opsin to form rhodopsin necessary for visual adaptation to darkness and normal function of the retina; it is required for normal bone development and epithelial tissue growth; probably acts as a cofactor in many metabolic reactions

Uses: Vitamin A deficiency

Dosage and routes:

- *Adult and child >8 yr:* PO 100,000-500,000 IU qd × 3 days, then 50,000 qd × 2 wk; dose based on severity of deficiency; maintenance 10,000-20,000 IU for 2 mo
- *Child 1-8 yr:* IM 17,500-35,000 IU qd × 10 days
- *Infant <1 yr:* IM 7500-15,000 IU × 10 days

Maintenance

- *Child 4-8 yr:* IM 15,000 IU qd × 2 mo
- *Child <4 yr:* IM 10,000 IU qd × 2 mo

Available forms include: Caps 10,000, 25,000, 50,000 IU; drops 5000 IU; inj 50,000 IU/ml

Side effects/adverse reactions:

▼ *ORAL: Gingival bleeding, dry/cracked lips*

CNS: Headache, increased intracranial pressure, intracranial hypertension, lethargy, malaise

GI: ***Jaundice,*** nausea, vomiting, anorexia, abdominal pain

EENT: Papilledema, exophthalmos

INTEG: Drying of skin, pruritus, increased pigmentation, night sweats, alopecia

MS: Arthraglia, retarded growth, hard areas on bone

META: Hypomenorrhea, hypercalcemia

Contraindications: Hypersensitivity to vitamin A, malabsorption syndrome (PO), pregnancy category X

Precautions: Impaired renal function

Pharmacokinetics:

PO/INJ: Stored in liver, kidneys, fat; excreted (metabolites) in urine, feces

DENTAL CONSIDERATIONS

General:

- Oral manifestation of side effects could indicate hypervitaminosis.
- May cause dry/peeling skin around lips; provide lip lubricant for patient comfort during dental treatment.

---

vitamin D (calcifediol [D3], calitriol [D_3], ergocalciferol [D_2], dihydrotachysterol [vitamin D analog], doxercalciferol, and alfacalcidol*)

Calciferol, Calcijex, Calderol, Deltalin, DHT, Drisdol, Hectorol, Hytakerol, Rocaltrol

🍁 One-Alpha, Ostoforte, Radiostol Forte

Drug class.: Fat-soluble vitamin

Action: Needed for regulation of calcium phosphate levels, normal bone development, parathyroid activity, neuromuscular functioning

Uses: Varies with the type of vitamin D selected but generally includes vitamin D deficiency, rickets, renal osteodystrophy, tetany, hypoparathyroidism, and hypophosphatemia; doxercalciferol is indicated for reduction of elevated intact parathyroid hormone (iPTH) levels for secondary hyperparathyroidism in patients receiving chronic renal dialysis

Dosage and routes:

- *Adult:* PO/IM 12,000 IU qd, then increased to 500,000 IU/day

• *Child:* PO/IM 1500/5000 IU qd × 2-4 wk; may repeat after 2 wk or 600,000 IU as single dose

Hypoparathyroidism

• *Adult and child:* PO/IM 200,000 IU given with 4 g calcium tab

Doxercalciferol

• *Adult:* PO at dialysis depending on iPTH levels; initial dose 10 μg 3 × wk

Available forms include: Tabs 400, 1000, 50,000 IU; caps 25,000, 50,000 IU; liq 8000 IU/ml; inj 500,000 IU/ml, 500,000 IU/5 ml; doxercalciferol caps 2.5 μg

Side effects/adverse reactions:

▼ *ORAL:* Metallic taste, dry mouth can be early signs of toxicity

CNS: ***Convulsions,*** fatigue, weakness, drowsiness, headache, psychosis

CV: Hypertension, dysrhythmias

GI: Nausea, vomiting, anorexia, cramps, diarrhea, constipation, decreased libido

GU: ***Hematuria, albuminuria, renal failure,*** polyuria, nocturia

INTEG: Pruritus, photophobia

MS: Decreased bone growth, early joint pain, early muscle pain

Contraindications: Hypersensitivity, hypercalcemia, renal dysfunction, hyperphosphatemia

Precautions: Cardiovascular disease, renal calculi, pregnancy category C, hyperphosphatemia

Pharmacokinetics:

PO/INJ: Half-life 7-12 hr, duration 2 mo; stored in liver; excreted in bile (metabolites), urine

Drug interactions of concern to dentistry:

• Decreased effects of vitamin D: phenobarbital

DENTAL CONSIDERATIONS

General:

• Sensitivity of eyes to dental light may indicate late toxicity.

• Monitor vital signs every appointment due to cardiovascular side effects.

Teach patient/family:

• That oral side effects are associated with early symptoms of overdose

vitamin E (alpha tocopherol)

Amino-Opti-E, Aquasol E, E-Complex 600, E-200 IU Softgels, E-400 IU, E-Vitamin Succinate, Liqui-E, Pheryl-E, Vita-Plus E, Weber Vitamin E

Drug class.: Vitamin E (fat-soluble vitamin)

Action: Needed for digestion and metabolism of polyunsaturated fats, decreased platelet aggregation; decreases blood clot formation; promotes normal growth and development of muscle tissue, prostaglandin synthesis; antioxidant effect protects against free radicals

Uses: Vitamin E deficiency, hemolytic anemia in premature neonates, prevention of retrolental fibroplasia

Dosage and routes:

Prophylaxis

• *Adult and adolescent:* PO 30 IU qd

Treatment

• *Adult and adolescent:* PO 60-75 IU/day

• *Child:* PO 1 IU/kg/day or 4-5 times the RDA

Available forms include: Caps

100, 200, 400, 500, 600, 1000 IU; 73.5, 147, 165 mg; tabs 200, 400 IU; 330 mg; drops 50 mg/ml

Side effects/adverse reactions:

CNS: Headache, fatigue

CV: Increased risk of thrombophlebitis

GI: Nausea, cramps, diarrhea

GU: Gonadal dysfunction

EENT: Blurred vision

INTEG: Sterile abscess, contact dermatitis

MS: Weakness

META: Altered metabolism of hormones (thyroid, pituitary, adrenal), altered immunity

Contraindications: None significant

Precautions: Pregnancy category A

Pharmacokinetics:

PO: Metabolized in liver, excreted in bile

Drug interactions of concern to dentistry:

• With doses >400 IU: increased action of oral anticoagulants

DENTAL CONSIDERATIONS

General:

• Determine why the patient is taking the drug.

---

warfarin sodium

(war'far-in)

Coumadin, Panwarfin, Sofarin

♣ Warfilone

Drug class.: Oral anticoagulant

Action: Interferes with blood clotting by indirect means; depresses hepatic synthesis of vitamin K–dependent coagulation factors (II, VII, IX, X)

Uses: Pulmonary emboli, deep vein thrombosis, MI, atrial dysrhythmias, to reduce risk of recurrent MI and thromboembolic events

Dosage and routes:

• *Adult:* PO/IV individualized for each patient depending on PT, can range from 1-10 mg

Available forms include: Tabs 1, 2, 2.5, 3, 5, 6, 7.5, 10 mg; inj 2 mg/5 ml

Side effects/adverse reactions:

▼ *ORAL: Gingival bleeding,* stomatitis, salivary gland pain/swelling

CNS: Fever

GI: Diarrhea, ***hepatitis,*** nausea, vomiting, anorexia, cramps

HEMA: ***Hemorrhage, agranulocytosis, leukopenia, eosinophilia***

GU: ***Hematuria***

INTEG: Rash, dermatitis, urticaria, alopecia, pruritus

Contraindications: Hypersensitivity, hemophilia, leukemia with bleeding, peptic ulcer disease, thrombocytopenic purpura, hepatic disease (severe), severe hypertension, subacute bacterial endocarditis, acute nephritis, blood dyscrasias, pregnancy category D, eclampsia, preeclampsia

Precautions: Alcoholism, elderly

Pharmacokinetics:

PO: Onset 12-24 hr, peak 1.5-3 days, duration 3-5 days, half-life 1.5-2.5 days; 99% bound to plasma proteins; metabolized in liver; excreted in urine, feces (active/inactive metabolites); crosses placenta

Drug interactions of concern to dentistry:

• Increased action: diflunisal, salicylates, propoxyphene, metronidazole, erythromycin, clarithromycin, ketaconazole, NSAIDs, indomethacin, chloral hydrate, tetracyclines, fluoroquinolones, acetaminophen

• Decreased action: barbiturates, carbamazepine

DENTAL CONSIDERATIONS

General:

• Question patients about their recent use of acetaminophen because acetaminophen has been shown to increase the INR to 4.0 or greater depending on the amount of acetaminophen taken. Treatment may need to be delayed. Additional use of acetaminophen will require close monitoring of INR values. (*JAMA* 279:657-662, 1998.)

• Patients on chronic drug therapy may rarely have symptoms of blood dyscrasias, which can include infection, bleeding, and poor healing.

• Consider local hemostasis measures to prevent excessive bleeding.

• Increase in bleeding with IM injections may occur.

Consultations:

• Medical consult should include partial prothrombin time, prothrombin time, or INR.

• For dental surgical procedures that may result in excessive bleeding, consider requesting dose reduction before dental treatment so that PT is no more than twice normal.

• In a patient with symptoms of blood dyscrasias, request a medical consult for blood studies and postpone dental treatment until normal values are reestablished.

Teach patient/family:

• Importance of good oral hygiene to prevent soft tissue inflammation

• Caution to prevent injury when using oral hygiene aids

• To report oral lesions, soreness, or bleeding to dentist

---

zafirlukast

(za-fir'loo-kast)

Accolate

Drug class.: Selective leukotriene receptor antagonist

Action: Competitive and selective receptor antogonist of leukotriene LD_4 and LTE_3, resulting in inhibition of bronchospasm and airway edema

Uses: Prophylaxis and chronic treatment of asthma

Dosage and routes:

• *Adult and child >12 yr:* PO 20 mg bid at least 1 hr before or 2 hr after meals

• *Child 7-11 yr:* PO 10 mg bid at least 1 hr before or 2 hr after meals

Available forms include: Tabs 10, 20 mg

Side effects/adverse reactions:

CNS: Headache, dizziness

GI: Nausea, diarrhea, abdominal pain, vomiting, dyspepsia

RESP: Infections

META: Elevation of ALT

MS: Asthenia, myalgia, back pain

MISC: Generalized pain, fever, accidental injury

Contraindications: Hypersensitivity

Precautions: Not for acute bronchospasm, food decreases bioavailability, pregnancy category B, lactation, patients <12 yr, hepatic impairment, liver enzyme elevation, elderly

Pharmacokinetics:
PO: Rapid absorption, peak plasma levels 3 hr, extensively metabolized, 90% fecal excretion, 10% urinary excretion, 99% plasma protein bound

Drug interactions of concern to dentistry:
• Increased PT with concurrent use of warfarin
• Reduced plasma levels: erythromycin, terfenadine, theophylline
• Increased plasma levels with aspirin

DENTAL CONSIDERATIONS
General:
• Midday appointments and a stress reduction protocol may be required for anxious patients.
• Avoid prescribing aspirin-containing products.
• Acute asthmatic episodes may be precipitated in the dental office. Sympathomimetic inhalants should be available for emergency use. A stress reduction protocol may be required.
• Be aware that aspirin or sulfite preservatives in vasoconstrictor-containing products can exacerbate asthma.
• Consider semisupine chair position for patients with respiratory disease and if GI side effects are a problem.

Consultations:
• Medical consult may be required to assess disease control in the patient.

Teach patient/family:
• Use of electric toothbrush if patient has difficulty holding conventional devices
• Importance of updating health and drug history if physician makes any changes in evaluation/drug regimens

zalcitabine
(zal-site'a-been)
Hivid

Drug class.: Synthetic pyrimidine antiviral

Action: Converted by cellular enzymes to active drug; functions as antimetabolite to inhibit replication of HIV in vitro

Uses: Used in combination with zidovudine in advanced HIV infection

Dosage and routes:
• *Adult:* PO 0.75 mg with 200 mg zidovudine q8h

Available forms include: Tabs 0.375, 0.75 mg

Side effects/adverse reactions:
▼ *ORAL: Oral ulcers, dry mouth, glossitis*
CNS: Peripheral neuropathy, headache, nervousness, fatigue, Bell's palsy
*CV: **Hypertension, syncope palpitation, tachycardia, CHF***
*GI: **Pancreatitis,*** nausea, dysphagia, diarrhea, GI pain, anorexia
HEMA: Epistaxis
*GU: **Renal failure,*** polyuria, renal calculus, abnormal renal function
EENT: Abnormal vision
INTEG: Rash, sweating, pruritus, dermatitis
MS: Muscle pain

Contraindications: Hypersensitivity

Precautions: Pregnancy category C, lactation, children <13 yr, renal impairment, hepatic impairment

Pharmacokinetics:
PO: Peak plasma levels following oral doses in 0.8-1.6 hr; phosphorylated form excreted in urine

(70%); food decreases rate of oral absorption

Drug interactions of concern to dentistry:

• Increased peripheral neuropathy: metronidazole, dapsone

DENTAL CONSIDERATIONS

General:

• Examine oral cavity for side effects if on long-term drug therapy.

• Monitor vital signs every appointment due to cardiovascular side effects.

• Palliative medication may be required for management of oral side effects.

• Assess salivary flow as a factor in caries, periodontal disease, and candidiasis.

• Prophylactic antibiotics may be indicated to prevent infection if surgery or deep scaling is planned.

• Patients may be more susceptible to infection and have delayed wound healing.

Consultations:

• Medical consult may be required to assess disease control and patient's ability to tolerate stress.

Teach patient/family:

• Importance of good oral hygiene to prevent soft tissue inflammation

• Caution to prevent injury when using oral hygiene aids

• That secondary oral infection may occur; must see dentist immediately if infection occurs

When chronic dry mouth occurs, advise patient:

• To avoid mouth rinses with high alcohol content due to drying effects

• Of need for daily home fluoride to prevent caries

• To use sugarless gum, frequent sips of water, or saliva substitutes

zaleplon

(za-lep'lan)

Sonata

Drug class.: Hypnotic

Action: Interacts with the GABA benzodiazepine receptor complex binding to the omega-1 receptor subunit

Uses: Short-term treatment of insomnia

Dosage and routes:

• *Adult:* PO 10 mg immediately before bedtime; dose should not exceed 20 mg

Elderly, debilitated, or smaller patient

• *Adult:* PO 5 mg immediately before bedtime

Available forms include: Caps 5, 10 mg

Side effects/adverse reactions:

▼ *ORAL: Dry mouth*

CNS: Headache, dizziness, amnesia, anxiety, paresthesia, somnolence, depression, nervousness

CV: Palpitation, arrhythmia, tachycardia, syncope

GI: Nausea, constipation, abdominal pain, dyspepsia

RESP: Bronchitis

HEMA: Anemia

GU: Dysmenorrhea, bladder pain, dysuria

EENT: Abnormal vision, ear pain, eye pain, conjunctivitis, dry eyes

INTEG: Pruritus, rash

META: Weight gain, gout, hypercholesterolemia

MS: Myalgia, asthenia

Contraindications: Hypersensitivity

Precautions: Abuse potential similar to benzodiazepines, elderly,

Z

debilitated, smaller patients adjust dose downward; pregnancy category C, lactation, children

Pharmacokinetics:

PO: Rapid absorption, bioavailability 30%, peak plasma levels 1 hr, wide tissue distribution, rapid hepatic metabolism (CYP3A4), excretion in urine; heavy, high-fat meal delays absorption significantly

Drug interactions of concern to dentistry:

• Caution when using dental drugs that inhibit or induce cytochrome P-450 enzymes

• CNS depression: all CNS depressant drugs

DENTAL CONSIDERATIONS

General:

• Assess salivary flow as a factor in caries, periodontal disease, and candidiasis.

• Determine why patient is taking the drug.

• Consider semisupine chair position for patient comfort if GI side effects occur.

Consultations:

• Medical consult may be required to assess disease control and patient's ability to tolerate stress.

Teach patient/family:

When chronic dry mouth occurs, advise patient:

• To avoid mouth rinses with high alcohol content due to drying effects

• To use daily home fluoride products for anticaries effect

• To use sugarless gum, frequent sips of water, or saliva substitutes

zanamivir

(za-nam'a-veer)

Relenza

Drug class.: Antiviral

Action: Inhibits neuraminidase, which is essential for replication of influenza type A and B viruses

Uses: Uncomplicated influenza in adults and children >12 yr with symptoms of no more than 2 days; more effective against influenza type A virus

Dosage and routes:

• *Adult and child >12 yr:* Inh 2 inhalations (total amount 10 mg) twice daily, 12 hr apart; 2 doses should be given on day 1 if at least 2 hr apart, then q12h thereafter; doses must be given not more than 2 days after onset of flu symptoms

Available forms include: Oral inh rotadisks packaged as a unit with inhaler sufficient for 5-day therapy

Side effects/adverse reactions:

CNS: Headache, dizziness

GI: Diarrhea, nausea, vomiting

RESP: Bronchitis, cough, bronchospasm (asthmatics)

HEMA: Lymphopenia, neutropenia

EENT: Sinusitis; ear, nose, and throat infections

INTEG: Urticaria

META: Elevation of liver enzymes, CPK

MS: Myalgia, arthralgia

MISC: Fever, malaise, fatigue

Contraindications: Hypersensitivity

Precautions: Teach use of inhaler to patient; chronic obstructive pulmonary disease or asthma does not preclude influenza vaccine, safety in high-risk medical conditions is unknown, pregnancy category B, lactation, children <12 yr

Pharmacokinetics:

ORAL INH: 4%-17% of inhaled dose is absorbed, peak serum levels 1-2 hr, low plasma protein binding (<10%), excreted unchanged in urine

Drug interactions of concern to dentistry:

• None reported

DENTAL CONSIDERATIONS

General:

• Acute influenza patients are unlikely to be seen in the dental office except for dental emergencies.

zidovudine

(zye-doe'vyoo-deen)

AZT, Novo-AZT

Apo-Zidovine, Retrovir

Drug class.: Antiviral thymidine analog

Action: Inhibits replication of viral DNA

Uses: Symptomatic HIV infections (AIDS, ARC), confirmed *P. carinii* pneumonia, or absolute CD4 lymphocytes <200/mm^3

Dosage and routes:

• *Adult:* PO 200 mg q4h with adjustment for severity; must stop treatment if severe bone marrow depression occurs; restart after bone marrow recovery; also given IV

Available forms include: Tabs 300 mg; caps 100 mg; syrup 50 mg/5 ml; inj 10 mg/ml

Side effects/adverse reactions:

ORAL: Taste changes, gingival bleeding, mucosal ulceration, swelling of lips or tongue, delayed healing, opportunistic infection

CNS: Fever, headache, malaise, diaphoresis, dizziness, insomnia, paresthesia, somnolence, chills, tremor, twitching, anxiety, confusion, depression, lability, vertigo, loss of mental acuity

GI: Nausea, vomiting, diarrhea, anorexia, cramps, dyspepsia, constipation, dysphagia, flatulence, rectal bleeding

RESP: Dyspnea

HEMA: ***Granulocytopenia, anemia***

GU: Dysuria, polyuria, frequency, hesitancy

EENT: Hearing loss, photophobia

INTEG: Rash, acne, pruritus, urticaria

MS: Myalgia, arthralgia, muscle spasm

Contraindications: Hypersensitivity

Precautions: Granulocyte count <1000/mm^3 or Hgb <9.5 g/dl, pregnancy category C, lactation, children, severe renal disease, severe hepatic function

Pharmacokinetics:

PO: Rapidly absorbed from GI tract, peak 0.5-1.5 hr; metabolized in liver (inactive metabolites); excreted by kidneys

Drug interactions of concern to dentistry:

• Toxicity: data are very limited; however, drugs that undergo metabolism involving glucuronidation may possibly delay the metabolism and subsequent excretion of zidovudine; these drugs include aspirin, acetaminophen, and indomethacin; other drugs that can cause granulocytopenia could increase the risk of toxicity

Z

• Decreased peak serum levels: clarithromycin

DENTAL CONSIDERATIONS

General:

• Examine for oral manifestations of opportunistic infections.

• Patients on chronic drug therapy may rarely have symptoms of blood dyscrasias, which can include infection, bleeding, and poor healing.

• Avoid dental light in patient's eyes; offer dark glasses for patient comfort.

• Place on frequent recall due to oral side effects.

Consultations:

• In a patient with symptoms of blood dyscrasias, request a medical consult for blood studies and postpone dental treatment until normal values are reestablished.

• Medical consult may be required to assess disease control in the patient.

Teach patient/family:

• Importance of good oral hygiene to prevent soft tissue inflammation

• Caution to prevent injury when using oral hygiene aids

• That secondary oral infection may occur; must see dentist immediately if infection occurs

---

zileuton

(zye-loo'ton)

Zyflo Filmtab

Drug class.: Leukotriene pathway inhibitor

Action: Inhibits the enzyme 5-lipoxygenase to interfere with synthesis of leukotrienes (LTB_4, LTC_4, LTD_4, and LTE_4), which contribute to inflammation, edema, mucous secretion, and bronchoconstriction

Uses: Prophylaxis and chronic treatment of asthma

Dosage and routes:

• *Adult:* PO 600 mg qid with meals and hs, daily dose 2400 mg

Available forms include: Tabs 600 mg

Side effects/adverse reactions:

CNS: Headache, dizziness, insomnia, somnolence, malaise

CV: Chest pain

GI: Abdominal pain, dyspepsia, nausea, constipation, flatulence, vomiting

HEMA: Lymphadenopathy, hyperbilirubinemia

GU: UTI, vaginitis

EENT: Conjunctivitis

INTEG: Pruritis

MS: Asthenia, myalgia, arthralgia, neck pain

MISC: Generalized pain, malaise, elevation liver enzymes, fever

Contraindications: Hypersensitivity; active liver disease or transaminase elevations greater than or equal to 3 times the upper limit

Precautions: Not for acute bronchospasm, status asthmaticus; theophyllin, warfarin, propranolol; hepatic impairment, pregnancy category C, lactation, children <12 yr, monitor ALT levels

Pharmacokinetics:

PO: Rapid absorption, peak plasma levels 1.7 hr, 93% bound to plasma proteins, metabolized, 94.5% excreted in urine

Drug interactions of concern to dentistry:

• Increased plasma levels of theophylline, propranolol

• Significant increase in PT when taking warfarin

DENTAL CONSIDERATIONS

General:

• Consider semisupine chair posi-

tion for patient comfort due to GI side effects of disease.

• Acute asthmatic episodes may be precipitated in the dental office. Sympathomimetic inhalants should be available for emergency use.

• Midday appointments and a stress reduction protocol may be required for anxious patients.

• Be aware that aspirin or sulfite preservatives in vasoconstrictor-containing products can exacerbate asthma.

Consultations:

• Medical consult may be required to assess disease control in the patient.

Teach patient/family:

• Importance of updating health and drug history if physician makes any changes in evaluation/ drug regimens

---

zolmitripan

(zole′my-tri-pan)

Zomig

Drug class.: Serotonin agonist

Action: A selective serotonin agonist for 5-HT_{1D} and 5-HT_{1B} serotonin receptors on intracranial blood vessels, trigeminal sensory nerves (cranial vessel constriction), and inhibition of proinflammatory neuropeptide release

Uses: Acute treatment of migraine with or without aura in adults

Dosage and routes:

• *Adult:* PO initial 2.5 mg or lower; if headache returns repeat dose in 2 hr not to exceed 10 mg in 24 hr; lack of response to first dose requires physician consult before taking second dose; safe use in treating more than 3 headaches in 30 days has not been established; doses of 5 mg cause an increase in side effects

Available forms include: Tabs 2.5, 5 mg

Side effects/adverse reactions:

▼ *ORAL: Dry mouth (5%)*

CNS: Dizziness, somnolence, warm sensation, hyperesthesia, paresthesia, dizziness, vertigo, numbness

CV: Chest pain, chest tightness, palpitation, ***serious cardiac events may occur (coronary artery spasm, myocardial ischemia, MI, ventricular tachycardia, ventricular fibrillation)***

GI: Nausea, dyspepsia, dysphagia

RESP: Bronchitis, hiccups

HEMA: Ecchymosis

GU: Hematuria, cystitis, frequency

EENT: Sweating, photosensitivity, pruritus, rash, dry eyes

MS: Myalgia, leg cramps, back pain; neck, jaw, and throat pain

MISC: Asthenia, allergy reaction

Contraindications: Hypersensitivity, ischemic heart disease (angina, MI), Prinzmetal's variant angina, uncontrolled hypertension, within 24 hr of use of ergotamine or other $5HT_1$ agonist, hemiplegic or basilar migraine, prophylactic therapy of migraine, Wolff-Parkinson-White syndrome, accessory conduction arrhythmias, MAO inhibitors

Precautions: Renal impairment, hepatic impairment, may cause coronary vasospasm, pregnancy category C, lactation, children, geriatric

Pharmacokinetics:

PO: Good absorption, peak plasma levels 2 hr; bioavailability 40%, metabolized to active *N*-desymethyl metabolite; half-life of metabolite 2-3 hr; plasma protein

Z

binding 25%; excreted mainly in urine (65%) and less in feces (30%)

Drug interactions of concern to dentistry:

• Potential serotonin crises: selective serotonin reuptake inhibitors, ergot-containing drugs (avoid use within 24 hr of taking this drug)

• Decreased plasma levels: cimetidine

DENTAL CONSIDERATIONS

General:

• This is an acute-use drug; thus it is doubtful that patients will come to the office if acute migraine is present.

• Be aware of patient's disease, its severity, and frequency when known.

• Advise patient if dental drugs prescribed have a potential for photosensitivity.

Consultations:

• If treating chronic orofacial pain, consult with physician of record.

• Medical consult may be required to assess disease control and patient's ability to tolerate stress.

Teach patient/family:

• That dryness of the mouth may occur when taking this drug

• To avoid mouth rinses with high alcohol content due to drying effects

• Importance of updating health and drug history if physician makes any changes in evaluation/drug regimens

zolpidem

(zole-pi'dem)

Ambien

Drug class.: Nonbarbiturate, nonbenzodiazepine sedative-hypnotic

Action: Presumed to interact with a subunit of the GABA-benzodiazepine receptor, binding only to the omega-1 subunit

Uses: Insomnia

Dosage and routes:

• *Adult:* PO 10 mg before bedtime

Available forms include: Tabs 5, 10 mg

Side effects/adverse reactions:

▼ *ORAL:* Dry mouth, taste alteration

CNS: Dizziness, daytime drowsiness, amnesia, headache

CV: ***Tachycardia, hypertension***

GI: Nausea, vomiting, dyspepsia

GU: Menstrual disorder, vaginitis, cystitis

EENT: Double vision, tinnitus

INTEG: Urticaria, acne

MS: Muscle pain

Contraindications: Hypersensitivity, ritonavir

Precautions: Pregnancy category B, lactation, altered reaction time, elderly, limit duration of use

Pharmacokinetics:

PO: Half-life 2.5 hr, peak plasma levels 1.6 hr; highly protein bound

Drug interactions of concern to dentistry:

• Increased CNS depression: alcohol, all CNS depressants, fluconazole, ketoconazole, itraconazole

DENTAL CONSIDERATIONS

General:

• Assess salivary flow as a factor in caries, periodontal disease, and candidiasis.

• Monitor vital signs every appointment due to cardiovascular side effects.

Consultations:

• Medical consult may be required to assess disease control in the patient.

Teach patient/family:

When chronic dry mouth occurs, advise patient:

• To avoid mouth rinses with high alcohol content due to drying effects

• Of need for daily home fluoride to prevent caries

• To use sugarless gum, frequent sips of water, or saliva substitutes

Appendixes

Appendix A

Abbreviations

ā before
aa of each
abd abdomen
ABGs arterial blood gases
ac before meals *(ante cibum)*
ACE angiotensin-converting enzyme
Ach acetylcholine
ACT activated coagulation time
ACTH adrenocorticotropic hormone
ad lib as desired
ADH antidiuretic hormone
ADP adenosine diphosphate
AIDS acquired immunodeficiency syndrome
aka also known as
ALT alanine aminotransferase, serum
ama against medical advice
amb ambulation
amp ampule
ANA antinuclear antibody
ant anterior
ANUG acute necrotizing ulcerative gingivitis
AP anteroposterior
APAP acetaminophen
APB atrial premature beats
APTT activated partial thromboplastin time
ARC AIDS-related complex
AROM active range of motion
ASA acetylsalicylic acid (aspirin)
asap as soon as possible
ASHD arteriosclerotic heart disease
AST aspartate aminotransferase, serum
AV atrioventricular
BAL blood alcohol level
BCG bicolor guiac test
bid twice a day *(bis in die)*
BM bowel movement
BMR basal metabolic rate
bol bolus
BP blood pressure
BPH benign prostatic hypertrophy
bpm beats per minute
BS blood sugar
BUN blood urea nitrogen
Bx biopsy
c̄ with
C Celsius (centigrade)
C section Cesarean section
Ca cancer, calcium
CAD coronary artery disease
cAMP cyclic adenosine monophosphate
cap capsule
cath catheterization or catheterize
CBC complete blood count
CBS chronic brain syndrome
CC chief complaint
cc cubic centimeter
CHF congestive heart failure

cm centimeter
CMV cytomegalovirus
CNS central nervous system
CO_2 carbon dioxide
CoA coenzyme A
c/o complains of
COPD chronic obstructive pulmonary disease
CPAP continuous positive airway pressure
CPK creatinine phosphokinase
CPR cardiopulmonary resuscitation
CrCl creatinine clearance
C&S culture and sensitivity
CSF cerebrospinal fluid
CV cardiovascular
CVA cerebrovascular accident
CVP central venous pressure
D&C dilation and curettage
del rel delayed release
DIC disseminated intravascular coagulation
DM diabetes mellitus
DOA dead on arrival
DOB date of birth
dr dram
dsg dressing
DVT deep vein thrombosis
D_5W 5% glucose in distilled water
dx diagnosis
ECG electrocardiogram (EKG)
EEG electroencephalogram
EENT ear, eye, nose, and throat
elixir elixir, hydroalcoholic solution containing an active drug(s)
ENDO endocrine systems
EPS extrapyramidal symptoms
ESR erythrocyte sedimentation rate
F Fahrenheit
FBS fasting blood sugar
FHT fetal heart tones
FIo_2 inspired oxygen concentration
FSH follicle-stimulating hormone
fx fracture
g gram
gal gallon
GI gastrointestinal
G6PD glucose-6-phosphate dehydrogenase
Ghb glycosylated emoglobin
gr grain
gtt drop
GTT glucose tolerance test
GU genitourinary
Gyn gynecology
H hydrogen
HbA1c lab test for glycosylated hemoglobin
Hct hematocrit
HCG human chorionic gonadotropin
HDL high-density lipoprotein
HDCV human diploid cell rabies vaccine
HEMA hematologic system
Hgb hemoglobin
H&H hematocrit and hemoglobin
H&P history and physical exam
5-HIAA 5-hydroxyindoleacetic acid
HMG-CoA 3-hydroxy-3-methylglutaryl–coenzyme A reductase
5-HT 5-hydroxytryptamine (serotonin)

H_2O water
HOB head of bed
HR heart rate
hr hour
hs at bedtime *(hora somni)*
hypo hypodermically
Hx history
ICU intensive care unit
I&D incision and drainage
IgG immunoglobulin G
IM intramuscular
inf infusion
inh inhalation
inj injection
INR international normalized ratio
INTEG relating to integumentary structures
I&O intake and output
IOP intraocular pressure
IPPB intermittent positive-pressure breathing
ITP idiopathic thrombocytopenic purpura
IUD intrauterine contraceptive device
IV intravenous
IVAC intravenous controller
IVP intravenous pyelogram
IVPB intravenous piggyback
K potassium
kg kilogram
L or l left
L liter
lat lateral
lb pound
LDH lactic dehydrogenase
LDL low-density lipoprotein
LE lupus erythematosus
LFT liver function tests
LH luteinizing hormone
LHRH luteinizing hormone–releasing hormone
liq liquid
LLQ left lower quadrant
LMP last menstrual period
LOC loss of consciousness
LR lactated Ringer's solution
LRI lower respiratory infection
LUQ left upper quadrant
m meter, minim
m^2 square meter
MAO monoamine oxidase
MCA motorcycle accident
META metabolic
mEq milliequivalent
mg milligram
μg microgram
MI myocardial infarction
min minute
mixt mixture
ml milliliter
mm millimeter
mo month
MS musculoskeletal
MVA motor vehicle accident
n nanogram
Na sodium
NC nasal cannula
neg negative
NIDDM non–insulin-dependent diabetes mellitus
NKA no known allergies
NMI no middle initial
noc nocturnal (night)
NPO nothing by mouth *(nil per os)*
NS normal saline
NSAID nonsteroidal antiinflammatory drug
NV neurovascular
O_2 oxygen
OBS organic brain syndrome
OD right eye *(oculum dexter)*
oint ointment
OOB out of bed
OR operating room
ORIF open reduction, internal fixation

OS left eye *(ocular sinister)*
os mouth
OTC over the counter
OU each eye *(oculum interque)*
oz ounce
p̄ after (post)
p pulse
$Paco_2$ arterial carbon dioxide tension (pressure tore)
Pao_2 arterial oxygen tension (pressure tore)
PAT paroxysmal atrial tachycardia
PBI protein-bound iodine
pc after meals *(post cibum)*
PCA patient-controlled analgesia
PCN penicillin
PCWP pulmonary capillary wedge pressure
PE physical examination
PEEP positive end-expiratory pressure
PERRLA pupils equal, round, react to light and accommodation
pH hydrogen ion concentration
PMS premenstural syndrome
PO by mouth *(per os)*
postop postoperatively
PP postprandial
ppm parts per million
preop preoperatively
prep preparation
prn as needed *(pro re nata)*
PT prothrombin time
PTT partial thromboplastin time
PVC premature ventricular contraction
q every
qAM every morning
qd every day
qh every hour
qid four times a day
qod every other day
qPM every night
qsad add a sufficient quantity
qt quart
q2h every 2 hours
q3h every 3 hours
q4h every 4 hours
q6h every 6 hours
q12h every 12 hours
r right
RAIU radioactive iodine uptake
RBC(s) red blood count or cell(s)
RDA recommended dietary allowance
rec rectal
REM rapid eye movement
RESP respiratory system
RLQ right lower quadrant
R/O rule out
ROM range of motion
RTI respiratory tract infection
RUQ right upper quadrant
Rx therapy, treatment, or prescription
s̄ without
SAN sinoatrial node
SC subcutaneous
SIADH syndrome of inappropriate antidiuretic hormone
sig patient dosing instructions on prescription label
SIMV synchronous intermittent mandatory ventilation

SL sublingual
SLE systemic lupus erythematosus
SMBG self-monitored blood glucose
SOB short of breath
sol solution
ss one half
stat at once
surg surgical
sus rel sustained release dose form
supp suppository
Sx symptoms
syr syrup, a highly concentrated sucrose solution containing a drug(s)
T temperature
T_3 triiodothyronine
T_4 thyroxine
tab tablet
TAH total abdominal hysterectomy
TBG thyroxine-binding globulin
tbsp tablespoon
TD transdermal
temp temperature
tid three times daily *(ter in die)*
time rel time release dose form
tinc tincture, alcoholic solution of a drug
TMD temporomandibular dysfunction
TMJ temporomandibular joint
top topical
TPN total parenteral nutrition
TPR temperature, pulse, respirations
TSH thyroid-stimulating hormone
tsp teaspoon
TT thrombin time
Tx treatment
U unit
UA urinalysis
URI upper respiratory infection
UTI urinary tract infection
UV ultraviolet
vag vaginal
VD venereal disease
VLDL very-low-density lipoprotein
VO verbal order
vol volume
VPB ventricular premature beats
VS vital signs
WBC white blood (cell) count
wk week
WNL within normal limits
wt weight
yr year
$>$ greater than
$<$ less than
$\neq$ not equal
$\uparrow$ increase
$\downarrow$ decrease
2° secondary

Appendix B

Drugs causing dry mouth

Drug category	Brand name	Generic name
ANOREXIANT	Adipex-P, Fastin, Ionamin	phentermine
	Anorex	phendimetrazine
	Mazanor, Sanorex	mazindol
	Tenuate, Tepanil	diethylpropion
ANTIACNE	Accutane	isotretinoin
ANTIANXIETY	Atarax, Vistaril	hydroxyzine
	Ativan	lorazepam
	BuSpar	buspirone
	Equanil, Miltown	meprobamate
	Librium	chlordiazepoxide
	Paxipam	halazepam
	Serax	oxazepam
	Sonata	zalephon
	Valium	diazepam
	Xanax	alprazolam
ANTIARTHRITIC	Arava	leflunomide
ANTICHOLINERGIC/ ANTISPASMODIC	Anaspaz	hyoscyamine
	Atropisol	atropine
	Banthine	methantheline
	Bellergal	belladonna alkaloids
	Bentyl	dicyclomine
	Darbid	isopropamide
	Daricon	oxyphencyclimine
	Ditropan	oxybutynin
	Donnatal, Kinesed	hyoscyamine atropine, phenobarbital, scopolamine
	Librax	chlordiazepoxide, clidinium
	Pamine	methscopolamine
	Pro-Banthine	propantheline
	Transderm-Scōp	scopolamine
ANTICONVULSANT	Felbatol	felbamate
	Lamictal	lamotrigine
	Neurontin	gabapentin
	Tegretol	carbamazepine

ANTIDEPRESSANT	Anafranil	clomipramine
	Asendin	amoxapine
	Celexa	citalopram
	Effexor	venlafaxine
	Elavil	amitriptyline
	Luvox	fluvoxamine
	Marplan	isocarboxazid
	Nardil	phenelzine
	Norpramin	desipramine
	Parnate	tranylcypromine
	Paxil	paroxetine
	Prozac	fluoxetine
	Sinequan	doxepin
	Tofranil	imipramine
	Wellbutrin	bupropion
	Zoloft	sertraline
ANTIDIARRHEAL	Imodium AD	loperamide
	Lomotil	diphenoxylate, atropine
	Motofen	difenoxin
ANTIHISTAMINE	Actifed	triprolidine with pseudoephedrine
	Atarax	hydroxyzine
	Benadryl	diphenhydramine
	Chlor-Trimeton	chlorpheniramine
	Claritin	loratadine
	Dimetane	brompheniramine
	Dimetapp	brompheniramine, phenylpropanolamine
	Phenergan	promethazine
	Pyribenzamine (PBZ)	tripelennamine
ANTIHYPERTENSIVE	Capoten	captopril
	Catapres	clonidine
	Coreg	carvedilol
	Ismelin	guanethidine
	Aceon	perindopril
	Minipress	prazosin
	Serpasil	reserpine
	Wytensin	guanabenz
	Vasotec	enalapril
ANTIINFLAMMATORY ANALGESIC	Dolobid	diflunisal
	Celebrex	celecoxib
	Feldene	piroxicam
	Motrin	ibuprofen
	Nalfon	fenoprofen
	Naprosyn	naproxen
	Vioxx	rofecoxib

ANTINAUSEANT	Antivert	meclizine
	Dramamine	diphenhydramine
	Marezine	cyclizine
ANTIPARKINSONIAN	Akineton	biperiden
	Artane	trihexyphenidyl
	Cogentin	benztropine mesylate
	Larodopa	levodopa
	Marflex	orphenadrine HCl
	Parsidol	ethopropazine
	Sinemet	carbidopa, levodopa
	Tasmar	tolcapone
ANTIPSYCHOTIC	Clozaril	clozapine
	Compazine	prochlorperazine
	Eskalith	lithium
	Haldol	haloperidol
	Mellaril	thioridazine
	Navane	thiothixene
	Orap	pimozide
	Risperdal	resperidone
	Sparine	promazine
	Stelazine	trifluoperazine
	Thorazine	chlorpromazine
	Triavil	amitriptyline, perphenazine
	Zyprexa	olanzapine
ANTISECRETORY	Aciphex	rabeprazole
ANTISPASMODIC	Detrol	tolterodine
ANTIVIRAL	Sustiva	efavirenz
BRONCHODILATOR	ephedrine (generic)	
	Isuprel	isoproterenol
	Proventil, Ventolin	albuterol
	Xopenex	levalbuterol
CNS STIMULANT	Dexedrine	dextroamphetamine
	Desoxyn	methamphetamine
DECONGESTANT	Ornade	phenylpropanolamine, chlorpheniramine
	Sudafed	pseudoephedrine
DIURETIC	Aldactone	spironolactone
	Diuril	chlorothiazide
	Dyazide, Maxzide, Dyrenium	triamterene, hydrochlorothiazide
	HydroDIURIL, Esidrix	hydrochlorothiazide
	Lasix	furosemide
	Midamor	amiloride

MIGRAINE	Amerge	naratriptan
	Maxalt	rizatriptan
MUSCLE RELAXANT	Flexeril	cyclobenzaprine
	Lioresal	baclofen
	Norflex, Disipal	orphenadrine
NARCOLEPSY	Provigil	modafinil
NARCOTIC ANALGESIC	Demerol	meperidine
	MS Contin	morphine
OPHTHALMIC	Azopt	brinzolamide
SEDATIVE	Dalmane	flurazepam
	Halcion	triazolam
	Restoril	temazepam

Appendix C

Controlled substances chart

Drugs	United States	Canada
Heroin, LSD, peyote, marijuana, mescaline, phencyclidine	Schedule I (CI)	Schedule H
Opium, fentanyl, morphine, meperidine, methadone, oxycodone (and its combinations), hydromorphone, codeine (single-drug entity), and cocaine	Schedule II (CII)	Schedule N
Short-acting barbiturates	Schedule II	Schedule C
Amphetamine and methylphenidate	Schedule II	Schedule G
Codeine combinations, hydrocodone combinations, glutethimide, paregoric, phendimetrazine, thiopental, testosterone, and other androgens	Schedule III (CIII)	Schedule F
Benzodiazepines (diazepam, midazolam, etc.), chloral hydrate, meprobamate, phenobarbital, propoxyphene (and combinations), pentazocine (and combinations), and methohexital	Schedule IV (CIV)	Schedule F
Antidiarrheals and antitussives with opioid derivatives	Schedule V (CV)	

Appendix D

FDA pregnancy categories

A Studies have failed to demonstrate a risk to the fetus in any trimester

B Animal reproduction studies fail to demonstrate a risk to the fetus; no human studies available

C Only given after risks to the fetus are considered; animal reproduction studies have shown adverse effects on fetus; no human studies available

D Definite human fetal risks; may be given in spite of risks if needed in life-threatening conditions

X Absolute fetal abnormalities; not to be used anytime during pregnancy because risks outweigh benefits

Appendix E

Drugs that affect taste

ALCOHOL DETOXIFICATION
disulfiram (Antabuse)

ALZHEIMER'S
donepezil (Aricept)

ANALGESICS (NSAIDS)
diclofenac (Voltaren)
etodolac (Lodine)
ketoprofen (Orudis)
meclofenamate (Meclofen)
sulindac (Clinoril)

ANESTHETICS (GENERAL)
midazolam (Versed)
propofol (Diprivan)

ANESTHETICS (LOCAL)
lidocaine transoral delivery system (Dentipatch)

ANOREXIANTS
diethylpropion (Tenuate)
mazindol (Mazanor)
phendimetrazine (Adipost)
phentermine (Ionamin)

ANTACIDS
aluminum hydroxide (Amphojel)
calcium carbonate (Tums)
lansoprazole (Prevacid)
magaldrate (Riapan)
omeprazole (Prilosec)
sucralfate (Carafate)

ANTIARTHRITIC
leflunomide (Arava)

ANTICHOLINERGICS
clidinium (Quarzan)
mepenzolate (Cantil)
methantheline (Banthine)
propantheline (Pro-Banthine)

ANTICONVULSANTS
fosphenytoin (Cerebyx)
phenytoin (Dilantin)
topiramate (Topamax)

ANTIDEPRESSANTS
amitriptyline (Elavil)
clomipramine (Anafranil)
desipramine (Norpramin)
doxepin (Sinequan)
fluoxetine (Prozac)
imipramine (Tofranil)
nefazodone (Serzone)
nortriptyline (Pamelor)
protriptyline (Vivactil)
sertraline (Zoloft)

ANTIDIABETICS
metformin (Glucophage)
tolbutamide (Orinase)

ANTIDIARRHEALS
bismuth subsalicylate (Pepto-Bismol)

ANTIEMETICS
dolasetron mesylate (Anazemet)

ANTIFUNGALS
griseofulvin (Fulvicin)
terbinafine (Lamisil)

ANTIGOUT
allopurinol (Zyloprim)
colchicine

ANTIHISTAMINE (H_1) ANTAGONISTS
azelastine (Astelin)
cetirizine (Zyrtec)

ANTIHISTAMINE (H_2) ANTAGONISTS
famotidine (Pepcid)

ANTIHYPERLIPIDEMICS
cerivistatin (Baycol)
clofibrate (Atromid-S)
fluvastatin (Lescol)

ANTIINFECTIVES
ethionamide (Trecator-SC)
levofloxacin (Levoquin)
lincomycin (Lincocin)
metronidazole (Flagyl)

ANTIINFLAMMATORY/ ANTIARTHRITIC
auranofin (Ridaura)
aurothioglucose (Solganal)
celecoxib (Celebrex)
rofecoxib (Vioxx)
sulfasalazine (Azulfidine)

ANTIPARKINSON
entacapone (Comtan)
levodopa (Larodopa)
levodopa-carbidopa (Sinemet)
pergolide (Permax)
pramipexole dihydrochloride (Mirapex)

ANTIPSYCHOTICS
lithium (Eskalith)
pimozide (Orap)
prochlorperazine (Compazine)
quetiapine fumarate (Seroquel)
risperidone (Risperdal)
triflupromazine (Vesprin)

ANTITHYROID
methimazole (Tapazole)
propylthiouracil

ANTIVIRALS
acyclovir (Zovirax)
amprenavir (Agenerase)
delavirdine mesylate (Rescriptor)
didanosine (Videx)
efavirenz (Sustiva)
foscarnet (Foscavir)
indinavir (Crixivan)
penciclovir (Denavir)
rimantadine (Flumadine)
ritonavir (Norvir)
saquinavir (Invirase)
valcyclovir (Valtrex)
zidovudine (Retrovir)

ANXIOLYTIC/SEDATIVES
chloral hydrate (Noctec)
estazolam (ProSom)
quazepam (Doral)
zolpidem (Ambien)

ASTHMA PREVENTIVES
cromolyn (Intal)
nedocromil (Tilade)

BRONCHODILATORS
albuterol (Proventil)
bitolterol (Tornalate)
ipratropium (Atrovent)
isoproterenol (Isuprel)
metaproterenol (Alupent)
pirbuterol (Maxair)
terbutaline (Brethine)

CALCIUM AFFECTING DRUGS
alendronate (Fosamax)
calcitonin (Calcimar)
etidronate (Didronel)

CANCER CHEMOTHERAPEUTICS

fluorouracil (Efudex)
levamisole (Ergamisol)
tamoxifen (Nolvadex)

CARDIOVASCULAR

amiodarone (Cordarone)
amlodipine (Norvasc)
bepridil (Vascor)
captopril (Capoten)
clonidine (Catapres)
diltiazem (Cardizem)
enalapril (Vasotec)
flecainide (Tambocor)
fosinopril (Monopril)
guanfacine (Tenex)
labetalol (Trandate)
losartan (Cozarr)
mecamylamine (Inversine)
mexiletine (Mexitil)
moricizine (Ethmozine)
nadolol (Corgard)
nifedipine (Procardia XL)
penbutolol (Levabol)
perindopril (Aceon)
propafenone (Rythmol)
quinidine (Cardioquin)
valsartan (Diovan)

CNS STIMULANTS

dextroamphetamine (Dexedrine)
methamphetamine (Desoxyn)

DECONGESTANT

phenylephrine (Neo-Synephrine)

DIURETICS

acetazolamide (Diamox)
methazolamide (Naptazine)
polythiazide (Renese)

GLUCOCORTICOIDS

budesonide (Rhinocort)
flunisolide (Aerobid)
rimexolone (Vexol)

GALLSTONE SOLUBILIZATION

ursodiol (Actigall)

HEMORHEOLOGIC

pentoxifylline (Trental)

IMMUNOMODULATORS

interferon alfa (Roferon-A)
levamisole (Ergamisol)

IMMUNOSUPPRESSANTS

azathioprine (Imuran)

METHYLXANTHINES

aminophylline (Somophyllin)
dyphylline (Dilor)
oxtriphylline (Choledyl)
theophylline (Theo-Dur)

NICOTINE CESSATION

nicotine polacrilex (Nicorette)

OPHTHALMICS

apraclonidine (Iopidine)
brimonidine (Alphagan)
brinzolamide (Azopt)
dorzolamide (Truspot)
olopatadine (Pantanol)

RETINOID, SYSTEMIC

acitretin (Soriatane)

SALIVARY STIMULANT

pilocarpine (Salagen)

SKELETAL MUSCLE RELAXANTS

baclofen (Lioresal)
cyclobenzaprine (Flexeril)
methocarbamol (Robaxin)

VITAMINS

calcifediol (vitamin D)
calcitriol (vitamin D)
dihydrotachysterol (vitamin D)
phytonadione (vitamin K)

Appendix F

Combination products

Accuretic: quinapril 10 mg with hydrochlorothiazide 12.5 mg, or quinapril 20 mg with hydrochlorothiazide 12.5 mg, or quinapril 20 mg with hydrochlorothiazide 25 mg

Aceta with Codeine, Tylenol with Codeine No. 3: acetaminophen 300 mg with codeine phosphate 30 mg

Actagen, Actifed, Allercon, Allerfrim, Aprodine, Cenafed Plus, Genac, Triposed: pseudoephedrine 60 mg with triprolidine HCl 2.5 mg

Adderall 5: amphetamine aspartate 1.25 mg, amphetamine sulfate 1.25 mg, dextroamphetamine saccharate 1.25 mg, and dextroamphetamine sulfate 1.25 mg

Adderall 10: amphetamine sulfate 2.5 mg, dextroamphetamine sulfate 2.5 mg, dextroamphetamine saccharate 2.5 mg, and dextroamphetamine sulfate 2.5 mg

Aggrenox: aspirin 25 mg with dipyridamole 200 mg

Ak-Trol Ointment, Dexasporin Ointment, Dexacidin Ointment: dexamethasone 1 mg, polymyxin B sulfate 10,000 U, and neomycin sulfate 3.5 mg/g

Ak-Trol, Maxitrol, Dexacidin Suspension: dexamethasone 1 mg, polymyxin B sulfate 10,000 U, and neomycin sulfate 3.5 mg/ml of supension

Aldactazide 25/25: spironolactone 25 mg with hydrochlorothiazide 25 mg

Aldactazide 50/50: spironolactone 50 mg with hydrochlorothiazide 50 mg

Aldoclor-150: methyldopa 250 mg with chlorothiazide 150 mg

Aldoclor-250: methyldopa 250 mg with chlorothiazide 250 mg

Aldoril-15: methyldopa 250 mg with hydrochlorothiazide 15 mg

Aldoril-25: methyldopa 250 mg with hydrochlorothiazide 25 mg

Aldoril D30: methyldopa 500 mg with hydrochlorothiazide 30 mg

Aldoril D50: methyldopa 500 mg with hydrochlorothiazide 50 mg

Allegra-D: fexofenadine 60 mg with pseudoephedrine HCl 120 mg

Allent, Bromfed, Endafed: pseudoephedrine HCl 120 mg with brompheniramine maleate 12 mg

Allerest Maximum Strength 12 Hour, Contac Maximum Strength 12 Hour, Drize, Ornade Spansules, Resaid, Rhinolar-EX 12 Hour and Triaminic-12: phenylpropanolamine hydrochloride 75 mg with chlorpheniramine maleate 12 mg

Aleve Cold and Sinus: naproxen sodium 220 mg with pseudoephedrine hydrochloride

Ambenyl Cough Syrup, Amgenal, Bromotuss/Codeine, Bromanyl Syrup: bromodiphenhydramine HCl 12.5 mg/5 ml with codeine phosphate 10 mg/5 ml

Anacin, Gensan: aspirin 400 mg with caffeine 32 mg

Anexsia 5/500, Bancap HC, Ceta-Plus, Co-Gesic, Dolacet, Duocet,

Hydrocet, Hydrogesic, Hy-Phen, Lorcet-HD, Lortab 5/500, Margesic H, Panacet 5/500, Stagesic, T-Gesic, Vicodin, Zydone: hydrocodone bitartrate 5.0 mg with acetaminophen 500 mg

Anexsia 7.5/650, Lorcet Plus: hydrocodone bitartrate 7.5 mg with acetaminophen 650 mg

Anexsia 10/660: hydrocodone bitartrate 10 mg with acetaminophen 660 mg

Antrocol Elixir: atropine sulfate 0.195 mg/5 ml with phenobarbital 16 mg/5 ml

Apresazide 25/25: hydralazine HCl 25 mg with hydrochlorothiazide 25 mg

Apresazide 50/50: hydralazine HCl 50 mg with hydrochlorothiazide 50 mg

Apresazide 100/50: hydralazine HCl 100 mg with hydrochlorothiazide 50 mg

Apri, Desogen, Ortho-Cept: desogestrel 0.15 mg with ethinyl estradiol 30 mg

Arthrotec: diclofenac 75 mg with misoprostol 200 µg; or diclofenac 50 mg with misoprostol 200 µg

Aspirin Free Excedrin, Bayer Select Maximum Strength Headache: acetaminophen 500 mg with caffeine 65 mg

Azo-Sulfisoxazole: sulfisoxazole 500 mg with phenazopyridine HCl 50 mg

Barbidonna: belladonna alkaloids, atropine sulfate 0.025 mg, hyoscyamine sulfate 0.1286 mg, scopolamine hydrobromide 0.0074 mg and phenobarbital 16 mg

Barbidonna No. 2: belladonna alkaloids, atropine sulfate 0.025 mg, hyoscyamine sulfate 0.1286 mg, scopolamine hydrobromide 0.0074 mg, and phenobarbital 32 mg

BC Powder: aspirin 650 mg with caffeine 32 mg, salicylamide 145 mg

BC Powder Arthritis Strength: aspirin 742 mg with caffeine 36 mg, salicylamide 222 mg

BC Tablets: aspirin 325 mg with caffeine 16 mg, salicylamide 95 mg

Bellergal-S, Phenerbel-S: ergotamine tartrate 0.6 mg with levorotatory belladonna alkaloids maleates 0.2 mg and phenobarbital 40 mg tablets

Benylin Adult: dextromethorphan hydrobromide 15 mg/5 ml

Benylin DM: dextromethorphan hydrobromide 10 mg/5 ml

Bromfed Tablets: pseudoephedrine HCl 60 mg with brompheniramine maleate 4 mg

Bromfed Capsules: pseudoephedrine HCl 120 mg with brompheniramine maleate 12 mg

Bromfenex-PD, Dallergy-JR, ULTRAbrom PD: pseudoephedrine HCl 60 mg with brompheniramine maleate 6 mg

Bromo-Seltzer: acetaminophen 325 mg, citric acid 2.224 g, sodium bicarbonate 2.871 g/capful measure

Brontex: codeine phosphate 10 mg with guaifenesin 300 mg tablets

Brontex Liquid: codeine phosphate 2.5 mg with guaifenesin 75 mg/5 ml

Butibel: belladonna extract 15 mg (0.187 mg of alkaloids of belladonna leaf) with butabarbital sodium 15 mg

Butibel Elixir: belladonna extract 15 mg with butabarbital sodium 15 mg in each 5 ml

Cafergot, Ercaf, and **Wigraine:** ergotamine tartrate 1 mg with caffeine 100 mg

Cafergot Suppositories: ergotamine tartrate 2 mg, caffeine 100 mg
Caladryl Clear: pramoxine HCl 1% with zinc acetate 0.1%, camphor 0.1%, alcohol 2%
Caladryl Lotion: pramoxine HCl 1% with calamine 8%, camphor 0.1%, alcohol 2.2%
Calcidrine Syrup: codeine 8.4 mg/5 ml with calcium iodide anhydrous 152 mg/5 ml
Capital with Codeine or **Tylenol with Codeine Elixir:** acetaminophen 120 mg/5 ml with codeine 12 mg/5 ml
Capozide 25/15: captopril 25 mg with hydrochlorothiazide 15 mg
Capozide 25/25: captopril 25 mg with hydrochlorothiazide 25 mg
Capozide 50/15: captopril 50 mg with hydrochlorothiazide 15 mg
Capozide 50/25: captopril 50 mg with hydrochlorothiazide 25 mg
Carisoprodol Compound, Sodol Compound, Soma Compound: carisoprodol 200 mg with aspirin 325 mg
Chardonna-2: belladonna extract 15 mg with phenobarbital 15 mg
Children's Cepacol: acetaminophen 160 mg/5 ml and pseudoephedrine 15 mg/5 ml
Chloraseptic (Vicks) Sore Throat Lozenges, benzocaine 6 mg with 10 mg menthol: **Children's Throat Spray,** phenol 0.5%: **Mouthrinse,** phenol 1.4%: **Children's Lozenges,** benzocaine 5 mg
Chlor-Trimeton 4 Hour Relief Tablets: pseudoephedrine sulfate 60 mg, chlorpheniramine maleate 4 mg
Chlor-Trimeton 12 Hour Relief Tablets: pseudoephedrine sulfate 120 mg with chlorpheniramine maleate 8 mg
Claritin-D ext. rel.: loratadine 5 mg with pseudoephedrine sulfate 120 mg
Claritin-D 24 Hour: loratadine 10 mg with pseudoephedrine sulfate 240 mg
CombiPatch: estradiol 0.05 mg with norethindrone 0.14 mg; estradiol 0.05 mg with norethindrone 0.25 mg
Combipres 0.1 mg: clonidine HCl 0.1 mg with chlorthalidone 15 mg
Combipres 0.2 mg: clonidine HCl 0.2 mg with chlorthalidone 15 mg
Combivent: albuterol sulfate 103 μg with ipratropium bromide 18 μg
Combivir: lamivudine 150 mg with zidovudine 300 mg
Comtrex Allergy-Sinus, Sine-off Sinus Medicine, Sinutab Maximum Strength Sinus Allergy: pseudoephedrine HCl 30 mg with chlorpheniramine maleate 2 mg and acetaminophen 500 mg
Comtrex Cough Formula Liquid: dextromethorphan hydrobromide 7.5 mg/5 ml with pseudoephedrine HCl 15 mg/5 ml and guaifenesin 50 mg/5 ml
Comtrex Liqui-Gels, Cold Relief Tablets, Triaminicol Multi-Symptom Cough and Cold Tablets: phenylpropanolamine HCl 12.5 mg with chlorpheniramine maleate 2 mg and dextromethorphan HBr 10 mg
Comtrex Maximum Strength Multi-Symptom Cold and Flu, Co-Apap, Multi-Symptom Tylenol Cold, Mapap Cold Formula: pseudoephedrine HCl 30 mg with chlorpheniramine maleate 2 mg and dextromethorphan HBr 15 mg
Comtrex Max Strength Multi-Symptom Cold and Flu Relief, Maximum Strength Comtrex Liqui-Gels: phenylpropanolamine

HCl 12.5 mg with chlorpheniramine maleate 2 mg, dextromethorphan HBr 15 mg and acetaminophen 500 mg

Contact Cough and Chest Cold: dextromethorphan hydrobromide 5 mg/5 ml, pseudoephedrine 15 mg/5 ml and guaifenesin 50 mg/ 5 ml

Contact Severe Cold and Flu Formula, Maximum Strength Comtrex Liqui-Gels: dextromethorphan hydrobromide 15 mg, phenylpropanolamine hydrochloride 12.5 mg, chlorpheniramine maleate 2 mg, and acetaminophen 500 mg

Contact Severe Cold and Flu Nightime: dextromethorphan hydrobromide 5 mg, pseudoephedrine HCl 10 mg, chlorpheniramine maleate 0.67 mg, and acetaminophen 167 mg

Contact 12 Hour Capsule: phenylpropranolamine HCl 75 mg and chlorpheniramine 8 mg

Corzide 40/5: bendroflumethiazide 5 mg with nadolol 40 mg

Corzide 80/5: bendroflumethiazide 5 mg with nadolol 80 mg

Cystex: methenamine 162 mg, sodium salicylate 162.5 mg, benzoic acid 32 mg

Darvocet-N 50, Propoxyphene Napsylate with Acetaminophen Tablets: acetaminophen 325 mg with propoxyphene napsylate 50 mg

Darvocet-N 100, Propacet 100: propoxyphene napsylate 100 mg with acetaminophen 650 mg

Darvon Compound-65 Pulvules: aspirin 389 mg with caffeine 32.4 mg, propoxyphene HCl 65 mg

Deconamine CX: hydrocodone bitartrate 5 mg with pseudoephedrine HCl 30 mg and guaifenesin 300 mg

Deconamine CX Liquid: hydrocodone bitartrate 5 mg with pseudoephedrine HCl 60 mg and guaifenesin 200 mg/5 ml

Deconamine SR, Deconomed SR, Rinade B.I.D, Kronofed-A, N D Clear, Novafed A, Time-Hist, Rescon ED, Pseudo-Chlor: pseudoephedrine hydrochloride with chlorpheniramine maleate 8 mg-Demi-Regroton: chlorthalidone 25 mg with reserpine 0.125 mg

Dimacol, Sudafed Cold and Cough Liquid Caps: pseudoephedrine hydrochloride 30 mg with dextromethorphan hydrobromide 10 mg and guaifenesin 100 mg Dimetane-DC Cough Syrup, Bromanate DC, Bromphen DC, Myphetane DC, Poly-Histine CS: phenylpropanolamine HCl 12.5 mg, brompheniramine maleate 2 mg and codeine phosphate 10 mg/5 ml

Dimetane-DX Cough Syrup, Bromatane DX, Bromophen DX, Bromarest DX, Bromfed DM, Myphetane DX: dextromethorphan hydrobromide 10 mg/5 ml with brompheniramine maleate 2 mg/5 ml, pseudoephedrine HCl 30 mg/5 ml

Dimetapp DM Elixir: phenylpropanolamine HCl 12.5 mg, brompheniramine maleate 2 mg, dextromethorphan hydrobromide 10 mg/5 ml

Dimetapp, Diametapp 4 Hour Liqui-Gel, Dimaphen, Vicks DayQuil Allergy Relief 4 Hour: phenylpropanolamine HCl 25 mg, brompheniramine maleate 4 mg

Diutensin-R: methyclothiazide 2.5 mg with reserpine 0.1 mg

Donnagel Liquid or tablets: 600 mg attapulgite per 15 ml or per tablet

Donnatal, Hyosophen, Malatal, Spasmolin: atropine sulfate 0.0194 mg, hyoscyamine sulfate 0.1037 mg, scopolamine hydrobromide 0.0065 mg, and phenobarbital 16.2 mg

Donnatal, Bellacane, Hyosophen, Susano Elixirs: belladonna alkaloids, atropine sulfate 0.0194 mg/5 ml, hyoscyamine sulfate 0.1037 mg/5 ml, scopolamine hydrobromide 0.0065/5 ml and phenobarbital 16.2 mg/5 ml

Donnatal Extentabs: belladonna alkaloids, atropine sulfate 0.0582 mg, hyoscyamine sulfate 0.3111 mg, scopolamine hydrobromide 0.0195 mg, and phenobarbital 48.6 mg

Drixomed: pseudoephedrine sulfate 120 mg with desbrompheneramine 6 mg

Drixoral Plus or Drixoral Cold and Flu Tablets: pseudoephedrine sulfate 60 mg, dextrobrompheniramine maleate 3 mg and acetaminophen 500 mg

Drixoral Cough and Congestion Capsules, Vicks 44 Non-Drowsy Cold and Cough LiquiCaps, Thera-Flu Non-Drowsy Flu, Cold and Cough Maximum: pseudoephedrine HCl 60 mg, dextromethorphan hydrobromide 30 mg

Duratuss, Entex PSE, Guaimax-D, Ru-Tuss DE, Zephrex LA: pseudoephedrine HCl 120 mg with guaifenesin 600 mg

Duratuss-G: guaifenesin 120 mg

Duratuss HD Elixir, Vanex Expectorant Liquid: pseudoephedrine HCl 30 mg with hydrocodone bitartrate 2.5 mg and guaifenesin 100 mg per 5 ml

Dyazide: hydrochlorothiazide 25 mg with triamterene 37.5 mg

Empirin with Codeine 30 mg (No. 3): aspirin 325 mg with codeine phosphate 30 mg

Empirin with Codeine 60 mg (No. 4): aspirin 325 mg with codeine phosphate 60 mg

Enduronyl: deserpidine 0.25 mg with methylclothiazide 5 mg

Enduronyl-Forte: deserpidine 0.5 mg with methylclothiazide 5 mg

Entex, Dura-Gest, Enomine: guaifenesin 200 mg, phenylephrine HCl 5 mg and phenylpropanolamine HCl 45 mg

Entex LA, Ami-TexLA, Guaipax, Exgest LA, Partuss LA, Rymed TR, Stamoist LA: guaifenesin 400 mg with phenylpropanolamine HCl 75 mg

E-Pilo and PE (products 1 through 6): epinephrine bitartrate 1% with pilocarpine HCl 1%, 2%, 3%, 4%, 6%

Equagesic, Micranin: meprobamate 200 mg with aspirin 325 mg

Esgic, Fioricet, Repan, Amaphen, Endolor, Femcet, Medigesic: acetaminophen 325 mg with butalbital 50 mg, caffeine 40 mg

Esgic-Plus: butalbital 50 mg with acetaminophen 500 mg and caffeine 40 mg

Esimil: guanethidine monosulfate 10 mg with hydrochlorothiazide 25 mg

Etrafon 2-10, Triavil 2-10: perphenazine 2 mg with amitriptyline HCl 10 mg

Etrafon, Triavil 2-25: perphenazine 2 mg with amitriptyline HCl 25 mg

Etrafon-A, Triavil 4-10: perphenazine 4 mg with amitriptyline HCl 10 mg

Etrafon-Forte, Triavil 4-25: perphenazine 4 mg with amitriptyline HCl 25 mg

Excedrin (Aspirin Free), Bayer Select Maximum Strength Headache Caplets, Excedrin Extra Strength: acetaminophen 500 mg and caffeine 65 mg
Excedrin Sinus Extra Strength, Bayer Select Head Cold, Bayer Select Maximum Strength Sinus Relief, Contact Nondrowsy Sinus, Dristan Cold Tablets, Maximum Strength Ornex, Maximum Strength Sine-Aid, Maximum Strength Sinutab without Drowsiness, Maximum Strength Tylenol Sinus, Maximum Strength Sudafed Sinus, Maximum Strength Dynafed, Tavist Sinus: pseudoephedrine HCl 30 mg with acetaminophen 500 mg
Excedrin Migraine: aspirin 250 mg with acetaminophen 250 mg, caffeine 65 mg
Excedrin PM Liquid: acetaminophen 167 mg with diphenhydramine HCl 8.3 mg/5 ml
Excedrin PM (caplets): acetaminophen 500 mg with diphenhydramine citrate 38 mg
Excedrin PM (liquigels): acetaminophen 500 mg with diphenhydramine HCl 25 mg
Femhrt 1/5: norethindrone acetate 1 mg with ethinyl estradiol 5 μg
Fioricet with Codeine: acetaminophen 325 mg, butalbital 50 mg, caffeine 40 mg, and codeine phosphate 30 mg
Fiorinal, Fiorgen PF, Lanorinal, Marnal: aspirin 325 mg with butalbital 50 mg, caffeine 40 mg
Fiorinal with Codeine No. 3: aspirin 325 mg with butalbital 50 mg, caffeine 40 mg, codeine phosphate 30 mg
Flexaphen: chlorzoxazone 250 mg with acetaminophen 300 mg
Goody's Extra Headache Powders: aspirin 520 mg with acetaminophen 260 mg and caffeine 32.5 mg per powder
Guaifenesin/PPA 75: guaifenesin 600 mg with phenylpropanolamine HCl 75 mg
Helidac: bismuth subsalicylate 262.4 mg with metronidazole 250 mg (tabs) plus tetracycline 500 mg (caps)
Humibid DM, Fenesin DM, Guaifenex DM, Guaifenex Rx PM, Iobid DM, Monafed DM, Muco-Fen-DM, Respa DM: dextromethorphan hydrobromide 30 mg with guaifenesin 600 mg
Humibid DM Sprinkles: dextromethorphan hydrobromide 15 mg with guaifenesin 30 mg
Hycodan, Tussigon: hydrocodone bitartrate 5 mg with homatropine methylbromide 15 mg and acetaminophen 500 mg
Hydrap-ES, Ser-Ap-Es, Tri-Hydroserpine, Marpres, Unipres: hydrochlorothiazide 15 mg with hydralazine 25 mg and reserpine 0.1 mg
HydroClear-Tuss, Hydrocodone GF Syrup, Atuss-EX: hydrocodone bitartrate 5 mg with guaifenesin 100 mg in each 5 ml
Hydropres-50, Hydro-Serp, Hydroserpine No. 2: reserpine 0.125 mg with hydrochlorothiazide 50 mg
Hydroserpine No. 1: reserpine 0.125 mg with hydrochlorothiazide 25 mg
Hyphed Syrup: hydrocodone bitartrate 2.5 mg with pseudoephedrine HCl 30 mg and chlorpheniramine maleate 2 mg in each 5 ml
Hyzaar: losartan potassium 50 mg with hydrochlorothiazide 12.5 mg
Iberet-500 Filmtabs, Generet-500: iron 105 mg, vitamins B_1 6 mg, B_2 6 mg, B_3 30 mg, B_5 10 mg,

B_6 5 mg, B_{12} 25 μg, and C 500 mg
Iberet-500 Liquid: iron 78.75 mg, vitamins B_1 4.5 mg, B_2 4.5 mg, B_3 22.5 mg, B_5 7.5 mg, B_6 3.75 mg, B_{12} 18.75 μg, and C 375 mg
Imodium Advanced: loperamide 2 mg and simethicone 125 mg
Inderide 40/25, Propranolol HCl, Hydrochlorothiazide Tablets 40/25: propranolol HCl 40 mg with hydrochlorothiazide 25 mg
Inderide 80/25, Propranolol HCl, Hydrochlorothiazide Tablets 80/25: propranolol HCl 80 mg with hydrochlorothiazide 25 mg
Inderide LA 80/50: propranolol HCl 80 mg with hydrochlorothiazide 50 mg
Inderide LA 120/50: propranolol HCl 120 mg with hydrochlorothiazide 50 mg
Inderide LA 160/50: propranolol HCl 160 mg with hydrochlorothiazide 50 mg
Iophen-C, Tussi-Organidin: codeine phosphate 10 mg/5 ml with iodinated glycerol 30 mg/5 ml
Iophen-DM, Tusso-DM, Tussi-Organidin DM: dextromethorphan hydrobromide 10 mg and iodinated glycerol 30 mg/5 ml
Legatrin PM: acetaminophen 500 mg with diphenhydramine hydrochloride 50 mg
Levsin with Phenobarbital Tablets, Bellacane: hyoscyamine sulfate 0.125 mg with phenobarbital 15 mg
Lexxel: enalapril maleate 5 mg with felodipine 5 mg
Lexxel 2: enalapril maleate 5 mg with felodipine 2.5 mg
Librax: clidinium bromide 2.5 mg with chlordiazepoxide HCl 5 mg
Lopressor HCT 50/25: metoprolol tartrate 50 mg with hydrochlorothiazide 25 mg
Lopressor HCT 100/25: metoprolol tartrate 100 mg with hydrochlorothiazide 25 mg
Lopressor HCT 100/50: metoprolol tartrate 100 mg with hydrochlorothiazide 50 mg
Lorcet-HD: hydrocodone bitartrate 5 mg with acetaminophen 500 mg
Lorcet Plus: hydrocodone bitartrate 7.5 mg with acetaminophen 650 mg
Lorcet 10/650: hydrocodone 10 mg with acetaminophen 650 mg
Lortab ASA, Alor 5/500: hydrocodone bitartrate 5 mg with aspirin 500 mg
Lortab 2.5/500: hydrocodone 2.5 mg with acetaminophen 500 mg
Lortab 5/500, Hydrocodone w/APAP: hydrocodone bitartrate 5 mg with acetaminophen 500 mg
Lortab 7.5/500: hydrocodone bitartrate 7.5 with acetaminophen 500 mg
Lortab Elixir: 2.5 mg hydrocodone with 120 mg acetaminophen in 5 ml
Lotensin HCT 20/12.5: benazepril 20 mg with hydrochlorothiazide 12.5 mg
Lotensin HCT 20/25: benazepril 20 mg with hydrochlorothiazide 25 mg
Lotrel 2.5/10: amlidopine 2.5 mg with benazepril 10 mg
Lotrel 5/10: amlidopine 5 mg with benazepril 10 mg
Lotrel 5/20: amlidopine 5 mg with benazepril 20 mg
Lotrisone: clotrimazole 1% and betamethasone dipropionate 0.05%
Maxzide-25 MG: triamterene 37.5 mg with hydrochlorothiazide 25 mg
Maxzide: hydrochlorothiazide 50 mg with triamterene 75 mg

Melagesic PM: acetaminophen 500 mg with melatononin 1.5 mg
Menogen: esterified estrogen 1.25 mg with methyltestosterone 2.5 mg
Menogen H. S.: esterified estrogen 0.625 mg with methyltestosterone 1.25 mg
Mepergan: meperidine HCl 25 mg/ml with promethazine HCl 25 mg/ml injection
Mepergan Fortis caps: meperidine HCl 50 mg with promethazine HCl 25 mg
Metatensin No. 2: reserpine 0.1 mg with trichlormethiazide 2 mg
Metatensin No. 4: reserpine 0.1 mg with trichlormethiazide 4 mg
Midol Maximum Strength Multi-Symptom Menstrual, Premsym PMS, Aspirin Free Excedrin Dual, Multi Symptom Pamprin, Lurline PMS, Aspirin Free Excedrin Dual: acetaminophen 500 mg with caffeine 60 mg, pamabrom 25 mg, and pyrilamine maleate 15 mg
Midol Regular Strength Multi-Symptom, Menoplex: acetaminophen 325 mg, phenytoloxamine citrate 30 mg with pyrilamine maleate 12.5 mg
Midol PM: acetaminophen 500 mg with diphenhydramine 25 mg
Minizide 1: prazosin HCl 1 mg with polythiazide 0.5 mg
Minizide 2: prazosin HCl 2 mg with polythiazide 0.5 mg
Minizide 5: prazosin HCl 5 mg with polythiazide 0.5 mg
Moduretic: amiloride HCl 5 mg with hydrochlorothiazide 50 mg
Motrin IB Sinus: ibuprofen 200 mg, pseudoephedrine 30 mg
Multisymptom Pamprin, Lurline PMS, Aspirin Free Excedrin Dual: acetaminophen 500 mg with caffeine 60 mg, pamabrom 25 mg, and pyrilamine maleate 15 mg
Murocoll-2: scopolamine hydrobromide 0.3%, phenylephrine hydrochloride 10% drops
MycoLog II: triamcinolone acetonide 0.1% and nystatin 100,000 units/gram (ointment or cream)
Mylanta Liquid: aluminum hydroxide 200 mg, magnesium hydroxide 200 mg, simethicone 20 mg
Naldecon CX Adult Liquid: codeine phosphate 10 mg/5 ml with guaifenesin 200 mg/5 ml and phenylpropanolamine HCl 12.5 mg/5 ml
Naldecon-DX Adult, Naldelate DX Adult: dextromethorphan hydrobromide 10 mg/5 ml with guaifenesin 100 mg/5 ml, phenylpropanolamine HCl 12.5 mg/5 ml
Naldecon-DX Children's Syrup: dextromethorphan hydrobromide 5.0 mg/5 ml with guaifenesin 100 mg/5 ml, phenylpropanolamine HCl 6.25 mg/5 ml
Naldecon EX Pediatric Drops: 50 mg/ml guaifenesin and 6.25 mg/ml phenylpropanolamine HCl
Norco: hydrocodone bitartrate 10 mg with aspirin 325 mg
Norgesic: orphenadrine citrate 25 mg with aspirin 385 mg, caffeine 30 mg
Norgesic Forte: orphenadrine citrate 50 mg with aspirin 770 mg, caffeine 60 mg
NyQuil Nighttime Cold/Flu Medicine, Nite Time Cold Formula, Nytcold, Genite: pseudoephedrine HCl 10 mg, doxylamine succinate 1.25 mg, dextromethorphan hydrobromide 5 mg, and acetaminophen 167 mg/5 ml
Onset: hydrocodone bitartrate 5 mg with acetaminophen 500 mgOrnex, Sinus Relief, Vicks DayQuil Sinus Pressure and Pain, No-Drowsiness Coldrine: pseu-

doephedrine HCl 30 mg with acetaminophen 500 mg

Orthoxicol Cough Syrup, Cheracol Cough Syrup: dextromethorphan hydrobromide 6.7 mg/5 ml with chlorpheniramine 1.3 mg/5 mg and phenylpropanolamine HCl 8.3 mg/5 ml

Palgic-D: pseudoephedrine HCl 90 mg with carbinoxamine maleate 8 mg

Pamprin Multi-Symptom: acetaminophen 400 mg with pamabrom 25 mg, pyrilamine maleate 12.5 mg

Pancof XP: hydrocodone bitartrate 2.5 mg with guaifenesin 100 mg and pseudoephedrine HCl 15 mg in each 5 ml

Parepectolin: attapulgite 600 mg/15 ml

Pediazole, Eryzole: erythromycin ethlysuccinate (equivalent to 200 mg of erythromycin) per 5 ml with sulfisoxazole acetyl (equivalent to 600 mg of sulfisoxazole) per 5 ml

Percocet (note now available in several strengths): **Percocet 2.5/325**: oxycodone hydrochloride 2.5 mg with acetaminophen 325 mg; **Percocet 5/325:** oxycodone hydrochloride 5 mg with acetaminophen 325 mg; **Percocet 7.5/500:** oxycodone hydrochloride 7. 5 mg with acetaminophen 500 mg; **Percocet 10/650:** oxycodone hydrochloride 10 mg with acetaminophen 650 mg

Percodan, Roxiprin: oxycodone hydrochloride 4.5 mg, oxycodone terephthalate 0.38 mg, and aspirin 325 mg

Percodan-Demi: aspirin 325 mg with oxycodone HCl 2.25 mg, oxycodone terephthalate 0.19 mg

Percogesic, Aceta-Gesic, Major-Gesic, Phenylgesic: acetaminophen 325 mg with phenyltoloxamine citrate 30 mg

Peri-Colace, Disanthrol, D-D-S Plus, Genasoft Plus, Peri-Dos, Pro-Sof Plus, Regulace: docusate sodium 100 mg with casanthranol 30 mg

Phenergan VC Syrup, Prometh VC Plain, Promethazine HCl VC: promethazine HCl 6.25 mg/5 ml with phenylephrine HCl 5 mg/5 ml

Phenergan with Codeine Syrup, Pentazine VC with Codeine Liquid, Prometh with Codeine Syrup, Pherazine with Codeine Syrup: promethazine hydrochloride 6.25 mg with codeine phosphate 10 mg, Phenergan with Dextromethorphan, Pherazine DM, Prometh with Dextromethorphan, Phenameth DM: dextromethorphan hydrobromide 15 mg/5 ml with promethazine HCl 6.35 mg/5 ml

Premphase: conjugated estrogens 0.625 mg with medroxyprogesterone acetate 5 mg

Prempro: conjugated estrogens 0.625 mg with medroxyprogesterone acetate 2.5 mg

Prevpac: lansoprazole 30 mg (2 caps), amoxicillin 500 mg (4 caps), and clarithromycin 500 mg (2 tabs)

Primaxin IM: imipenem 500 mg with cilastatin 500 mg; imipenem 750 mg with cilastatin 750 mg for injection

Primaxin IV: imipenem 250 mg with cilastatin 250 mg; imipenem 500 mg with cilastatin 500 mg for injection

Prinzide: lisinopril 10 mg with hydrochlorothiazide 12.5 mg

Prinzide 25: lisinopril 20 mg with hydrochlorothiazide 25 mg

Profen LA, Coldloc, Dura-Vent, Guaifenex PPA 75, SINUvent:

phenylpropanolamine HCl 75 mg with guaifenesin 600 mg

Pyridium Plus: phenazopyridine HCl 150 mg with hyoscyamine hydrobromide 0.3 mg and butabarbital 15 mg

Rauzide: bendroflumethiazide 4 mg with rauwolfia serpentina powdered 50 mg

Rebetron: ribavirin, interferon alfa-2b

Regroton: reserpine 0.25 mg with chlorthalidone 50 mg

Renese-R: reserpine 0.25 mg with polythiazide 2 mg

Rhinocaps: phenylpropranolamine hydrochloride 20 mg with acetaminophen 162 mg and aspirin 162 mg

Rifamate: isoniazid 150 mg with rifampin 300 mg

Rifater: isoniazid 50 mg with rifampin 120 mg and pyrazinamide 300 mg

Robaxisal: methocarbamol 400 mg with aspirin 325 mg

Robitussin-DM, Cheracol-D, Genatuss DM, Halotussin DM, Mytussin DM: dextromethorphan hydrobromide 10 mg/5 ml with guaifenesin 100 mg/5 ml

Ru-Tuss Expectorant Liquid, Rhinosyn-X Liquid: pseudoephedrine hydrochloride 30 mg with destromethorphan hydrobromide 10 mg and guaifenesin 100 mg

Rynatan: azatadine maleate 1 mg with pseudoephedrine sulfate 120 mg

Singlet for Adults Tablets, Simplet Tablets, TheraFlu Cough and Cold Medicine Powder: pseudoephedrine HCl 60 mg, chlorpheniramine maleate 4 mg, and acetaminophen 650 mg

Sinutab Without Drowsiness: pseudoephedrine HCl 30 mg with acetaminophen 325 mg

Sudafed 12 Hour Caplets: pseudoephedrine HCl 120 mg

Synalgos-DC: aspirin 356.4 mg with caffeine 30 mg and dihydrocodeine bitartrate 16 mg

Talacen: pentazocine HCl 25 mg with acetaminophen 650 mg

Talwin Compound Caplets: aspirin 325 mg with pentazocine HCl 12.5 mg

Tarka 1:240: trandolapril 1 mg with verapamil 240 ml

Tarka 2:180: trandolapril 2 mg with verapamil 180 ml

Tarka 2:240: trandolapril 2 mg with verapamil 240 ml

Tarka 4:240: trandolapril 4 mg with verapamil 240 ml

Tavist-D: phenylpropanolamine HCl 75 mg with clemastine fumarate 1.34 mg

Teczem: enalapril maleate 5 mg with diltiazem maleate 180 mg

Teen Midol: acetaminophen 400 mg with pamabrom 25 mg

Tenoretic 50: atenolol 50 mg with chlorthalidone 25 mg

Tenoretic 100: atenolol 100 mg with chlorthalidone 25 mg

Terra-Cortril Suspension: hydrocortisone acetate 1.5% and oxytetracycline HCl 0.5%

Thiosulfil Forte: sulfamethizole 500 mg

Timentin Inj: ticarcillin disodium 3 g with clavulanate potassium 100 mg

Timolide 10/25: timolol maleate 10 mg with hydrochlorothiazide 25 mg

TracTabs 2X: methenamine 120 mg, methylene blue 6 mg, phenyl salicylate 30 mg, atropine 0.06 mg, hyoscyamine SO_4 0.03 mg, benzoic acid 7.5 mg

Triad: butalbital 50 mg with acetaminophen 325 mg and caffeine 40 mg

Triaminic-DM Syrup: dextromethorphan hydrobromide 5 mg/5 ml with phenylpropanolamine HCl 6.25 mg/5 ml

Triavil 4-50: perphenazine 4 mg and amitriptyline HCl 50 mg

TriHemic 600: iron 115 mg, vitamin B_{12} 25 μg, vitamin C 600 mg, folic acid 1 mg, and intrinsic factor 75 mg

Trinalin Repetabs: pseudoephedrine HCl 120 mg with azatadine maleate 1 mg

Trinsicon, Feotrinsic, Foltin, Livitrinsic-F, Contrin: iron 110 mg, vitamin B_{12} 15 μg, vitamin C 75 mg, folic acid 0.5 mg, and intrinsic factor 240 mg

Triple Sulfa, Gyne-Sulf, Sultrin Tripple Sulfa, Trysul, Dayto Sulf, V.V.S.: sulfathiazole 3.42%, sulfacetamide 2.86%, and sulfabenzamide 3.7% vaginal cream

Tritec: ranitidine bismuth citrate 400 mg

Tussafed HC Syrup: hydrocodone bitartrate 2.5 mg with phenylephrine HCl 7.5 mg and guaifenesin 50 mg in each 5 ml

Tussi-Organidin DM NR: guaifenesin 100 mg with dextromethorphan HBr 10 mg/5 ml

Tylenol Children's Cold Tablets: 7.5 mg pseudoephedrine HCl with 0.5 mg chlorpheniramine maleate and acetaminophen 80 mg

Tylenol Flu Night Time Maximum Strength (powder): pseudoephedrine HCl 60 mg, diphenhydramine HCl 50 mg, and acetaminophen 1000 mg dissolved in 6 oz hot water

Tylenol Multi-Symptom Hot Medication (powder): pseudoephedrine HCl 60 mg, chlorpheniramine maleate 4 mg, dextromethorphan hydrobromide 30 mg with acetaminophen 650 mg dissolved in 6 oz hot water

Tylenol PM Extra Strength: acetaminophen 500 mg with diphenhydramine 25 mg

Tylenol with Codeine No. 2: acetaminophen 300 mg with codeine phosphate 15 mg

Tylenol with Codeine No. 3: acetaminophen 300 mg with codeine phosphate 30 mg

Tylenol with Codeine No. 4: acetaminophen 300 mg with codeine phosphate 60 mg

Tylox, Roxicet 5/500, Roxilox: acetaminophen 500 mg with oxycodone HCl 5 mg

Unasyn Inj: ampicillin sodium 1 g with sulbactam sodium 500 mg; ampicillin sodium 2 g with sulbactam sodium 1 g

Uniretic 7.5: moexipril 7.5 mg with hydrochlorothiazide 12.5 mg

Uniretic 15: moexipril 15 mg with hydrochlorothiazide 25 mg

Unisom Nighttime Sleep Aid: doxylamine succinate 25 mg

Unisom With Pain Relief: diphenhydramine HCl 50 mg with acetaminophen 650 mg

Urised, Uritin, Atrosept, Dolsed, UAA, Uridon Modified: methenamine 40.8 mg, phenyl salicylate 18.1 mg, atropine 0.03 mg, hyoscyamine 0.03 mg, and methylene blue 5.4 mg

Urisedamine: methenamine mandelate 500 mg with hyoscyamine 0.15 mg

Vanquish Caplets: aspirin 227 mg with acetaminophen 194 mg, caffeine 33 mg, and buffers

Vaseretic 5-12.5: enalapril maleate 5 mg with hydrochlorothiazide 12.5 mg

Vaseretic 10-25: enalapril maleate 10 mg with hydrochlorothiazide 25 mg
Vicks Children's NyQuil Nighttime Cough/Cold Liquid, Vicks Children's Cough/Cold Liquid: pseudoephedrine HCl 10 mg, chlorpheniramine maleate 0.67 mg, dextromethorphan hydrobromide 5 mg/5 ml
Vicks Cough Silencers: dextromethorphan hydrobromide 2.5 mg with benzocaine 1 mg lozenges
Vicks Formula 44D, Cough and Decongestant Liquid: dextromethorphan hydrobromide 10 mg/5 ml with pseudoephedrine HCl 20 mg/5 ml
Vicks Formula 44M, Cold, Flu and Cough Capsules, AlkaSeltzer Plus Cold and Cough, Genacol: dextromethorphan hydrobromide 10 mg with chlorpheniramine 2 mg, pseudoephedrine HCl 30 mg, and acetaminophen 250 mg
Vicodin: acetaminophen 500 mg with hydrocodone bitartrate 5.0 mg
Vicodin-ES: acetaminophen 750 mg with hydrocodone bitartrate 7.5 mg
Vicodin-HP: acetaminophen 660 mg with hydrocodone bitartrate 10 mg
Vicoprofen: hydrocodone bitartrate 7.5 mg with ibuprofen 200 mg
Wigraine, Cafergot, Ercaf: ergotamine tartrate 1 mg and caffeine 100 mg
Wigraine Suppositories, Cafatine, Cafetrate: ergotamine tartrate 2 mg, caffeine 100 mg
Zestoretic 10/12.5: lisinopril 10 mg with hydrochlorothiazide 12.5 mg
Zestoretic 20/12.5, Prinzide 12.5: lisinopril 20 mg with hydrochlorothiazide 12.5 mg
Zestoretic 20/25, Prinzide 25: lisinopril 20 mg with hydrochlorothiazide 25 mg
Ziac 2.5: bisoprolol fumarate 2.5 mg with hydrochlorothiazide 6.25 mg
Ziac 5: bisoprolol fumarate 5.0 mg with hydrochlorothiazide 6.25 mg
Ziac 10: bisoprolol fumarate 10 mg with hydrochlorothiazide 6.25 mg
Ziradyl Lotion: diphenhydramine HCl 1% with zinc oxide 2%, alcohol 2%, camphor, and parabens
Zosyn: piperacillin 2 g with tazobactam 0.25 gm; piperacillin 3 g with tazobactam 0.375 mg and piperacillin 4 g with tazobactam 0.5 g in vials for IV administration
Zydone: hydrocodone bitartrate 5 mg and acetaminophen 400 mg; or hydrocodone bitartrate 7.5 mg and acetaminophen 400 mg; or hydrocodone bitartrate 10 mg and acetaminophen 400 mg

Appendix G

Dose calculations by weight

Manufacturer-recommended doses are based on extensive clinical trials and are usually intended for the average, healthy adult male of an average weight and age. Thus age, sex, weight, and chronic diseases of the major organs of metabolism (liver) and excretion (kidney) may affect the usual safe and effective FDA-approved dose recommendations. Creatine clearance, peak and trough blood levels, and symptomatic patient response are often used to titrate doses for a given therapeutic effect. Dentists seldom treat the infant, but doses for the pediatric and geriatric patient require an adjustment downward from the usual adult dose. The geriatric patient may be particularly susceptible to effects produced by CNS depressants or drugs that affect renal function. No reliable general rule for dose calculations can supplant clinically derived doses, and many drug monographs now list doses for children based on a mg/kg or mg/lb basis. Children's doses have also been based on a downward reduction of adult doses as determined by body surface area and weight. Clark's rule has been used for many years as a general guide for calculating children's doses.

Clark's Rule:

$$\frac{\text{Child's weight (lb)}}{150} \times \text{Adult dose} = \text{Child's dose}$$

weight lb/kg chart

1 kg = 2.2 lb

kilograms (kg)	pounds (lb)
10	22
20	44
25	55
30	66
35	77
40	88
45	99
50	110
55	121
60	132

Appendix H

Herbal and nonherbal remedies

Black cohosh
(Cimicifuga racemosa, Cimicifugae racemosae rhizoma)
Other names: Black snakeroot, baneberry
Class: Herbal remedy
Major ingredients: The active chemicals are described as triterpene glycosides (acetin, 27-deoxyacetin) along with tannins, a variety of acidic compounds, isoflavones, fatty acids, and a volatile oil. The fresh and dried rhizomes are the portion of the plant used.

Claimed actions: Estrogen-like action, suppression of luteinizing hormone release, and interaction with estrogen receptors.
Uses: It is used for the symptoms of premenstrual and dysmenorrhea disorders and menopausal-associated hot flashes, vaginal dryness, water retention, and related complaints. Most of the pharmacologic studies are from the laboratory, but some clinical testing seems to support a role in reducing menopausal symptoms. Its use should be avoided in pregnancy and lactation.
Administration: Generally available in extracts for oral administration.
Side effects: GI complaints have been reported. Higher doses may cause more significant GI complaints, visual disturbances, lowered blood glucose levels, and CNS side effects such as dizziness. Use for longer than 6 months not recommended.
Dental considerations:
Ask why the product is being used. Evidence is lacking, but there is theoretically a chance that patients taking oral anticoagulants, aspirin, or NSAIDs could show increased bleeding times.
Drug interactions: No dental drug interactions are reported.

Chamomile
(Matricaria chamomilla, Matricaria recutita, Anthemis nobilis, and Matricariae flos)
Other names: common chamomile, German chamomile
Class: Herbal remedy
Major ingredients: Volatile oil containing alpha-bisabolol and other bisabolol derivatives (chamazulene, apigenin), various flavonoids, umbelliferone (a coumarin-like ingredient), and many other components. The portion of the plant used is the dried flower.

Claimed actions: Antiinflammatory, antispasmodic, antibacterial, carminative, and to promote wound healing.
Uses: It has been used to treat inflammation and spasm in the GI tract; topically for inflammation, burns, wounds, and infections of the skin and mucous membranes (including the oral cavity); topi-

cally for anogenital inflammation, as a deodorant, and for a variety of other complaints. There are some data in laboratory models to support the antiinflammatory activity.
Administration: It is available in a variety of dose forms, including teas, infusions (external use), a mouth rinse, and oral dose forms.
Side effects: Slight risk of contact dermatitis: possible cross allergies with ragweed.
Dental considerations:
Ask why the product is being used. Evidence is lacking, but there is theoretically a chance that patients taking oral anticoagulants could show increased bleeding times.
Drug interactions: Risk of increased sedation with CNS depressants. The GI activity of this herb might affect the absorption of some orally administered drugs.

Chaste tree, Chaste berry
(Vitex agnus-castus, angi casti fructrus)
Other names: Chaste tree fruit, monk's pepper, chaste tree
Class: Herbal remedy
Major ingredients: Iridoid glycosides (agnuide and aucubin), flavonoids, progestins, testosterone, and multiple essential oils. The portion of the plant used is the dried, ripe fruit.

Claimed actions: Inhibition of the release of prolactin through a proposed action on dopamine receptors, although not shown in human studies. It may also be antiandrogenic.
Uses: Premenstrual ailments, irregular menstrual cycle complaints, and breast pain. Also used in menopausal symptoms. There is a possible risk of increased ovulation and pregnancy in some women. Should be used with caution when other progestins/estrogens are used. Avoid use in pregnancy and lactation.
Administration: Extracts of the crushed fruit for oral administration.
Side effects: Usually minor but can include skin rashes, dry mouth, and headaches.
Dental considerations:
Ask why the product is being used.
Drug interactions: No dental drug interactions are reported. Dopamine receptor antagonists may block some herbal effects.

Chondroitin sulfate
Other names: Chondroitin
Class: Nonherbal remedy
Major ingredient: Chondroitin sulfate is a mucopolysaccharide, that is, a glycosaminoglycan (GAG). It is found in mammalian cartilaginous tissue and is believed to play a role in flexibility. It is highly viscous and related chemically to sodium hyaluronate.

Claimed actions: It has useful viscoelastic properties suitable for use in selected types of ocular surgery, usually in combination with sodium hyaluronate. Orally administered GAGs are believed to concentrate in cartilage. Chrondocytes use GAGs to form a new cartilage matrix. It may also inhibit leukocyte elastase where high concentrations are associated with rheumatoid arthritis. Other properties may include bringing synovial

fluid into the joint. All of these may contribute to reduced inflammatory activity in joints. Serum lipid–lowering and antithrombogenic effects have also been suggested.
Uses: Chrondrotin in an ophthalmic solution has been used to treat dry eyes. In combination with sodium hyaluronate it is used to support ocular surgery during cataract removal and lens implantation surgery. Its use in cardiovascular diseases remains in doubt. Its most popular use is in arthritis. Limited clinical studies seem to indicate that it is somewhat less effective than NSAIDs.
Administration: A variety of oral dose forms are available, many in combination with glucosamine. Professionally used ophthalmic preparations are also available.
Side effects: Long-term side effects are unknown. GI complaints may be reported on occasion.
Dental considerations:
Ask why the product is being used. Arthritic patients may also be taking aspirin, NSAIDs, or arthritic disease modifying drugs in addition to chondroitin. Question patient about other antiarthritic drugs used, including OTC drugs.
Drug interactions: None reported with dental drugs.

Dong quai
(Angelica sinensis)
Other names: Chinese angelica, dang-gui
Class: Herbal remedy
Major ingredients: It contains a variety of coumarins (oxypeucdeanin, osthol, and others), an essential oil, phytoextrogens, polysaccharides, lactones, and even vitamins E and B_{12}. The portion of the plant used is the roots.

Claimed actions: Vasodilation, antispasmodic in blood vessels, CNS stimulation, and immunosuppressant and antiinflammatory properties. The mechanism of action of these effects is unclear.
Uses: It is used in Chinese herbal medicine in combination with other herbs. Uses include dysmenorrhea, other menstrual problems, and menopausal symptoms. Other uses include arthritis, hypertension, and ulcers. However, significant clinical studies are lacking. The remedy does not appear in the German Commission E Monographs. Avoid use during pregnancy and lactation.
Administration: Administered orally as in infusion, a tincture, or a chewable root.
Side effects: Photosensitization and some GI complaints including a laxative action are reported. Avoid during pregnancy and nursing.
Dental considerations:
Ask why the product is being used. Evidence is lacking, but there is theoretically a chance that patients taking oral anticoagulants, aspirin, or NSAIDs could show increased bleeding times.

Drug interactions: No dental drug interactions reported; its use with coumarin anticoagulants or calcium channel blockers is not recommended.

Echinacea

(Echinacea angustifolia, Echinacea purpurea, and Echinacea pallida)

Other names: American cone flower, Kansas snakeroot, purple cone flower

Class: Herbal remedy

Major ingredients: Caffeic acid glycoside (echinacoside), alkylamides (echinacein and others), essential oils (humulene and others), a variety of flavonoids, and many other components. As with any plant the contents vary with the species, the parts of the plant used, and if dried or fresh. The portion of the plant used is the flower, other aboveground parts, and even the roots.

Claimed actions: Improved wound healing, stimulation of the immune system (some laboratory data suggest an increase in macrophage phagocytic activity and numbers of neutrophils), antibacterial, antiviral, and antiinflammatory activity. It may act as a nonspecific stimulator to the immune system, including macrophages and T-lymphocytes.

Uses: It has been used to enhance would healing, for *Candida* infections, as supportive therapy for common colds and upper respiratory infections, and lower urinary tract infections. Other uses include rheumatoid arthritis and as supportive use in colon cancer. Efficacy in prevention of colds and upper respiratory infections is not supported. Recent data do not support its use for common colds.

Contraindications: Should not be used in patients with autoimmune diseases or progressive infectious diseases, including tuberculosis, multiple sclerosis, leukocytosis, AIDS, HIV infection, and collagen diseases. *Caution:* Use beyond 8 consecutive weeks can suppress immunity.

Administration: It is available in a variety of preparations for internal (oral administration) and external use. Parenteral dose forms are available in Germany. Products are intended for oral or topical administration.

Side effects: Generally limited to parenteral doses only. Fatigue, headache, and dizziness were reported with oral doses. Possible risk of cross-allergic reaction with chamomile or ragweed.

Dental considerations:
Ask why it is being used. Drug interactions: Use beyond 8 consecutive weeks could cause hepatic toxicity and should not be used with other hepatotoxic drugs (ketoconazole). May decrease effectiveness of immunosuppressants.

Evening Primrose Oil

(Oenothera biennis)

Other names: Evening primrose

Class: Herbal remedy

Major ingredients: The oil is a mixture of fatty acids, including linoleic acid (50%-80%), gamma-linolenic acid (GLA, 6%-11%), and smaller amounts of other fatty acids, including palmitic acid, oleic acid, and stearic acid. Other ingredients include tannin, sitosterol, and trace minerals. The portion of the plant used is the seeds.

Claimed actions: Antiatherosclerotic, relief of premenstrual tension, relief of mastalgia, and antiinflammatory actions for arthritis and dermatologic conditions. The fatty acids contained in the oil may function like essential oils and act as precursors of prostaglandins that help regulate metabolic functions.

Uses: It is used for reduction of serum cholesterol and triglycerides. A single study using GLA appeared to show a significant lowering of serum cholesterol, but another study did not. Weight reduction claims are also made. Laboratory trials describing a decrease in platelet aggregation have not been clinically tested. Value in PMS shows some modest benefits after repeated use. Relief of cyclic breast pain may be better than placebo. Data do not support a reduction in rheumatoid disease destruction of tissues, but may have some effect in relieving symptoms. Claims are also made that GLA is effective in controlling symptoms of atopic dermatitis. This herb is not listed in the German Commission E monographs.

Administration: It is available for oral administration in capsules.

Side effects: Few side effects are noted and occur only occasionally. They generally include GI complaints, including GI upset and nausea.

Dental considerations:
Ask why the product is being used.

Drug interactions: No dental drug interactions are reported. One reference recommended that the oil not be used in patients taking drugs that lower the seizure threshold (e.g., phenothiazines).

Feverfew

(Tanacetum parthenium, Chrysanthemum parthenium)

Other names: Feather few, Feverfew leaf, bachelor's button

Class: Herbal remedy

Major ingredients: Sesquiterpene lactones (parthenolide 85%), volatile oils (camphor, *trans*-chrysanthylacetate), flavonoids (luteolin, apdgenin), and many other constituents. The portion of the plant used is the leaves.

Claimed actions: Antiinflammatory, may decrease platelet aggregation (laboratory studies), and reduces histamine release. Other actions include inhibition of prostaglandin synthesis and decrease in serotonin release from platelets. It is not listed in the German Commission E monographs.

Uses: Prophylactic use in migraine headaches, rheumatoid arthritis, stimulation of menstruation. It has also been used in folk medicine to control fever, as an external anti-

septic, and even a mouth rinse following extractions. Avoid use during pregnancy and lactation.
Side effects: Oral products produce few complaints; chewing the leaves may lead to oral ulcerations, swelling of circumoral tissues. Potential risk of increased bleeding time.
Administration: It is available in many oral dose forms or used to make an infusion.
Dental considerations:
Ask why product is being used.
In patients taking warfarin or other oral anticoagulant, inquire about bleeding history.
Inquire about unusual bleeding episodes following dental treatment.
Drug interactions: Avoid drugs that affect platelet action, such as aspirin and NSAIDs; they may reduce effectiveness. Advise patient not to take this herb for 2-3 weeks before surgery.

Garlic
(Allium Sativum)
Other names: Allium, poor man's treacle
Class: Herbal remedy
Major ingredients: A volatile oil containing several sulfur compounds, a sulfur containing amino acid identified as alliin. With grinding alliin is converted to allicin (responsible for the typical odor of garlic). Many other constituents are also present, including minute quantities of trace minerals, betacarotene, and vitamins. The portion of the plant used is whole, fresh or dried, garlic clove and oil of garlic.

Claimed action: Antibacterial, lipid-lowering activity, inhibition of platelet aggregation, antihypertensive, antioxidant, and a preventative for age-related vascular disorders.
Uses: It has been used to treat a wide array of bacterial, fungal, and viral infections. Data suggest it is about 1% as effective as penicillin in vitro. Use in oral fungal infections remains in doubt. Data show a limited reduction in cholesterol, reduction in blood pressure, and a decrease in platelet aggregation. The use of garlic in cancer prevention is controversial. Long-term effects are unknown.
Administration: It is available in a variety of oral dose forms; however, the whole garlic clove is believed to contain the highest concentration of allicin, the major active ingredient.
Side effects: The taste and odor of garlic is by far the most common complaint. Rarely GI symptoms may occur with larger doses. Halitosis and burning of the mouth have been reported.
Dental considerations:
Ask why the product is being used.
Inquire about unusual bleeding episodes following dental treatment.
Drug interactions: Evidence is lacking, but there is always a chance that patients taking oral anticoagulants, aspirin, or NSAIDs could show increase bleeding time. Advise patient not to take this herb for 2-3 weeks before surgery.

Ginger

(Zingiber Officinale, Zingiberis rhizoma)

Other names: Ginger root

Class: Herbal remedy

Major ingredients: The root contains a volatile oil and other chemicals termed *pungent principles.* These latter compounds are collectively known as gingerols, shogaols, and gingerdiols. The portion of the plant used is the root.

Claimed actions: Motion sickness prevention, promotion of salivary and gastric secretions, positive inotropic action, and antiinflammatory effects have all been claimed for this herb.

Uses: The most common uses include prevention of motion sick ness and in dyspepsia. It has also been used for morning sickness of pregnancy and in rheumatoid arthritis. Galanolactone, an active ingredient, has been reported to have serotonin (5-HT) antagonist activity, and gingerols may have a positive inotropic effect. There is a difference of opinion about its safe use in pregnancy and lactation with the German Commission E monographs warning against its use. Patients with gallstones should not take ginger.

Administration: Only the rhizome (root) of the plant is used. The German Commission E reference lists the dose at 2-4 g daily.

Side effects: Generally not reported except for toxic doses that could include CNS depression and arrhythmia.

Dental considerations:

Ask why the product is being used.

Drug interactions: None reported. Evidence is lacking, but there is theoretically a chance that patients taking oral anticoagulants, aspirin, or NSAIDs could show increased bleeding times.

Gingko

(Gingko biloba, Gingko folium)

Other names: Maidenhair tree, ginkyo

Class: Herbal remedy

Major ingredients: Common ingredients with claimed pharmacologic activity include multiple flavonoids (biobetin, ginkgetin), flavone glycosides (quercetin), bioflavones, terpenoids (ginkolides A, B, and C), and bilobalide. The portion of the plant used is the leaf.

Claimed actions: Improvement in blood flow in the microcirculation, inhibition of development of traumatically or toxic induced cerebral edema, improved hypoxic tolerance in cerebral tissues, reduction in retinal edema, increased memory performance, inhibition of age-related reduction in muscarinic receptors, and antagonism of platelet-activating factor (PAF). May also have monoamine oxidase inhibition properties.

Uses: It has been used to treat cerebral insufficiency, Alzheimer's dementia and other forms of dementia, circulatory disorders associated with diabetes, memory deficits, vertigo, tinnitus, and impotency associated with use of selective serotonin reuptake inhibitors. There are some data to support these uses. Benefits for exercise performance are not verified. It use is contraindicated during pregnancy and lactation.

Administration: Capsules and tablets of leaf extracts are available for use. Doses range from 120 to 240 mg of dry extract for 8 weeks for chronic diseases. Use for longer than 3 months requires reevaluation of benefits.
Side effects: May include GI complaints, headaches, and allergic reactions. Use with caution in patients with hypertension. One report of oral ulcerations is noted.
Dental considerations:
Ask why the product is being used. Inquire about unusual bleeding episodes following dental treatment.
Drug interactions: There is some evidence for anticoagulant activity with gingko; monitor or use antiplatelet drugs such as aspirin or NSAIDS with caution. Discontinue gingko use 2 weeks before surgery and general anesthesia. *Caution:* Concurrent use with MAO inhibitors and tricyclics.

Ginsing
(Panax quinquefolium, Panax ginsing)
Class: Herbal remedy
Major ingredients: Constituents vary with the species of ginsing used. Contains steroid-like compounds called ginsenosides or panaxosides. Other ingredients include a volatile oil and flavonoids along with smaller quantities of other ingredients.

Claimed actions: Effects vary from CNS stimulation to depression. Improves resistance to stress in laboratory models, but there is a lack of evidence in humans. There are also claims of decreased platelet aggregation and increased memory and concentration.
Uses: Improvement of stamina and to enhance performance, a tonic and "adaptogen."
Administration: The root is use for teas and various other oral preparations.
Side effects: Not well documented but may include insomnia, diarrhea, and skin rash. However, adulterants included with ginsing products may increase risk for other side effects.
Dental considerations:
Ask why the product is being used.
Drug interactions: No specific dental drug interactions are reported, but ginsing may have monoamine oxidase inhibition properties. Discontinue use of ginsing 2 weeks before general anesthesia.

Glucosamine sulfate
Other names: Chitosamine, glucosamine
Class: Nonherbal remedy
Major ingredient: Glucosamine sulfate, an aminomonosaccharide (2-amino-2-deoxyglucose), is a component of mucopolysaccharides and mucoproteins. Other salt forms may also be used.

Claimed actions: Glucosamine is used in the synthesis of glycoproteins and glycosaminoglycans (GAGs). It is formed in the body from glucose through intermediary metabolic steps to be incorporated into GAGs, which are essential for cartilage function in joints.
Uses: It is used to treat the signs and symptoms of osteoarthric disease. Other uses have included

other inflammatory disorders, including tendinitis and rheumatoid arthritis. It has been clinically studied in comparison to NSAIDs. Some reports indicate equivalency with NSAIDs, but there is considerable doubt about its overall value in osteoarthritis. Nonetheless, patients indicated relief of pain and increased mobility. Oral, IV, IM, and intraarticular routes have been used to study glucosamine's effectiveness. These studies may lack rigid testing for effect in inflammatory joint diseases.
Administration: The usual dose is 500 mg three times daily.
Side effects: Side effects are uncommon but can include GI effects such as nausea, heartburn, diarrhea, and epigastric pain. CNS side effects are also rarely observed; they may include headache, insomnia, and drowsiness. However, arthritic patients may be taking aspirin, NSAIDs, or disease-modifying osteoarthritis drugs in addition to glucosamine and chondroitin. Question patient about other antiarthrtic drugs used, including OTC drugs.
Dental considerations:
Ask why the product is being used.
Drug interactions: No dental drug interactions are documented.

Goldenseal
(Hydrastis canadensis)
Other names: Eye root, yellow root, turmeric root
Class: Herbal remedy
Major ingredients: Contains the isoquinoline alkaloids hydrastine and beberine, other related alkaloids, and a volatile oil.

Claimed actions: Astringent and antiseptic. May also stimulate the secretion of bile and may have laxative action. Hydrastine has been shown to cause vasoconstriction in peripheral vessels. Berberine may have some antibacterial actions. This herb is not included in the German Commission E monographs.
Uses: It has been used in the treatment of eye infections or irritations, mucous membrane infections, and herpes labialis. It has also been used in the treatment of traveler's diarrhea and giardiasis. It is contraindicated for use in pregnancy and lactation.
Administration: Dose forms could not be documented, but it may be used in herbal product combinations.
Side effects: Safe in usual doses; adverse effects are more often observed with toxic doses (may include hypertension, convulsions, and breathing difficulties).
Dental considerations:
Ask why the product is being used.
Drug interactions: None reported.

Hawthorn

(Crataegus oxyancantha, Crataegi folim cum flore, C. monogyna, and C. Laevigata)

Other names: English hawthorn, maybush

Class: Herbal remedy

Major ingredients: Flavonoids (hyperoside, vitexin-rhamnose, rutin, and proanthocyanidins) with vasodilating properties, as well as inhibition of vasoconstriction. Proanthocyanidins are reported to block angiotensin-converting enzyme (ACE). It also contains tyramine, a biogenic amine. The plant parts used include the flowers, leaves, fruits, and mixtures of other plant parts.

Claimed actions: Laboratory studies indicate positive inotropic effects, increased coronary and myocardial perfusion, and reduced peripheral vascular resistance. Dilation of coronary and peripheral blood vessels has also been reported. This information is based on laboratory studies only. Some ingredients may cause CNS depression.

Uses: Hypertension, reduction in anginal pain, decrease in cardiac sufficiency, and cardiotonic. It is approved in Germany as a prescription drug for mild cardiac insufficiency and bradyarrhythmias. Other uses include atherosclerosis.

Administration: It is available in oral dose forms as an extract and plant parts for brewing teas.

Side effects: No contraindications or side effects are listed. At least one reference offered a caution when used with other drugs that may affect cardiac function.

Dental considerations: Ask why the product is being used. Monitor vital signs in patients with cardiovascular disease.

Kava

(Piper methysticum, Piperis methystrici rhizoma)

Other names: Kava-Kava, kew, tonga

Class: Herbal remedy

Major ingredients: Kava lactones (kava alpha-pyrones), including methysticin, kawain, and others. The plant part used is the dried rhizomes.

Claimed actions: These lactones have demonstrable pharmacologic activity on the CNS. Reported actions include sedation, muscle relaxation, and anticonvulsive and antispasmodic effects.

Uses: It has been used for a variety of complaints, including the relief of tension, stress, insomnia, and anxiety. An intoxicating effect has also been reported. Mechanism of actions range from GABA receptor modification to dopamine antagonist activity. It has also been used for a variety of other applications ranging from promotion of wound healing to gonorrhea treatment. There is little doubt the lactones are pharmacologically active, but the therapeutic value remains to be established. A local anesthetic action is also claimed.

Administration: Products for oral administration are available; in some areas the kava-kava is chewed. Use should be limited to no more than 3 months. It should not be used in patients with endogenous depression or Parkinson's disease or during pregnancy and lactation.

Side effects: Continued use results in discoloration of hair, skin, and nails. GI complaints may occasionally accompany use. Chewing kava-kava can result in circumoral numbness. Patients using kava-kava may have reduced alertness.

Dental considerations:
Ask why the product is being used.

Drug interactions: Use caution when other CNS depressants are given, including other herbal remedies with antidepressant or sedative activity. One report suggests avoiding benzodiazepines in patients using Kava.

Ma-Huang

(Ephedra Sinica, Ephedra herba)

Other names: Ephedra, Mormon tea, Desert herb

Class: Herbal remedy

Major ingredients: Contains ephedrine; some species also contain pseudoephedrine. Other components may include norepinephrine. The plant parts used are the dried young branches harvested in the fall, although some species may not contain these active alkaloids.

Claimed actions: Ephedrine has both direct and indirect actions on the sympathetic nervous system. It has direct effects on adrenergic receptors, and its indirect action is one of releasing stored catecholamines (norepinephrine) from presynaptic nerve terminals. This is well established, and ephedrine is used as a sympathomimetic. It is orally effective with a longer duration of action than epinephrine. CNS-stimulating effects are also suggested with ephedrine.

Uses: It is used for bronchospasm in asthma and other bronchospastic diseases. It acts as a cardiac stimulant with increases in blood pressure. It is also used to decrease appetite (anorexiant) and in the treatment of narcolepsy.

Administration: Various oral preparations are available, and it is also used in teas. Doses should be carefully controlled and followed to avoid excessive sympathomimetic effects.

Side effects: Hypertension, tachycardia, restlessness, headache, irritability, arrhythmias, hyperglycemia, and other related actions due to excessive or prolonged sympathetic stimulation. It should not be used in combination with St. John's wort.

Dental Considerations:
Ask why this product is being used. If it is being used to treat asthma or bronchitis, the same precautions as for any asthmatic patient should be observed. If it is being used as an appetite suppressant, ask the patient if he or she has previously taken Fen-Phen and follow appropriate guidelines for management. Monitor vital signs every appointment due to cardiovascular side effects.

Drug interactions: Patients on high doses of Ma-Huang could possibly show exaggerated responses to injected catecholamines. Avoid the use of drugs that enhance the action of epinephrine on the cardiovascular system. Patients should avoid combinations of Ma-Huang with cardiac glycosides, halothane, guanethidine, and MAO inhibitors.

Saw Palmetto

(Serenoa repens, Sabal fructus)

Other names: Sabal, cabbage palm, saw palmetto berry

Class: Herbal remedy

Major ingredients: Contains various sitosterols (phytosterols) such as beta-sitosterol and other sitosterol compounds, flavonoids, polysaccharides, and free fatty acids. The portion of the plant used is the ripe, dried fruit.

Claimed actions: It is reported to be antiandrogenic, antiinflammatory, and may have some low-level estrogenic activity. The antiandrogenic activity is suggested to occur by inhibition of the enzyme testosterone-5-alpha-reductase. This action prevents the conversion of testosterone to dihydrotestosterone, the active androgenic hormone. Some data support blockade of dihydrotestosterone to receptors in the cell nucleus. Limited data seem to support the estrogenic effects. The antiinflammatory effects remain doubtful.

Uses: This herbal product has been used in the treatment of symptoms associated with benign prostatic hypertrophy, in particular urinary difficulties. Clinical trials show better results than placebo with claims of comparative results to prescription medications. There is no direct effect on reduction of the size of the prostate gland. Improvement in urinary symptoms may be somewhat similar to finasteride (Proscar).

Administration: It is available for oral administration as the herb, in teas, or in extracts.

Side effects: Few side effects are reported with usual doses. Headache and GI side effects, including diarrhea with higher doses, may occur. Whether it can influence other androgens or even show estrogenic effects in women is not clear. Avoid use in pregnancy and in women of childbearing age.

Dental considerations:
Ask why the product is being used.

Drug interactions: No dental drug interactions are reported.

St. John's wort

(Hypericum perforatum, Hyperici herba)

Other names: Hypericum, kaimath weed, John's wort

Class: Herbal remedy

Major ingredients: Contains quinoids (hypericin, pseudohypericin), flavonoids (hyperside, quercitin, rutin), bioflavonoids, and a volatile oil. The pharmacologically active component is established as hypericin. The portions of the plant used are the aboveground parts harvested during the flowering season.

Claimed actions: The primary actions are antidepressant, antiinflammatory, and antimicrobial. Hypericin may act as a selective serotonin reuptake inhibitor or a monoamine oxidase inhibitor.

Uses: It is used for the treatment of symptoms of depression; data indicate that it may be equal to or slightly less effective than the tricyclic antidepressant amitriptyline. Hypericin is soon to be evaluated as a drug for depression. The volatile oil seems to increase the healing of burns. It has been suggested to have some effect against herpes simplex viruses and HIV. The efficacy remains to be established. Extracts may have some antibacterial properties. It has also been used for symptoms of dyspepsia.

Administration: A variety of oral preparations are available, and it is also used as an infusion.

Side effects: Side effects are generally minimal, but photosensitization, headache, nervousness, restlessness, hypomania, and constipation have been noted. It should be used with caution in severely depressed patients. Its safety during pregnancy and lactation is unknown. Avoid use in patients with a history of seizure disorders or migraine.

Dental considerations:
Ask why the product is being used.

Drug interactions: It should be used only with caution in patients taking other antidepressive medications, including MAO inhibitors, tricyclic antidepressants, and selective serotonin reuptake inhibitors. It has been suggested that a risk of serotonin syndrome could occur with these antidepressants. Avoid indirect-acting sympathomimetics. Discontinue use 2 weeks before general anesthesia. Other drugs suggested to interact include metronidazole, caffeine, theophylline, and iron salts. Avoid dental drugs with a potential for photosensitivity.

Valerian

(Valeriana officinalis, Valerianae radix)

Other names: Valerian root, Indian valerian

Class: Herbal remedy

Major ingredients: Valepotriates (isovaltrate and others), a volatile oil (bornyl isovalerenate and isovalerenic acid), sesquiterpenes, and multiple other substances. Pharmacologically active components are not identified with any certainty. The portions of the plant used are the fresh underground parts and roots.

Claimed actions: Sedation, reduction in nervousness, sleep promoting, and antispasmodic.

Uses: It is used for restlessness, sleeping disorders, and insomnia. Other uses include agitation associated with menstrual activity, colic, stomach cramps, and uterine spasticity. Laboratory data suggest that it may increase GABA levels at synapses. Antispasmodic properties are not well defined. Limited clinical evidence suggest some improvement in sleep. It has also been used externally by adding to bath water.

Administration: It is available for oral use in a variety of oral products, including tinctures, infusions, and extracts.

Side effects: Generally not observed in usual doses. GI complaints, headache, sleeplessness, mydriasis, excitability, and cardiac disturbances may occur with long-term use.

Dental considerations:
Ask why the product is being used.

Drug interactions: Although no interactions are reported, monitor patients for increased sedation when using other CNS depressants.

Yohimbe bark

(Pausinystalia yohimbe)

Other names: Yohimbe cortex

Class: Herbal

Major ingredients: The principal alkaloid is yohimbine (quebrachine) with lesser amounts of stereoisomers of yohimbine along with other alkaloids, including corynantheidine and allo-yohimbine. It also contains a variety of plant tannins. The portion of the plant used is the dried bark of the trunk and branches of the tree.

Claimed actions: The major effects of this drug are due to yohimbine. Do not confuse the prescription drug yohimbine with yohimbe. Yohimbine has α_2-adrenergic antagonist activity. Presynapatic α_2-receptors regulate norepinephrine release. In a feedback-type action, antagonism of these receptors is associated with greater norepinephrine release. It may also dilate blood vessels; claims are made for a calcium channel blocking action and inhibition of monoamine oxidase enzymes.

Uses: It has been used to treat erectile dysfunction, as an aphrodisiac, for exhaustion, and even for orthostatic hypotension. Limited data concern yohimbine and not yohimbe. Yohimbine has not been approved for this application. According to the German Commission E monographs, yohimbe's effectiveness is not documented and it is not recommended.

Administration: Limited products are available and usually in combination with other ingredients.

Side effects: Usual doses produce few side effects; however, in large doses significant adverse effects are reported. These include increased salivation, anxiety, hallucinations, exanthema, nervousness, irritability, tachycardia, and sweating. Other effects may also be observed. Cardiac failure, which could be fatal, is reported. Contraindicated in patients with hepatic or renal impairment and psychiatric disorders.

Dental considerations:
Ask why the product is being used.

Drug interactions: No specific dental drug interactions are reported, but it may have MAO inhibitory action. Avoid use of indirect-acting sympathomimetics and tricyclic antidepressants.

BIBLIOGRAPHY

Blumenthal M et al: *The complete German Commission E monographs,* Austin, 1998, American Botanical Council.

DerMarderosian A, editor: *The review of natural products,* St Louis, 1996, Facts and Comparisons.

Miller LG: Herbal medicinals: selected clinical considerations focusing on known or potential drug-herb interactions, *Arch Intern Med* 158(20):2200-2211, 1998.

Natural medicines comprehensive database, Stockton, CA, 1999, Pharmacist's Letter/Prescriber's Letter, Therapeutic Research Faculty.

Nonherbal dietary supplements, *Pharmacist's Letter* 98(4), 1998.

O'Hara MA et al: A review of 12 commonly used medicinal herbs, *Arch Fam Med* 7:523-536, 1998.

PDR for herbal remedies, Montvale, NJ, 1998, Medical Economics.

Therapeutic use of herbs, continuing education booklets part 1 and part 2, Stockton, CA, 1998, Pharmacist's Letter.

Appendix I

Selected references

Advisory Statement: Antibiotic prophylaxis for dental patients with total joint replacements, *JADA* 128:1004-1008, July 1997.

Borea G et al: Tranexamic acid as a mouthwash in anticoagulant-treated patients undergoing oral surgery, *Oral Surg Oral Med Oral Pathol* 75:29-31, 1993.

Cohen DM, Bhattacharyya I, Lydiatt WM: Recalcitrant oral ulcers caused by calcium channel blockers: diagnosis and treatment considerations, *JADA* 130:1611-1618, November 1999.

Dajani AS et al: Prevention of bacterial endocarditis: recommendations by the American Heart Association, *JADA* 128:1142-1151, August 1997.

Drug interaction facts, updated bimonthly, St Louis, Facts and Comparisons.

Facts and comparisons, St Louis, updated monthly, Facts and Comparisons.

Gage TW: New drugs and drug products approved in 1998, *Texas Dental Journal* 116:18-31, September 1999.

Gahart BL: *2000 Intravenous medications,* ed 16, St Louis, 1999, Mosby.

Halevy S, Shai A: Lichenoid drug eruptions, *J Am Acad Dermatol* 29:249-255, 1993.

Hardman JG et al: *Goodman and Gilman's the pharmacological basis of therapeutics,* ed 9, New York, 1996, McGraw-Hill.

Little JW, Falace DA: *Dental management of the medically compromised patient,* ed 5, St Louis, 1997, Mosby.

The medical letter, handbook of adverse drug interactions, New Rochelle, NY, 1999, The Medical Letter.

The medical letter on drugs and therapeutics, vols 40 and 41, New Rochelle, NY, 1998-1999, The Medical Letter.

1999 Mosby's GenRX, ed 9, St Louis, 1999, Mosby.

Physicians' desk reference, ed 53, Montvale, NJ, 1999, Medical Economics.

Rees TD: Oral effects of drug abuse, *Crit Rev Oral Biol Med*3(3):163-184, 1992.

Rees TD: Systemic drugs as a risk factor for periodontal disease initiation and progression, *Compendium* 16:20-42, 1995.

Shulman JD, Wells LM: Acute fluoride toxicity from ingesting home-use dental products in children birth to 6 years of age, *J Public Health Dent* 57(3):150-158, 1997.

Skidmore-Roth L: *2000 Mosby's nursing drug reference,* St Louis, 1999, Mosby.

Souto JC et al: Oral surgery in anticoagulated patients without reducing the dose of oral anticoagulant, *J Oral Maxillofac Surg* 54:27-32, 1996.

United States Pharmacopeial Convention: *Drug information for the health care professionals USPDI,* ed 17, Rockville, Md, 1997, The Convention.

United States Pharmacopeial Convention: *USP Dictionary of USAN and International Drug Names 1998,* Rockville, Md, 1998, The Convention.

Valsecchi R, Cainelli T: Gingival hyperplasia induced by erythromycin, *Acta Derm Venereol (Stockh)* 72:157, 1992.

Westbrook P et al: Reversal of nifedipine-induced gingival hyperplasia by the calcium channel blocker, isradipine, *J Dent Res* 74(S1):208, 1995.

Whal MJ: Altering anticoagulant therapy: a survey of physicians, *JADA* 127:625-638, 1996.

Whal MJ: Myths of dental surgery in patients receiving anticoagulant therapy, *JADA* 131:77-81, 2000.

Wright JM: Oral manifestations of drug reactions, *Dent Clin North Am* 28:529-543, 1984.

Zelickson BD, Rogers RS: Oral drug reactions, *Dermatol Clin* 5:695-708, 1987.

Generic and Trade Name Index

Index

A

abacavir, 10
abacavir sulfate, 19
Abbreviations, 725-729
Abenol, 21-22
Abitrate, 157-158
absorbable gelatin sponge, 13, 20
acarbose, 6, 20-21
Accolate, 10, 14, 713-714
Accupril, 8, 582-583
Accuretic, 739
Accutane, 12, 349-350, 730
Accutane-Roche, 349-350
Aceon, 8, 521-523, 731, 738
Aceta-Gesic, 747
acetaminophen, 4, 21-22
Aceta with Codeine, 739
Acetazolam, 22-23
acetazolamide, 5, 12, 13, 22-23, 738
acetazolamide sodium, 22-23
acetohexamide, 6, 24-25
Achromycin, 16, 649-651
Acid Control, 263-264
Aciphex, 13, 586-587, 732
acitretin, 12, 25-26, 738
Actagen, 739
Actifed, 731, 739
Actigall, 5, 13, 702, 738
Actimmune, 14, 340-341
Actinex, 11, 399
Actiprofen, 328-330
Actiq (lozenges), 268-269
Actisite, 16, 651
Actonel, 7, 600
Actos, 6, 541-542
Actron, 354-356
ACU-dyne, 547-548
acyclovir, 10, 737
acyclovir sodium, 26-27
acyclovir (topical), 10, 26
Adalat, 476-477
Adalat CC, 476-477
Adalat FT, 476-477
Adalat PA, 476-477
Adderall 5, 739
Adderall 10, 739
Adipex-P, 531-532, 730
Adipost, 525-526, 736
Adrenalin, 4, 11, 16, 238-239
Adrenalin Chloride, 238-239
ADRENERGIC AGONISTS, 4
Adsorbocarpine, 537
Advil, 328-330
Aerobid, 277-278, 738
Aerobid Inhalant, 13
Aerobid-M, 277-278
Aerodine, 547-548
Aerolate Sr, 652-653
Aeroseb-Dex, 191
Aerosporin, 4
Aerosporin (ophthalmic), 14, 544-545
Afrin, 11, 505
Afrin Children's Nose Drops, 505
Aftate, 671
Agenerase, 10, 50-51, 737
Aggrenox, 739
Agrylin, 15, 51-52
A-Hydrocort, 320-322
Airet, 28-29
Akarpine, 537
AKbeta, 368-369
AK-Con Ophthalmic, 463-464
AK-Dex, 192-193
AK-Homatropine, 316-317
Akineton, 5, 9, 84-85, 732
Akne-mycin, 242
AKPro, 213
AK-Sulf, 627-628
AK-Tob, 665
Ak-Trol, 739
Ak-Trol Ointment, 739
Ak-Zol, 22-23
Ala-Cort, 322-323
alatrofloxacin, 12
Albalon, 463-464
Albert Glyburide, 303-304
albuterol, 10, 28-29, 732, 737
ALCOHOL DETOXIFICATION DRUGS, 736
Alconefrin, 533-534
Aldactazide 25/25, 739
Aldactazide 50/50, 739
Aldactone, 12, 623-624, 732
Aldara, 13, 332

Entries can be identified as follows: generic name, Trade Name, DRUG CATEGORY, *Combination Product.*

Aldoclor-150, 739
Aldoclor-250, 739
Aldomet, 8, 428-430
Aldoril-15, 739
Aldoril-25, 739
Aldoril D30, 739
Aldoril D50, 739
alendronate, 7, 737
alendronate sodium, 29-30
Alesse, 493-495
Alesse-21, 493-495
Alesse-28, 493-495
Aleve, 464-465
Aleve Cold and Sinus, 739
alfacalcidol, 710-711
Alferon N, 13, 338-339
alitretinoin, 12, 30
AlkaSeltzer Plus Cold and Cough, 750
Alkeran, 11, 405-406
Allegra, 7, 271
Allegra-D, 739
Allent, 739
Aller-Chlor, 137-138
Allercon, 739
Allercort, 13, 322-323
Allerdryl, 211-212
Allerest Eye Drops, 463-464
Allerest Maximum Strength 12 Hour, 739
Allerest 12 Hour Nasal, 505
Allerfrim, 739
Allergy Drops, 463-464
AllerMax, 211-212
AllerMed, 211-212
Alloprin, 30-31
allopurinol, 7, 9, 30-31, 737
allopurinol sodium, 30-31
Alocril (ophthalmic solution), 466-467
Alomide, 14
Alomide Ophthalmic, 385
Alor 5/500, 745
Alora, 247-248
ALPHA-ADRENERGIC ANTAGONISTS, 8
Alpha-Baclofen, 69-70
Alphaderm, 322-323
Alphagan, 13, 88-89, 738
alpha tocopherol, 711-712
Alphatrex, 77-78
alprazolam, 5, 31-32, 730
alprostadil, 12, 15, 32-33
Alrex, 393
Alrex (optic), 15
Alrex (topical), 13
Altace, 8, 588-590
Alti-Bromocriptine, 89-90
Alti-Clonazepam, 160-161
Alti-Valproic, 703-705
aluminum hydroxide, 736
aluminum magnesium complex, 396-397
Alupent, 11, 417-418, 737
ALZHEIMER'S DRUGS, 4, 11, 736
amantadine, 9, 10
amantadine HCl, 33-34
Amaphen, 743
Amaryl, 6, 300-302
ambenonium, 11, 14
ambenonium chloride, 34-35
Ambenyl Cough Syrup, 739
Ambien, 5, 720-721, 737
Amcort, 684-686
Amen, 403-404
Amerge, 14, 456-466, 733
Americaine, 73-74
Amersol, 328-330
A-MethaPred, 431-432
amethopterin, 426-427
Amgenal, 739
Amicar, 13, 36-37
Amigesic, 609-610
amiloride, 12, 732
amiloride HCl, 35-36
aminocaproic acid, 13, 36-37
aminoglutethimide, 11, 37-38
AMINOGLYCOSIDES (TOPICAL), 4
Amino-Opti-E, 711-712
aminophylline, 10, 16, 38-39, 738
amiodarone, 6, 738
amiodarone HCl, 39-40
Ami-TexLA, 743
amitriptyline, 6, 731, 732, 736
amitriptyline HCl, 40-42
amlexanox, 10, 42
amlodipine, 5, 8, 738
amlodipine besylate, 43-44
amoxapine, 6, 44-45, 731
amoxicillin, 15
amoxicillin/clavulanate, 15
amoxicillin/clavulanate potassium, 45-46

Entries can be identified as follows: generic name, Trade Name, DRUG CATEGORY, *Combination Product.*

amoxicillin trihydrate, 46-48
Amoxil, 15, 46-48
amphetamine, 734
Amphojel, 736
amphotericin B, 7, 48
ampicillin/ampicillin sodium/ ampicillin trihydrate, 15, 48-50
Ampicin, 48-50
amprenavir, 10, 50-51, 737
AMYOTROPHIC LATERAL SCLEROSIS DRUGS, 4
Anacin, 739
Anacobin, 172-173
Anadrol, 12
Anadrol-50, 505-506
Anaflex, 4, 9
Anaflex 750, 609-610
Anafranil, 6, 158-160, 731, 736
anagrelide, 15
anagrelide hydrochloride, 51-52
ANALGESICS, 4, 731, 736
Anapolon 50, 505-506
Anaprox, 9, 15, 464-465
Anaprox DS, 464-465
Anaspaz, 327-328, 730
Anazemet, 736
Ancalixir, 528-529
Ancef, 11, 113-114
Ancobon, 7, 274-275
Ancotil, 274-275
Andro-100, 647-648
Andro-Cyp, 647-648
androgens, 734
Android-F, 281-282
Andro LA, 647-648
Andronate, 647-648
Andropository, 647-648
Andryl 200, 647-648
Anergan, 566-567
ANESTHETICS, 4, 736
Anexate, 276-277
Anexsia 5/500, 739-740
Anexsia 7.5/650, 740
Anexsia 10/660, 740
ANGIOTENSIN-CONVERTING ENZYME INHIBITORS, 8
ANGIOTENSIN II RECEPTOR ANTAGONISTS, 8
Anorex, 730
ANOREXIANTS, 4, 730, 736
Anorex SR, 525-526
Ansaid, 14, 285-286
Antabuse, 4, 217, 736
ANTACIDS, 4, 736
ANTAGONISTS, 4
ANTIACNE DRUGS, 730
ANTIANGINALS, 4-5
ANTIANXIETY DRUGS, 5, 730
ANTIARTHRITIC DRUGS, 9, 730, 736, 737
ANTIASTHMATICS, 5
ANTICARIES DRUGS, 5
ANTICHOLELITHICS, 5
ANTICHOLINERGICS, 5, 730, 736
ANTICOAGULANTS, 5
ANTICONVULSANTS, 5-6, 730, 736
ANTIDEPRESSANTS, 6, 731, 736
ANTIDIABETICS, 6, 736
ANTIDIARRHEALS, 6, 731, 734, 736
ANTIDYSRHYTHMICS (ANTIARRHYTHMICS), 6
ANTIEMETICS, 7, 736
Antiflex, 496
ANTIFUNGALS, 736
ANTIGOUT DRUGS, 7, 737
Antihist-1, 152
ANTIHISTAMINES, 5, 7, 731
ANTIHYPERCALCEMICS, 7
ANTIHYPERLIPIDEMICS, 8, 737
ANTIHYPERTENSIVES, 8, 731
ANTIINFECTIVES, 8, 9, 737
ANTIINFLAMMATORIES, 9, 731, 737
ANTIMALARIALS, 9
ANTINAUSEANTS, 732
ANTIPARKINSONIAN DRUGS, 9, 732, 737
ANTIPSYCHOTICS, 9-10, 732, 737
ANTISECRETORY DRUGS, 732
Antispas, 200-201
ANTISPASMODICS, 730, 732
ANTITHYROID DRUGS, 10, 737
ANTITUBERCULARS, 10
Anti-Tuss, 306-307
ANTITUSSIVES, 10, 734
Antivert, 732
Antivert 25, 401-402
Antivert 50, 401-402
ANTIVIRALS, 10, 732, 737
Antrocol Elixir, 740
Anturan, 632-633

Entries can be identified as follows: generic name, Trade Name, DRUG CATEGORY, *Combination Product.*

Anturane, 16, 632-633
Anusol HC, 322-323
ANXIOLYTIC/SEDATIVES, 737
Anzemet, 7, 217-218
Apacet, 21-22
Aphthasol, 10, 42
APHTHOUS STOMATITIS DRUGS, 10
Apo-Acetazolamide, 22-23
Apo-Allopurinol, 30-31
Apo-Alpraz, 31-32
Apo-Amitripytline, 40-42
Apo-Amoxi, 46-48
Apo-Ampi, 48-50
Apo-Atenol, 56-58
Apo-Benzotropine, 74-76
Apo-Bromocriptine, 89-90
Apo-C, 54-55
Apo-Carbamazepine, 105-106
Apo-Cefaclor, 111-112
Apo-Cephalex, 123-124
Apo-Chlorazepate, 163-164
Apo-Chlordiazepoxide, 131-132
Apo-Chlorpromaide, 140-141
Apo-Chlorthalidone, 141-142
Apo-Cimetidine, 146-147
Apo-Clonazepam, 160-161
Apo Cloxi, 165-166
Apo-Diazepam, 196-197
Apo-Diclo, 197-199
Apo-Diflunisal, 205-206
Apo-Diltaz, 209-210
Apo-Dimenhydrinate, 210-211
Apo-Dipyridamole, 214
Apo-Doxy, 225-226
Apo-Erythro, 242-244
Apo-Erythro-EC, 242-244
Apo-Erythro-ES, 242-244
Apo-Erythro-S, 242-244
Apo-Famotidine, 263-264
Apo-Fluphenazine, 282-284
Apo-Flurazepam, 284-285
Apo-Flurbiprofen, 285-286
Apo-Folic, 290-291
Apo-Furosemide, 296-297
Apo-gain, 445-446
Apo-Gemfibrozil, 299-300
Apo-Glyburide, 303-304
Apo-Guanethidine, 309-310
Apo-Haloperidol, 313-315
Apo-Hydro, 318-319
Apo-Hydroxyzine, 326-327
Apo-Ibuprofen, 328-330
Apo-Imipramine, 330-332
Apo-Indomethacin, 335-336
Apo-Ipravent, 341-342
Apo-ISDN, 347-348
Apo-K, 546-547
Apo-Keto, 354-356
Apo-Keto-E, 354-356
APO-Loperamide, 388-389
Apo-Lorazepam, 390-391
Apo-Megestrol, 405
Apo-Meprobamate, 413-414
Apo-Methyldopa, 428-430
Apo-Metoclop, 433-434
Apo-Metoprolol, 436-437
Apo-Metronidazole, 437-439
Apo-Napro-Na, 464-465
Apo-Napro-Na DS, 464-465
Apo-Naproxen, 464-465
Apo-Nifed, 476-477
Apo-Nitrofurantoin, 479
Apo-Nizatidine, 481-482
Apo-Oxazepam, 501
Apo-Oxitriphylline, 502-503
Apo-Pen-VK, 514-515
APO-Perphenazine, 523-524
Apo-Piroxicam, 543-544
Apo-Prednisone, 553-554
APO-Primidone, 557-558
Apo-Propranolol, 572-574
Apo-Quinidine, 583-585
Apo-Ranitidine, 590
Apo-Selegiline, 613-615
Apo-Sucralfate, 626-627
Apo-Sulfamethoxazole, 629-630
Apo-Sulfatrim, 630-631
Apo-Sulfinpyrazone, 632-633
Apo-Sulfisoxazole, 633-634
Apo-Sulin, 634-635
Apo-Tamoxifen, 639-640
Apo-Tetra, 649-651
Apo-Theo-LA, 652-653
Apo-Thioridazine, 654-656
Apo-Timol, 661-663
Apo-Timop, 663-664
Apo-Tolbutamide, 667-668
Apo-Triazo, 687-688
Apo-Trifluoperazine, 689-690
Apo-Trihex, 692-693
Apo-Trimip, 697-698
Apo-Verap, 708-709
Apo-Zidovine, 717-718

Entries can be identified as follows: generic name, Trade Name, DRUG CATEGORY, *Combination Product.*

Appecon, 525-526
APPETITE SUPPRESSANTS, 10
apraclonidine, 13, 52-53, 738
Apresazide 25/25, 740
Apresazide 50/50, 740
Apresazide 100/50, 740
Apresoline, 8, 317-318
Apri, 740
Aprodine, 739
Aquachloral, 5
Aquachloral Supprettes, 129-130
AquaMEPHYTON, 16, 536
Aquasol A, 16, 709-710
Aquasol E, 16, 711-712
Aralen, 9
Aralen HCl, 133-134
Aralen Phosphate, 133-134
Arava, 9, 363-364, 730, 736
ardeparin, 5
ardeparin sodium, 53-54
Aricept, 4, 11, 219-220, 736
Aristocort, 13, 684-686
Aristocort A, 686
Aristocort C, 686
Aristocort D, 686
Aristocort Forte, 684-686
Aristocort Intraarticular, 684-686
Aristocort Intralesional, 684-686
Aristocort R, 686
Aristospan Intralesional, 684-686
Armour Thyroid, 658
Arrestin, 695
Artane, 9, 692-693, 732
Arthritis Foundation Pain Reliever, 55-56
Arthropan, 9, 144-145
Arthrotec, 740
Articulose-50, 551-553
Articulose LA, 684-686
ASA, 55-56
Asacol, 13, 414-415
ascorbic acid, 54-55
ascorbic acid calcipotriene, 16
Ascorbicap, 54-55
Asendin, 6, 44-45, 731
Asmalix, 652-653
A-Spas, 200-201
aspirin, 4, 9, 14, 55-56
aspirin clopidogrel, 15
Aspirin Free Anacin Maximum Strength, 21-22
Aspirin Free Excedrin, 21-22, 740
Aspirin Free Excedrin Dual, 746
aspirin probenecid, 16
Astelin, 7, 66, 737
ASTHMA DRUGS, 10, 737
AsthmaHaler, 238-239
Asthma Nefrin, 238-239
Asulfidine-En-Tabs, 631-632
Atacand, 8, 102-103
Atarax, 5, 7, 326-327, 730, 731
Atasol, 21-22
atenolol, 4, 8, 56-58
Ativan, 5, 390-391, 730
atorvastatin, 8, 11
atorvastatin calcium, 58
atovaquone, 9, 15, 58-59
Atretol, 105-106
Atridox, 15, 227
Atrigel, 16
Atromid-S, 8, 157-158, 737
Atropair, 61
atropine, 5, 730, 731
Atropine Care, 61
atropine sulfate, 59-60
atropine sulfate (optic), 14, 15, 61
Atropine Sulfate S.O.P., 61
Atropisol, 61, 730
Atrosept, 749
Atrovent, 11, 341-342, 737
A/T/S, 242
Atuss-EX, 744
Augmentin, 15, 45-46
auranofin, 61-62, 737
auranofin gold, 9
aurothioglucose, 9, 737
aurothioglucose/gold sodium thiomalate, 62-63
Avandia, 6, 607-608
Avapro, 8, 342-343
Aventyl, 485-486
Avirax, 26-27
Avita, 682
Avlosulfon, 184
Avonex, 13, 338-339
Axid, 7, 481-482
Axid AR, 481-482
Aygestin, 12, 482-483
azatadine, 7
azatadine maleate, 63-64
azathioprine, 14, 64-65, 738
azelaic acid, 12, 65-66
azelastine, 7, 737
azelastine HCl, 66

Entries can be identified as follows: generic name, Trade Name, DRUG CATEGORY, *Combination Product.*

Azelex, 12, 65-66
azithromycin, 14, 66-68
Azmacort, 13
Azmacort Oral Inhaler, 682-683
Azopt, 13, 89, 733, 738
Azo-Standard, 525
Azo-Sulfisoxazole, 740
AZT, 10, 717-718
Azulfidine, 13, 631-632, 737

B

Baby Anbesol, 73-74
Baby Orajel, 73-74
Baby Orajel Nighttime, 73-74
bacampicillin, 15
bacampicillin HCl, 68-69
baclofen, 16, 69-70, 733, 738
Bactocill, 497-498
Bactrim, 15, 16, 630-631
Bactroban, 8, 455-456
Bactroban Nasal 2%, 455-456
Balminil, 306-307, 576-577
Bancap HC, 739-740
Banflex, 496
Banophen, 211-212
Banthine, 5, 421-422, 730, 736
Barbidonna, 740
Barbidonna No. 2, 740
Barbita, 528-529
BARBITURATES, 5, 10, 734
Baridium, 525
Baycol, 8, 11, 125-126, 737
Bayer Select, 328-330
Bayer Select Head Cold, 744
Bayer Select Maximum Strength Headache, 740
Bayer Select Maximum Strength Headache Caplets, 744
Bayer Select Maximum Strength Sinus Relief, 744
BC Powder, 740
BC Powder Arthritis Strength, 740
BC Tablets, 740
becaplermin, 16, 70-71
Beclodisk, 71-72
Becloforte, 71-72
beclomethasone, 13
beclomethasone dipropionate, 71-72
Beclovent, 71-72
Beconase AQ Nasal, 71-72
Beconase Inhalation, 71-72
Bedoz, 172-173
Beepen-K, 514-515
Bellacane, 743, 745
belladonna alkaloids, 730
Bellergal, 730
Bellergal-S, 740
Benadryl, 5, 7, 9, 10, 211-212, 731
benazepril, 8, 72-73
Benemid, 9, 16, 558-559
Bentovate-1/2, 77-78
Bentyl, 5, 200-201, 730
Bentylol, 200-201
Benuryl, 558-559
Benylin Adult, 195-196, 740
Benylin Cough, 211-212
Benylin Decongestant, 576-577
Benylin DM, 740
Benylin-E, 306-307
Benylin Pediatric, 195-196
Benzacot, 695
Benzamycin, 242
benzocaine gel, 73-74
benzocaine liquid 20%, 73-74
benzocaine ointment/paste 20%, 73-74
benzocaine spray 20%, 73-74
benzocaine (topical), 4, 73-74
Benzodent, 73-74
BENZODIAZEPINES, 5, 734
benzonatate, 10, 74
benztropine, 5, 9
benztropine mesylate, 74-76, 732
Bepadin, 76-77
Bepen, 77-78
bepridil, 5, 8, 738
bepridil HCl, 76-77
BETA-ADRENERGIC ANTAGONISTS, 4-5, 8
Betadine, 8, 547-548
Betagan, 13
Betagan Liquifilm, 368-369
Betaloc, 436-437
betamethasone/betamethasone acetate/ betamethasone sodium phosphate, 13, 78-80
betamethasone benzoate/ betamethasone dipropionate/ betamethasone valerate, 77-78
Betapace, 6, 621-622
Betapen-VK, 514-515
Beta-Tim, 663-664
Betatrex, 77-78
Beta-Val, 77-78
Betaxin, 653-654

Entries can be identified as follows: generic name, Trade Name, DRUG CATEGORY, *Combination Product.*

betaxolol, 8, 13
betaxolol HCl, 80-81
betaxolol HCl (optic), 81-82
betaxolol (optic), 15
bethanechol, 11
bethanechol chloride, 82
Betimol, 663-664
Betnelan, 78-80
Betnesol, 78-80
Betoptic, 13, 15, 81-82
Betoptic S, 81-82
Bewon, 653-654
Biamine, 653-654
Biaxin, 14, 150-151
bicalutamide, 11, 83
Bi-cillin, 15
Bicillin L-A, 513-514
Biocef, 123-124
Biodine, 547-548
Bio-Gan, 695
BioTab, 225-226
biperiden, 5, 9, 732
biperiden HCl, 84-85
biperiden lactate, 84-85
Bismatrol, 85
Bismatrol Extra Strength, 85
Bismed, 85
bismuth subsalicylate, 6, 85, 736
bisoprolol, 8
bisoprolol fumarate, 85-87
bitolterol, 10, 737
bitolterol mesylate, 87-88
black cohosh, 752
Bleph-10, 627-628
Blocadren, 8, 14, 661-663
Bonamine, 401-402
Bonine, 7, 401-402
Bontril PDM, 525-526
Breonesin, 306-307
Brethaire, 645-646
Brethine, 11, 645-646, 737
Brevicon, 493-495
Bricanyl, 645-646
brimonidine, 13, 738
brimonidine tartrate, 88-89
brinzolamide, 13, 733, 738
brinzolamide (optic), 89
Bromanyl Syrup, 739
Bromarest DX, 742
Bromatane DX, 742
Bromfed, 739
Bromfed Capsules, 740
Bromfed DM, 742
Bromfed Tablets, 740
Bromfenex-PD, 740
bromocriptine, 9
bromocriptine mesylate, 89-90
Bromophen DX, 742
Bromo-Seltzer, 740
Bromotuss/Codeine, 739
Bromphen, 90-91
brompheniramine, 7, 731
brompheniramine maleate, 90-91
Bronalide, 277-278
BRONCHODILATORS, 10-11, 732, 737
Bronitin Mist, 238-239
Bronkaid Mist, 238-239
Bronkaid Mistometer, 238-239
Bronkometer, 11
Brontex, 740
Brontex Liquid, 740
Bucladin-S, 7
buclizine, 7
budesonide, 13, 91-93, 738
bumetanide, 12, 93-94
Bumex, 12, 93-94
bupivacaine, 4
bupivacaine HCl (local), 94-96
bupropion, 6, 16, 731
bupropion hydrochloride, 96-97
BuSpar, 5, 97-98, 730
buspirone, 5, 730
buspirone HCl, 97-98
busulfan, 11, 98-99
butenafine, 7, 99
Butibel, 740
Butibel Elixir, 740
butoconazole, 7
butoconazole nitrate, 100
butyrophenone, 9
Bydramine, 211-212

C

Cafatine, 750
Cafergot, 740, 750
Cafergot Suppositories, 741
Cafetrate, 750
Caladryl Clear, 741
Caladryl Lotion, 741
Calan, 5, 8, 708-709
Calan SR, 708-709
Calcidrine Syrup, 741
calcifediol, 710-711, 738

Entries can be identified as follows: generic name, Trade Name, DRUG CATEGORY, *Combination Product.*

Calciferol, 16, 710-711
Calcijex, 710-711
Calcilean, 315-316
Calcimar, 7, 100-101, 737
Calciparine, 315-316
calcipotriene, 100
calcitonin (human)/calcitonin (salmon), 7, 100-101, 737
calcitriol, 738
CALCIUM AFFECTING DRUGS, 737
calcium carbonate, 736
CALCIUM CHANNEL ANTAGONISTS, 5, 8
Calderol, 710-711
calitriol, 710-711
Calm-X, 210-211
camphorated opium tincture, 6, 102
CANCER CHEMOTHERAPEUTICS, 11, 738
candesartan, 8
candesartan cilexetil, 102-103
Canesten, 164-165
Cantil, 5, 406-407, 736
Capital with Codeine, 741
Capoten, 8, 104-105, 731, 738
Capozide 25/15, 741
Capozide 25/25, 741
Capozide 50/15, 741
Capozide 50/25, 741
capsaicin, 12, 103-104
Capsin, 103-104
captopril, 8, 104-105, 731, 738
Capzasin-P, 103-104
Carafate, 13, 626-627, 736
Carbacot, 425-426
carbamazepine, 5, 105-106, 730
Carbex, 613-615
carbidopa, 732
Carbocaine, 4, 411-412
Carbocaine with Neo-Cobefrin, 411-412
Carbolith, 384-385
Cardene, 5, 8, 473-474
Cardene IV, 473-474
Cardene SR, 473-474
CARDIAC GLYCOSIDES, 11
Cardioquin, 583-585, 738
CARDIOVASCULAR DRUGS, 738
Cardizem, 5, 8, 209-210, 738
Cardizem CD, 209-210
Cardizem SR, 209-210
Cardura, 8, 221-222
carisoprodol, 16, 107
Carisoprodol Compound, 741
Carmol-HC, 322-323
carteolol, 8, 13, 15, 107-109
carteolol HCl, 109
Cartia XT, 209-210
Cartrol, 8, 107-109
carvedilol, 8, 109-111, 731
Casodex, 11, 83
Cataflam, 197-199
Catapres, 8, 161-162, 731, 738
Catapres-TTS, 161-162
Caverject, 12, 15, 32-33
CCNU, 387-388
Cebid, 54-55
Ceclor, 11, 111-112
Ceclor CD, 111-112
Cecon, 54-55
Cedax, 11, 119-120
Cedocard-SR, 347-348
CeeNU, 11, 387-388
cefaclor, 11, 111-112
cefadroxil, 11, 112-113
Cefanex, 123-124
cefazolin, 11
cefazolin sodium, 113-114
cefdinir, 11, 114-115
cefepime, 11, 115-116
cefixime, 11, 116-117
cefpodoxime, 11
cefpodoxime proxetil, 117-118
cefprozil, 11
cefprozil monohydrate, 118-119
ceftibuten, 11, 119-120
Ceftin, 11, 121-122
cefuroxime, 11
cefuroxime axetil, 121-122
Cefzil, 11, 118-119
Celebrex, 9, 14, 122-123, 731, 737
celecoxib, 9, 14, 122-123, 731, 737
Celestoderm-V/2, 77-78
Celestone, 13, 78-80
Celestone Extended Release, 78-80
Celestone Phosphate, 78-80
Celestone Soluspan, 78-80
Celexa, 6, 149-150, 731
CellCept, 14, 456-457
Celontin, 6, 427-428
Cemill, 54-55
Cenafed, 576-577
Cenafed Plus, 739

Cena-K, 546-547
Cenestin, 12, 249
Cenocort A-40, 684-686
Cenocort Forte, 684-686
CENTRAL NERVOUS SYSTEM STIMULANTS, 11, 732, 738
cephadrine, 11
cephalexin, 11, 123-124
CEPHALOSPORINS, 11
cephradine, 124-125
Cerebyx, 5, 295-296, 736
Cerespan, 508-509
cerivastatin, 8, 11, 737
cerivastatin sodium, 125-126
CES, 248-249
Cetamide, 627-628
Cetane, 54-55
Ceta-Plus, 739-740
cetirizine, 7, 737
cetirizine hydrochloride, 126-127
Cevi-Bid, 54-55
cevimeline, 16, 127-128
chamomile, 752-753
Chardonna-2, 741
chaste tree/chaste berry, 753
Chenix, 5, 128-129
chenodiol, 5, 128-129
Cheracol Cough Syrup, 747
Cheracol-D, 748
Children's Advil, 328-330
Children's Apo-Ibuprofen, 328-330
Children's Cepacol, 741
Children's Lozenges, 741
Children's Motrin Oral Drops, 328-330
Children's Sufedrin, 576-577
Children's Throat Spray, 741
Chlo-Amine, 137-138
chloral hydrate, 5, 129-130, 734, 737
chlorambucil, 11, 130-131
Chloraseptic (Vicks) Sore Throat Lozenges, 741
Chlorate, 137-138
chlordiazepoxide, 5, 730
chlordiazepoxide HCl, 131-132
chlorhexidine, 8, 10, 15
chlorhexidine gluconate, 132-133
chlorhexidine gluconate chip, 133
chloroquine, 9
chloroquine HCl/chloroquine phosphate, 133-134
chlorothiazide, 12, 135-136, 732
Chlorphed, 90-91
chlorphenesin, 16
chlorphenesin carbamate, 136-137
chlorpheniramine, 7, 731, 732
chlorpheniramine maleate, 137-138
Chlorpromanyl, 138-140
chlorpromazine, 7, 9, 732
chlorpromazine HCl, 138-140
chlorpropamide, 6, 140-141
chlorthalidone, 12, 141-142
Chlor-Trimeton, 7, 137-138, 731
Chlor-Trimeton 4 Hour Relief Tablets, 741
Chlor-Trimeton 12 Hour Relief Tablets, 741
Chlor-Tripolon, 137-138
chlorzoxazone, 16, 142-143
Cholaxin, 658
Choledyl, 11, 16, 502-503, 738
Choledyl SA, 502-503
CHOLESTEROL LOWERING AGENTS, 11
cholestyramine, 8, 143-144
CHOLINERGIC AGONISTS, 11
choline salicylate, 9, 144-145
CHOLINESTERASE INHIBITORS, 11
chondroitin sulfate, 753-754
Cibacalcin, 100-101
Cibalith-S, 384-385
ciclopirox, 7
ciclopirox olamine, 145
cilostazol, 15, 145-146
cimetidine, 7, 146-147
Cinalone 40, 684-686
Cinobac, 16, 147-148
Cinonide 40
cinoxacin, 16, 147-148
Cin-Quin, 583-585
Cipro, 12, 148-149
ciprofloxacin, 12, 148-149
Cipro IV, 148-149
cisapride, 13
citalopram, 6, 731
citalopram hydrobromide, 149-150
Citanest, 4, 554-556
Citanest Forte with epinephrine, 554-556
citrovorum factor, 364-365
Claripex, 157-158
clarithromycin, 14, 150-151

Entries can be identified as follows: generic name, Trade Name, DRUG CATEGORY, *Combination Product.*

Claritin, 7, 390, 731
Claritin-D ext. rel., 741
Claritin-D 24 Hour, 741
Claritin RediTabs, 390
Clavulin, 45-46
Clear Eyes, 463-464
clemastine fumarate, 7, 152
Cleocin, 14, 153-155
Cleocin Pediatric, 153-155
C-Lexin, 123-124
clidinium, 5, 730
clidinium bromide, 152-153
Climara, 247-248
clindamycin, 14
clindamycin HCl/clindamycin palmitate HCl/clindamycin phosphate, 153-155
clindium, 736
Clinoril, 9, 15, 634-635, 736
clobetasol, 13
clobetasol propionate, 155
clocortolone, 13
clocortolone pivalate, 156
Cloderm, 13, 156
clofazimine, 9, 156-157
clofibrate, 8, 157-158, 737
Clomid, 12, 158
clomiphene, 12
clomiphene citrate, 158
clomipramine, 6, 158-160, 731, 736
Clonapam, 160-161
clonazepam, 5, 160-161
clonidine, 8, 731, 738
clonidine HCl/clonidine transdermal, 161-162
clopidogrel bisulfate, 162-163
clorazepate dipotassium, 5, 163-164
Clotriaderm, 164-165
clotrimazole, 7, 164-165
cloxacillin, 15
cloxacillin sodium, 165-166
Cloxapen, 165-166
clozapine, 9, 166-167, 732
Clozaril, 9, 166-167, 732
Co-Apap, 741
Cobex, 172-173
cocaine, 734
codeine, 4, 10, 167-168, 734
codeine combinations, 734
codeine sulfate/codeine phosphate, 167-168
Codimal-A, 90-91
Codoxy, 504-505
Cofatrim Forte, 630-631
Cogentin, 5, 9, 74-76, 732
Co-Gesic, 739-740
Cognex, 4, 11, 636-638
colchicine, 7, 9, 168-169, 737
Cold and Cough Maximum, 743
Coldloc, 747-748
Cold Relief Tablets, 741
Colestid, 8, 169-170
colestipol, 8
colestipol HCl, 169-170
Combination products, 739-750
Combi-Pak, 164-165
CombiPatch, 741
Combipres 0.1 mg, 741
Combipres 0.2 mg, 741
Combivent, 741
Combivir, 741
Compazine, 7, 9, 561-563, 732, 737
Compoz, 211-212
Comtan, 9, 236-237, 737
Comtrex Allergy-Sinus, 741
Comtrex Cough Formula Liquid, 741
Comtrex Liqui-Gels, 741
Comtrex Maximum Strength Multi-Symptom Cold and Flu, 741
Comtrex Max Strength Multi-Symptom Cold and Flu Relief, 741-742
Congest, 248-249
Conjec-B, 90-91
Conjugated Estrogen CDS, 248-249
conjugated estrogens, 12
conjugated estrogens, synthetic, 12
Contac Maximum Strength 12 Hour, 739
Contact Cough and Chest Cold, 742
Contact Nondrowsy Sinus, 744
Contact Severe Cold and Flu Formula, 742
Contact Severe Cold and Flu Nightime, 742
Contact 12 Hour Capsule, 742
Contrin, 749
Controlled substances chart, 734
Cophene-B, 90-91
Cordarone, 6, 39-40, 738
Cordarone IV, 39-40
Cordran, 13, 284

Entries can be identified as follows: generic name, Trade Name, DRUG CATEGORY, *Combination Product.*

Cordran SP, 284
Coreg, 8, 109-111, 731
Corgard, 4, 8, 458-460, 738
Coronex, 347-348
Cortacet, 322-323
Cortaid, 322-323
Cort-Dome, 322-323
Cortef, 13, 320-323
Cortenema, 320-322
Corticaine, 322-323
Corticreme, 322-323
Cortifair, 322-323
Cortiform, 320-322
cortisone, 13
cortisone acetate, 170-171
Cortone, 13, 170-171
Cortril, 322-323
Corzide 40/5, 742
Corzide 80/5, 742
Cotanal-65, 571-572
Cotarim, 630-631
Cotazym, 507-508
Cotazyme, 13
Cotazyme-65B, 507-508
Cotazym-S, 507-508
co-trimazole, 630-631
Coumadin, 5, 712-713
Cozaar, 8, 391-392, 738
Cramp End, 328-330
Crixivan, 10, 334-335, 737
cromolyn, 14, 737
cromolyn sodium, 171-172
Crystamine, 172-173
Crysti-12, 172-173
Crystodigin, 6, 11, 206-207
Curretab, 403-404
Cutivate, 13, 288
cyanocobalamin, 16, 172-173
Cyanoject, 172-173
cyclizine, 7, 732
cyclizine HCl/cyclizine lactate, 173-174
cyclobenzaprine, 16, 733, 738
cyclobenzaprine HCl, 174-175
Cycloflex, 174-175
Cyclomen, 182-183
cyclophosphamide, 175-176
cycloserine, 10, 176-177
cyclosporine, 14, 177-178
Cycrin, 403-404
Cyklokapron, 13, 678-679
Cylert, 11, 510
Cylert Chewable, 510
Cyomin, 172-173
cyproheptadine, 7
cyproheptadine HCl, 178-178
Cystex, 742
Cystospaz-M, 327-328
Cytadren, 11, 37-38
Cytomel, 12, 381-382
Cytotec, 13, 15, 447-448
Cytovene, 10, 298-299
Cytovene IV, 298-299
Cytoxan, 11, 175-176

D

daclizumab, 14,179-180
Dalacin C Flavored Granules, 153-155
Dalalaone DP, 192-193
Dalalone LA, 192-193
Dalaone, 192-193
Dalcaine, 377-379
Dallergy-JR, 740
Dalmane, 5, 284-285, 733
dalteparin, 5
dalteparin sodium, 180-181
danaparoid, 5, 181-182
danazol, 12, 182-183
Danocrine, 12, 182-183
Dantrium, 16, 183-184
Dantrium Intravenous, 183-184
dantrolene, 16
dantrolene sodium, 183-184
Dapa, 21-22
dapsone, 184
dapsone metronidazole, 9
Darbid, 730
Daricon, 730
Darvocet-N 50, 742
Darvocet-N 100, 742
Darvon, 4, 571-572
Darvon Compound-65 Pulvules, 742
Darvon-N, 4, 571-572
Datril, 21-22
Daypro, 9, 15, 499-500
Dayto Sulf, 749
Dazamide, 22-23
DDAVP, 12, 188-189
DDAVP Nasal Spray, 188-189
DDAVP Rhinal Tube, 188-189
DDAVP Rhinyl Nasal Solution, 188-189
DDAVP Spray, 188-189
ddI, 10, 201-202

Entries can be identified as follows: generic name, Trade Name, DRUG CATEGORY, *Combination Product.*

DDS, 184
D-D-S Plus, 747
Decaderm, 13, 191
Decadrol, 192-193
Decadron, 192-193
Decadron DosePak, 192-193
Decadron LA, 192-193
Decadron Phosphate, 191, 192-193
Decaject, 192-193
Decaject-LA, 192-193
Decaspray, 191
Declomycin, 16, 186-187
Deconamine CX, 742
Deconamine CX Liquid, 742
Deconamine SR, 742
DECONGESTANTS, 11, 732, 738
Deconomed SR, 742
Dehist, 90-91
Delatest, 647-648
Delatestryl, 647-648
delavirdine, 10
delavirdine mesylate, 184-186, 737
Del-Mycin, 242
Delta-Cortef, 13, 551-553
Deltalin, 710-711
Deltasone, 553-554
Delta-Tritex, 686
Demadex, 12, 674-675
demeclocycline, 16
demeclocycline HCl, 186-187
DEMENTIA/ALZHEIMER'S DRUGS, 11
Demerol, 4, 407-408, 733
Demicort, 322-323
Demulen 1/35, 493-495
Demulen 1/50, 493-495
Denavir, 10, 512-513, 737
Dentipatch, 736
DentiPatch, 4, 379-380
Denture Orajel, 73-74
Depacon, 703-705
Depakene, 6, 10, 703-705
Depakote, 5, 14, 703-705
Depakote Sprinkle, 703-705
depAndro, 647-648
depMedalone 40, 431-432
depMedalone 80, 431-432
Depo-Estradiol, 246-247
Depogen, 246-247
Depoject, 431-432
Depo-Medrol, 431-432
Deponit, 480-481
Depo-Prodate, 431-432
Depo-Provera, 403-404
Depotest, 647-648
Depo-Testosterone, 647-648
Depropred 40, 431-432
Depropred 80, 431-432
Dermabet, 77-78
Dermacort, 322-323
Dermarest, 322-323
DERMATOLOGIC DRUGS, 12
Dermatop, 13
Dermatop Emollient Cream, 550-551
Dermovate, 155
Dermtex HC, 322-323
Deronil, 192-193
desipramine, 6, 731, 736
desipramine HCl, 187-188
desmopressin, 12
desmopressin acetate, 188-189
Desogen, 493-495, 740
desogestrel, 493-495
desonide, 13, 189-190
DesOwen, 13, 189-190
desoximetasone, 13, 190-191
Desoxyn, 4, 10, 11, 420-421, 732, 738
Desoxyn Gradumet, 420-421
Desyrel, 6, 680-681
Detensol, 572-574
Detrol, 5, 671-672, 732
Dexacen-4, 192-193
Dexacen LA-8, 192-193
Dexacidin Ointment, 739
Dexacidin Suspension, 739
Dexadron, 13
dexamethasone, 13, 191-193
dexamethasone acetate, 192-193
dexamethasone sodium phosphate, 191, 192-193
Dexaone, 192-193
Dexasone, 192-193
Dexasone-LA, 192-193
Dexasporin Ointment, 739
Dexchlor, 193-194
dexchlorpheniramine, 7
dexchlorpheniramine maleate, 193-194
Dexedrine, 11, 194-195, 732, 738
Dexedrine Spansules, 194-195
Dexone, 192-193
Dexone LA, 192-193
dextroamphetamine, 11, 732, 738
dextroamphetamine sulfate, 194-195

Entries can be identified as follows: generic name, Trade Name, DRUG CATEGORY, *Combination Product.*

dextromethorphan, 10
dextromethorphan hydrobromide, 195-196
DextroStat, 194-195
Dey-Dos Racepinephrine, 238-239
d4t, 10, 625-626
DHPG, 298-299
DHT, 208-209, 710-711
DHT Intensol, 208-209
DHT Oral Solution, 208-209
DiaBeta, 6, 303-304
Diabinese, 6, 140-141
Diamine TD, 90-91
Diamox, 5, 12, 13, 22-23, 738
Diapid, 12, 396
Diarr-Eze, 388-389
Diastat, 196-197
Diazc, 196-197
Diazemuls, 196-197
diazepam, 5, 196-197, 730, 734
Diazepam Intensol, 196-197
Dibenzyline, 8, 529-530
diclofenac, 14, 197-199, 736
dicloxacillin, 15
dicloxacillin sodium, 199-200
dicyclomine, 5, 730
dicyclomine HCl, 200-201
didanosine, 10, 201-202, 737
dideoxyinosine, 201-202
Didronel, 7, 260, 737
Didronel IV, 260
diethylpropion, 4, 10, 730, 736
diethylpropion HCl, 202-203
Difenac, 197-199
difenoxin, 731
difenoxin/atropine, 6
difenoxin HCl with atropine sulfate, 203-204
diflorasone, 13
diflorasone diacetate, 204
Diflucan, 7, 273-274
diflunisal, 9, 14, 205-206, 731
Digest 2, 463-464
Digitaline, 206-207
digitoxin, 6, 11, 206-207
digoxin, 6, 11, 207-208
dihydrotachysterol, 16, 208-209, 710-711, 738
Dilacor XR, 209-210
Dilantin, 6, 534-536, 736
Dilantin Infatabs, 534-536
Dilantin Kapseals, 534-536
Dilatrate-SR, 347-348
Dilaudid, 4, 323-324
Dilaudid HP, 323-324
Dilocaine, 377-379
Dilor, 11, 16, 229-230, 738
Dilor-400, 229-230
diltiazem, 5, 8, 738
diltiazem HCl, 209-210
Dimacol, 742
Dimaphen, 742
Dimelor, 24-25
dimenhydrinate, 7, 210-211
Dimetane, 7, 90-91, 731
Dimetane-DX Cough Syrup, 742
Dimetane Extentabs, 90-91
Dimetapp, 731, 742
Dimetapp Allergy, 90-91
Dimetapp DM Elixir, 742
Dimetapp 4 Hour Liqui-Gel, 742
Dinate, 210-211
Dioval, 246-247
Diovan, 8, 705, 738
Dipentum, 13, 490-491
Diphen, 211-212
Diphenhist, 211-212
diphenhydramine, 5, 7, 9, 10, 731, 732
diphenhydramine HCl, 211-212
diphenoxylate, 731
diphenoxylate/atropine, 6
diphenoxylate HCl with atropine sulfate, 212-213
Diphenylan, 534-536
dipivefrin, 13, 15
dipivefrin HCl, 213
Dipridacot, 214
Diprivan, 4, 569-571, 736
Diprolene, 13, 77-78
Diprolene AF, 77-78
Diprosone, 77-78
dipyridamole, 15, 214
dirithromycin, 14, 214-215
Disalcid, 609-610
Disanthrol, 747
Disipal, 733
disodium cromoglycate, 171-172
disopyramide/disopyramide phosphate, 6, 215-216
disulfiram, 4, 217, 736
Ditropan, 5, 503-504, 730
Ditropan XL, 503-504
Diuchlor H, 318-319

Entries can be identified as follows: generic name, Trade Name, DRUG CATEGORY, *Combination Product.*

Diulo, 434-435
DIURETICS, 12, 732, 738
Diuril, 12, 135-136, 732
divalproex, 5, 14
Dixarit, 161-162
DM Syrup, 195-196
Dobryx, 225-226
Doktors, 533-534
Dolacet, 739-740
dolasetron, 7
dolasetron mesylate, 217-218, 736
Dolgesic, 328-330
Dolobid, 9, 14, 205-206, 731
Dolophine, 4, 419-420
Dolsed, 749
Dom-Valproic, 703-705
donepezil, 4, 11, 736
donepezil HCl, 219-220
dong quai, 754
Donnagel Liquid or tablets, 742
Donnatal, 730
Donnatal Elixir, 743
Donnatal Extentabs, 743
Donnatal Hyosophen, 743
Donovex, 16
Dopamet, 428-430
Dopar, 369-370
Doral, 5, 580-581, 737
Dorcol, 576-577
dornase alfa, 14, 220
dorzolamide, 13, 738
dorzolamide HCl, 221
Dose calculations by weight, 751
Dovonex, 100
doxazosin, 8
doxazosin mesylate, 221-222
doxepin, 5, 6, 12, 731, 736
doxepin HCl, 223-224
doxepin HCl (topical), 222-223
doxercalciferol, 16, 710-711
Doxy-Caps, 225-226
Doxycin, 225-226
doxycycline, 15, 16
doxycycline hyclate (dental/systemic), 224-225
doxycycline hyclate/doxycycline calcium, 225-226
doxycycline hyclate gel, 227
DPE, 213
Dramamine, 7, 210-211, 732
Dramamine II, 401-402
Dramanate, 210-211
Dreison-1/4, 284
Drenison, 284
DriCort, 322-323
Drisdol, 710-711
Dristan Cold Tablets, 744
Dristan 12 Hour, 505
Drixomed, 743
Drixoral Cold and Flu Tablets, 743
Drixoral Cough, 195-196
Drixoral Cough and Congestion Capsules, 743
Drixoral Plus, 743
Drize, 739
dronabinol, 227-229
Droxia, 325-326
Drugs
  dosage calculations for, 751
  and dry mouth, 730-733
  and taste, 736-738
Dry mouth, drugs causing, 730-733
Dull-C, 54-55
Duocet, 739-740
Duo-Trach Kit, 377-379
Dura Estrin, 246-247
Duragesic, 4
Duragesic 25, 50, 75, 100 Transdermal Patches, 268-269
Dura-Gest, 743
Duralith, 384-385
Duralone 40, 431-432
Duralone 80, 431-432
Duramist Plus, 505
Duramorph PF, 454-455
Duranest, 4, 258-260
Duranest MPF, 258-260
Duranest with Epinephrine, 258-260
Duraquin, 583-585
Duratest, 647-648
Duration, 505, 533-534
Duratuss, 743
Duratuss-G, 743
Duratuss HD Elixir, 743
Dura-Vent, 747-748
Duricef, 11, 112-113
Duvoid, 82
D-Vert, 401-402
Dyancin, 444-445
Dyazide, 732, 743
Dycill, 199-200
Dyclone, 14, 229
dyclonine hydrochloride, 4, 229
Dymelor, 6, 24-25

Entries can be identified as follows: generic name, Trade Name, DRUG CATEGORY, *Combination Product.*

Dynabac, 14, 214-215
Dynacin, 225-226
DynaCirc, 8, 351-352
Dynafed IB, 328-330
Dynapen, 15, 199-200
dyphylline, 11, 16, 229-230, 738
Dyrenium, 12, 686-687, 732
Dysep HB, 263-264

E

Easprin, 55-56
E-Base, 242-244
echinacea, 755
EC Naprosyn, 464-465
E-Complex 600, 711-712
econazole, 7
econazole nitrate, 230
Ecostatin, 230
Ecotrin, 55-56
Ectosone Mild, 77-78
E-Cypronate, 246-247
Edecrin, 12, 251-252
Edecrin Sodium, 251-252
Edex, 32-33
EES 200, 242-244
EES 400, 242-244
EES Granules, 242-244
efavirenz, 10, 230-232, 732, 737
Effexor, 6, 706-708, 731
Effexor XR, 706-708
Effidac24, 576-577
Efodine, 547-548
Efudex, 12, 279-280, 738
E-200 IU Softgels, 711-712
E-400 IU, 711-712
Elavil, 6, 40-42, 731, 736
Eldepryl, 9, 613-615
Elixophyllin, 652-653
Eltor 120, 576-577
Eltroxin, 375
Emadine, 7, 13, 232
emedastine, 7, 13
emedastine difumarate (optic), 232
Emo-Cort, 322-323
Empirin, 55-56
Empirin with Codeine 30 mg (No. 3), 743
Empirin with Codeine 60 mg (No. 4), 743
E-Mycin, 242-244
enalapril, 8, 731, 738
enalapril maleate, 232-234
Enbrel, 9, 250-251
Endafed, 739
Endep, 40-42
ENDOCRINE DRUGS, 12
Endodan, 504-505
Endolor, 743
Endur-Acin, 472-473
Enduronyl, 743
Enduronyl-Forte, 743
Enomine, 743
enoxacin, 12, 234-235
enoxaparin, 5
enoxaparin sodium, 235-236
entacapone, 9, 236-237, 737
Entex, 743
Entex LA, 743
Entex PSE, 743
Entrophen, 55-56
Enzymase, 507-508
ephedrine, 4, 11, 732
ephedrine sulfate, 237-238
Epiferin, 238-239
E-Pilo and PE, 743
Epinal, 238-239
epinephrine/epinephrine bitartrate/ epinephrine HCl, 4, 11, 16, 238-239
epinephrine inhalation, 11
EpiPen Auto-Injector, 238-239
EpiPen Jr., 238-239
Epitol, 105-106
Epival, 703-705
Epivir, 10, 359-360
Epivir HBV, 359-360
Eppy/N, 238-239
eprosartan, 8, 239-240
Equagesic, 743
Equanil, 5, 413-414, 730
Ercaf, 740, 750
ERECTILE DYSFUNCTION DRUGS, 12
Ergamisol, 14, 366-367, 738
ergocalciferol, 710-711
ergoloid mesylate, 11, 240
Ergomar, 240-241
Ergostat, 240-241
ERGOT ALKALOIDS, 12
ergotamine tartrate, 240-241
Eridium, 525
Erybid, 242-244
Eryc, 242-244
Erycette, 242
Erygel, 242

Entries can be identified as follows: generic name, Trade Name, DRUG CATEGORY, *Combination Product.*

Erymax, 242
EryPed, 242-244
Ery-sol, 242
Ery-Tab, 242-244
Erythra-Derm, 242
Erythro, 242-244
Erythrocin, 14, 242-244
Erythrocin Stearate, 242-244
Erythrocot, 242-244
Erythromid, 242-244
erythromycin, 14
erythromycin base/erythromycin estolate/erythromycin ethylsuccinate/erythromycin gluceptate/erythromycin lactobionate/erythromycin stearate, 242-244
Erythromycin Filmtabs, 242-244
erythromycin (ophthalmic), 15, 241
erythromycin (topical), 8, 242
Erytroderm (topical), 8
Eryzole, 747
Esclim, 247-248
Esgic, 743
Esgic-Plus, 743
Esidrix, 318-319, 732
Esimil, 743
Eskalith, 10, 384-385, 732, 737
Eskalith CR, 384-385
estazolam, 5, 244, 737
esterified estrogens, 12, 245
Estinyl, 12, 253-254
Estivin-II, 463-464
Estrab, 12
Estrace, 12, 246-247
Estraderm, 12, 247-248
estradiol/estradiol cypionate/estradiol valerate, 12, 246-247
estradiol transdermal, 12, 247-248
Estragyn LA, 246-247
Estratab, 245
Estro-Cyp, 246-247
Estrofem, 246-247
estrogenic substances, conjugated, 12, 248-249
estrogens, 12
estrogens A, conjugated synthetic, 249
Estroject-LA/Delestrogen, 246-247
estropipate, 12, 249-250
Estrostep, 493-495
Estrostep-21, 493-495
Estrostep Fe, 493-495
etanercept, 9, 250-251
ethacrynate, 12
ethacrynate sodium/ethacrynic acid, 251-252
ethambutol, 10
ethambutol HCl, 252-253
ethinyl estradiol, 12, 253-254, 493-495
ethionamide, 10, 254-255, 737
Ethmozine, 6, 453-454, 738
ethopropazine, 5, 9, 255-256, 732
ethosuximide, 5, 256-257
ethotoin, 5, 257-258
ethynodiol diacetate, 493-495
Etibi, 252-253
etidocaine, 4
etidocaine HCl, 258-260
etidronate, 7, 737
etidronate disodium, 260
etodolac, 9, 14, 260-262, 736
Etrafon, 743
Etrafon 2-10, 743
Etrafon-A, 743
Etrafon-Forte, 743
Euflex, 287
Euglucon, 303-304
Eulexin, 12, 287
Euthroid, 12
Euthyrox, 375
evening primrose oil, 756
Evista, 7, 12
E-Vitamin Succinate, 711-712
Evoxac, 127-128
Excedrin (Aspirin Free), 744
Excedrin Extra Strength, 744
Excedrin IB, 328-330
Excedrin Migraine, 744
Excedrin PM (caplets), 744
Excedrin PM Liquid, 744
Excedrin PM (liquigels), 744
Excedrin Sinus Extra Strength, 744
Exelderm, 7, 627
Exgest LA, 743
Exovac, 16
EXPECTORANTS, 10, 12
EZE-DS, 142-143

F

famciclovir, 10, 262
famotidine, 7, 263-264, 737
Famvir, 10, 262
Fareston, 11, 673-674

Entries can be identified as follows: generic name, Trade Name, DRUG CATEGORY, *Combination Product.*

Fastin, 531-532, 730
felbamate, 5, 264-265, 730
Felbatol, 5, 264-265, 730
Feldene, 9, 15, 543-544, 731
felodipine, 5, 8, 265-266
FemCare, 164-165
Femcet, 743
Femhrt 1/5, 744
Femiron, 270-271
Femizole, 164-165
Femogex, 246-247
FemPatch, 247-248
Femstat, 7, 100
Femstat 3, 100
FemStat One, 100
Fenesin, 306-307
Fenesin DM, 744
fenofibrate, 8
fenofibrate (micronized), 266-267
fenoprofen, 9, 14, 731
fenoprofen calcium, 267-268
fentanyl, 734
fentanyl transdermal, 4, 268-269
Feosol, 14, 270-271
Feostat, 270-271
Feotrinsic, 749
Fergon, 270-271
Fer-in-Sol, 270-271
Fero-Grad, 270-271
Fero-Gradumet, 270-271
Ferospace, 270-271
Ferralet, 270-271
Ferralyn, 270-271
ferrous fumarate/ferrous gluconate/ ferrous sulfate, 14, 270-271
Fertinic, 270-271
feverfew, 756
fexofenadine, 7
fexofenadine HCl, 271
finasteride, 12, 14, 15, 271-272
Fiorgen PF, 744
Fioricet, 743
Fioricet with Codeine, 744
Fiorinal, 744
Fiorinal with Codeine No. 3, 744
FK506, 638-639
Flagyl, 9, 14, 437-439, 737
Flagyl 375, 437-439
Flagyl ER, 437-439
Flagyl IV RTU, 437-439
Flavorcee, 54-55
flavoxate, 16
flavoxate HCl, 272
flecainide, 738
flecainide acetate, 6, 272-273
Flexaphen, 744
Flexeril, 16, 174-175, 733, 738
Flexoject, 496
Flomax, 15, 640-641
Flonase, 13, 288
Florinef, 13
Florinef Acetate, 275-276
Florone, 13, 204
Florone E, 204
Flovent (inhaler), 288
Floxin, 12, 487-488
Floxin IV, 487-488
fluconazole, 7, 273-274
flucytosine, 7, 274-275
fludrocortisone, 13
fludrocortisone acetate, 275-276
Flumadine, 10, 598-599, 737
flumazenil, 4, 276-277
flunisolide, 13, 277-278, 738
Fluocin, 278-279
fluocinonide, 13, 278-279
Fluonex, 278-279
Fluor-A-Day, 618-620
Fluoritabs, 618-620
Fluoroplex, 279-280
FLUOROQUINOLONES, 12
fluorouracil, 11, 738
fluorouracil (topical), 279-280
Fluotic, 618-620
fluoxetine, 6, 280-281, 731, 736
fluoxymesterone, 12, 281-282
fluphenazine, 9
fluphenazine decanoate/fluphenazine enanthate/fluphenazine HCl, 282-284
Flura-Drops, 618-620
flurandrenolide, 13, 284
flurazepam, 5, 733
flurazepam HCl, 284-285
flurbiprofen, 14, 15, 285-286
flurbiprofen sodium, 287
Flurodex Karidium, 618-620
flutamide, 11, 287
Flutex, 686
fluticasone (inhalant), 13
fluticasone propionate, 288
fluticasone (topical), 13
fluvastatin, 8, 11, 737
fluvastatin sodium, 288-289

Entries can be identified as follows: generic name, Trade Name, DRUG CATEGORY, *Combination Product.*

fluvoxamine, 6, 731
fluvoxamine maleate, 289-290
FoilleCort, 322-323
FOLATE ANTAGONISTS, 13
Folex, 11, 12
folic acid, 16, 290-291
folinic acid, 364-365
Foltin, 749
Folvite, 16, 290-291
Formulex, 200-201
Fortovase, 10
Fosamax, 7, 29-30, 737
foscarnet, 10, 737
foscarnet sodium/phosphonoformic acid, 291-292
Foscavir, 10, 291-292, 737
fosfomycin, 16
fosfomycin tromethamine, 293
fosinopril, 8, 293-295, 738
fosphenytoin, 5, 736
fosphenytoin sodium, 295-296
Fotovase, 610-611
Fragmin, 5, 180-181
Froben, 285-286
Froben SR, 285-286
5-FU, 279-280
Fulvicin, 736
Fulvicin P/G, 305-306
Fulvicin U/F, 305-306
Fumasorb, 270-271
Fumerin, 270-271
Fungizone Oral Suspension, 48
Fungizone (topical), 7
Furadantin, 16, 479
Furalan, 479
Furatoin, 479
furosemide, 12, 296-297, 732
Furoside, 296-297

G

gabapentin, 5, 297-298, 730
Gabitril, 6, 658-660
GALLSTONE SOLUBILIZATION DRUGS, 738
ganciclovir, 10, 298-299
Gantanol, 16, 629-630
Gantrisin, 16
Garamycin Ophthalmic, 300
Garamycin (optic), 4, 15
garlic, 757
Gastrocrom, 171-172
GASTROESOPHAGEAL REFLUX DRUGS, 13
GASTROINTESTINAL DRUGS, 13
Gastrosed, 327-328
GeeGee, 306-307
Gelfoam, 13, 20
gemfibrozil, 8, 299-300
Gemonil, 410-411
Genabid, 508-509
Genac, 739
Genacol, 750
Genahist, 211-212
Gen-Allerate, 137-138
Genaphed, 576-577
Genasoft Plus, 747
Genaspor, 671
Genatuss, 306-307
Genatuss DM, 748
Gen-Cefazolin, 113-114
Gen-Cimetidine, 146-147
Gen-Clonazepam, 160-161
Generet-500, 744-745
Gen-Famotidine, 263-264
Gen-Fibro, 299-300
Gen-Glybe, 303-304
Genite, 746
Gen-Minoxidil, 445-446
Genoptic, 300
Genoptic SOP, 300
Genora 0.5/35, 493-495
Genora 1/35, 493-495
Genora 1/50, 493-495
Genpril, 328-330
Gen-Ranitidine, 590
Gen-Salbutamol, 28-29
Gensan, 739
Gen-Selegiline, 613-615
Gentacidin, 300
Gentak, 300
gentamicin (optic), 15
gentamicin sulfate (ophthalmic), 300
Gen-Tamoxifen, 639-640
gentamycin ophthalmic, 4
Gen-Timolol, 663-664
Gen-Triazolam, 687-688
Genuine Bayer, 55-56
Gen-Xene, 163-164
Geridium, 525
Gerimal, 240
GG-Cen, 306-307

Entries can be identified as follows: generic name, Trade Name, DRUG CATEGORY, *Combination Product.*

ginger, 758
gingko, 758
ginseng, 759
GLAUCOMA TREATMENT, 13
Glaucon, 238-239
glimepiride, 6, 300-302
glipizide, 6, 302-303
GLUCOCORTICOIDS, 13, 738
Glucophage, 6, 418-419, 736
glucosamine sulfate, 759
Glucotrol, 6, 302-303
Glucotrol XL, 302-303
Glu-K, 546-547
glutethimide, 734
glyburide, 6, 303-304
glycopyrrolate, 5, 304-305
Glycotuss, 306-307
Glynase PresTab, 303-304
Glyset, 6, 443
Glytuss, 306-307
goldenseal, 760
gold sodium thiomalate, 9
Goody's Extra Headache Powders, 744
Gravol, 210-211
Gravol L/A, 210-211
Grifulvin V, 305-306
Grisactin Ultra, 305-306
griseofulvin, 7, 736
griseofulvin microsize/griseofulvin ultramicrosize, 305-306
Grisovin-FP, 305-306
Gris-PEG, 305-306
guaifenesin, 10, 12, 306-307
Guaifenesin/PPA 75, 744
Guaifenex DM, 744
Guaifenex PPA 75, 747-748
Guaifenex Rx PM, 744
Guaimax-D, 743
Guaipax, 743
guanabenz, 8, 731
guanabenz acetate, 307
guanadrel sulfate, 308-309
guanethidine, 731
guanethidine sulfate, 309-310
guanfacine, 8, 738
guanfacine HCl, 310-311
Guiatuss, 306-307
Gylate, 306-307
Gynecort, 322-323
Gyne-Lotrimin, 164-165
Gyne-Lotrimin 3, 164-165
Gyne-Lotrimin Combination Pack, 164-165
Gynergen, 240-241
Gyne-Sulf, 749
Gynogen, 246-247

H

Habitrol, 16, 475-476
halazepam, 5, 311-312, 730
halcinonide, 13, 312
Halcion, 5, 687-688, 733
Haldol, 9, 313-315, 732
Haldol LA, 313-315
halobetasol, 13
halobetasol propionate, 312-313
Halofed, 576-577
Halog, 13, 312
Halog-E, 312
haloperidol/haloperidol decanoate, 9, 313-315, 732
Halotestin, 12, 281-282
Halotussin DM, 748
Haltran, 328-330
hawthorn, 761
Hectorol, 16, 710-711
Helidac, 744, 437-439
Helidac Chewable, 85
Helidac Therapy, 649-651
Hemocyte, 270-271
HEMORHEOLOGIC DRUGS, 738
HEMOSTATICS, 13
heparin/heparin calcium/heparin sodium, 5, 315-316
Heparin-Leo, 315-316
Hep Lock, 315-316
Hep-Lock U/P, 315-316
Herbal/nonherbal remedies, 752-764
heroin, 734
Herplex Liquifilm, 330
Herplex (optic), 15
Herplex (topical), 10
Hexadrol, 192-193
Hexadrol Phosphate, 192-193
Hexadrol Therapeutic Pack, 192-193
Hiprex, 16, 423-424
Hip-Rex, 423-424
Histaject Modified, 90-91
HISTAMINE ANTAGONISTS, 7, 737
Histanil, 566-567
Histerone-50, 647-648
Histerone-100, 647-648
HIV DRUGS, 10

Entries can be identified as follows: generic name, Trade Name, DRUG CATEGORY, *Combination Product.*

Hivid, 10, 714-715
homatropine hydrobromide (optic), 14, 15, 316-317
HTCZ, 318-319
Humalin 30/70, 337-338
Humalin 50/50, 337-338
Humalin U Ultralente, 337-338
Humalog, 337-338
Humibid, 10, 12
Humibid DM, 744
Humibid DM Sprinkles, 744
Humibid LA, 306-307
Humibid Sprinkle, 306-307
Humulin 70/30, 337-338
Humulin L, 337-338
Humulin N, 337-338
Humulin-R, 337-338
Humulin-U, 337-338
Hurricaine, 4, 73-74
Hycodan, 10, 319-320
Hycodan Tussigon, 744
Hydeltrasol, 551-553
Hydeltra TBA, 551-553
Hydergine, 11, 240
Hydergine LC, 240
Hyderm, 322-323
hydralazine, 8
hydralazine HCl, 317-318
Hydramine, 211-212
Hydrap-ES, 744
Hydrate, 210-211
Hydrea, 11, 325-326
Hydril, 211-212
Hydrocet, 740
Hydro-Chlor, 318-319
hydrochlorothiazide, 12, 318-319, 732
Hydrochlorothiazide Tablets 40/25, 745
Hydrochlorothiazide Tablets 80/25, 745
HydroClear-Tuss, 744
hydrocodone, 10
hydrocodone bitartrate, 319-320
hydrocodone combinations, 734
Hydrocodone GF Syrup, 744
Hydrocodone w/APAP, 745
hydrocortisone/hydrocortisone acetate/ hydrocortisone buteprate/ hydrocortisone butyrate/ hydrocortisone valerate, 13, 322-323
hydrocortisone/hydrocortisone acetate/ hydrocortisone cypionate/ hydrocortisone sodium succinate/ hydrocortisone sodium phosphate, 13, 320-322
Hydrocortone, 320-322
Hydrocortone Acetate, 320-322
Hydrocortone Phosphate, 320-322
Hydro-D, 318-319
HydroDIURIL, 12, 318-319, 732
Hydrogesic, 740
hydromorphone, 4, 734
hydromorphone HCl, 323-324
Hydropres-50, 744
Hydro-Serp, 744
Hydroserpine No. 1, 744
Hydroserpine No. 2, 744
Hydrostat IR, 323-324
Hydro-Tex, 322-323
hydroxocobalamin, 172-173
hydroxychloroquine, 9
hydroxychloroquine sulfate, 324-325
hydroxyurea, 11, 325-326
hydroxyzine, 5, 7, 730, 731
hydroxyzine HCl/hydroxyzine pamoate, 326-327
Hygroton, 12, 141-142
Hylorel, 8, 308-309
hyoscyamine, 5, 730
hyoscyamine atropine, 730
hyoscyamine sulfate, 327-328
Hyosophen Elixir, 743
Hyphed Syrup, 744
Hy-Phen, 740
Hytakerol, 16, 208-209, 710-711
Hytone, 322-323
Hytrin, 8, 15, 643-644
Hytuss, 306-307
Hytuss 2X, 306-307
Hyzaar, 744
Hyzine, 326-327

I

Iberet-500 Filmtabs, 744-745
Iberet-500 Liquid, 745
Ibifon, 328-330
IBU, 328-330
Ibuprin, 328-330
ibuprofen, 9, 14, 328-330, 731
Ibuprohm, 328-330
I-deprenyl, 613-615
idoxuridine-idu (ophthalmic), 330

Entries can be identified as follows: generic name, Trade Name, DRUG CATEGORY, *Combination Product.*

idoxuridine (optic), 15
idoxuridine (topical), 10
Iletin, 337-338
Iletin II, 337-338
Iletin II NPH, 337-338
Iletin NPH, 337-338
Ilotycin, 15, 242-244
Ilotycin Ophthalmic, 241
Ilozyme, 507-508
IMDUR, 348-349
imipramine, 6, 731, 736
imipramine HCl/imipramine pamoate, 330-332
imiquimod, 13, 332
Imitrex, 14, 635-636
IMMUNOMODULATORS, 13-14, 738
IMMUNOSUPPRESSANTS, 14, 738
Imodium, 388-389
Imodium A-D, 6, 388-389, 731
Imodium Advanced, 745
Impril, 330-332
Imuran, 14, 64-65, 738
Indameth, 335-336
indapamide, 12, 332-333
Inderal, 4, 6, 8, 14, 572-574
Inderal LA, 572-574
Inderide 40/25, 745
Inderide 80/25, 745
Inderide LA 80/50, 745
Inderide LA 120/50, 745
Inderide LA 160/50, 745
indinavir, 10, 737
indinavir sulfate, 334-335
Indocid, 335-336
Indocid SR, 335-336
Indocin, 9, 14, 335-336
Indocin SR, 335-336
indomethacin/indomethacin sodium trihydrate, 9, 14, 335-336
INH, 345-346
insulin/insulin lispro, 6, 337-338
Intal, 14, 171-172, 737
interferon alfa, 738
interferon alfa-2a/interferon alfa-2b/interferon alfa-n1/interferon alfa-n3/interferon beta-1a, 11, 13, 338-339
interferon gamma-1b, 14, 340-341
Intron A, 11, 13, 338-339
Inversine, 8, 400-401, 738
Invirase, 10, 610-611, 737
Iobid DM, 744
Iodex-P, 547-548
Ionamin, 4, 10, 531-532, 730, 736
Iophen-C, 745
Iophen-DM, 745
Iopidine, 52-53, 738
ipratropium, 11, 737
ipratropium bromide, 341-342
irbesartan, 8, 342-343
Ircon, 270-271
Irospan, 270-271
Ismelin, 8, 309-310, 731
ISMO, 4, 348-349
Iso-Bid, 347-348
Isocaine, 411-412
Isocaine/Levonordefrin, 411-412
isocarboxazid, 6, 343-344, 731
isoetharine, 11, 344-345
isoetharine HCl, 344-345
Isonate, 347-348
isoniazid, 10, 345-346
isopropamide, 730
isoproterenol, 4, 11, 732, 737
isoproterenol HCl/isoproterenol sulfate, 346-347
Isoptin, 708-709
Isoptin SR, 708-709
Isopto Atropine, 14, 15, 61
Isopto Carpine, 13, 15, 537
Isopto Cetamide, 627-628
Isopto Homatropine, 14, 15, 316-317
isorbide dinitrate, 4
isorbide mononitrate, 4
Isordil, 4, 347-348
Isordil Titradose, 347-348
isosorbide dinitrate, 347-348
isosorbide mononitrate, 348-349
Isotamine, 345-346
Isotrate, 347-348
isotretinoin, 12, 349-350, 730
isoxsuprine, 15
isoxsuprine HCl, 350-351
isradipine, 8, 351-352
Isuprel, 4, 11, 346-347, 732, 737
Isuprel Mistometer, 346-347
itraconazole, 7, 352-353
I-Tropine, 61

J

Janest-28, 493-495

Entries can be identified as follows: generic name, Trade Name, DRUG CATEGORY, *Combination Product.*

K

K^+ 10, 546-547
Kadian, 454-455
Kalium, 546-547
Kaochlor, 546-547
Kaon, 546-547
Kaon-Cl, 546-547
Kaopectate II, 388-389
Karigel, 620-621
kava, 761
KayCiel, 546-547
Kayelixir, 546-547
K^+ Care ET, 546-547
K-Dur, 546-547
Keflex, 11, 123-124
Keftab, 123-124
Kefzol, 113-114
K-Electrolyte, 546-547
Kemadrin, 9, 563-564
Kenacort, 684-686
Kenacort Diacetate, 684-686
Kenaject-40, 684-686
Kenalog, 13, 686
Kenalog-10, 684-686
Kenalog-40, 684-686
Kenalog-H, 686
Kenalog in Orabase, 686
Kendral-Ipratropium, 341-342
Kenonel, 686
Keppra, 6, 367-368
Kerlone, 8, 80-81
ketoconazole, 7, 353-354
ketoprofen, 9, 15, 354-356, 736
ketorolac/ketorolac tromethamine/ ketorolac tromethamine injection, 15, 356-357
ketotifen, 7, 15
ketotifen fumarate, 357
Key-Pred 25 and 50, 551-553
Key-Pred-SP, 551-553
K-Ide, 546-547
Kinesed, 730
K-Lease, 546-547
Klonopin, 5, 160-161
K-Lor, 546-547
Klor-Con 8, 546-547
Klor-Con 10, 546-547
Klor-Con/EF, 546-547
Klotrix, 546-547
K-Lyte, 546-547
K-Norm, 546-547
Konakion, 536
Kronofed-A, 742
K-Tab, 546-547
Ku-Zyme HP, 507-508

L

labetalol, 8, 357-359, 738
Lamictal, 5, 360-361, 730
Lamisil, 7, 644-645, 736
Lamisil AT, 645
Lamisil Derma-Gel, 645
lamivudine, 10, 359-360
lamotrigine, 5, 360-361, 730
Lamprene, 9, 156-157
Lanacort, 322-323
Laniazid, 10, 345-346
Lanophyllin, 652-653
Lanorinal, 744
Lanoxicaps, 207-208
Lanoxin, 6, 11, 207-208
lansoprazole, 13, 361-362, 736
Largactil, 138-140
Larodopa, 9, 369-370, 732, 737
Lasix, 12, 296-297, 732
Lasix Special, 296-297
latanoprost, 13, 362-363
L-Caine, 377-379
Ledercillin-VK, 514-515
leflunomide, 9, 363-364, 730, 736
Legatrin PM, 745
Lemoderm, 322-323
Lemoderm Cortate, 322-323
Lente Iletin II, 337-338
Lentel, 337-338
Leponex, 166-167
Lescol, 8, 11, 288-289, 737
leucovorin, 11
leucovorin calcium, 364-365
Leukeran, 130-131
LEUKOTRIENE PATHWAY INHIBITORS, 14
LEUKOTRIENE RECEPTOR ANTAGONISTS, 14
Levabol, 738
levalbuterol, 11, 732
levalbuterol HCl, 365-366
levamisole, 14, 738
levamisole HCl, 366-367
Levaquin, 12, 372-373
Levate, 40-42
Levatol, 8, 510-512
Levbid, 327-328
levetiracetam, 6, 367-368

Entries can be identified as follows: generic name, Trade Name, DRUG CATEGORY, *Combination Product.*

Levite, 493-495
Levlen, 493-495
levobunolol, 13
levobunolol HCl, 368-369
levocabastine, 7, 15
levocabastine HCl, 369
levodopa, 9, 369-370, 732, 737
levodopa-carbidopa, 9, 371-372, 737
levofloxacin, 12, 372-373, 737
levomethadyl acetate, 4
levomethadyl acetate HCl, 373-374
levonorgestrel, 12, 493-495
levonorgestrel implant, 374-375
Levoquin, 737
Levora, 493-495
Levo-T, 375
Levothroid, 375
levothyroxine, 12
levothyroxine sodium, 375
Levoxyl, 375
Levsin, 5, 327-328
Levsinex, 327-328
Levsin with Phenobarbital Tablets, 745
Lexxel, 745
Lexxel 2, 745
L-Homatropine, 316-317
Librax, 730, 745
Libritabs, 131-132
Librium, 5, 131-132, 730
Licon, 278-279
Lidemol, 278-279
Lidex, 13, 278-279
Lidex-E, 278-279
lidocaine, 4, 6
lidocaine HCl (cardiac), 376
lidocaine HCl (local), 377-379
lidocaine HCl (topical), 379
lidocaine (topical), 4
lidocaine transoral, 4, 379-380, 736
Lidoject, 377-379
Lidopen Auto-Injector, 376
Lincocin, 14, 380-381, 737
lincomycin, 14, 737
lincomycin HCl, 380-381
Lincorex, 380-381
LINCOSAMIDES, 14
Lioresal, 16, 69-70, 733, 738
liothyronine, 12
liothyronine sodium, 381-382
liotrix, 12, 382
Lipitor, 8, 11, 58
lipodine, 13
Liquaemin Sodium, 315-316
Liquamenin Sodium PF, 315-316
Liquid Pred, 553-554
Liqui-E, 711-712
Liqui-Gels, 328-330
Liquiprin, 21-22
lisinopril, 8, 383-384
Lithane, 384-385
lithium, 732, 737
lithium carbonate/lithium citrate, 10, 384-385
Lithizine, 384-385
Lithobid, 384-385
Lithonate, 384-385
Lithotabs, 384-385
Livitrinsic-F, 749
Livostin, 7, 15, 369
Livostin Nasal, 369
Locoid Cream, 322-323
Locoid Ointment, 322-323
Lodine, 9, 14, 260-262, 736
Lodine XL, 260-262
lodoxamide, 14
lodoxamide tromethamine, 385
Loestrin 21, 493-495
Loestrin Fe, 493-495
Lofene, 212-213
Logen, 212-213
lomefloxacin, 12
lomefloxacin HCl, 385-386
Lomocort, 212-213
Lomotil, 6, 212-213, 731
lomustine, 11, 387-388
Loniten, 8, 445-446
Lonox, 212-213
Lo/Ovral, 493-495
Loperacap, 388-389
loperamide, 6, 731
loperamide HCl, 388-389
Lopid, 8, 299-300
Lopresor SR, 436-437
Lopressor, 4, 8, 436-437
Lopressor HCT 100/25, 745
Lopressor HCT 100/50, 745
Lopressor HCT 50/25, 745
Loprox, 7, 145
Lopurin, 30-31
Lorabid, 11, 389-390
loracarbef, 11, 389-390
loratadine, 7, 390, 731

Entries can be identified as follows: generic name, Trade Name, DRUG CATEGORY, *Combination Product.*

lorazepam, 5, 390-391, 730
Lorazepam Intensol, 390-391
Lorcet 10/650, 745
Lorcet-HD, 740, 745
Lorcet Plus, 740, 745
Lortab 2.5/500, 745
Lortab 5/500, 740, 745
Lortab 7.5/500, 745
Lortab ASA, 745
Lortab Elixir, 745
losartan, 8, 738
losartan potassium, 391-392
Losec, 491-492
Losopan, 396-397
Lotemax, 393
Lotemax (optic), 15
Lotemax (topical), 13
Lotensin, 8, 72-73
Lotensin HCT 20/12.5, 745
Lotensin HCT 20/25, 745
loteprednol etabonate (optic), 393
loteprednol (optic), 15
loteprednol (topical), 13
Lotrel 2.5/10, 745
Lotrel 5/10, 745
Lotrel 5/20, 745
Lotrimin, 164-165
Lotrisone, 745
lovastatin, 8, 11, 394
Lovenox, 5, 235-236
Loxapac, 394-396
loxapine, 9
loxapine succinate/loxapine HCl, 394-396
Loxitane, 9, 394-396
Loxitane-C, 394-396
Loxitane IM, 394-396
Lozide, 332-333
Lozol, 12, 332-333
LSD, 734
Ludiomil, 6, 397-398
Lufyllin, 229-230
Lufyllin-400, 229-230
Luminal, 5, 6, 10
Luminal Sodium, 528-529
Luride Lozi-Tabs, 618-620
Lurline PMS, 746
Luvox, 6, 289-290, 731
Lyderm, 278-279
lypressin, 12, 396
Lysodren, 11, 448-449

M

Maalox Antidiarrheal, 388-389
Macrobid, 479
Macrodantin, 479
MACROLIDES, 14
magaldrate, 4, 396-397, 736
ma-huang, 762
Major-Gesic, 747
Malatal, 743
MALE PATTERN BALDNESS DRUGS, 14
Mallisol, 547-548
Malogen, 647-648
Malogex, 647-648
Mandelamine, 423-424
Maolate, 16, 136-137
Mapap Cold Formula, 741
maprotiline, 6
maprotiline HCl, 397-398
Marcaine, 4, 94-96
Marcaine Hydrochloride with Epinephrine, 94-96
Marcillin, 48-50
Marezine, 7, 173-174, 732
Marflex, 732
Margesic H, 740
marijuana, 734
Marinol, 227-229
Marnal, 744
Marplan, 6, 343-344, 731
Marpres, 744
Marthritic, 609-610
masoprocol, 11, 399
MAST CELL STABILIZERS, 14
Matulane, 11, 560-561
Mavik, 8, 677-678
Maxair, 11, 542-543, 737
Maxalt, 14, 603-604, 733
Maxalt-MLT, 603-604
Maxaquin, 12, 385-386
Maxeran, 433-434
Maxiflor, 204
Maximum Strength Anbesol, 73-74
Maximum Strength Comtrex Liqui-Gels, 741-742
Maximum Strength Dynafed, 744
Maximum Strength Orajel, 73-74
Maximum Strength Ornex, 744
Maximum Strength Sine-Aid, 744
Maximum Strength Sinutab without Drowiness, 744

Entries can be identified as follows: generic name, Trade Name, DRUG CATEGORY, *Combination Product.*

Maximum Strength Strength Tylenol Sinus, 744
Maximum Strength Sudafed Sinus, 744
Maxipime, 11, 115-116
Maxitrol, 739
Maxivate, 77-78
Maxzide, 732, 745
Maxzide-25 MG, 745
Mazanor, 4, 10, 399-400, 730, 736
mazindol, 4, 10, 399-400, 730, 736
Measurin, 55-56
Mebaral, 6, 410-411
mecamylamine, 8, 738
mecamylamine HCl, 400-401
meclizine, 7, 732
meclizine HCl, 401-402
Meclofen, 736
meclofenamate, 15, 402-403, 736
Meclomen, 15, 402-403
Medigesic, 743
Medihalder-Epi, 238-239
Medihaler-Ergotamine, 240-241
Medihaler-Iso, 346-347
Medipren, 328-330
Mediquell, 195-196
Medralone 40, 431-432
Medralone 80, 431-432
Medrol, 13, 431-432
Medrol Dosepak, 431-432
medroxyprogesterone, 12
medroxyprogesterone acetate, 403-404
Med Tamoxifen, 639-640
Med Timolol, 663-664
MedValproic, 703-705
mefenamic acid, 15, 404-405
Megace, 11, 405
Megacillin, 513-514
megestrol, 11
megestrol acetate, 405
Melagesic PM, 746
Mellaril, 9, 654-656, 732
melphalan, 11, 405-406
Menadol, 328-330
Menest, 245
Meni-D, 401-402
Menogen, 746
Menogen H.S., 746
Menoplex, 746
Mentax, 7, 99
mepenzolate, 5, 736
mepenzolate bromide, 406-407
Mepergan, 746
Mepergan Fortis caps, 746
meperidine, 4, 4, 733, 734
meperidine HCl, 407-408
mephenytoin, 6, 408-409
mephobarbital, 6, 410-411
Mephyton, 536
mepivacaine, 4
mepivacaine HCl, 411-412
meprobamate, 5, 413-414, 730, 734
Meprolone, 431-432
Mepron, 9, 15, 58-59
Meprospan 200/400, 413-414
mercaptopurine, 11, 414
Merezine, 7
Meridia, 4, 10, 616-617
mesalamine, 13, 414-415
Mesantoin, 6, 408-409
Mesasal, 414-415
mescaline, 734
mesoridazine, 9
mesoridazine besylate, 415-417
Mestinon, 11, 14, 578-579
Mestinon SR, 578-579
mestranol, 493-495
Metadate ER, 430-431
Metaderm Mild, 77-78
Metaderm Regular, 77-78
metaproterenol, 11, 737
metaproterenol sulfate, 417-418
Metatensin No. 2, 746
Metatensin No. 4, 746
metformin, 6, 736
metformin HCl, 418-419
methadone, 4, 734
methadone HCl, 419-420
Methadose, 419-420
methamphetamine, 4, 10, 11, 732, 738
methamphetamine HCl, 420-421
methantheline, 5, 730, 736
methantheline bromide, 421-422
methazolamide, 12, 13, 422-423, 738
methazolamine, 13
methenamine, 16
methenamine hippurate/methenamine mandelamine, 423-424
methimazole, 10, 424-425, 737
methocarbamol, 16, 425-426, 738
methohexital, 734

Entries can be identified as follows: generic name, Trade Name, DRUG CATEGORY, *Combination Product.*

methotrexate/methotrexate sodium, 9, 11, 12, 426-427
methscopolamine, 730
methsuximide, 6, 427-428
methyldopa/methyldopate, 8, 428-430
Methylin, 430-431
methylphenidate, 11, 734
methylphenidate HCl, 430-431
methylprednisolone/ methylprednisolone acetate/ methylprednisolone sodium succinate, 13, 431-432
METHYLXANTHINES, 738
methysergide, 14
methysergide maleate, 432-433
Meticorten, 13, 14, 553-554
metoclopramide, 7, 13
metoclopramide HCl, 433-434
metolazone, 12, 434-435
metoprolol, 4, 8
metoprolol tartrate, 436-437
Metric 21, 437-439
Metro IV, 437-439
metronidazole/metronidazole HCl, 14, 437-439, 737
Mevacor, 8, 11, 394
mexiletine, 6, 738
mexiletine HCl, 439-440
Mexitil, 6, 439-440, 738
Miacalcin Nasal Spray, 100-101
mibefradil, 8
Micardis, 8, 642
Micatin, 7, 440
miconazole, 7
Miconazole-7, 440
miconazole nitrate, 440
Micranin, 743
Micro-K, 14, 546-547
Micronase, 303-304
Micronor, 482-483
Microzide, 318-319
Midamor, 12, 35-36, 732
midazolam, 4, 5, 734, 736
midazolam HCl, 440-442
Midol IB, 328-330
Midol Maximum Strength Multi-Symptom Menstrual, 746
Midol PM, 746
Midol Regular Strength Multi-Symptom, 746
miglitol, 6, 443
MIGRAINE DRUGS, 14, 733
Milontin, 6, 530-531
Milophene, 158
Miltown, 5, 413-414, 730
Mims Atropine, 61
MINERALS, 14
Minidyne, 547-548
Minims Homatropine, 316-317
Minipress, 8, 549-550, 731
Minitran, 480-481
Minizide 1, 746
Minizide 2, 746
Minizide 5, 746
Minocin, 16, 444-445
minocycline, 16
minocycline HCl, 444-445
minoxidil, 8, 12, 14, 445-446
Minoxigaine, 445-446
Miocarpine, 537
Mio-rel, 496
Mirapex, 9, 548-549, 737
Mircette, 493-495
mirtazapine, 6, 446-447
misoprostol, 13, 15, 447-448
mitotane, 11, 448-449
Moban, 9, 451-452
Moban Concentrate, 451-452
Mobenol, 667-668
modafinil, 11, 449-450, 733
Modecate, 282-284
Modecate concentrate, 282-284
Modicon, 493-495
Moditen Enanthate, 282-284
Moditen HCl, 282-284
Moduretic, 746
moexipril, 8
moexipril hydrochloride, 450-451
molindone, 9
molindone HCl, 451-452
Mol-Iron, 270-271
Monafed DM, 744
Monistat, 7
Monistat 3, 440
Monistat-7, 440
Monistat-Derm, 440
MONOAMINE OXIDASE INHIBITORS, 6
Monodox, 225-226
Mono-Gesic, 609-610
Monoket, 348-349
Monopril, 8, 293-295, 738
montelukast, 10, 14

montelukast sodium, 452-453
Monurol, 16, 293
moricizine, 6, 453-454, 738
morphine, 4, 733, 734
morphine sulfate, 454-455
MOS, 454-455
Motofen, 6, 203-204, 731
Motrin, 9, 14, 328-330, 731
Motrin IB, 328-330
Motrin IB Sinus, 746
Mouthrinse, 741
6-MP, 414
M-Prednisol 40, 431-432
M-Prednisol 80, 431-432
MS Contin, 4, 454-455, 733
mtx, 426-427
Muco-Fen-DM, 744
MUCOLYTICS, 14
Multipax, 326-327
MULTIPLE SCLEROSIS DRUGS, 14
Multi Symptom Pamprin, 746
Multisymptom Pamprin, 746
Multi-Symptom Tylenol Cold, 741
mupirocin/mupirocin calcium, 8, 455-456
Murocoll-2, 746
Muro's Opcon, 463-464
MUSCLE RELAXANTS, 733
Muse, 32-33
Myambutol, 10, 252-253
MYASTHENIA GRAVIS DRUGS, 14
Mycelex, 7
Mycelex-7, 164-165
Mycelex-G, 164-165
Mycelex Lozenges, 164-165
Mycelex Twin Pack, 164-165
Myciguent, 4
Myclo-Gyne, 164-165
Mycobutin, 10, 593-594
MycoLog II, 746
mycophenolate, 14
mycophenolate mofetil, 456-457
Mycostatin, 7, 486-487
MYDRIATIC DRUGS, 14
My-E, 242-244
Myidone, 557-558
Mykrox, 434-435
Mylanta-AR, 263-264
Mylanta Liquid, 746
Myleran, 11, 98-99
Mymethasone, 192-193
Myochrysine, 9
Myolin, 496
Myotrol, 496
Myphetane DX, 742
Myrosemide, 296-297
Mysoline, 6, 557-558
Mytelase, 11, 14, 34-35
Mytussin DM, 748
M-Zole 3, 440

N

nabumetone, 9, 15, 457-458
nadolol, 4, 8, 458-460, 738
Nadopen-VK, 514-515
Nadostine, 486-487
Nafazair, 463-464
naftifine, 7
naftifine HCl, 460
Naftin, 7, 460
Naldecon CX Adult Liquid, 746
Naldecon DX Adult, 746
Naldecon-DX Children's Syrup, 746
Naldecon EX Pediatric Drops, 746
Naldelate DX Adult, 746
Nalfon, 14, 267-268, 731
Nalfon 200, 267-268
nalmefene, 4
nalmefene HCl, 460-461
naloxone, 4
naloxone HCl, 461-462
naltrexone, 4
naltrexone HCl, 462-463
naphazoline, 15
naphazoline HCl, 463-464
Naphcon, 15, 463-464
Naphcon Forte, 463-464
Naprelan, 464-465
Naprosyn, 9, 15, 464-465, 731
Naprosyn-E, 464-465
Naprosyn Oral Suspension, 464-465
Naprosyn SR, 464-465
naproxen/naproxen sodium, 9, 15, 464-465, 731
naratriptan, 14, 733
naratriptan HCl, 456-466
Narcan, 4, 461-462
NARCOLEPSY DRUGS, 733
NARCOTIC ANALGESICS, 14, 733
Nardil, 6, 526-528, 731
Nasacort AQ Nasal Spray, 682-683

Nasahist-B, 90-91
Nasalcrom, 171-172
Nasal Decongestant Spray, 505
Nasalide, 277-278
Natulan, 560-561
Navane, 9, 656-657, 732
Naxen, 464-465
N D Clear, 742
ND-StatrRevised, 90-91
NebuPent, 9, 515-516
Necon, 493-495
Necon 0.5/35, 493-495
Necon 1/35, 493-495
Necon 1/50, 493-495
nedocromil, 14, 737
nedocromil sodium, 466-467
nefazodone, 6, 736
nefazodone HCl, 467-468
nelfinavir, 10
nelfinavir mesylate, 468-470
Nelfon, 9
Nelova 0.5/35E, 493-495
Nelova 1/35E, 493-495
Nelova 1/50, 493-495
Nelova 10/11, 493-495
Nembutal, 5, 10
Nembutal Sodium, 518-519
Neo-Codema, 318-319
Neo-Estrone, 245
Neofer, 270-271
neomycin, 4
Neoquess, 327-328
Neoral, 177-178
Neosar, 175-176
neostigmine, 11, 14
neostigmine bromide/neostigmine methylsulfate, 470-471
Neo-Synephrine, 11, 16, 738
Neo-Synephrine (nasal), 533-534
Nephro-Fer, 270-271
Neptazane, 12, 422-423, 738
Neptazine, 13
Nervine SleepAid, 211-212
Nervocaine, 377-379
Nestrex, 579-580
Neuroforte-R, 172-173
Neurontin, 5, 297-298, 730
Neutracare, 620-621
Neutrexin, 13, 15, 695-696
nevirapine, 10, 471
Nia-Bid, 8, 472-473
Niac, 472-473
Niacels, 472-473
niacin, 8, 16, 472-473
niacinamide, 472-473
Niacor, 472-473
Niaspan, 472-473
nicardipine, 5, 8
nicardipine HCl, 473-474
Nico-400, 472-473
Nicobid, 472-473
Nicoderm, 475-476
NicoDerm CQ, 475-476
Nicolar, 472-473
Nicolid, 16
Nicorette, 16, 474-475, 738
Nicorette DS, 474-475
nicotinamide, 472-473
NICOTINE CESSATION DRUGS, 738
nicotine polacrilex, 16, 474-475, 738
nicotine transdermal system/nicotine spray, 16, 475-476
Nicotinex, 472-473
nicotinic acid, 472-473
Nicotrol, 475-476
Nicotrol NS ProStep, 475-476
nifedipine, 5, 8, 476-477, 738
Nilstat, 486-487
nisoldipine, 8, 477-479
Nite Time Cold Formula, 746
NITRATES, 4
Nitro-Bid, 480-481
Nitro-Bid IV, 480-481
Nitrocap T.D., 480-481
Nitrocine, 480-481
Nitro-Dur II, 480-481
nitrofurantoin/nitrofurantoin macrocrystals, 16, 479
Nitrogard, 480-481
nitroglycerin, 4, 480-481
Nitroglyn, 480-481
NITROIMIDAZOLES, 14
Nitrol, 480-481
Nitrolin, 480-481
Nitrolingual, 480-481
Nitrong, 480-481
Nitrong SR, 480-481
NitroQuick, 480-481
Nitrospan, 480-481
Nitrostat, 480-481
nizatidine, 7, 481-482
Nizoral, 7, 353-354

Entries can be identified as follows: generic name, Trade Name, DRUG CATEGORY, *Combination Product.*

Nizoral Shampoo, 353-354
Noctec, 737
Nolvadex, 639-640, 738
NONSTEROIDAL ANTIINFLAMMATORIES, 4, 14-15
No Pain-HP, 103-104
Norco, 746
Nordette, 493-495
Norethin 1/35E, 493-495
Norethin 1/50M, 493-495
norethindrone/norethindrone acetate, 12, 482-483, 493-495
Norflex, 16, 496, 733
norfloxacin, 12, 483-484
Norfranil, 330-332
Norgesic, 746
Norgesic Forte, 746
norgestimate, 493-495
norgestrel, 12, 484-485, 493-495
Norinyl, 493-495
Normiflo, 5, 53-54
Normodyne, 8, 357-359
Noroxin, 12, 483-484
Norpace, 6, 215-216
Norpace CR, 215-216
Norplant System, 12, 374-375
Norpramin, 6, 187-188, 731, 736
Nor-Pred TBA, 551-553
Nor-QD, 482-483
nortriptyline, 6, 736
nortriptyline HCl, 485-486
Norvasc, 5, 8, 43-44, 738
Norvir, 10, 602-603, 737
Nostril, 533-534
Nostrilla, 505
Novafed, 576-577
Novafed A, 742
Novaldex, 11
Nova moxin, 46-48
Nova-Rectal, 518-519
Novasen, 55-56
Novo-Alprazol, 31-32
Novo-Ampicillin, 48-50
Novo-Atenolol, 56-58
Novo-AZT, 717-718
NovoBetament, 77-78
Novo-Butamide, 667-668
Novo-Carbamaz, 105-106
Novo-Chlorhydrate, 129-130
Novo-Chlorpromazine, 138-140
Novo-Cimetidine, 146-147
Novo-Clopate, 163-164
Novo-Cloxin, 165-166
Novo-Cromolyn, 171-172
Novo-Difenac, 197-199
Novo-Difenac SR, 197-199
Novo-Diflunisal, 205-206
Novo-digoxin, 207-208
Novo-Diltiazem, 209-210
Novo-Dimenate, 210-211
Novo-Dipam, 196-197
Novodipiradol, 214
Novo-Doxepin, 223-224
Novodoxylin, 225-226
Novo-Erythro, 242-244
Novoferrogluc, 270-271
Novoferrosulfa, 270-271
Novofibrate, 157-158
Novoflupam, 284-285
Novo-Flurazine, 689-690
Novo-Flurbiprofen, 285-286
Novo-Folacid, 290-291
Novofumar, 270-271
Novo-Gemfibrozil, 299-300
Novo-Glyburide, 303-304
Novo-Hydrazide, 318-319
Novohydrocort, 322-323
Novo-Hydroxyzin, 326-327
Novo-Hylazin, 317-318
Novo-Keto-EC, 354-356
Novolente-K, 546-547
Novo-Lexin, 123-124
Novolin 70/30, 337-338
Novolin ge 30/70, 337-338
Novolin ge 50/50, 337-338
Novolin ge Lente, 337-338
Novolin ge NPH, 337-338
Novolin ge Toronto, 337-338
Novolin ge Ultralente, 337-338
Novolin L, 337-338
Novolin N, 337-338
Novolin R, 337-338
Novo-Lorazem, 390-391
Novomedopa, 428-430
Novo-Metformin, 418-419
Novo-Methacin, 335-336
Novometoprol, 436-437
Novo-Naprox, 464-465
Novo-Naprox Sodium, 464-465
Novo-Naprox Sodium DS, 464-465
Novo-Niacin, 472-473
Novonidazole, 437-439
Novo-Nifedin, 476-477
Novopentobarb, 518-519

Entries can be identified as follows: generic name, Trade Name, DRUG CATEGORY, *Combination Product.*

NovoPen-VK, 514-515
Novoperidol, 313-315
Novo-Pheniram, 137-138
Novo-Pindol, 540-541
Novo-Pirocam, 543-544
Novo-Poxide, 131-132
Novopramine, 330-332
Novo-Pranol, 572-574
Novo-Profen, 328-330
Novopropamide, 140-141
Novopyrazone, 632-633
Novoquindin, 583-585
Novo-Ranitidine, 590
Novoreserpine, 592-593
Novo-Ridazine, 654-656
Novo-Rythro, 242-244
Novo-Rythro EnCap, 242-244
Novo-Salmol, 28-29
Novosecobarb, 612-613
Novo-Selegiline, 613-615
Novosemide, 296-297
Novosorbide, 347-348
Novo-Soxazole, 633-634
Novospiroton, 623-624
Novo-Sundac, 634-635
Novo-Tamoxifen, 639-640
Novotetra, 649-651
Novo-Thalidone, 141-142
Novo-Timol, 661-663
Novo-Timolol, 663-664
Novo-Tolmetin, 670-671
Novo-Trimel, 630-631
Novo-Trimipramine, 697-698
Novo-Triolam, 687-688
Novotriptyn, 40-42
Novo-Valproic, 703-705
Novo-Veramil, 708-709
Novoxapam, 501
NP-27, 671
NPH Iletin I and II, 337-338
NPH-N, 337-338
NTS, 480-481
NTZ Long-Acting, 505
Nu-Alpraz, 31-32
Nu-Amox, 46-48
Nu-Ampi, 48-50
Nu-Carbamazepine, 105-106
Nu-Cephalex, 123-124
Nu-Cimet, 146-147
Nu-Cloxi, 165-166
Nu-Cotrimox, 630-631
Nu-Diclo, 197-199
Nu-Dilitaz, 209-210
Nu-Famotidine, 263-264
Nu-Flurbiprofen, 285-286
Nu-Gemfibrozil, 299-300
Nu-Glyburide, 303-304
Nu-Ibuprofen, 328-330
Nu-Indo, 335-336
Nu-Loperamide, 388-389
Nu-Loraz, 390-391
Nu-Medopa, 428-430
Nu-Metop, 436-437
Nu-Nifed, 476-477
Nu-Pen-VK, 514-515
Nu-Pirox, 543-544
Nuprin, 328-330
Nu-Prox, 464-465
Nu-Ranit, 590
Nu-Selegiline, 613-615
Nu-Tetra, 649-651
Nu-Timol, 663-664
Nutracort, 322-323
Nu-Triazo, 687-688
Nu-Valproic, 703-705
Nu-Verap, 708-709
Nyaderm, 486-487
Nydrazid, 345-346
NyQuil Nighttime Cold/Flu Medicine, 746
nystatin, 7, 486-487
Nystex, 486-487
Nytcold, 746
Nytol Quickcaps, 211-212

O

Obalan, 525-526
Obe-Nix, 531-532
Obestine-30, 531-532
Obezine, 525-526
Oby-Cap, 531-532
Ocupress, 13, 15, 109
Octamide, 433-434
Octocaine, 377-379
Octocaine with Epinephrine, 377-379
Octosim, 188-189
Ocu-Carpine, 537
Ocufen, 15, 287
Ocuflox, 15, 488
Ocuflox Ophthalmic Solution, 488
Ocu-Sul, 627-628
Ocu-tropine, 61
ofloxacin, 12, 15, 487-488
Ogen, 12, 249-250

olanzapine, 9, 488-490
olopatadine, 7, 738
olopatadine HCl, 490
olopatadine (optic), 15
olsalazine, 13
olsalazine sodium, 490-491
omeprazole, 13, 491-492, 736
Omnicef, 11, 114-115
Omnipen, 15, 48-50
Omnipen-N, 48-50
ondansetron, 7
ondansetron HCl, 492-493
One-Alpha, 710-711
Onset, 746-747
OPHTHALMIC DRUGS, 733, 738
Ophtho-Dipivefrin, 213
opium, 734
Optimine, 7, 63-64
Orabase-B, 73-74
Orabase Baby, 73-74
Orabase Gel, 73-74
Oracort, 686
Oradexan, 192-193
Orajel, 73-74
Orajel Mouth Aid, 73-74
oral contraceptives, 12, 493-495
Oralone, 686
Oraminic II, 90-91
Orap, 9, 539-540, 732, 737
Orasone, 553-554
Orbenin, 165-166
Oretic, 318-319
Orfo, 496
Organidin NR, 306-307
Orgaran, 5, 181-182
Orinase, 6, 667-668, 736
Orlaam, 4, 373-374
orlistat, 10, 495
Ormazine, 138-140
Ornade, 732
Ornade Spansules, 739
orphenadrine, 16, 733
orphenadrine citrate, 496
orphenadrine HCl, 732
OrthoCept, 493-495
Ortho-Cept, 740
Ortho-Cyclen, 493-495
Ortho-Est, 249-250
Ortho-Novum 1/35, 493-495
Ortho-Novum 1/50, 493-495
Ortho-Novum 7/7/7, 493-495
Ortho-Novum 10/11, 493-495
Ortho Tri-Cyclen, 493-495
Orthoxicol Cough Syrup, 747
Orudis, 9, 15, 354-356, 736
Orudis-E, 354-356
Orudis KT, 354-356
Orudis-SR, 354-356
Oruvail, 354-356
oseltamivir, 10
oseltamivir phosphate, 497
OSTEOPOROSIS DRUGS, 7
Ostoforte, 710-711
Ovcon 35, 493-495
Ovcon-50, 493-495
Ovral, 493-495
Ovrette, 12, 484-485
oxacillin, 15
oxacillin sodium, 497-498
Oxandrin, 12, 498-499
oxandrolone, 12, 498-499
oxaprozin, 9, 15, 499-500
oxazepam, 5, 501, 730
oxidized cellulose, 13, 501-502
oxtriphylline, 11, 16, 502-503, 738
oxybutynin, 5, 730
oxybutynin chloride, 503-504
Oxycel, 501-502
oxycodone, 4, 504-505, 734
OxyContin, 504-505
oxymetazoline, 11
oxymetazoline HCl, 505
oxymetholone, 12, 505-506
oxyphencyclimine, 730

P

Pacerone, 39-40
paclitaxel, 11, 506-507
Pain Doctor, 103-104
Pain X, 103-104
Palafer, 270-271
Palgic-D, 747
Palmiron, 270-271
Pamelor, 6, 485-486, 736
Pamine, 730
Pamprin IB, 328-330
Pamprin Multi-Symptom, 747
Panacet 5/500, 740
Panadol, 21-22
Pancof XP, 747
Pancrease, 507-508
Pancrease MT 4, 507-508
pancrelipase, 13, 507-508
Pandel, 13, 322-323

Entries can be identified as follows: generic name, Trade Name, DRUG CATEGORY, *Combination Product.*

Panmycin, 649-651
Panretin, 12, 30
Panshapem, 531-532
Pantanol, 738
Panwarfin, 712-713
papaverine, 15
papaverine HCl, 508-509
Paraflex, 16, 142-143
Parafon Forte DSC, 142-143
paregoric, 6, 102, 734
Parepectolin, 747
Parlodel, 9, 89-90
Parlodel SnapTabs, 89-90
Parnate, 6, 679-680, 731
paroxetine, 6, 509-510, 731
Parsidol, 5, 9, 255-256, 732
Parsitan, 255-256
Partuss LA, 743
Patanol, 7, 15, 490
Pathocil, 199-200
Pavabid, 508-509
Pavacels, 508-509
Pavacot, 508-509
Pavagen, 508-509
Pavarine, 508-509
Pavased, 508-509
Pavatine, 508-509
Pavatym, 508-509
Paverolan, 508-509
Paxil, 6, 509-510, 731
Paxil CR, 509-510
Paxipam, 311-312, 730
PBZ, 7, 698-699, 731
PBZ-SR, 698-699
PCE Dispertab, 242-244
Pedaject-50, 551-553
Pedalone TBA, 551-553
Pedia Care Allergy Formula, 137-138
PediaCare Infant's, 576-577
Pediaflor, 618-620
Pediapred, 551-553
Pediazole, 747
Pedicort-RP, 551-553
Pedi-Dent, 618-620
Peganone, 5, 257-258
pemoline, 510
Penbritin, 48-50
penbutolol, 8, 510-512, 738
penciclovir, 10, 737
penciclovir cream, 512-513
Penecort, 322-323
Penetrex, 12, 234-235
Penglobe, 68-69
penicillin G benzathine, 15, 513-514
PENICILLINS, 15
penicillin V potassium/penicillin V, 15, 514-515
Pentacarinat, 515-516
Pentam 300, 15, 515-516
pentamidine/pentamidine isethionate, 9, 15, 515-516
Pentasa, 414-415
Penta-Valproic, 703-705
Pentazine, 566-567
Pentazine VC with Codeine Liquid, 747
pentazocine, 4, 734
pentazocine HCl/pentazocine lactate, 516-517
pentobarbital/pentobarbital sodium, 5, 10, 518-519
pentoxifylline, 15, 16, 519-520, 738
Pen-Vee K, 514-515
Pepcid, 7, 263-264, 737
Pepcid AC Acid Controller, 263-264
Pepcid IV, 263-264
Pepcid RPD, 263-264
PEPTIDE ANTIINFECTIVES, 15
Pepto-Bismol, 6, 85, 736
Pepto-Bismol Maximum Strength, 85
Pepto Diarrhea Control, 388-389
Peptol, 146-147
Percocet, 504-505, 747
Percocet 2.5/325, 747
Percocet 5/325, 747
Percocet 7.5/500, 747
Percocet 10/650, 747
Percocet-Demi, 504-505
Percodan, 504-505, 747
Percodan-Demi, 747
Percogesic, 747
Percolone, 504-505
pergolide, 9, 737
pergolide mesylate, 520-521
Periactin, 7, 178-178
Peri-Colace, 747
Peridex, 8, 10, 132-133
Peridol, 313-315
Peri-Dos, 747
PeriGard, 8
perindopril, 8, 731, 738
perindopril erbumine, 521-523
PerioChip, 15, 133

Entries can be identified as follows: generic name, Trade Name, DRUG CATEGORY, *Combination Product.*

PERIODONTAL SPECIALTY PRODUCTS, 15
PerioGard, 132-133
Periostat, 15, 16, 224-225
PERIPHERAL VASCULAR DISEASE DRUGS, 15
Permapen, 513-514
Permax, 9, 520-521, 737
Permitil, 282-284
Permitil Concentrate HCl, 282-284
perphenazine, 9, 523-524, 732
Persantine, 15, 214
Pertofrane, 187-188
Pertussin CS and ES, 195-196
pethidine, 407-408
peyote, 734
Phenameth, 566-567
Phenazine, 566-567
Phenazo, 525
Phenazodine, 525
phenazopyridine, 16
phenazopyridine HCl, 525
Phencen-50, 566-567
phencyclidine, 734
phendimetrazine, 4, 10, 730, 734, 736
phendimetrazine tartrate, 525-526
Phendry, 211-212
phenelzine, 731
phenelzine sulfate, 6, 526-528
Phenerbel-S, 740
Phenergan, 5, 7, 566-567, 731
Phenergan Fortis, 566-567
Phenergan Plain, 566-567
Phenergan VC Syrup, 747
Phenergan with Codeine Syrup, 747
Phenetron, 137-138
phenobarbital, 5, 6, 10, 528-529, 730, 734
PHENOTHIAZINES, 9
phenoxybenzamine, 8
phenoxybenzamine HCl, 529-530
phensuximide, 6, 530-531
Phentercot, 531-532
phentermine, 4, 10, 730, 736
phentermine HCl/phentermine resin, 531-532
phentolamine, 8
phentolamine mesylate, 532-533
Phentride, 531-532
phenylephrine, 11, 16, 738
phenylephrine HCl (nasal), 533-534
Phenylgesic, 747
phenylpropanolamine, 731, 732
Phenytex, 534-536
phenytoin, 6, 736
phenytoin sodium/phenytoin sodium extended/phenytoin sodium prompt, 534-536
Pherazine with Codeine Syrup, 747
Pheryl-E, 711-712
Phyllocontin, 38-39
Phyllocontin-350, 38-39
phytonadione, 16, 536, 738
Pilagan, 537
Pilocar, 537
pilocarpine, 13, 16, 738
pilocarpine HCl (oral), 537-538
pilocarpine HCl/pilocarpine nitrate (optic), 537
pilocarpine (optic), 15
Piloptic, 537
Pilostat, 537
pimoline, 11
pimozide, 9, 539-540, 732, 737
pindolol, 8, 540-541
pioglitazone, 6, 541-542
pirbuterol, 11, 737
pirbuterol acetate, 542-543
piroxicam, 9, 15, 543-544, 731
Pitrex, 671
Plaquenil, 9
Plaquenil Sulfate, 324-325
PLATELET AGGREGATION INHIBITORS, 15
Plavix, 15, 162-163
Plegine, 525-526
Plendil, 5, 8, 265-266
Pletal, 15, 145-146
PMS-Baclofen, 69-70
PMS Benzotropine, 74-76
PMS-bismuth subsalicylate, 85
PMS Carbamazepine, 105-106
PMS-Cephalexin, 123-124
PMS-Chloral Hydrate, 129-130
PMS-Cimetidine, 146-147
PMS-Clonazepam, 160-161
PMS-Cyproheptadine, 178-178
PMS Diazepam, 196-197
PMS-Dimenhydrinate, 210-211
PMS Haloperidol, 313-315
PMS-Hydromorphone, 323-324
PMS-Isoniazid, 345-346
PMS-Levothyroxine, 375

Entries can be identified as follows: generic name, Trade Name, DRUG CATEGORY, *Combination Product.*

PMS-Lithium Carbonate, 384-385
PMS-Lithium Citrate, 384-385
PMS-Loperamide Hydrochloride, 388-389
PMS-Methylphenidate, 430-431
PMS-Metoclopramide, 433-434
PMS-Oxtriphylline, 502-503
PMS Perphenazine, 523-524
PMS-Piroxicam, 543-544
PMS-Primidone, 557-558
PMS Prochlorperazine, 561-563
PMS-Procyclidine, 563-564
PMS-Propranolol, 572-574
PMS-Pyrazinamide, 577-578
PMS-Sodium Chromglycate, 171-172
PMS-Sulfasalazine, 631-632
PMS-Theophylline, 652-653
PMS-Trifluoperazine, 689-690
PMS-Trihexyphenidyl, 692-693
PMS-Valproic Acid, 703-705
PNEUMOCYSTIC PNEUMONITIS DRUGS, 15
Pneumopent, 515-516
Polaramine, 7, 193-194
Polaramine Repetabs, 193-194
Polocaine, 411-412
Polocaine/Levonordefrin, 411-412
Polocaine MPF, 411-412
Polycillin, 48-50
Polycillin-N, 48-50
Polydine, 547-548
Polymox, 46-48
polymyxin, 15
polymyxin B ophthalmic, 4
polymyxin B sulfate (ophthalmic), 544-545
polythiazide, 12, 545-546, 738
Ponstan, 404-405
Ponstel, 15, 404-405
Pontocaine, 4, 648-649
Pontocaine Cream, 648-649
Posicor, 8
potassium bicarbonate/potassium acetate/potassium chloride/ potassium gluconate/potassium phosphate, 14, 546-547
povidone iodine, 8, 547-548
PP-Cap, 571-572
pramipexole, 9
pramipexole dihydrochloride, 548-549, 737
Prandase, 20-21
Prandin, 6, 590-592
Pravachol, 8, 11, 549
pravastatin, 8, 11
pravastatin sodium, 549
prazosin, 8, 731
prazosin HCl, 549-550
Precose, 6, 20-21
Predalone-50, 551-553
Predate S, 551-553
Predcor-25 and 50, 551-553
Predcor-TBA, 551-553
Predicort-50, 551-553
prednicarbate, 13, 550-551
Prednicen-M, 553-554
prednisolone/prednisolone acetate/ prednisolone phosphate/prednisolone tebutate, 13, 551-553
Prednisol TBA, 551-553
prednisone, 13, 14, 553-554
Prednisone Intensol, 553-554
Pregnancy categories, 735
Prelone, 551-553
Prelu-2, 4, 10, 525-526
Premarin, 12, 248-249
Premphase, 747
Prempro, 747
Premsym PMS, 746
Prevacid, 13, 361-362, 736
Prevalite, 143-144
Preventil, 737
Prevex B, 77-78
Prevex-HC, 322-323
Prevident, 620-621
Prevident 5000 Plus, 620-621
Prevpac, 747
Priftin, 10, 595-597
prilocaine, 4
prilocaine hydrochloride, 554-556
Prilosec, 13, 491-492, 736
Primabalt, 172-173
primaquine, 9
primaquine phosphate, 556-557
Primatene Mist Suspension, 238-239
Primatine, 11
Primatine Mist, 238-239
Primaxin IM, 747
Primaxin IV, 747
primidone, 6, 557-558
Principen, 48-50
Prinivil, 8, 383-384
Prinzide, 747

Entries can be identified as follows: generic name, Trade Name, DRUG CATEGORY, *Combination Product.*

Prinzide 12.5, 750
Prinzide 25, 747, 750
Probalan, 558-559
Pro-Banthine, 5, 568-569, 730, 736
Probate, 413-414
probenecid, 9, 558-559
procainamide, 6
procainamide HCl, 559-560
Procan SR, 559-560
procarbazine, 11
procarbazine HCl, 560-561
Procardia, 5, 476-477
Procardia SL, 476-477
Procardia XL, 8, 476-477, 738
prochlorperazine, 7, 9, 732, 737
prochlorperazine edisylate/ prochlorperazine maleate, 561-563
Procnbid, 559-560
Procyclid, 563-564
procyclidine, 9
procyclidine HCl, 563-564
Procytox, 175-176
Profen LA, 747-748
Prograf, 14, 638-639
Prolixin, 9
Prolixin Concentrate, 282-284
Prolixin Decanoate, 282-284
Prolixin Enanthate, 282-284
promazine, 9, 732
promazine HCl, 564-566
promethazine, 5, 7, 731
promethazine HCl, 566-567
Promethazine HCl VC, 747
Prometh VC Plain, 747
Prometh with Codeine Syrup, 747
Promine, 559-560
Pronestyl, 6, 559-560
Pronestyl SR, 559-560
Propacet 100, 742
propafenone, 6, 567-568, 738
Propanthel, 568-569
propantheline, 5, 730, 736
propantheline bromide, 568-569
Propecia, 14, 271-272
Propine C, 13, 15
Propine C Cap B.I.D., 213
propofol, 4, 569-571, 736
propoxyphene, 734
propoxyphene napsylate/propoxyphene HCl, 4, 571-572
Propoxyphene Napsylate with Acetaminophen Tablets, 742
propranolol, 4, 6, 8, 14
propranolol HCl, 572-574
Propranolol HCl, 745
Propulsid, 13
propylthiouracil, 10, 574-575, 737
Propyl-Thyracil, 574-575
Prorazin, 561-563
Prorex, 566-567
Proscar, 12, 15, 271-272
Pro-Sof Plus, 747
ProSom, 5, 244, 737
PROSTAGLANDINS, 15
Prostaphlin, 15, 497-498
PROSTATE HYPERPLASIA DRUGS, 15
ProStep, 16
Prostigmin, 11, 14
Prostigmin Bromide/Prostigmin, 470-471
Protilase, 507-508
Protostat, 437-439
protriptyline, 6, 736
protriptyline HCl, 575-576
Proventil, 10, 28-29, 732
Proventil HFA, 28-29
Proventil Repetabs, 28-29
Provera, 12, 403-404
Provigil, 11, 449-450, 733
Proviodine, 547-548
Proxipam, 5
Prozac, 6, 280-281, 731, 736
Pseudo-Chlor, 742
pseudoephedrine, 11, 732
pseudoephedrine HCl/pseudoephedrine sulfate, 576-577
Pseudogest, 576-577
Psorcon, 204
ptu, 574-575
Pulmacort Turbuhaler, 91-93
Pulmozyme, 14, 220
Purinethol, 11, 414
Purinol, 30-31
PVFK, 514-515
pyrazinamide, 10, 577-578
Pyribenzamine, 731
Pyridiate, 525
Pyridium, 16, 525
Pyridium Plus, 748
pyridostigmine, 11, 14
pyridostigmine bromide, 578-579
pyridoxine, 16
pyridoxine HCl, 579-580

Q

Q-Profen, 328-330
quanadrel, 8
quanethidine, 8
Quarzan, 5, 152-153, 736
quazepam, 5, 580-581, 737
Questran, 8, 143-144
Questran Lite, 143-144
quetiapine, 9
quetiapine fumarate, 581-582, 737
Quibron-T, 652-653
Quinaglute, 6, 583-585
Quinalan, 583-585
quinapril, 8, 582-583
Quinate, 583-585
Quinidex Extentabs, 583-585
quinidine, 6, 738
quinidine gluconate/quinidine polygalacturonate/quinidine sulfate, 583-585
quinine, 9
quinine sulfate, 585-586
Quinora, 583-585
quinupristin/dalfopristin, 586

R

rabeprazole, 13, 732
rabeprazole sodium, 586-587
Radiostol Forte, 710-711
raloxifene, 7, 12
raloxifene hydrochloride, 587-588
ramipril, 8, 588-590
ranitidine, 7, 590
Rauzide, 748
Reactine, 126-127
Rebetron, 748
Regitine, 8, 532-533
Reglan, 7, 13, 433-434
Regonol, 578-579
Regranex, 16
Regranex Gel, 70-71
Regroton, 748
Regulace, 747
Regular Iletin I, 337-338
Regular Iletin II, 337-338
Regular Purified Pork Insulin, 337-338
Relafen, 9, 15, 457-458
Relaxazone, 142-143
Relenza, 10, 716-717
Remeron, 6, 446-447
Remular, 142-143
Remular-S, 142-143
Renedil, 265-266
Renese, 12, 545-546, 738
Renese-R, 748
Renova, 682
repaglinide, 6, 590-592
Repan, 743
Rep-Pred 40, 431-432
Rep-Pred 80, 431-432
ReQuip, 9, 605-607
Resaid, 739
Rescon ED, 742
Rescriptor, 10, 184-186, 737
Reserfia, 592-593
reserpine, 7, 592-593, 731
Respa DM, 744
Respbid, 652-653
resperidone, 732
Restoril, 5, 642-643, 733
Resyl, 306-307
Retin-A, 12, 682
Retin-A Regimen Kit, 682
retinoic acid, 682
RETINOIDS, SYSTEMIC, 738
Retrovir, 10, 717-718, 737
Revex, 4, 460-461
ReVia, 4, 462-463
Rezulin, 6, 699-700
R-Gel, 103-104
Rheumatrex, 9, 426-427
Rhinalar, 277-278
Rhinall, 533-534
Rhinocaps, 748
Rhinocort, 738
Rhinocort Inhalant, 13
Rhinocort Nasal Inhaler, 91-93
Rhinolar-EX 12 Hour, 739
Rhinosyn-X Liquid, 748
Rhodis, 354-356
Rhodis-E, 354-356
Rho-Loperamide, 388-389
Rhotrimine, 697-698
riboflavin, 16, 593
Ridaura, 9, 61-62, 737
rifabutin, 10, 593-594
Rifadin, 10, 594-595
Rifadin IV, 594-595
Rifamate, 748
rifampin, 10, 594-595
rifapentine, 10, 595-597
Rifater, 748
Rilutek, 4, 597-598
riluzole, 4, 597-598

Entries can be identified as follows: generic name, Trade Name, DRUG CATEGORY, *Combination Product.*

Rimactane, 594-595
rimantadine, 10, 737
rimantadine HCl, 598-599
rimexolone, 13, 599, 738
Rinade B.I.D., 742
Riopan, 4, 396-397, 736
Riopan Extra Strength, 396-397
risedronate, 7
risedronate sodium, 600
Risperdal, 9, 600-602, 732, 737
risperidone, 9, 600-602, 737
Ritalin, 11, 430-431
Ritalin SR, 430-431
ritonavir, 10, 602-603, 737
Rivotril, 160-161
rizatriptan, 14, 733
rizatriptan benzoate, 603-604
RMS, 454-455
Robaxin, 16, 425-426, 738
Robaxin 750, 425-426
Robaxisal, 748
Robidex, 195-196
Robidone, 319-320
Robidrine, 576-577
Robigesic, 21-22
Robinul, 5, 304-305
Robinul Forte, 304-305
Robitet, 649-651
Robitussin, 10, 306-307
Robitussin-DM, 748
Robitussin Pediatric, 195-196
Rocaltrol, 710-711
Rofact, 594-595
rofecoxib, 9, 15, 604-605, 731, 737
Roferon-A, 11, 13, 738
Roferon A, 338-339
Rogaine, 12, 14
Rogaine for Men, 445-446
Rogaine for Women, 445-446
Rogitine, 532-533
Romazicon, 4, 276-277
Romyin, 242
ropinirole, 9
ropinirole HCl, 605-607
rosiglitazone, 6
rosiglitazone maleate, 607-608
Rota caps, 71-72
Roubac, 630-631
Rounax, 21-22
Rowasa, 414-415
Roxanol, 454-455
Roxanol SR, 454-455
Roxicet 5/500, 749
Roxicodone, 4, 504-505
Roxicodone Intensol, 504-505
Roxicodone SR, 504-505
Roxilox, 749
Roxiprin, 504-505, 747
Rubesol, 172-173
Rubramin, 16
Rubramin PC, 172-173
Rufen, 328-330
Ru-Tuss DE, 743
Ru-Tuss Expectorant Liquid, 748
Rymed TR, 743
Rynacrom, 171-172
Rynatan, 748
Rythmodan, 215-216
Rythmodan-LA, 215-216
Rythmol, 6, 567-568, 738

S

St. John's wort, 763
Sal-Adult, 55-56
Salagen, 16, 537-538, 738
Salazopyrin EN-Tab, 631-632
Salflex, 609-610
Sal-Infant, 55-56
SALIVARY STIMULANTS, 16, 738
salmeterol, 10
salmeterol xinafoate, 608-609
Salofalk, 414-415
salsalate, 4, 9, 609-610
Salsitab, 609-610
Sal-Tropine, 5, 59-60
Sandimmune, 14, 177-178
Sandimmune SGC, 177-178
SangCya, 177-178
Sanorex, 399-400, 730
Sansert, 14, 432-433
saquinavir, 10, 737
saquinavir mesylate, 610-611
SAS-500, 631-632
saw palmetto, 763
scopolamine, 7, 730
scopolamine tolterodine, 5
scopolamine (transdermal), 611-612
SD Deprenyl, 613-615
secobarbital/secobarbital sodium, 5, 10, 612-613
Seconal, 5, 10, 612-613
SEDATIVE-HYPNOTICS, 5, 733, 737

Entries can be identified as follows: generic name, Trade Name, DRUG CATEGORY, *Combination Product.*

Sedatuss, 195-196
selegiline, 9
selegiline HCl, 613-615
Selestoject, 78-80
Semilente Iletin I, 337-338
Sensorcaine, 94-96
Sensorcaine-MPF, 94-96
Sensorcaine-MPF with Epinephrine, 94-96
Sensorcaine with Epinephrine, 94-96
Septra, 16, 630-631
Ser-Ap-Es, 744
Serax, 5, 501, 730
Serentil, 9, 415-417
Serentil Concentrate, 415-417
Serevent, 10, 608-609
Serevent Diskus, 608-609
Seromycin, 10
Seromycin Pulvules, 176-177
Serophene, 158
Seroquel, 9, 581-582, 737
SEROTONIN-SPECIFIC REUPTAKE INHIBITORS, 6
Serpasil, 8, 731
Sertan, 557-558
sertraline, 6, 615-616, 731, 736
Serzone, 6, 467-468, 736
Shogan, 566-567
Shovite, 172-173
sibutramine, 4, 10, 616-617
Siladryl, 211-212
sildenafil, 12
sildenafil citrate, 617-618
Simiron, 270-271
Simplet Tablets, 748
simvastatin, 8, 618
Sinemet, 9, 371-372, 732, 737
Sinemet CR, 371-372
Sine-off Sinus Medicine, 741
Sinequan, 5, 6, 223-224, 731, 736
Sinex, 533-534
Sinex Long-Lasting, 505
Singlet for Adults Tablets, 748
Singulair, 10, 14, 452-453
Sinutab Maximum Strength Sinus Allergy, 741
SINUvent, 747-748
SKELETAL MUSCLE RELAXANTS, 16, 738
Skelid, 7, 660-661
Sleep-Eze-D, 211-212
Slo-Bid, 652-653
Slo-Niacin, 472-473
Slo-Phyllin, 652-653
Slow-Fe, 270-271
Slow-K, 546-547
SMOKING CESSATION DRUGS, 16
SMZ/TMP, 630-631
sodium fluoride, 5, 14, 618-620
sodium fluoride (topical), 620-621
Sodium Sulamyd, 627-628
Sodol Compound, 741
Sofarin, 712-713
Solazine, 689-690
Solfoton, 528-529
Solganal, 9, 62-63, 737
Solu-Cortef, 320-322
Solu-Flur, 618-620
Solu-Medrol, 431-432
Solurex, 192-193
Solurex-LA, 192-193
Soma, 16, 107
Soma Compound, 741
Sominex Formula, 211-212
Somnol, 284-285
Somophyllin, 10, 16, 738
Sonata, 5, 715-716, 730
Sorbitrate, 347-348
Sorbitrate SA, 347-348
Soriatane, 12, 25-26, 738
Sotacor, 621-622
sotalol, 6
sotalol HCl, 621-622
sparfloxacin, 12, 622-623
Sparine, 9, 564-566, 732
Spasmoban, 200-201
Spasmolin, 743
Spectazole, 7, 230
Spectrobid, 15, 68-69
Spectro-Homatropine, 316-317
spironolactone, 12, 623-624, 732
Sporanox, 7, 352-353
S-P-T, 658
Stagesic, 740
Stamoist LA, 743
stanozolol, 12, 624-625
Staticin, 242
stavudine, 10, 625-626
Stelazine, 9, 689-690, 732
Stemetic, 695
Stemetil, 561-563
Sterapred, 553-554
Stieva-A, 682

Entries can be identified as follows: generic name, Trade Name, DRUG CATEGORY, *Combination Product.*

Stieva-A Forte, 682
Stimate, 188-189
Stimate Nasal Spray, 188-189
Storzolamide, 22-23
Strifton Forte DSC, 142-143
sucralfate, 13, 626-627, 736
Sudafed, 11, 576-577, 732
Sudafed Cold and Cough Liquid Caps, 742
Sudafed Liquid, 576-577
Sudafed 12 Hour, 576-577
Sudafed 12 Hour Caplets, 748
Sulamyd (optic), 15
Sulamyd Sodium, 16
Sular, 8, 477-479
sulconazole, 7
sulconazole nitrate, 627
Sulcrate, 626-627
sulfacetamide, 15
sulfacetamide sodium, 16, 627-628
Sulfair, 627-628
sulfamethizole, 16, 628-629
sulfamethoxazole, 16, 629-630
sulfamethoxazole/trimethoprim, 15, 16, 630-631
Sulfare-Forte, 627-628
sulfasalazine, 13, 631-632, 737
Sulfatrim, 630-631
Sulfex, 627-628
sulfinpyrazone, 16, 632-633
sulfisoxazole, 16, 633-634
Sulfizole, 633-634
SULFONAMIDES, 16
sulindac, 9, 15, 634-635, 736
Sultrin Triple Sulfa, 749
sumatriptan, 14
sumatriptan succinate, 635-636
Sumycin, 649-651
Supasa, 55-56
Supeudol, 504-505
Suprax, 11, 116-117
Surgicel, 13, 501-502
Surmontil, 6, 697-698
Susano Elixir, 743
Sus-Phrine Suspension, 238-239
Sustiva, 10, 230-232, 732, 737
Symadine, 33-34
Symmetrel, 9, 10, 33-34
Synacort, 322-323
Synalgos-DC, 748
Syn-Clonazepam, 160-161
Syn-Diltiazem, 209-210
Synercid I.V., 586
Synflex, 464-465
Synflex DS, 464-465
Syn-Nadolo, 458-460
Syn-Pindolol, 540-541
Synthroid, 12, 375

T

T_3, 381-382
T_4, 375
Tabrex, 15
Tac-3, 684-686
tacrine, 4, 11
tacrine HCl, 636-638
tacrolimus, 14, 638-639
Tagamet, 7, 146-147
Tagamet HB (OTC), 146-147
Tagamet HB 200 (OTC), 146-147
Talacen, 748
Talwin, 516-517
Talwin Compound Caplets, 748
Talwin NX, 4, 516-517
Tambocor, 6, 272-273, 738
Tamiflu, 10, 497
Tamofen, 639-640
Tamone, 639-640
Tamoplex, 639-640
tamoxifen, 11, 738
tamoxifen citrate, 639-640
tamsulosin, 15
tamsulosin HCl, 640-641
Tapazole, 10, 424-425, 737
Tarka 1:240, 748
Tarka 2:180, 748
Tarka 2:240, 748
Tarka 4:240, 748
Tasmar, 9, 668-669, 732
Taste, drugs affecting, 736-738
Tavist, 7, 152
Tavist-1, 152
Tavist-D, 748
Tavist Sinus, 744
Taxol, 11, 506-507
tazarotene, 12
tazarotene topical, 641
Tazorac, 12, 641
T-Diet, 531-532
Tebamide, 695
Tebrazid, 577-578
Teczem, 748
Teen Midol, 748
Tegamide, 695

Entries can be identified as follows: generic name, Trade Name, DRUG CATEGORY, *Combination Product.*

Tegopen, 15, 165-166
Tegretol, 5, 105-106, 730
Tegretol Chewtabs, 105-106
Tegretol CR, 105-106
Tegretol XR, 105-106
Telachlor, 137-138
Teldrin, 137-138
telmisartan, 8, 642
temazepam, 5, 642-643, 733
Temovate, 13, 155
Temovate Emollient Cream, 155
Temovate Gel, 155
Tempra, 21-22
Tenex, 8, 310-311, 738
Ten-K, 546-547
Tenoretic 50, 748
Tenoretic 100, 748
Tenormin, 4, 8, 56-58
Ten-Tab, 202-203
Tenuate, 4, 10, 202-203, 730, 736
Tenuate Dospan, 202-203
Tepanil, 202-203, 730
Teramine, 531-532
Terazol, 7
Terazol 3, 646
Terazol 7, 646
terazosin, 8, 15
terazosin HCl, 643-644
terbinafine, 7, 736
terbinafine HCl, 644-645
terbutaline, 11, 737
terbutaline sulfate, 645-646
terconazole, 7, 646
Terfluzine, 689-690
Terra-Cortril Suspension, 748
Tessalon, 10, 74
Testaderm, 647-648
Testamone-100, 647-648
Testaqua, 647-648
Testex, 647-648
Testoject, 647-648
Testoject-50, 647-648
Testone LA, 647-648
testosterone/testosterone cypionate/ testosterone enanthate/ testosterone propionate, 12, 647-648, 734
Test-PA, 647-648
Testred Cypionate, 647-648
tetracaine/tetracaine HCl (topical), 4, 648-649
TETRACYCLICS, 6
tetracycline fiber, 16
tetracycline periodontal fiber, 651
TETRACYCLINES, 16
tetracycline/tetracycline HCl, 16, 649-651
Tetracyn, 649-651
Teveten, 8, 239-240
T-Gen, 695
T-Gesic, 740
Thalitone, 141-142
Theo-24, 652-653
Theobid, 652-653
Theoclear, 652-653
Theo-Dur, 11, 16, 652-653, 738
Theo-Dur Sprinkle, 652-653
Theolair, 652-653
theophylline ethylenediamine, 38-39
theophylline/theophylline sodium glycinate, 11, 16, 652-653, 738
Theovent, 652-653
TheraFlu Cough and Cold Medicine Powder, 748
Thera-Flu Non-Drowsy Flu, 743
Theramycin-Z, 242
thiamine, 16
thiamine HCl, 653-654
thiethylperazine, 7
thiethylperazine maleate, 654
thiopental, 734
thioridazine, 9, 732
thioridazine HCl, 654-656
Thiosulfil Forte, 16, 628-628, 748
thiothixene, 9, 656-657, 732
thioxanthene, 9
Thorazine, 7, 9, 138-140, 732
Thor-Prom, 138-140
3TC, 10, 359-360
Thyrar, 658
thyroid, 12
Thyroid Strong, 658
thyroid usp (desiccated), 658
Thyrolar, 382
L-thyroxine sodium, 375
tiagabine, 6
tiagabine HCl, 658-660
Tiamate, 209-210
Tiazac, 209-210
Ticlid, 15, 660
ticlopidine, 15, 660
Ticon, 695
Tigan, 7, 695
Tilade, 14, 466-467, 737

Entries can be identified as follows: generic name, Trade Name, DRUG CATEGORY, *Combination Product.*

tiludronate, 7
tiludronate disodium, 660-661
Time-Hist, 742
Timentin Inj, 748
Timodal, 663-664
Timolide 10/25, 748
timolol, 8, 13, 14, 15
timolol maleate, 661-664
Timoptic, 13, 15
Timoptic Solution, 663-664
Timoptic-XE, 663-664
Tinactin, 7, 671
Ting, 671
Tipramine, 330-332
tizanidine, 14
tizanidine HCl, 664-665
tobramycin ophthalmic, 4, 15, 665
Tobrex, 4, 665
tocainide, 6
tocainide HCl, 665-666
Tofranil, 6, 330-332, 731, 736
Tofranil-PM Capsules, 330-332
tolazamide, 6, 666-667
tolbutamide, 6, 667-668, 736
tolcapone, 9, 668-669, 732
Tolectin, 9, 15, 670-671
Tolectin DS, 670-671
Tolinase, 6, 666-667
tolmetin, 9, 15
tolmetin sodium, 670-671
tolnaftate, 7, 671
Tol-Tab, 667-668
tolterodine, 732
tolterodine tartrate, 671-672
Tonocard, 6, 665-666
Topamax, 6, 672-673, 736
Topicort, 13, 190-191
Topicort LP, 190-191
Topicort Mild, 190-191
Topilene, 77-78
topiramate, 6, 672-673, 736
Topisone, 77-78
Toprol XL, 436-437
Topsyn, 278-279
Toradol, 15, 356-357
Torecan, 7, 654
toremifene, 11
toremifene citrate, 673-674
Tornalate, 10, 87-88, 737
torsemide, 12, 674-675
Totacillin, 48-50
Totacillin-N, 48-50
TracTabs 2X, 748
tramadol, 4
tramadol HCl, 675-676
Trancot, 413-414
Trandate, 357-359, 738
trandolapril, 8, 677-678
tranexamic acid, 13, 678-679
Transderm-Nitro, 480-481
Transderm Scop, 7, 611-612, 730
Transderm-V, 611-612
Tranxene, 5, 163-164
Tranxene-SD, 163-164
tranylcypromine, 731
tranylcypromine sulfate, 6, 679-680
Traveltabs, 210-211
Traxene T-Tab, 163-164
trazodone, 6
trazodone HCl, 680-681
Trazon, 680-681
Trecator, 10
Trecator-SC, 254-255, 737
Trendar, 328-330
Trental, 15, 16, 519-520, 738
tretinoin, 12, 682
Trexan, 462-463
Triacet, 686
Triad, 749
Triadapin, 223-224
Triaderm, 686
Trialodine, 680-681
Triam-A, 684-686
triamcinolone acetonide, 682-683
triamcinolone acetonide (topical), 686
triamcinolone (inhalant), 13
triamcinolone topical, 13
triamcinolone/triamcinolone acetonide/ triamcinolone diacetate/ triamcinolone hexacetonide, 13, 684-686
Triam Forte, 684-686
Triaminic-12, 739
Triaminic-DM Syrup, 749
Triaminicol Multi-Symptom Cough and Cold Tablets, 741
Triamolone 40, 684-686
Triamonide 40, 684-686
triamterene, 12, 686-687, 732
Trianide, 686
Triavil, 732
Triavil 2-10, 743
Triavil 2-25, 743

Entries can be identified as follows: generic name, Trade Name, DRUG CATEGORY, *Combination Product.*

Triavil 4-10, 743
Triavil 4-25, 743
Triavil 4-50, 749
triazolam, 5, 687-688, 733
Triban, 695
Tribenzagan, 695
Tricor, 8
TriCor, 266-267
TRICYCLICS, 6
Tri-derm, 686
Tridesilon, 189-190
Tridil, 480-481
Tridione, 6, 693-694
trifluoperazine, 9, 732
trifluoperazine HCl, 689-690
triflupromazine, 7, 9, 737
triflupromazine HCl, 690-692
trifluridine, 15, 692
TriHemic 600, 749
Trihexane, 692-693
Trihexy, 692-693
trihexyphenidyl, 9, 732
trihexyphenidyl HCl, 692-693
Tri-Hydroserpine, 744
Trikacide, 437-439
Tri-Kort, 684-686
Trilafon, 9, 523-524
Tri-Levlen, 493-495
Trilog, 684-686
Trilone, 684-686
trimethadione, 6, 693-694
trimethobenzamide, 7, 695
trimetrexate, 13, 15
trimetrexate glucuronate, 695-696
trimipramine, 6
trimipramine maleate, 697-698
Trimox, 46-48
Trinalin Repetabs, 749
Tri-Norinyl, 493-495
Trinsicon, 749
Triostat, 381-382
tripelennamine, 7, 731
tripelennamine HCl, 698-699
Triphasil, 493-495
Triple Sulfa, 749
Triposed, 739
triprolidine with pseudoephedrine, 731
Triptil, 575-576
Triptone Caplets, 210-211
Tristoject, 684-686
Tritec, 749
Trivora, 493-495
troglitazone, 6, 699-700
trovafloxacin, 12
trovafloxacin mesylate/alatrofloxacin mesylate, 700-701
Trovan, 12, 700-701
Trovan IV, 12
Trovan I.V., 700-701
Truphylline, 38-39
Trusopt, 13, 221, 738
Trysul, 749
T-Stat, 242
Tums, 736
Tussafed HC Syrup, 749
Tussi-Organidin, 745
Tussi-Organidin DM, 745
Tussi-Organidin DM NR, 749
Tusso-DM, 745
Tusstat, 211-212
12 Hour Sinarest, 505
Tylenol, 21-22
Tylenol Arthritis Extended Relief, 21-22
Tylenol Children's Cold Tablets, 749
Tylenol Flu Night Time Maximum Strength (powder), 749
Tylenol Multi-Symptom Hot Medication (powder), 749
Tylenol PM Extra Strength, 749
Tylenol with Codeine Elixir, 741
Tylenol with Codeine No. 2, 749
Tylenol with Codeine No. 3, 739, 749
Tylenol with Codeine No. 4, 749
Tylox, 504-505, 749

U

U-500, 337-338
UAA, 749
Ulcidine-HB, 263-264
UL-RAbrom PD, 740
Ultracaine, 377-379
Ultralente, 337-338
Ultralente I, 337-338
Ultram, 4, 675-676
Ultrase MT, 507-508
Ultravate, 13, 312-313
Unasyn Inj, 749
Uni-Bent Unisom, 211-212
Unicort, 322-323
Uni-Dur, 652-653
Uniphyl, 652-653
Unipres, 744

Entries can be identified as follows: generic name, Trade Name, DRUG CATEGORY, *Combination Product.*

Uniretic 7.5, 749
Uniretic 15, 749
Unisom Nighttime Sleep Aid, 749
Unisom With Pain Relief, 749
Univasc, 8, 450-451
Urabeth, 82
Urecholine, 11, 82
Urex, 423-424
URICOSURICS, 16
Uridon, 141-142
Uridon Modified, 749
URINARY TRACT INFECTION DRUGS, 16
Urised, 749
Urisedamine, 749
Urispas, 16, 272
Uritin, 749
Uritol, 296-297
Urodine, 525
Urogesic, 525
Urozide, 318-319
ursodiol, 5, 13, 702, 738
Ursofalk, 702

V

valacyclovir, 10, 737
valacyclovir HCl, 702-703
Valadol, 21-22
Valergen, 246-247
valerian, 764
Valisone, 77-78
Valisone Reduced Strength, 77-78
Valium, 5, 196-197, 730
Valnac, 77-78
valproic acid/valproate sodium/ divalproex sodium, 6, 10, 703-705
valsartan, 8, 705, 738
Valtrex, 10, 702-703, 737
Vanadom, 107
Vancenase AQ, 71-72
Vancenase AQ Forte, 71-72
Vancenase Nasal, 71-72
Vanceril, 71-72
Vanceril 84 μg Double Strength, 71-72
Vanceril DS, 71-72
Vanceril Inhalant, 13
Vancocin, 15, 705-706
vancomycin, 15
vancomycin HCl, 705-706
Vanex Expectorant Liquid, 743
Vanquish Caplets, 749
Vantin, 11, 117-118
Vaponefrin, 238-239
Vascor, 5, 8, 76-77, 738
Vaseretic 10-25, 750
Vaseretic 5-12.5, 749
VasoClear, 463-464
Vasocon, 463-464
VASOCONSTRICTORS, 16
Vasodilan, 15, 350-351
Vasotec, 8, 232-234, 731, 738
Vasotec IV, 232-234
V-Cillin K, 15, 514-515
Vectrin, 444-445
Veetids, 514-515
Velosef, 11, 124-125
Velosulin Human BR, 337-338
Veltane, 90-91
venlafaxine, 6, 731
venlafaxine HCl, 706-708
Ventlin Nebules, 28-29
Ventodisk, 28-29
Ventolin, 10, 28-29, 732
Ventolin Rotacaps, 28-29
verapamil/verapamil HCl, 5, 8, 708-709
Verelan, 708-709
Versed, 4, 5, 440-442, 736
Vertab, 210-211
Vesant, 546-547
Vesprin, 7, 9, 690-692, 737
Vexol, 13, 599, 738
V-Gan, 566-567
Viagra, 12, 617-618
Vi-Atrol, 212-213
Vibal, 172-173
Vibedoz, 172-173
Vibramycin, 16, 225-226
Vibra-Tabs, 225-226
Vicks Children's Cough/Cold Liquid, 750
Vicks Children's NyQuil Nighttime Cough/Cold Liquid, 750
Vicks Cough Silencers, 750
Vicks DayQuil Allergy Relief 4 Hour, 742
Vicks Formula 44D Cough and Decongestant Liquid, 750
Vicks Formula 44M Cold, Flu and Cough Capsules, 750
Vicks 44 Non-Drowsy Cold and Cough LiquiCaps, 743
Vicodin, 740, 750
Vicodin-ES, 750

Vicodin-HP, 750
Vicoprofen, 750
vidarabine (ophthalmic), 15, 709
vidarabine (topical), 10
Videx, 10, 201-202, 737
Viokase, 507-508
Vioxx, 9, 15, 604-605, 731, 737
Vira-A Ophthalmic, 709
Vira-A (optic), 15
Vira-A (topical), 10
Viracept, 10, 468-470
Viramune, 10, 471
Viridium, 525
Virilon IM, 647-648
Viroptic, 15
Viroptic Ophthalmic Solution, 692
Visken, 8, 540-541
Vistaril, 5, 7, 326-327, 730
Vistaril IM, 326-327
Vitabee, 172-173
Vita-C, 54-55
vitamin A, 16, 709-710
vitamin A acid, 682
vitamin B_1, 16, 653-654
vitamin B_2, 16, 593
vitamin B_3, 472-473
vitamin B_6, 16, 579-580
vitamin B_9, 16, 290-291
vitamin B_{12}, 172-173
vitamin $B_{12}a$, 172-173
vitamin C, 54-55
vitamin D, 16, 710-711, 738
vitamin D_2, 710-711
vitamin D_3, 16, 710-711
vitamin D analog, 710-711
vitamin E, 16, 711-712
vitamin K, 738
vitamin k_1, 536
VITAMINS, 16, 738
Vita-Plus E, 711-712
Vitrasert implant, 298-299
Vivactil, 6, 575-576, 736
Vivelle, 247-248
Vivelle-Dot, 247-248
Vivol, 196-197
Volmax, 28-29
Voltaren, 14, 197-199, 736
Voltaren Rapide, 197-199
Voltaren Suppositories, 197-199
Voltarin XR, 197-199
Voltarten SR, 197-199
V.V.S., 749

W

warfarin, 5
warfarin sodium, 712-713
Warfilone, 712-713
Weber Vitamin E, 711-712
Weh-less, 525-526
Wellbutrin, 6, 96-97, 731
Wellbutrin SR, 96-97
Wellcovorin, 11, 364-365
Wellferon, 13, 338-339
Wescort Cream, 322-323
Westcort Ointment, 322-323
Westroid, 658
Wigraine, 740, 750
Wigraine Suppositories, 750
Winpred, 553-554
Winstrol, 12, 624-625
Wintrocin, 242-244
WOUND REPAIR DRUGS, 16
Wymox, 46-48
Wytensin, 8, 307, 731

X

Xalatan, 13, 362-363
Xanax, 5, 31-32, 730
Xanax TS, 31-32
XANTHINES AND XANTHINE DERIVATIVES, 16
Xenical, 10, 495
Xopenex, 11, 365-366, 732
Xylocaine, 4
Xylocaine (cardiac), 376
Xylocaine Cardiac, 6
Xylocaine (local), 377-379
Xylocaine-MPF, 377-379
Xylocaine (topical), 4
Xylocaine Viscous, 379
Xylocaine with Epinephrine, 377-379
Xylocard, 376

Y

yohimbe bark, 765

Z

Zaditor, 7, 15, 357
zafirlukast, 10, 14, 713-714
Zagam, 12, 622-623
zalcitabine, 10, 714-715
zaleplon, 5, 715-716, 730
Zanaflex, 14, 664-665
zanamivir, 10, 716-717
Zantac, 7, 590

Entries can be identified as follows: generic name, Trade Name, DRUG CATEGORY, *Combination Product.*

Zantac 75, 590
Zantac 75 EFFERdose, 590
Zantac 150 GELdose, 590
Zantac-C, 590
Zantac EFFERdose, 590
Zantryl, 531-532
zapine, 732
Zarontin, 5, 256-257
Zaroxolyn, 12, 434-435
Zeasorb-AF, 671
Zebeta, 8, 85-87
Zelitrex (Europe), 702-703
Zenapax, 14, 179-180
Zephrex LA, 743
Zerit, 10, 625-626
Zestoretic 10/12.5, 750
Zestoretic 20/12.5, 750
Zestoretic 20/25, 750
Zestril, 8, 383-384
Ziac 2.5, 750
Ziac 5, 750
Ziac 10, 750
Ziagen, 10, 19
zidovudine, 10, 717-718, 737
ZilaDent, 73-74
zileuton, 10, 14, 718-719
Ziradyl Lotion, 750
Zithromax, 14, 66-68
Zocor, 8, 618
Zofran, 7, 492-493
Zofran ODT, 492-493
Zolicef, 113-114
zolmitripan, 14, 719-720
Zoloft, 6, 615-616, 731, 736
zolpidem, 5, 720-721, 737
Zomig, 14, 719-720
Zonalon, 12, 222-223
Zostrix, 12, 103-104
Zostrix-HP, 103-104
Zosyn, 750
Zovia 1/35E, 493-495
Zovia 1/50E, 493-495
Zovirax, 10, 26-27, 737
Zyban, 16, 96-97
Zydone, 740, 750
Zyflo, 10, 14
Zyflor Filmtab, 718-719
Zyloprim, 7, 9, 30-31, 737
Zymase, 507-508
Zyprexa, 9, 488-490
Zyprexaolan, 732
Zyrtec, 7, 126-127, 737

* Proamantine:
generic: Midodrine HCL
for orthostatic hypotension.

American Dental Association Advisory Statement for Patients with Total Joint Replacement

PATIENTS AT POTENTIAL INCREASED RISK OF HEMATOGENOUS TOTAL JOINT INFECTION*

IMMUNOCOMPROMISED/IMMUNOSUPPRESSED PATIENTS

- Inflammatory arthropathies: rheumatoid arthritis, systemic lupus erythematosus
- Disease-, drug-, or radiation-induced immunosuppression

OTHER PATIENTS

- Insulin-dependent (type 1) diabetes
- First 2 years following joint placement
- Previous prosthetic joint infections
- Malnourishment
- Hemophilia

**Based on Ching and colleagues, Brause, Murray and colleagues, Poss and colleagues, Jacobson and colleagues, Johnson and Bannister and Jacobson and colleagues.*

SUGGESTED ANTIBIOTIC PROPHYLAXIS REGIMENS*

PATIENTS NOT ALLERGIC TO PENICILLIN: CEPHALEXIN, CEPHRADINE, OR AMOXICILLIN

2 g orally 1 hour before dental procedure

PATIENTS NOT ALLERGIC TO PENICILLIN AND UNABLE TO TAKE ORAL MEDICATIONS: CEFAZOLIN OR AMPICILLIN

Cefazolin 1 g or ampicillin 2 g intramuscularly or intravenously 1 hour before the procedure

PATIENTS ALLERGIC TO PENICILLIN: CLINDAMYCIN

600 mg orally 1 hour before the dental procedure

PATIENTS ALLERGIC TO PENICILLIN AND UNABLE TO TAKE ORAL MEDICATIONS: CLINDAMYCIN

600 mg IV 1 hour before the procedure

**No second doses are recommended for any of these dosing regimens.*

Advisory Statements from ADA and AAOP. Antibiotic prophylaxis for dental patients with total joint replacements, *JADA* 128:1004-1008, July 1997. Reprinted by permission of ADA Publishing Co., Inc.